Brunnstrom's Clinical Kinesiology

SIXTH EDITION

Brunnstrom's Clinical Kinesiology

SIXTH EDITION

Revised by

Peggy A. Houglum, PhD, PT, ATC
Associate Professor
Athletic Training
Rangos School of Health Sciences
Duquesne University
Pittsburgh, Pennsylvania

Dolores B. Bertoti, MS, PT
Associate Professor and Chair,
Allied Health and Human Services
Alvernia University
Reading, Pennsylvania

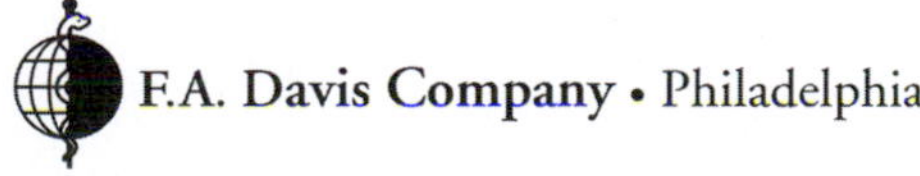

F.A. Davis Company • Philadelphia

F. A. Davis Company
1915 Arch Street
Philadelphia, PA 19103
www.fadavis.com

Printed in the United States of America

Last digit indicates print number: 10 9 8 7 6 5 4 3 2 1

Senior Acquisitions Editor: T. Quincy McDonald
Manager of Content Development: George W. Lang
Senior Developmental Editor: Jennifer A. Pine
Art and Design Manager: Carolyn O'Brien

Library of Congress Cataloging-in-Publication Data

Houglum, Peggy A., 1948-
Brunnstrom's clinical kinesiology. — 6th ed. / revised by Peggy A. Houglum, Dolores B. Bertoti.
p. ; cm.
Clinical kinesiology
Includes bibliographical references and index.
ISBN 978-0-8036-2352-1
I. Bertoti, Dolores. II. Brunnstrom, Signe. Brunnstrom's clinical kinesiology. III. Title. IV. Title: Clinical kinesiology.
[DNLM: 1. Kinesiology, Applied. 2. Joints—physiology. 3. Movement. 4. Muscle Contraction. 5. Muscles—physiology. WE 103]

612.7′4—dc23

2011041199

For Joel & Rita, Pam & Bob, Joan & Steve, Deanna & Dan: I am very blessed to call you relatives and most grateful to call you friends.
—Peg

In celebration of 25 years as a Breast Cancer survivor, I joyfully dedicate my work on this book in thanksgiving for the blessings in my life; my loving family, Willy, Christopher, and Beth; and to Mom, who taught all of my brothers and sisters and I the beauty of love for each other: Jack, Carol, Mary, John, Vince, Karina, Andrew, Dien, Pat, Mary, Michael, Mary Pat, Tim, Andrea, and Maureen.
—Dolores

Preface

When Dolores and I were invited by F. A. Davis to rewrite *Brunnstrom's Clinical Kinesiology*, we were honored to be considered to undertake the project. In our own respective programs half a country apart, we each "grew up" with this text, as it was a required textbook for each of us in our professional education programs.

Although the world of fiction contains several classical novels, from *Oliver Twist* to *Catcher in the Rye,* there are very few textbooks, especially in the health professions, that withstand the test of time and fall within the category of "classics." However, *Brunnstrom's Clinical Kinesiology* is, indeed, one such textbook. The mere fact that it is celebrating its Golden Anniversary year of publication is evidence of its stand-alone presence in the world of health care. It was originally written by Signe Brunnstrom when there were few textbooks in kinesiology and little research on the topic. Her text began as a teaching manual for her students at Columbia University and evolved into a book through a grant from the Office of Vocational Rehabilitation. It was her desire to provide kinesiological information from a clinical perspective to assist professionals in their own performance in the field of rehabilitation.

Her desire to meet the needs of professionals in rehabilitation continues to be met today in this new and updated version of her original textbook. We have included information based on new evidence, applications based on new techniques, and chapters based on new knowledge to expand Brunnstrom's original text to move her original idea of providing clinical applications of kinesiology to rehabilitation into the 21st century.

Dolores and I first met when we spent an intensive and productive weekend together developing a proposal for this immense project. We instantly hit it off and have been on the same wavelength throughout the past 4 years as this project has moved from vision to reality.

Our goal for this revision has been to keep the classic Brunnstrom touch in this text while moving its information into the 21st century. We also wanted to maintain Brunnstrom's idea of this text as a book of useful information that aids students and clinicians in their understanding of body movement and its application in the clinical world. If there is one criticism of many of today's kinesiology texts, it is that much of the information includes biomechanical calculations and engineering perspectives rather than a clinical perspective. Although there are individuals who prefer to include these calculations and information, there are also many who find such information unnecessary for students becoming health care professionals.

Therefore, we have preserved Signe Brunnstrom's perspective of approaching kinesiology from a clinical perspective throughout this text. We have included only essential calculations when they are necessary, as the goal of this text is to provide clinical applications of kinesiology rather than biomechanics. For this reason, you will find this text thinner than other kinesiology texts. The kinesiology presented in this book is pertinent to those individuals who perform as health care providers of individuals in need of rehabilitation treatments, prevention techniques, and corrective exercises.

It has been 50 years since Signe Brunnstrom's first edition was published and students began learning from her wealth of information. The fact that this text continues to contribute to the education of health care students today speaks to the scholarship, foresight, and richness that Signe Brunnstrom infused within in it 50 years ago. She appreciated the unique simplicity of the body with its complexity of movement and wanted other clinicians to share in her appreciation of how wondrously it works. We do, too, and hope that this edition provides you with the enrichment and appreciation of body motion the way Signe Brunnstrom's early editions did for us. We will let you decide if we have accomplished this goal.

Peggy A. Houglum
Dolores B. Bertoti

Biographical Sketch of Signe Brunnstrom, 1898–1988

Anna Signe Sofia Brunnstrom was born at Karlberg Castle (the Swedish Military Academy) in Stockholm, Sweden, on January 1, 1898. She was the second daughter of Captain Edvin Brunnstrom and his wife Hedwig. She died in Darien Convalescent Center in Darien, Connecticut, on February 21, 1988. During the 90 years of her life, she served in many capacities. She was a master clinician, scholar, translator, researcher, educator, author, lecturer, mentor, traveller, and humanitarian. Her reputation as a physical therapist was known worldwide.

At age 16, she entered Uppsala College, where she studied sciences, history, geography, and gymnastics. In 1917, she passed the required examination to enter the Royal Institute for Gymnastics in Stockholm. The Institute was founded by fencing master Per Henrik Ling in 1813. Ling developed a system of medical gymnastics, called "Swedish exercises" that spread across Europe and later into the United States. His exercises were unusual at the time because hands-on resistance or assistance was applied by the therapist. Ling's techniques became the foundation for many of the treatment approaches that Miss Brunnstrom would use in her future work. At the Institute, she excelled in calisthenics and graduated on May 30, 1919, with the title of "Gymnastikdirektor."

In 1920, Miss Brunnstrom went to Berne, Switzerland, to work with a physical therapist. A year later, she established her own "Sjugymnastik Institute" in Lucerne. There she gained a reputation as a therapist treating disabled children with scoliosis and poliomyelitis. She also established an evening program for working women in need of remedial exercise.

She left Switzerland in 1927 and travelled to New York City, where she accepted a position in exercise therapy at the Hospital for the Ruptured and Crippled (later to be renamed the Hospital for Special Surgery). Fourteen Scandinavians worked in the physiotherapy department, and Miss Brunnstrom became the person to whom they all looked for advice as a generous and patient friend. To make ends meet during the depression years, Miss Brunnstrom became a physical training instructor in the gymnasium of the Metropolitan Life Insurance Company. There she applied her ideas about physical education for working women and started special remedial exercise classes. She worked for Metropolitan on and off for 20 years and also offered "Swedish massage" to private patients, received referrals from physicians, and taught exercise classes at New York University.

In 1931, Miss Brunnstrom was admitted to Barnard College, where she took nine credits in chemistry and three credits in English. Recognizing that she could successfully handle American university work, she then enrolled at New York University, where as a part-time student she earned a Master's degree in physical education and a Master of Arts degree in education.

On November 26, 1934, at age 36, Anna Signe Sofia Brunnstrom became a citizen of the United States of America and officially had her name changed to Signe Brunnstrom.

Only 6 years after she came to New York, her first article in English, "Faulty Weight Bearing with Special Reference to Position of the Thigh and Foot" (Physiother. Rev. 15 [3], 1935), was published. This article was the forerunner of 22 clinical articles; several book chapters; three voluminous research reports; numerous abstracts and book reviews (including many translations of classic European work); several films; and three major textbooks on prosthetic training, kinesiology, and hemiplegia movement therapy. She also read and translated the works of major European and American scientists and brought them to the kinesiology literature. These scientists included Blix, Borelli, Bethe and Franke, Braune and Fisher, Elfman, Duchenne, Fick, Inman, Marey, Magus, and the Weber brothers.

Signe Brunnstrom remains one of the most productive contributors to the body of physical therapy knowledge. Through her students and writings, she has left a great legacy to practicing physical and occupational therapists.

In 1938, Miss Brunnstrom was appointed an instructor of therapeutic exercise at New York University. She taught there until 1942 and later in 1948, when she joined the faculty of the Institute for Rehabilitation Medicine as a research associate working on a suction socket study sponsored by the Veterans Administration and NYU.

In the spring of 1941, with the United States still not drawn into World War II, Miss Brunnstrom applied through the American Red Cross to serve as a civilian physical therapist in a military hospital. She was assigned to the physical therapy department at Sheppard Field, Texas, with the Army Air Corps. She left Texas 2 years later, hoping to enlist in the US Army Medical Specialist Corps, but was refused because of her age (she was 45). She then enlisted in the US Navy, and in 1943 reported to the Navy Hospital at Mare Island, California, as the officer in charge of physical therapy. It was there, while working with a young naval medical officer, Dr. Henry Kessler, that she made major contributions to the rehabilitation of amputees. After the war, Dr. Kessler founded the well-known Kessler Institute of Rehabilitation in West Orange, New Jersey. Miss Brunnstrom was discharged from the Navy in 1946 with the rank of lieutenant.

After the war, Miss Brunnstrom participated in prosthetic research at the University of California and New York University. In addition, she was Director of Professional Education at the Kessler Institute. She was also a clinical consultant at the Burke Foundation in White Plains, New York, the New York State Rehabilitation Hospital at West Haverstraw, and the Veterans Administration; she was also a visiting instructor at Stanford University in California. In 1951, she was awarded a Fulbright Lectureship to Greece, where she worked on developing a school of physical therapy and trained aides to carry out amputee exercise programs. Throughout this time, Miss Brunnstrom was in great demand to conduct continuing education courses, seminars, and workshops.

From 1955 through 1971, one of Miss Brunnstrom's many professional activities was teaching kinesiology to physical and occupational therapy students at the College of Physicians and Surgeons, Columbia University, New York. A teaching grant from the US Office of Vocational Rehabilitation enabled her to prepare a laboratory manual for the students. The manual was developed into the textbook *Clinical Kinesiology,* which was published in 1962. This was the first American kinesiology text to be written for physical and occupational therapy students. Before this time, most kinesiology textbooks were oriented to physical education and athletic activities.

Signe Brunnstrom received numerous honors and awards, including the US Navy Medal of Merit in 1945, the Marian Williams Research Award presented by the American Physical Therapy Association (APTA) in 1965, the University Citation of the State University of New York at Buffalo (equivalent to an honorary doctorate) in 1973, and an appointment to honorary membership in the Union of Swedish Physical Therapists in 1974. In 1987, the Board of Directors of APTA renamed the Award for Excellence in Clinical Teaching in her honor. The award is now known as the Signe Brunnstrom Award for Excellence in Clinical Teaching.

—Jay Schleichkorn, PhD, PT

Contributors

Christopher R. Carcia, PhD, PT, SCS, OCS
Associate Professor
Department of Physical Therapy
Rangos School of Health Sciences
Duquesne University
Pittsburgh, Pennsylvania

Ingrid Provident, EdD, OTR/L
Assistant Professor
Occupational Therapy
College for Continuing and Professional Studies
Chatham University
Pittsburgh, Pennsylvania

Reviewers

Leigh Ann Adams, MSEd, ATC
Head Athletic Trainer
Department of Athletics
Emory & Henry College
Emory, Virginia

Jennifer Austin, PhD, ATC
Assistant Professor; Director, Athletic Training Education Program
Department of Exercise and Sport Sciences
Colby-Sawyer College
New London, New Hampshire

Samantha Boudreau, MS, ATC
Assistant Athletic Trainer/Instructor
Department of Kinesiology/Athletic Training
Charleston Southern University
North Charleston, South Carolina

Jason Christopher Craddock, EdD, ATC, CSCS
Program Coordinator, Athletic Training Education
Department of Physical Therapy and Human Performance
Florida Gulf Coast University
Fort Myers, Florida

Amy L. Everitt, EdD, ATC
Professor
Department of Sport and Movement Science
Salem State College
Salem, Massachusetts

Eric J. Fuchs, PhD, ATC, EMT-B
Director, Athletic Training Education Program/Assistant Professor
Department of Exercise and Sports Science
Eastern Kentucky University
Richmond, Kentucky

Xristos K. Gaglias, MA, ATC
Curriculum Director
Athletic Training Education
Stony Brook University
Ridge, New York

Traci Gearhart, PhD, ATC, LAT
Director, Athletic Training Education/Associate Professor
Department of Sport Sciences
Wingate University
Wingate, North Carolina

Bonnie M. Goodwin, MESS, ATC
Chair; ATEP Program Director; Assistant Professor; Assistant Athletic Trainer
Department of Health & Sport Sciences
Capital University
Columbus, Ohio

Brian Michael Hatzel, PhD, ATC
Associate Professor and Chairperson
Movement Science Department
Grand Valley State University
Grand Haven, Michigan

Joseph G. Hayes, Jr., PT, DPT, OCS
Assistant Professor of Physical Therapy
Department of Physical Therapy
Touro College
Commack, New York

Paul Higgs, ATC, LAT, CSCS
Head Athletic Trainer
Department of Athletics
Georgia College
Milledgeville, Georgia

Troy L. Hooper, MPT, ATC, LAT
Assistant Professor
Master of Athletic Training Program
Texas Tech University Health Sciences Center
Lubbock, Texas

Elizabeth Jewell, MA, ATC, LAT
Clinical Coordinator, Athletic Training Education Program
Department of Physical Education and Recreation
North Carolina Central University
Durham, North Carolina

Sherri L. Jones, MS, ATC, LAT
Associate Professor/Athletic Training Education Program Curriculum Director
Department of Education
King College
Bristol, Tennessee

Louis V. Lepak, PT, DPT, MPH, CWS
Assistant Professor
Rehabilitation Sciences
University of Oklahoma
Jenks, Oklahoma

Gary Eugene McIlvain, EdD, ATC/LAT
Associate Professor/ATEP Director
School of Kinesiology
Marshall University
Ashland, Kentucky

John Mercer, PhD
Associate Professor
Department of Kinesiology and Nutrition Sciences
University of Nevada, Las Vegas
Las Vegas, Nevada

Roger D. Newman-Norlund, PhD
Assistant Professor (TT)
Department of Exercise Science
University of South Carolina
Columbia, South Carolina

Doreen M. Stiskal, PT, PhD
Chair
Department of Physical Therapy
Seton Hall University
South Orange, New Jersey

Marilyn Strawbridge, EdD, CSCS
Professor
College of Education
Butler University
Indianapolis, Indiana

Benito J. Velasquez, DA, ATC, LAT
Associate Professor
School of Human Performance & Recreation
The University of Southern Mississippi
Hattiesburg, Mississippi

Luis Velez, MA, ATC, CSCS
Assistant Athletic Trainer/Instructor
School of Health, Exercise, and Sport Science
Lenoir-Rhyne University
Hickory, North Carolina

Stacy Walker, PhD, ATC
Assistant Professor
School of Physical Education, Sport, and Exercise Science
Ball State University
Muncie, Indiana

Marc Willey, PhD, OTR/L, CHT
Assistant Professor
Department of Occupational Therapy
University of Central Arkansas
Conway, Arkansas

Curtis Williams, MBA, ATC
Professor/Head Athletic Trainer
Department of Education
Oklahoma Wesleyan University
Bartlesville, Oklahoma

Acknowledgments

From Peggy Houglum:

There are many people who have been invaluable to me throughout this project. I would be remiss if I did not recognize them. First, I must thank Dolores Bertoti for agreeing to co-author this text with me; she and I have seen this text's potential from the start and have approached its development and completion with the same vision throughout the process. It has been a pleasure to work with my new friend. A special thank you goes to members of Duquesne University's Rangos School of Health Sciences. Members of the school are a close community of professionals who are not only colleagues but also friends; without their direct or indirect contributions, this book could not have been written. Within the university, I am most grateful to Dr. Greg Frazer, Rangos School Dean, who always supports his faculty in our endeavors, and Provost Pearson, who supports and encourages all university faculty. A very special thank you is owed to my Department Chair, Dr. Paula Turocy, and my colleague Dr. Jason Scibek, who took over my teaching load, burdening themselves with an unusual overload so I could take a sabbatical to finish this text. Susan Venditti, our Administrative Assistant, has always "had my back"; she is a professional's professional and assisted me in more ways than I can count, even when I wasn't present in the department. Dr. Christopher Carcia, PT, created an outstanding spine chapter, made a great contribution to the hip and pelvis chapter, and is responsible for the fine ancillaries that accompany this text. Dr. Ingrid Provident, OTR/L, the author of the hand and wrist chapter and the chapter on kinesiology applications of the upper extremity in ADLs, made complex topics easily understandable. Jennifer Pine, Developmental Editor, deserves special recognition for her patience with me and Dolores for our never-ending, "Just one more change" requests, for her yeoman's attention to detail that caught our omissions, and for her exceptional ability to maintain an even keel when I am sure all she wanted to do was strangle one or both of us. Pete Houdak and Bonnie Virag, two Duquesne University students, spent hours posing as models during a nearly week-long photo shoot; thanks to them for donating their bodies to this text. Members of Graphic World Inc. put together the final product. Two members finalized this edition: Rose Boul, Senior Art Coordinator, and Grace Onderlinde, Production Editor, provided needed persistence, perseverance, and patience in the creation of what you now hold in your hands. Liz Schaeffer, Developmental Editor and Electronic Products Coordinator for F. A. Davis, managed, directed, and coordinated with wonderful clarity and vision the creation and production of the fine digital resources that accompany this text. We believe that these resources are a marvelous and unique complement to the text, which provides students with alternatives to understanding what could otherwise be difficult concepts to grasp. Putting together a textbook requires much more than authors with an idea. An entire legion of qualified experts is necessary; we believe that we have, among the throng that has participated in this project, some of the very best.

From Dolores Bertoti:

This work would not have been possible without the support of so many friends and colleagues. I am appreciative of the support from both the administration and my fellow faculty and students at Alvernia University, including a reduction in teaching during the semester when I was buried deep in the research and writing process. My academic dean, Dr. Karen Thacker, never missed an opportunity to ask me how the book was coming, and she shared in my professional excitement throughout the long process. I am especially grateful to my faculty colleagues in Athletic Training who proofread and offered me feedback when the chapters were being developed: Dr. Tom Porrazzo, Dr. Kim Stoudt, and Mr. Jay Mensinger. I would also like to acknowledge the invaluable insights my Kinesiology students offered as they read and reacted to portions of the text; they are who I wrote this book for and are my biggest support. I had images of their eager faces before me during the days of seemingly endless writing; they truly motivated me. Two students traveled to Duquesne to participate in the photo shoot, Courtney Renshaw and Mike Lloyd; Chris Burkert helped me out locally with additional photos. Our developmental editor, Jennifer Pine, was an absolute pleasure to work with and I am grateful for her continual encouragement and kind "nudging" to meet deadlines. Most importantly, I am honored to have had the opportunity to work with Peg Houglum on this text. She is an amazing scholar and surely a champion in the field. I truly have been privileged to work with her.

Brief Contents

Unit One: Basic Concepts 1

CHAPTER 1: Basic Concepts in Kinesiology: Kinematics 2
CHAPTER 2: Mechanical Principles: Kinetics 28
CHAPTER 3: The Movement System: Nerve and Muscle Physiology and the Control of Human Movement 82
CHAPTER 4: Muscle Activity and Strength 125

Unit Two: Upper Quarter 159

CHAPTER 5: Shoulder Complex 161
CHAPTER 6: Elbow and Forearm Complex 217
CHAPTER 7: Wrist and Hand 254
Ingrid Provident, EdD, OTR/L, and Peggy A. Houglum, PhD, PT, ATC
CHAPTER 8: Head, Neck, and Trunk 314
Christopher R. Carcia, PhD, PT, SCS, OCS

Unit Three: Lower Quarter 369

CHAPTER 9: Pelvis and Hip 370
Dolores B. Bertoti, MS, PT, and Christopher R. Carcia, PhD, PT, SCS, OCS
CHAPTER 10: Knee 423
CHAPTER 11: Ankle and Foot 474

Unit Four: Functional Activities 533

CHAPTER 12: Stance and Gait 535
CHAPTER 13: Kinesiology Applications in Daily Functional Activities 593
CHAPTER 14: Kinesiology Applications of Upper Extremity Activities of Daily Living 617
Ingrid Provident, EdD, OTR/L, and Peggy A. Houglum, PhD, PT, ATC
CHAPTER 15: Sports and Recreation 634

Contents

Unit One: Basic Concepts 1

CHAPTER 1 Basic Concepts in Kinesiology: Kinematics 2
Clinical Scenario 3
Historical Perspective: A Glance at the Past 3
Introduction 3
Kinesiology Terminology 4
Human Movement: Kinetics and Kinematics 5
Planes of Motion and Axes of Motion 5
Segment and Body Motion 6
Naming Movements at Joints 6
Osteokinematics: Joint Motion in Terms of Position and Type 9
Definition 10
Description of Types of Motion 10
Degrees of Freedom 11
Clinical Goniometry 11
End Feel 14
Kinematic Chains 16
Arthrokinematics: Joint Surface Motion 17
Definition 17
Types of Joints 17
Joint Structure 18
Basic Arthrokinematic Joint Motions 20
Close-Packed and Open-Packed Joint Positions 24
Clinical Applications 24
Summary 25
Clinical Scenario Solution 25
Discussion Questions 25
Lab Activities 26
References 27

CHAPTER 2 Mechanical Principles: Kinetics 28
Clinical Scenario 29
Introduction 29
Determinants of Motions 29
Types of Motion 29
Location of Motion 30
Magnitude of Motion 30

Direction of Motion 30
Rate of Motion and Change of Motion 31
Forces 31
Types of Forces 31
Newton's Laws of Motion 33
Force Vectors and Their Considerations 35
Composition of Forces 36
Levers 37
First-Class Lever 38
Second-Class Lever 39
Third-Class Lever 39
Mechanical Advantage 39
Static Equilibrium 40
Torque 40
Parallel Force Systems 43
Resolution of Forces 45
Forces Acting at Angles 45
Laws of the Right Triangle 49
Force Applications to the Body 51
Weight and Center of Gravity (Center of Mass) 52
Levers and Muscle Activity 57
Free Body Diagrams 60
Calculation of Muscle and Joint Forces 61
Applying Resistances to the Body 69
Clinical Application of Concepts 70
Pulleys 70
Leverage Factor 73
Stretching vs. Joint Mobilization 73
Pressure 74
Summary 75
Clinical Scenario Solution 75
Discussion Questions 75
Lab Activities 76
References 81
CHAPTER 3 The Movement System: Nerve and Muscle Physiology and the Control of Human Movement 82
Clinical Scenario 83
Introduction 83
Physiology of Excitable Tissue: Nerve and Muscle 84

Nervous System Anatomy Overview 86
Nervous System Classifications 86
Nerve Fibers 87
Muscular System 90
Structure of Skeletal Muscle 90
Muscle Fiber Types 96
The Motor Unit 98
Joint, Tendon, and Muscle Receptors 99
Joint Receptors 99
Golgi Tendon Organs 100
Muscle Spindles 100
Kinesthesia and Proprioception 105
Movement or "Motor" Control 107
Dynamic Systems Approach to Understanding Motor Control 108
Motor Control at the Spinal Region 108
Motor Control within the Brainstem 109
Cerebral Motor Centers 109
Intermediate Control Centers 111
Integration of Motor Control to Produce Functional Movement 112
Functional Applications and Clinical Considerations 113
Muscle Weakness 113
Abnormal Muscle Tone 115
Coordination Problems 115
Involuntary Movements 116
Common Pathological Conditions Affecting Movement System Function 116
Peripheral Nerve Injury 118
Cerebral Palsy 118
Cerebrovascular Accident 119
Basal Ganglia Disorders 119
Cerebellar Disorders 119
Summary 119
Clinical Scenario Solution 119
Discussion Questions 120
Lab Activities 120
References 120

CHAPTER 4 Muscle Activity and Strength 125

Clinical Scenario 126

Introduction 126

Muscle Activity 126

Recording Muscle Activity 126

Muscle Activation 127

Muscle Anatomic Activity 128

Muscle Functional Activity 129

Muscle Characteristics 131

Viscosity 131

Elasticity and Extensibility 131

Stress-Strain 133

Creep 134

Muscle Strength 134

Muscle Size 135

Fiber Architecture 135

Passive Components 136

Length-Tension Relationships and Physiological Length of Muscle 137

Moment Arm 138

Speed of Contraction 139

Active Tension 140

Age and Gender 141

Passive Excursion of Muscles 141

Passive Insufficiency 142

Tendon Action of Muscle 143

Active Excursion of Muscles 144

Active Insufficiency 144

Leverage and Length-Tension Interactions 145

Positive and Negative Work 146

Open Kinetic Chain versus Closed Kinetic Chain 149

Factors Affecting Maximum Isometric Muscle Force 150

Exercise-Induced Muscle Injury 151

Delayed-Onset Muscle Soreness 151

Hamstring Strain 151

Summary 152

Clinical Scenario Solution 152

Discussion Questions 152

Lab Activities 153

References 154

Unit Two: **Upper Quarter** 159

CHAPTER 5 **Shoulder Complex** 161

Clinical Scenario 162

Introduction 162

Bones 162

Manubrium 163

Clavicle 163

Scapula 163

Humerus 165

Joints 166

Definition of Shoulder Girdle Movements 167

Sternoclavicular Joint 170

Acromioclavicular Joint 173

Scapulothoracic Joint 175

Glenohumeral Joint 176

Resting and Close-Packed Positions of the Shoulder Complex Joints 183

The Bicipital Groove 183

Scapulohumeral Rhythm 183

Muscles of the Shoulder Complex 185

Scapular Stabilizer Muscles of the Shoulder Complex 185

Glenohumeral Stabilizing Muscles of the Shoulder 191

Large Muscle Movers of the Shoulder 197

Function of Muscles of the Shoulder Complex 200

Passive and Dynamic Stabilization of the Glenohumeral Joint 200

Synergistic Muscle Actions 203

Muscle Forces and Moment (Lever) Arm Lengths 205

Muscle Activity during Functional Motions 207

Functional Deficiency Applications 208

Summary 210

Clinical Scenario Solution 210

Discussion Questions 211

Lab Activities 211

References 213

CHAPTER 6 Elbow and Forearm Complex 217

Clinical Scenario 218

Introduction 218

Bones 219

Humerus 219

Ulna 220

Radius 221

Joints 221

Humeroulnar and Humeroradial Joints 221

Radioulnar Articulations 229

Muscles 232

Elbow Flexors 232

Elbow Extensors 240

Forearm Supinators 240

Forearm Pronators 242

Functional Movement and the Muscles of the Elbow/Forearm Region 243

Muscles as Agonists, Antagonists, and/or Synergists 244

Selection of Muscles in Functional Movement: Synergistic Contractions 244

One-Joint and Multijoint Muscles of the Elbow and Forearm 245

Typical Elbow and Forearm Muscular Function: Summary and Comparisons 245

Closed Kinematic Chain Motion at the Elbow Complex 247

Analyses of Muscle Activity during Common Functional Movements 248

Placing the Hand behind the Head 248

Pulling 248

Summary 249

Clinical Scenario Solution 250

Discussion Questions 250

Lab Activities 250

References 252

CHAPTER 7 Wrist and Hand 254

Ingrid Provident, EdD, OTR/L, and Peggy A. Houglum, PhD, PT, ATC

Clinical Scenario 255

Introduction 255

Bones 255

Wrist 256

Hand 258

Phalanges 259

Joints 259

Wrist 259

Hand 259

Fingers and Thumb 260

Soft Tissue Supporting Structures 262

Muscles 266

Muscles Acting on the Wrist 266

Muscles Acting on the Digits 276

Extensor Mechanism 280

Motions 288

Motions of the Wrist 288

Motions of the Fingers 290

Functional Movements of the Wrist and Hand 291

Types of Grasp 291

Strength of Grip 293

Grasping 295

Intrinsic-Plus and Intrinsic-Minus Positions 302

Abduction and Adduction of Digits 2 to 5 302

Balanced Forces 303

Fingers 305

Thumb 305

Synergic Action of Wrist Muscles in Movements of the Thumb and Little Finger 307

Peripheral Nerves of the Wrist and Hand 307

Peripheral Nerve Innervations 307

Peripheral Nerve Injuries 308

Summary 310

Clinical Scenario Solution 310

Discussion Questions 311

Lab Activities 311

References 312

CHAPTER 8 Head, Neck, and Trunk 314

Christopher R. Carcia, PhD, PT, SCS, OCS

Clinical Scenario 315

Introduction 315

Bones 315
Normal Curves of the Vertebral Column 315
Nonpalpable Structures 316
Palpable Structures 317
Vertebral Joints, Ligaments, and Motions 321
Vertebral Motions 321
Anterior Vertebral Joint Elements 322
Posterior Vertebral Joint Elements 324
Cervical Region 326
Thoracic Region 327
Lumbar Region 329
Sacrum 331
Sacroiliac Joint 331
Symphysis Pubis 335
Coccygeal Joints 335
Pelvic Balance 335
Muscles 335
Anterior Cervical Muscles 336
Posterior Cervical Muscles 341
Posterior Thoracic and Lumbar Muscles 342
Anterior and Lateral Trunk Muscles 343
Functions of the Head, Neck, and Trunk Muscles 351
Balancing of the Head and the Vertebral Column 352
Trunk Motions and Stabilization of the Vertebrae 352
Forward Bending and Lifting (Knees Extended) 355
Squat Lifting 357
Functional Activities (Muscles of the Extremities and Trunk) 358
Breathing and Coughing 359
Temporomandibular Joints 359
Motions of the Temporomandibular Joint 359
Muscles 360
Temporomandibular Dysfunction 361
Summary 362
Clinical Scenario Solution 362
Lab Activities 363
References 364

Unit Three: Lower Quarter 369

CHAPTER 9 **Pelvis and Hip** 370

Dolores B. Bertoti, MS, PT, and Christopher R. Carcia, PhD, PT, SCS, OCS

Clinical Scenario 371

Introduction 371

Bones 371

- *Pelvis* 372
- *Femur* 374
- *Biomechanical Angulations of the Femur* 375
- *Biomechanical Angulations of the Acetabulum* 378

Joints 379

- *Pelvis* 379
- *Hip Joint* 380
- *Osteokinematics* 382
- *Arthrokinematics* 388
- *Soft Tissue at the Hip Joint* 388

Muscles 389

- *Flexors* 390
- *Adductors* 402
- *Extensors* 403
- *Abductors* 403
- *Lateral Rotators* 405
- *Medial Rotators* 406

Factors Affecting the Roles of the Muscles of the Pelvis and Hip 406

- *Muscle Line of Pull and Leverage* 407
- *Muscular Sufficiency: Multi-Joint versus Single-Joint Muscles* 407
- *Weight-bearing and Nonweight-bearing Functions of Hip Muscles* 408

Analysis of Muscle Activity at Pelvis and Hip 408

- *Analysis of Sagittal Plane Motion at the Hip and Pelvis* 408
- *Analysis of Frontal Plane Motion and Control at the Hip and Pelvis* 411
- *Analysis of Transverse Plane Motion at the Hip and Pelvis* 415

Summary 417

Clinical Scenario Solution 418

Discussion Questions 418

Lab Activities 418

References 420

CHAPTER 10 Knee 423
Clinical Scenario 424
Introduction 424
Bones 425
Femur 425
Tibia 426
Patella 427
Joints 428
Tibiofemoral Joint 428
Patellofemoral Joint 439
Q Angle 441
Muscles 441
Knee Extensors 442
Knee Flexors 449
Tibial Rotators 450
Functions of Muscles of the Knee 451
Knee Extensors 451
Knee Flexors 452
One-Joint and Two-Joint Muscles Acting at the Knee 453
Joint Forces 456
Tibiofemoral Joint Forces 456
Patellofemoral Joint Forces 458
Torque of Muscles Acting at the Knee 460
Interaction of Muscles and Ligaments in Function 462
Sensory Innervation and Reflexes 463
Static and Dynamic Connections 463
Muscle Protection of Ligaments 463
Summary 464
Clinical Scenario Solution 464
Discussion Questions 464
Lab Activities 465
References 466
CHAPTER 11 Ankle and Foot 474
Clinical Scenario 475
Introduction 475
Bones 475
Leg Bones 475
Tarsal Bones 477
Metatarsal Bones 479
Phalanges 479

Joints 480
Motion Terminology 480
Tibiofibular Joints 480
Talocrural Joint 482
Subtalar Joint 489
Transverse Tarsal Joint 492
Tarsometatarsal Joints 495
Intermetatarsal Joints 496
Metatarsophalangeal and Interphalangeal Joints 497
Muscles of the Ankle and Foot 497
Posterior Group of Muscles 497
Lateral Group of Muscles 505
Anterior Group of Muscles 507
Intrinsic Muscles of the Foot 510
Function of Leg and Foot Muscles and Joints 511
Pronation and Supination 517
Arches of the Foot 520
Loading of the Foot 523
Deformities of the Foot 524
Summary 526
Clinical Scenario Solution 526
Discussion Questions 526
Lab Activities 527
References 529

Unit Four: Functional Activities 533

CHAPTER 12 Stance and Gait 535
Clinical Scenario 536
Introduction 536
Stance Posture 536
Forces Required to Maintain Stance 537
Postural Sway 539
Balance of Forces Occurring in Symmetric Stance: Functional Applications 540
Recovery Strategies 542
Walking Gait 543
Gait Terminology 543
Functional Tasks of Gait 545
Kinematics of Gait 546

Kinetics of Gait 554
Muscles of Gait 556
Gait Analysis 561
Developmental Aspects of Gait: Life Span Changes 565
Immature Walking 565
Mature Walking 565
Gait Changes in the Older Adult 567
Gait Efficiency 567
Determinants of Gait 567
Challenges to Gait Efficiency 568
Running Gait 574
Phases 575
Kinematics 576
Changes at Different Speeds 579
Muscle Activity at the Hip, Knee, and Ankle in Running 580
Kinetics of Running 583
Summary 584
Clinical Scenario Solution 585
Discussion Questions 585
Lab Activities 586
References 587
CHAPTER 13 Kinesiology Applications in Daily Functional Activities 593
Clinical Scenario 594
Introduction 594
Mobility 594
Floor Mobility: Rolling and Floor-to-Stand 594
Sit-to-Stand Transfer 599
Occupational and Daily Activities 602
Lifting Tasks 602
Household Tasks 604
Occupational Tasks 606
Clinician Activities 609
Patient Protective Measures: Spotting during Ambulation 610
Clinician Ergonomics: Manual Resistance 612
Summary 614
Clinical Scenario Solution 614
Discussion Questions 615

Lab Activities 615
References 616
CHAPTER 14 Kinesiology Applications of Upper Extremity Activities of Daily Living 617
Ingrid Provident, EdD, OTR/L, and Peggy A. Houglum, PhD, PT, ATC
Clinical Scenario 618
Introduction 618
Functional Applications 618
Activities Requiring Primarily Shoulder Complex Movement 618
Activities Requiring Primarily Elbow Movement 623
Activities Requiring Primarily Forearm Movement 626
Activities Requiring Primarily Wrist Movement 629
Summary 631
Clinical Scenario Solution 631
Discussion Questions 632
Lab Activities 632
References 633
CHAPTER 15 Sports and Recreation 634
Clinical Scenario 634
Introduction 635
Sports Activities 636
Baseball Pitching 636
Fast Pitch Softball Pitching 641
Soccer Instep Kick 644
Freestyle Swimming 647
Leisure Activities 652
Golf Swing 652
Tennis Serve 656
Cycling 660
Summary 663
Clinical Scenario Solution 663
Discussion Questions 663
Lab Activities 664
References 664
Glossary 668
Index 687

Introduction

This book is written with a strong clinical base and perspective. The minimal biomechanical elements in this book are included only to allow an understanding of the clinical importance of these applications. The book is written with the intent of direct application of information to clinical, functional, and practical use. To that end, throughout the chapters there are *Practice Points*. These are special inserts that are related to the topic at hand and provide special clinical insight, information, or application of the topic discussed. The experience of the authors enables these "tidbits" of clinical reality to bring meaning to the information presented. The start of each chapter presents a *Clinical Scenario*. These clinical scenarios are again addressed at the end of the chapter, after the reader has acquired insight and information that assists him or her in realizing the significance of the scenario. Clinical relevance of information is repeated throughout the chapters to encourage students to see why it is important to know and understand the concepts presented throughout the text. The end of each chapter includes two types of exercises: discussion questions and lab activities. The discussion questions are thought-provoking as well as reminders of the more important take-home points of the chapter. The lab activities may be performed in small groups or individually and are intended to apply hands-on elements of the lessons within the chapter.

Since this is likely an introductory text for individuals seeking to eventually move into biomechanics, we have introduced mathematical formulas and concepts in English, not metric, values. We realize that most professional publications require metric values, but since many students have yet to progress in their careers to realize the significance or size of the numbers in terms of force or applications made either to or by the body, we prefer to put these formulas in the more familiar terms of the English measurement system.

Information in this text is divided into four units. Each unit contains specific information that falls under the umbrella of a single element within kinesiology. Kinesiology is broken down into these units to allow the reader to build on the information obtained in one unit to better understand the next, successive unit. The first unit is basic to understanding the other units of the book. It deals with the basic information that is relevant to the understanding of how the body functions from a kinesiological perspective. Chapter 1 provides information on the basic structure and function of joints and muscles as well as planes and directions of motion. Chapter 2 involves the physical concepts that produce forces and torque, create levers, and how these impact body movement. Although it discusses physics concepts, it does so with a clinical approach, placing little emphasis on the mathematical methodology and more emphasis on the functional application. To provide a total perspective on body movement, Chapter 3 includes information on muscles and how they are constructed, how they function neurologically, and how they utilize energy for motion. Motor control and the body's ability to function dynamically through the interaction of multiple systems are presented. Chapter 4 is the final chapter of this unit, and it presents the various types of muscle contractions and how their functions change during motion. Whereas Chapter 3 discusses muscle function from a neurological approach, Chapter 4 discusses muscle's mechanical features, how changing length of muscle and altering angles of joints changes a muscle's ability to perform. It also looks at the main physical factors that determine muscle strength.

The second and third units utilize information from the first unit to develop a clinical understanding of how the body performs from a kinesiological perspective. These two units are divided into upper and lower extremities with the axial skeleton placed between them. Each of these chapters within these two units approaches its specific body segment in similar fashion: The bones and joints are presented and followed by a review of the muscles. Once this basic information is provided, how the segment functions is addressed, providing details that are unique for each body segment. Chapter 5 presents information on the shoulder complex. Chapter 6 delves into the elbow and forearm. Chapter 7 is written by an occupational therapist and deals with the complexities of the wrist and hand. Chapter 8 provides information on the axial skeleton and is written by a physical therapist with expertise on the spine. Chapters 9, 10, and 11 provide information on the hip, knee, and foot and ankle, respectively.

Unit 4, the final section of this text, puts all of the information in the previous three units into practical application for activities from those we perform on a daily basis to specific sport and leisure activities.

It provides the reader with application of the concepts introduced in the first unit and combines them with information about the specific body segments provided in the second and third units to create a total picture of kinesiology. Most clinicians are required to utilize their kinesiological knowledge to provide appropriate plans of care for the individuals they treat. After separating kinesiology into small tidbits to allow the reader to grasp the information, this last unit puts it all together to create the complete picture of what kinesiology is and how it is used in health care. Chapter 12 presents information on posture, stance, and gait. Topics include the joint motions, muscle activity, and forces seen in normal gait; the development and changes that occur in normal gait; and pathological gaits commonly seen clinically. It also goes beyond walking gait and analyzes running gait. Chapter 13 provides kinesiological analysis of activities of daily living. Sequences of movement, joint requirements, and muscle activity are analyzed for daily activities such as moving around on the floor, moving from sitting to standing, and lifting; analyses of examples of work and household tasks are also provided. Chapter 14, written by an occupational therapist, provides special attention to upper extremity tasks and their analysis. Upper extremity tasks in this chapter are divided into tasks of the shoulder girdle, elbow, forearm, and wrist to provide the reader with in-depth analysis of common activities performed by these joints. Analysis of sports movements is the topic of Chapter 15. Sports are divided into competitive and recreational sports and are all commonly occurring activities at all levels of competition and within the greatest age range of participants.

As was mentioned, this book takes a strong clinical approach to kinesiology. It is not a biomechanics book, but a kinesiology text that presents information that is directly applicable to the concerns, needs, and functions of clinicians. It is meant to serve the purpose of providing present and future clinicians with the ability to appreciate human motion, understand relevant kinesiological application, and produce successful treatment results.

INTRODUCTION TO

Unit 1: Basic Concepts

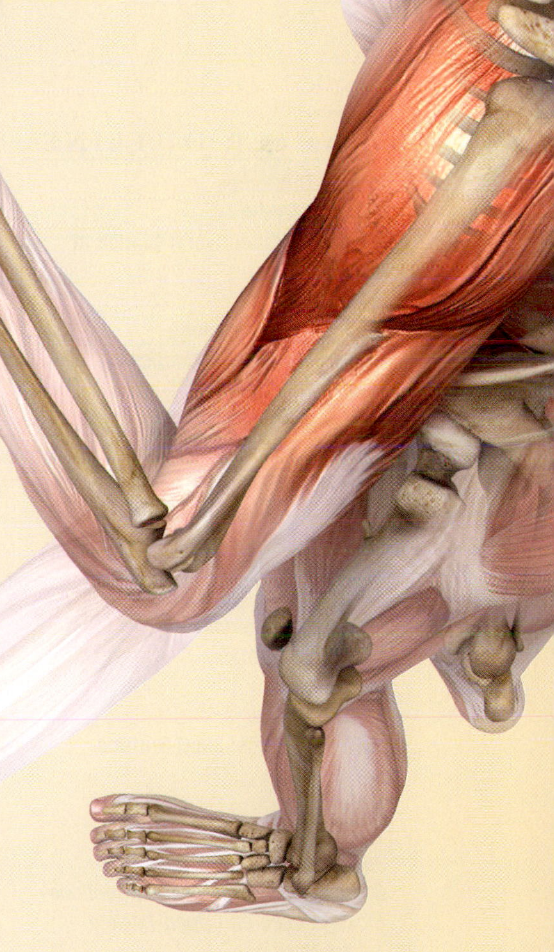

The first unit of the text introduces you to the basics of kinesiology. Chapter 1 provides information on the kinematics of kinesiology. Information is presented on planes of motion and axes within the body, various kinds of joints and their classifications, kinematic chain concepts, open- and close-packed positions of the joints, degrees of freedom of joints, and why this information is important to the understanding of clinical kinesiology.

Chapter 2 introduces kinetics. Kinetics deals with forces. Within this chapter, the types of forces applied to the body are discussed along with Newton's Laws of Motion, and vectors. Included in vectors is an expanded discussion on composition or makeup of forces. Additionally, various levers and torques and how they occur in the body are presented. To add to the understanding of force applications in functional applications, how the body deals with these forces and how clinicians are able to estimate these forces are discussed.

Chapter 3 moves into the physiology of the neuromuscular system and how the unique interactions between the neural and muscle systems allow the body to respond to stimulations within the environment. A discussion of muscle fiber structure, types, motor units, nerve fibers, and joint receptors is presented in an effort to further understand the dynamic interrelationship between these systems.

Chapter 4 provides information on muscle strength—specifically, the types of muscle contraction, how the muscles function against gravity and outside forces, and how the structure and physiology of muscle determine strength output of any muscle. A brief discussion on how strength is measured is also presented.

Basic Concepts in Kinesiology: Kinematics

"Never be afraid to try something new. Remember, amateurs built the ark. Professionals built the Titanic."
—Author Unknown

CHAPTER OUTLINE

Learning Outcomes
Clinical Scenario
Historical Perspective: A Glance at the Past
Introduction
Kinesiology Terminology
Human Movement: Kinetics and Kinematics
Planes of Motion and Axes of Motion
Segment and Body Motion
Naming Movements at Joints
Osteokinematics: Joint Motion in Terms of Position and Type
Definition
Description of Types of Motion
Degrees of Freedom
Clinical Goniometry
End Feel
Kinematic Chains
Arthrokinematics: Joint Surface Motion
Definition
Types of Joints
Joint Structure
Basic Arthrokinematic Joint Motions
Close-Packed and Open-Packed Joint Positions
Clinical Applications
Summary
Clinical Scenario Solution
Discussion Questions
Lab Activities
References

LEARNING OUTCOMES

This chapter provides the basic information required to begin a study of kinesiology. By the end of this chapter, you should be able to:

- ❑ Use basic kinesiology terminology when describing movement of the body and the body segments in space;
- ❑ Define kinematics, osteokinematics, and arthrokinematics and give examples of the use of each of these terms and their relevance to studying kinesiology;
- ❑ Identify the cardinal planes of the body and be able to demonstrate movement in each of the three cardinal planes—sagittal, frontal, and transverse—and the axes for these motions;
- ❑ Describe the different types of motion, such as translatory and rotary, and relate these to motions within the human body;
- ❑ Describe and define joint motion in terms of degrees of freedom, joint structural type and amount, and direction of motion;
- ❑ Define and describe the common materials found in joints and summarize their functional significance to joint structure—joint capsule, synovial fluid, ligament, and bursa;
- ❑ Describe and give examples of joints classified as uniaxial, biaxial, and triaxial and define degrees of freedom;
- ❑ Describe and cite examples of movements in an open and a closed kinematic chain;
- ❑ Describe and cite examples of the different types of arthrokinematic surface motions that occur between joint surfaces—rolling, spinning, sliding;
- ❑ Describe and cite examples of different joint shapes and explain the concave-convex principle;

- ❑ Define and give examples of close-packed and open-packed joint positions and describe compression compared to distraction of those joint surfaces and how these factors are relevant to joint function;
- ❑ Explain the functional and clinical relevance of demonstrating competence in describing joint motion and human movement in kinematic terms.

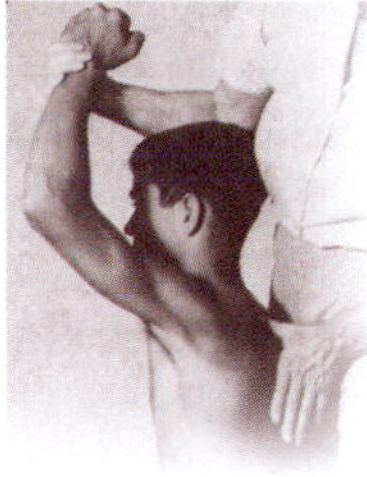

CLINICAL SCENARIO

Jamie, a clinician in the health professions, is attending her son's Little League game when another player appears to have hurt his finger. Jamie watches with concern from the sidelines as the volunteer coach, who happens to be the insurance man in Jamie's neighborhood, calmly announces that the finger is just "jammed." He proceeds to start to minister to the little boy, telling him to stay still and he will "pull it out." Jamie is facing a dilemma. What is the best course of action and how should Jamie go about it?

Historical Perspective: A Glance at the Past

Welcome to a study of Kinesiology! You are about to embark on an adventure that will expand your knowledge of the human body and provide you with an appreciation of the beauty of human movement. Kinesiology is not a one-dimensional study that requires you to learn lists of facts about anatomical structure; rather, it is literally the study of *movement.* This journey will require you to be *actively* engaged in your learning process. Part of your learning will be through your own movement and the movements of your peers. As a new student in kinesiology, you are joining the ranks of many others, for kinesiology has a very long and impressive history.

Studying kinesiology actually dates back to ancient Greece to the times of Aristotle and Hippocrates; as you may recall, ancient Greece is often associated with the Olympic Games and the Greeks' enthusiasm for athletic performance and sports. Later, famous anatomist and physician Claudius Galen (131–201 AD) advanced the knowledge of kinesiology by studying two human skeletons on display in Alexandria and dissecting hundreds of pigs and apes. Based on such scrutinizing study, he produced intricate descriptive analyses of the human form; his detailed descriptions of the musculature of the hand are very close to what is still known to be accurate today. During the second century, Galen introduced terms that we still use today and will discuss in these first chapters; his terms include words such as diarthrosis, synarthrosis, agonist, and antagonist that will become very familiar to you as you move through the chapters in this book. During the early phase of the Renaissance, Leonardo da Vinci (1452–1519) emerged as one of the greatest artists of all times, well known, even today, for his beautiful artistic depictions of the human body. He dissected hundreds of bodies so that he could gain an understanding of the musculature and form of the human body; we see that knowledge and appreciation expressed in his artwork (Fig. 1.1A). Da Vinci was soon followed by Galileo (1564–1642) and then Giovanni Borelli (1608–1679). These scientists gave mathematical expression to the events related to human movement and wrote of the mechanics of muscle action, equilibrium as it relates to the center of gravity, the relationship between muscle force and its angle of application, and the relation of the moments of rotation to lever arms in the body.[1]

So, let us proceed to not only understand but also appreciate the findings of these early investigators. Following the findings of these early enthusiasts of human movement, others have continued to improve and evolve our knowledge of how the body moves. By the time you have completed this text, you will join the list of distinguished individuals who have come to understand and appreciate human movement.

Introduction

You know already that kinesiology is the study of human motion and has been studied for several centuries. Today, kinesiology has used the findings from over the centuries combined with modern technology to create a highly sophisticated means of analysis of

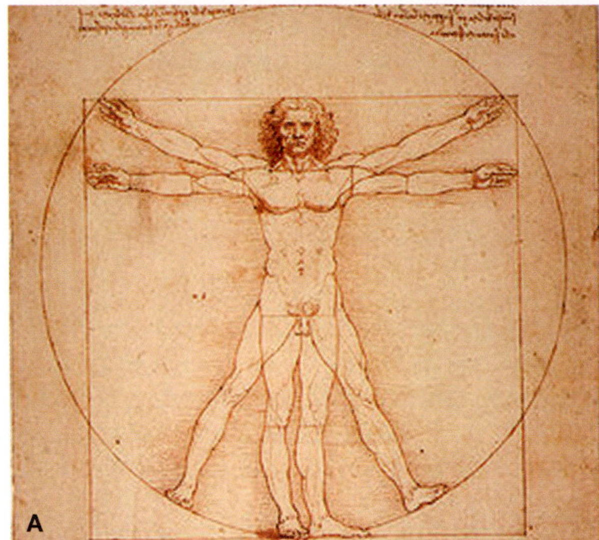

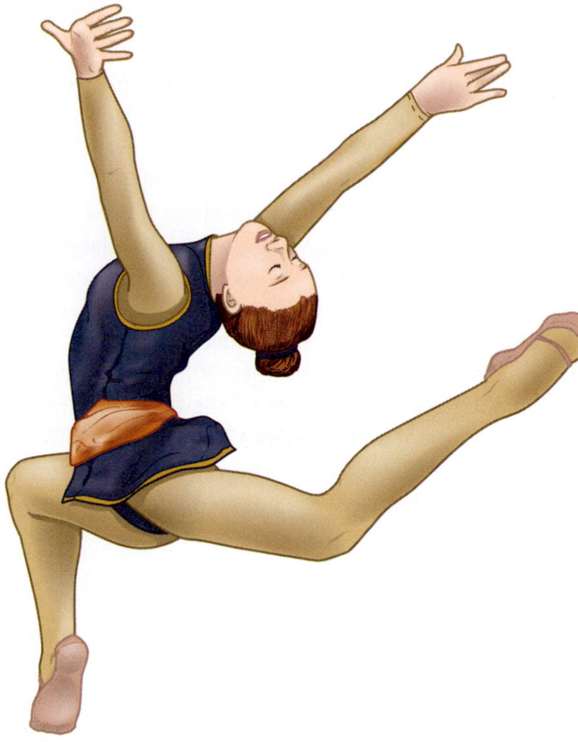

Figure 1.1 From ancient times until the present day, an appreciation of the beauty of the human form in motion has always captivated the attention of artists, scientists, health professionals, and athletes.

human movement. This scientific evolutionary study of simple as well as complex motions evolves from pondering numerous questions: How does a person walk? What joints and muscles are involved in throwing, reaching, climbing, swinging a golf club, getting dressed, driving a vehicle, brushing your teeth? How much motion is required at each of the joints to execute efficient and effective movements? What is the sequence of muscle requirements used in the simple act of shaking a person's hand?

This inquiry into human motion evolved from purely art to a mixture of art and science, combining theories and principles gleaned from anatomy, physiology, anthropology, physics, mechanics, and biomechanics. **Biomechanics** is the application of the principles of mechanics to the living human body. Kinesiology is actually a combination of art and science; it involves an appreciation of the beauty of human movement with an understanding of the scientific principles that provide that movement. Clinical kinesiology is the application of kinesiology to environments of the health care professional.

The purpose of studying clinical kinesiology in health care is to understand movement and the forces acting on the human body and to learn how to manipulate these forces to prevent injury, restore function, and provide optimal human performance. This text presents the basics of kinesiology with an emphasis on clinical application for the health care professional.

Although humans have always been able to see and feel posture and motion, the forces affecting motion (gravity, muscle tension, external resistance, and friction) are never seen. These forces acting on the body are fundamental to human motion and to the ability to modify it. The human body assumes many diverse positions (Fig. 1.2A,B,C). To discuss human movement, it is imperative that we use a common language. If you were to embark on a study of computer science, it would be necessary for you to learn language that includes terms such as "hard drive," "bytes," "disc space," and "flash drive," to name a few examples. The same is true when embarking on a study of kinesiology: A common language is essential for understanding the topic and communicating with others. Some of the terms in this text may be familiar to you and others may not. To assist you in understanding these terms, there is a glossary for all bold-faced terms at the end of this text with indications of where the term is first used and defined within the text. It may be helpful to refer to this glossary throughout your readings.

Kinesiology Terminology

Movement is the essence of kinesiology. Within the study of movement are two terms that are used to further delineate this study of human movement. These terms are defined first.

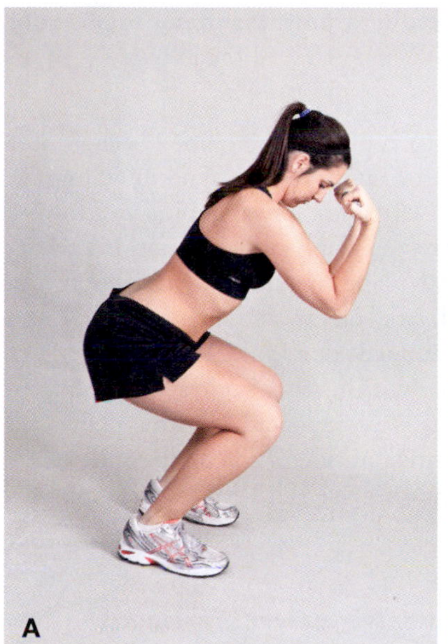

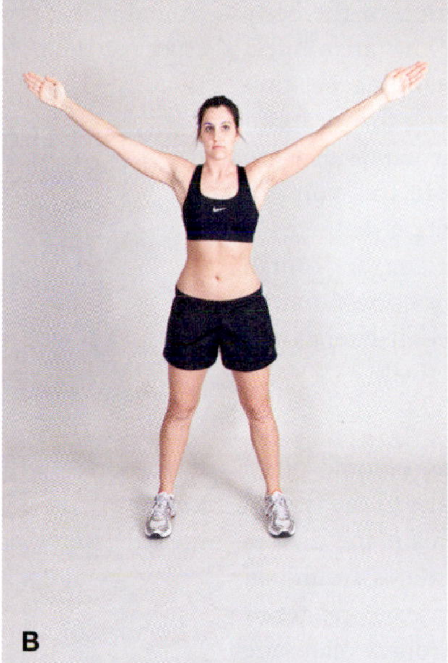

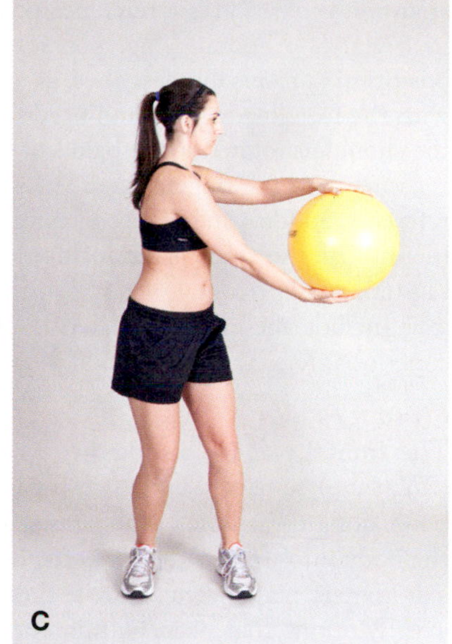

Figure 1.2 Examples of the variety of joint and segment positions that the human body can assume during functional activity: A) demonstrates flexion and extension positions of joints; B) emphasizes motions of abduction and adduction; and C) illustrates rotation. A view of these positions in three dimensions is even more complex.

Human Movement: Kinetics and Kinematics

Much of the terminology we use is derived from one of two sub-studies of human movement: kinetics or kinematics. **Kinetics** concentrates on the forces that produce or resist the movement. **Kinematics**, on the other hand, deals with types of motion or movement without regard for the forces that produce that motion. When discussing kinematics, we include descriptors such as the type of motion, the direction of the motion, and the quantity of the motion. Quantity of motion is discussed in units such as degrees of motion or the amount of linear distance a body or segment moves. A kinematic description of human movement features the position and movement of the body segment, including the joints and their relationship to each other and to the external world. This description may highlight the movement of a single point on the body, the position of several segments on an extremity, or the position or motions of a single joint and its adjacent joint surfaces. Kinematics uses the three-dimensional system used in mathematics and physics to describe the orientation of the body and its segments in space. The use of this system helps us identify and predict motion of the body and its segments.

Kinematics is further subdivided into two subtopics according to the specific focus of motion—osteokinematics and arthrokinematics. **Osteokinematics** concerns the movements of the bony partners or segments that make up a joint, and **arthrokinematics** focuses specifically on the minute movements occurring within the joint and between the joint surfaces. This chapter describes and discusses elements of kinematics and how to study, describe, and assess human movement using the descriptive language of osteokinematics and arthrokinematics. Before we can begin a discussion on osteokinematics and arthrokinematics, let us identify other terms basic to the understanding of human motion. Kinetics and the forces related to the production of human movement is the content of the next chapter.

Planes of Motion and Axes of Motion

The body and its segments move in planes of motion around axes of motion. The human body moves in three planes of motion in the world. These planes of motion are called **cardinal planes** of motion (Fig. 1.3). The three axes around which these planes rotate, in physics terms, are x, y, and z. These axes, depicted in Figure 1.3, are the x or medial-lateral axis runs side to side and is located in the frontal plane; the y or vertical axis runs up and down or superior-inferior and is in a transverse plane; and the z or anterior-posterior axis runs from front to back and is in the sagittal plane.[2] All movement can be described as occurring along a plane of motion and around that plane of motion's axis.

These axes of motion are also described in functional terms in reference with the **anatomical position**. The anatomical position is a reference position of the body in a static, or nonmoving, position. The anatomical position is universally described as a standing position with the feet, knees, body, and head facing forward, and the shoulders rotated so the palms of the hands also face forward with the fingers extended. From this point of reference, motion and planes of motion are defined. As mentioned, the three planes of motion are the frontal, sagittal, and horizontal planes, and their corresponding axes include the anterior-posterior, medial-lateral, and superior-inferior axes of motion, respectively.

Frontal Plane

The **frontal** plane is also known as the **coronal** plane (XY plane), so named because it is parallel to the frontal bone along the coronal skull suture. This plane divides the body into front and back parts. It rotates around an axis that is perpendicular to it: the anterior-posterior axis. Motions that occur within the frontal plane are (Fig. 1.3):

- Abduction and adduction (hip, shoulder, digits)
- Ulnar and radial deviation (a type of abduction/adduction at the wrist)
- Lateral flexion or bending (neck, trunk)

In summary, these motions occur within the frontal plane and around an axis that lies at right angles to the frontal plane, proceeding from the anterior to posterior aspect of the body.

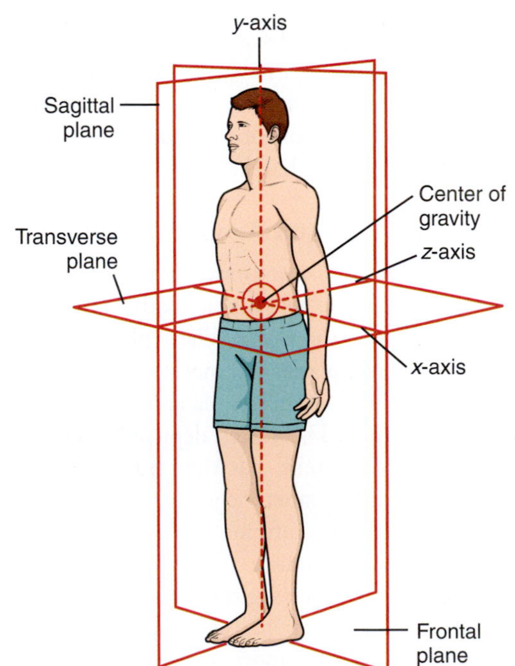

Figure 1.3 The three cardinal planes and axes of the body as seen in standing in anatomical position.

Sagittal Plane

The **sagittal plane** (YZ plane) is so named because it is parallel to the sagittal suture of the skull, dividing the body into right and left sides. Photographically, this is a side view. The clearest examples of joint motions occurring in the sagittal plane are defined as flexion and extension (neck, trunk, elbow and many others) and dorsiflexion and plantarflexion (ankle).

These motions within the sagittal plane pivot around an axis that is perpendicular to this plane and traverses from the medial side of the body to the lateral side of the body (x-axis). This axis of motion is a medial-lateral axis.

Horizontal Plane

The **horizontal** or **transverse** plane is so named because it is parallel to the horizon and the floor (XZ plane). It divides the body into upper and lower parts. Rotations occur in this plane around a longitudinal or y-axis. As with other axes relative to their plane of motion, this axis lies perpendicular to the transverse plane in a cephalocaudal direction and is referred to in physics as the y-axis and in kinesiology as a superior-inferior axis, vertical axis, or longitudinal axis. Motions that occur within the transverse plane are:

- Medial and lateral rotation (hip and shoulder)
- Pronation and supination (forearm)
- Eversion and inversion (foot)

Segment and Body Motion

Some of the terms used to describe motions in the previous section may be foreign to you. In this section, they are defined and specific segments providing these motions are identified. All human movement is defined in terms of planes and axes of motion.

Naming Movements at Joints

Since joints are the articulations between two bony partners or segments, the naming of joints follows a very simple convention. We name joints by using the names of the two bones that form the joint, typically by naming the proximal bone first. For example, the articulation at the wrist is between the distal radius and proximal row of carpal bones; hence, the wrist joint is the radiocarpal joint. Descriptive directional terminology is used to describe the type of movements seen between the two articulating joint segments as described below (Fig. 1.4).

Flexion is a bending movement so that one bone segment moves toward the other and a decrease in the

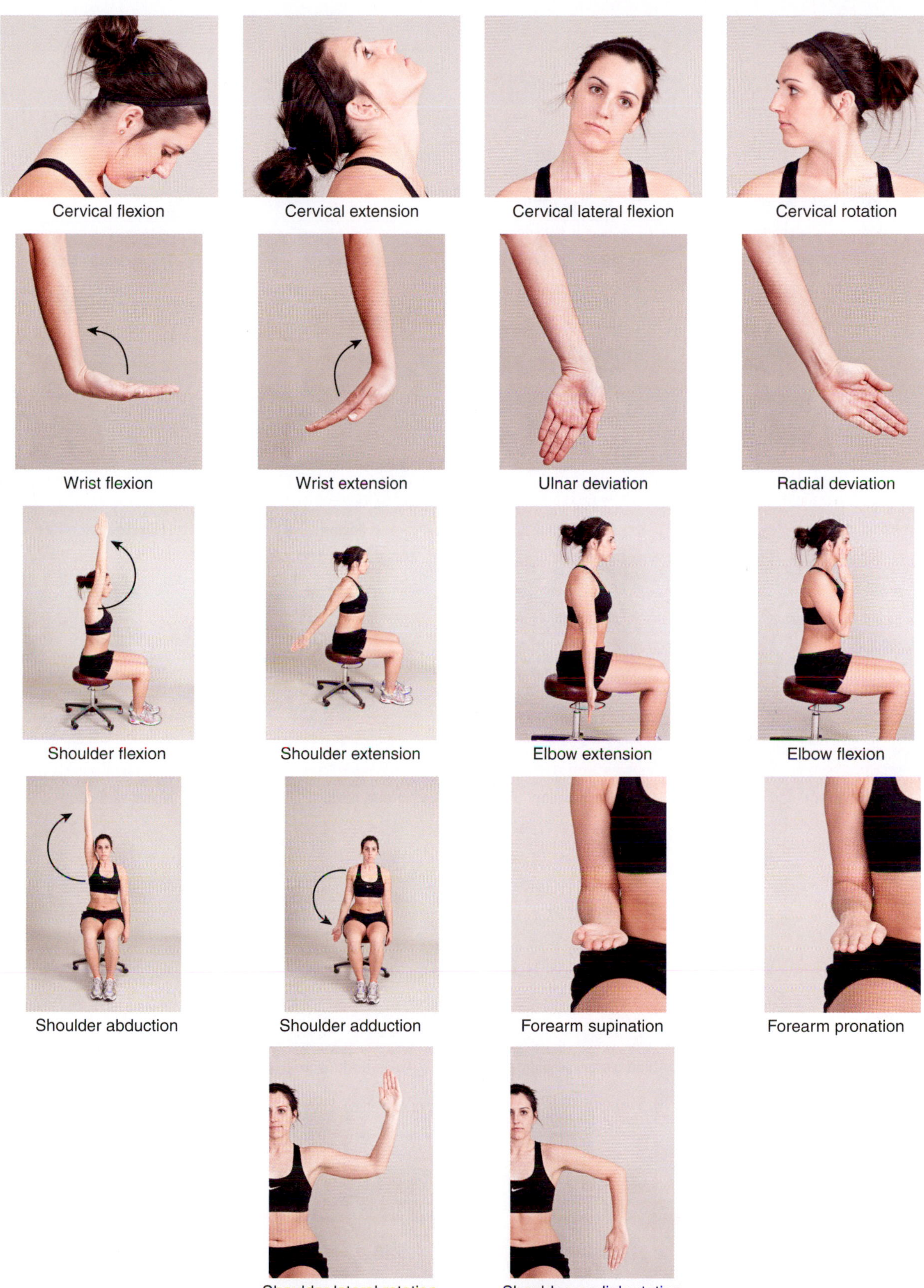

Figure 1.4 Types of joint movement.

Continued

Trunk rotation

Trunk lateral flexion

Trunk flexion

Trunk extension

Hip abduction

Hip adduction

Hip flexion

Hip extension

Hip medial rotation

Hip lateral rotation

Knee flexion

Knee extension

Ankle dorsiflexion

Ankle plantarflexion

Ankle adduction

Ankle abduction

Ankle inversion

Ankle eversion

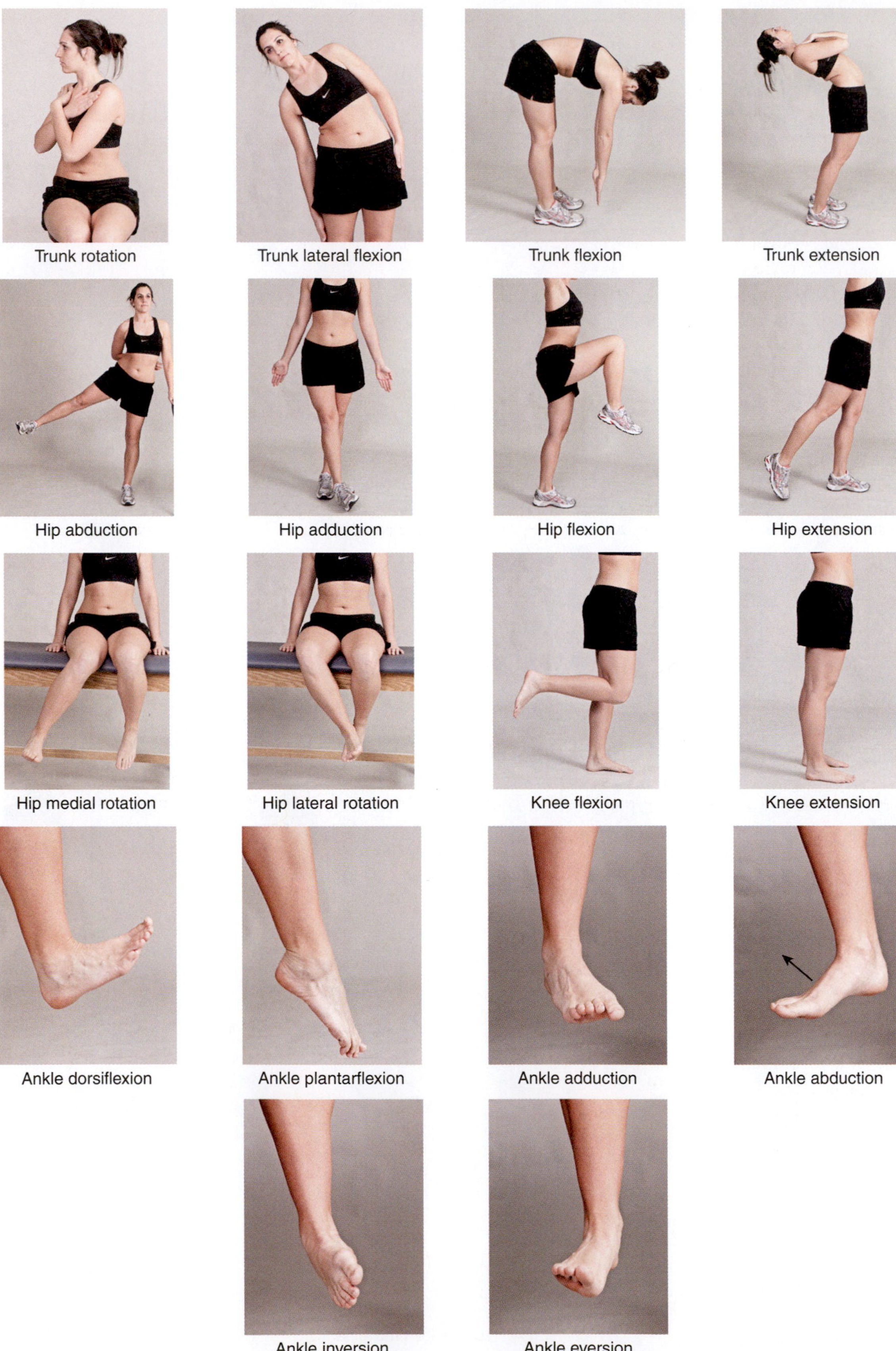

Figure 1.4—cont'd

angle of the joint occurs in the sagittal plane around a medial-lateral axis. Conversely, flexion's countermovement partner in the opposite direction but along the same plane is extension. **Extension** is the movement of one bone segment away from the other bone, producing an increase in the joint angle. If extension goes beyond the anatomic reference position, it is called **hyperextension**. For example, at the elbow (we now will use the correct kinesiology naming system and call it the "humeroulnar" joint), when the anterior surface of the forearm approximates the anterior surface of the upper arm, the joint moves into flexion. Please note that flexion of the humeroulnar joint may be accomplished either by flexion of the forearm toward the arm, as in bringing a cup to your mouth, or by flexion of the arm toward the forearm, as in performing a chin-up. Since the joint segments producing movement may change their role as the moving segment or the stationary segment, it is so important to always know the reference points so an accurate description of motion is possible.

Flexion is labeled differently for some specific joints or segments. Flexion movement of the ankle (talotibial) joint, for example, occurs as the dorsum of the foot moves toward the anterior surface of the tibia, but this motion is called **dorsiflexion** rather than flexion. At this same joint, extension movement in which the foot's dorsum moves away from the tibia is called **plantarflexion.**

Abduction is a position or motion of a segment away from the midline, and **adduction** is a position or motion toward the midline. Abduction and adduction occur in the frontal plane around an anterior-posterior axis. Usually, when we talk about midline, we mean the midline of the body. In the fingers and toes, however, the reference for midline is different; the middle finger in the hand is the midline for the fingers, and the second toe is the midline in the foot. In the fingers and toes, movement toward those midline reference points is called adduction and motion away from them is called abduction. As with flexion and extension, the wrist (radiocarpal) joint also has unique terms for some of its abduction-adduction motions. Adduction is called **ulnar deviation** or **ulnar flexion** because it is a sideways motion moving the little finger toward the ulna, and abduction is called **radial deviation** or **radial flexion** because it is a sideways motion moving the thumb toward the radius. Another example of a change in motion terminology involves the axial skeleton. A sideways movement of the neck or trunk within the frontal plane is not abduction or adduction, but **lateral flexion**; this term is further clarified by referring to the direction of motion as either right lateral flexion or left lateral flexion.

Rotation is movement of a bony segment around a longitudinal or vertical axis in the transverse plane. Rotation is further clarified by naming its direction so that **medial** (or internal) **rotation** is a turning toward the midline or inward, and **lateral** (or external) **rotation** is turning toward the side or away from the midline. In this text, we will adhere to the terms lateral and medial rotation as the preferred terms rather than external and internal rotation since they more accurately describe the movements. Examples of these types of rotation occur at the hip and shoulder. **Pronation** is a specific term used to describe the rotation into a palm-down position of the forearm. **Supination** is the partnered specific term used to describe the rotation into a palm-up position of the forearm. Supination and pronation are terms also used in describing movement of the foot, but these terms related to foot motion are presented in more detail in Chapter 11. **Inversion** and **eversion** are additional terms used to describe specific types of rotational movements in the foot. These specific motions are also described in detail in Chapter 11.

Retraction and **protraction** are movements along a line parallel to the ground such as we will see when we study the movements of the scapula in Chapter 5 and when we study pelvic motion in Chapter 9.

Special Cases

We have already presented some changes from the "usual" terms that are unique to specific joints. There are also cases in which terms change because the location of the plane of motion changes. Such a case involves the thumb. The thumb is a special case because its normal position is rotated 90° from the plane of the hand. Therefore, motions of flexion and extension occur in the frontal plane rather than the sagittal plane, and abduction and adduction occur in the sagittal plane rather than the frontal plane (see Fig. 7.8). Two additional examples of special cases are forearm supination and pronation with the elbow in flexion and hip medial rotation and lateral rotation with the hip in flexion. As the forearm rotates, the motion no longer occurs on a longitudinal axis but on an anterior-posterior axis, and likewise, the flexed hip also rotates on an anterior-posterior axis. A good foundation of understanding of body motion and position is vital to understanding how these planes and axes of movements change with changes in position. These concepts will be presented throughout the text.

Osteokinematics: Joint Motion in Terms of Position and Type

This section of the chapter describes movement from an osteokinematic perspective in kinematic terms.

Osteokinematic motion is what we easily visualize and feel as the bones move during functional activities. Osteokinematic motion is described using the terms just discussed.

Definition

Osteokinematics regards the movements of our bony levers through their ranges of motion. This motion is produced by muscles. Osteokinematics describes the movement that occurs between the shafts of two adjacent bones as the two body segments move with regard to each other. Examples of osteokinematic motion are the forearm flexing toward the humerus at the elbow or the tibia increasing the angle with the femur during extension of the knee. Osteokinematic motions are described as taking place in one plane of the body (frontal, sagittal, or transverse) and around their corresponding axes.

Description of Types of Motion

The body and its segments move one of two ways: Motion is either translatory or rotary. These motions are defined and explained in this section.

Translatory Motion

In **translatory**, or **linear**, motion, the motion occurs along or parallel to an axis. Linear motion means that all points on the moving object travel the same distance, in the same direction with the same velocity, and at the same time. An example of translatory motion is an elevator moving straight up and down within an elevator shaft. This movement is in a straight line. It is also called **rectilinear.**

Curvilinear is another subset of linear motion in which the object travels in a curved path such as that which occurs when tossing a ball to a friend. Thus, any point on the object can be used to describe the path of the total object.

In the human body, there are few examples of true translatory, or linear, joint motions. The closest example of a motion that is translatory or linear is the sliding of the carpal bones next to each other. These concepts are presented in Chapter 7.

Rotary Motion

In **rotary,** or **angular,** motion, the motion occurs in a circle around an axis. Rotary movements occur around an axis or a pivot point, so every point on the object attached to the axis follows the arc of a circle. Individual points on the object move at different velocities, and the velocity of each point is related to its distance from the axis of motion. An example of this is a game of "crack the whip," commonly played on ice skates. The person who is the anchor is the center of motion, or the axis. The last person on the end of the "whip" moves much faster than those individuals closer to the center because the distance he must travel is farther, and yet all members of the "whip" complete one revolution at the same time. The same concept is true when you bat a ball; the end of the bat moves much faster than the shoulders at the axis end, so the ball can be hit with the bat a lot farther than it can be thrown with the arm.

In simplified terms, joint motions occur around an axis and are rotary, whereby every point on a bony segment adjacent to the joint follows the arc of a circle, the center of which is the joint axis. Rotary motions take place about a fixed or relatively fixed axis, and the pivot point for this angular or rotary motion is called the **axis of rotation,** located within or near the surface of the joint. For example, with the humerus stabilized in elbow flexion and extension, the forearm rotates around the axis of the elbow joint. Individual points on the forearm segment move at different velocities, with the velocity of each point related to its distance from the axis of motion; the farther the distance from the axis of motion, the greater the velocity of that point (Fig. 1.5).

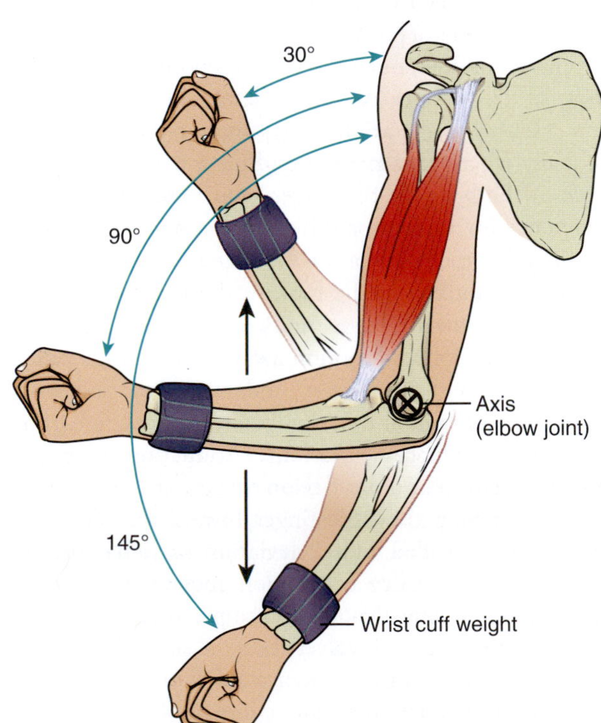

Figure 1.5 Motion at a joint depicted as angular motion. Note the difference in distance traveled at varying points in the body segment.

Impact of Translatory and Rotary Motion

Functional motion involves a combination of linear and rotary movements. In walking, the trunk and the body as a whole move in a forward direction to create a translatory movement of the body forward, but this forward body motion is produced by rotary motion of the hip, knee, and ankle. The upper extremity combines rotary motions at the shoulder, elbow, radioulnar, and wrist joints to provide a translatory path for a baseball during a pitch. In order to closely study functional movement, it is crucial that we analyze each specific joint's unique contribution to the overall movement pattern of the extremity or body as a whole. As we will see in the sections that follow, motions at joints are dictated by the shape and congruency of the articulating joint surfaces, exerted forces, and the number of planes within which they move.

Degrees of Freedom

The ability of the body to transform joint angular motion into efficient translatory motion of body segments involves the degrees of freedom of motion.[3,4] **Degrees of freedom** is the number of planes within which a joint moves. Given that the body and its segments move in three planes of motion, the degrees of freedom are maximal at three degrees as well. When studying the following section, refer to Figure 1.6 and Table 1–1 to see a summary of joint structure and function.

Joints that move in one plane around one axis have one degree of freedom. These joints are **uniaxial** (moving around a single axis) and include two types because of their structural anatomy: **hinge** or **pivot**. Examples of uniaxial hinge joints are the interphalangeal and elbow joints, which perform motions of flexion and extension in the sagittal plane around the medial-lateral axis. The radioulnar joint is another uniaxial joint that permits supination and pronation within the transverse plane around a longitudinal or vertical axis. In summary, uniaxial joints are restricted to an arc of motion in a single plane around a single axis.

If a joint moves around two axes, the segments moves in two planes, and the joint has two degrees of freedom of motion. These joints are **biaxial** and include three structural types: **condyloid, ellipsoidal**, and **saddle**. The root word of "condyloid"—"condyle"—means knuckle, so a condyloid-joint shape is a spherical convex surface partnered with an opposing concave surface, as seen in the metacarpophalangeal joints of the hand (your knuckles) and the metatarsophalangeal joints of the foot. An ellipsoidal structure has a spindle-like shape in which one somewhat flattened convex surface articulates with a fairly deep concave surface such as seen at the radiocarpal joint at the wrist. Both condyloid and ellipsoidal joints permit flexion-extension within the sagittal plane around the medial-lateral axis and abduction-adduction within the frontal plane around an anterior-posterior axis. A saddle joint is a biaxial joint in which each bony partner has a concave and convex surface oriented perpendicular to each other, like a rider in a saddle. The carpometacarpal joint of the thumb is a saddle joint, but this joint is actually a modified biaxial joint that is discussed in Chapter 7.

Ball-and-socket joints, such as the hip and glenohumeral joints, are **triaxial** and have three degrees of freedom. Movement takes place about three main axes, all of which pass through the joint's center of rotation. At the hip and shoulder, the axes of motion are similar: The axis for flexion-extension has a medial-lateral direction; the axis for abduction-adduction has an anterior-posterior direction; and the axis for rotation courses in a superior-inferior direction in the anatomical position. Three degrees of freedom of motion are the greatest number of degrees of motion a joint can possess. Figure 1.6 depicts the various joint structural types.

Unless otherwise stated, joint motion occurs with the proximal segment fixed and the distal segment moving. For example, when the elbow flexes or extends, the proximal segment of the joint (humerus) is fixed or stabilized as the distal segment (forearm) moves.

It is through the summation of two or more joints and their degrees of freedom that body segments may gain sufficient degrees of freedom to produce complex yet smooth functional movement. An example of a well-coordinated, successive movement combination is circumduction. **Circumduction** is a motion in which the moving segment follows a circular path. Circumduction occurs in triaxial joints and is actually a combination of straight planes motions.

Normal function involves motion in combined planes and axes. The multiple degrees of freedom of the body's segments permit a wide selection of movement patterns. In the simple movement of rising from a supine to a standing position, 21 different combinations of the arm, leg, and head-trunk components have been documented in healthy young adults.[5]

Clinical Goniometry

Goniometry (Gr. *gonia,* angle, and *metron,* measure) is a valuable clinical measurement used to define the quantity of joint motion, either actively or passively. Since it measures the relative position of two bony segments, goniometry is a way to measure and record the osteokinematic motion available at the joint. Although sophisticated joint motion analysis equipment is available

Synarthrodial Joints

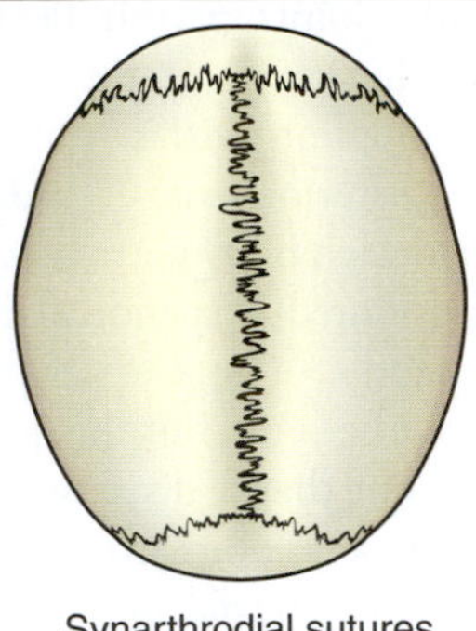

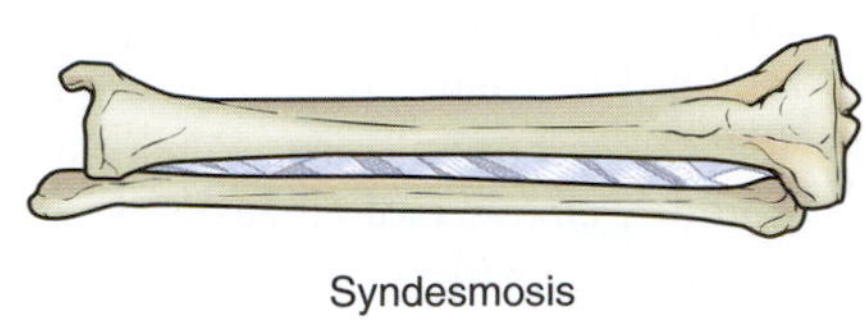

Amphiarthrodial Joints

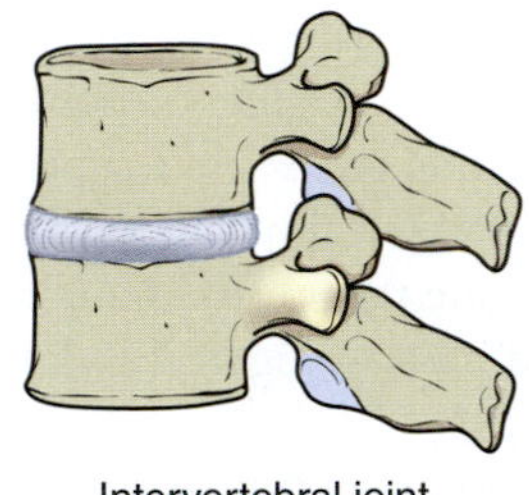

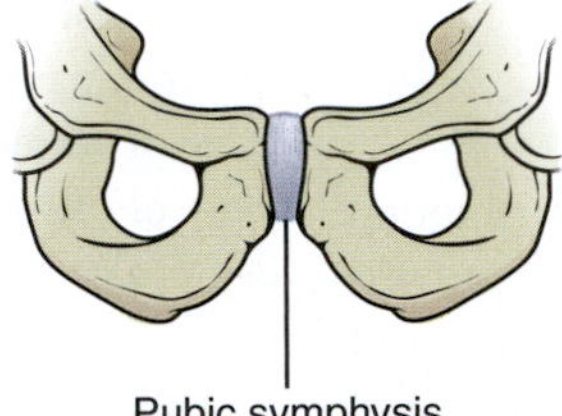

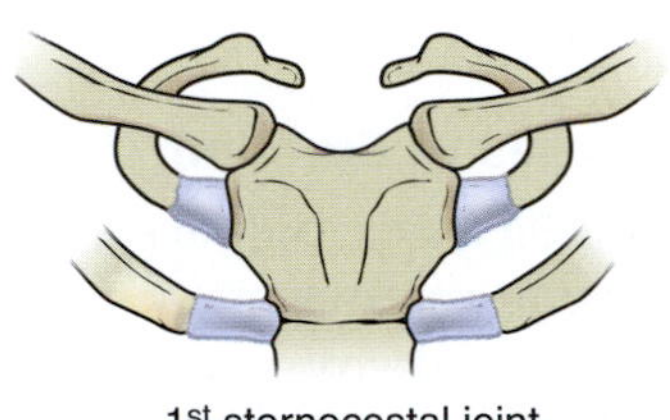

Diarthrodial (Synovial) Joints

Uniaxial Joints

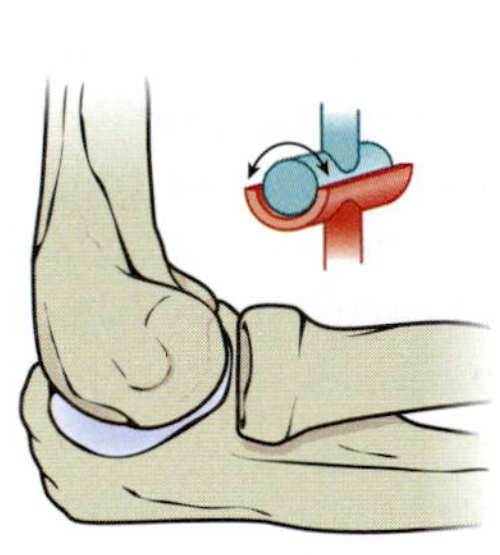

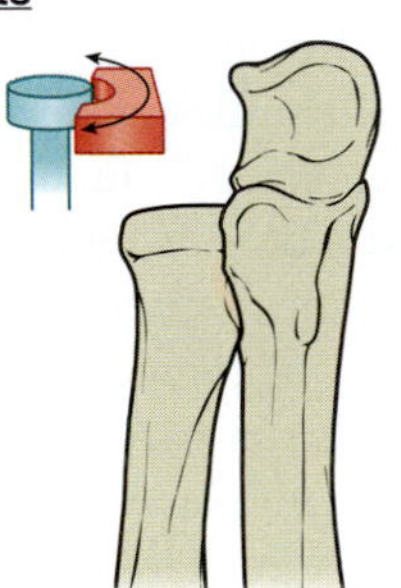

Triaxial Joints

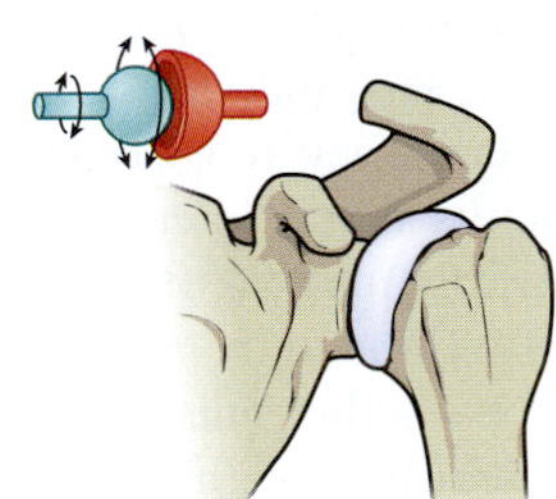

Biaxial Joints

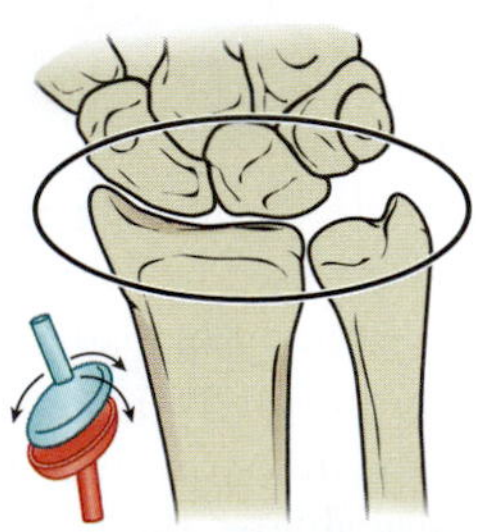

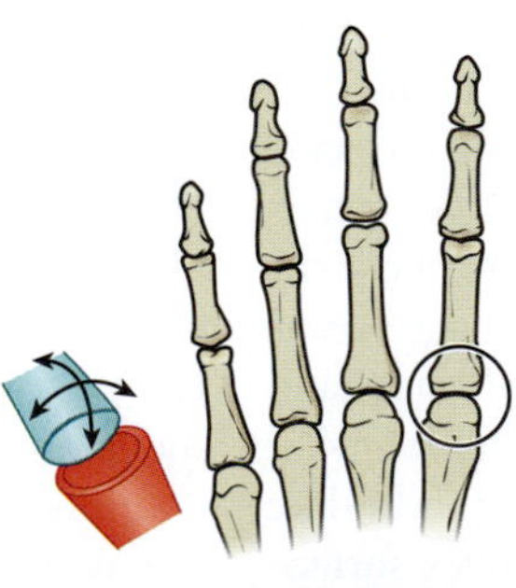

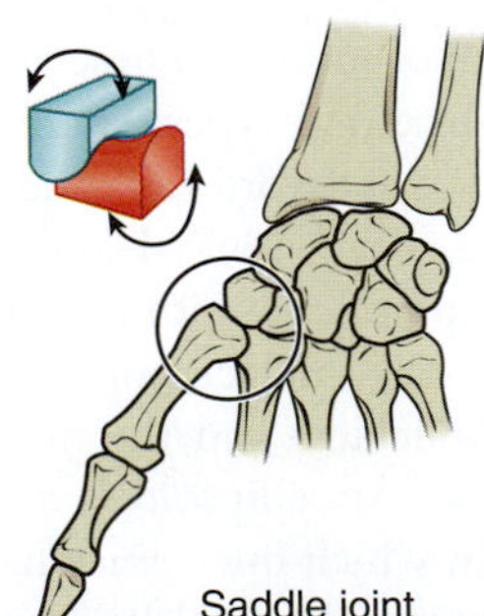

Figure 1.6 Various joint structure types: synarthrodial, amphiarthrodial, and diarthrodial (synovial); hinge, condyloid, ellipsoidal, saddle, pivot, and ball and socket.

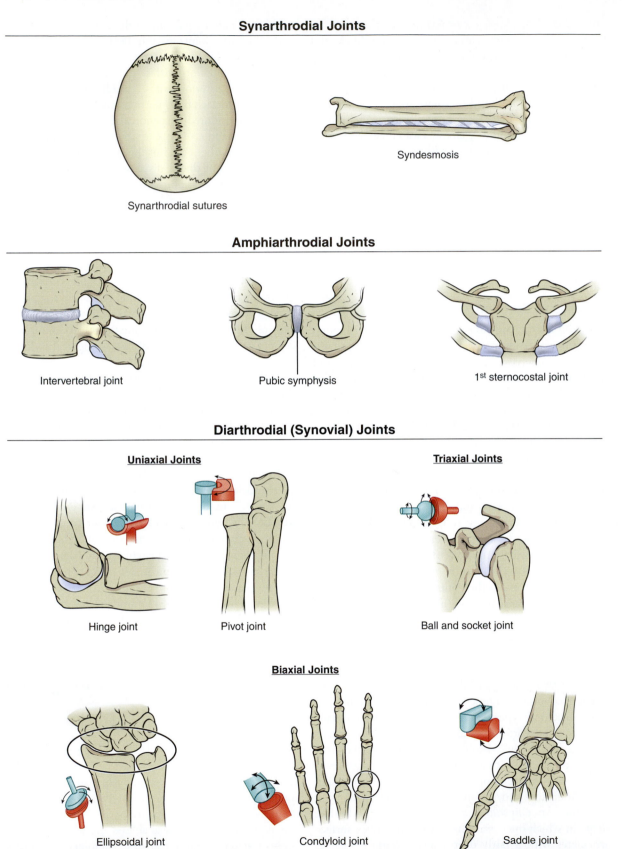

TABLE 1–1 | JOINT CLASSIFICATION BY STRUCTURE AND FUNCTION

Type	Structure/ Shape	Primary Function	Motion	Example
I. Synarthrosis Syndesmosis	Fibrous	Stability, shock absorption and force transmission	Very slight	Tibiofibular articulation
II. Amphiarthrosis	Cartilaginous	Stability with specific and limited mobility	Limited	Pubic symphysis Intervertebral joints 1st sternocostal joint
III. Diarthrosis	Synovial w/ligaments	Mobility	Free according to degrees of freedom	
a. Nonaxial	Irregular plane surfaces	Contributory motion	Gliding	Between carpal bones between tarsal bones
b. Uniaxial 1° freedom				
	Hinge (ginglymus: Greek: hinge)	Motion in sagittal plane	Flexion, extension	Elbow, interphalangeal joints of fingers and toes, knee, ankle
	Pivot Trochoid: Greek: wheel shape)	Motion in transverse plane	Supination, pronation, inversion, eversion	Forearm, subtalar joint of foot, atlas on axis
c. Biaxial 2° freedom				
	Condyloid : Generally spherical convex surface paired with a shallow concave surface	Motion in sagittal and frontal planes	Flexion and extension, abduction and adduction	Metacarpophalangeal joints in hand and foot
	Ellipsoidal: Somewhat flattened convex surface paired with a fairly deep concave surface	Motion in sagittal and frontal planes	Flexion and extension, radial and ulnar deviation	Radiocarpal joint at wrist
	Saddle: Each partner has a concave and convex surface oriented perpendicular to each other; like a rider in a saddle	Motion in sagittal and frontal planes with some motion in transverse plane	Flexion and extension, abduction and adduction, opposition of thumb	Carpometacarpal joint of thumb
d. Triaxial 3° freedom	Ball and socket: a spherical type "ball" paired with a concave cup	Motion in all three planes: sagittal, frontal and transverse	Flexion and extension, abduction and adduction, rotation (medial and lateral)	Shoulder, hip

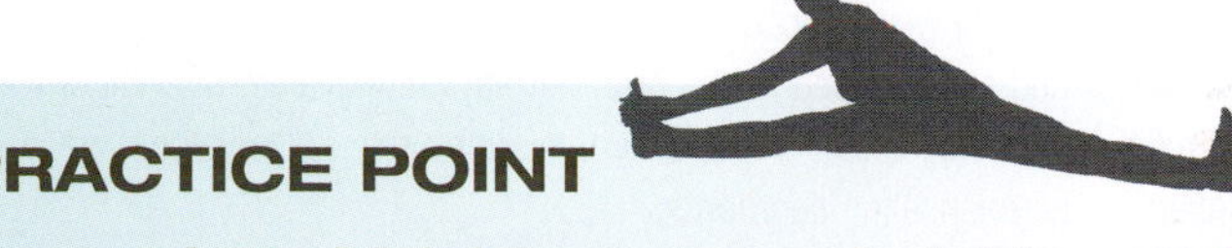

PRACTICE POINT

When range of motion is limited, there is a corresponding limitation in body segment function. This functional outcome increases impairment and risk of injury and decreases optimal function. Sometimes even loss of motion in one degree of freedom is severely disabling, as would occur in a finger joint of a professional typist, violinist, or baseball pitcher.

in clinical laboratories, a manual **goniometer** is the most frequently used tool. A goniometer looks like a protractor with two arms hinged at a fulcrum, or axis. The arms of the goniometer are placed parallel to the joint's two body segments with the goniometer's axis superimposed on the joint (Fig. 1.7). The goniometer measures the body joint's range of motion in each plane of movement, such as glenohumeral flexion, hip abduction, and forearm supination. For details on the techniques of goniometry, there are several comprehensive texts available on the topic such as the text by Norkin and White.[2]

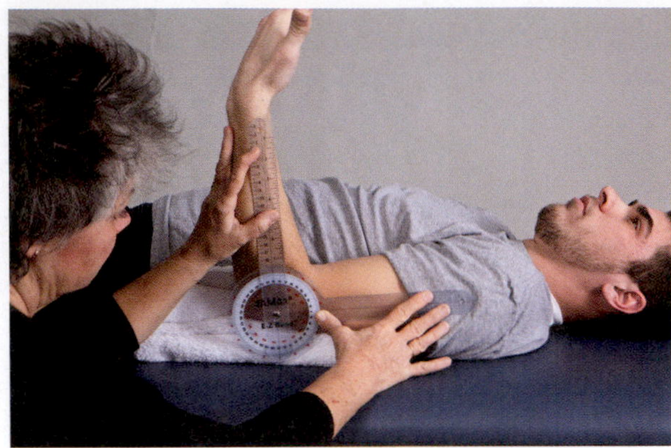

Figure 1.7 Application of a goniometer to measure the position of the elbow in the sagittal plane. The stationary arm of the goniometer is aligned parallel to the long axis of the subject's arm. The moving arm of the goniometer is aligned parallel to the long axis of the forearm, and the axis or fulcrum of the goniometer is placed over the axis of the elbow joint.

Goniometric measurement is a useful tool for the health care professional in assessing and recording progress or change in motion during treatment of pathological conditions. Many textbooks provide values for normal adult range of motion, but standardized normal tables comparing all the variables involved such as age, sex, body build, and type of motion (active or passive) have not been established. Table 1–2 displays goniometric values that may be used as guidelines for the approximate normal joint range of motion in normal adults. Because of individual variations in build and body type, it is useful to use these standardized values as a reference, but it is most important to use the individual's own "normal" for reliable comparison by measuring the uninvolved, or contralateral, extremity segment, assuming that it is present and unimpaired. In Table 1–2, the values in bold type are rounded numbers that are convenient to remember as the amount of normal motion for the extremity joints. The values in parentheses are the range of *average* normal motions reported in several sources.[6-12]

Normal individual ranges of motion vary with bony structure, muscular development, body fat, ligamentous integrity, gender, and age. Slender individuals and those with normal joint laxity may have more range of motion than those who have greater muscular development or who are obese. For example, Dubs and Gschwend[13] measured index finger hyperextension in over 2000 people and found wide variability, from 100° to 10°. They found that joint laxity was greater in females than in males and decreased with age. Males showed a more rapid decrease in range during adolescence and a greater overall decrease compared to their female counterparts. The ranges of motion of some joints during infancy and childhood may differ markedly from the average adult values.

End Feel

When a normal joint is moved passively to the end of its range of motion, resistance to further motion is palpated by the examiner. First described by Cyriax,[14] this resistance is called the **end feel** and is normally dictated by the joint's structure. Resistance is described as hard,

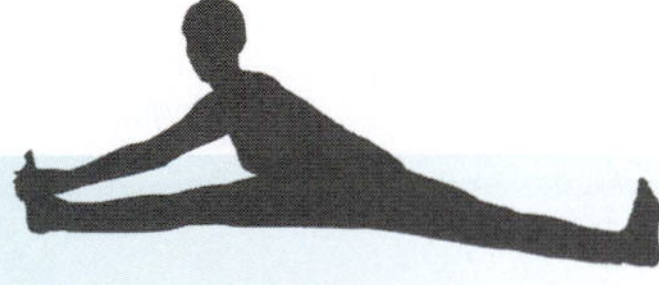

PRACTICE POINT

Pathologic limitations of joint motion, such as caused by edema, pain, or soft tissue shortening, restrict normal function. Contributions to functional movement from multiple segments and joints within an extremity are an advantage used to maintain function during isolated joint impairment. For example, the person who cannot fully pronate the forearm can still have normal hand function by compensatory increases in wrist, elbow, shoulder, and even trunk motions. A person with a stiff knee can walk using compensatory motions of the ankle, hip, back, or the opposite lower extremity. Such compensation, however, occurs at a price of increased energy expenditure and/or increased stress on other structures. Years of compensatory use may result in repetitive microtrauma and dysfunction in the compensating segments.

TABLE 1–2 | SUMMARY RANGES OF JOINT MOTION

SHOULDER	flexion **0° to 180°** (150° to 180°) extension **0°** hyperextension **0° to 45°** (40° to 60°) abduction **0° to 180°** (150° to 180°) medial rotation **0° to 90°** (70° to 90°) lateral rotation **0° to 90°** (80° to 90°)
ELBOW	flexion **0° to 145°** (120° to 160°) extension **0°**
FOREARM	supination **0° to 90°** (80° to 90°) pronation **0° to 80°** (70° to 80°)
WRIST	neutral when the midline between flexion and extension is 0° and when forearm and third metacarpal are in line flexion **0° to 90°** (75° to 90°) extension **0° to 70°** (65° to 70°) radial deviation/abduction **0° to 20°** (15° to 25°) ulnar deviation/adduction **0° to 30°** (25° to 40°)
FINGERS	MCP flexion **0° to 90°** (85° to 100°) MCP hyperextension **0° to 20°** (0° to 45°) MCP abduction **0° to 20°** MCP adduction **0°** PIP flexion **0° to 120°** (90° to 120°) DIP flexion **0° to 90°** (80° to 90°) IP extension **0°**
THUMB	MCP flexion **0° to 45°** (40° to 90°) MCP abduction and adduction (NEGLIGIBLE) IP flexion **0° to 90°** (80° to 90°)
HIP	flexion **0° to 120°** (110° to 125°) hyperextension **0° to 10°** (0° to 30°) abduction **0° to 45°** (40° to 55°) adduction **0°** (30° to 40° across midline) lateral rotation **0° to 45°** (40° to 50°) medial rotation **0° to 35°** (30° to 45°)
KNEE	flexion **0° to 120°** (120° to 160°) extension **0°**
ANKLE\FOOT	neutral with foot at a right angle to the leg and knee flexed plantarflexion **0° to 45°** (40° to 50°) dorsiflexion **0° to 15°** (10° to 20°) inversion and eversion (see Chapter 11).
TOES	MTP flexion **0° to 40°** (30° to 45°) MTP hyperextension **0° to 80°** (50° to 90°) MTP abduction (slight) IP flexion **0° to 60°** (50° to 80°) IP extension **0°**

The values in bold type are round numbers that are convenient to remember in estimating the amount of normal motion typically present. The values in parentheses are the ranges of average normal motion reported in several sources.

KEY:
DIP = distal interphalangeal joint
IP = interphalangeal joint
MCP = metacarpophalangeal joint
MTP = metatarsophalangeal joint
PIP = proximal interphalangeal joint

SOURCES: American Academy of Orthopaedic Surgeons, 1965; Departments of the Army and Air Force, 1968; Kendall, Kendall, and Wadsworth, 1971; Daniels and Worthingham, 1986; Gerhardt and Russe, 1975; and Kapandji, 1982 and 1987.

firm, or soft. A **hard,** or **bony, end feel** is felt when motion is stopped by contact of bone on bone, as in elbow extension when the olecranon process of the ulna moves snugly into the olecranon fossa of the humerus. A **firm,** or **capsular, end feel** is one in which the limitation feels springy because it occurs from the resistance encountered from the capsular, or ligamentous, structures. Wrist flexion is an example of firm end feel. A **soft end feel** is felt at the end of available range of motion when soft tissues approximate each other, such as when the muscle bulk of the arm contacts the fleshy muscle bulk of the forearm at the end of elbow flexion. All of these end feels are normal and dictated by the structure of the joint.

Pathologic end feels occur either at a different place in the range of motion than expected or have an end feel that is not characteristic of the joint. An **empty end feel** is a pathologic type denoting pain on motion but absence of resistance. An empty end feel is present when the joint lacks normal soft tissue stability and a supporting structure is not intact, which is indicative of serious joint injury. Normal end feels are pathologic if they occur when they should not. For example, a bony end feel that occurs in knee flexion because of a bone fragment within the joint is not normal, nor is a soft end feel in elbow extension because of excessive edema.

Kinematic Chains

In kinesiology, a combination of several joints uniting successive segments constitutes a **kinematic chain.** In the human body, movement occurs because of this combination of multiple joints working cooperatively to produce the desired outcome. For instance, reaching for a book on a shelf in the library is an example of this concept as the arm is a chain of joints from the scapula, thorax, shoulder, elbow, forearm, and wrist to the fingers and thumb that all work together in this movement chain to produce the desired motion. We can take this example a step further, and also identify the links from the neck, trunk, pelvis, and lower limbs that may be used to reach for a book on a top shelf. In this example, the links within the upper extremity are free to move (open) and offer the necessary mobility to execute the task. However, the lower extremity joints are fixed (closed) but equally important to this task.

It is important to recognize that human movements are combinations of open and closed kinetic chain movements. These kinetic or kinematic chains are used to describe or analyze a movement skill. Kinematic chains are either open kinematic chains (OKC) or closed kinematic chains (CKC).

Open and Closed Kinematic Chains

In an **open kinematic chain (OKC),** the distal segment of the chain moves in space whereas in a **closed kinematic chain (CKC),** the distal segment is fixed, and proximal parts move.[15] Open chain motion occurs when reaching for an object, bringing the hand to the mouth, or kicking a ball (Fig. 1.8A). In open chain motions, segment motion is not dependent on another segment, so one segment can either move or not move, regardless of what other segments in the chain are doing. Open chain movements are highly variable since all of the participating joints are free to contribute any number of degrees of motion to the entire unit's movement. Open chain movements are required for many skilled extremity movements, and because the variability is so high, stability is sacrificed for mobility and risk of unskilled movement and even risk of injury can be a factor. Open chain movements also produce faster motion than closed chain movements.

Equally important to daily function are closed chain motions. Closed chain motions occur when the distal

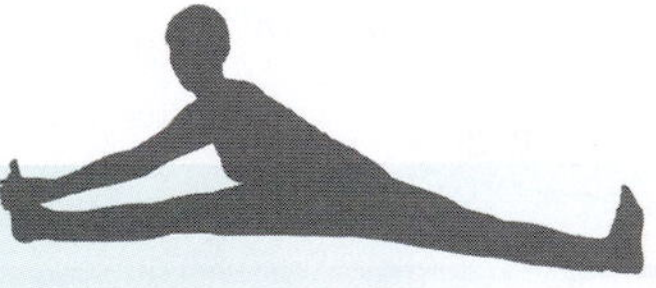

PRACTICE POINT

From the thorax to the finger, at least 19 degrees of freedom in planar motions can be identified.[15] Such freedom of motion constitutes the mechanical basis for performance of skilled manual activities and the versatility of the upper extremity. In the lower extremity and trunk, there are 25 or more degrees of freedom between the pelvis and the toe. The sum total of these joints and degrees of freedom allow a number of daily functions, from permitting the foot to adjust to an irregular or slanting surface to maintaining the body's center of gravity within the small base of support of one planted foot. Debating the *exact* number of degrees of freedom in a complete kinematic chain is really not necessary for clinical purposes. However, such realization provides additional appreciation for the extreme complexity and demands of the body by even simple movements in daily function. What an incredible masterpiece the human body is!

segment is fixed and the proximal segments move. Closed chain motion occurs during activities such as a chin-up, push-up, standing from a seated position, or a half-squat exercise (Fig. 1.8B). Movement of one segment in closed chain motion requires all the segments to move. When the ankle starts to move, the knee and hip must also move; the ankle is unable to move independently of the other two joints in the lower extremity. When a person uses the armrest of a chair to assist in rising from the chair (or performs a push-up), the hand is fixed and the forearm and shoulder move in relation to the hand, the arm moves away from the forearm (elbow extension), and the arm moves toward the trunk (shoulder adduction). Closed kinematic chain activities do not have the speed of motion that open chain activities produce, but they do provide more power and strength for functional activities.

Both open and closed kinematic chain motions occur in different segments during functional body motion as in Figures 1.2 and 1.8. Most activities of the human body involve a combination of open and closed chain events. Walking is a good example; we are in a closed chain position when we place our weight on the limb and in an open chain activity when the limb swings forward.

A

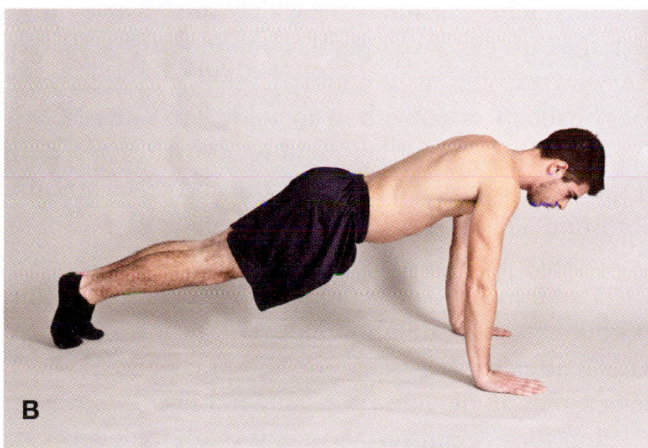

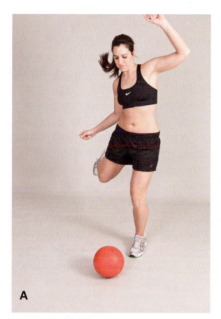

Figure 1.8 A) As the player winds up to kick the ball, the distal segments of the upper extremities are free to move (open kinematic chain), the distal end of the right lower extremity is also in an open chain, whereas the distal end of the left lower extremity is fixed in stance (closed kinematic chain). B) In performing a push-up, the distal segments at both the upper and lower extremities are fixed (closed kinematic chain).

Arthrokinematics: Joint Surface Motion

Although human joints have been compared with geometric shapes and mechanical joints such as the hinge, pivot, plane, sphere, and cone, the exquisite motions and capabilities of human joints are much more complicated than these simple geometric comparisons. The fact that no human joint throughout the body has yet been replicated satisfactorily by any joint replacement design is testimony to the complication and sophistication of the body's joints. The phenomenal superiority of human joints to man-made joints is due not only to the physiologic capacities of biologic joints, such as low coefficient of friction, presence of sensation and proprioceptive feedback, and dynamic growth responses to wear and use, but also to the mechanical complexities of human joints.

Definition

Whereas osteokinematics is concerned with the movement of the shafts of the bones and is primarily under voluntary control, arthrokinematics is concerned with how the two articulating joint surfaces actually move on each other. One of the factors that provides for the complexity of human joints is their arthrokinematic movements. Although these motions are not voluntary, they are vital for normal joint function and mobility.

Types of Joints

Joints can be classified structurally and functionally by describing the type and amount of motion allowed. You will see that structure and function are intimately related: Structure allows for functional purpose in movement and the functional requirement actually dictates the structure. Functionally, some types of joints are primarily responsible for providing stability whereas others offer primarily mobility.

Joint Structure

Arthrology (Gr. *arthron,* joint) is the study of the classification, structure, and function of joints. Joint structure and function are intimately related, as we shall see in the following sections which clearly demonstrate that understanding the anatomy or structure of a joint lends itself to understanding how that joint will function and vice versa. The most common and simplest joint classification system focuses on the structure of joints with three main types identified: **synarthrosis, amphiarthrosis,** and **diarthrosis** (Table 1–1).

Synarthrodial Joints

Joints whose primary purpose is to offer stability are joints which are largely fibrous in structure. These joints are synarthroses (noun, plural) or synarthrodial joints (adjective). These names should be easy to remember because as you know, the prefix *syn* comes from Greek meaning "together" or "joined,"[16] very descriptive of the function of this type of joint. Think of other uses of that prefix in words you have commonly used before such as synonym (words with like meaning). These joints are bound by fibrous connective tissue, known for its strength, and the fit between the two bony segments is very tight, with the joint surfaces highly congruent. Examples of a synarthrodial joint structure are the sutures of the skull; they are very stable and fit very tightly, like perfectly matched puzzle pieces. Synarthrodial joints are further divided into other main subtypes that further illustrate this relationship between structure and function.

A **syndesmosis joint** is a synarthrodial joint such as the joints between the radius and ulna and between the tibia and fibula. Syndesmosis joints are joined by a strong interosseous membrane, in which the close relationship of these pairs of bones next to each other is highly desirable with little or no mobility allowed.

Another example is the tight fit of a tooth in its socket; this is a synarthrodial **gomphosis** joint. The overall functions of synarthrodial joints are to maximize stability and allow force dissipation over highly congruent joint connecting surfaces.

Amphiarthrodial Joints

Joints that provide both stability and mobility are called amphiarthrosis (noun) or amphiarthrodial joints (adjective). The prefix *amphi* comes from Greek meaning "on both sides" or "double,"[16] very descriptive of the function of this type of joint. Think of other uses of that prefix in words you have commonly used before such as amphitheatre (partly under cover and partly outside) and amphibian (lives sometimes on land and sometimes in water). Amphiarthrodial joints are hallmarked by a cartilaginous structure with combinations of both fibrous and hyaline (or articular) cartilage and typically have a disc between the bony partners. The disc serves to tighten the fit between the two bony partners and to offer shock absorption. Examples of amphiarthrodial joints include the intervertebral joints of the spine, the pubic symphysis, and the first sternocostal joint. All of these joints offer a great deal of stability and a very specific or limited amount of mobility. The pubic symphysis, for example, is stable most of the time but during pregnancy, the disc is softened and its supporting ligaments become lax gradually by hormonal changes so that when delivery is imminent, the joint provides the required mobility to allow for the birth of the baby.

Diarthrodial Joints

Joints whose purpose is primarily to provide mobility are called a diarthrosis (noun) or diarthrodial joints (adjective). The prefix *di* meaning "twice, double or two,"[16] is descriptive of the fact that, functionally, this type of joint provides almost all of our joint mobility; these joints have several anatomical features which ensure necessary stability while still permitting mobility for function. The key structural component of diarthrodial joints is that they all have a joint capsule. This capsule connects the distal end of one joint segment to the proximal end of the other joint segment. The capsule maintains a small amount of fluid, called synovial fluid, within the joint space. For this reason, diarthrodial joints are also called **synovial joints.**

Joint Capsule

Although joint capsules vary widely in size and thickness, the capsules have several common features. Picture the joint capsule as a double-layered and somewhat baggy balloon, often with many folds. The outer layer is thicker than the inner layer and is primarily comprised of dense irregular fibrous tissue, called the **stratum fibrosum.** This makes sense since fibrous tissue occurs in areas requiring strength. The fibrous outer layer offers additional joint stability and protects the joint. Within its folds are multiple joint neural receptors. These afferent receptors are proprioceptors, which detect joint angle, joint position, and changes in joint position for the central nervous system. Joint proprioceptors are discussed further in Chapter 3. The inner synovial layer is thinner, highly vascular and known as the **stratum synovium.** It produces and secretes a pale, viscous **synovial fluid** into the joint space. Synovial fluid constantly nourishes and lubricates the mobile joint surfaces.

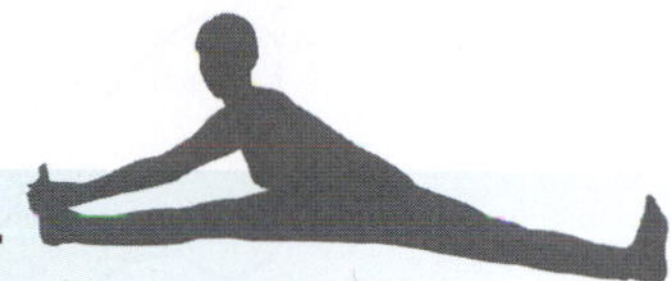

PRACTICE POINT

The anatomy of the joint capsule demonstrates an interesting contrast and shows how structure and function are closely tied. The inner capsular layer has a rich vascular supply is important for nourishment for the joint surfaces; however, this layer is poorly innervated. On the other hand, the outer synovial layer is laden with innervating joint receptors, which are important for detecting joint position and motion. Imagine what happens with any pathology accompanied by joint swelling, such as an acute sprain or even the pronounced and chronic swelling at the ankles seen in people with congestive heart failure. The swelling expands the joint capsule, causing it to distend and distort the afferent joint receptors, rendering them less sensitive to detecting joint position and movement. Imagine the functional consequences of such a problem and the importance of balance and proprioceptive training during rehabilitation. In the case of the elderly person with chronic joint swelling, think of the risk of falls and the need for balance retraining. In the case of a basketball player who sprains the ankle and suffers injury to the joint proprioceptors, do you think that this may increase the risk of re-injury or reduce the athlete's ability to run or jump safely?

Diarthrodial joint and synovial joint are interchangeable terms. These joints are the most common type of human joint and are subdivided and classified by the number of axes about which they move. The number of axes of these joints is determined by the structure of the bony joint surfaces, a factor that further demonstrates the ever-present relationship between structure and function. The classification system of uniaxial, biaxial and triaxial joints and their types has been previously described. Table 1–1 presents an overall summary of joint classification by structure and function.

The surfaces of these synovial joints are not purely geometric with flat, cylindrical, conic, or spherical designs. All joint surfaces are described as either **ovoid** (egg-shaped) or **sellar** (L., saddle) in shape.[17, 18] Most synovial joints are ovoid. In an ovoid shape, the radius of curvature varies from point to point.[19] The ovoid articular surfaces of two bones forming a joint create a convex-concave paired relationship. The concave-convex joint relationship may range from "nearly planar," as in the carpal and tarsal joints, to "nearly spheroid," as in the glenohumeral and hip joints. In engineering, the convex curvature is called the "male" component, and the concave curvature is called the "female" component. The center of rotation is in the convex component at some distance from the joint surface. In most cases, the ovoid surface of one bone in a pair is larger than its companion, as clearly seen in the glenohumeral joint (Fig. 1.9). This structural arrangement permits a large range of motion with an economy of articular surface and reduction in the size of the joint. Some joints are called sellar joints because they resemble the matching of a rider in a saddle (reciprocal reception). As mentioned, each joint surface has both convex and concave curvatures that are perpendicular to each other (Fig. 1.10) and are matched with oppositely designed joint surfaces in its partner segment. Examples of sellar joints include the carpometacarpal joint of the thumb, the sternoclavicular joint, and the ankle (talocrural joint).

Other Materials Found in Synovial Joints

Materials commonly found associated with synovial joints include cartilage, ligaments, articular discs, the joint capsule, synovial fluid, and bursae. The joint capsule and synovial fluid have been previously described, but the following descriptions highlight some of the unique features of these other important joint structures.

There are three types of cartilage: fibrous, hyaline or articular, and elastic. These are all described in basic anatomy texts. For our purposes here, it is useful to remember that fibrous cartilage is known for its strength and shock absorption potential whereas hyaline cartilage is very smooth and actually slippery. Hyaline cartilage is also known as articular cartilage because it covers the ends of the articulating ends of the bones forming the joints. Joints may also contain fibrocartilaginous discs; the menisci at the knee are examples. These fibrocartilaginous discs serve to improve the fit between the joint's bony surfaces and to absorb some of the impact forces imparted to the joints. Occasionally, one surface of the joint, for example in the hip and shoulder, may be rimmed with a fibrous labrum, which forms a ring or lip around the outer edge of the

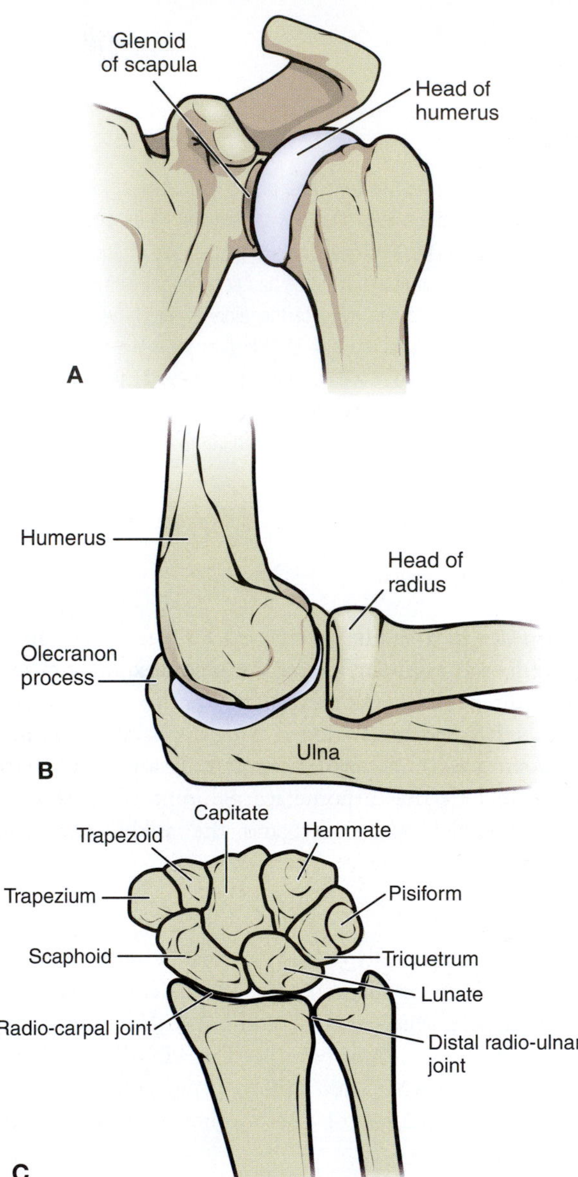

Figure 1.9 Examples of concave-convex relationships of joint surfaces redrawn from radiographs: A) Glenohumeral joint of the shoulder (anterior-posterior view); B) Humeroulnar joint of the elbow (lateral view); C) Radiocarpal and midcarpal joints of the wrist (anterior-posterior view).

concave joint partner, deepening it and enhancing the joint's stability.

As you know from your study of anatomy, ligaments connect bone to bone. Their purpose is to add stability, to limit joint motion within a specific plane, and to prevent extreme motion which could cause injury. They are named usually by their location and the bones they connect. Since ligaments stop end-range motion by becoming taut when motion occurs in directions opposite to their position, it is often easy to predict their function if we know the ligament's name and location. For example, the palmar radiocarpal ligament is located on the palmar (anterior) surface of the wrist joint; therefore, it will prevent excessive wrist extension. Another example is the knee's medial collateral ligament; since it is on the medial aspect of the knee, part of its purpose is to prevent the tibia from moving laterally from its alignment with the femur. Some ligaments are actually blended within the joint capsule to strengthen the capsule and provide it with additional reinforcement and stability. These ligaments are called intracapsular ligaments. Ligaments not meshed with the capsule are extracapsular ligaments.

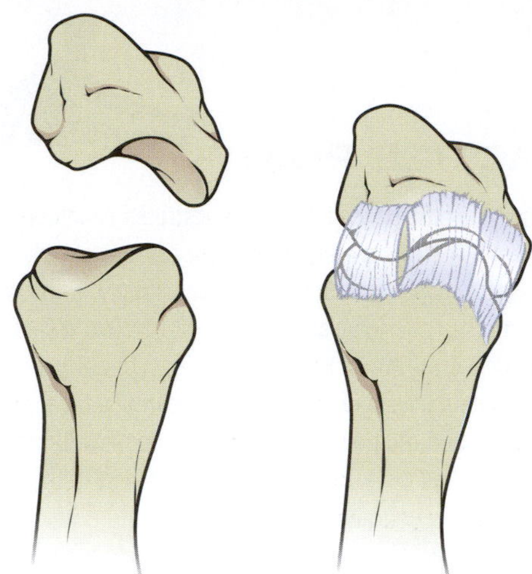

Figure 1.10 Sellar joint with concave and convex surfaces of each bone (carpometacarpal joint of the thumb).

A **bursa** is a fluid-filled sac whose purpose is to reduce friction between structures and offer additional protection or shock absorption between joint surfaces. We have many bursae within our bodies; some joints have several whereas other joints have only a few. For example, the olecranon bursa that is located at the elbow reduces friction between the olecranon process and the surface the elbow leans on, and it also absorbs shock every time the elbow moves into or locks in extension. Bursae are usually independent structures, but they can also be continuous with the synovial membrane of a joint capsule, as is the case of the suprapatellar bursa at the anterior knee joint.[20] At times, the body will create additional bursae in response to the demands put upon it. These acquired bursae are great examples of how the body adapts its structure to meet the demands of function. Tendons attach muscle to bone and are sometimes enveloped in a bursal sheath, called a tendon sheath.

Basic Arthrokinematic Joint Motions

How a synovial joint moves is a function of the structural configuration of each of the articulating surfaces and how

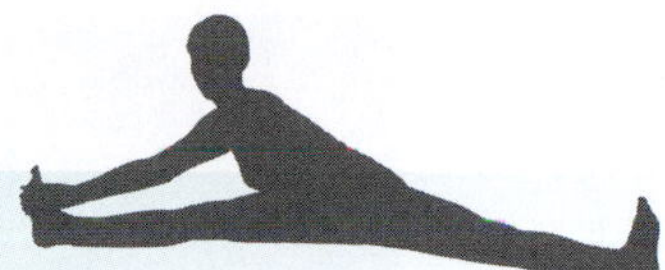

PRACTICE POINT

It is important to differentiate between joint **dislocation** and joint **subluxation.** A dislocation quite literally means that the two bony segments forming a joint are completely disassociated from each other. Such an injury usually means that significant damage to the capsule has occurred. Dislocation usually occurs secondary to acute trauma. In cases of shoulder or hip dislocations, the labrum may also be torn. A subluxation, on the other hand, occurs when there is a separation of the two bony partners, and the joint partners are partially disassociated from each other. Subluxation may occur over time, such as in hip subluxation in children with cerebral palsy or shoulder subluxation in persons with hemiplegia secondary to a cerebrovascular accident, or it may occur acutely when a joint suffers profound forces sufficient to disrupt some of the stabilizing elements but not enough to separate the joint segments entirely. Acute subluxation occurs most commonly in sports; in these cases, the partially disassociated segment usually spontaneously relocates.

they move on each other. Once again, we will see that structure and function are intimately related: Structure will allow for the joint's functional purpose, and the function can be achieved because of the joint's structural characteristics. Although we have seen that the main osteokinematic movements at joints are rotary in nature, it is important to note that when surfaces move or rotate around each other, the joint surfaces also undergo simultaneous arthrokinematic motions. When a joint moves in an arthrokinematic movement, three types of basic motion can occur between the two surfaces: (1) rolling or rocking, (2) sliding or gliding, and (3) spinning.[19] Most joint movements involve a combination of these motions. As previously mentioned, when a joint moves, usually one of the joint surfaces is stable and the other surface moves on this relatively fixed base.[21]

Rolling (or **rocking)** is a rotary, or angular, motion in which each subsequent point on one surface contacts a new point on the other surface, such as in "rolling" a ball across the floor (Fig. 1.11). **Sliding** (or **gliding)** is a translatory, or linear, motion in which the movement of one joint surface is parallel to the plane of the adjoining joint surface, such as when a figure skater "glides" across the ice. In sliding or gliding, one point of reference (the skate blade) contacts new points across the adjacent surface (the ice). **Spinning,** as in "spinning" a top, is a rotary, or angular, motion in which one point of contact on each surface remains in constant contact with a fixed location on the other surface. Most normal joint movement has some combination of rolling, sliding, and spinning. The knee joint shows this most clearly. If there were only a rolling of the condyles of the femur on the tibial plateau, the femur would roll off the tibia and the knee would dislocate (Fig. 1.11A). Instead, when the femur extends on the fixed tibia, as it does when an individual rises from a seated to a standing position, the femoral condyles slide as they roll and so maintain contact with the tibial condyles (Fig. 1.11B). In the last few degrees of knee extension in a closed kinetic chain, the femur spins (medially rotates on the tibia) to achieve full knee extension. This combination of roll, slide, and spin allows a large range of motion within a joint while using a small articular surface. If a joint possessed only one of these arthrokinematic motions, its range of motion would be limited or its joint surfaces would need to be larger to accomplish the same range of motion.

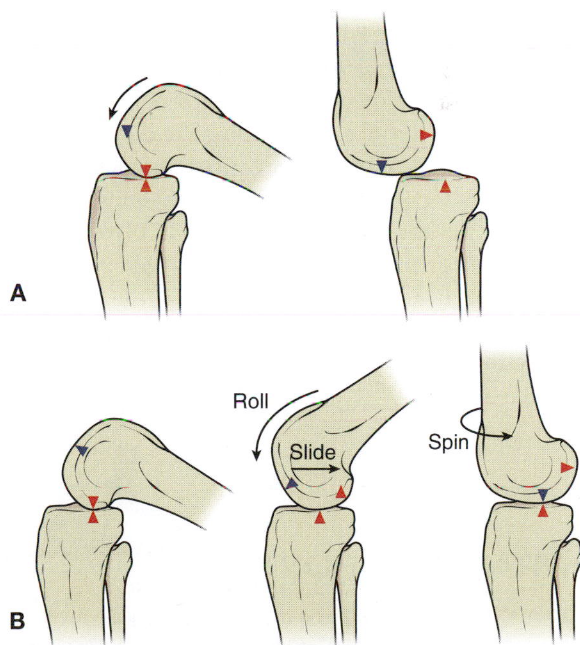

Figure 1.11 Movements of joint surfaces: A) Pure rolling or hinge motion of the femur or the tibia would cause joint dislocation; B) Normal motion of the knee demonstrates a combination of rolling, sliding, and spinning in the last 20° of extension (terminal rotation of the knee).

In order for the articular surfaces to have voluntary and full active control of joint motion, these arthrokinematic movements must be present.[21] In other words, large osteokinematic motions, such as flexion or abduction, must be accompanied by small simultaneous arthrokinematic motions that amount to only a few millimeters of translatory motion or full range of motion is not possible. These small arthrokinematic motions are called **accessory movements,** component movements,[22] or **joint play.**[23] Without these accessory motions, normal physiologic motion is not possible.

In addition to roll, slide, and spin, there are other accessory movements that may also be considered either joint play or arthrokinematic motions. These include the translatory motions of joint compression and joint distraction. During these accessory motions, the joint surfaces are moved together to approximate each other or are pulled away in traction from each other, respectively. Sometimes compression or distraction occurs between the joint surfaces by virtue of the forces exerted by muscles acting across the joint surfaces, as we shall see in Chapter 6 when discussing the pull of the brachioradialis muscle attaching near the wrist joint. In other cases, compression or distraction is produced by an externally applied force such as when a clinician distracts a joint as part of a joint mobilization technique or in the application of either manual or mechanical external traction to the spine. Compression may facilitate joint proprioceptors and improve joint stability. Distraction may assist in synovial fluid circulation within a joint and increase joint mobility.

However slight, these passive translations that occur in most joints are described by defining the direction of the translation. Three directions are most commonly identified: anterior–posterior, medial–lateral, and superior–inferior. The amount of translation is often used to test the integrity of the ligaments.[17] One example is distraction or separation of joint surfaces at the metacarpophalangeal joint (Fig. 1.12). In addition to distraction, normal synovial joint surfaces may undergo lateral glide, anterior-posterior glide, and rotation. These motions cannot be performed voluntarily by the subject but require relaxation of muscles and the application of passive movement by a clinician. These small motions are routinely performed by clinicians during the evaluation and treatment of joint motion problems.

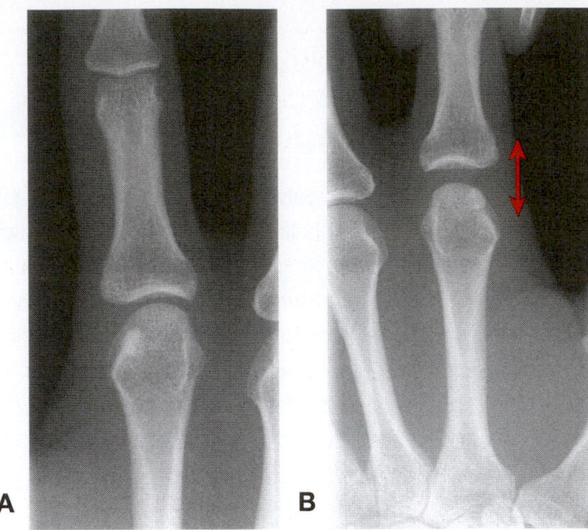

Figure 1.12 Radiograph of the metacarpophalangeal joint of the index finger: A) at rest; and B) at the limit of long-axis distraction. The relationship of the articulating surfaces of the bones in B should be compared with their relationship with the joint at rest. Arrow indicates the direction of pull by the examiner.

Joint Shapes as They Pertain to Arthrokinematic Motion

The shapes of joint surfaces range from flat to curved, with most joint surfaces curved and having one surface relatively convex in shape and its partner relatively concave.[17] At some joints, such as the hip, this concave-convex relationship is quite dramatic. At other joints, the convex-concave relationship is more subtle, such as in the interphalangeal joints of the fingers. In spite of the range from obvious to subtle configurations, however, the arthrokinematic movement of joint surfaces relative to the movement of the shaft of the bones (osteokinematics)

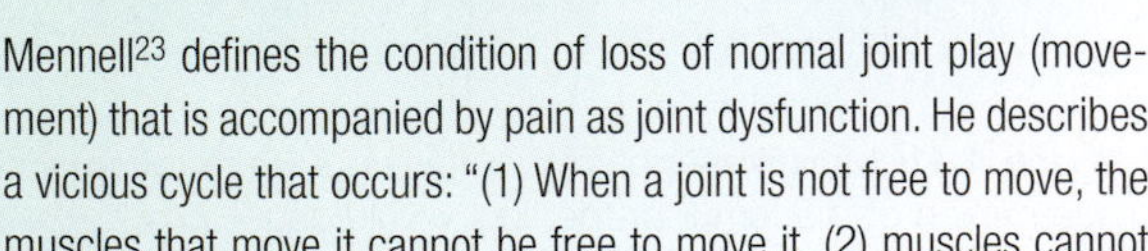

PRACTICE POINT

Mennell[23] defines the condition of loss of normal joint play (movement) that is accompanied by pain as joint dysfunction. He describes a vicious cycle that occurs: "(1) When a joint is not free to move, the muscles that move it cannot be free to move it, (2) muscles cannot be restored to normal if the joints which they move are not free to move, (3) normal muscle function is dependent on normal joint movement, and (4) impaired muscle function perpetuates and may cause deterioration in abnormal joints."[23]

follows a principle related to its mechanical properties known as the **convex-concave principle**. Although it has been biomechanically demonstrated not to be a steadfast rule at all joints,[24-27] this principle states that if the bone with the convex joint surface moves on the bone with the concave surface, the convex joint surface slides in the direction opposite to the bone segment's rolling motion (Figs. 1.11 and 1.13). If the bone with the concave surface moves on the convex surface, the concave articular surface slides in the same direction as the bone segment's roll does. The proximal interphalangeal joint of the index finger is used as an example in Figure 1.13. When flexion of this joint occurs at the proximal phalanx, points on this bone's convex joint surface move in a direction that is opposite to that of the shaft of the proximal phalanx (Fig. 1.13B). On the other hand, if the concave surface of the middle phalanx moves on the fixed proximal phalanx, the joint surface of the middle phalanx moves in the same direction as the moving middle phalanx (Fig. 1.13C).

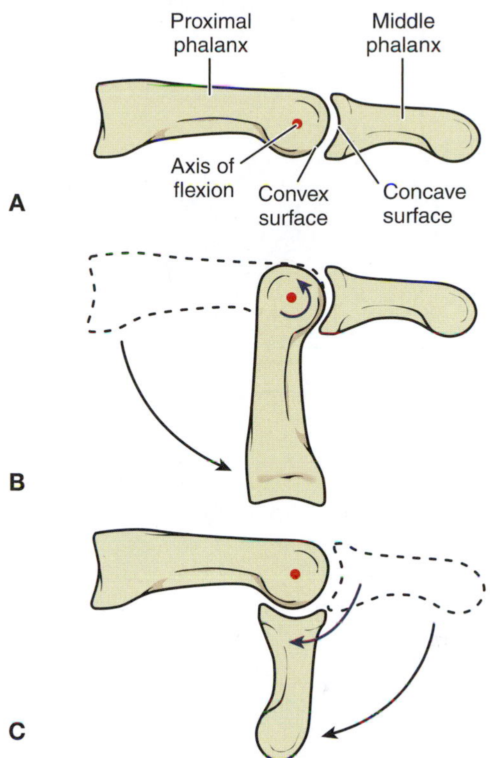

Figure 1.13 Lateral view of the proximal interphalangeal joint of the index finger (A) in extension and (B & C) in flexion. In B, when the bone with the convex joint surface moves into flexion, the joint surface slides in an opposite direction to the motion of the shaft of the bone. In C, when the bone with the concave joint surface moves into flexion, the joint surface moves in the same direction as the shaft of the bone. (Black arrow denotes the rolling of the bony segment; green arrow denotes the sliding of the joint surface.)

Joint Axes in Function

Because of the incongruity of joint surfaces and the motions of roll, slide, and spin, human joint axes are complex. A joint's axis does not remain stationary like a mechanical door hinge; rather, the center axis of a human joint moves as the joint position changes, usually following a curvilinear path (Fig. 1.14). This change in position of the center of axis of rotation is called the instantaneous axis of rotation. The largest movement of this axis occurs in the knee, elbow, and wrist. In addition, the joint's *instantaneous axes or rotations* are seldom exactly perpendicular to the long axes of the bones but are frequently oblique. This is particularly noticeable, for example, as when the little finger is flexed into the palm. The tip of the finger points to the base of the thumb rather than to the base of the fifth metacarpal. In another example, when the elbow is extended from full flexion with the forearm in supination, the forearm

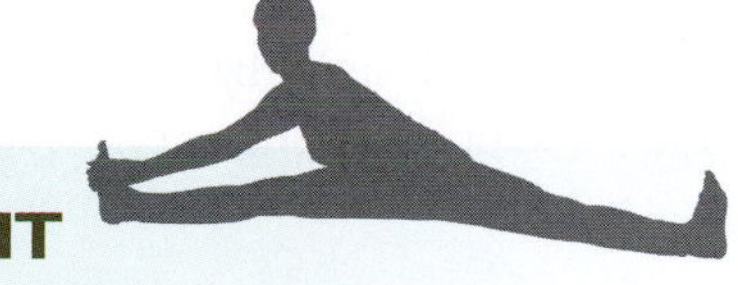

PRACTICE POINT

These oblique axes and changing positions of the joint centers of rotation create challenges and necessitate compromise when mechanical appliances and joints are applied to the body, as in goniometry, orthotic devices, and exercise equipment. Mechanical appliances usually have a fixed axis of motion that is perpendicular to the moving part. When the mechanical and anatomic parts are coupled, perfect alignment can occur at only one point in the range of motion. At other points in the range of motion, the mechanical appliance may bind and cause pressure on the body part, or it may force the human joint in abnormal directions. Thus, the placement of mechanical joints is critical where large ranges of motion are desired. Although many advances have been made, the search continues for mechanical joints that more nearly approximate the complexity of human joints.

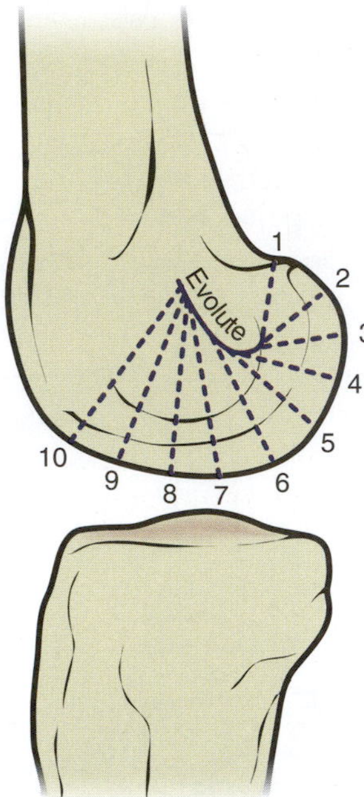

Figure 1.14 Changing radius of curves of the femoral condyles. The axis of motion for flexion and extension moves: number 1 represents the radius for curvature in flexion and number 10, the radius in extension.

laterally deviates 0 to 20°. This lateral deviation of the forearm from the humerus is called the carrying angle and is discussed in Chapter 6 (see Fig. 6-2).

Close-Packed and Open-Packed Joint Positions

The surfaces of a joint's segments usually match each other perfectly in only one position of the joint. This point of congruency (coinciding exactly) is called the **close-packed position.**[19] When in this position, (1) the maximum area of surface contact occurs, (2) the attachments of the ligaments are farthest apart and under tension, (3) capsular structures are taut, and (4) the joint is mechanically compressed and difficult to distract (separate). In all other positions, the joint surfaces do not fit perfectly and are incongruent; these are called **open-packed,** or **loose-packed,** positions. In the open-packed positions, the ligamentous and capsular structures are slack, and the joint surfaces may be distracted several millimeters. Open-packed positions allow the necessary motions of spin, roll, and slide typically with an increase in accessory movements and decreased joint friction. The position at which there is the least congruency and at which the capsule and ligaments are loosest or most slack is the **resting position.** The resting position is unique for each joint type but usually occurs when the joint is positioned near its midrange. The resting position is often used as the preferred joint position when joint mobilizations are applied to a joint to gain mobility, especially during earlier treatment sessions (Fig. 1.15).

The close-packed position is usually at one extreme in the joint's range of motion. For example, the close-packed position is in full extension for the elbow, wrist, hip, and knee; dorsiflexion for the ankle; and full flexion for the metacarpophalangeal joints. In these positions, the joint's capsule and ligaments are taut, and the joint has great mechanical stability with reduced need for muscle forces to maintain the position. For example, when the metacarpophalangeal joints are in 90° of flexion, lateral motion (abduction) cannot occur. This is an advantage in gripping when muscle forces can be directed to finger flexion rather than being needed to also keep the fingers from spreading. The hips and knees are in their close-packed positions in extension. This close-packed position of these joints permits erect standing with little or no contraction of the muscles of the hips or knees. When an individual "rests" on the joint ligaments rather than using muscle force to maintain a position, energy expenditure is reduced.

Clinical Applications

Application of arthrokinematic principles is basic to the assessment of the integrity of joint structures and use of joint mobilization techniques in the treatment of **hypomobile** or painful soft tissues. Normally, ligaments and capsular structures limit passive accessory motions in open-packed positions. If a ligament ruptures, the ligament no longer provides motion control so the joint may be **hypermobile.** If joint soft tissue structures are in an acute inflammatory stage, the joint's accessory motion will be painful and hypomobile. Some angular joint motions, such as wrist flexion and extension, occur because of an exquisite coordination of several joints. The wrist has at least 12 articulations between the midcarpal and radiocarpal joints that must all function properly for full wrist movement to occur (see Fig. 1.9C). In a person with pain and limitation of wrist flexion, localization of the impairment is made by a thorough and carefully detailed evaluation, including assessment of the accessory movements at each of these articulations.

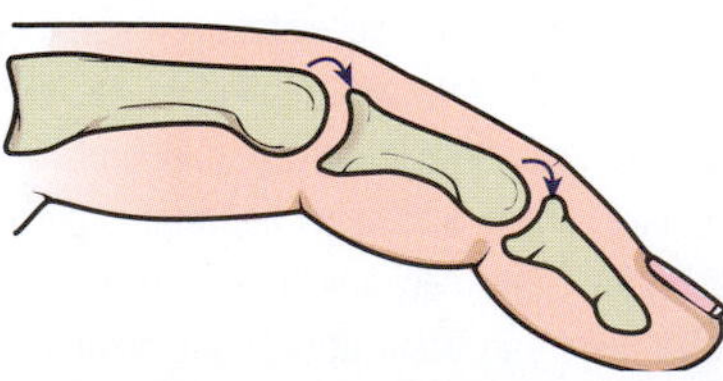

Figure 1.15 A normal interphalangeal joint in resting position.

Joint surface relationships must be appreciated by the clinician when motion of the joint is limited and exercise is used to increase motion. For example, if scar tissue formation affecting the skin, capsule, tendon, or ligaments interferes with interphalangeal joint flexion and limits finger flexion, the clinician must be able to accurately treat the problem. When the concave base of the phalanx cannot flex, a stretch force applied distally on the phalanx may pry the joint so that anterior tissues are overstretched while posterior tissues are compressed. This could result in further injury to joint structures. In such a case, a gentle distraction force applied close to the joint and in line with the joint's surface provides for a better treatment outcome (Fig. 1.12B).

Summary

This opening chapter is a foundational chapter for the study of kinesiology. The main focus of this chapter is describing and analyzing human movement in *kinematic* terms: Movement is studied by looking at the type, direction and amount of motion, both at the segment level and the body as a whole as we move about, engaged in functional activity. Kinematics is further subdivided into osteokinematics, which describes the movement of one bone on another, and arthrokinematics, which describes the actual gliding motions of joint articular surfaces on each other. Joints offer varying amounts of movement or degrees of freedom, according to how many planes they can move in as they rotate about an axis. A joint classification system is reviewed which presents the amount of motion and the structure of the joint simultaneously so that this common-sense approach to describing movement is simplified. Examples of how these kinematic concepts and principles relate to functional movements are described throughout the chapter.

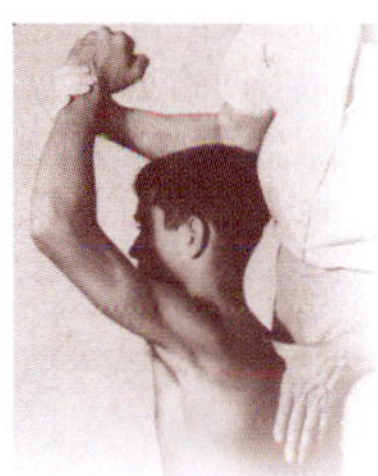

CLINICAL SCENARIO SOLUTION

Jamie realizes that although the volunteer coach is trying to be helpful, he does not have the knowledge or training required to administer any intervention for this little boy. She knows that she not only must be diplomatic and tactful, but must also be clear to the coach about the possible consequences. Since the coach knows her, he is receptive to her approach. Jamie acknowledges his devotion to his players as a volunteer coach, but she gives him a very brief yet descriptive summary of the complexity of joint structure. He immediately recognizes the wisdom of simply giving the boy first aid, limited to supplying an ice pack, and recommends that his parents seek medical attention.

Discussion Questions

1. How are both stability and mobility achieved by the human body through joint structure?
2. How are joint structure and function interrelated? Give some examples to illustrate.
3. Why is it clinically important to adhere to a universal terminology system when describing human movement?
4. What is the value of using the anatomical position as a convention when describing joint motion?
5. What are the pros and cons of open and closed chain exercises? What is the functional relevance of both?

Lab Activities

Osteokinematics

1. With a partner, use Figures 1.3 and 1.4 to guide you in performing and observing motions in all the planes. Remember to perform each motion starting from stance in the anatomical position. Observe from the front while your partner performs frontal plane motions at the neck, trunk, shoulder, elbow, wrist, fingers, hip, knee, ankle, and toes. Identify the direction of the axis of motion. Repeat for motions in the sagittal plane, viewing from the side, and in the horizontal or transverse plane.
2. Describe and demonstrate the motions available at all of the joints in the body, using proper osteokinematic terminology such as what plane and axis (axes) are involved, the name of the motion, the anatomic joint name and joint type, and the number of degrees of freedom engaged. Use Figure 1.4 and Table 1–1 as a guide.
3. With a partner or a group, design and lead a dance or exercise warm-up routine by calling out for the active movement of different joints. Call out the motion and the approximate degrees of motion by using Figure 1.4 and Tables 1–1 and 1–2 to guide you.
4. Although covered in detail in other coursework and texts, use a universal goniometer and Table 1–1 to visualize the osteokinematic bony segment motions and to visualize generally the available motions at joints in different planes.
5. Describe and demonstrate normal range of motion of joints and their normal end feels.
6. Perform open and closed chain motions. Based on your new knowledge gained in this chapter, combined with your previous study of anatomy, describe joint motions, muscles activated, and types of muscle contractions.
7. With a partner or a small group, devise and demonstrate open and closed chain functional activities or potential exercises for the shoulder, elbow, wrist, hip, knee, and ankle. Compare and contrast.

Arthrokinematics

1. Using a disarticulated bone set or skeleton, find examples of the different types of joints: synarthrodial (including a syndesmosis), amphiarthrodial, diarthrodial (including all of the types of uniaxial, biaxial and triaxial joints). Use Table 1–1 as a guide. Compare and contrast these joint types with a specific focus on how different structures afford stability, mobility and combinations of both stability and mobility.
2. Perform normal joint motions using a disarticulated bone set or skeleton to visualize and study basic joint motions. As you move the joints, look closely at the joint surfaces and note when you observe the following motions: a) rolling or rocking; b) sliding or gliding; and c) spinning. Observe the convex-concave principle by noting the directions of the articular surface and the shaft when the bone with the convex surface is moved and when the bone with the concave surface is moved.
3. Demonstrate joint stability in close-packed positions and joint mobility in open-packed positions. Examine the joint surfaces as they move and make note of when the joint surfaces are either compressed or distracted. When moving different joints through varying points in their range, apply an external manual compression or distraction force and discuss the clinical implications.
4. Have your partner sit at a table or desk so that the forearm and palm are supported and the fingers are hanging over the edge. The examiner should sit in front or to the side of the subject and should hold the second metacarpal (index finger) between the thumb and fingers of one hand and the first phalange of the index finger with the other hand. The subject *must* relax the forearm and hand throughout the following activities:
   a. Convex-concave principle: Hold the metacarpal still and passively move the phalange from flexion to extension several times. Visualize the directions of motion of the articular surface and the shaft. Next, hold the phalange still and move the metacarpal into flexion and extension to visualize movements (Fig. 1.12).
   b. Close-packed and open-packed joint positions: Hold the metacarpal still and move the phalange. Notice that in extension of the joint, medial-lateral motion into abduction and adduction are present (open-packed position), but in 90° of flexion, the joint surfaces feel more congruent and the joint is more stable, with limited medial-lateral mobility (close-packed position).

c. Accessory motion or joint play: Keep the metacarpal stabilized so that it cannot move, keep the joint in an open-packed position and keep the subject relaxed while gently performing the following passive motions:

i. Distraction: Gently pull the phalange distally 1 to 2 mm. Subject can palpate the joint space with other finger (Fig. 1.12).

ii. Rotation: Gently rotate the phalange in each direction.

iii. Anterior and posterior glides: The examiner's thumb must be on the dorsal surface of the base of the phalange and forefinger on the palmar surface. The phalange is gently moved passively up and down without any angular motion (i.e., flexion or extension). Note that these motions cannot be performed actively by the subject and that they cannot be performed passively in the close-packed position or if the subject is not relaxed.

References

1. Hirt S. What is Kinesiology? A Historical Review. *The Physical Therapy Review* 35(8):1–11, 1955.
2. Norkin CC, White DJ. *Measurement of Joint Motion: A Guide to Goniometry*, 3 ed. Philadelphia: FA Davis, 2003.
3. Reuleaux F. *Theoretische Kinematik*. Braunschweigh: F. Vieweg & Son, 1875.
4. Fischer O. *Kinematik Organischer Gelenke*. Braunschweig: R Vierweg; 1907.
5. Van Sant A. Rising from a supine position to erect stance. *Physical Therapy* 68:185, 1988.
6. Kapandji IA. *The Physiology of the Joints, Vol 1, Upper Limb*. 5 ed. Edinburgh: Churchill Livingstone, 1982.
7. *American Academy of Orthopaedic Surgeons: Joint Motion Method of Measuring and Recording*. Chicago: American Academy of Orthopaedic Surgeons,1965.
8. *Departments of the Army and the Air Force: Joint Motion Measurement TM 8-640/AFP 160-14.* Washington, DC: Department of the Army,1968.
9. Kendall HO, Kendall FP, Wadsworth GE. *Muscles: Testing and Function*, 2 ed. Baltimore: Williams & Wilkins, 1971.
10. Daniels L, Worthingham C. *Muscle Testing: Techniques of Manual Examination*, 5 ed. Philadelphia: WB Saunders, 1986.
11. Gerhardt JJ, Russe OA. *International SFTR Method of Measuring and Recording Joint Motion*. Bern, Switzerland: Hans Huber, Year Book Medical Publishers, 1975.
12. Kapandji IA. *The Physiology of the Joints, Vol 2, Lower Limb*, 5 ed. Edinburgh, Scotland: Churchill Livingstone, 1987.
13. Dubs L, Gschwend N. General joint laxity: Quantification and clinical relevance. *Archives of Orthopaedic and Trauma Surgery* 107:65, 1988.
14. Cyriax J, Cyriax P. *Illustrated Manual of Orthopaedic Medicine*, 1 ed. London: Butterworth-Heinemann, 1983.
15. Steindler A. *Kinesiology of the Human Body Under Normal and Pathological Conditions*. Springfield, IL: Charles C Thomas, 1955.
16. *Tabers Cyclopedic Medical Dictionary,* 20 ed. Philadelphia: FA Davis Company, 2005.
17. Neumann DA. *Kinesiology of the Musculoskeletal System: Foundations for Physical Rehabilitation*. St. Louis: Mosby Inc, 2002.
18. Levangie PK, Norton CC. *Joint Structure & Function: A Comprehensive Analysis*, 4th ed. Philadelphia: FA Davis, 2005.
19. MacConaill MA, Basmajian JV. *Muscles and Movements: A Basis for Human Kinesiology*. Baltimore: Williams & Wilkins, 1969.
20. Muscolino JE. *Kinesiology: The Skeletal System and Muscle Function*. St. Louis: Mosby Inc, 2006.
21. Levangie P, Norkin CC. *Joint Structure and Function A Comprehensive Analysis*, 4 ed. Philadelphia: F A Davis, 2005.
22. Maitland GD. *Peripheral Manipulation*, 2 ed. Boston: Butterworths, 1977.
23. Mennell JM. *Joint Pain: Diagnosis and Treatment Using Manipulative Techniques*. Boston: Little, Brown & Co, 1964.
24. Novotny JE, Beynnon BD, Nichols CE. Modeling the stability of the human glenohumeral joint during external rotation. *Journal of Biomechanics* 33:345–354, 2000.
25. Novotny JE, Nichols CE, Beynnon BD. Normal kinematics of the unconstrained glenohumeral joint under coupled moment loads. *Journal of Shoulder and Elbow Surgery* 7(6):629–639, 1998.
26. Soslowsky LJ, Flatow EL, Bigliani L. Quantification of in situ contact areas at the glenohumeral joint: a biomechanical study. *Journal of Orthopaedic Research* 10:524–534, 1992.
27. Oatis CA. *Kinesiology: The Mechanics & Pathomechanics of Human Movement*, 2 ed. Philadelphia: Lippincott Williams & Wilkins, 2008.
28. Fick R. *Anatomie und Mechanik der Gelenke: Teil III, Spezielle Gelenk und Muskel Mechanik*. Jena: Fisher, 1911.

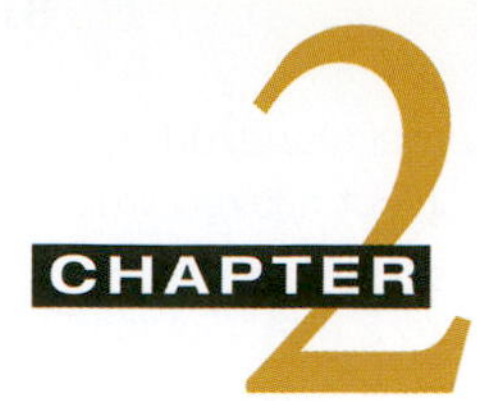

Mechanical Principles: Kinetics

"Give me a lever long enough and a fulcrum on which to place it and I shall move the world."

—Archimedes, 287 BC–212 BC

Greek mathematician, physicist, engineer, inventor, and astronomer

CHAPTER OUTLINE

Learning Outcomes
Clinical Scenario
Introduction
Determinants of Motions
Types of Motion
Location of Motion
Magnitude of Motion
Direction of Motion
Rate of Motion and Change of Motion
Forces
Types of Forces
Newton's Laws of Motion
Force Vectors and Their Considerations
Composition of Forces
Levers
First-Class Lever
Second-Class Lever
Third-Class Lever
Mechanical Advantage
Static Equilibrium
Torque
Parallel Force Systems
Resolution of Forces
Forces Acting at Angles
Laws of the Right Triangle
Force Applications to the Body
Weight and Center of Gravity (Center of Mass)
Levers and Muscle Activity
Free Body Diagrams

LEARNING OUTCOMES

This chapter identifies the mechanical and physics principles of force applications that are relevant to human movement. By the end of the chapter, you should be able to:

- ❑ Identify the four forces that act upon the body;
- ❑ Explain the three classes of levers and provide an example of each in the human body;
- ❑ List Newton's laws of motion and distinguish how they apply to the human body;
- ❑ Identify the elements of a force vector diagram and explain the tangential force and its significance in joint motion;
- ❑ Describe a free body diagram and its function in kinesiology;
- ❑ Explain why muscle and joint reaction forces are often larger than the external forces applied to the body;
- ❑ Ascertain the ratio formulas for a right triangle;
- ❑ Describe the differences between force and torque;
- ❑ Provide a clinical example of the applications of Newton's laws of motion;
- ❑ Offer a clinical example of how to alter a quadriceps exercise to increase resistance provided to a patient without increasing the weight.

Calculation of Muscle and Joint Forces
Applying Resistances to the Body
Clinical Application of Concepts
Pulleys
Leverage Factor
Stretching vs. Joint Mobilization
Pressure
Summary
Clinical Scenario Solution
Discussion Questions
Lab Activities
References

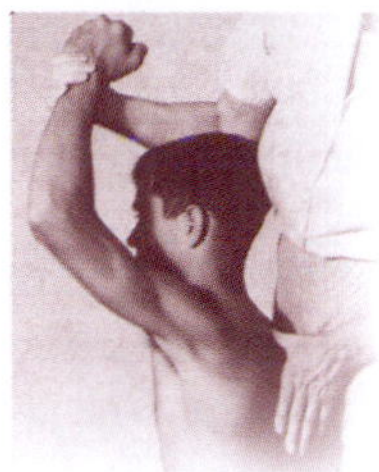

CLINICAL SCENARIO

William wished he had paid more attention to his physics professor during his sophomore year. He is now taking a kinesiology class that he really enjoys, but he does not recall much of the physics concepts his current professor is now reviewing. He is lost when Professor Violet starts discussing how bones are levers and muscles provide torque to move them. He is not sure he even remembers the difference between torque and force. As Professor Violet continues her presentation, William is intrigued when she states that we can change the amount of work a muscle must do just by changing where we apply the force against that muscle. William wonders, "How can that be?" and "What does that have to do with physics?"

Introduction

So that we understand how muscles and their neural innervations create motion, we need to investigate how they respond when the body segments experience outside forces applied to them. **Kinetics** deals with forces that produce, stop, or modify motion of either the body as a whole or the individual body segments. **Kinematics**, as you learned in Chapter 1, deals with motion of the body and/or its segments without regard to the forces acting to produce those motions. This chapter advances from the ideas of the movements you learned in the first chapter to how those movements occur through the application of various forces. Forces within the body and forces outside the body both affect how a body moves. Muscles produce forces to move our body. Many factors influence how the muscles function to provide us with the mobility, ability, and variability we have to interact with our environment, meet the demands our bodies face, and perform meaningful activity. Fortunately, there are laws of motion that help us anticipate performance needs. Throughout this chapter, we will investigate these laws and see how they influence movement and outcomes. Understanding how these laws determine both body motion and environmental factors will help us understand movement of the body's segments that will be studied in subsequent chapters. A note of caution for those with a phobia of physics: This chapter contains some basic physics applications, but they will be explained sufficiently to make sense and will be applied only when necessary to further your understanding of the clinical application of how laws of motion are relevant to the body and our interests as clinicians.

Determinants of Motions

Before we can appreciate force applications, we must be able to describe body motion. Motion is simply the displacement of a body or one of its segments from one point to another. Five variables determine and describe body or segmental motion:

1) Type of motion;
2) Location of the motion;
3) Magnitude of the motion;
4) Direction of the motion; and
5) Rate of motion or rate of change at which the motion occurs.

Let us take a brief look at each of these variables. An understanding of these principles may provide for a greater understanding of the forces acting on the body.

Types of Motion

As was mentioned in Chapter 1, because the body is made up of rigid segments that are connected together by joints, there are two types of motion that occur in the body: translatory motion and rotary motion. **Translatory motion** occurs as a linear displacement. In other words, movement is in a straight line. For example, translatory motion occurs when you reach across your desk to pick up a pencil. Your arm, forearm, wrist, and hand move in a straight motion across the desk. Whenever there is translatory motion in the body, some rotation movement usually accompanies it. For example, as you reach across the desk for a pencil, the forearm, wrist, and hand are moving in a straight line, but the shoulder is rotating. **Rotary motion** is movement of a rigid segment around an axis. This is also known as angular displacement. In true rotary motion, the axis is fixed so each part of the rigid segment that rotates around the axis moves through the same angle at the same time. In the body, true rotary motion does not usually occur because there is some shifting of the axis (joint) during motion. As you may have already realized, body movement is a combination of linear and rotary motions. Walking is a good example: The entire body moves from one point to another in a straight line, but rotary motions of the hip, knee, and ankle accomplish this body movement.

Location of Motion

Because the body is three-dimensional, we must create a frame of reference for body movement in three dimensions. These three dimensions, or axes, of movement were presented in Chapter 1. You recall that the x-axis, also called the coronal axis, frontal axis or mediolateral (left-to-right) axis, is the horizontal axis, whereas the y-axis is the vertical axis, or longitudinal axis, and the z-axis is the sagittal axis, or anterior-posterior axis. Body motion occurs around these axes within their planes of motion. A plane of motion is perpendicular to the axis of motion around which it rotates.

Body segmental movements occur within these three planes of motion. Each segment is variable in how many of these planes it is able to move. The number of planes in which a segment moves is primarily dependent upon the shape of the joint, so each joint's planes of movement will be discussed as we go through each segment in subsequent chapters.

Magnitude of Motion

Distance is how far a force moves a body. This is also known as the magnitude a body or segment is displaced. It is measured in either linear or rotary distance. Linear distance is measured in meters or feet. Rotary distance is measured in degrees (as in degrees of a circle) and is described as **range of motion** when discussing joint motion. A full circle of motion is 360°.

Direction of Motion

Since body motion occurs around joint axes, let's first address rotary motion. If we refer to the axes of movement, it is easier to understand the directions of movement. Motion has a positive and a negative component. Similar to a common graph, moving along the x-axis toward the right is positive and toward the left is negative. Moving along the y-axis upward is positive and downward is negative. Finally, moving along the z-axis toward the front or anteriorly is positive and moving backward or posteriorly is negative. In the anatomical position, movement in the x-axis (medial-lateral axis) occurs in the sagittal plane and provides flexion and extension; movement on the z-axis (anterior-posterior axis) occurs in the frontal planes and includes abduction and adduction; and rotation motions occur on the y-axis (superior-inferior or vertical axis) in the transverse plane.

Now, let's jump from rotary to translatory motion. We already know that translatory motion is also produced by the body and its segments. As with rotary motion, translatory motion can occur along any of the three axes of motion. Linear motion, however, is described according to both the axis of motion in which it occurs and whether the motion is going toward a positive or a negative direction. For example, translatory motion is positive if it occurs as motion to the right along the medial-lateral axis (x-axis), forward motion along the AP (z-axis), and upward motion along the vertical axis (y-axis). Negative motions occur in opposite directions on these axes.

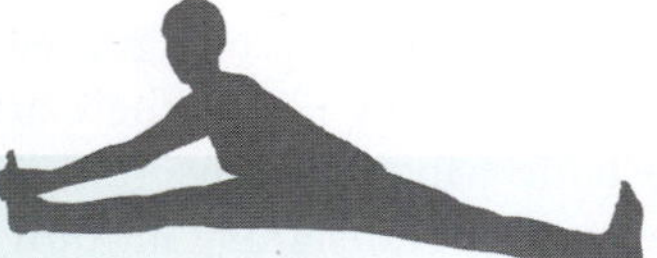

PRACTICE POINT

Movement of planes around axes can be a difficult concept to grasp, so perhaps this activity may make it more understandable for you: Take a piece of paper, poke a hole in its center, and place a pencil in the hole; you now have an axis (pencil) and a plane of movement (paper). Position the pencil in one of the three axes of motion and rotate the paper around the pencil to see the movement that occurs in each plane. Identify both the axis you have the pencil in and the plane of motion in which the paper is rotating. The plane of motion is always perpendicular to the axis of motion. Place the pencil in each axis of motion and identify each plane of motion within which the paper moves while spinning around an axis.

Rate of Motion and Change of Motion

When motion occurs, the rate of motion is an important consideration. **Velocity** is the rate at which a body or segment moves. In translatory motion, it is measured in meters or feet per second (m/s, ft/s, respectively), but in rotary motion the measurement is degrees per second (°/s). **Acceleration** is the rate at which a change in velocity occurs. Acceleration can be either a positive or a negative number. If it is positive, the segment is moving faster and faster, but if it is negative, the segment is slowing down more and more. If the motion is linear, the measurement is m/s per second or ft/s per second (m/s^2 or ft/s^2, respectively). If the motion is rotary, the measurement is °/s per second ($°/s^2$). We have already discussed the definition of force. However, when we talk about motion occurring around an axis, force is called **torque.** Therefore, torque is merely force applied in an arc of motion around an axis.

Forces

Kinetics is the study of forces acting on the body. Motion occurs because of these forces. When we discuss forces, there are several words commonly used to describe forces and their effects. **Displacement** is the motion of a body or segment that occurs when force is applied. A **force** is a push or a pull that produces displacement. Forces have two dimensions—magnitude and direction. In other words, an applied force is going to have a certain magnitude or quantity, say 5 pounds, *and* will also have a certain direction of movement, say upward, if you lift an object overhead. Perhaps the easiest way to visualize a push or a pull is to imagine a tug-of-war (Fig. 2.1). If both teams pull on the rope with the same force, no movement of the rope occurs. The system is balanced because both forces are equal; this is a state of **equilibrium.** If the forces are unbalanced as one team pulls harder or one team slips, movement will occur in the direction of the stronger force.

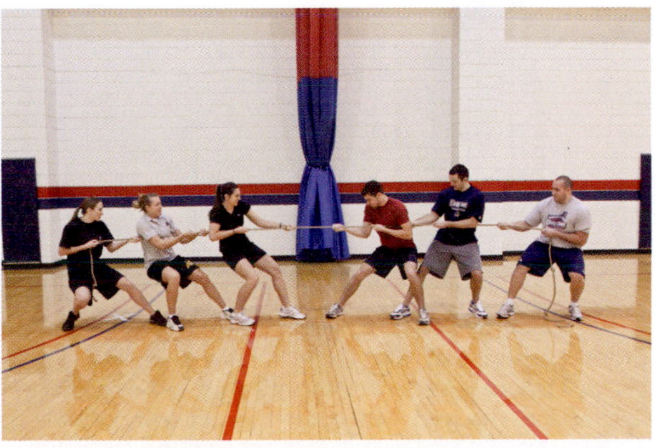

Figure 2.1 Forces at equilibrium in a tug-of-war.

Types of Forces

Whenever the body moves, it encounters forces. From a functional standpoint, four primary sources of force affect body movement:

- **Gravity.** The most prevalent force that all structures encounter is gravity. Gravitational force is commonly referred to as the "weight" of an object, body, or body segment. If an appliance or object is attached to a body segment—such as a dumbbell in a hand or a cast on a leg—that object increases the weight (or pull of gravity) of that segment. Since gravity is an important factor in body motion, it is discussed in more detail below.
- **Muscles.** Muscles produce forces on their bone segments by either active contraction or passive stretching. Muscle force provides motion of body segments and of the entire body.
- **Externally applied resistances.** These devices are numerous and are whatever the muscles must work against to produce motion. Examples of externally applied resistances include exercise pulleys, manual resistance, doors, or windows.
- **Friction.** Friction is the resistance to movement between two objects that are in contact with each other. Friction can be advantageous or disadvantageous by providing stability if optimum, retarding motion if excessive, and leading to instability if inadequate

Forces act on a mass. "Mass" and "weight" are terms that are often interchanged, but they are not the same. A **mass** is the amount of matter contained within an object, whereas **weight** is the force of gravity acting on the object. Weight is actually the pull of gravity with an acceleration force of 32 ft/sec/sec or 32 ft/s^2 (9.8 m/sec/sec or 9.8 m/s^2). If you weigh yourself at sea level at the equator, your weight will be greater than if you weigh yourself on the top of Mount Everest because, although your mass has not changed, the pull of gravity is less when it is farther from the center of the earth so your weight is less. The confusion comes with the labels that are interchangeably used to incorrectly describe mass and weight. Mass is measured in kilograms (kg), but the term is often used to identify weight. In the US system, few people are familiar with the correct term for mass, so "pounds" is identified with mass when, in fact, it is a measure of force (gravity's force). However seldom used, the proper US term for mass is **slug**. One slug is equal to 14.59 kg. When used as mass, 1 pound is equal to 0.031 slugs. **Newtons** is the term for force in the metric system: 9.8 Newtons is equivalent to 1 kgf (kilogram-force). See Tables 2–1 and 2–2 for definitions and conversions between the metric and US systems.

A **moment** is the result of force acting at a distance from the point of motion, or the axis. In mathematical terms, a moment (M) is the product of this distance (d) and the force (F): M = d × F. In translational forces, d is the length of the **lever arm** (or the perpendicular distance from the force vector to the center of motion), but in rotary forces, the lever arm is the **moment arm** (or the perpendicular distance from the force vector to the joint's axis of motion). If we look at the moment formula, we can see why distance of a force from an axis of motion is important in determining a force application. For example, if we have a mass of 10 pounds (4.45kg) with its distance to the center of motion at 12 in. (30cm), we know that it has a force-arm of 10 lb × 12 in. (4.45 kg × 30 cm), or 120 in.-lb (133.5 kg-cm). However, if the lever arm were shortened to 6 in. (15cm), the force arm would decrease to 60 in.-lb, or 66.75 kg-cm. If we apply this formula to a rotary motion, how moment arm length influences force becomes even clearer. As an example, imagine a 5-lb (2.27-kg) weight placed at the ankle on a lower extremity that weighs 25 lb (11.36 kg) as in Figure 2.2. The distance from the ankle (where the 5-lb weight is attached) to the hip (the axis of motion) is 3.5 ft (3.15m). Therefore, the amount of force required of the hip flexors to lift the leg and ankle weight is 3.5 ft × (5 lb + 25 lb), or 1.067 m × (2.27 kg + 11.34 kg). In order to lift the leg with the weight attached, the hip flexors must create a moment of 105 ft-lb or 14.52 m-kg. However, if the knee is flexed with the distance from the weight to the hip at 3 ft (0.91 m), then the hip flexor's moment requirement is 90 ft-lb, or 12.39 m-kg.

Forces are expressed as a combination of their magnitude and rate of change in direction, or acceleration. If we look at the formula for force, it may make more sense. The mathematical formula for force is $F = m \times a$, where F is the amount of force created, m is the mass of the object, and a is the acceleration of the object. Force

TABLE 2–1 | CONVERSION FACTORS

Mass	
1 slug (sg)	= 14.59 kilograms (kg)
1 gram (gm)	= 0.001 kilogram (kg)
Force	
1 pound (lb)	= 4.448 Newtons (N)
1 Newton (N)	= 0.225 pound (lb)
1 dyne	= 0.00001 Newton (N)
1 pound (lb)	= 0.45 kilogram (kg)*
1 kilogram (kg)*	= 2.2 pound (lb)
Distance	
1 foot (ft)	= 0.3048 meter (m)
1 inch (in)	= 2.54 centimeters (cm)
1 centimeter (cm)	= 0.01 meter (m)
Torque (bending moment)	
1 foot-pound (ft-lb)	= 1.356 Newton-meters (N-m)
1 dyne-centimeter (dyne-cm)	= 0.0000001 Newton-meter (N-m)

*The kilogram is a unit of mass, but it is commonly used as a unit of force instead of the correct unit, Newton.

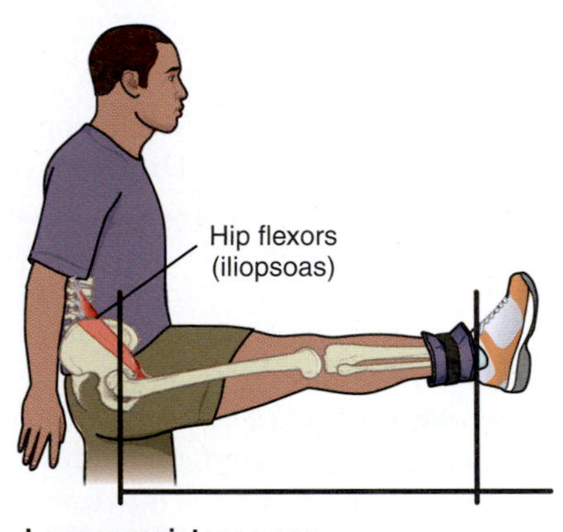

Longer resistance arm

Hip flexors
(iliopsoas)

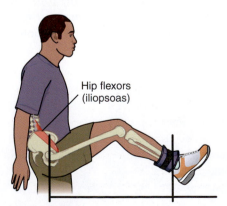

Shorter resistance arm

Figure 2.2 Changing the length of the lever arm changes the force requirements. With the knee flexed, the lever arm length of the amount of force pulling against the muscles lifting the leg reduces, so the muscle does not have to work as hard to lift the leg and cuff weight.

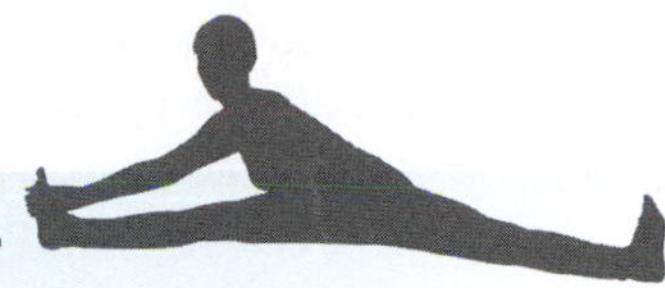

PRACTICE POINT

In a clinical situation, if a patient does not have enough muscle strength to overcome an external resistance, such as a cuff weight, an easy way to reduce the external resistance is to shorten the cuff weight's moment arm. The other more obvious way is to reduce the weight and maintain the weight's position at the more distal point on the extremity; however, if the lightest cuff weight available was 5 lb, its force could be easily adjusted by changing its placement on the extremity.

is expressed in either British units (sometimes called US units) or metric units. Since the metric system is the system most scientists and professional publications use, metric units are also referred to as the International System of Units (SI). The US system uses ounces, pounds, feet, and inches whereas the SI system uses grams, kilograms, meters, and centimeters. We will provide both in this text to make it easier to appreciate forces. Based on the formula for force, we know that forces are expressed with two components, mass and acceleration. In SI units, we see mass expressed as Newtons (N), and in US units, it is pounds (lb or #); 1 pound = 4.448 Newtons. Since force is a combination of mass and acceleration, forces are labeled as Newton-meter per second^2 (N-m/s^2) or foot-pound/second^2 (ft-lb/s^2) in SI or US units, respectively.

Newton's Laws of Motion

Sir Isaac Newton (1643–1727) was a mathematician who identified and articulated the laws that govern all motion. He observed that when forces were applied to an object, motion of that mass could be predicted. These three fundamental laws governing motion that we continue to use today deal with inertia, acceleration, and action-reaction.

Newton's First Law of Motion: Inertia

Newton's first law of motion states that **if a body is at rest, it will remain at rest, and if a body is in uniform motion, it will remain in motion, until an outside force acts upon it.**[1] The property of a body that resists change in motion or equilibrium is defined as **inertia.** Therefore, this law is the law of inertia, and sometimes you may see it called the law of equilibrium. As strange as it may seem, they are essentially the same: One label looks at this law of motion from what occurs because of this law and the other takes the perspective of what must be overcome. Let's take a look first at this law from an inertia perspective before we see it from an equilibrium view. We know from physics that **inertia** is the reluctance of a body to change its current state, whether it is stationary or moving uniformly. For example, if you want to move a file cabinet from one side of your desk to the other, it takes a lot more force to initiate the cabinet's movement than it does once you get it moving. That is inertia. Inertia is what must be overcome in order to cause a change in the body's (in this case, the file cabinet's) position.

Individuals who refer to Newton's first law of motion as a law of equilibrium take the perspective of what must be disturbed to satisfy the law. When a body is at rest, it is in a state of static equilibrium: The forces are all equal so no motion is occurring. For example, a 1500-lb car parked in the driveway is in static equilibrium because gravity is pulling down at 1500-lb and the driveway is pushing up at 1500-lb. When a body is in a uniform motion, it is in a state of dynamic equilibrium because it is moving at a uniform rate; if the car's cruise control is set at 50 miles per hour (mph), then the car is moving uniformly over the road at a constant pace, or uniform rate. In either the static or dynamic equilibrium case here, acceleration is not occurring, so the car's acceleration is zero. If, however, a force is applied to the car in either static or dynamic equilibrium, equilibrium is no longer present, and the body's acceleration is no longer zero. For example, if the car moving at 50 mph is suddenly hit from behind by another vehicle going 70 mph, the car is now going faster than 50 mph, causing acceleration to occur because an outside force affected its uniform motion. Let's take another example: A hockey puck sitting undisturbed on an ice rink is in static equilibrium because the weight or force of the puck pushing down on the ice is balanced by an equal force of the ice pushing up on the puck. After the puck is struck (accelerated) by an outside force, this outside force accelerates the puck to move in a lateral direction. Once the puck moves, it is again in equilibrium (this time, dynamic equilibrium) and moves in a uniform direction and at a uniform velocity until other forces are impressed upon it. These outside forces include either friction between the ice and puck to decelerate the puck's velocity or collision with a stick or wall to change the puck's direction and velocity.

In its simplest terms, Newton's first law of motion may be stated this way: A force is required to start a motion, to change direction or speed of a motion, and to stop a motion. In mathematical terms, the law states:

$$\Sigma F = 0$$

In this formula, F is force and Σ (sigma) is the total sum of all the forces. All of these forces equal zero so the object is in equilibrium. There can be several forces acting on a body, but in our example of the puck sitting on the ice, there are only two—the downward force, or weight, of the puck on the ice, and the force equal to that coming from the upward force of the ice. If the total forces are not equal, $\Sigma F \neq 0$, then the body is accelerating or decelerating.

Translatory applications of this law can be disastrous when a person is transported in a wheelchair, on a stretcher, or in an automobile, and the vehicle is stopped suddenly. If the person is not attached to the vehicle (e.g. by a seat belt), the body continues forward until stopped by another force ("If a body is in uniform motion, it will remain in motion, until an outside force acts upon it"). Seat belts or restraining straps are recommended, and frequently required, to prevent injuries caused by abrupt stops of wheelchairs and stretchers, as well as of automobiles. Whiplash neck injuries from rear-end collisions of automobiles occur because the automobile seat and the person's body are impelled forward as a unit while the unsupported head remains at rest. The violent stretching of the neck structures then produces a force to rapidly "whip" the head and neck first into flexion, then extension, with resulting injury to both posterior and anterior structures of the head and neck.

Newton's Second Law of Motion: Acceleration

The same force or forces acting on different bodies cause the bodies to move differently. Newton's second law of motion states: **The acceleration (a) of a body is proportionate to the magnitude of the net forces (F) acting on it and inversely proportionate to the mass (m) of the body.** As an equation, it is expressed as:

$$a \propto \frac{F}{m}$$

More simply stated, a greater force is required to move (or stop the motion of) a large mass than a small one. Let's expand on an example we had with Newton's first law of motion. According to this second law of motion, we know that the larger the mass (the bigger the body), the more force it takes to move it if it is stopped or stop it if it is moving. This time, you have a full two-drawer file cabinet and a full four-drawer file cabinet to move. It is much easier to move the two-drawer file cabinet across the floor than the four-drawer file cabinet. According to Newton's second law of motion, to cause acceleration of the file cabinets, it takes more force to move the larger four-drawer than the smaller two-drawer file cabinet.

This law is pertinent in clinical situations. For example, let us assume you have two patients with a grade 5/5 in gastrocnemius strength, but the first patient is a 250-lb football player and the second patient is a 100-lb dancer. Although their strength grades are both normal, you should not expect each of them to lift 250 lb in a heel-raise exercise.

Newton's Third Law of Motion: Action-Reaction

Newton's third law of motion states that **for every action force there is an equal and opposite reaction force.** This means that whenever one body applies a force to another body, that second body provides an equal force in the exact opposite direction with equal magnitude as the first body; one body or object provides the action and the other provides the reaction force. The easiest way to discuss this law is to present an example: If you hold your notebook in your hand, there are two equal forces acting on it—your arm muscles to keep the notebook in the position you desire it to be and gravity pulling it to the ground. The forces acting on the

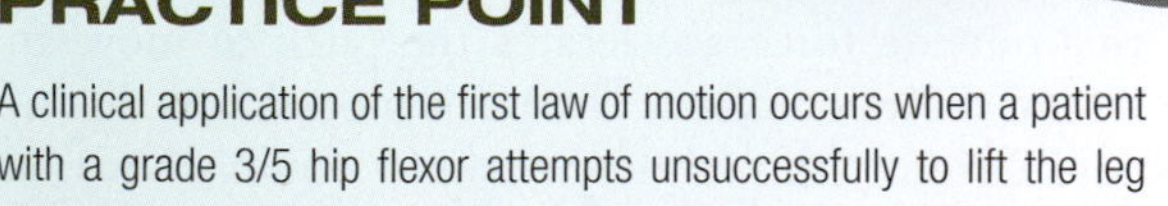

PRACTICE POINT

A clinical application of the first law of motion occurs when a patient with a grade 3/5 hip flexor attempts unsuccessfully to lift the leg upward to perform a straight leg raise. The patient may be able to complete the motion if the clinician begins the motion; in this case, the clinician overcomes inertia and the patient is then able to lift the leg unaided.

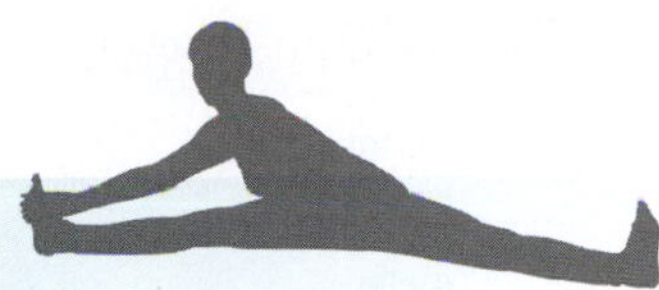

PRACTICE POINT

A clinical application of the law of inertia occurs with changes in the mass of a segment for an individual. When a lower extremity mass increases, such as a cast on the leg, greater muscle force is required to start and stop the leg swing when walking. In patients with muscle weakness (inability to develop adequate muscle force), one of the important considerations is to keep the mass of appliances (such as splints and adapted equipment) as light as possible to reduce the muscle force requirements necessary to move or control them.

notebook are equal since the book has not fallen to the floor and you have not changed the position of the notebook. Another example: If two football linemen push each other and neither moves, they are abiding by the law that states for every action there is an equal and opposite reaction. Player A produces an action force toward player B, and player B provides an equal reaction force toward player A. Until one overtakes the other, they are abiding by Newton's third law of motion. One more example demonstrates how large masses and small masses interact. When a basketball player jumps up for a rebound, he pushes off the ground and the ground pushes back at him. The earth's mass is so much larger than the basketball player's mass that the player moves upward into the air as the earth pushes back; however, since the player is so small compared to the earth, the player's mass does not affect the earth's movement.

Force Vectors and Their Considerations

Because forces applied by or to the body have both magnitude and direction (two dimensions), they are vector forces. Items that have only magnitude, or one dimension, are scalar quantities, such as 2 cars, 5 miles, or 7 vertebrae. As mentioned earlier, a vector force is expressed as moments. Vector forces can be expressed both graphically and mathematically (Fig. 2.3). Graphically, force vectors are represented by an arrow. The start of the arrow represents the point of attachment of the force on a body, or where it is applied. The arrowhead indicates the direction of the force. The shaft is the line of action of the force, and its length is drawn to a scale representing the magnitude of the force. The force system is located in space by placement on a rectangular coordinate system, with forces directed either up or to the right given a positive (+) sign, and forces directed either down or to the left given a negative (–) sign. The magnitudes of the forces are expressed in pounds, Newtons (N), or dynes (Table 2–2).

Force Vector Diagrams

Vector forces can be combined when more than one force is applied to a body or segment. The combination of these vectors will result in a new vector, called the **resultant vector.** By adding or subtracting two or more forces, their combined effect creates a single resultant force. This resultant force is the simplest force that results when all of the forces act together. If two or more forces act along a line or parallel lines, the forces are added to find the single resultant force. To simplify and

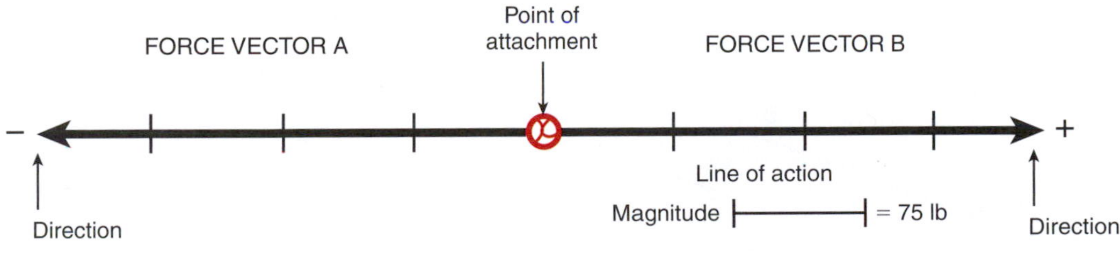

FORCE A = −300 lb
FORCE B = +300 lb

Figure 2.3 Forces have magnitude and direction. This graphic representation of a tug-of-war demonstrates that forces occur as a result of the magnitude, or amount of pull, each person provides and the direction in which each person pulls. As long as the total magnitudes are equal in opposite directions, no motion occurs.

TABLE 2–2 | SYSTEMS COMMONLY USED TO EXPRESS WEIGHTS AND MEASURES

System	Mass	Force	Distance	Torque	Time
B.E./U.S.	slug	pound	foot	lb-ft	sec
S.I.	kg	Newton	meter	N-m	sec
cgs	gram	dyne	cm	dyne-cm	sec

B.E. = British Engineering (foot, pound, sec); S.I. = International System of Units; cgs = centimeter, gram, second

better visualize the magnitude and direction of such multiple forces, the process of **composition of forces** is used. Look at Figure 2.4A to see two vectors, *A* and *B*. If we combine the vectors, we place one vector with its tail attached to the head of the first vector to establish a resultant vector in Figure 2.4B. In this example, we see that the vectors are going in the same direction so their forces and magnitudes are combined to create the resultant vector that continues in the same direction but with a much greater force magnitude. In Figure 2.5A, we see three vectors, but this time they are not in the same direction. However, we can still combine them, but this time the resultant vector is the line between the first tail and the last head, as is seen in Figure 2.5B.

Composition of Forces

Several forces often act on the body simultaneously. If we apply the concepts in the previous paragraph to the body in a practical situation, the composition of forces may become more meaningful. In Figure 2.6, we see a number of forces acting on the leg. In this figure, the forces include the weights of the leg, the weight boot, and the weight on the boot. Since all three of these forces are in the same direction, we can draw the sum of these forces to scale as seen in Figure 2.6B and 2.6C or add the forces together (Fig. 2.6D) since we know that

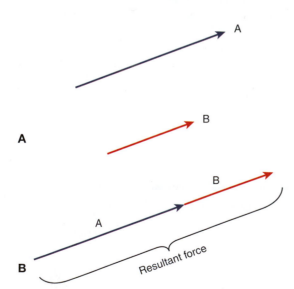

Figure 2.4 Two vector forces are added together when they are in the same direction. As in the tug-of-war, when forces occur in the same direction, their magnitudes are added together.

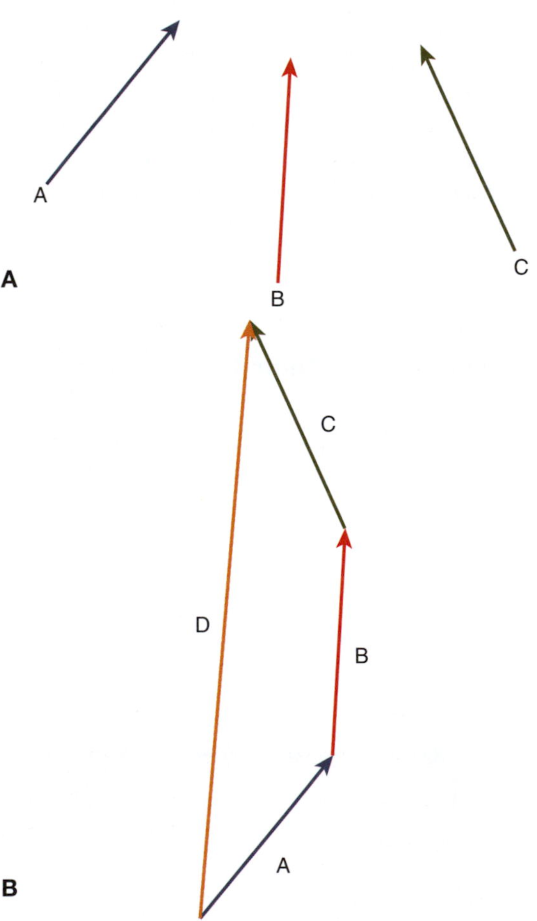

Figure 2.5 Multiple vector forces that are in different directions may still be added together. The tail (or start) of one force vector is added to the head (or end of the magnitude and direction) of another force vector until all of the force vectors are summed together.

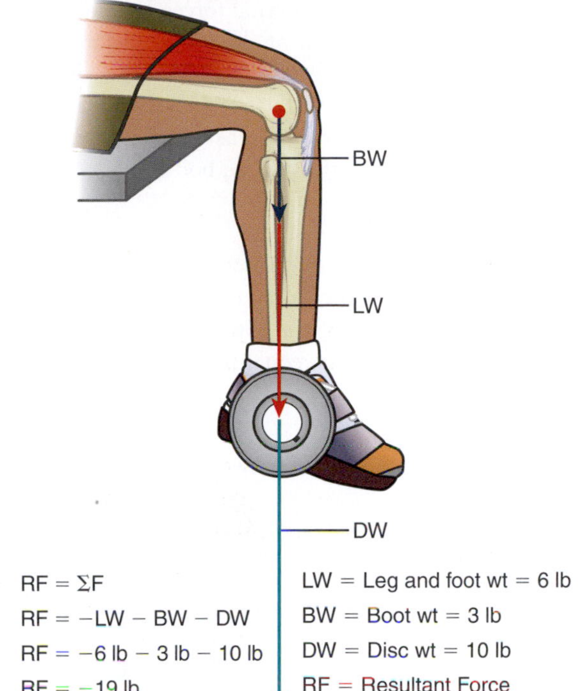

Figure 2.6 Forces acting at the knee joint when the subject is sitting with a weight at the ankle. The algebraic composition of the resultant force is given (negative sign indicates that the direction of the force is down).

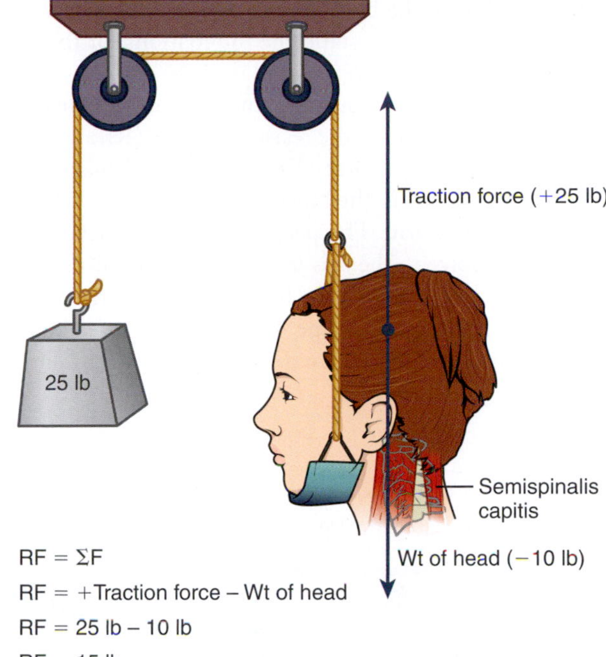

Figure 2.7 Resultant vector force when forces oppose each other. The weight of the head produces a downward force whereas the traction produces an upward force. A counterbalance force of 10 lb from the traction unit eliminates the downward force of the weight of the head, so the actual traction force applied to the cervical spine is 15 lb.

the sum of the individual forces is the total force (RF = ΣF). In both methods, the resultant force is the same. Since the knee joint is not moving with these forces pulling on it, we know that the resultant force is equal in force and opposite in direction to the forces of the joint's ligaments, fascia, and capsule, which are holding the joint in place. If these soft tissue structures were unable to provide an equal force to these distracting forces, the joint would dislocate. When the body segment is stable and no motion occurs, the forces are in balance or in equilibrium. In such a case, the sum of the forces is zero (the positive forces equal the negative forces).

Levers

Muscles apply forces that produce movement of the body's levers. A simple machine that consists of a rigid bar that rotates around an axis, or fulcrum, is a **lever.** In biomechanics, the principles of levers assist in visualizing the more complex system of forces that produce

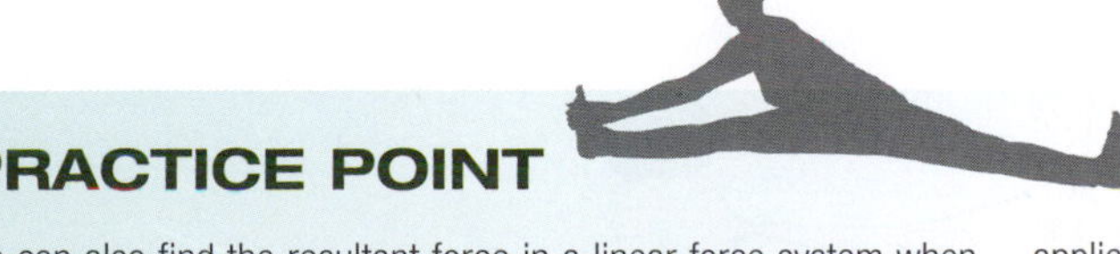

PRACTICE POINT

We can also find the resultant force in a linear force system when the forces act in opposite directions. In the clinical example in Figure 2.7, we see a patient receiving cervical traction. The traction force in this example is 25 lb (111N), but the weight of the head and neck (10 lb) reduces the amount of traction force actually applied. In this case, the effective upward traction force on the cervical spine is really 15 lb (67 N). Since weight of the head is approximately 10 pounds, any traction weight less than that will not provide sufficient counterbalance weight to produce effective cervical traction.

rotary motion in the body. Reducing body segments to levers helps us to understand the foundations for therapeutic applications in treatment.

The three elements of mechanical levers include the axis (A) and two forces, the resistance force (R), and the moving (or holding) force (F). The perpendicular distance from the axis to the line of action of the resistance is the **resistance arm**. The perpendicular distance from the moving force to the axis is the **force arm**. Lever systems in the body include the body segment as the lever and the joint as the axis. The forces acting on the body segment include the external forces as the resistance force and the muscles, or internal forces, as the moving force. The relative position of the axis, resistance arm, and force arm to one another define the different classes of levers. Figure 2.8 illustrates each of the classes of levers discussed below as well as a common example and an example within the human body.

First-Class Lever

First-class levers, such as a seesaw or balance scale (Fig. 2.8A, B), gain either force or distance, depending on the relative lengths of the force arm and the resistance arm. If two forces are equal on either side of a first

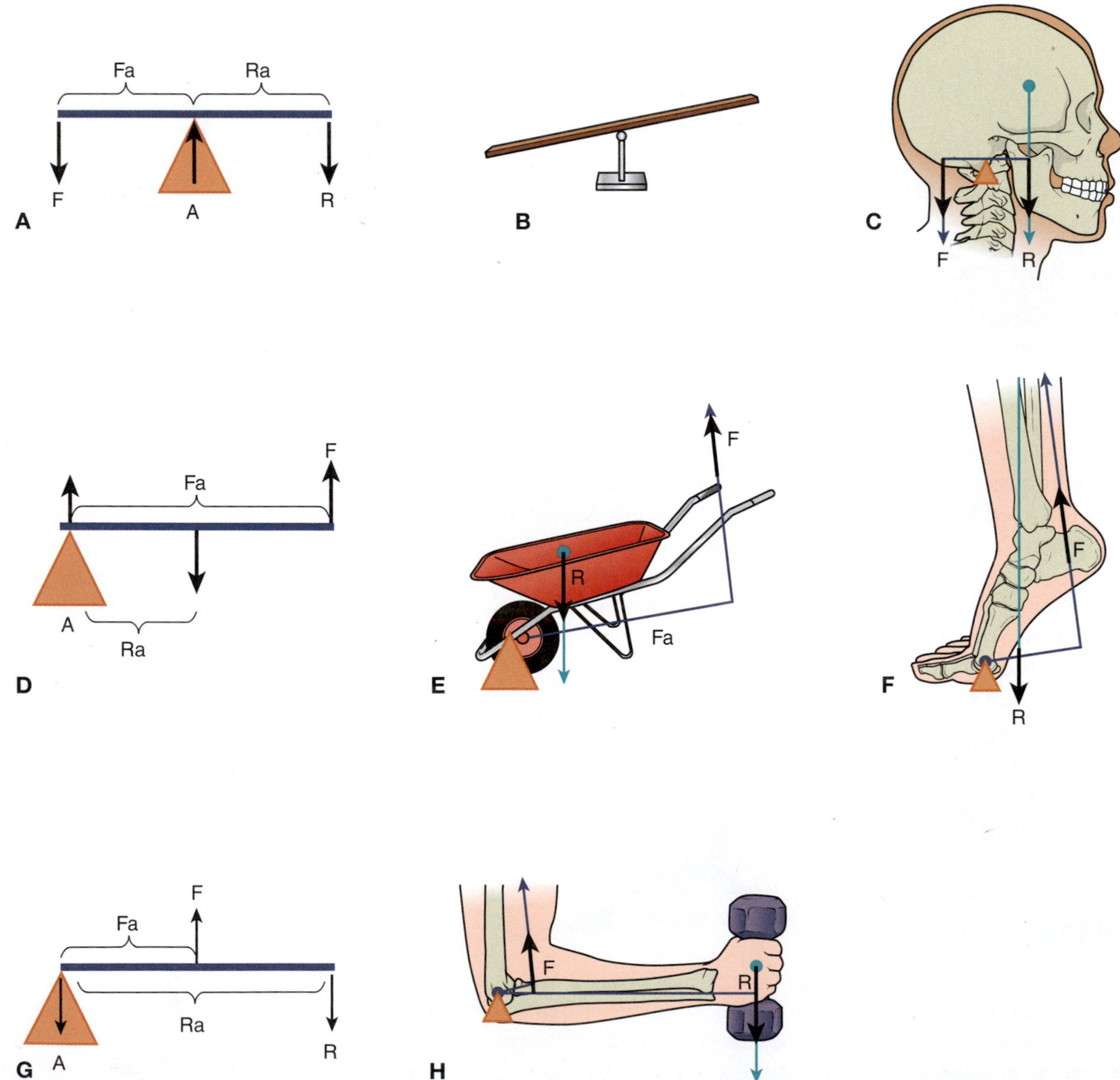

Figure 2.8 Classes of levers are represented in geometry, common activities or tools, and the body: A–C = first class; D–F = second class; G–H = third class. F = Force; Fa = force arm; R = resistance; Ra = resistance arm.

class lever, the force with the longer arm (distance from the force to the axis) has the advantage. This class of lever is commonly seen on a seesaw in which individuals of unequal size can balance each other by moving the larger individual closer to the axis to shorten that individual's lever arm (Fig. 2.8B). An example of a first-class lever system in the body is the atlanto-occipital joint (axis), in which the weight of the head (resistance) is balanced by neck extensor muscle force (Fig. 2.8C). The side from the axis that has the advantage is the one with the greater product of the larger force and the longer arm length. If both have equal forces with equal lever arm lengths or an equal product of force and lever arm length, then the system is in equilibrium.

Second-Class Lever

In second-class levers, the point of resistance application lies between the force and the axis so the lever arm of the resistance is always shorter than the lever arm of the force (Fig. 2.8D). Second-class levers, therefore, provide a force advantage so large weights can be supported or moved by a smaller force. The wheelbarrow (Fig. 2.8E) is an example of this type of lever. Even the deeper anterior and shallower posterior shape of a wheelbarrow is designed so that the heaviest load (more cargo room in the front of the container) is carried farthest from the handles and closest to the axis of motion (wheel) so the person moving it has the mechanical advantage, even when the load is very heavy. A person standing on the balls of the feet is an example of a second-class lever in the body (Fig. 2.8F). Unfortunately, there are not many second-class levers in the body; the body rarely has a mechanical advantage over the resistance forces it encounters.

Third-Class Lever

Third-class levers have the point of force application located between the resistance and the axis (Fig. 2.8G). The third-class lever is most common in the human body. In this lever, the resistance arm is always longer than the force arm, so the mechanical advantage lies with the resistance force. This arrangement is designed to produce speed of the distal segment and move a small weight a long distance. Thus, in the human body, a small amount of shortening of a muscle (such as the brachialis) causes a large arc of motion at the joint (elbow in this example) to position the end of the segment (the hand) in a large range of positions. This type of lever occurs in most **open-chain motions** of the extremities. An open-chain motion occurs during a nonweight-bearing activity when the distal part of the extremity is free to move and movements at one joint do not influence the other joints of the extremity. Examples of an open-chain motion include:

- The deltoid acting on the glenohumeral joint to elevate the arm from the side;
- The flexor digitorum profundus closing the interphalangeal joints around a ball;
- The extensor carpi radialis extending the wrist in a wave;
- The anterior tibialis dorsiflexing the ankle joint to lift the foot off the floor;
- The biceps and brachialis flexing the elbow to bring a cup to the mouth.

All of these muscles produce large ranges of motion with relatively less muscle motion (Fig. 2.8G).

All three types of levers demonstrate that what is gained in excursion is lost in force and, conversely, what is gained in force is lost in motion. In essence, a lever creates an advantage of either force or distance in motion. The classification of levers as first-, second-, or third-class solely depends on the relative positions of the axis, weight, and force to each other. If the axis is central, the lever class is I; if the resistance is central, the lever class is II; and if the force is central, the lever class is III.

Mechanical Advantage

Mechanical advantage (MA) of a lever refers to the ratio between the length of the force arm and the length of the resistance arm. Therefore, the equation is:

$$MA = \frac{\text{Force Arm Length}}{\text{Resistance Arm Length}}$$

The ratio for a lever system with arm lengths equal for the force and the resistance is 1. The ratio for lever systems with a longer force arm than a resistance arm is greater than 1, and the ratio for lever systems with a longer resistance arm than a force arm is less than 1. The higher the quotient of the ratio, the greater the mechanical advantage is. An increase in the force arm length or a decrease in the resistance arm length results in a greater mechanical advantage. Keep in mind that mechanical advantage has to do only with arm length; a longer arm length will make a task easier, regardless of the amount of force that is working. For example, if Force A has a shorter arm length than Resistance B, Force A is going to have to always work harder against Resistance B, regardless of the amount of force produced by Resistance B. On the other hand, if Force A has a longer arm length, it will never have to work as hard as Resistance B. To clarify further, let us take these examples and apply numbers to them. If Force A's arm length is 1 ft and Resistance B's arm length is 2 ft, it would not matter if Force A was 10 lb or 30 lb; Resistance B would still not have to produce as much force to be equal to Force A. This is so since Force A at 10 lb × 1 ft will produce 10 ft-lb, but Resistance B would have to be only 5 lb (5 lb × 2 ft = 10 ft-lb) to create a force equal to Force A. If Force A was 30 lb, then it would create (30 lb × 1 ft) 30 ft-lb of force; however, in order to equal Force A, Resistance B would only have to be 15 lb (15 lb × 2 ft).

Assuming forces to be equal in magnitude, the mechanical advantage lies with the force that has the longer lever arm in first-class levers. In second-class levers, the force will always have a greater mechanical advantage because its lever arm is always longer than the resistance arm. However, in third-class levers, the reverse is true; the resistance force always has the mechanical advantage since its lever arm is always longer than the force arm. In clinical application to body segments, whenever the force arm of the working muscle is shorter than the resistance arm of the segment moved by the muscle, the muscle must exert more force to lift the segment. On the contrary, when the muscle's force arm is longer than the resistance arm of the segment, the muscle does not have to work as hard to lift the body part. As mentioned, most muscles in the body work as third-class levers; this means that muscles will usually need to produce more force to move the segment than the weight of the extremity it is lifting.

Static Equilibrium

In the fundamental Newtonian equation F = ma, F represents the sum or resultant of **all the forces** acting on the body or segment. When that body or segment is not moving, it is in the state of static equilibrium and acceleration is zero ($\Sigma F = 0$). Remember that since a force has two dimensions, we must consider both its magnitude and its direction. If clockwise force is positive and counterclockwise force is negative and we know that joints move in an arc, then we also know the force's directions. Static equilibrium equations for the forces on the three-lever systems in Figure 2.8 can be written in the following manner (using positive and negative signs for direction):

Static equilibrium:	$\Sigma F = 0$
First-class lever:	$\Sigma F = -F + R = 0$
Second-class lever:	$\Sigma F = -F + R = 0$
Third-class lever:	$\Sigma F = -F + R = 0$

(Refer to Figure 2.8 for the abbreviations.)

Thus, if two of these forces are known, the unknown third force can be calculated.

Since clinical forces are usually dynamic and continually changing as a segment moves through its range of motion, they are very difficult to calculate; therefore, static equilibrium is usually used to estimate forces applied to the body at a specified joint position. We present a few formulas in this chapter and explain how they are used to help you to understand and appreciate the forces that occur clinically. These forces are important since they affect our daily patient treatments. For example, the force between the joint surfaces at the ankle in standing when standing on one leg is greater than the entire body weight. This fact is true because the line-of-gravity line of the body falls not through the ankle joint, but slightly anterior to the lateral malleolus. Therefore, the person is prevented from falling forward by the gastrocnemius-soleus muscle's contraction force pulling on the tibia. As we see in Figure 2.9, the combined downward pulls of gravity and the contraction of the muscle provide compression force on the ankle. Without going into the specific computations to get the answer, it is sufficient to realize that a muscle creates a compression force on the joint when it contracts so the total amount of force on the joint is more than just the body's weight.

Torque

As has been mentioned, torque is force which is applied around an axis; therefore, torque produces joint motion. Similar to the formula for force, torque (τ), or moment

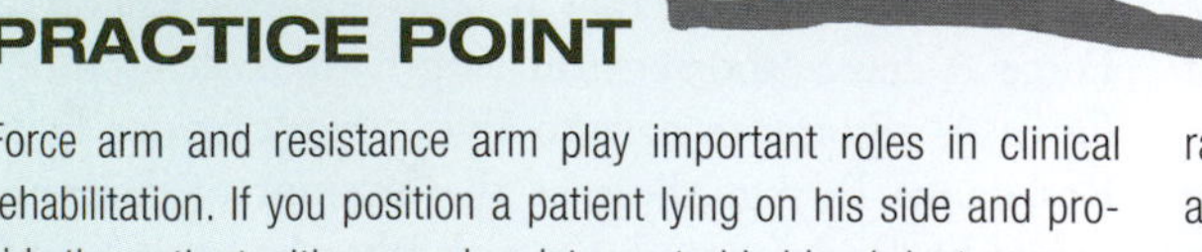

PRACTICE POINT

Force arm and resistance arm play important roles in clinical rehabilitation. If you position a patient lying on his side and provide the patient with manual resistance to his hip abductors, your force arm will be longer if you apply your resistance at his ankle rather than at his knee. Positioning your hand at the ankle will allow you to provide appropriate resistive force without exerting as much effort as would be required of you with your hand on the patient's knee.

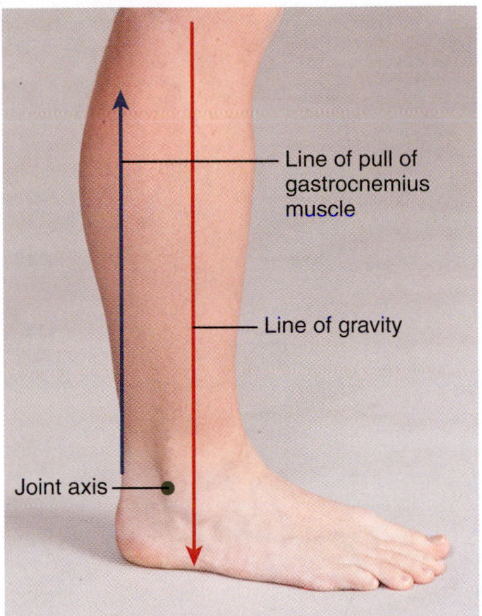

Figure 2.9 When a muscle contracts, it adds to the forces being applied to a joint. When standing, the posterior calf muscles contract to hold the body upright and increase joint compressive forces on the ankle (talocrural) joint.

(when force is applied around an axis), is the product of a force times the perpendicular distance (d) from its line of action to the axis of motion (or its potential motion if the object is currently stationary):

$$\tau = F \cdot d.$$

Since body segments move around joints and the joints are the axis of that movement, the muscles and forces acting on the body produce torque and the lever arms of these forces and muscles are moment arms. Therefore, the "d" in the formula is the moment arm length from the point where the force is applied on the body segment to that segment's joint. Before we move to the body, let us use a common example to see how the torque formula applies to an every day activity. We can use an example of opening a large, heavy door to see the torque formula's application and why distance is important. If you push a heavy door at its center, it requires much more force to open the door than if you push it at a point farthest from the door's hinges (axis). Less force is required to open the door when you apply your force farther from the hinges because your moment arm is longer. Another example demonstrating the importance of force arm lengths and torque is a seesaw: A 50-lb (222 N) child can balance a 100-lb (445 N) child if the lever arm distance for the 50-lb child is twice the length of the lever arm distance for the 100-lb child ($\tau = F \cdot d$). If the seesaw was long enough on the lighter child's end, the resistance of the 100-lb child could be balanced by the 50-lb child's fingertip pressure on his end of the seesaw!

In Figure 2.10 the subject is holding an exercise weight in the hand with the shoulder in three positions of flexion. At the shoulder, the torque produced by the weight varies with the perpendicular distance from the

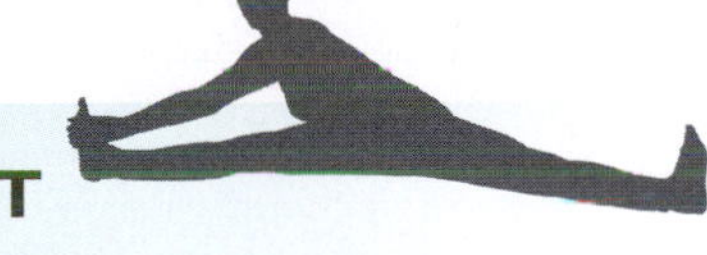

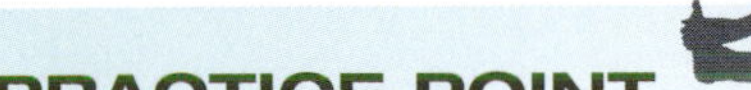

PRACTICE POINT

If a patient we are treating for ankle arthritis has pain when he uses a golfer's lift to retrieve his golf ball out of the hole after he has putted, it may be easier to explain to the patient why he has pain and how to alter his lift if we have this knowledge of increased joint forces that occurs during single limb stance.

Clinicians often use torque principles in testing the strength of muscles (manual muscle testing) and in applying manual resistive exercises. For example, when testing the strength of the elbow flexors, the clinician applies resistance at the wrist rather than on the mid-forearm. Wherever the clinician provides resistance, the torque produced by the patient's elbow flexors is the same. The resistance required by the clinician to match the patient's force, however, is approximately one-half less at the wrist than at the mid-forearm because of the longer resistance arm.

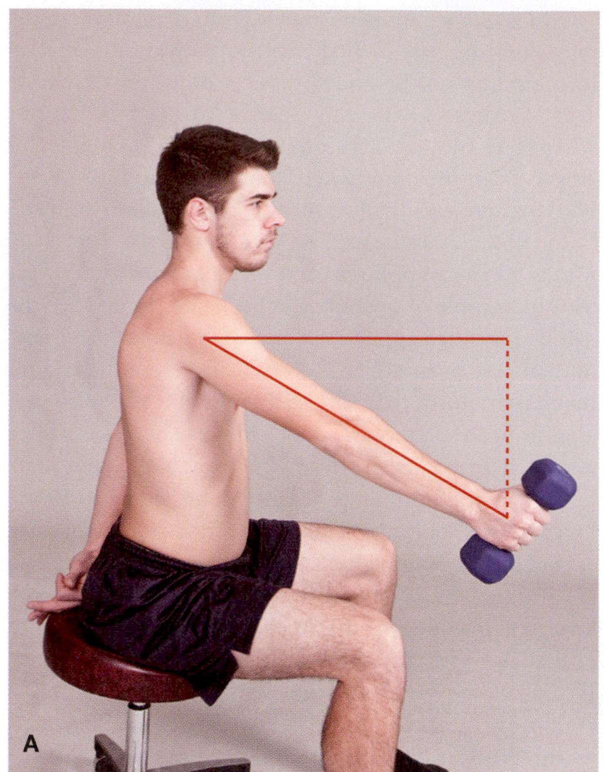

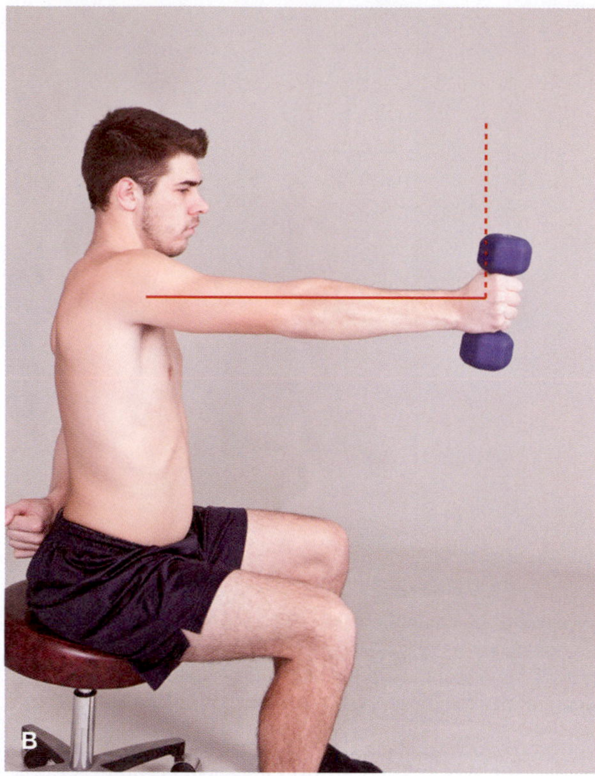

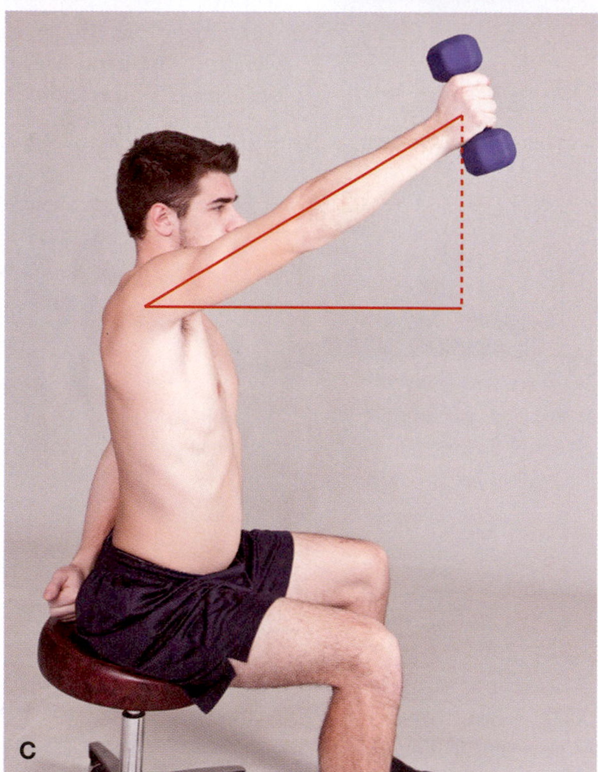

Figure 2.10 Variation of the resistance torque at the shoulder when a 10-lb weight is held in the hand and the shoulder is flexed to 60°, 90°, and 120°.

line of action of the force (weight) to the joint axis. The perpendicular distance is the resistance arm. Thus, the torque produced by the weight increases as the hand moves away from the body (Fig. 2.10A). The weight's torque reaches its maximum at 90° of shoulder flexion (Fig. 2.10B) The weight's torque decreases again as shoulder flexion continues to the end range (Fig. 2.10C). As a rule, when the line of pull of a force is 90°, or perpendicular to its moment arm, it produces its greatest resistance.

Parallel Force Systems

A parallel force system occurs when all of the forces acting on a segment are parallel to each other. They can be in the same or opposite directions. These forces are added together. However, keep in mind that they may have a plus or minus sign in front of them, depending on their direction of application. For example, if force A is moving an object to the right, upward, or clockwise, it is a positive force, but if the force is moving an object to the left, downward, or counterclockwise, it is a negative force (Fig. 2.11). Since we know the static equilibrium formulas for torque ($\Sigma\tau = 0$) and force ($\Sigma F = 0$), we can use equations to find unknown forces. For example, the forces on the forearm in the diagram in Figure 2.12 can be used to calculate the muscle force. The torque produced by each force ($\tau = F \times d$) is substituted into the equilibrium formula ($\Sigma F = 0$), so the formula becomes $(\tau M) + (\tau x) + (\tau W) = 0$ where τM is the muscle torque, τx is torque of the weight of the forearm and hand, and τW is the torque of the weight of the object in the hand. Then positive and negative signs are assigned. **In the torque equation, these signs show the turning effect of the force on the coordinate system and not the direction of the force.** If a torque produces or tends to produce a clockwise motion of the coordinate system, the sign is positive. If a torque tends to produce a counterclockwise motion, it is negative.

So, now the formula becomes:

$$-(\tau M) + (\tau x) + (\tau W) = 0.$$

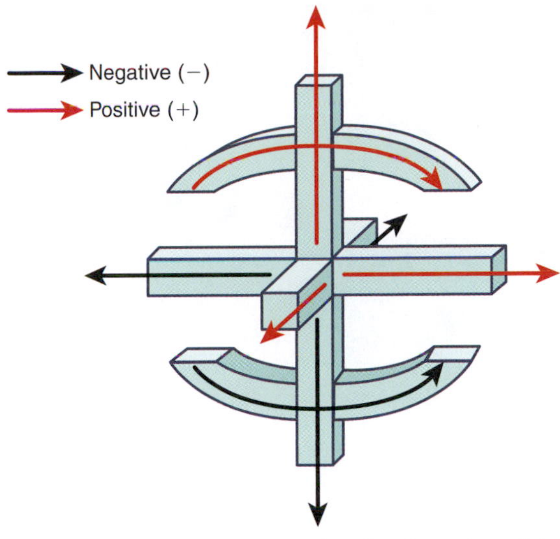

Figure 2.11 Positive and negative directions of parallel forces. Forces moving an object to the right, upward, or clockwise are positive whereas forces moving an object to the left, downward, or counterclockwise are negative.

We can now insert the number values for each of the letters:

$$-(2\text{ in} \times M) + (6\text{ in} \times 3\text{ lb}) + (12\text{ in} \times 10\text{ lb}) = 0.$$

When we solve for each parentheses, we get:

$$-(2\text{ in} \times M) + (18\text{ in.-lb}) + (120\text{ in.-lb}) = 0.$$

The equation is then solved for the (M), the muscle force:

Moving − (2 in × M) to the right side of the equation makes it a positive number.

Combining the two remaining parentheses on the left side, and then dividing that total by the 2 inches:

The answer is 69 lb.

Therefore, with this forearm at 90° and the hand holding a 10-lb object, the elbow flexors must exert 69 pounds of force to maintain the position with the weight!

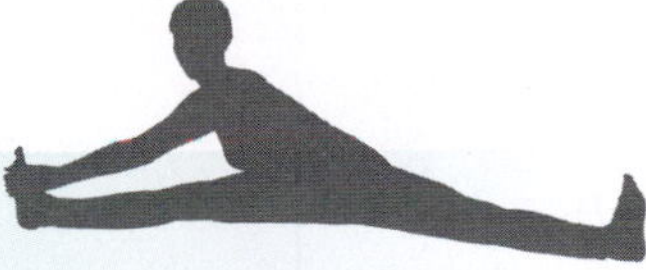

PRACTICE POINT

Clinically, reducing torque is important in lifting and carrying to prevent strain or injury to the person lifting. For example, in the two- or three-person lift and transfer of a patient from bed to stretcher or wheelchair, instructions include sliding the patient close to the bodies of the lifters before attempting to lift the patient. The next instruction is to lift and quickly roll the patient toward the lifters' chests. The moves of first sliding and then rolling the patient bring the patient's center of gravity closer to the center of gravity of the lifters, thus reducing the torque and likelihood of injury from excessive strain.

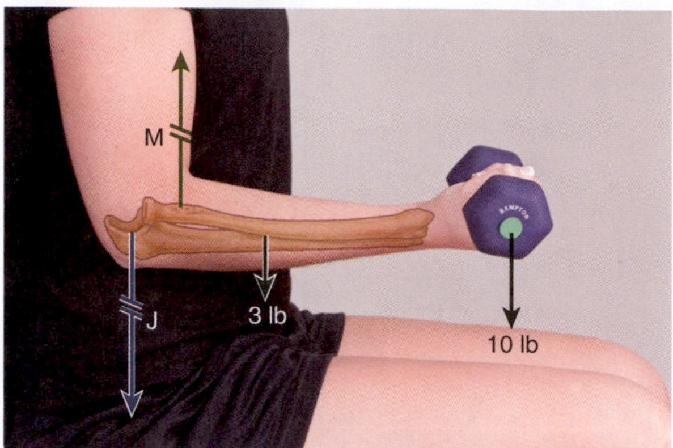

10 lb = Weight of object
3 lb = Weight of forearm and hand
M = Muscle force (contraction of the elbow flexors)
J = Joint force (reaction force of the humerous on the ulna)

Figure 2.12 Forces on the forearm when holding a 10-lb weight in the hand.

Although this is a theoretical example, the model helps us estimate and appreciate the forces applied to the body which must be overcome by the muscles to either maintain a position or provide motion. As with the illustration we just went through, most of the body's levers are third-class levers. This means that the muscles must generate and the joints must tolerate very large forces to hold or move a small, distally-placed resistance. In the shoulder flexion diagram in Figure 2.10, we see that the torque of the resistance changes as the shoulder goes through its range of motion. This change occurs because the moment arm length varies as the shoulder moves. The resistance torque is at a maximum of 20 ft-lb when the extremity is horizontal. If the shoulder stops at any point in its range of motion, the system is in equilibrium; at each point where motion stops the shoulder flexor muscles must produce a torque equal to the resistance torque ($\Sigma\tau = 0$). The moment arm of the muscles is, however, only a few inches long. Therefore, the muscles must exert significantly greater forces to hold the weight at any point in the motion. For example, with the resistance torque greatest at 90°, or the horizontal position, the muscles' torque must be more than 10 times the resistance torque.

On the other hand, the first-class lever system is energy efficient, so smaller muscle forces are able to support larger resistances. For example, Figure 2.13 illustrates standing on one foot. Although the lever system is different, the formulas used to determine forces acting on the system are the same. For those who wish to take on a challenge and see if you can

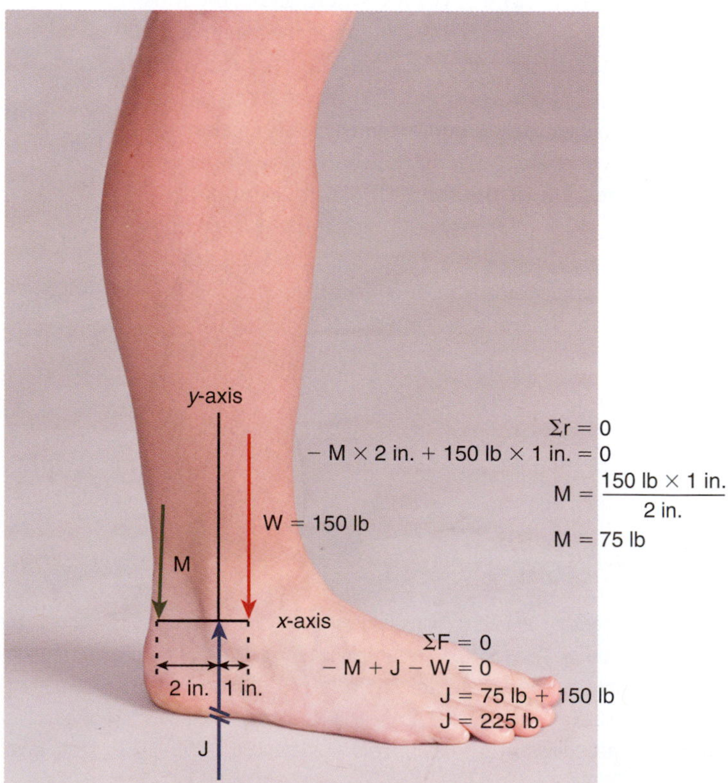

Figure 2.13 Diagram and equations for the forces on the tibia during unilateral stance with approximate calculations of the magnitudes of the muscle (M) and joint compression (J) forces.

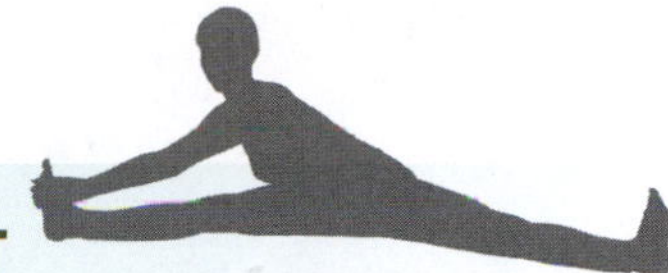

PRACTICE POINT

Clinical application of this concept of moment arms is important in splint design and construction. Figure 2.14 illustrates the forces applied by a forearm splint designed to provide dynamic assistance to finger extension (by a rubber band). Shortening the forearm lever arm (Fig. 2.14B) increases pressures on the wrist and forearm. Designing optimal splint lengths is important in reducing joint compression forces.

solve the problem, the formulas, values, and diagrams are listed in the illustration. However, for those who wish to merely appreciate the results, the next few sentences explain the forces required of the muscles, those applied to the joint, and their explanations. For an individual with a body weight of 150 lb (the resistance force) a counterforce of 75 lb must be produced from the calf muscles. In this case, the muscles are not working as hard as in the elbow example because their moment arm is twice as long as that of the resistance arm. However, the amount of force compressing the tibia on the talus is 225 lb, much more than the body's weight.

If the distance from the axis of motion of either the resistance arm or the muscle's moment arm changes, the magnitude of the forces also changes. Lengthening a lever arm increases the forces applied to the body and thereby increases pressure on the joint. For example, if the person sways forward slightly so the line of gravity falls 2 inches in front of the ankle's axis of motion, the muscle force requirement increases to 200 lb and the joint compression force boosts to 300 lb. Just imagine how much more these forces are magnified if the individual is heavier.

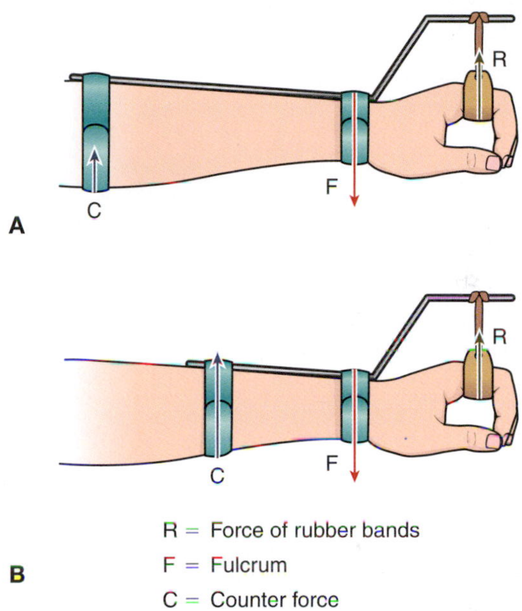

Figure 2.14 A) Forearm splint for assisting finger extension with the forces exerted on the forearm and hand by the splint. B) Increase in counterforce C (and consequently in F) when the splint's forearm lever arm is reduced in length.

Resolution of Forces

Many of the forces that occur in or on the body are applied at angles to the segment rather than in a parallel system. Figure 2.15 shows an example in which the forces (W is the weight force, M is the muscle force, and J is the joint reaction force) are neither parallel to each other nor perpendicular to the moment arm. Resolution of a force can help us understand these types of force applications. **Resolution of a force** breaks down the force into its two component forces. We can use this resolution to (1) visualize the effect of such angular forces on the body, (2) determine the torque produced by the forces, and (3) calculate the magnitude of unknown muscle and joint forces. This process is based on the mathematical principle that any number can be represented by two or more different numbers (e.g., 7 can be represented by 6 + 1 or 5 + 2). Since a force vector is a number, we can also extend that principle to state that any vector can be represented by two or more vectors. Resolution of a force vector, then, is the division of a vector into two or more component vectors. **Component vectors** are the forces whose combined magnitudes and directions produce a single vector known as the resultant vector.

Forces Acting at Angles

The resultant forces of a vector force in the same plane acting at angles to each other cannot be found by simple addition or subtraction; unfortunately, they must be

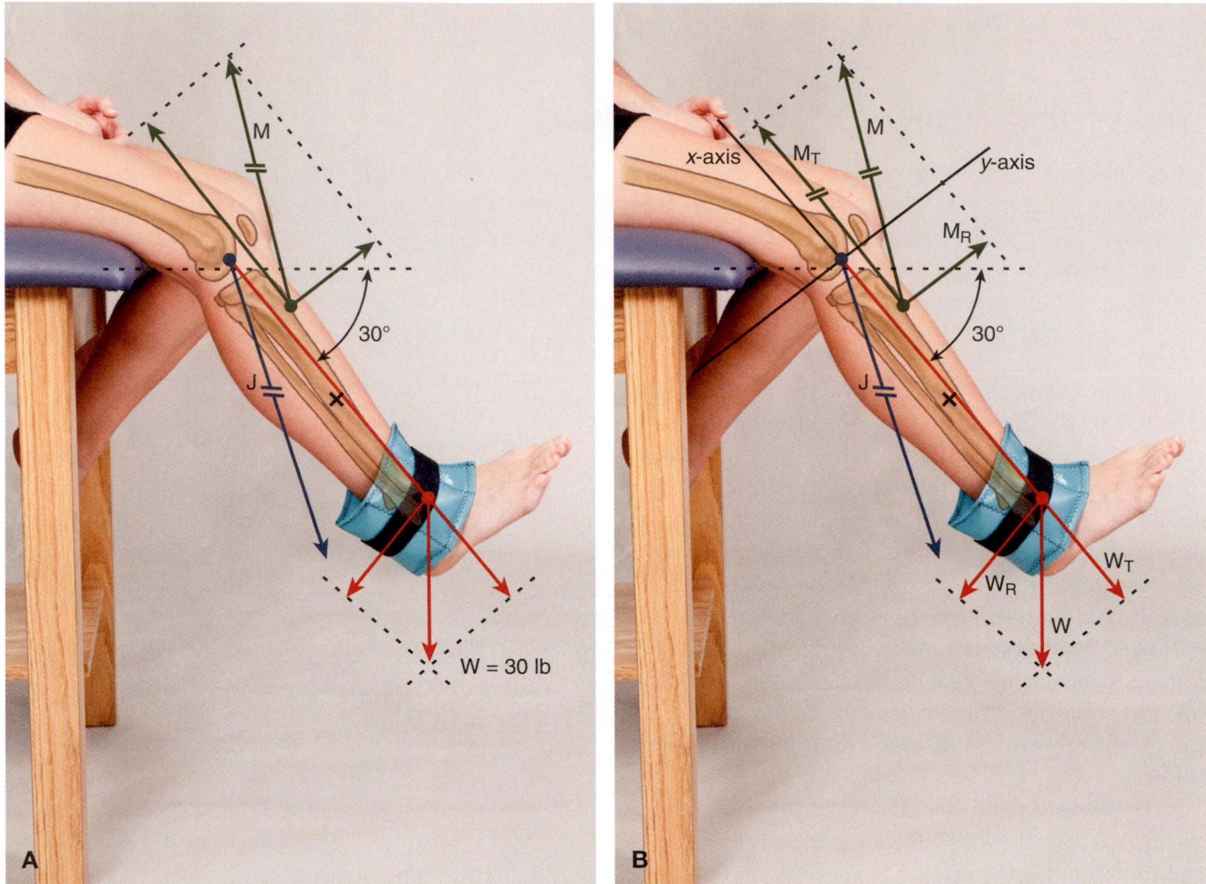

Figure 2.15 Forces acting on the leg (tibia) when the seated subject has an exercise weight on the foot and the knee is in 30° of flexion. **A)** A diagram of the resolution of the weight and muscle forces acting on the knee. **B)** The muscle (M) and weight (W) forces are each composed of a tangential force. In this case, the muscle's tangential force compresses the joint and the weight's tangential force distracts the joint. Component forces perpendicular to the segment always produce rotation of that segment.

found using either graphs or trigonometry. If two forces are pulling from the same point, the resultant force can be found graphically by constructing a parallelogram. The resultant force is the diagonal of the parallelogram, not the sum of the two forces. This is a **concurrent force system**. In other words, the result of the two forces will create a resultant force, and this resultant force will be a combination of both original forces with its origin at the same site as the two original forces. Lines drawn parallel to the original forces create a parallelogram. When the force vectors are to scale, the line crossing through the center of the parallelogram from the starting point of the vectors is the resultant vector's force magnitude and direction. For example, look at Figure 2.16. There are two forces acting in different directions from the same point. When a parallelogram is drawn with these force vectors, the line running through its center from their point of application is the resultant force (Fig. 2.17). If you have ever used a slingshot or a bow and arrow, you have used this concept.

As the angle between the two forces increases, the resultant force decreases, reaching a minimum when the forces are in line with each other and acting in directly opposite directions, when the angle between them becomes 180°; this is essentially a parallel system with one force positive and the other negative. Conversely, as the angle between the forces becomes smaller, the resultant force increases. When the angle becomes zero, the forces are in line with each other (or parallel) and in the same direction, so the resultant force is the sum of the two forces.

Since the component vectors produce the resultant vector and the center of motion for body segments is a joint, then we know that the two existing vectors that produce the resultant vector act to either rotate a segment or move the segment away from or toward the joint. Let's imagine an example and draw a diagram to make this point clearer. The diagram is seen in Figure 2.22. The knee is flexed at a 45° angle. In addition to the muscle contracting to hold the joint in place, there are two other forces acting on the knee:

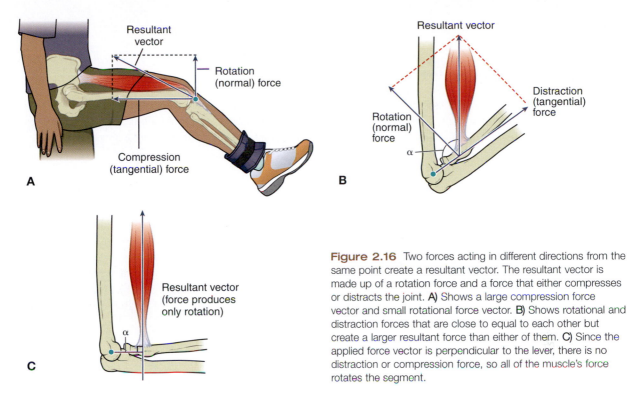

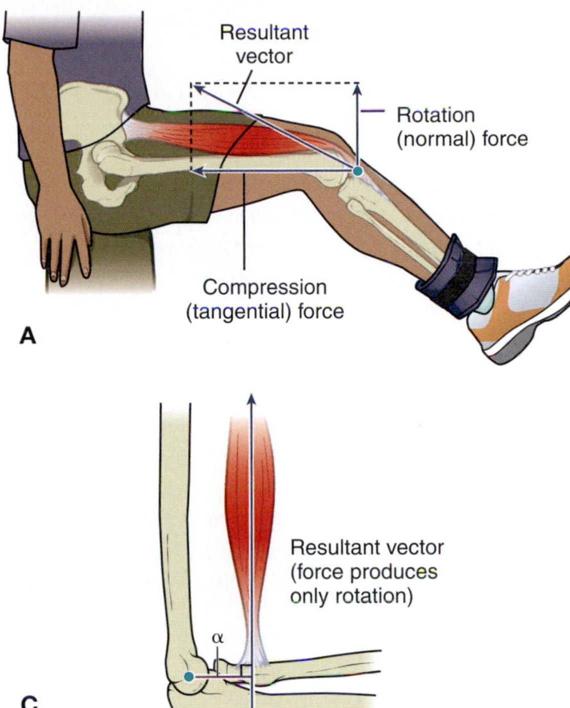

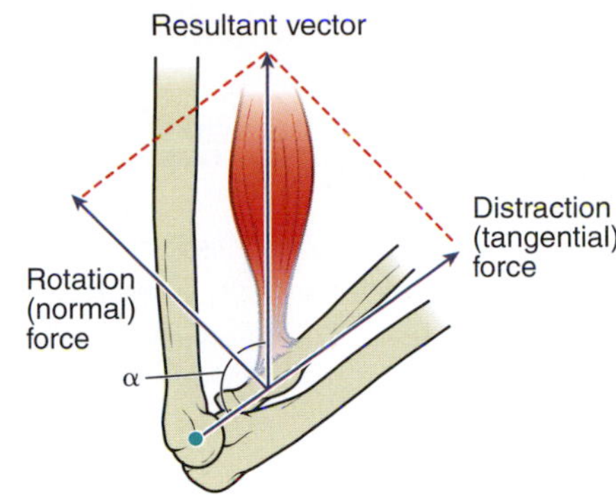

Figure 2.16 Two forces acting in different directions from the same point create a resultant vector. The resultant vector is made up of a rotation force and a force that either compresses or distracts the joint. A) Shows a large compression force vector and small rotational force vector. B) Shows rotational and distraction forces that are close to equal to each other but create a larger resultant force than either of them. C) Since the applied force vector is perpendicular to the lever, there is no distraction or compression force, so all of the muscle's force rotates the segment.

the leg weight and a cuff weight. For each force, one component vector will rotate the segment. The other component force for each of the forces applied will either pull the segment toward the joint, as seen by the muscle's tangential force or away from the joint as seen by the leg and cuff weights' tangential forces in the same figure. The vector producing rotation is the **normal force** vector and the compression or distraction vector is the **tangential force** vector. If a force vector is perpendicular to the body segment, then all of the force created by the resultant vector produces only rotation and does not produce any tangential force (see Fig. 2.16C). In essence, both component vectors are parallel and in the same direction when the resultant force vector is at 90°

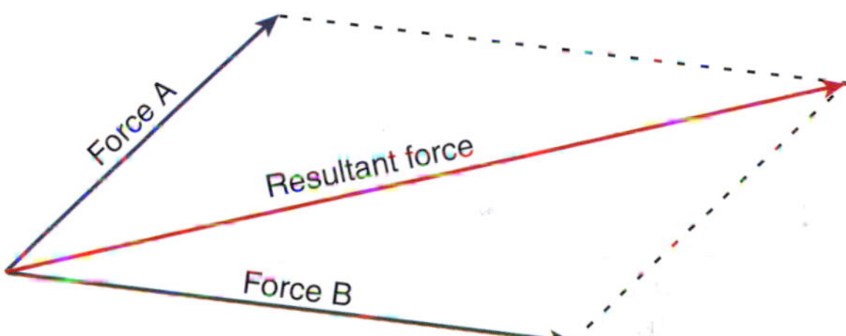

Figure 2.17 A parallelogram is made up of two vector forces, and their resultant force demonstrates graphically how two force vectors acting on one point create a resultant vector force.

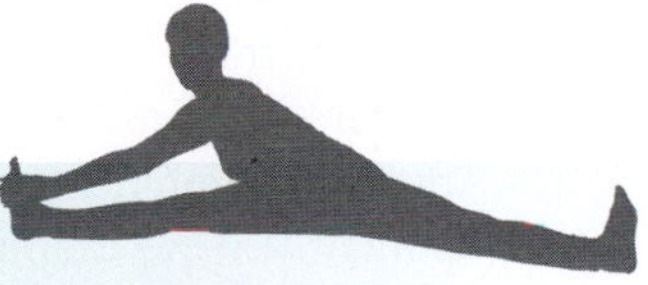

PRACTICE POINT

There are many concurrent force systems throughout the body. A good clinical example is the deltoid muscle. As is seen in Figure 2.18, the anterior and posterior portions of the muscle insert on the deltoid tuberosity from different directions. When they pull with equal force, however, their resultant force causes the arm to elevate into abduction. Balance of the three deltoid portions provide for optimal shoulder elevation in the sagittal plane. Other clinical examples of the body combining muscle angles to create greater resultant forces are seen in the gastrocnemius and trapezius, as demonstrated in Figure 2.19. Although sections of these muscles lie in different directions, when they work together, they are able to produce a greater force at a new angle which lies between the two heads. In some ways, this design allows muscles to have greater strength than they would with only one fiber direction.

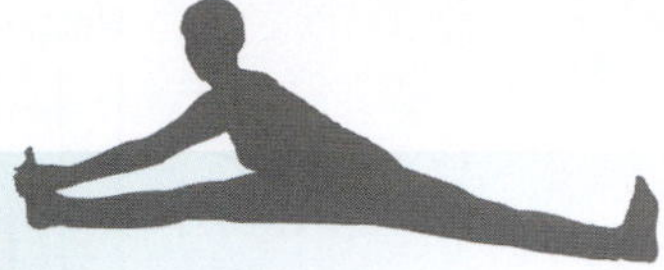

PRACTICE POINT

Figure 2.20 is a good example of how resultant forces increase or decrease as the angle becomes smaller or larger, respectively. If the patient moves toward the head of the bed, the angle between the ropes becomes smaller, and the traction force increases. If the patient moves toward the foot of the bed, the angle between the ropes becomes larger, and the traction force decreases.

Another clinical example of this concept occurs at the patellofemoral joint. When in standing, the force vector of the quadriceps and the patellar ligament are in opposite directions, so they cancel each other out, producing no resultant vector. It makes a difference in how deep a squat exercise is performed. As demonstrated in Figures 2.21A and B, as the depth of the squat and the knee flexion angle increases, the resultant force becomes greater, compressing the patella with more and more force against the femur. If a volleyball player has patellofemoral pain syndrome, she may be required to be able to perform a 90° squat, but until you are able to resolve her pain, it may be necessary to limit her squat exercises to a pain free motion.

to the body segment. Figure 2.20 demonstrates that the force vectors change, depending on the position of the segment and angle created at the joint. This factor is something to keep in mind when determining where in the range of motion the greatest gravitational resistance occurs. This topic of changing body positions to alter gravitational resistance is discussed later.

In the example in Figure 2.15, a coordinate system is on the leg so its x-axis coincides with the long axis of the tibia. The quadriceps muscle force (M) and the resistance (weight) force (W) are resolved into their rectangular components. As has been discussed, the **perpendicular component** (of M or W) is the **rotary component** or the **normal force.** It is that part of the muscle's or resistance's force which causes rotary motion of the segment around the axis. In the example, the quadriceps muscle (M), with its line of pull at an acute angle to the tibia, must produce a relatively large force to create a large enough rotary component (M_R) to move the knee in extension. Conversely, the weight (W) acting at an acute angle to the long axis of the segment resists extension of the knee—not with the full force of 30 lb, but only with its rotary component (W_R) of the W force. Only when the weight is at a 90° angle (perpendicular) to the segment is the rotary force the entire magnitude of the weight (W force). Since a rotary component is always perpendicular to the long axis, the measurement of distances to calculate torque ($\tau = F \cdot d$) is simplified. In this example, torque of the weight force is found by multiplying the rotary component (W_R) by the actual weight arm distance of the lever. Recall that the tangential component vector of a force causes either compression or distraction of a joint, depending on the direction of that component. In the example shown in Figure 2.15, a large part of the tension produced by the quadriceps muscle (M) is directed toward the femur causing compression of the tibia against the femur. When such a component compresses a joint (M_T), it is sometimes called the *stabilizing component* of the muscle force (M). On the other hand, the tangential component of the weight (W_T) causes distraction of the joint surfaces; this type of force is also known as the *distracting component*. As with

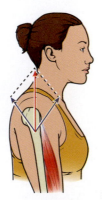

Figure 2.18 Similar to the parallelogram, anterior and posterior deltoid muscles work together to produce a resultant force to abduct the humerus.

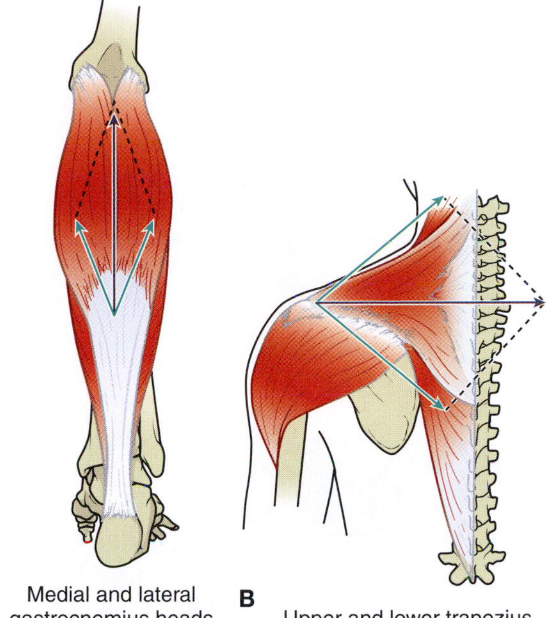

Figure 2.19 There are several muscles within the body that have multiple directions of insertions and, therefore, are able to provide greater force in a new direction. Two examples include the medial and lateral gastrocnemius heads (A) and upper and lower trapezius (B), which exhibit greater force in an altered direction that works to the body's advantage.

the normal components, the magnitudes of both the distracting and stabilizing tangential components can vary from 0% to 100% of the total force, depending on the joint's position. The magnitudes of the stabilizing and distracting components are inversely related: as one approaches 0%, the other approaches 100%.

Laws of the Right Triangle

Calculating forces using graphics is not always practical or convenient. Vector forces can also be determined using trigonometry. Right-angle triangle trigonometry provides us with all the information we need to determine body vectors. From your high school days, you recall these basic trigonometric factors (Fig. 2.23 and 2.24):

- **The Pythagorean theory**: The hypotenuse equals the square root of the sum of the squares of the other two sides. Written mathematically with C as the hypotenuse, or the side opposite to the right angle, and A and B as the other two sides of a right triangle:

$$C = \sqrt{A^2 + B^2}$$

- **SOH – CAH – TOA**: As this mnemonic of the sine, cosine, and tangent laws is described, look at Figure 2.24. A division is a ratio of the numerator to the denominator, so each of these relationships between a right triangle's sides is actually a ratio. These abbreviations relate to a right-angle triangle and the angle, theta (θ), relative to the relationship of sides of a right triangle:
- SOH: **Sine** of theta equals the side **Opposite** to the right angle divided by the **Hypotenuse** side of the triangle.
- CAH: **Cosine** of theta equals the side **Adjacent** to the right angle divided by the **Hypotenuse** side of the right angle.
- TOA: **Tangent** of theta equals the side **Opposite** to the right angle divided by the side **Adjacent** to the right angle.

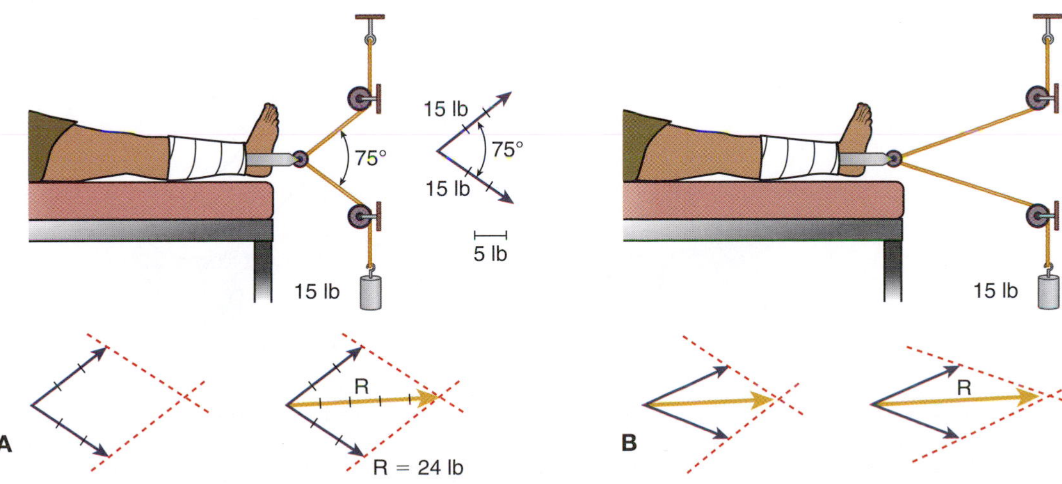

Figure 2.20 Resultant force changes with a change in the angle of the component forces. The resultant traction force applied to a limb changes with a change in the parallelogram formed by the traction unit. The resultant force is the diagonal from the origin of the forces. A) The resultant force vector is smaller with a larger angle between the two pulley lines. B) When the angle between the pulley lines becomes more acute, the resultant vector force, or distraction force, on the leg increases.

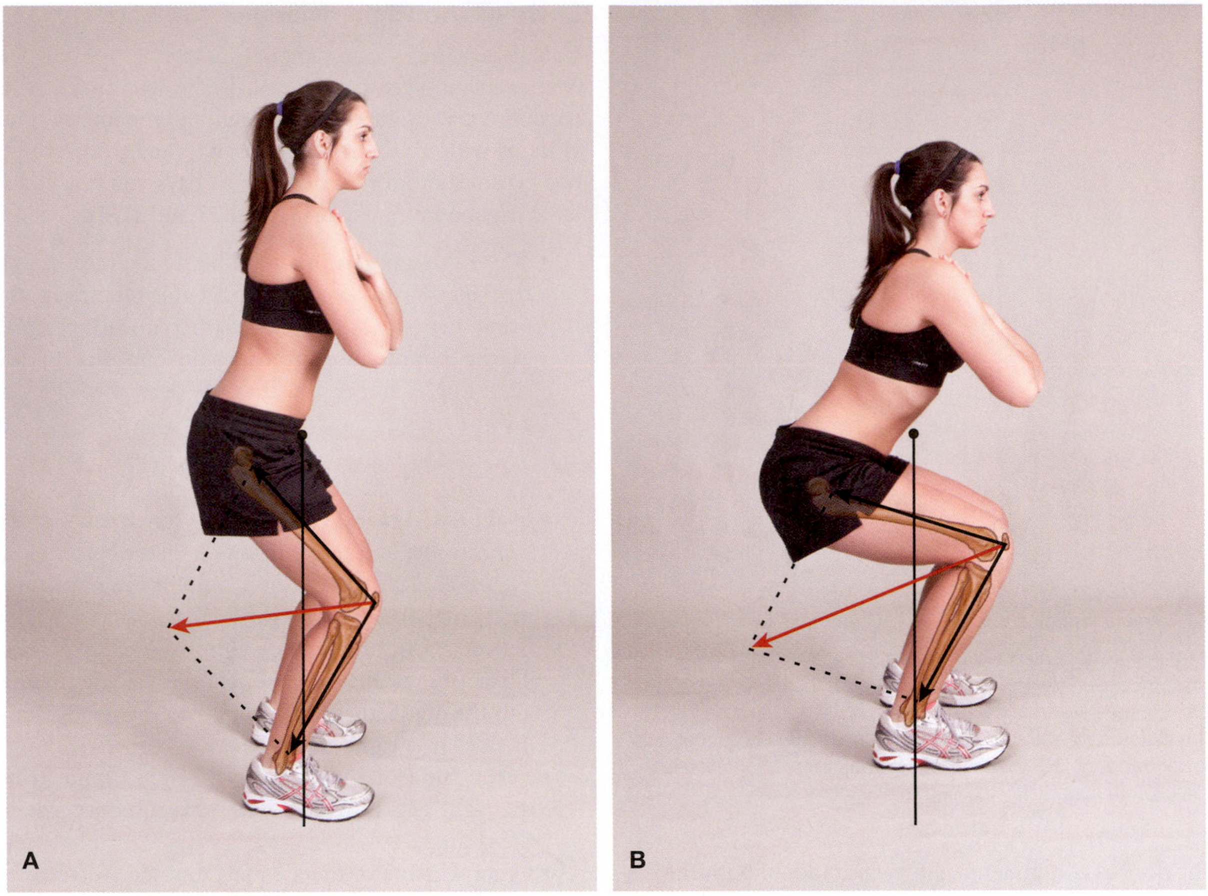

Figure 2.21 Resultant force vectors using parallelograms may also be applied to the patellofemoral joint. As the squat angle changes—A) half squat; B) full squat—the compression pressure of the patella against the femur increases because of the resultant vector produced by the quadriceps muscle and patellar ligament.

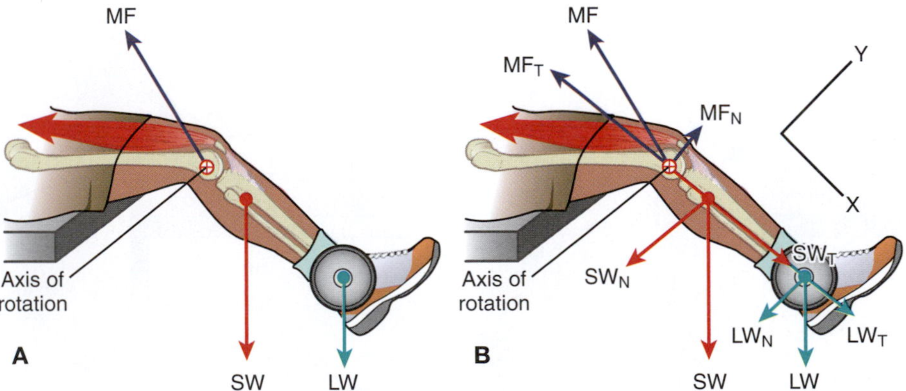

Figure 2.22 A force is created by component vectors. These component vectors rotate a joint and either distract or compress a joint. With the free body diagram is superimposed on the leg, the formula used includes M as the muscle, M_T for tangential force, M_N for rotational force, W for the weight boot, WT for the tangential force, WN for the rotational force, L for the leg weight, L_T for the tangential force, and L_N for the rotational force.

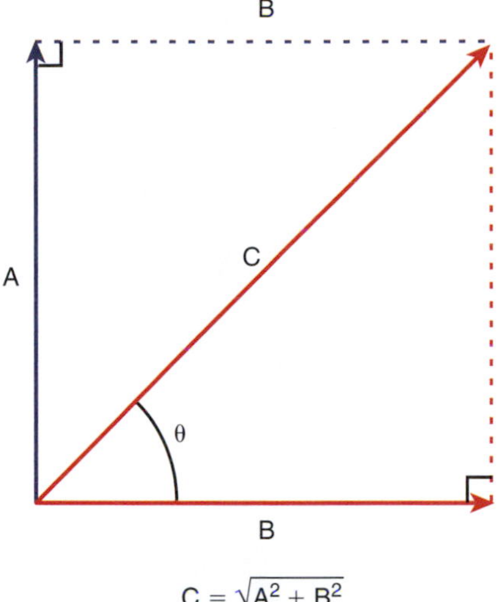

Figure 2.23 Pythagorean theory of a right triangle: the length of the opposite side to the right angle is the square root of the sum of the squares of the two adjacent sides of the right angle.

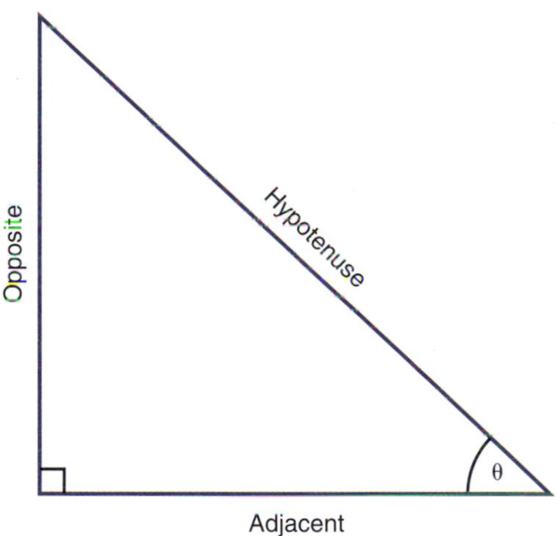

Figure 2.24 SOH-CAH-TOA. These three formulas are used to calculate the magnitudes of torques and unknown forces impacting muscle activity and joint structures. S= sine; C= cosine; T= tangent; O= opposite; A= adjacent; H=hypotenuse. In each case, the middle letter is the numerator and the third letter is the denominator in the ratio.

In mathematical terms, these formulas look like this:

$$\text{Sin } \theta = \frac{\text{Opposite side}}{\text{Hypotenuse side}} \quad \text{Cos } \theta = \frac{\text{Adjacent side}}{\text{Hypotenuse side}}$$

$$\text{Tan } \theta = \frac{\text{Opposite side}}{\text{Adjacent side}}$$

We can use these laws of the right triangle to calculate the magnitudes of the torques and unknown muscle and joint forces and further appreciate the impact these forces have on treatment and rehabilitation. A rectangle can be divided into two right triangles. If we create a rectangle using component and resultant vectors, the resultant force is the hypotenuse (Fig. 2.23). The ratios of the sides and hypotenuse of the right triangle are always the same for any same angle. Table 2–3 lists the ratio values for several angles. For example, the value of 0.500 is the sine of a 30° angle; this means that the opposite side is one-half the length (or magnitude) of the hypotenuse. Therefore, if either the values of one side and one angle or the values of two sides are known, the remaining sides and angles can be found.

Using these formulas, then, we can calculate either any angle of torque or the amount of torque applied either by the muscles or to the body by other forces. It is important to grasp these concepts since we must deal with them whenever we treat injuries. Although trigonometry tends to make some people apprehensive, we will keep these concepts simple and make them clinically applicable.

Force Applications to the Body

Clinically, several methods are used to reduce the effect of weight on a joint. If we reduce the weight on a joint, we will reduce the forces applied to an injured segment or joint. When a body part is positioned and supported to move in a plane parallel to the earth, the effects of gravity are reduced so a muscle weaker than 3/5 is able to move a segment. Movement in this plane is frequently called "gravity-free," "gravity-eliminated," or "gravity-minimized" motion. The weight of the body or segments

TABLE 2–3 | USEFUL TRIGONOMETRIC FUNCTIONS AND RATIOS OF COMMON ANGLES (FOR OTHER ANGLES, THE READER SHOULD REFER TO TABLES OF NATURAL TRIGONOMETRIC FUNCTIONS)

Angle	sin	cos	tan
0°	0.000	1.000	0.000
10°	0.174	0.985	0.176
20°	0.342	0.940	0.364
30°	0.500	0.866	0.577
45°	0.707	0.707	1.000
60°	0.866	0.500	1.732
70°	0.940	0.342	2.747
80°	0.985	0.174	5.671
90°	1.000	0.000	∞

may be suspended from above by slings and springs or supported from below, thereby permitting weak muscles to exercise or painful joints to be unloaded.[2] Another weightless environment is the therapeutic pool, where Archimedes' principle of buoyancy is used: **A body submerged in a liquid is buoyed up by a force equal to the weight of the liquid displaced.** Because gravity is reduced in aquatic exercises, they are frequently and successfully used in several rehabilitation situations. Aquatic exercises are used rather than land exercises to reduce the resistance of gravity with weak muscles; very painful joints that are unable to function with land exercises are often successfully moved in water; or nonweight-bearing segments can be unloaded of weight to permit pain-free activities, walking, running, and other aquatic exercises.

Weight and Center of Gravity (Center of Mass)

We know that gravity is a force that acts on all bodies. Therefore, gravity is a force that we must understand as well as appreciate its impact on the body and body segment's motion.

Center of Gravity or Center of Mass

To determine how gravity affects a body segment, we must locate the center from which gravity's force acts. The **center of gravity (COG)** of an object or body is the theoretical point around which the mass of the object is balanced. It is around this center that gravity acts. This point is also called the **center of mass (COM)** (Fig. 2.25). If you could place your fingertip directly under the COG of an object, it would remain balanced on your fingertip. This COM is the point of origin for gravity's vector force. It is easier to find in symmetrical objects than it is in asymmetrical objects. The center of gravity of symmetrical objects occurs in the geometric center of the object, but in asymmetrical objects, it may even occur outside the mass. For example, if you stood on one leg with the other leg lifted and extended behind you while you were flexed at your waist with your arms overhead, your COG would lie outside your body, probably somewhere in front of your thighs and below your torso. Figure 2.26 shows changes in the COM with changes in body positions and with the additions of appliances. COM and COG are used interchangeably throughout this text.

The center of gravity of the body as a whole is the sum of the centers of gravity of individual segments. Knowledge of the location of the segmental centers of gravity and the approximate weight of the segments is clinically useful in adjusting exercise loads, applying traction, and balancing parts of the body. Figure 2.25 indicates the COG of the body as well as the body segments when in the anatomical position. Body segment parameters have been determined on cadavers.[3,4] For specific details, refer to the original studies or to Drillis et al.[5]

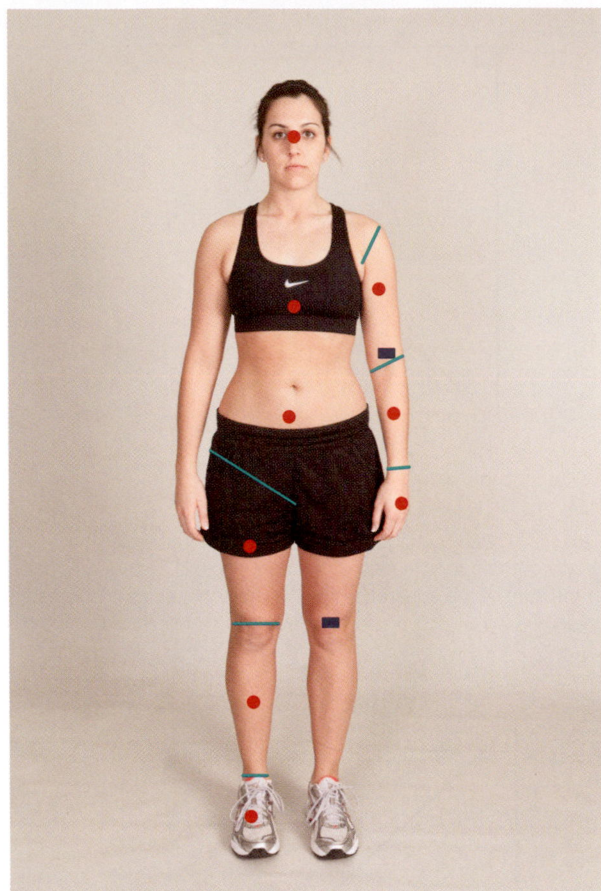

Figure 2.25 Location of the center of gravity of the body and of the body's segments. Red circles indicate COM of each segment. Rectangles indicate COM of each extremity. The circle below the navel indicates the body's COM.

The center of gravity of the extended upper extremity is just above the elbow joint, and that of the extended lower extremity is just above the knee joint. The arm, forearm, thigh, and leg are larger proximally, and thus their individual centers of gravity lie closer to the proximal end. This point is approximately $^4/_9$ (45%) of the length of the segment, measured from the proximal end.

The center of gravity of the head, arms, and trunk (HAT) is located anterior to the border of the 11th thoracic vertebra and just below the xiphoid process of the sternum.[6] The weight of HAT is approximately equal to 60% of the body weight. In Figures 2.27A and B, note the increased distance from the hip joint to the line of the center of gravity of HAT as forward inclination increases. This position requires increasingly more force

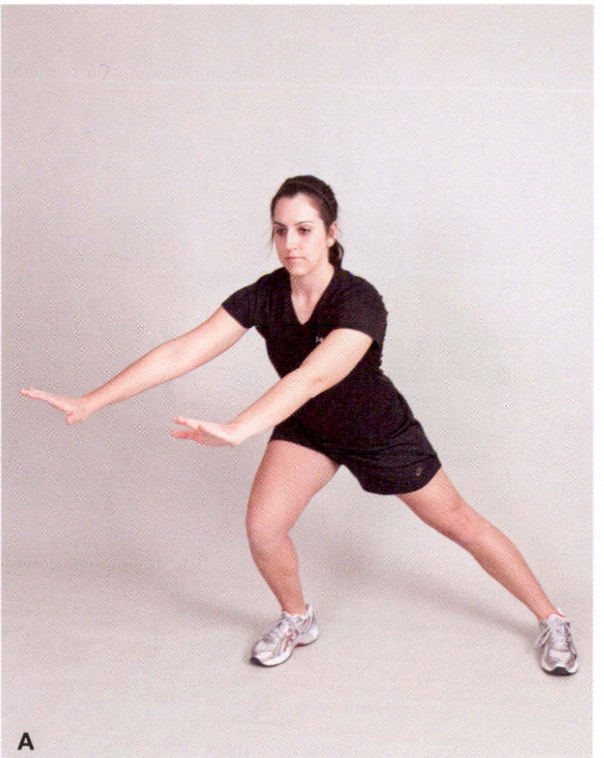

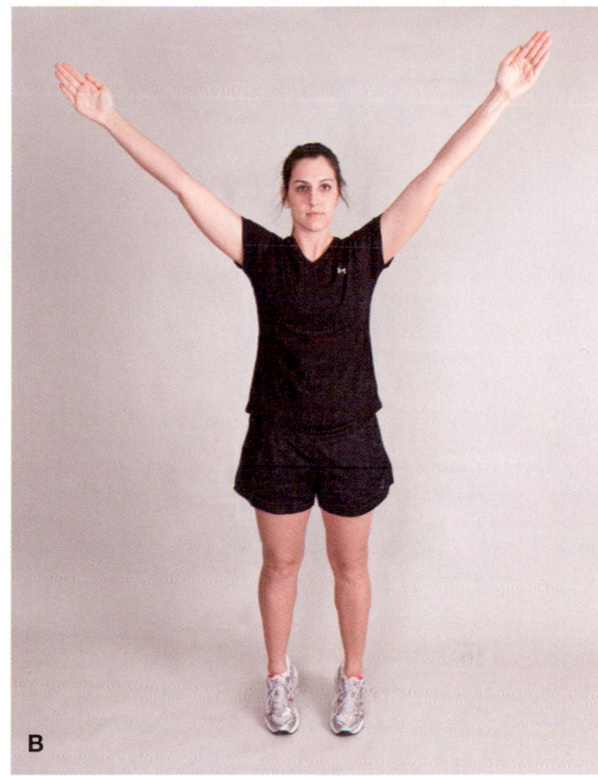

Figure 2.26 Changes in the body's center of gravity occurs with changes in positions. Sometimes the body's center of gravity lies within the body and sometimes it lies outside of it.

in the back and hip extensor muscles to support the weight of the trunk.

The **center of gravity of the adult body in the anatomic position is slightly anterior to the second sacral vertebra,**[4] or approximately 55% of a person's height.[7] The center-of-gravity mark usually falls near the level of the anterior-superior iliac spines. Variations in body proportions and weight distribution cause alterations in the location of this point. It is usually slightly higher in men than in women, because men tend to have broader shoulders, while women tend to have broader hips.

A change in the position of individual segments causes a change in the position of the center of gravity of the extremity and the body as a whole. When the extremity is flexed, the center of gravity moves proximally and to a point on a line between individual segments centers (Fig. 2.29). Deliberate movement of the center of gravity of segments is frequently used in therapeutic exercise to alter the resistive torque (weight times its perpendicular distance to the axis of motion) of an extremity. For example, shoulder flexion against gravity is easier to perform when the elbow is flexed than when the elbow is extended. A sit-up exercise is

PRACTICE POINT

In patients with paralysis of the hip musculature such as paraplegics and tetraplegics, control of the center of gravity of HAT is essential for stability in sitting. Stability of HAT during upper extremity motions requires an additional external support. In a wheelchair, this may be gained by holding onto parts of the chair (Fig. 2.28).

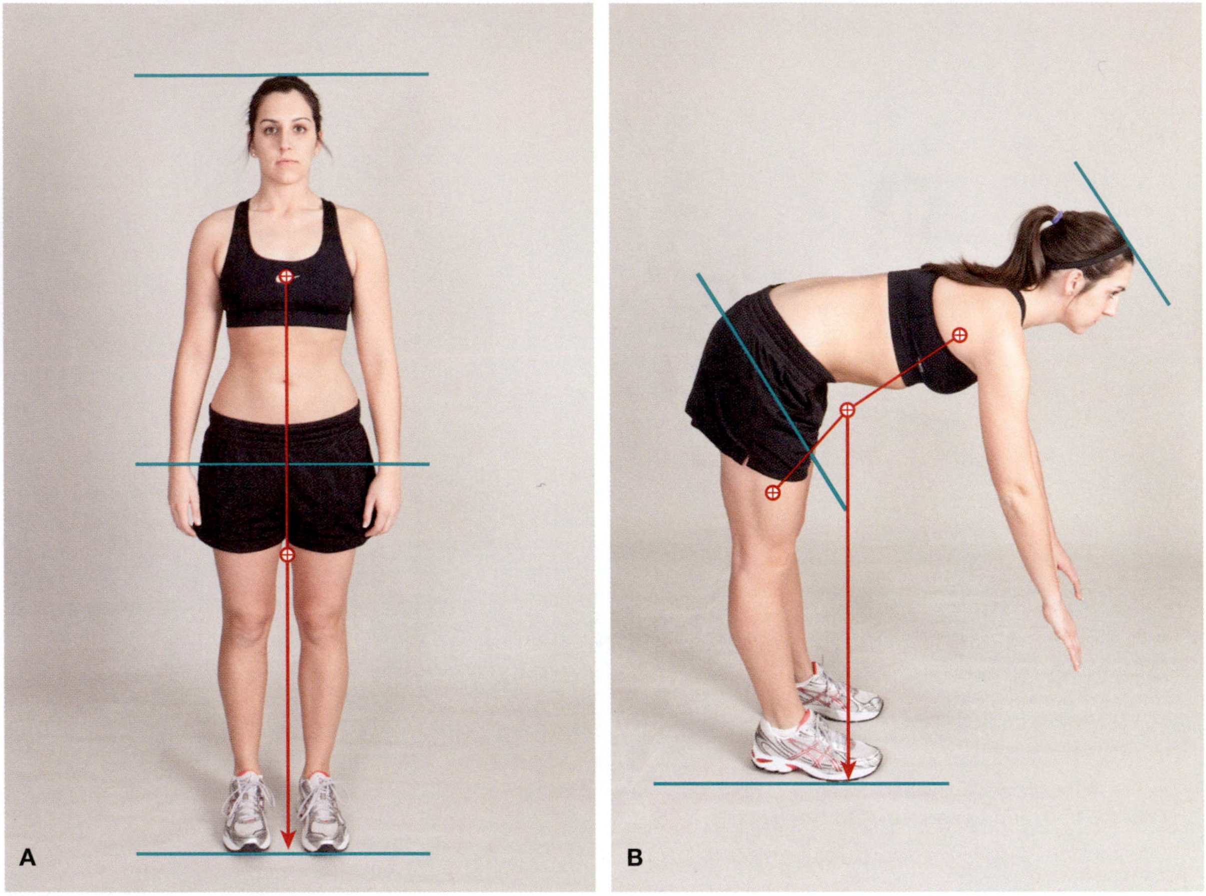

A

B

Figure 2.27 As the center of gravity of the head, arms and trunk (HAT) moves in front of the hips, the resistance arm of the HAT increases, so back and hip extensor muscles must increase their force to support the HAT weight.

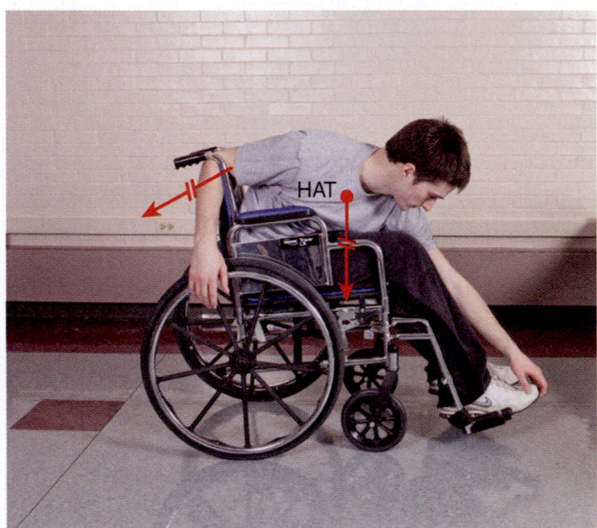

Figure 2.28 Methods of stability and control of the center of gravity of the head, arms, and trunk (HAT) in persons with hip and trunk muscle paralysis, such as spinal cord injuries. Here, the person hooks the arm around the handlebar so the elbow flexors can be used to lower and raise the trunk.

easiest to perform when the arms are at the sides, and it becomes progressively more difficult when the arms are folded on the chest or the hands are placed on top of the head. Changing the torque of the lower extremities provides a method for altering the difficulty of abdominal muscle exercises. In the supine position, the abdominal muscles contract to stabilize the pelvis when the legs are raised. The resistance that the abdominal muscles must meet decreases by flexing the lower extremities before lifting the lower extremities; the resistance reduces even more by raising only one leg. The magnitude of the decrease in torque is illustrated in Figure 2.29. Although the weight of the single extremity is the same in both positions, the center of gravity has moved from 15 in. (37 cm) from the hip joint axis to 8 in. (20 cm); therefore, the torque has been reduced from 360 in.-lb (40.6 N) to 192 in.-lb (21.7 N). This decrease in torque not only reduces the stabilization force required of the abdominal muscles but also reduces the force that the hip flexor muscles must generate to raise the extremity.

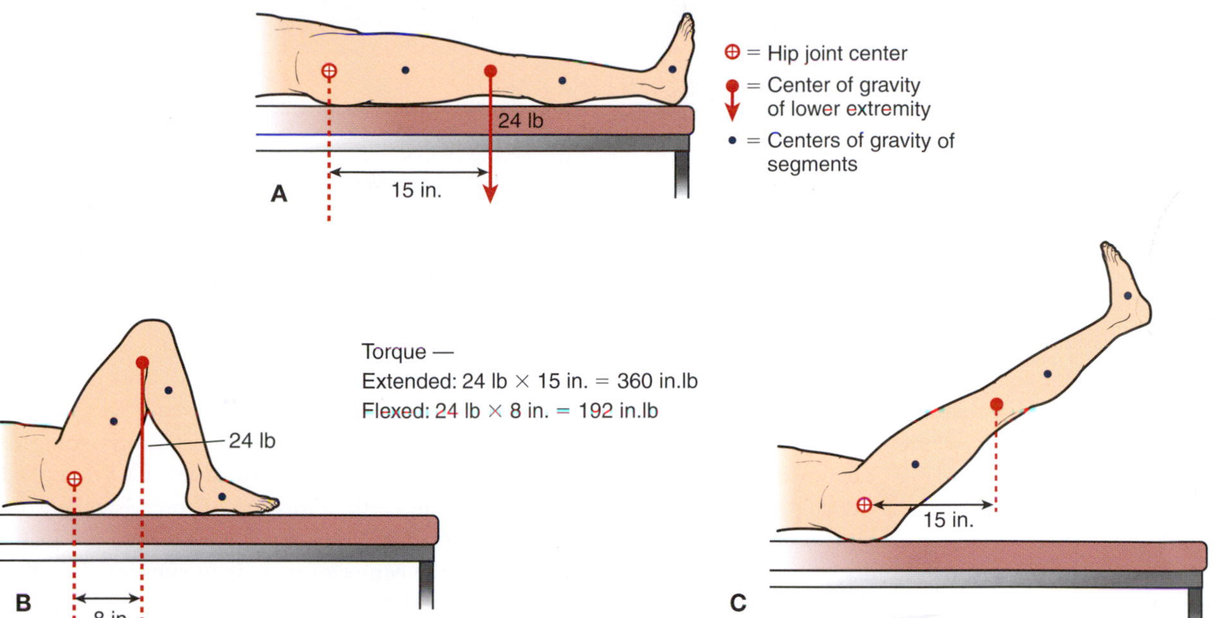

Figure 2.29 Alteration of the torque of the lower extremity by changing the position of individual segments. **A)** The leg is fully extended, so its resistance arm is 15 inches; **B)** With the hip and knee flexed, the lower extremity's COG moves proximally, so the resistance arm is now 8 inches. **C)** If the individual raises the legs off the table, how much force the abdominals must produce to stabilize the trunk will depend on the position of the hips and knees and how far the lower extremity COGs are from the axis of motion.

The center of gravity of a solid object, such as a brick or a ball, is not difficult to visualize. The human body, however, has many irregularly shaped segments, so its center of gravity is more difficult to determine. To further complicate matters, as the positions of the segments change, so does the center of gravity of the body as a whole. A patient with muscle weakness can collapse in a fraction of a second if the gravity line moves outside the base of support. Knowledge of where and how the force of gravity acts on the body (and its segments) is important clinically to facilitate motion, change exercise loads, and balance parts.

Stable, Unstable, and Neutral Equilibrium

If the center of gravity of a body is disturbed slightly and the body tends to return the center of gravity to its former position, the body is in **stable equilibrium.** Rocking while sitting in a rocking chair is an example of stable equilibrium. If the center of gravity does not return but seeks a new position, the body falls. The body is then in a state of **unstable equilibrium,** such as may occur if a person sitting on a narrow-based stool leans forward. Examples of **neutral equilibrium** include a rolling ball or a person who is propelled in a wheelchair. Neutral equilibrium occurs when the center of gravity is displaced, but it remains at the same level; that is, it neither falls nor returns to its former position.

The degree of stability (resistance to being overthrown) of a body depends on four factors:

1) Height of the center of gravity above the base of support;
2) Size of the base of support;
3) Location of the gravity line within the base of support; and
4) Weight of the body.

Changing any one or more of these factors either improves or reduces stability. Stability is enhanced by a low center of gravity, wide base of support, gravity's line over the center of the support, and heavy weight. On the other hand, stability is diminished if the center of gravity is elevated, the base of support is narrowed, the line of gravity falls outside the center of support, or the object's weight is reduced.

Any deviation from the anatomic position causes the center of gravity to move. If the arms are folded on the chest or raised overhead, the center of gravity rises. If the subject flexes the head, trunk and hips, the center of gravity moves toward the feet. Because the body's center of gravity is relatively high, an erect person is in a position of unstable equilibrium. Only a small force is needed to cause displacement of the body. This may be a good or a bad factor. It is a good factor in that it does not take much force to initiate walking. On the other

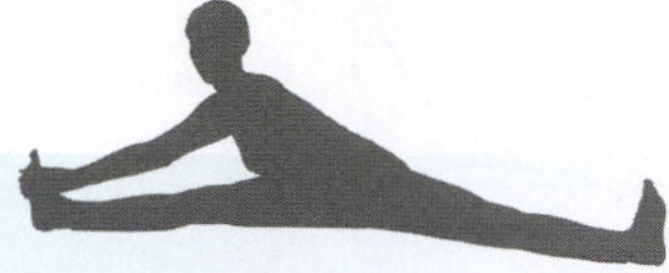

PRACTICE POINT

The size of football linemen and the crouched positions they take with a wide forward-backward stance promote stability and resistance to being overthrown by an opponent. Instability, on the other hand, is enhanced by a high center of gravity, narrow base of support, and light weight as exemplified by the positions and moves of football running backs.

hand, the body may be at risk for falling if other factors are not present. Fortunately, falling is prevented by an intact and automatic neuromuscular system, which maintains the body's center of gravity within its base of support. Therefore, walking is actually a sequence of disturbing and catching the center of gravity. Uncertainty in the person's ability to control and balance the body may cause the individual to widen the distance between their feet to increase the base of support or walk with the knees flexed to lower the center of gravity; however, such a change in center of gravity requires greater energy and may promote further loss of balance. For example, the novice downhill snow skier sits back rather than leans forward on the skis. People who attempt to walk in a dark and unfamiliar place usually tend to flex the hips and knees or spread their feet apart, as do patients who are unsure of their balance. The clinician is responsible for providing both the physical and psychological support to help patients learn to perform motor tasks safely and effectively.

Not only does the center of gravity change with motions, but it can also change with additions to or subtractions from the body segments. If the COG changes, the line of gravity also changes. For example, if an individual has a cast on the right leg, the additional weight of the leg will shift the COG to the right, and along with it, the LOG (line of gravity) will also adjust to that side. An individual with a leg amputation above the knee has an elevated and laterally adjusted COG, so in the standing position, this individual may be at greater risk for falling until he or she adjusts to the change in COG and LOG positions. When you carry your heavy suitcase home for a long holiday, the suitcase adds weight to the side of your body on which you are carrying it, so your COG is shifted to that side. To stop yourself from falling over to that side, you shift your trunk to the opposite side so the combined weight of your body and the heavy suitcase is within your base of support.

Base of Support

Since gravity is a force vector, it must not only have an axis (center of motion) from which it is applied, but it must also have dimension (magnitude) and direction. The dimension, or magnitude, is the weight of the body or segment. The direction of gravity is always going to be a vertically downward pull from the COM toward the center of the earth. This line of force is called the **line of gravity (LOG).** A body is stable when the LOG runs through the center of its base of support. A body's **base of support (BOS)** is the area within the points of contact of the body and any object the individual relies on for support. For example, if you stand with your feet shoulder-width apart, your base of support is the area under your feet and the area of the floor between your feet as seen in Figure 2.30. If the patient with a cast on the leg in the paragraph above uses crutches to ambulate, then that individual is more stable because his BOS includes the area between the feet and extends to include the points of contact of the crutches and the floor area between the crutches and feet. The larger the base of support, the more stable an object is (since it would take more to move the COG outside the BOS), and contrarily, a smaller BOS makes an object less stable. That is one reason why it is more difficult to stand on one leg than on two. If the COM falls outside the BOS, the object is unstable and falls unless either the BOS moves under the object or a force overcomes gravity to maintain the object's position. Standing on one leg is more difficult because not only is the BOS smaller, but it also takes less motion to move the COM outside the BOS.

Increased stability occurs with a larger base of support. A larger base of support makes it more difficult to lose balance or be overthrown by outside forces. When outside forces are delivered from a lateral direction, it is more difficult to maintain the LOG and COG over the BOS. If we anticipate the force, however, we can provide for a more stable base to accept the oncoming force. For example, if you anticipate a force coming at you in a forward-backward (A-P) direction, you place your feet in that direction with one foot in front of you and the other behind so you are in a better position to maintain your COM within your base of support. Likewise, if a force is directed to you from the side, you

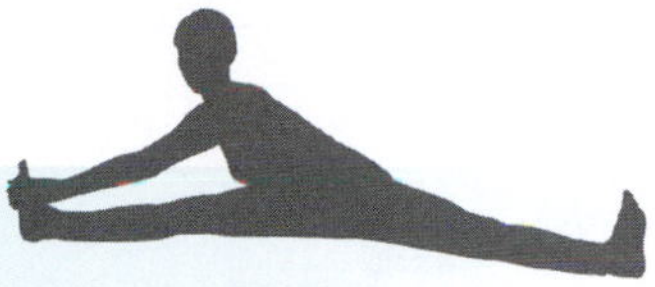

PRACTICE POINT

You can demonstrate the importance of the size of the base of support with a partner. Have your partner stand with his or her feet together and see how much force you must apply to move him or her off balance. Now have your partner stand with the feet farther apart and repeat your attempts to push him or her off balance. With the feet apart, the BOS is much larger so the COM does not move out of the BOS as easily when the BOS is smaller. How would a patient use this concept if he had balance difficulties and did not use assistive devices to walk?

will widen your BOS from left to right to maintain your COM and LOG within your BOS. We can apply this concept to a common experience: If you stand when riding a crowded bus or train, you will place your feet in a position with one toward the front of the vehicle and the other toward the back of the vehicle since that is the direction of the vehicle's stop and start forces.

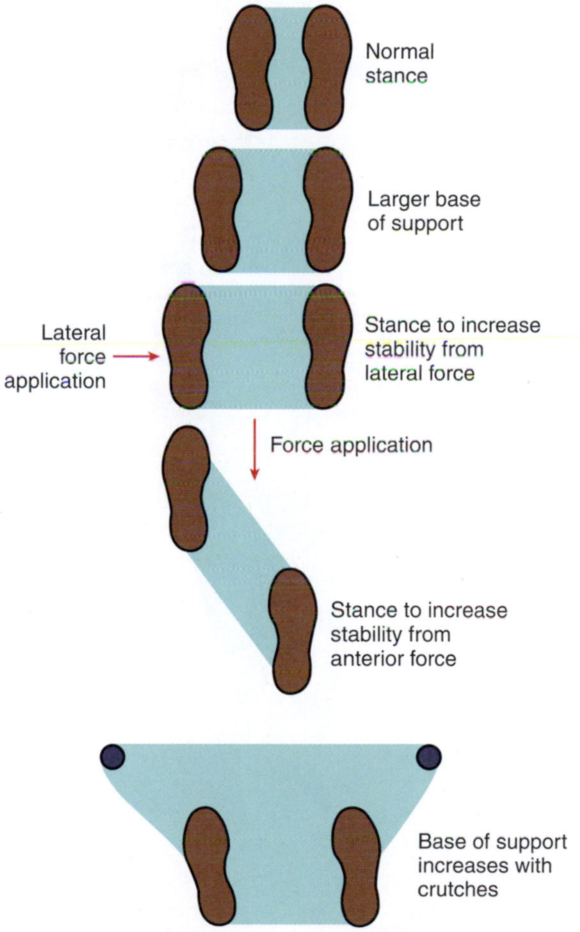

A large base of support is sometimes advantageous and sometimes not advantageous. For example, a weight lifter who lifts a large Olympic bar with several weight plates on it over his head should have a broad base of support to provide himself the stability required to hold the weight overhead and maintain his weight and that of the bar within his BOS. Likewise, a wrestler who does not want to be thrown by an opponent will also create for himself a large base of support (Fig. 2.31A) On the other hand, a volleyball player who must move quickly out of her base of support does not want a large base from which to move (Fig. 2.31B); movement must occur suddenly and in any direction, so the player must be ready. A large base of support for this player prolongs her time within her stable base and delays her response to meet the ball.

Figure 2.30 Variations in the base of support. The base of support includes the area between the feet and any object that the individual is holding onto or leaning against. With feet close together, the area between and including the feet is smaller compared to when the feet are spread apart. Individuals using crutches expand their base of support significantly since their base of support now extends to the area between the crutches and the body.

Levers and Muscle Activity

Since most of the levers throughout the body are third class, muscles must work harder than resistance forces to provide desired motion. In essence, the lever arm lengths, or moment arms, of muscles are shorter than the resistance arm lengths, or moment arms, of forces working against the muscle, so muscles must produce more force than the resistance force. Let us use the biceps brachii as an example. It attaches to the forearm very near the elbow joint; however, the center of mass of the forearm and hand lies distally to the mid-forearm, considerably farther than the insertion of the biceps brachii from the elbow joint. Therefore, the biceps must work much harder to lift the weight of the forearm and hand than it would if it inserted more distally on the forearm than the forearm's COM. In order for a person to lift a 10-lb weight in a curl, the biceps (disregarding other elbow flexor muscles for this example) must produce a total of 81.55 lb (Fig. 2.32).

As clinicians, we can use this concept to our advantage. Using a previous example, if we provide a patient with manual resistance, applying our force to the distal end of the segment will be to our advantage because we

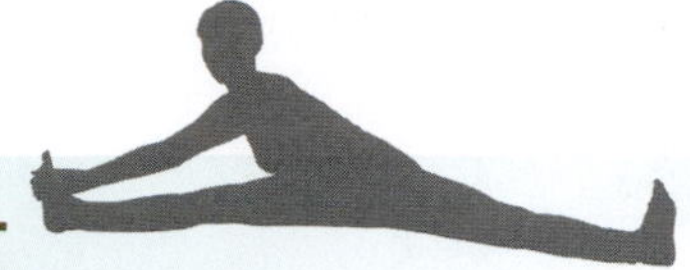

PRACTICE POINT

To apply these COG and BOS concepts, use your partner once again. Have your partner stand erect with the feet shoulder-width apart. Notice how much force is required to push your partner off his or her BOS when you apply your force from side-to-side. Now, with the feet in the same position and keeping the heels on the floor, have your partner squat to lower his or her COM. Repeat the push and notice how much more force is required to move your partner off balance. We see these concepts commonly used in daily and sport activities. For example, a football lineman stands in a crouched position with the hips and knees flexed to lower the COM and the feet are spread apart in a forward-backward stance to increase the BOS, and the player aligns himself for the A-P directed forces so his opponent has a more difficult time overtaking him. Identify how this concept could be used with a patient you are treating if this patient was a football lineman. What if your patient was a cashier; what instructions would you provide to improve her stability at her work?

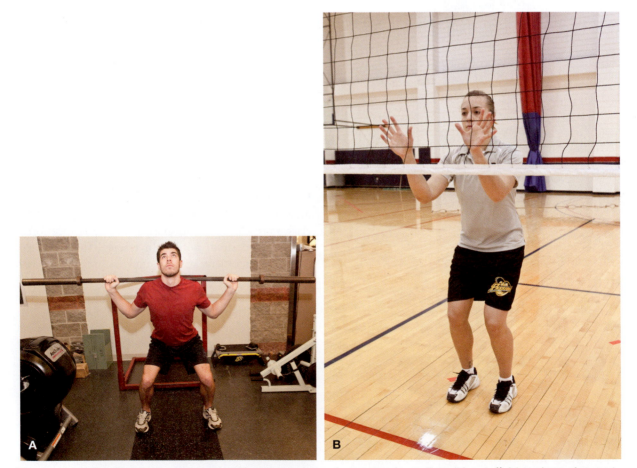

Figure 2.31 Sometimes it is advantageous to have a large base of support and sometimes it is not. **A)** A large base of support provides stability and is necessary, especially when supporting a heavy weight. **B)** If rapid movement is required, a small base of support allows the individual to move rapidly out of his or her base of support and is advantageous during some sports activities that require rapid changes in direction or movement.

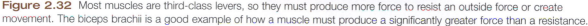

MF × Muscle movement arm = External forces × External movement arm

$$MF = \frac{EF \times EMA}{MMA}$$

$$\frac{(10\ \text{lb} \times 14\ \text{in.}) + (3.3\ \text{lb} \times 7\ \text{in.})}{2\ \text{in.}}$$

$$\frac{140\ \text{lb} + 23.1\ \text{in.}}{2\ \text{lb}} = 81.55\ \text{lb}$$

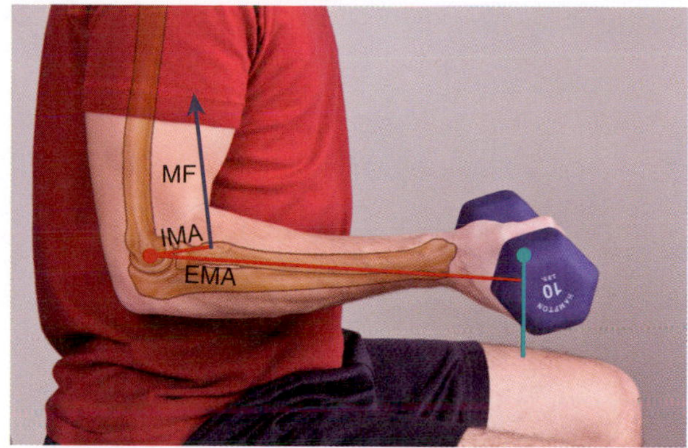

Figure 2.32 Most muscles are third-class levers, so they must produce more force to resist an outside force or create movement. The biceps brachii is a good example of how a muscle must produce a significantly greater force than a resistance.

will not work as hard as the patient must work to deliver an appropriate amount of resistance during the exercise. We can also use this concept to alter an exercise without changing much of the exercise itself. For example, if a patient is unable to perform a straight leg raise because the hip flexors lack sufficient strength, instructing the patient to flex the knee slightly will shorten the resistance arm so the exercise can be performed. As the patient's strength increases, the knee may be positioned in full extension to provide additional resistance.

Although third-class levers of the body require large forces exerted by muscles, they also provide for a tremendous amount of motion during activity. Although the biceps does not have a force advantage, it is able to provide movement of the elbow with little of its own motion. In other words, the biceps does not have to shorten very far to produce a large arc of motion for the hand. This concept is similar to a group of children playing "crack the whip." They all travel in a circle with the same angular displacement and angular velocity, but their linear velocity and displacement is very different from one another. The children closer to the axis do not move as much linearly, but the children farther from the center of motion must move much faster to keep up with the angular displacement of those closer to the center (Fig. 2.34).

Therefore, the body's levers appear to be more designed for speed of motion than for strength. When implements such as golf clubs, baseball bats, tennis racquets, or paddles are attached to the distal upper extremity, speed of motion translates into additional forces and greater results for desired activities. Throwing a ball is another example of upper extremity forces providing greater motion and speed of motion. Kicking a soccer ball, football, or running involve these same concepts in the lower extremity. The longer the segment, the greater the angular velocity, so if an implement is used, such as a tennis racquet, the object (tennis ball) will travel farther and faster because of the increased length of the lever arm and consequent increased speed of angular motion (Fig. 2.35).

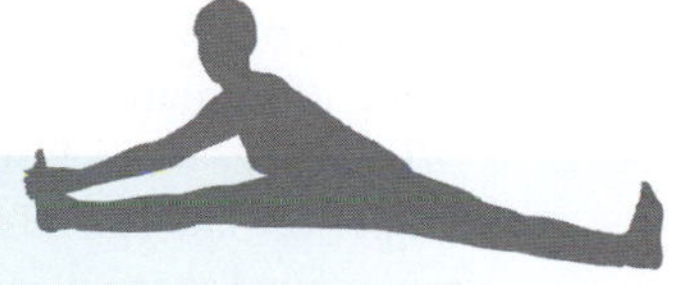

PRACTICE POINT

Understanding the impact of lever arm lengths is also important in performing proper body mechanics, such as in lifting techniques. Proper lifting includes bringing an object to be lifted close to the body before the lift is performed. Making this preparation reduces the lever arm of the object being lifted so its resistance arm is reduced. This maneuver applies less stress to body segments and allows for safer mechanics. As seen in Figure 2.33A, the individual bending over in a stoop-bend creates a long lever arm for the weight of the head, arms and trunk, and lifted object. A contrast, however, occurs in Figure 2.33B, in which there is a drastic reduction in the forces applied to the back with the more proper squat technique that shortens the resistance arm of the head, arms and trunk, and object lifted.

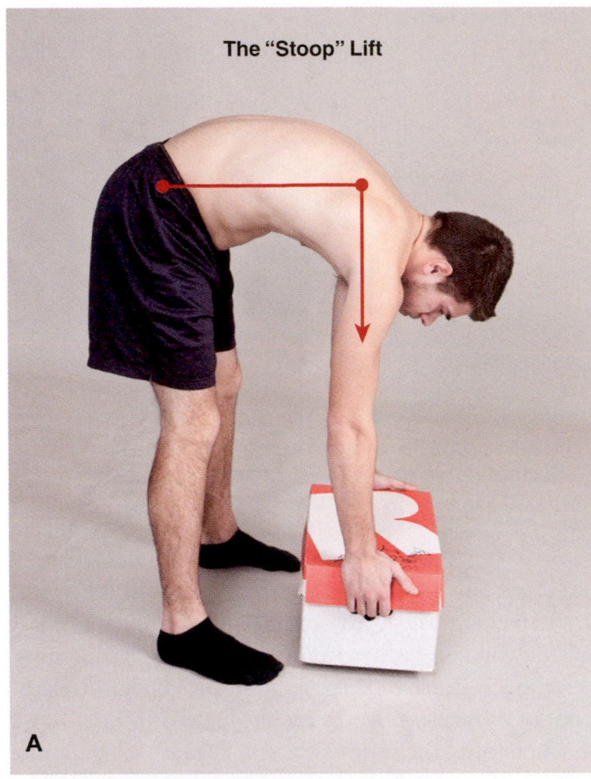

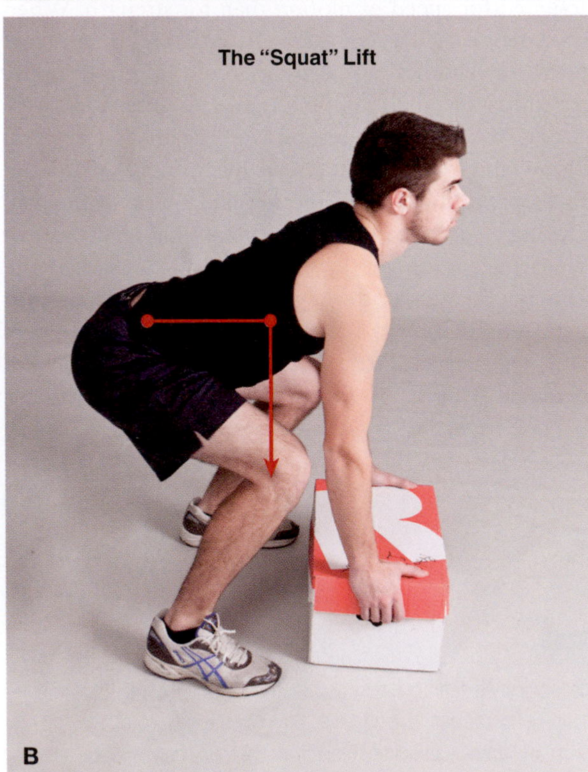

Figure 2.33 Using proper body mechanics includes moving objects close to the body. In (A) the object has a long lever arm and will place a much greater force on the body than the object in (B) when it is brought closer to the body so its lever arm is shortened.

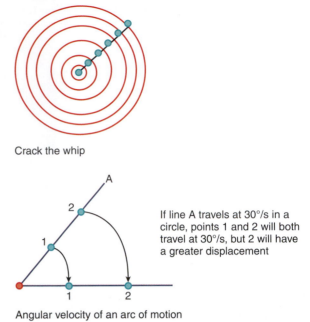

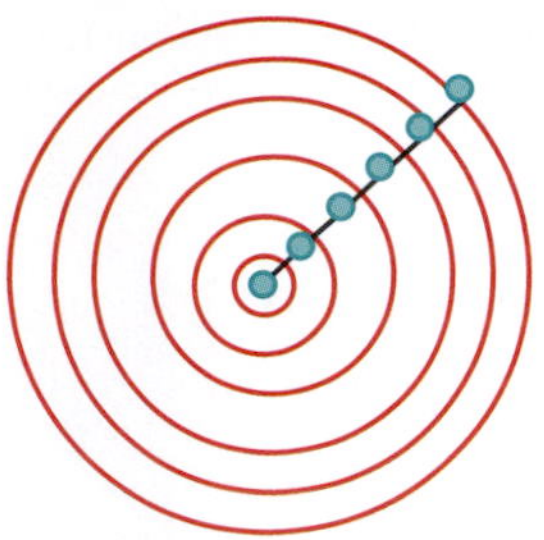

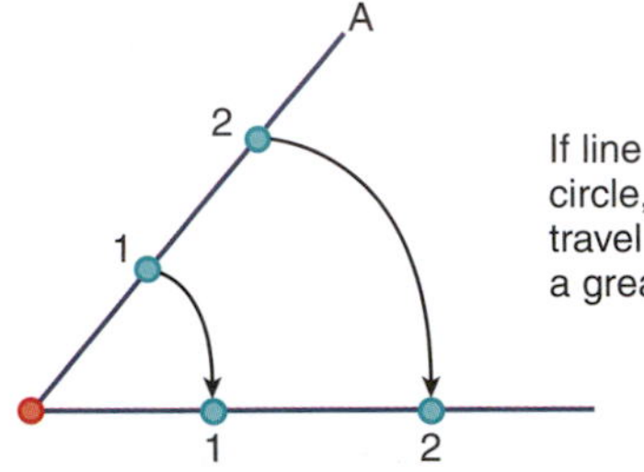

Figure 2.34 Angular velocity is the same on a line moving around an axis, but the linear velocity is much faster for those points farther from the axis of motion. In order to continue on a circular path, the point farthest from the center of motion must travel in its arc at a faster rate than points closer to the center of motion.

Free Body Diagrams

Now that we appreciate levers and forces a little more, let us take the next step in understanding how these mechanical constructs affect our daily movements. This section deals with the applications of various sciences including geometry, mathematics, and calculus. Before you panic, realize that the applications used here are basic and fully explained so they will be easy to understand. These calculations are necessary because it is important to realize the quantity of forces the body must produce as well as withstand during both daily activities and rehabilitation. Once you complete this section, you will realize that these concepts are not as difficult to grasp as you thought. You will also gain a greater appreciation of human activity and performance.

To realize muscle requirements for human activity and performance, it is easiest if we use engineering diagrams called **space diagrams**, or **free body diagrams**. Free body diagrams are simplified drawings of the body with the force vectors acting on the body or a segment. We have already used these diagrams in simplified versions earlier in this chapter. When we study forces and torques applied to the body, we must recall that these forces and torques have two dimensions, so we need to consider both their direction of application and the magnitude of those forces and torques applied to a body segment.

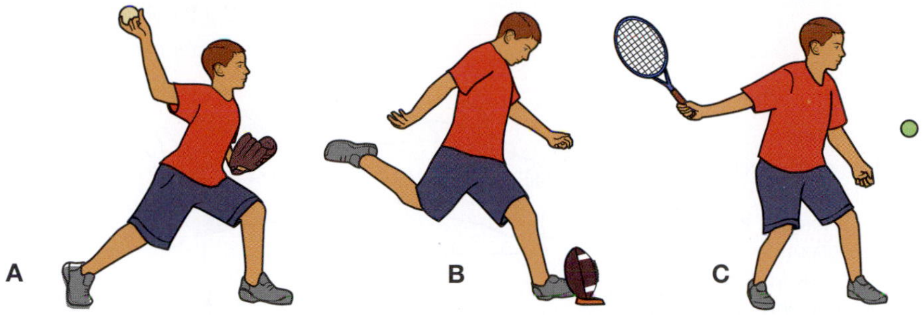

Figure 2.35 Increased speed of motion with increased angular velocity in the extremities with and without implements. A) Throwing a ball uses the summation of forces from the trunk and upper extremity to increase angular velocity of the ball. B) Kicking a ball, utilizing the combined forces from the trunk and lower extremity, increases angular velocity of the football. C) A racquet in the hand with elbow near extension adds even more angular velocity to the ball when it is hit by the racquet.

When we draw a free body diagram, we first identify the body segment studied. Let us take a simplified example first. Figure 2.36 shows a lower extremity. We then identify the forces acting on the segment. In this example, there are internal and external forces. The internal forces are the muscle forces acting on the segment. In this case, it is the hip flexors. The external forces are those forces acting against the muscles. In Figure 2.36, the external forces include the weight of the limb (gravity) and the cuff weight around the ankle. Since the limb is not moving, the forces are static. This means that the internal and external forces are in equilibrium. Without movement, the forces are equal to each other in order for the extremity to be held in its position off the table. In other words, the muscle force required to hold the leg off the table is equal to the total of the gravitational pull on the limb (limb weight) and the cuff weight. In this example, gravity is pulling clockwise and the hip flexor muscles are pulling counterclockwise on the hip. As you recall, torque is the product of the mass and its distance from the axis of movement, so the formula must include the amount of the force and the distance the center of mass is from the axis. The distance between the point where a force is applied and the axis of motion is a moment arm. An **internal moment arm** is the perpendicular distance from the joint's axis to the muscle. Similarly, an **external moment arm** is the perpendicular distance from the joint's axis to the external force or the segment's center of gravity. External forces include the weight of the segment and any other forces working against the muscle. Since no movement is occurring in Figure 2.36, all of the torques together equal zero. The upward torque of the muscles must equal the total downward pull of gravity on the weight of the leg and the cuff weight. Since we know that the weight of the leg of a 150-lb person is about 25 lb (see Table 2–4) and the distances for the COM are provided, we can determine the amount of torque required by the hip flexors to maintain the leg off the table with a 5-lb weight attached at the ankle.

Now, see if you can determine the muscle force required in Figure 2.37. In this figure, determine what the forces acting on the forearm are with a dumbbell weight in the hand. The vectors are labeled with force units if known. Although the problem is solved for you in the figure, try to solve it yourself before looking at the answer.

Calculation of Muscle and Joint Forces

Force is unidirectional and torque is bidirectional. As we have mentioned, force is expressed in pounds or kilograms. Torque, on the other hand, is expressed as foot-pounds or meter-kilograms. Force and torque impact both muscles and joints. This section takes a look at both.

Muscles

As mentioned, the torque applied to a body segment includes internal and external torques. The internal torque is the sum of all the torques provided by muscles acting on the segment. The external torque is the sum of all the external resistance acting on the segment. Since torque is a product of the moment arm and the mass, we must have some information before we can determine all of the internal and external torques. We can orient the forces according to x- and y-axes. In a free body diagram, the x-axis is in line with the length of the segment, and the y-axis is perpendicular to that body segment. When the segment is in a static position, all the forces and torques are equal and counterbalance each other. In computational language, since $\Sigma F_x = 0$ and $\Sigma F_y = 0$, therefore $\Sigma T = 0$. In these formulas, $\Sigma(F_x$ is the sum of all the forces acting on the x-axis, ΣF_y is the sum of all the forces acting on the y-axis, and ΣT is the sum of all of the torques acting on the segment.

All the forces in a static segment add up to zero because there is no motion. If the segment moves, then one force must be greater than another to produce movement. Since the segment is in a static position, all

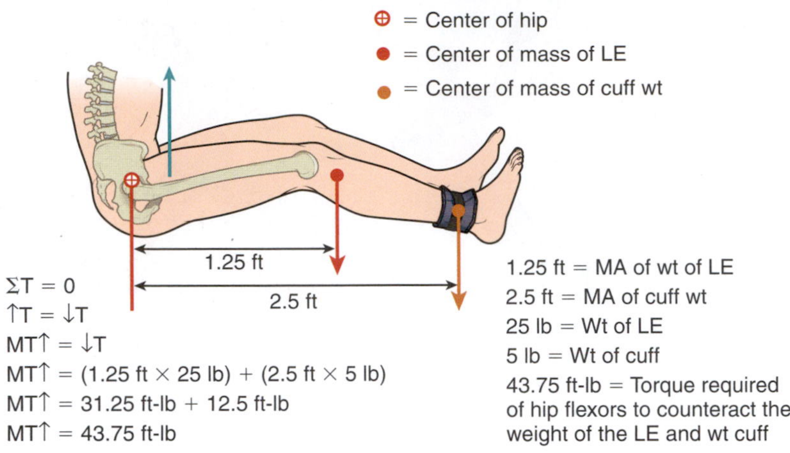

Figure 2.36 Clinical application of vector forces working against each other. Placing a weight on the end of an extremity increases the vector force of the resistance considerably. If a patient is unable to lift the extremity with the added weight, shortening the resistance arm by placing the weight closer to the axis of motion may allow the patient to lift the resistance successfully. LE = Lower extremity; MA = moment arm; MT = muscle torque; T = torque; Wt = weight.

TABLE 2–4 | AVERAGE WEIGHT OF BODY SEGMENTS AND ANATOMIC LOCATION OF CENTER OF GRAVITY OF INDIVIDUAL BODY SEGMENTS OF A MAN WEIGHING 150 LB

Segment Weights and Percentage of Total Body Weight	Approximate Anatomic Location of Centers of Gravity
***Head:* 10.3 lb (6.9%)**	*Head.* In sphenoid sinus, 4 mm beyond anterior inferior margin of sella. (On lateral surface, over temporal fossa on or near nasion-inion line.)
***Head and neck:* 11.8 lb (7.9%)**	*Head and neck.* On inferior surface of basioccipital bone or within bone 23 ± 5 mm from crest of dorsum sellae. (On lateral surface, 10 mm anterior to supratragal notch above head of mandible.)
***Head, neck, and trunk:* 88.5 lb (59.0%)**	*Head, neck, and trunk.* Anterior to 11th thoracic vertebra.
UPPER LIMB	**(Just above elbow joint)**
Arm: 4.1 lb (2.7%)	*Arm.* In medial head of triceps, adjacent to radial groove; 5 mm proximal to distal end of deltoid insertion.
Forearm: 2.4 lb (1.6%)	*Forearm.* 11 mm proximal to most distal part of pronator teres insertion; 9 mm anterior to interosseus membrane.
Hand: 0.9 lb (0.6%)	*Hand (in rest position).* On axis of metacarpal III, usually 2 mm deep to volar skin surface. 2 mm proximal to proximal transverse palmar skin crease, in angle between proximal transverse and radial longitudinal crease.
Upper limb: 7.3 lb (4.9%) *Forearm and hand:* 3.3 lb (2.2%)	
Lower Limb	**(Just above knee joint)**
Thigh: 14.5 lb (9.7%)	*Thigh.* In adductor brevis muscle (or magnus or vastus medialis), 13 mm medial to linea aspera, deep to adductor canal, 29 mm below apex of femoral triangle, and 18 mm proximal to most distal fibers of adductor brevis.
Leg: 6.8 lb (4.5%)	*Leg.* 35 mm below popliteus, at posterior part of posterior tibialis; 16 mm above proximal end of Achilles tendon; 8 mm posterior to interosseus membrane.
Foot: 2.1 lb (1.4%)	*Foot.* In plantar ligaments, or just superficial in adjacent deep foot muscles; below proximal halves of second and third cuneiform bones. On a line between ankle joint center and ball of foot in plane of metatarsal II.
Lower limb: 23.4 lb. (15.6%) *Leg and foot:* 9.0 lb. (6.0%)	
Entire Body	**(Anterior to second sacral vertebra)**

SOURCE: Williams M, and Lissner HR. *Biomechanics of Human Motion.* Philadelphia: WB Saunders, 1962, p 15 (with permission).

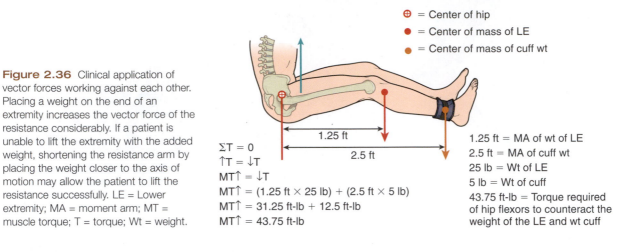

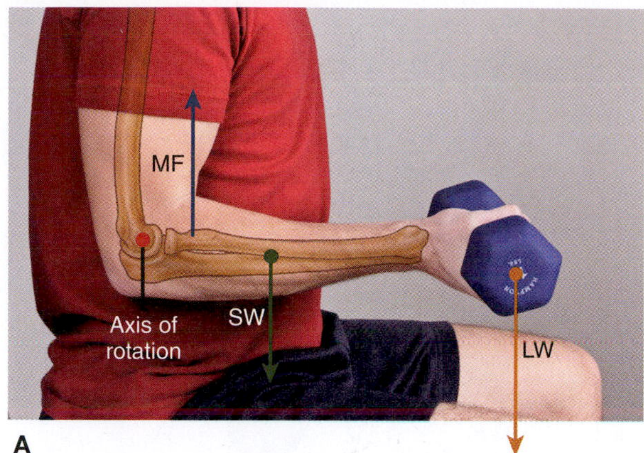

A

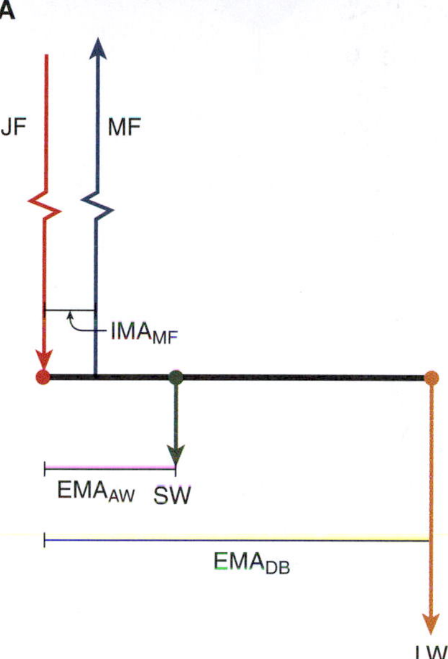

MF = Muscle force = unknown
AW = Arm weight force = 7.4 lb
DB = Dumbbell force = 5 lb
IMA_{MF} = Internal moment arm of muscle force (0.33 ft)
EMA_{AW} = External moment arm of arm weight (0.83 ft)
EMA_{DB} = External moment arm of dumbbell weight (1.67 ft)

Solution:

$\Sigma F = 0$

Internal torque = external torque

$MF \times IMA_{MF} = (AW \times EMA_{AW}) + (DB \times EMA_{DB})$

$MF(0.33\text{ ft}) = (7.4\text{ lb} \times 0.83\text{ ft}) + (5\text{ lb} \times 1.67\text{ ft})$

$MF(0.33\text{ ft}) = 6.14\text{ ft-lb} + 8.35\text{ ft-lb}$

$MF = \dfrac{14.49\text{ ft-lb}}{0.33\text{ ft}}$

$MF = 43.90\text{ lb}$

B

Figure 2.37 Computation of forces using a free body diagram. A) Holding the elbow flexed with a weight in the hand creates resistance forces, pulling the arm and weight down against an equal muscle force maintaining the elbow position. B) To calculate these forces, it is often easier with the aid of a body diagram with the specific values included in the diagram.

the forces, and hence, all the torques, are balanced; the positive forces equal the negative forces, and the internal torques equal the external torques.

The internal and external moment arms may change length as the joint moves through its range of motion. The long axis of the segment arm is the x-axis and the perpendicular distance to the moment arm is the y-axis. If we know the angle of pull of either the muscle or the resistance arm, we can determine their resultant torques (muscle or resistance torque) by using the known vectors and the sine, cosine, or tangent rules of a right triangle. Let's use Figure 2.38 to see how these formulas work for us. Once we draw a free body diagram as in Figure 2.38B and identify the x-axis and y-axis, we can see each of the forces acting on the body segment. In this example, the deltoid is the internal (muscle) force providing a torque that is equal to the combination of the weight of the arm and the dumbbell. In a 150-lb person, the entire arm and hand weigh 7.4 lb (3.4 kg). We know that the dumbbell in this example weighs 5 lb (2.25 kg). We also know that the COM of the upper extremity is just proximal to the elbow joint, 0.83 ft (0.25 m) from the shoulder joint axis. The COM of the dumbbell is in the palm, 1.67 ft (0.508m) from the shoulder joint axis. The insertion point of the deltoid muscle is on the deltoid tuberosity of the humerus, 0.33 ft (0.102 m) from the shoulder joint axis. According to the diagram, the angle between the downward force of gravity on the arm and on the dumbbell and the long axis of the arm is 45°. We can now plug these numbers into the formula for static torque:

$\Sigma T = 0$; therefore, internal torque = external torque

so

$$MF_R \times IMA_{MF} = (AW_R \times EMA_{AW}) + (DB_R \times EMA_{DB})$$

Plugging in the numbers, we get

$$MF_R = \frac{[(\cos 45^\circ \times 7.4\text{ lb}) \times (0.83\text{ ft})] + [(\cos 45^\circ \times 5\text{ lb}) \times (1.67\text{ ft})]}{0.33\text{ ft}}$$

($\cos 45^\circ = .707$)

Plugging in the cos 45° allows us to solve the equation:

$$MF_R = \frac{(5.23\text{ lb} \times 0.83\text{ ft}) + (3.54\text{ lb} \times 1.67\text{ lb})}{0.33\text{ ft}}$$

MF_R = Rotational torque of the muscle
IMA_{MF} = Internal moment arm of the muscle force
AW_R = Rotational torque of the forearm weight
EMA_{AW} = External moment arm of the forearm weight
DB_R = Rotational torque of the dumbbell
EMA_{DB} = External moment arm of the dumbbell

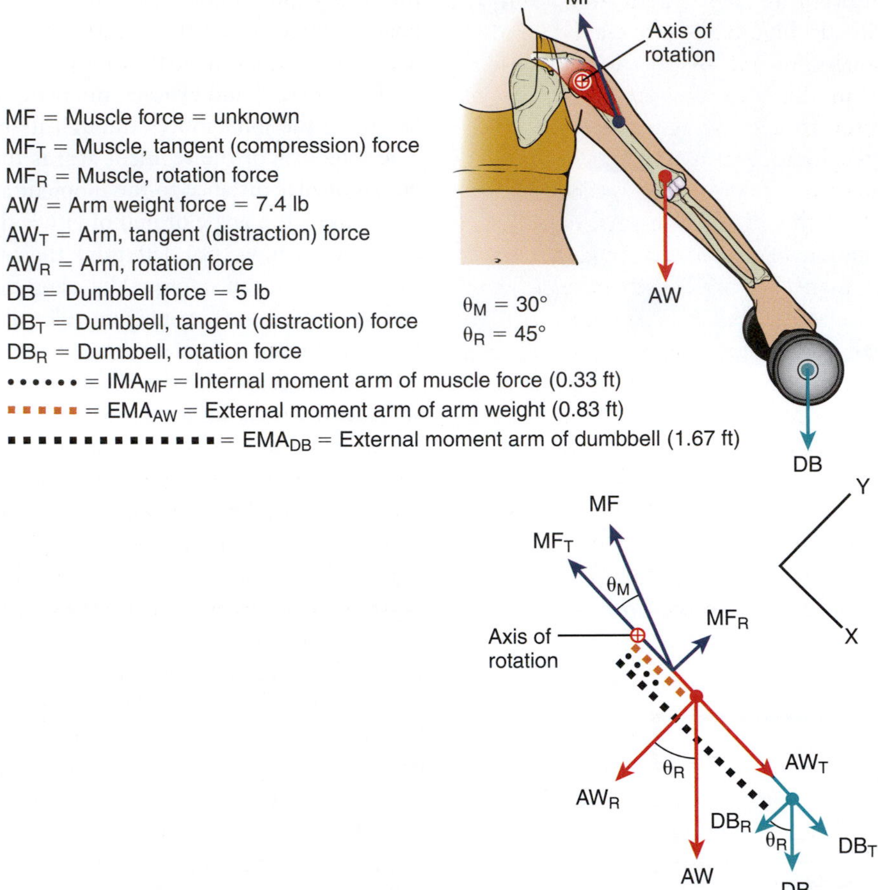

Figure 2.38 Computation of force components using a free body diagram. Additional calculations are required when the angles created by the forces are not parallel or perpendicular, as often occurs in the human body.

The rotational torque of the muscle to hold the segment in its current position is:

$$MF_R = 31.06 \text{ lb}$$

Now that we know the rotational torque of the deltoid muscle, we can calculate the other forces of the deltoid muscle.

The deltoid's resultant vector force is:

$$MF = \frac{MF_R}{\sin 30^\circ} \rightarrow MF = \frac{31.06 \text{ lb}}{.500} \rightarrow MF = 62.12 \text{ lb}$$

The deltoid's tangential vector force (in this case, the compressive force toward the joint) is:

$$MF_T = \frac{MF}{\cos 30^\circ} \rightarrow MF_T = \frac{62.12 \text{ lb}}{.866} \rightarrow MF_T = 71.73 \text{ lb}$$

If we convert the measurements to IU (1 lb = 4.448 N), the torques produced by the deltoid are 319.06 N in MF_T (compressive), 276.31 N in MF (resultant), and 138.15 N in MF_R (rotational) forces when the arm is at 45° of abduction and lifting a 5-lb weight.

Based on the computations we just performed, you can once again see that the force required of the muscles is greater than the external forces. As previously mentioned, this is the case in most body segments because the muscles moving against those external forces usually lie closer to the joint than the point where the external forces are applied. This arrangement makes the muscle moment arms shorter than the external force arms; muscle output must be greater than the external forces to make up for these differences.

As can be seen from the images in Figure 2.39, when a joint changes position, the angles of pull of both internal and external forces also change. Not only do the angles of pull change, but changes in vector force production occur as the segment moves through its range of motion. In Figure 2.39, we see the rotational vector component of the biceps changing as the elbow is placed in different positions. Likewise, its compression vector forces also change. As has been mentioned, the resultant force is made up of a combination of two forces, one that provides rotation and the other that provides either distraction or compression to the joint. The closer to perpendicular the resultant force is to the segment, the more of its force is directed toward rotation. When the resultant force is at 90° to the segment, all of its force only rotates the segment and none of its force distracts or compresses the joint. Since computation of forces is made with static conditions, these concepts of changing vector and resultant forces apply to both internal and external forces.

Joints

Although we cannot accurately measure forces directly applied to joint surfaces, it is important to at least estimate this information so clinicians may reduce stresses to injured or damaged joints. Joints encounter forces applied to them because of muscle contractions, gravity, external resistance, and friction. Understanding the causes and the results of these joint forces forms a major basis for the rationale of therapeutic exercise and rehabilitation. The primary forces applied to the joints may produce joint distraction, as when holding a suitcase in the hand (Fig. 2.40A), applying traction, or placing exercise weights on a dependent extremity (Fig. 2.40B). In distraction cases, ligaments and joint capsules experience tension placed on them. Most activities, however, produce compression of joint surfaces. Compression is readily appreciated in weight-bearing joints in sitting, standing, or walking (Fig. 2.40C). What healthy individuals do not always appreciate is the magnitude of joint compression forces that occur with these activities, as well as those forces that occur with active muscle contraction and functional activities. The joint force (J) is the **joint reaction force** of the

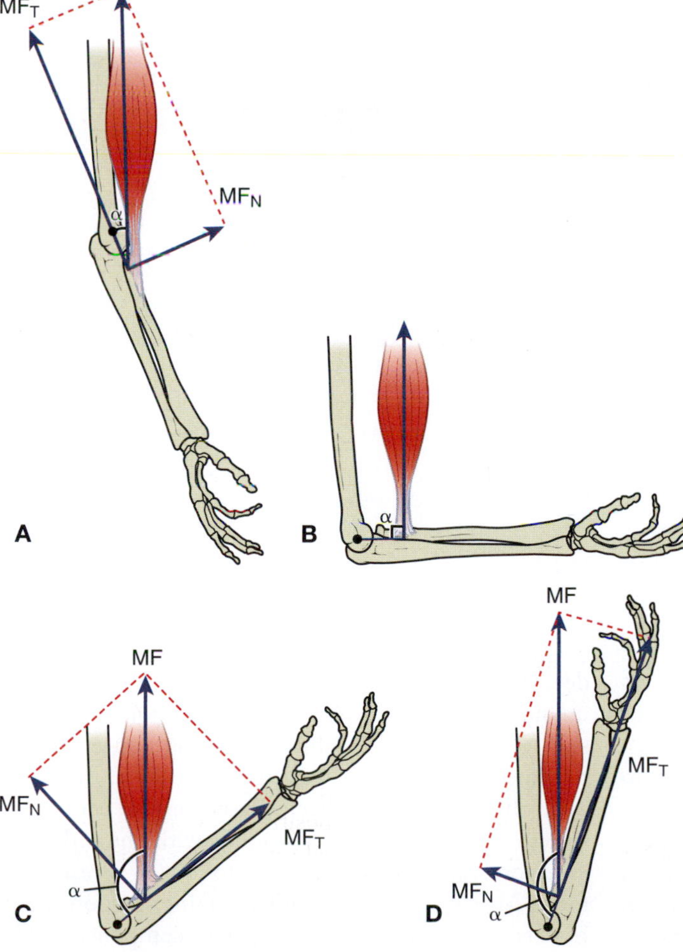

Figure 2.39 Muscle vectors and moment arms change with changes in joint positions. These images demonstrate that moment arm lengths change as the joint moves through its range of motion, resulting in changes in muscle force requirements throughout the motion.

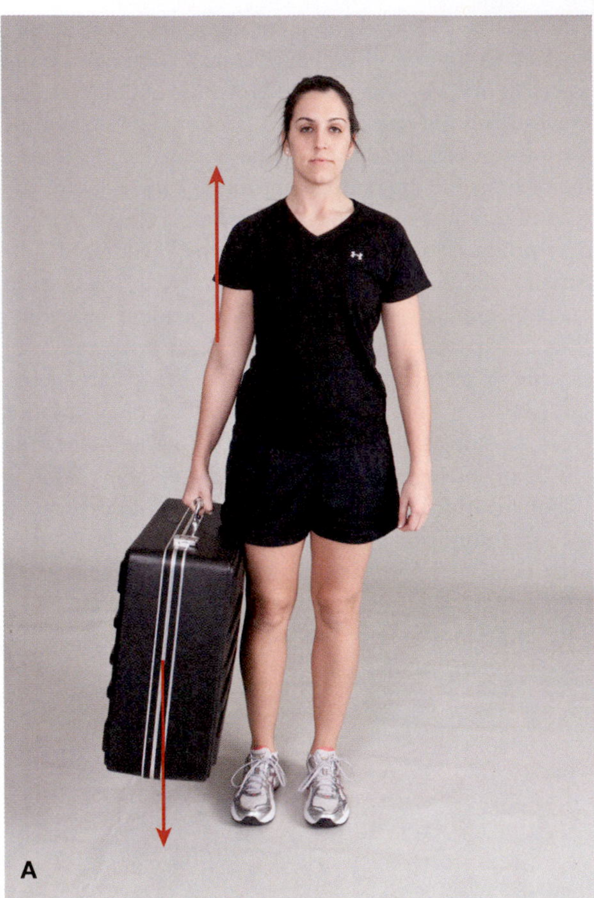

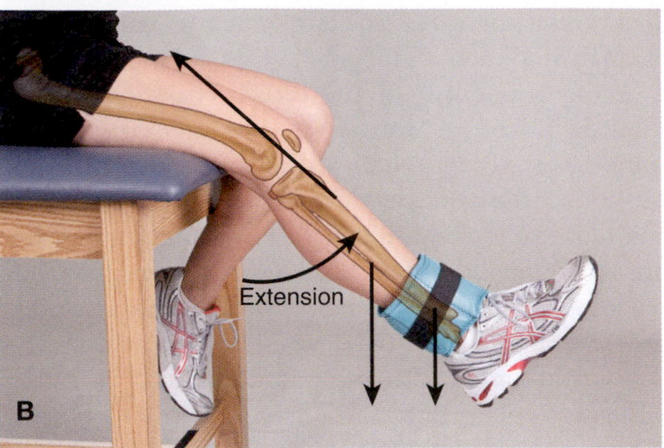

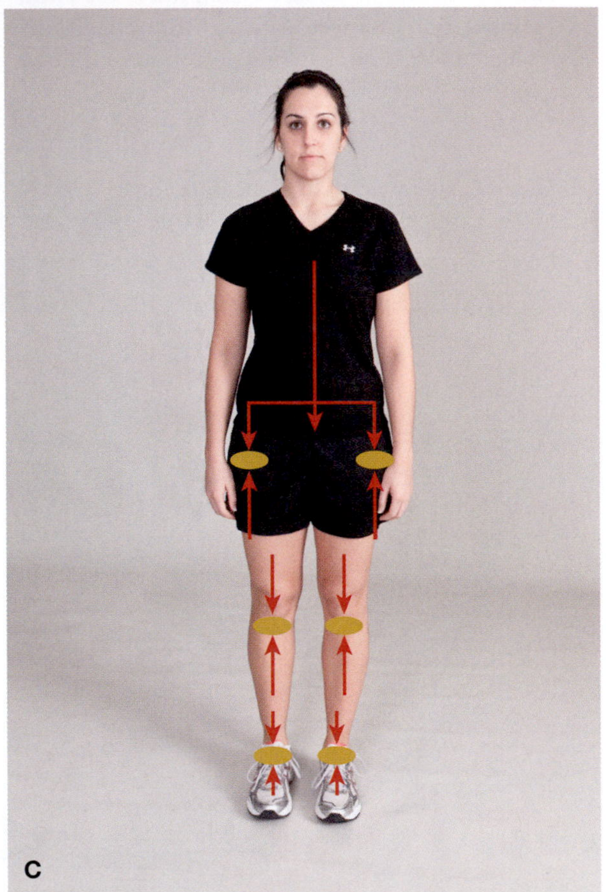

Figure 2.40 Traction and compression forces occur at joints producing stress to joints and their support structures. External and internal forces applied to joints sometimes produce traction to the joint and other times compression of the joint results.

mating joint surfaces. In joint pathologies such as arthritis, function is lost because such large compressive forces cause excruciating pain.

You may not realize it, but we already know how to calculate these joint reaction forces. This information can be obtained using the equilibrium formulas ($\Sigma F = 0$ and $\Sigma t = 0$), composition and resolution of forces, and the trigonometric ratios of the right triangle. An example of this process is seen in Figure 2.41, which demonstrates how to find the magnitude of the unknown quadriceps muscle and knee joint compression forces when the subject is sitting and extending the knee with a 30-lb weight on the foot. In Figure 2.41, this example has been placed on the coordinate system with the origin coinciding with the unknown joint force, and each of the three forces (W = resistance force, M = muscle force, and J = joint reaction force) has been resolved into perpendicular components. The

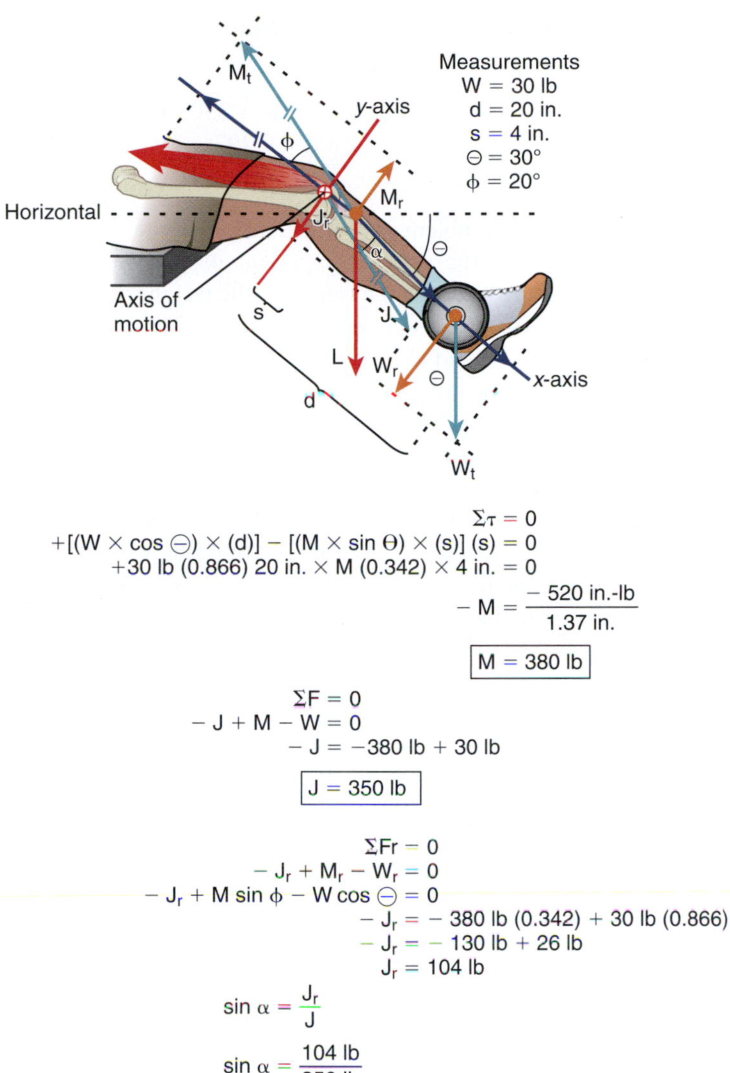

$$\Sigma\tau = 0$$
$$+[(W \times \cos \ominus) \times (d)] - [(M \times \sin \Theta) \times (s)]\ (s) = 0$$
$$+30 \text{ lb } (0.866)\ 20 \text{ in.} \times M\ (0.342) \times 4 \text{ in.} = 0$$
$$-M = \frac{-520 \text{ in.-lb}}{1.37 \text{ in.}}$$
$$\boxed{M = 380 \text{ lb}}$$

$$\Sigma F = 0$$
$$-J + M - W = 0$$
$$-J = -380 \text{ lb} + 30 \text{ lb}$$
$$\boxed{J = 350 \text{ lb}}$$

$$\Sigma Fr = 0$$
$$-J_r + M_r - W_r = 0$$
$$-J_r + M \sin \phi - W \cos \ominus = 0$$
$$-J_r = -380 \text{ lb } (0.342) + 30 \text{ lb } (0.866)$$
$$-J_r = -130 \text{ lb} + 26 \text{ lb}$$
$$J_r = 104 \text{ lb}$$
$$\sin \alpha = \frac{J_r}{J}$$
$$\sin \alpha = \frac{104 \text{ lb}}{350 \text{ lb}}$$
$$\sin \alpha = 0.297$$
$$\boxed{\alpha = 17°}$$

Figure 2.41 Free body diagram used to calculate joint reaction force. Once the internal and external forces are determined, the joint reaction forces may be calculated. Although not often specifically determined in the clinic, knowing what positions relieve joint compression forces are helpful when clinicians advise patients on activities to reduce joint forces.

diagram is labeled and the measured weight, angles, and distances are indicated. The approximate magnitudes of the muscle force (M = 380 lb) and joint force (J = 350 lb), as well as the direction of the joint force (α = 17°), are found using the equilibrium formulas and trigonometric ratios we have already seen. The following equations are arranged to show a step-by-step solution to the same problem. They illustrate the details of the relationships and provide solutions or explanations to parts of the problem, such as the rotary force of the weight, the torque of the resistance, or the muscle force.

The rotary component (W_r) of the 30-lb weight must be found first, so we use the formula for resolution of forces:

$$W_r = W \times \cos 30°$$
$$W_r = 30 \text{ lb} \times 0.866$$
$$W_r = 26 \text{ lb}$$

To find the torque produced by the weight (τ_w), we use the formula for torque:

$$\tau_w = W_r \times d$$
$$\tau_w = 26 \text{ lb} \times 20 \text{ in.}$$
$$\tau_w = 520 \text{ in.-lb}$$

To find the torque that the muscle must produce (τ_m) we use the equilibrium formula:

$$\Sigma\tau = 0\tau_w - \tau_m = 0$$
$$\tau_m = \tau_w$$
$$\tau_m = 520 \text{ in.-lb}$$

Before we can find the force in the muscle (M), we must know the rotary component M_r. We use the formula for torque to find the magnitude of the rotary component of the muscle (M_r):

$$\tau_m = M_r \times s$$
or
$$\tau_m \div s = M_r$$
$$M_r = 520 \text{ in.-lb} \div 4 \text{ in.}$$
$$M_r = 130 \text{ lb}$$

Once we have M_r, we can find the muscle force (M), using trigonometric ratio formulas of a right triangle. We know from sine tables that the sine of a 20° angle is 0.342:

$$\sin 20^\circ = M_r \div M$$
$$M = M_r \div \sin 20^\circ$$
$$M = 130 \text{ lb} \div 0.342$$
$$M = 380 \text{ lb}$$

To find the approximate magnitude of the joint reaction force (J), we can use the equilibrium formula and plug in the numbers we now have:

$$\Sigma F = 0$$
$$-J - M + W = 0$$
$$-J = -380 \text{ lb} + 30 \text{ lb}$$
$$J = 350 \text{ lb}$$

To find the angle of application for J, we must find one of the components of J. If, at equilibrium, the sum of the forces is zero, then the sum of the rectangular components must also be zero:

$$\Sigma F_y = 0$$
$$-J_r - M_r + W_r = 0$$

To find the magnitude of J, we can use the equilibrium formula:

$$-J_r = -M_r + W_r$$
$$-J_r = -130 \text{ lb} + 26 \text{ lb}$$

$$\Sigma F_x = 0 \text{ or } \Sigma F_y = 0.$$
$$J_r = 104 \text{ lb}$$

To find the angle of the joint force, we use the trigonometric formula for sine:

$$\sin\alpha = J_r \div J$$

We then look in the table of sines and cosines to find the degree of the angle:

$$\sin\alpha = 104 \text{ lb} \div 350 \text{ lb}$$
$$\sin\alpha = 0.297$$
$$\alpha = 17^\circ$$

If this problem were calculated with the knee in full extension, the rotary component of the weight (W_r) would be larger, so the torque of the weight (τ_w) and the muscle's torque (τ_m), the muscle force (M), and the joint force (J) would also increase. On the other hand, if the angle of the knee joint were increased to 60°, the values of W_r, τ_w, τ_m, M, and J would all be less.

Note that to make these calculations the first time around a little easier, the weight of the leg and foot was omitted in this problem. Now that you are more familiar with the process, we can add this factor into the calculations to obtain a more accurate answer of the total estimated force required of the leg to lift the weight cuff and the leg and the subsequent force applied to the hip joint. The weight of the leg and foot (w) is approximately 9 lb acting at its center of gravity, which is 8 inches from the origin of the coordinate system in a vertical direction. When this force is added, the corrected equilibrium equations still have the total torques at zero, so, as you would expect, the muscle force requirement is greater and the forces acting on the joint are also greater. The following calculations demonstrate how this occurs:

A. Solving first for M: $\Sigma\tau = 0$

$$[(30 \text{ lb} \times 0.866) \times 20 \text{ in}] + [(9 \text{ lb} \times 0.866) \times 8 \text{ in} -$$
$$[(M \times 0.342) \times 4 \text{ in}] = 0$$
$$M = 425 \text{ lb}$$

B. Then, finding J: $\Sigma F = 0$

$$-J - 425 \text{ lb} + 30 \text{ lb} - 9 \text{ lb} = 0$$
$$J = 386 \text{ lb}$$

The vector equation $\Sigma F = 0$ has been used to simplify equations for finding the joint forces (J). However, using this formula introduces a 2% error into this problem. Since this is a clinical kinesiology text, we feel it is more important to realize that forces applied by the muscles against relatively mild resistance impart high loads to joints than to identify precise calculations.

However, for those who desire to identify the exact calculations, we will not keep you in suspense. Finding the precise joint compression forces requires finding both of the components of J, then solving using the Pythagorean Theorem: $J = \sqrt{Jx^2 + Jy^2}$. Completing this calculation, J is 357 lb when the weight of the leg is neglected and 396 lb when the weight of the leg is included. For examples of calculations in other activities, positions, and joint areas and for calculation of forces in dynamics, refer to LeVeau[8] and Soderberg.[9]

Applying Resistances to the Body

Now that you have an idea of how forces act on the body and its segments, you can quickly realize why this information is important to appreciate. Clinically, the external resistances encountered by the body include the forces produced by casts, braces (orthoses), book bags, plates of food, pulleys, dumbbells, crutches, doors, exercise equipment, or manual resistance by a clinician. Although these forces may be small, they are usually applied on the distal portion of the extremity and, therefore, exert relatively large torques that the muscles must match during an isometric activity and overcome if motion is to occur. The clinician who has knowledge of these forces will be able to manipulate and adapt them for optimal results in a patient's rehabilitation program. For example, if the objective is to give resistive exercise to a particular muscle, a resistive torque should be selected that most nearly matches the torque that the muscle is capable of developing. However, if the objective is to assist functional use of a very weak muscle, the resistance torque should be made as small as possible.

Since gravity affects all objects, we must be aware of its effects on patient positioning and application of outside forces on injured segments. Items such as dumbbells or books behave in the same manner as weights of body segments because gravity always pulls downward in a vertical direction on all objects. The maximum resistance torque of an extremity's weight occurs when the extremity or segment is horizontal. In this position, the perpendicular distance from the action line of the force of gravity to the axis of motion is the longest (see Fig. 2.39). At all other points in the range of motion, the resistance torque is less.

Weights applied to the extremities frequently exert traction on joint structures, which may or may not be desirable. If we recall the composition of forces, we know that when a force is directed parallel to gravity, or directly downward, all of the force will be a distraction force on the joint. Thus, with the elbow in Figure 2.39 in extension with the patient standing, the weight of the arm acts entirely as a distracting force and does not have a rotary component. Codman's pendulum exercises are used early in shoulder rehabilitation to improve shoulder motion and are based on this effect.[10] To perform Codman's, the patient bends over, flexing at the hips and supporting himself with the opposite forearm on a table top. This position places the shoulder in a position of flexion. The extremity is passively swung as a pendulum using weight transfer from left to right lower extremities so that the hand describes larger and larger circles within the pain-free range. The distracting component of the arm's weight promotes the downward movement of the head of the humerus on the glenoid fossa so that shoulder flexion and abduction may occur; joint distraction with this passive motion also enhances synovial circulation within the joint. A cuff weight may be attached to the patient's wrist to provide additional traction force.

In some pathologic conditions, the effect of the distracting component of a weight is unwanted because it may cause pain and further stress or damage to joint structures. For example, in an anterior cruciate ligament sprain of the knee, weights attached to the foot for the purpose of strengthening the quadriceps muscles are contraindicated, especially in the early aspects of the rehabilitation program. In such cases, alternative methods of strengthening must be used that do not stress the joint or ligament.

On the other hand, joint compression may also be either advantageous or contraindicated. Patients whose joint proprioception has been diminished because of

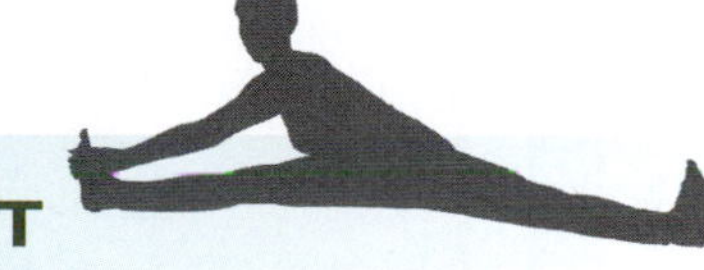

PRACTICE POINT

Knowing that the maximum resistance torque of gravity changes throughout a joint's range of motion can be an important realization in a patient's rehabilitation. For example, if we have a patient lift a dumbbell in shoulder flexion, we must first decide where in the range of motion we want maximum resistance to occur before we can position him for the exercise. If we want gravity's maximum effect occurring at the start of the motion, the patient is positioned supine. However, if we want the maximum resistance at the end of the motion, we will position him in prone. On the other hand, if we want maximum effects of gravity to be at midrange, we position the patient either standing or sitting.

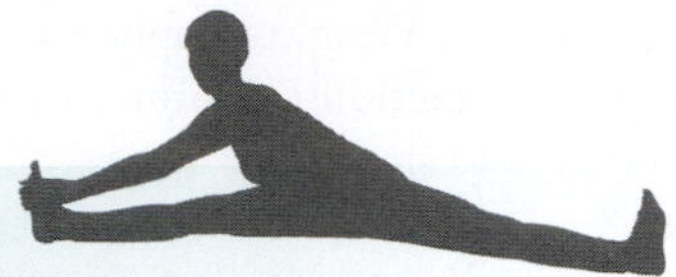

PRACTICE POINT

Mild joint distraction that does not disrupt or stress joint structures may actually assist in pain relief of ligamentous injuries. Grades I and II joint mobilizations provide mild distraction within a nonstressful range that does not stretch a joint's soft tissue structures but stimulate the cutaneous receptors to relieve pain.[11]

either joint injury or intra-articular swelling may be at risk for recurring injury if proprioception is not restored. Weight-bearing activities are among the exercises that are used to regain joint proprioception. Such activity has been demonstrated to facilitate these receptors.[12] Joint compressive activities for the shoulder could include weight-bearing activities such as push-ups or nonweight-bearing activities such as side-lying shoulder abduction exercises to 45°.

Clinical Application of Concepts

Many externally applied forces, which may occur with manual resistance, exercise pulleys, crutch-walking, propelling a wheelchair, or opening a door, do not act in a vertical direction as do weights attached to the body. Instead, the forces exert effects that vary according to angle at which they are applied. Like other forces, these forces will also have either a distracting or stabilizing component in addition to their rotational component. In pulley systems, the angle of application changes as the body part moves through its range of motion (Fig. 2.42). Each change in the angle (or direction) of the force causes a change in the magnitude of the rotary component of that force. In essence, the resistance torque will vary at different points of the range of motion. It is important to remember that a torque's greatest magnitude occurs when their direction of application is at a right angle or 90° to the segment or extremity.

Pulleys

Pulleys are used in both strength exercises and traction of body segments to change the direction of a force; these pulleys are single fixed pulleys. A pulley can also be used to increase or decrease the magnitude of a force; these pulleys are moveable pulley systems and are sometimes referred to as block-and-tackle systems.

Single Fixed Pulley

The line of action of a force may be changed by means of a pulley (Fig. 2.43). A force (F), acting in a downward direction, is used to move a weight in an upward direction. When pulleys are fixed, they do not provide any mechanical advantage to the force but only change its direction. This principle is illustrated by the cervical traction example (see Fig. 2.7). A single fixed pulley is often used in strengthening exercises as seen in Figure 2.43B.

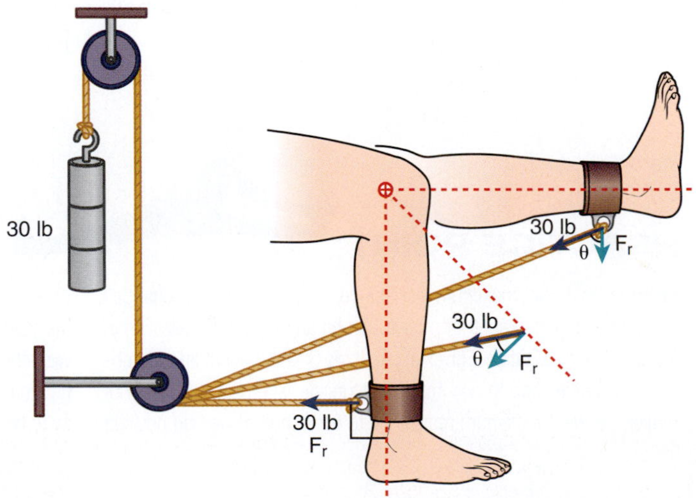

Figure 2.42 A pulley provides various resistance forces within a joint's range of motion. The greatest resistance occurs when the line of the pull of the pulley system forms a 90° angle with the body segment when the entire force is applied as a rotary component.

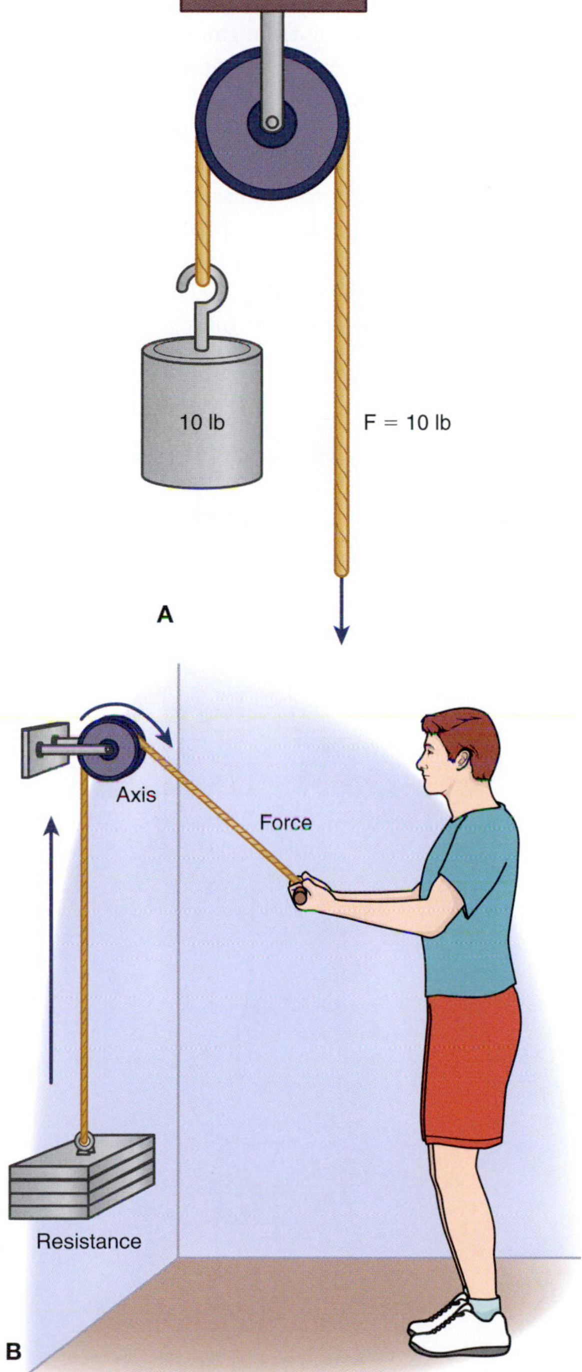

Figure 2.43 A fixed pulley system changes direction of a force's pull without providing any mechanical advantage. This may be useful clinically when it is desirable to create more or less force as a specific range of motion.

Movable Pulley

If a weight is attached to a movable pulley (Fig. 2.44A), half of the weight is supported by the rope attached to the stationary hook and half by the rope on the other side of the pulley. Therefore, the mechanical advantage of the force (F) is 2. The rope, however, must be moved twice the distance that the weight is raised, and what is gained in force is lost in distance. The leg traction systems in Figure 2.44B is an example of how a moveable

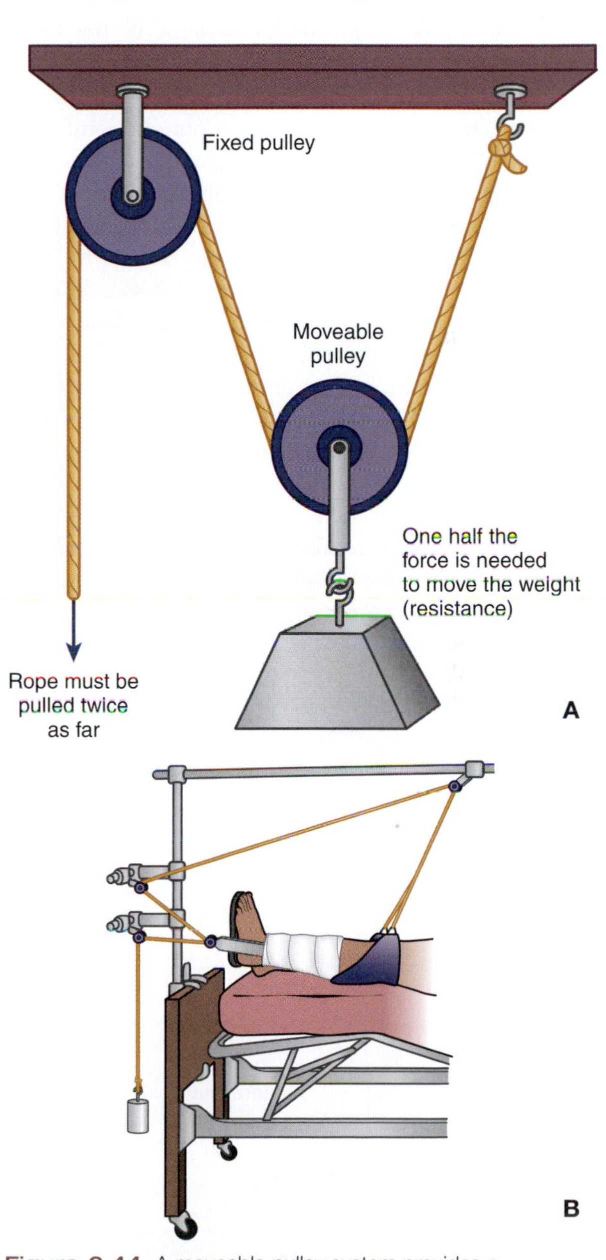

Figure 2.44 A moveable pulley system provides a mechanical advantage to either increase or decrease forces. **A)** A moveable pulley will make it easier to lift a heavy object. **B)** A moveable pulley is used to increase joint distraction without requiring a heavy load to be effective.

pulley is used to reduce weights and still provide adequate force. The pulley at the foot is "movable," and the pulleys on the bedpost are fixed. Since the pulley at the foot receives the force from two parts of the rope, this pulley in turn exerts greater than 15 lb of traction on the leg. In the exercise system in Figure 2.43B, the pulley is fixed, so it only changes the direction of the force and not the magnitude.

Anatomic Pulleys

There are several single pulley systems in the body. These single pulley systems may change the course of a tendon or improve a muscle's mechanical advantage by increasing its force arm distance from the joint. The medial malleolus at the ankle changes the angle of pull of the long toe flexor tendons and tibialis posterior tendon. The peroneal tubercle on the lateral calcaneous and the lateral malleolus provide the same task for the peroneus longus and brevis tendons (Fig. 2.45). Another pulley system involving the tendons of the long finger flexors is found on the palmar side of the phalanges. When the flexor digitorum profundus and superficialis contract, their tendons rise from the joint axes. The tendons are held down by seven pulley-like loops that also cause deflection of the tendons with movement. Although angles of muscle pulls may change because of their pulley mechanism, the force vector of the muscle remains straight. The muscle's line of action is usually from the immediate point of attachment of the muscle to the bone and extends into space according to the magnitude of the force. The vector is straight and does not follow the anatomic directions of the entire muscle.

An example of anatomic pulleys that improve muscle torque is the patella (Fig. 2.46). The quadriceps torque increases significantly because the patella moves the muscle's tendon away from the knee joint, thereby increasing the quadriceps' moment arm length.[13] The quadriceps and patellar tendons not only improve the torque production of the quadriceps, but they also change the tendon's direction of pull as the knee flexes. Other pulleys that improve muscle force include the calcaneus, femoral neck and phalangeal condyles. The calcaneus provides a 2-inch lever arm distance for the gastroc-soleus muscles (Fig. 2.47). The neck of the femur places the hip abductor muscles several inches

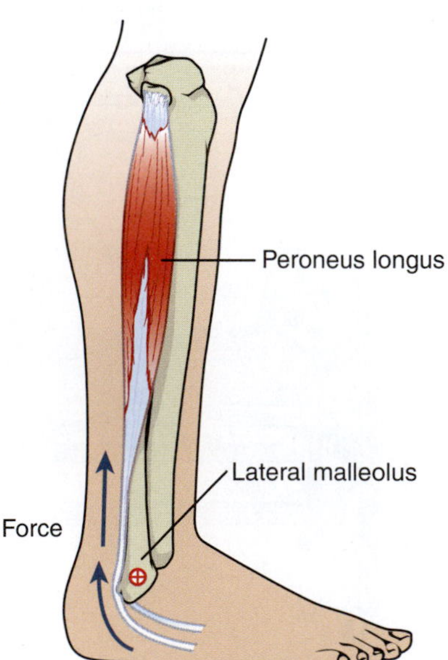

Figure 2.45 The body has several pulleys to change directions of pull of muscles throughout the body. An example is the lateral malleolus and peroneal tubercle, which provide a change of pull of the peroneal tendons at the ankle.

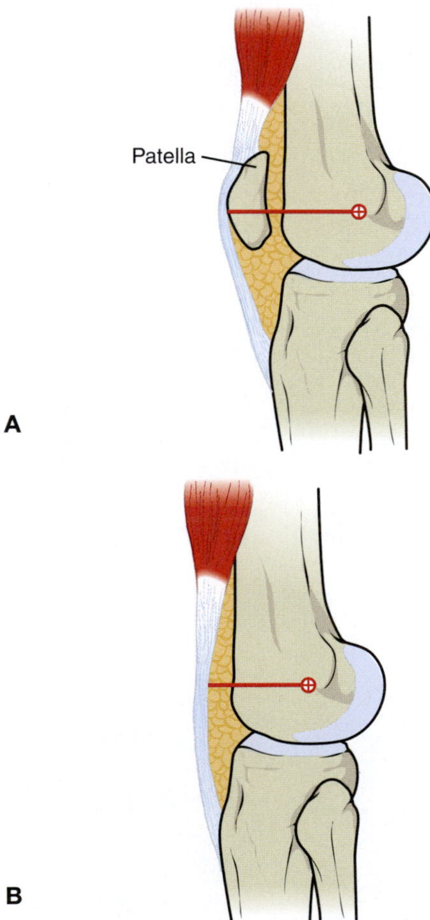

Figure 2.46 Anatomic pulleys change a muscle's angle of pull and improve torque production of muscles. **A)** The patella moves the quadriceps away from the center of motion to improve the quadriceps's torque and change the angle of the muscle's pull. **B)** Without a patella, the quadriceps is not able to provide as much torque since it lies closer to the center of motion.

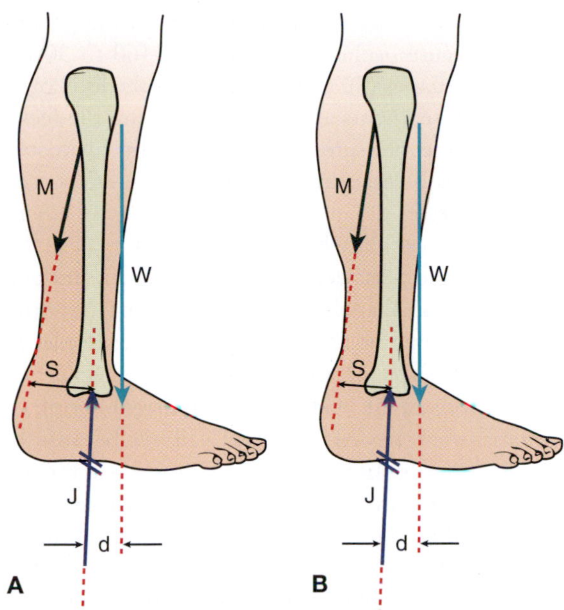

Figure 2.47 The calcaneus changes the angle of pull of the Achilles and increases its torque by moving the tendon away from the center of motion. **A)** A normal calcaneus. **B)** A short calcaneus reduces the moment arm of the Achilles tendon.

away from the hip joint. The condyles of the phalanges increase the force arm distances of the finger flexors. Small changes in these processes, as may occur with disease, injury, or surgery, can cause marked changes in the torque that a muscle can produce.

Leverage Factor

Mechanically, the greater the perpendicular distance between the muscle's line of action and the joint's center (moment arm distance), the greater the rotational component produced by the muscle at that joint. This principle is sometimes called the **leverage factor** of muscles. Bony processes thus play an important role in providing force arm distances for the muscles and in increasing the angle of attachment of tendon to bone.

The leverage factor or principle is an important consideration in a muscle whose moment arm distance changes as movement occurs, since its torque output will also change at different points in the range of motion. We can look at the biceps brachii as a good example of this change in leverage principle (Fig. 2.39). When the elbow is extended, the action line of the biceps brachii is closest to the joint center. As the elbow flexes toward 90°, the muscle's line of action moves away from the joint axis until it reaches its maximum distance from the axis of motion at 90°. Continuing past 90° into more flexion, the line of action of the biceps brachii begins to return closer to the joint as the elbow reaches 120° of flexion. Thus, **for the same force of muscle contraction, the biceps brachii muscle produces the most torque at 90° of elbow flexion.** The muscle is least effective as an elbow flexor when the elbow is in extension. Although the leverage factor affects the torque output of all muscles, the effect varies with specific muscles, joints, and motions. The biceps brachii, brachioradialis, and hamstring muscles show this effect more than other muscles such as the triceps brachii, deltoid, or gastrocnemius-soleus, where the perpendicular distance to the joint axis shows minimal changes throughout the range of motion.

Stretching vs. Joint Mobilization

Passive stretching exercises to increase joint motion after fractures, surgery, or joint pathologies have long been considered contraindicated by many clinicians and physicians. Biomechanically, there are sound reasons for this caution. Force that is applied on the distal end of a bone has a long lever arm that applies significant joint stress because of its mechanical advantage over the injured joint. This mechanical advantage amplifies the force applied to the joint by 10 to 20 times. For example, if a clinician

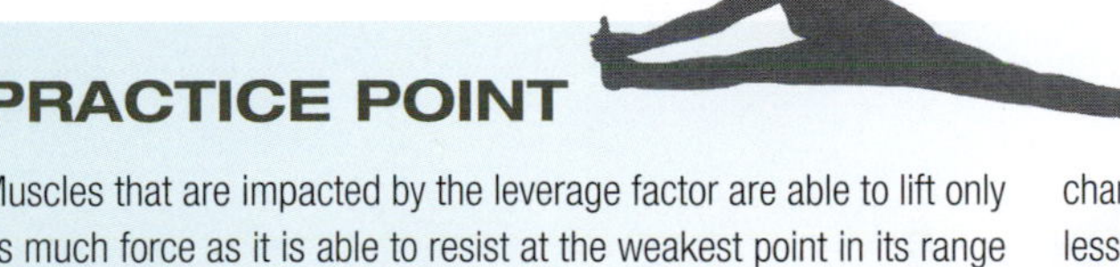

PRACTICE POINT

Muscles that are impacted by the leverage factor are able to lift only as much force as it is able to resist at the weakest point in its range of motion. For example, if the biceps brachii is able to resist a maximum force of 10 lb at 90° of elbow flexion, it will not be able to resist that much force as its moment arm becomes lesser or greater in different ranges of elbow motion. Unless the resistance torque also changes through the motion, the biceps resistance will have to be less than 10 lb if the patient is to move the elbow through its full range of motion against a constant resistance. If you provide a patient with manual resistance to the biceps, you will find that you must provide more resistance when the patient's elbow reaches 90° than at motions closer to extension and full flexion positions.

passively stretched a knee or an elbow with only 10 lb (4.5 kg) of force and applied that force 10 inches (25 cm) from the joint center, the result would be the same as if a force of 50 lb applied 2 inches from the joint center or a 100-lb force at 1 inch away from the joint was used.

On the other hand, joint mobilization applications following arthrokinematic principles are frequently indicated in pathologic conditions to relieve pain and restore normal joint motions. Some biomechanical commonalities of the basic mobilization techniques are that:

- The direction of the applied force follows the normal arthrokinematics of that joint.
- The magnitude of the force is carefully controlled to be gentle and compatible with the underlying pathology—"No forceful movement must ever be used and no abnormal movement must ever be used."[14]
- Motions of the joint surfaces are small, ranging from barely perceptible to a few millimeters in distance.

Achievements of such precision and control are gained by using very short force arms. In most instances, the force is applied very near the joint.

Pressure

To simplify biomechanical problems, forces are depicted as acting at their midpoint on a body. The tissues of the body, however, could not tolerate the pressures created by these point forces. In most cases, the application of forces on the skin, muscles, joint surfaces, and bones is over a larger area to reduce pressure.

Pressure is a function of the applied force per unit area (P = F/A) and is reported in pounds per square inch (PSI) or kilograms per square centimeter. Thus, if a 10-lb force is applied to a body over an area of 1 square inch, the pressure is 10 PSI, but if the same force is applied over an area of 2 square inches, the pressure is reduced to 5 PSI. Pressure in liquids, such as blood in the arteries and veins, is recorded in millimeters of mercury (Hg). One PSI is approximately equal to 50 mm Hg and is about the magnitude of the pressure it takes to cause occlusion of arterioles (60 to 30 mm Hg) and capillaries (30 to 10 mm Hg) at the level of the heart. When segments are dependent, as are the feet in standing, these pressures are increased by hydrostatic pressure. This pressure can be felt and the effects seen when one presses down on the fingernail and blanches (occludes) the capillary beds.

Skin, muscles, fasciae, ligaments, cartilage, and bone respond to optimal applications of pressure with normal growth and functional hypertrophy. For example, the skin on the soles of the feet becomes thicker and tougher with weight-bearing and walking. The soles of an infant's foot are soft and lack calluses because the infant does not yet bear weight and pressure on the feet. On the other hand, excessive pressure causes tissue injury, including blisters, corns, calluses, "stone bruises," ulcers, wounds, and stress fractures. The length of time that a pressure is applied to the tissue is also a determining factor in injury. Even a low pressure such as 1 PSI applied over several hours can lead to necrosis of tissue. This type of injury can occur from something as innocuous as a wrinkle in the sock or a tight shoe. People who have compromised neural systems become even more susceptible to these injuries since they are unable to detect discomfort or pain. Patients in this category include patients with spinal cord injuries, peripheral nerve injuries, diabetes, or Hansen's disease.

Pressure on an area is reduced by changing one of three factors:

- A decrease in the magnitude of the force;
- An increase the area of application; or
- A decrease the time of application.

Usually only one or possibly two of these factors can be changed while maintaining appropriate function. Decreasing the magnitude of a force occurs if the resistance arm length changes. For example, lengthening a forearm brace from midforearm length to just below the elbow improves the brace's force arm so less force is required at the point of application (Fig. 2.48). An

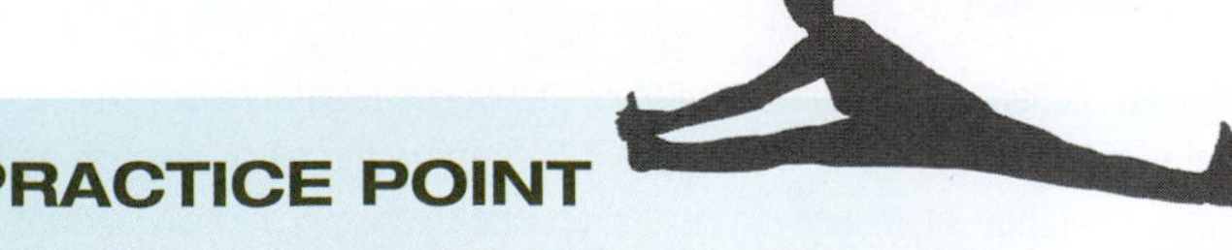

PRACTICE POINT

Pressure differences are also relevant during manual resistance activities. Using a closed hand rather than a hand with the fingers apart provides a more comfortable point of resistance application for the patient. Moreover, when providing massage techniques, using the entire flat surface of the hands rather than just the finger pads is much more comfortable for the patient.

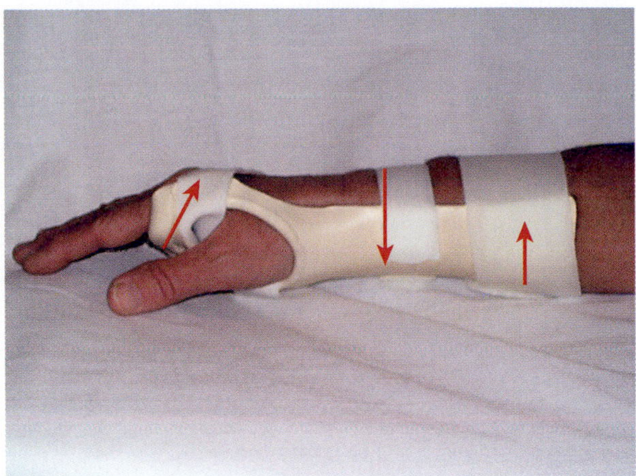

Figure 2.48 Pressure decreases on a surface when the pressure is applied over a larger surface area.

example of distributing a force over larger areas is using a convoluted foam mattress cover or a waterbed for sleeping. An example of decreasing the time that the force is felt occurs when a night splint is worn only half the night as opposed to the entire night; the results are less effective.

SUMMARY

Forces and their influence on body movement have been presented in this chapter. Differences between translational and rotary forces, Newton's three laws of motion, and the three types of levers were discussed related to their impact on body movement and function. Moment arms and torque change as joints move through their range of motions. Gravity is a primary consideration in any movement. When the body or a body segment moves over a surface, friction is also a force that impacts movement. This chapter presented free body diagrams and mathematical equations that are used by biomechanics to determine forces acting on the body and forces applied by the body. Clinical kinesiologists are more concerned about the appreciation of these forces and how to impact them in clinical situations rather than determining precise forces.

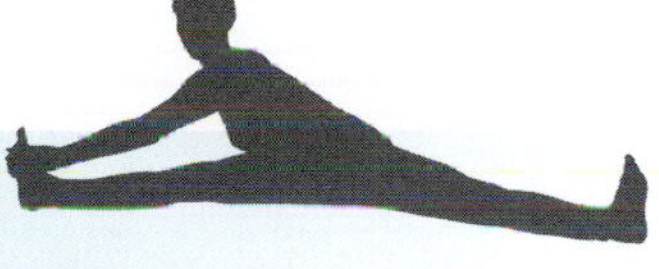

PRACTICE POINT

When an orthotic, a splint, or a brace, is applied on a patient, it is important to check the skin for areas of redness. Red areas indicate that there is excessive pressure on that area; the longer the redness remains the more pressure the soft tissue has endured. The orthosis should be altered to prevent any areas of redness. If not corrected, the areas of redness may lead to soft tissue breakdown and ulcer development.

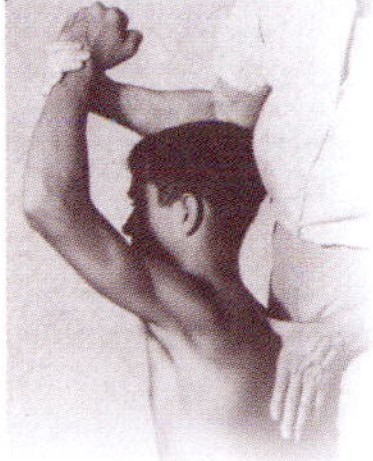

CLINICAL SCENARIO SOLUTION

As Professor Violet explained the relationship between the work the body's muscles produce and the forces they must overcome, William gained an appreciation of not only the body as a machine but also how changing body positions can alter how forces are directed. William has gained an understanding of the relationship between where a muscle inserts on a bone and what it must overcome before it is able to move its body part. He now sees the true value of understanding how physical laws of motion and using the body's segments as different levers is important in making clinical decisions such as how to position a patient for exercise or how to make a movement either easier or more difficult for the patient.

Discussion Questions

1. List six rotary motions and six translatory motions the body performs on a daily basis. What are the main differences in how these motions are performed by the body?

2. Although motions are discussed in terms of the planes and axes around which they occur, the planes and axes of a motion may change if the individual repositions a particular segment. For example, in the anatomic position, hip rotation occurs in a transverse plane around a vertical axis. What happens to the plane and axis of motion if the subject is sitting? What other joints and motions may change their axes and planes of motion if the segment's position changes?
3. If you have only one 5-lb cuff weight to use to strengthen a patient with a lower extremity injury, how are you able to provide progressive resistance using only that cuff weight?
4. There are far more third-degree levers in the body than either first- or second-degree levers. An example of one was provided earlier in the chapter, but how many other first- and second-degree levers are you able to identify?
5. Since forces are two dimensional in that they have a direction and a magnitude, the forces that are applied either to the body or by the body also have these two dimensions. When a force is applied perpendicular to the lever arm that is attached to an axis, all of the force is used to rotate the arm around the axis. How does the force change when it is not applied perpendicular to the lever arm? In other words, what is the affect of the force on the axis and its lever arm?
6. If a cuff weight is added to the wrist, what happens to the extremity's center of mass? How does that affect how the muscles that lift the arm? Can you think of another example in the body where this principle may be applied?

Lab Activities

1. In order to move objects or the body in space, the angular motion that occurs at the joints must produce linear motion. Observe a subject and describe the angular motion that occurs in order to accomplish the described linear movement.
   - **A.** Pushing a book across the surface of a table
     - **a.** Glenohumeral joint:
     - **b.** Humeroulnar joint:
   - **B.** Kicking a ball
     - **a.** Hip joint:
     - **b.** Knee joint:
   - **C.** Swimming using the breast stroke
     - **a.** Glenohumeral joint
     - **b.** Knee joint
2. While lying prone, isometrically contract the hamstrings at 0°, 45°, 90°, and 120° of knee flexion while your partner provides you with maximal resistance. Compare the force production at each of these angles. Describe why these differences occur.
3. Levers and forces: Make a three-point lever system using a board about 40 inches long and 6 inches wide. Mark the center of the board and 6-inch intervals on either side. Support the board on either end 18 inches from the center by triangular pieces of wood on bathroom scales and zero the scales.

   Place a 10-lb round or square weight on the center of the board. Call the force on the left A, the one in the center B, and the one in the right C. Draw a free body diagram of the lever (remove the scales and weight and replace with force vectors), and label the force vectors with their letters and with the known forces (use round numbers).

   Add 10 more pounds at the center of the lever. What is the relationship of the forces between A, B, and C? Write this as an equation using positive and negative signs, and then substitute the pound values of the forces to check it. Move the weight B to the right 6 inches. Does this relationship still hold? Move the weight back to the center and move the scale C in 6 inches. Same relationship? Notice that change in the magnitude of one force or change in the length of a force arm produces changes in the magnitude of the other two forces but the sum of the forces remains (equilibrium equation: $\Sigma F = 0$).

4. Draw parallelograms of the following component vector diagrams. Insert the resultant vector. What can you say to explain the resultant vector for each of the diagrams?

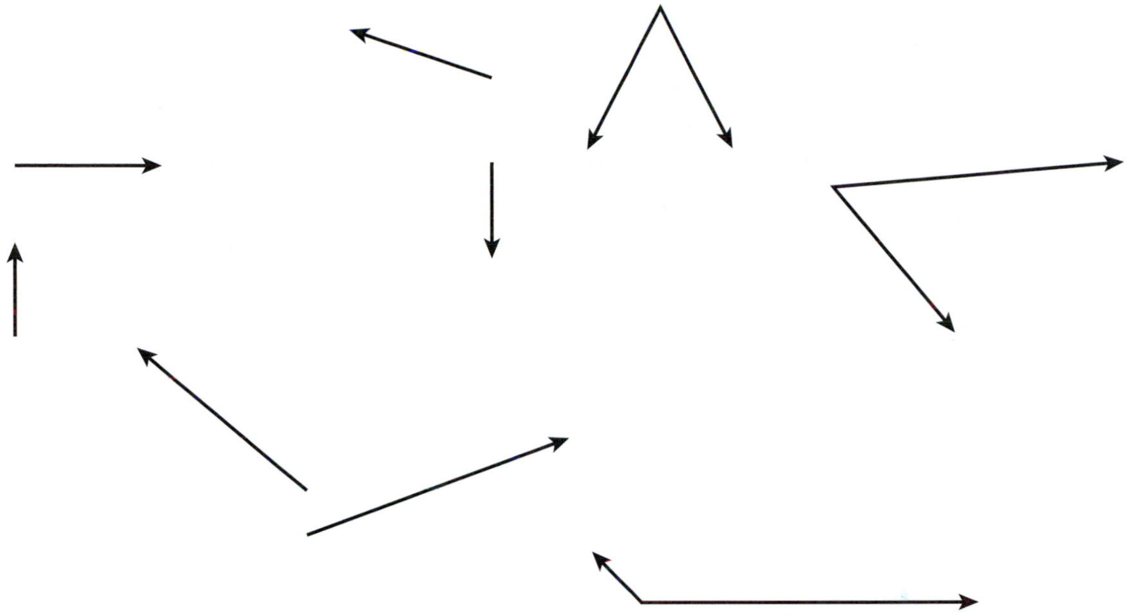

5. Calculate the force required by the muscle to hold the dumbbell in place in the figure below.

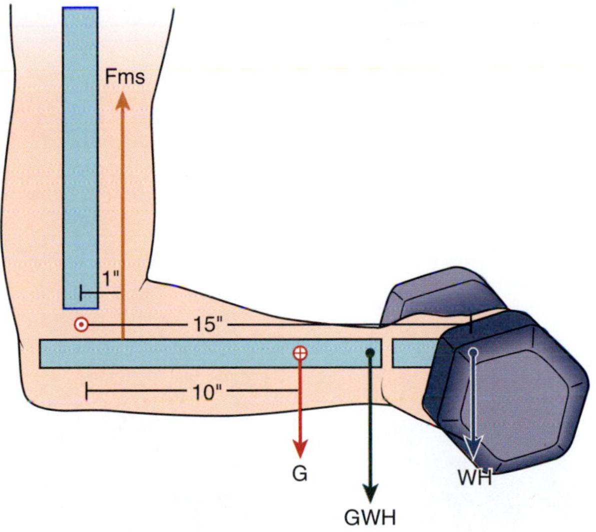

Dumbbell = 15 lb
G (forearm) = 8 lb
WH (wrist & hand) = 1.5 lb

6. Why is it impossible to do the following party tricks without cheating?
   - **A.** Stand with back and heels touching a wall and bend forward from the hips to touch the floor. Return to the upright position without falling or moving the feet.
   - **B.** Stand facing the edge of an open door with nose and abdomen touching the edge, the feet straddling the door, and the hands to the sides. Attempt to rise up on the toes.

   Observe what body motions occur to keep the center of gravity within the base of support when these activities are performed without the impediments.
7. Describe the movements of the body's center of gravity from sitting to standing.
8. The following exercises are to be performed in the sitting position with the elbow extended:

   Perform shoulder flexion to 90° with a 5 lb weight held in the hand.
   Perform shoulder flexion to 90° with a 5 lb cuff weight placed above the elbow.
   Which motion is easier to perform? Why?
9. List in order of difficulty these three push-up positions. Explain what makes one more difficult than the next.

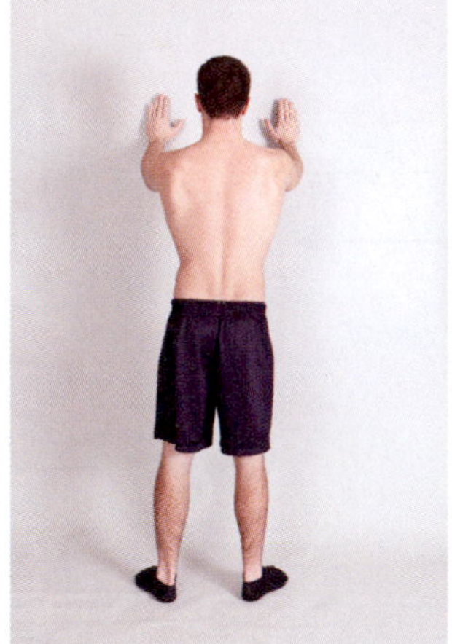
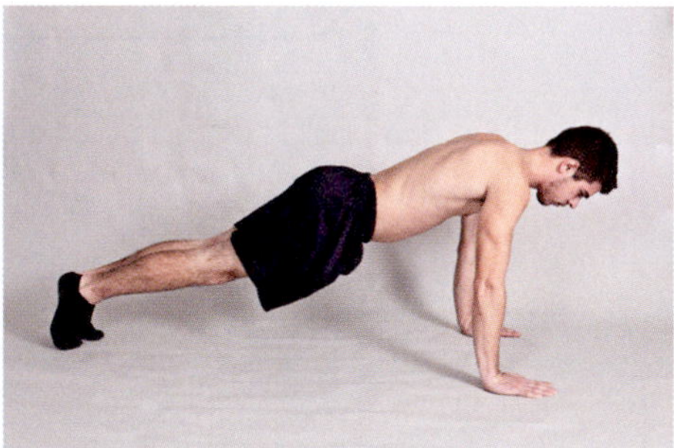
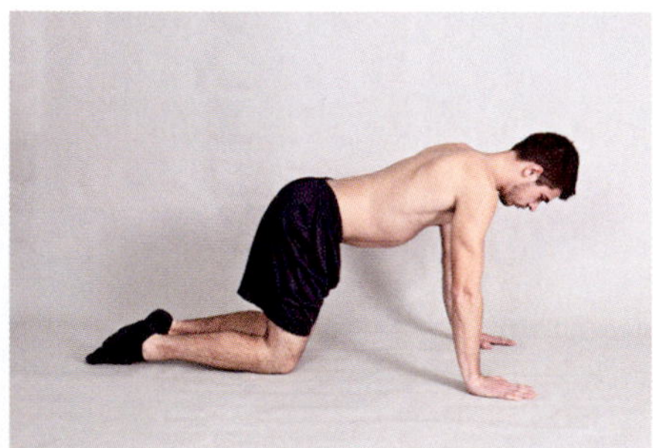

10. Explain why the punching bag will not fall over, regardless of how hard it is hit or from what angle it is hit.

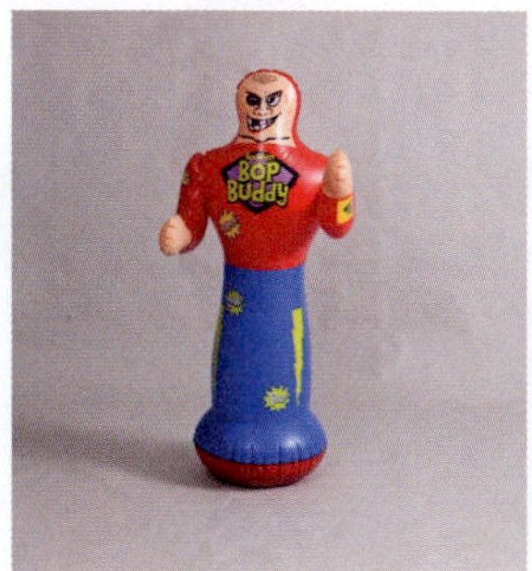

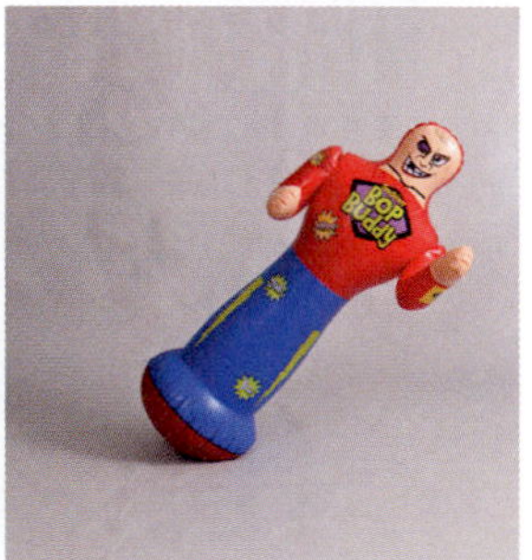

11. Diagram out the vector forces to demonstrate the difference in compressive forces acting on the patella in the two different positions below. What clinical implications does this have?

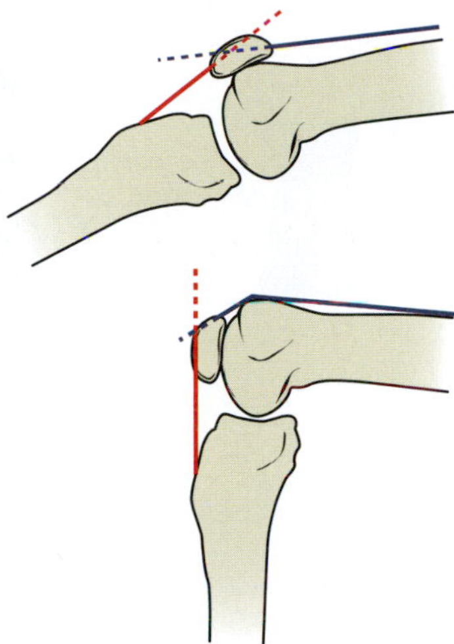

12. Draw the vector force for the combined efforts of the sternal and clavicular portions of the pectoralis major. What shoulder motion results?

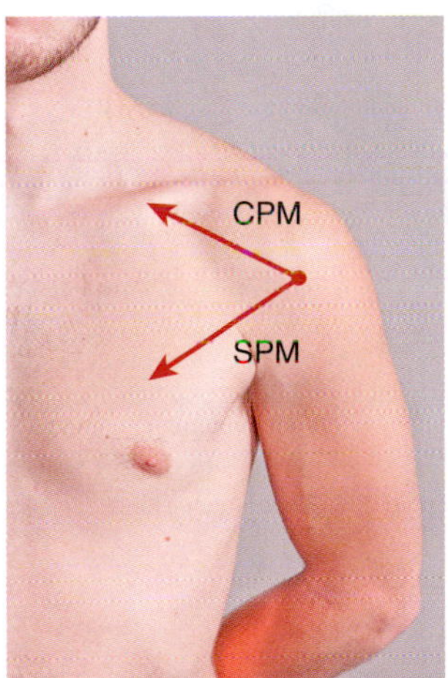

13. Indicate in each of the drawings below where you estimate the COG to be for each of the figures.

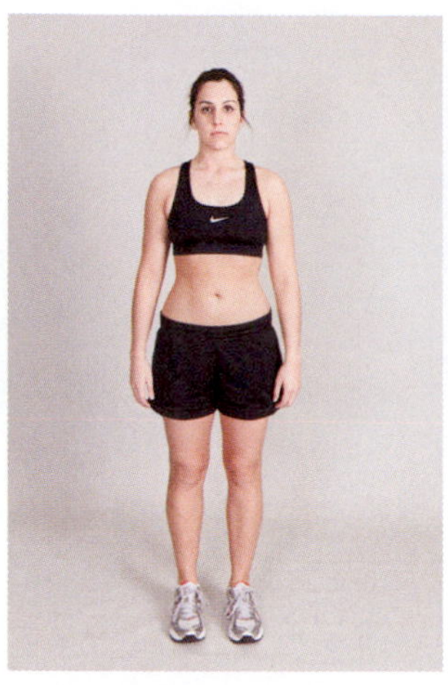
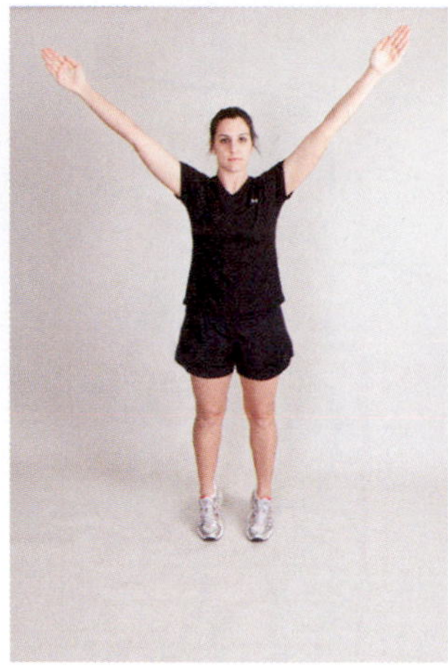
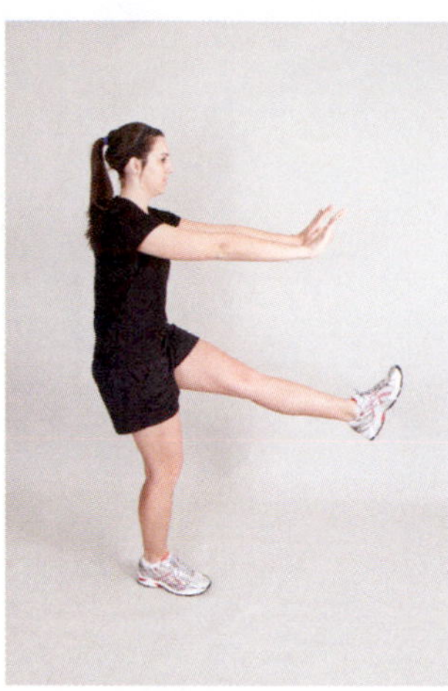
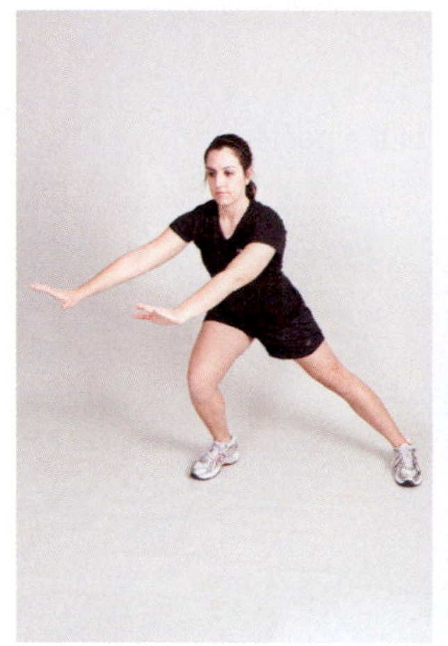
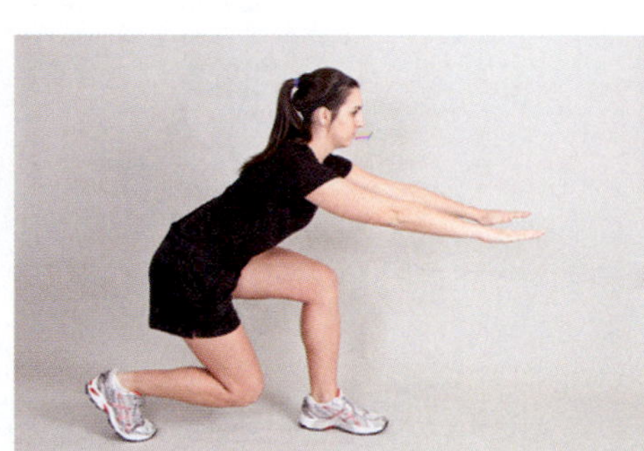
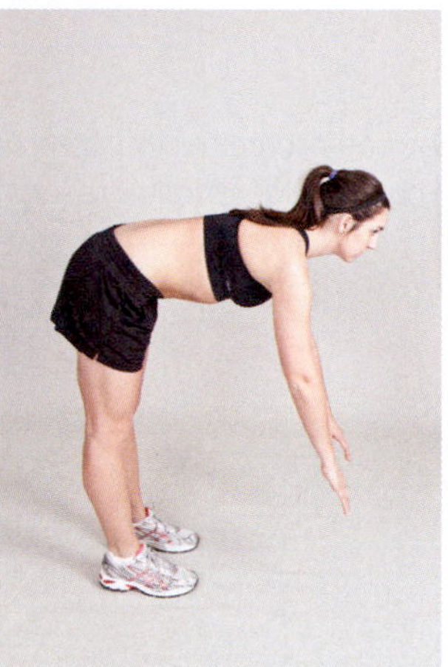

14. Based on these two drawings of the deltoid, in which position would the muscle produce more force to elevate the arm? Why?

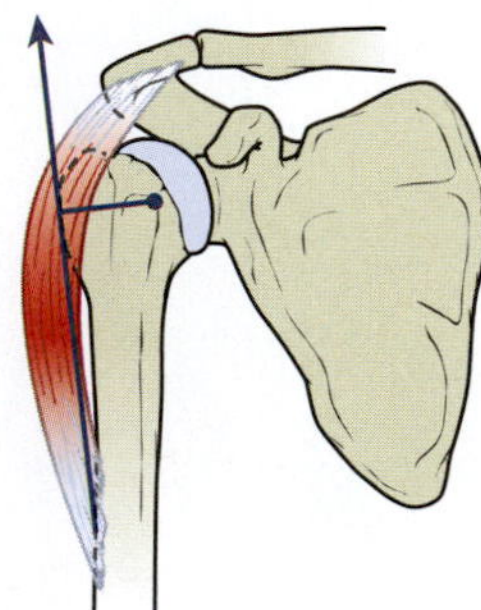
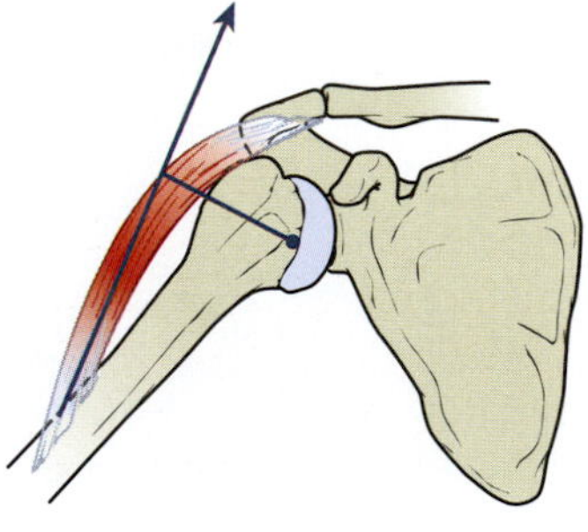

15. Since torque forces have a rotational and nonrotational component, identify for each of the angles below, the rotational and nonrotational components.

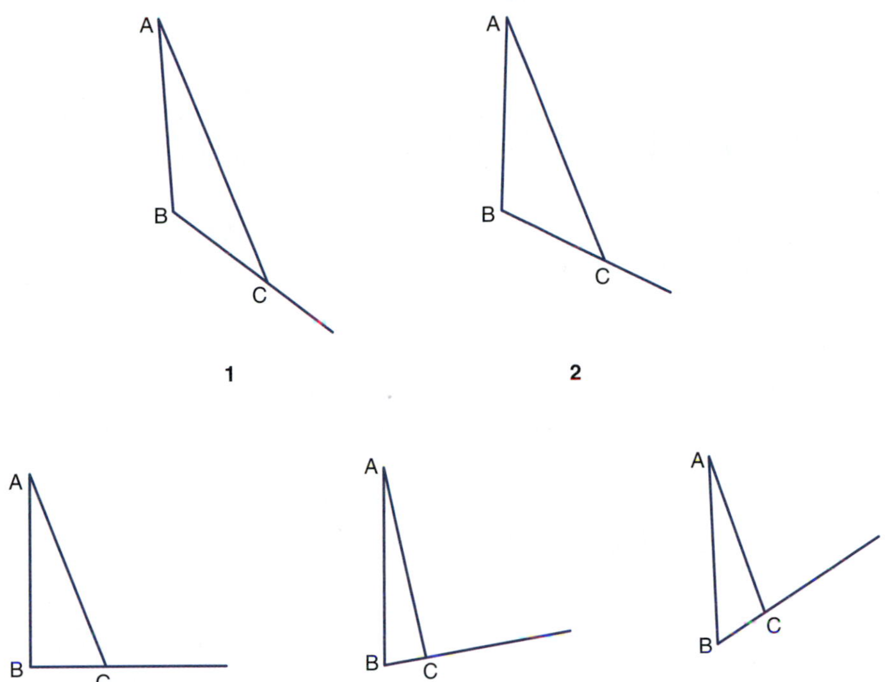

Which diagram(s) has all its torque force devoted to rotation? Which diagram(s) has its nonrotational force attempting to dislocate the joint? Which diagram(s) has its non-rotational force attempting to stabilize the joint?

References

1. Resnick D, Halliday R. *Physics for Students of Science and Engineering*. New York: John Wiley & Sons, 1963.
2. Kelsey DD, Tyson E. A new method of training for the lower extremity using unloading. *Journal of Orthopaedic and Sports Physical Therapy* 19(4):218–223, 1994.
3. Dempster WT. Space requirements of the seated operator. US Department of Commerce, Office of Technical Services: 55–159, 1955.
4. Braune W, Fischer O. *On the Centre of Gravity of the Human Body*. Berlin: Springer-Verlag, 1984.
5. Drillis R, Contini R, Bluestein M. Body segment parameters: A survey of measurement techniques. *Artificial Limbs* 25:44–66, 1964.
6. Elftman H. Knee action and locomotion. *Bulletin of the Hospital for Joint Diseases* 16(2):103–110, 1955.
7. Hellebrandt FA, Tepper RH, Braun GL. Location of the cardinal anatomical orientation planes passing through the center of weight in young adult women. *American Journal of Physiology* 121:465, 1938.
8. LeVeau BF, ed. *William & Lissner's Biomechanics of Human Motion,* 3 ed. Philadelphia: W.B. Saunders, 1992.
9. Soderberg G. *Kinesiology: Application to Pathological Motion*. Baltimore: Williams & Wilkins, 1986.
10. Zohn DA, Mennell J. *Musculoskeletal Pain: Diagnosis and Physical Treatment*. Boston: Little, Brown & Co, 1976.
11. MacDonald CW, Whitman JM, Cleland JA, Smith M, Hoeksma HL. Clinical outcomes following manual physical therapy and exercise for hip osteoarthritis: A case series. *Journal of Orthopaedic and Sports Physical Therapy* 36(8):588–599, 2006.
12. Konradsen L. Factors contributing to chronic ankle instability: Kinesthesia and joint position sense. *Journal of Athletic Training* 37(4):381–385, 2002.
13. Grelsamer RP, Klein JR. The biomechanics of the patellofemoral joint. *Journal of Orthopaedic and Sports Physical Therapy* 28:286–298, 1998.
14. Mennell JM. *Joint Pain: Diagnosis and Treatment Using Manipulative Techniques*. Boston: Little, Brown & Co, 1964.

The Movement System: Nerve and Muscle Physiology and the Control of Human Movement

"The key to success is discipline. Teens don't want to hear that. They think that they can just snap their fingers, and voila! But with discipline come knowledge, coordination, balance, muscle memory, confidence — things that make it possible to hit the bulls-eye three times in a row."
—*Carlos Santana, musician, 1947*

CHAPTER OUTLINE

Learning Outcomes
Clinical Scenario
Introduction
Physiology of Excitable Tissue: Nerve and Muscle
Nervous System Anatomy Overview
Nervous System Classifications
Nerve Fibers
Muscular System
Structure of Skeletal Muscle
Muscle Fiber Types
The Motor Unit
Joint, Tendon, and Muscle Receptors
Joint Receptors
Golgi Tendon Organs
Muscle Spindles
Kinesthesia and Proprioception
Movement or "Motor" Control
Dynamic Systems Approach to Understanding Motor Control
Motor Control at the Spinal Region
Motor Control within the Brainstem

LEARNING OUTCOMES

This chapter provides an overview of nerve and muscle interaction and how they function together. After reading this chapter, you should be able to:

- ❑ Describe the properties of irritability, excitability, and transmission that are the unique capabilities of nerve and muscle tissue;
- ❑ Give an overview of the nervous system's physiological, anatomical, and functional divisions and explain their functions;
- ❑ Describe the basic structure of skeletal muscle and how skeletal muscle contracts;
- ❑ Describe the different types of muscle fibers and their contribution to functional movement;
- ❑ Describe the function of proprioceptors—Golgi tendon organ, joint receptors, and muscle spindle—and explain how they contribute to human movement control;
- ❑ Define and describe what motor control means;
- ❑ Describe the functional contributions to motor control from the spinal region, the brainstem, the cerebellum, the basal ganglia, and the motor cortex, and summarize the functional consequences of damage to those areas;
- ❑ Describe the following common movement system impairments—weakness, abnormal muscle tone, coordination problems, and involuntary movements.

Cerebral Motor Centers
Intermediate Control Centers
Integration of Motor Control to Produce Functional Movement
Functional Applications and Clinical Considerations
Muscle Weakness
Abnormal Muscle Tone
Coordination Problems
Involuntary Movements
Common Pathological Conditions Affecting Movement System Function
Peripheral Nerve Injury
Cerebral Palsy
Cerebrovascular Accident
Basal Ganglia Disorders
Cerebellar Disorders
Summary
Clinical Scenario Solution
Discussion Questions
Lab Activities
References

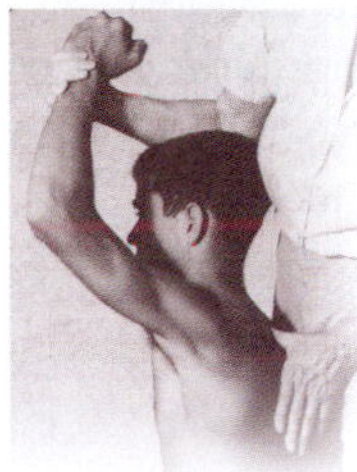

CLINICAL SCENARIO

Joseph is a 5-year old child with spastic diplegic cerebral palsy. He has spasticity in both lower extremities and weakness in his trunk, but he is able to ambulate around school and home using a walker. While playing outside, he fell, landing his elbow onto a broken glass bottle and partially severed his left ulnar nerve at the medial epicondyle. Jay, his clinician, needs to explain to Joseph's mother the differences between the weakness that he is displaying in his left hand and the weakness and spasticity that is present in his legs.

Introduction

Since this is a clinical kinesiology textbook, you may wonder what a chapter whose primary information regards physiology and movement theory is doing in such a text. As clinicians, it is important for us to understand how the body works, what makes it work, and how we can influence how it works in the exercise and rehabilitation programs we create for our patients. Since kinesiology is the study of human movement, we must appreciate the elements that produce motion. Human movement occurs as a result of an intimate relationship between anatomy and physiology. This chapter presents information relevant to the connections between these two systems; melding this chapter's information with the subsequent chapters will provide you with a clear understanding and appreciation of human movement.

Providing a basic understanding of neural physiology for the development and appreciation of the kinesiological functions in human performance is the goal of this chapter. We will first identify the basic physiology of uniquely excitable nerve and muscle tissue. Then, the building blocks of the components of the neuromuscular system—neurons, skeletal muscle, and sensory receptors—are described, and we will discuss how the entire system is dynamically organized to produce functional, purposeful movement. This information is followed by an overview of all of the central motor control areas with a focus on their functional contributions to movement. A discussion of movement impairments and their functional consequences follows and concludes with a discussion of clinical considerations, including a brief summary of some of the more common impairments resulting from motor control dysfunction. Impairment of the central and peripheral nervous systems are compared and contrasted. Some of the material in this chapter may serve as a quick review for those who have previously studied the anatomy and physiology of the neuromuscular system. For those who have not had the benefit of such courses, textbooks on human anatomy and physiology and neuroscience may be consulted for a more complete explanation of the functions of the neuromuscular system.

Purposeful movement is a fundamental characteristic of human behavior. Coordinated human movement is the result of an orchestration of muscles acting on the bony skeleton; this orchestration is organized by the nervous system and refined by multiple sensory mechanisms to produce mechanical responses. Human movement requires activation and integration of multiple parts of multiple systems within a split second. Movement is not the result of one single muscle acting across one joint but is an integrated system of the brain and body that responds, executes, interprets, and adjusts to continual feedback. The use of the term "system" is appropriate in discussions of body motion. A "system" is an assemblage or combination of parts that form a functioning unit. Viewing human movement as a system made up of several contributing elements such as the nervous, muscular, skeletal, and sensory systems allows us to study both structure and function simultaneously. What we usually think of as separate systems are actually components of a larger system that provides desired and purposeful outcomes. In other words, those structures or systems that contribute to more than one function are actually a part of more than one purposeful system.[1]

Therefore, the human **movement system** involves the functional interaction of structures that contribute to the act of moving.[2] Included in these structures are the nervous system's somatosensory and relay components that facilitate the skeletal and muscular systems.[3,4] The body's movement system changes throughout the life cycle in response to growth, maturation, aging, disease, or environmental demands.

Movement occurs through biomechanical responses to this neurological input. These biomechanical responses include skeletal muscle contractions that move the body's system of levers and pulleys which are formed by bones, tendons, and ligaments. A person's individuality is expressed by his or her own pattern of muscular contractions. These individually unique manifestations include facial expressions, body postures, fine motor skill performances such as typing or playing a musical instrument, and gross motor activities such as walking and running. The individual with a normal functioning neuromusculoskeletal system has a remarkable ability to develop just the right amount of muscle force needed to perform an endless variety of motor tasks—from placing a contact lens in one's eye to carrying a heavy load of textbooks to class.

Whatever the muscle activity, it is accomplished through intricate communication between the musculoskeletal and nervous systems. An elaborate nervous system provides fine control of muscle contractions over a wide range of lengths, tensions, speeds, and loads. The nervous system is very complex and has myriad responsibilities, including a variety of sensory and motor functions. The sensory nervous system provides accurate and timely information about the status of each body part and their environmental surroundings through its **afferent** (L. *ad,* to, plus *ferre,* to carry) receptors. Incoming sensory information from these afferent receptors travels to various parts of the nervous system where it is accepted, interpreted, and responded to in context with information previously stored in the brain. Once the nervous system has processed the afferent information, its **efferent** (L. *ex,* out, plus *ferre,* to carry) motor nerve impulses send a response to selected muscles or muscle groups to produce desired movements. Thus, the end product—desired movement—is achieved through the collaborative interaction and coordination of primarily the motor and sensory systems.

The body's ability to produce an appropriate response relies on numerous factors. These factors include the ability of muscles to develop graded amounts of active tension; the ability of the cardiovascular, respiratory, and digestive systems to provide the ingredients that fuel the contractile process; and the ability of the nervous system to regulate the rate and amount of contraction needed to accurately move certain body parts while stabilizing and inhibiting other parts. This entire process from afferent stimulation to motor response occurs within milliseconds.

Physiology of Excitable Tissue: Nerve and Muscle

As you learned in physiology, all living cells are surrounded by membranes formed by a continuous phospholipid bilayer. Embedded throughout these membranes are proteins with various characteristics. This section briefly reviews cell physiology to refresh your memory of the topics relevant to neuromuscular function as they relate to and further add to your understanding of kinesiology.

Uniquely, both nervous and muscular tissue membranes are excitable; that is, their membranes are irritable and thereby sensitive to electrochemical change. Furthermore, this excitability can be communicated between the tissues and from one region or system to another. Because of this unique characteristic, nerve cells and muscle cells are not only excitable but are also able to transmit this electrochemical information to produce movement. Before we discuss the specific interworking between the nervous and muscular systems, we need to understand how these tissues work.

Differences in electrical potential exist across the membranes of all living cells. Fluids bathe the inside and outside of each cell. These intracellular and extracellular fluids contain negatively and positively charged particles, called ions. The ions are predominantly negative inside the cell and positive outside the cell. This imbalance of ions from one side of a cell membrane to the other is called a **potential difference.** Two factors are responsible for the ability of a cell to maintain a potential difference across its membrane:

- The cell membrane has selective permeability. This means that it is relatively impermeable to certain ions and more permeable (lets ions pass through the membrane) to others. However, the permeability of the membrane to an ion can be increased

transiently by certain chemical substances released by nerve endings, as is discussed later.
- The cell can actively move ions across the membrane to maintain a required resting potential.

The potential inside a cell membrane is measured relative to the fluid just outside the membrane (Fig. 3.1). Under resting conditions when no action is occurring, the membrane potential, aptly called the **resting potential,** is negative. Nerve cells, muscle cells, and sensory receptors maintain a negative resting potential in the range of −60 to −90 mV (average = −85mV) between the inside and outside of their membranes.

A neuron innervating skeletal muscle and the skeletal muscle itself each possess membrane characteristics that allow them to react when a stimulus is provided. This ability to react to a stimulus is called **irritability.** Once nervous and muscular tissues react to a stimulus, the cell's membrane changes its resting potential and it becomes more positive. This process is called **depolarization.** When the nerve or muscle cell membranes are depolarized, they become *excitable* and transmit the electrochemical impulse along their membranes, so that the depolarization propagates, or moves, along the cell's membrane. When this depolarization continues to be transmitted, this impulse, is known as an **action potential**. Action potentials are the *language,* or the electrochemical messages, that are then propagated through the movement system. Let's examine this process step by step.

Think of a light switch turning on a ceiling light; when the switch is moved to the "on" position, a signal is sent through the electrical wire to the light bulb. The body reacts to a stimulus in a similar manner. A sufficient stimulus (electrical, mechanical, chemical, or thermal) applied to a nerve or muscle cell causes the cell membrane to be more permeable to certain ions. This increased permeability results in a rapid exchange of previously separated positive and negative ions as the stimulus moves across the membrane. This rapid ion movement causes the membrane to become more positively charged, or depolarized (Fig. 3.1). The flow of current between immediately adjacent regions serves to excite the polarized region ahead of the current, with the result that this region now contributes a greatly amplified electric signal. With subsequent adjacent regions becoming excited, the action potential propagates or spreads down the length of the axon without a change in its amplitude (intensity) as it moves along the axon. In other words, the excitation that is produced by a stimulus produces a wave of electrochemical activity that moves rapidly along nerve and muscle fibers and is associated with local changes in the electrical potential of each of the fibers. An action potential transmitted over a nerve fiber is a *nerve impulse,* whereas an action potential conducted over a muscle fiber is a *muscle impulse.* Immediately after depolarization, an active process, termed **repolarization,** returns the membrane to its resting potential.

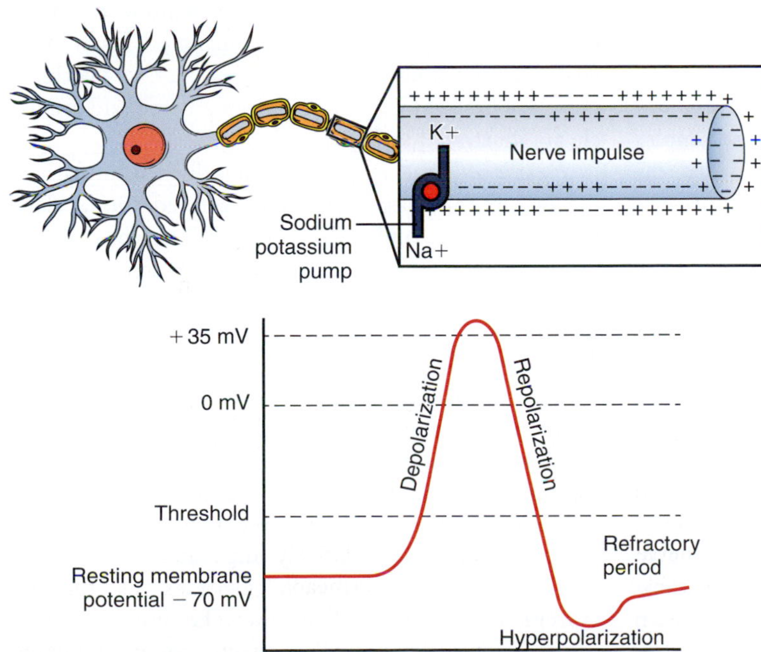

Figure 3.1 Generation of an action potential.

Neurons send "control signals" to other neurons or to muscles by releasing small amounts of chemicals termed **neurotransmitters.** Each time a nerve impulse arrives at the **synapse** (Gr. *synapsis,* a connection), a junction between nerves or at the junction between a motor neuron and a muscle fiber, neurotransmitters are released at the synapse. The chemical synapse between two neurons may be either excitatory or inhibitory. Excitatory synapses cause depolarization of the postsynaptic membrane to produce an action potential. In contrast, inhibitory synapses result in a **hyperpolarization** (more negative potential) of the postsynaptic membrane. This inhibition increases the voltage requirement so it is more difficult to create an action potential.[5]

Nervous System Anatomy Overview

Now that we understand how nerves and muscles "talk" to each other, let's examine the anatomical components of the nervous and muscular systems before we investigate how they work together in a functional movement system.

Nervous System Classifications

The most basic structure of the nervous system is the neuron. Neurons have many different shapes and sizes, depending on their location and functions in the nervous system. A typical neuron consists of a cell body containing the nucleus; several short radiating processes called dendrites; and one long process, the axon, which terminates in twig-like branches. The axon may also have branches or collaterals projecting along its course. The axon, together with its covering, or sheath, forms the nerve fiber.

Beyond comprehending the neuron, the nervous system becomes very complex. To make such a complex system easier to understand, science has divided the nervous system into smaller units. Because the nervous system performs so many functions and is comprised of various structures, it can be divided using a variety of methods. The most common methods used to discuss the nervous system include physiological, anatomical or functional divisions. *Physiologically*, the nervous system is divided into the somatic and visceral nervous systems. The somatic system includes all of the receptors and nerves that innervate muscles and skin. The visceral system is the autonomic system that is further subdivided into the sympathetic and parasympathetic systems. Further discussion of physiology is available in human physiology texts. This text, however, focuses on anatomical and functional classifications of the nervous system as they relate to movement.

Anatomically, the nervous system is divided into the central nervous system (CNS) and the peripheral nervous system (PNS). The central nervous system is composed of the brain and spinal cord and includes all of the nerves that communicate with each other within those areas. These neural structures are enclosed within the bony vertebral column and skull. On the other hand, the peripheral nervous system includes the cranial nerves, the afferent sensory nerves to the spinal cord and the efferent motor neurons from the spinal cord to the muscles. A cross section of a thoracic spinal cord segments and locations of major motor and sensory tracts are illustrated in Figure 3.2. The term **tract** describes a group of axons with common origin, function, and termination. The name of a tract often indicates the general origin and destination of the axons which make up the tract. For example, the spinocerebellar tracts convey sensory impulses from the spinal cord to the cerebellum. Likewise, axons in the corticospinal tract descend from the cerebral cortex and terminate within the spinal cord. General anatomic features of the neural pathways transmitting from the brain to individual muscle fibers are also illustrated schematically in Figure 3.2. Axons of **upper motor neurons** are located in the cerebral cortex and descend in the spinal cord. These upper motor neurons form axonal bundles as corticospinal pathways or tracts. Corticospinal tracts are in the lateral and medial portions of the spinal cord (Fig. 3.2) and are the lateral and medial corticospinal tract, respectively. The axons of the corticospinal tracts make synaptic contact, usually via interneurons, with **lower motor neurons.** Lower motor neurons are in the ventral horn gray matter of the spinal cord. Each lower motor neuron innervates a set of muscle fibers within a muscle. These connections between a nerve and a muscle are illustrated in Figure 3.2.

Functionally, the nervous system is divided similarly to the anatomically based system but with additional clarification. For example, the peripheral nervous system includes afferent and efferent nerves. In functional terms, the afferent system includes all nerves associated with the transmission of sensory information into the CNS. Afferent nerves includes peripheral axons, often called primary or first order afferents, originating from the receptors and entering into the dorsal horn of the spinal cord. Once in the spinal cord, afferent signals synapse and continue transmission within the central nervous system via second and third order afferents at various neural regions between the spinal cord and cortex.

The efferent system includes nerves that regulate movement and motor behavior. The initial efferent nerves within the central nervous system are upper

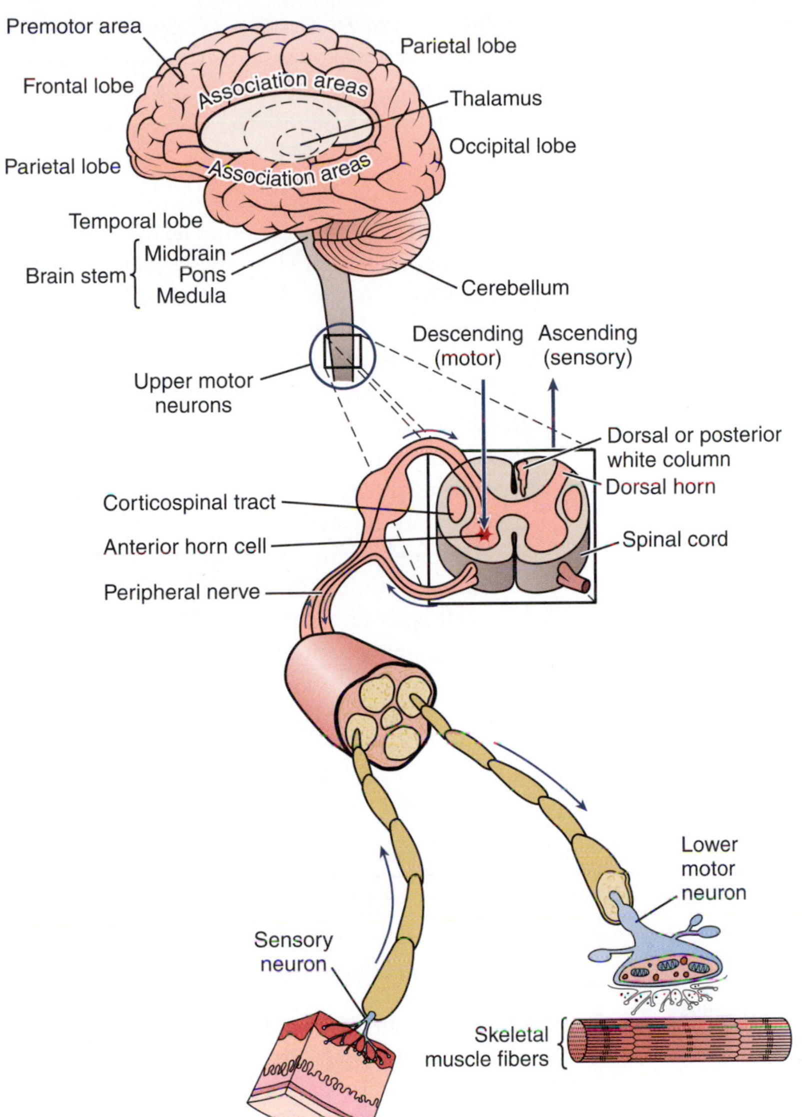

Figure 3.2 Major structures involved in the transmission of impulses to activate skeletal muscle fibers; central and peripheral components of the descending (motor) pathways from the cerebral cortex to the spinal cord and to muscles; cross section of the spinal cord at the thoracic level, illustrating the central gray matter and the peripheral white matter with ascending and descending tracts. Peripheral nerve fibers are enlarged to illustrate sensory and motor components. Note that structures and tracts exist on both the left and right sides; for simplicity, however, only one side is illustrated.

motor neurons since their connections, cell bodies, and axons lie within the brain and spinal cord. **Interneurons** are those neurons within the ventral horn and intermediate areas of the spinal cord. Interneurons transmit efferently to alpha and gamma lower motor neurons. Alpha and gamma lower motor neurons innervate extrafusal muscle fibers and intrafusal muscle fibers, respectively; muscle fibers are discussed in more detail later in this chapter. Interneurons function as a neural *bridge* between the upper and lower motor neurons.

Nerve Fibers

As we know, neurons are the functional structure of the nervous system. Afferent and efferent nerves must relay messages quite rapidly if they are to perform their responsibilities effectively. The motor and sensory nerves are wrapped with a myelin sheath to provide for this necessary transmission speed. Myelin is a white lipid substance that insulates the neural axon. Along this myelin sheath are regular indentations the length of the axon; these are nodes of Ranvier, named after a French histologist, Louis Ranvier (1835–1922). The myelin sheath increases the speed of neural transmission by allowing the excitation to jump along the axon from one node of Ranvier to the next rather than flowing to make contact with the entire axon. Characteristics of sensory and motor neurons are depicted in Figure 3.3.

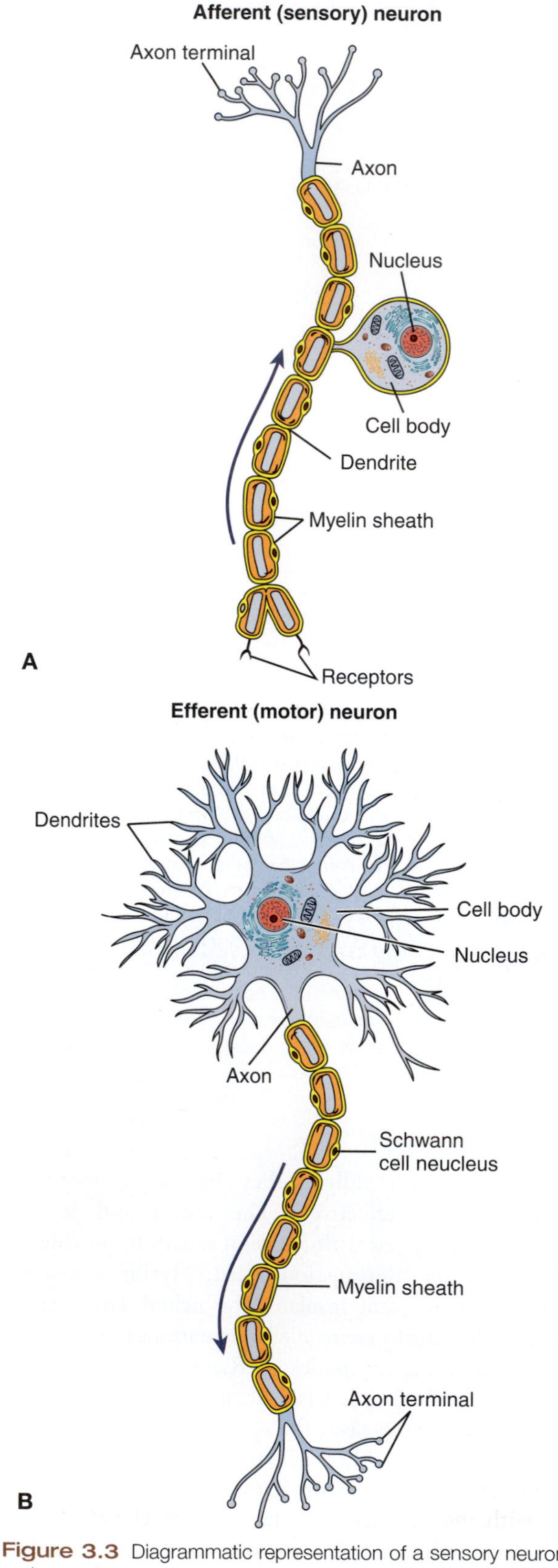

Figure 3.3 Diagrammatic representation of a sensory neuron and a motor neuron.

Nerve Fibers in the Peripheral Nervous System

A peripheral nerve trunk coming off the spinal cord is composed of many nerve fibers, both sensory and motor (Fig. 3.2). Functionally, peripheral nerves include the following fibers:

- Sensory nerves are functionally referred to as afferent nerve fibers. Their cell bodies lie in special **ganglia**. Sensory fibers carry impulses arising from various receptors in the skin, muscles, and special sense organs to the central nervous system, where the impulses are interpreted.
- Motor nerve fibers are functionally referred to as efferent nerve fibers. These motor fibers conduct impulses from the spinal cord to skeletal muscle fibers for voluntary muscle activity control. Their cell bodies are located in the gray matter of the spinal cord and brainstem. Lower motor neuron is the term used to describe a motor (efferent) nerve whose cell body and axon originate in the ventral horn of the spinal cord and synapse directly onto skeletal muscle. It is also often referred to as the *final common path* between the nervous system and the muscular system.
- Autonomic neurons are concerned with the involuntary control of glandular activities and smooth muscles, including smooth muscles surrounding arterioles and venules within muscles. Comprehensive explanations of the autonomic nervous system are beyond the scope of this text but may be found in physiology and neuroscience textbooks.

Classification of Motor and Sensory Nerve Fibers on the Basis of Axonal Diameter in the Peripheral Nervous System

When histologists and anatomists began studying the characteristics of the nervous system, neurons supplying various motor and sensory structures in the body were classified according to the diameter of their axons. Their classification system remains in use today (Table 3–1). The largest axons are classified as type A, and the smallest fibers are C; those of intermediate diameter are referred to as type B. Both A and B fibers are myelinated, whereas C fibers are unmyelinated. Type A fibers are further divided, based on fiber diameter. Type A subdivisions include type A-alpha (α), type A-beta (β), type A-gamma (γ), and type A-delta (δ).

The reason classification according to size is important has to do with the speed of nerve conduction. The speed at which a nerve impulse travels along the length of an axon is related to the diameter of the axon and whether it is enclosed in a myelin sheath. Larger axons conduct impulses at a faster velocity. This makes intuitive

TABLE 3–1 | NERVE FIBER TYPES

Fiber Type	Fiber Diameter (μm)	Conduction Velocity (m/sec)	Peripheral Organ	Function
A-alpha (α) (motor)	12–20	70–120	Skeletal muscle	Motor, skeletal muscle efferent
A-alpha Ia (sensory)	12–20	70–120	Muscle spindle afferent	Proprioception
A-alpha Ib (sensory)	12–20	70–120	Golgi tendon organs afferent	Proprioception
A-Beta II (sensory)	5–12	30–70	Muscle spindle and touch/pressure receptors	Touch, pressure, vibration
A-gamma (γ) (motor)	3–6	15–30	Intrafusal muscle fibers of muscle spindle	Motor, muscle spindle efferent
A-delta (δ) (sensory)	2–5	12–30	Skin	Pain and temperature afferent
B fibers	1–3	3–15	Autonomic Sympathetic	Autonomic efferent
C fibers IV	.5–1	.5–2	Skin, autonomic postganglionic	Pain and temperature afferent

Source: Bertoti, DB. *Functional Neurorehabilitation Across the Life Span.* Philadelphia: F. A. Davis Company, 2004. Reprinted with permission from F. A. Davis Company.[1]

sense, and a simple comparison helps us understand this concept. If you compare the largest-diameter nerve to a garden hose and the smallest-diameter nerve to a straw, it is much faster to move one gallon of water through the hose than through the straw. As we have already discussed, adding a myelin sheath causes the axon to conduct an impulse even faster. Type Aα are the largest myelinated axons (diameter = 20 μm) and conduct an impulse at a maximum velocity of approximately 120 m/s. The longest sensory and motor axons extend from the lumbar spinal cord segments to the foot muscles, a distance of approximately 1 meter in an adult of average height. Therefore, a minimum of 8 msec (0.008 second) is needed for a nerve impulse to travel the length of type Aα axon. As seen in Table 3–1, the smallest nerve fibers, type C (0.5 μm in diameter), convey nerve impulses from sensory endings in the skin that appear to produce sensations of pain when stimulated. Pain impulses are conducted at a velocity of approximately 0.5 m/s.

Classification of Sensory Fibers on the Basis of Fiber Origin within the Peripheral Nervous System

Afferent nerve fibers within the peripheral nervous system may also be classified according to the type of sensory receptor from which impulses are conducted. This method includes four groups. The first group (group I) is subdivided into subgroups Ia and Ib. Group Ia fibers carry impulses from the primary sensory receptor in muscles, the **muscle spindle**. Group Ib fibers carry impulses from sensory receptors located in tendons and are referred to as **Golgi tendon organs (GTO)**. The Golgi tendon organs are located at the interface of a muscle with its tendon. Diameters of group Ia and Ib fibers are approximately 12 to 20 mm. Muscle spindles and Golgi tendon organs are type A-α fibers. Group II fibers are equivalent to type A-β in diameter size (4 to 12 μm) and carry impulses from the secondary receptors in the muscle spindle.[6] The structure and function of muscle spindles and GTOs are described in the section on receptors.

Classification of Motor Fibers on the Basis of Fiber Destination within the Peripheral Nervous System

Efferent nerve fibers are classified into two groups based on which muscle fiber that they innervate. Alpha (α) motor neurons innervate **extrafusal** skeletal muscle. **Gamma (γ) motor neurons** innervate the contractile element called the **intrafusal** (within the spindle) **muscle fibers**. As the name indicates, the intrafusal muscle fibers lie within the muscle spindle while extrafusal muscle fibers are normal skeletal muscle fibers.

Nerve Fibers in the Central Nervous System

As with the peripheral nervous system classifications, the CNS also has different methods of classifying the nerves which comprise it. Within the central nervous system, nerves are classified typically by their physical characteristics such as size or shape. For example, the giant cortical neuron is so named for its size, and a pyramidal neuron is named for the shape of its cell body.

Another way of classifying neurons references their function. For example, the *association* neuron is a neuron within the association cortices of the brain. These nerves communicate with each other within the brain and literally create associations between neural areas, similar to the bridging function of the interneurons within the spinal cord; hence, their name—**association neurons**.

As previously mentioned, all sensory and motor axons travel in tracts within the CNS. Recall that tracts consist of bundled axons and are named for their origin, location and destination. Because many nerve fibers are covered with a myelin sheath, tracts appear white in unstained histologic sections; therefore, the term **white matter** is used to describe areas in the central nervous system that contain predominantly fiber tracts. Within various regions of the central nervous system, aggregations of anatomically and functionally related neurons (cell bodies) are distinguished from one another, and these aggregates are referred to as **nuclei** or **ganglia.** Regions of the central nervous system in which nerve cell bodies are concentrated appear gray in color because they are not covered with myelin; these sections are referred to as **gray matter.** The central region of the spinal cord contains nerve cell bodies (gray matter) surrounded by tracts of myelinated axons (white matter) (Fig. 3.2). Some tracts carry ascending or sensory impulses whereas others carry descending motor impulses. In the cerebrum, the cell bodies and tract positions reverse; the cortex appears gray because cell bodies of cortical neurons lie in the superficial surface layers. Tissue beneath the gray matter is white because here is where the myelinated axons that connect cortical neurons with other regions of the CNS are located.

Upper motor neurons lie within the central nervous system and carry impulses from the brain to motor neurons in the spinal cord, and **lower motor neurons** of the peripheral nervous system transmit motor impulses from the spinal cord to activate skeletal muscle fibers. Some neurons, termed **interneurons,** reside entirely within the spinal cord and transmit impulses from one neuron to the dendrites or cell body of another neuron nearby.

Most neurons discharge nerve impulses intermittently; that is, the neurons exhibit a level of firing even while at "rest." The frequency of discharge is modified by the influence of other neurons. Both facilitatory and inhibitory stimuli are continually transmitted from motor centers in the brain to interneurons throughout the spinal cord. Motor neurons receive synaptic connections from thousands of other neurons. Whether a given motor neuron becomes more active or less active depends on the net effect of all the facilitatory and inhibitory stimuli that arrive at the motor neuron at any given instant.

Afferent nerves also have various possible connections when they enter the spinal cord. After entering through the dorsal horn of the spinal cord, the sensory axon may give off a branch that synapses with interneurons in the spinal cord. However, the main fiber usually ascends through the spinal cord to synapse with other neurons in the central nervous system. A peripheral neuron with an uninterrupted axon like this is a **first order neuron.** Sensory neurons that receive synaptic input from a peripheral sensory neuron (first order neuron) and then carry the impulse to the brainstem and other lower centers in the central nervous system are **second order neurons.** Second order neurons frequently transmit the impulse to **third order neurons,** which are located in higher centers of the central nervous system.

Muscular System

Cognizant that the nervous and sensory systems constantly coordinate and refine our movements, we next examine muscles in terms of their structure and function. Like nerves, muscles are also excitable and respond dynamically; similarly, just as an action potential occurs as a single excitation and response of a nerve, a muscle twitch results as a single excitation and response of a muscle. (Fig. 3.4).

Structure of Skeletal Muscle

Just as the neuron is the basic element of the nervous system, the muscle fiber is at the core of the muscular system. Although very different from neurons, muscle fibers are also complex in their structure.

Muscle and Muscle Fiber Structure

Each segment of the body contains several skeletal muscles (Fig. 3.5A). A muscle is surrounded by a thin connective tissue covering called **epimysium**. The epimysium helps to keep each muscle separate from adjacent muscles. If we delve into a muscle, we see that another connective tissue layer called perimysium subdivides the muscle. **Perimysium** divides a muscle into sections within the entire muscle. Each subsection of a muscle is a fasciculus (Fig. 3.5B). If we move deeper into the muscle's **fasciculi,** we realize that they are made up of lots of muscle fibers. The muscle fibers are the basic structure of muscle. **Muscle fibers** are **muscle cells**

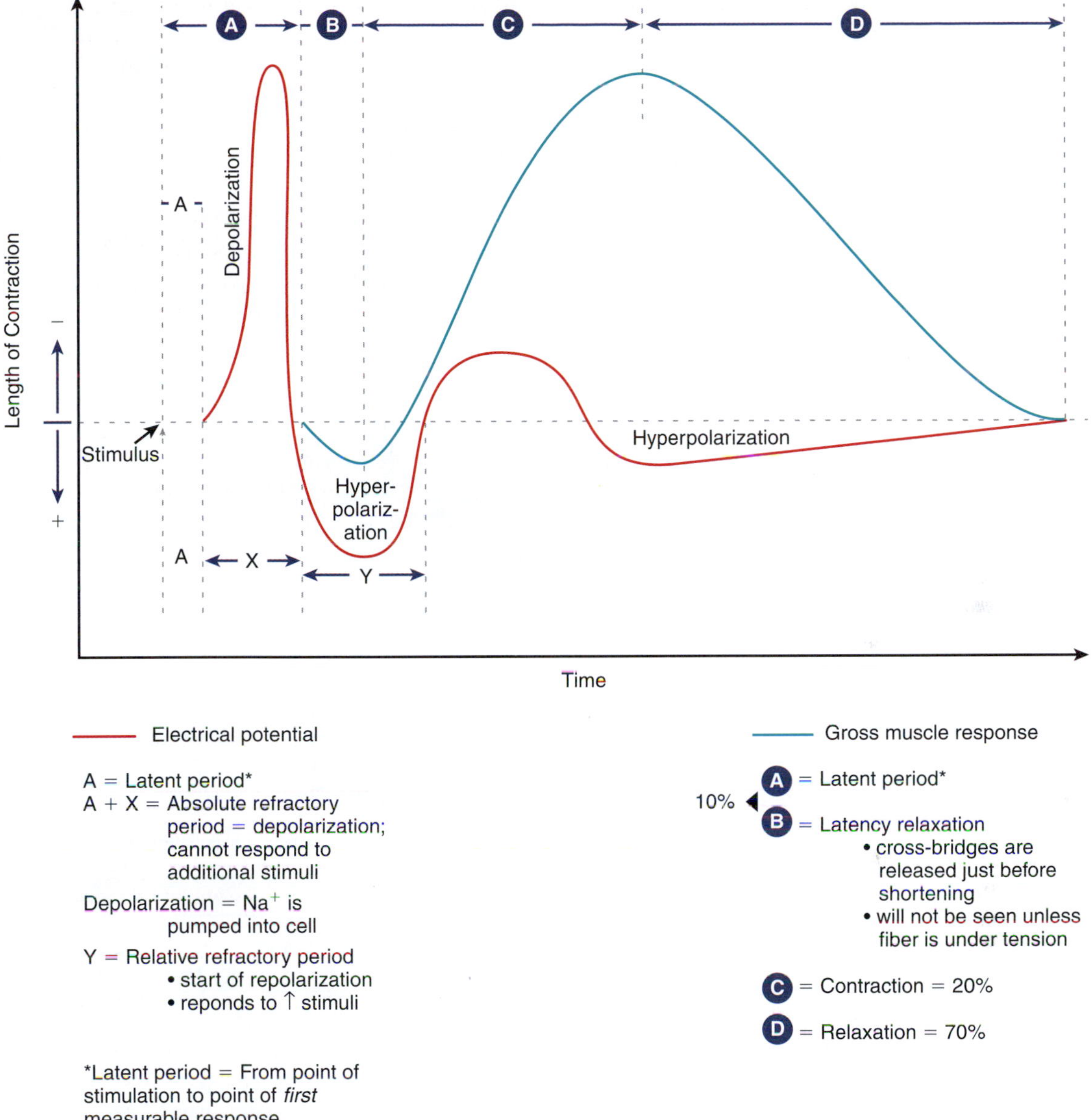

Figure 3.4 Time relationship of the electrical, chemical, and mechanical responses in a simple muscle twitch.

(Fig. 3.5C). Each muscle fiber is made up of multiple rod-like myofibrils, spanning the entire length of the muscle fiber (Fig. 3.5D). **Myofibrils** are bundles of filaments within a muscle fiber; myofibrils are also called **myofilaments.** The length of a muscle fiber varies from a few millimeters to many millimeters. The diameter of an individual muscle fiber ranges from 10 to 100 **micrometers (μm).** Each muscle cell has several nuclei. Each myofibril has a covering or membrane, the **sarcolemma,** and is composed of a gelatin-like substance, sarcoplasm (Fig. 3.5C). Hundreds of muscle fibers and other vital structures, such as mitochondria and the sarcoplasmic reticulum, are imbedded in the sarcoplasm. Mitochondria serve as "tiny factories" where metabolic processes occur.

A myofibril (Fig. 3.5D) is composed of units, and each unit is referred to as a **sarcomere.** A sarcomere lies between two Z-lines. Between these two Z-lines are many myofilaments. **Myofilaments** are made up of fine threads of two protein molecules, **actin** (thin filaments) and **myosin** (thick filaments) (Fig. 3.5E). These two filaments provide skeletal muscle with the appearance of

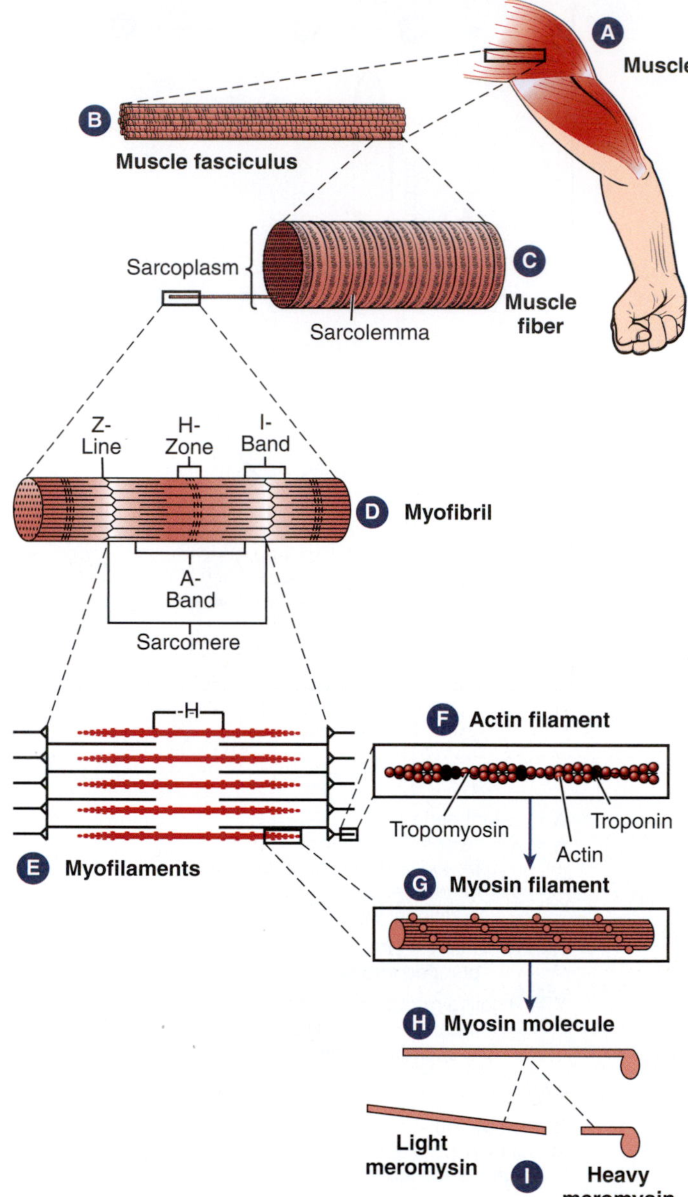

Figure 3.5 Diagram of the organization of skeletal muscle at rest, from **A)** the gross to **E)** the molecular levels. **F, G,** and **H** are cross sections of the myofibrils at the levels indicated. **I** is a diagram of the composition of the myofilaments. (Adapted from Bloom, W, and Fawcett, DW: *A Textbook of Histology,* ed 10. WB Saunders, Philadelphia, 1975, p 306.)

light and dark striations, which is why skeletal muscle is referred to as "striated" muscle. The striations are alternate bands of light and dark light-refractive materials that, when viewed under a microscope, are seen to be alternately lighter and darker bands (Figs. 3.5D).

The darker band in skeletal muscles, referred to as the anisotropic or A-band, contains both actin and myosin filaments (Fig. 3.5F–I). In the three-dimensional arrangement of these filaments, six actin filaments surround each myosin and three myosin filaments (Fig. 3.5) surround each actin filament. A-bands have an isotropic middle zone: the H-band which contains only myosin filaments (Fig. 3.5D, G). The lighter band in skeletal muscle—the isotropic or I-band—contains only actin filaments and is bisected vertically by a Z-line (Fig. 3.5D, F). One end of each actin myofilament within the I-band is anchored to the Z-line.

The thin actin filaments of the I-bands contain two proteins, troponin and tropomyosin (Fig. 3.5F). Actin is polymerized (linked together) to form two-stranded filaments that are twisted together (Fig. 3.5F) to form part of the actin filament. Tropomyosin is a rod-shaped molecule and composed of two separate polypeptide chains that are wound around each other to form a long,

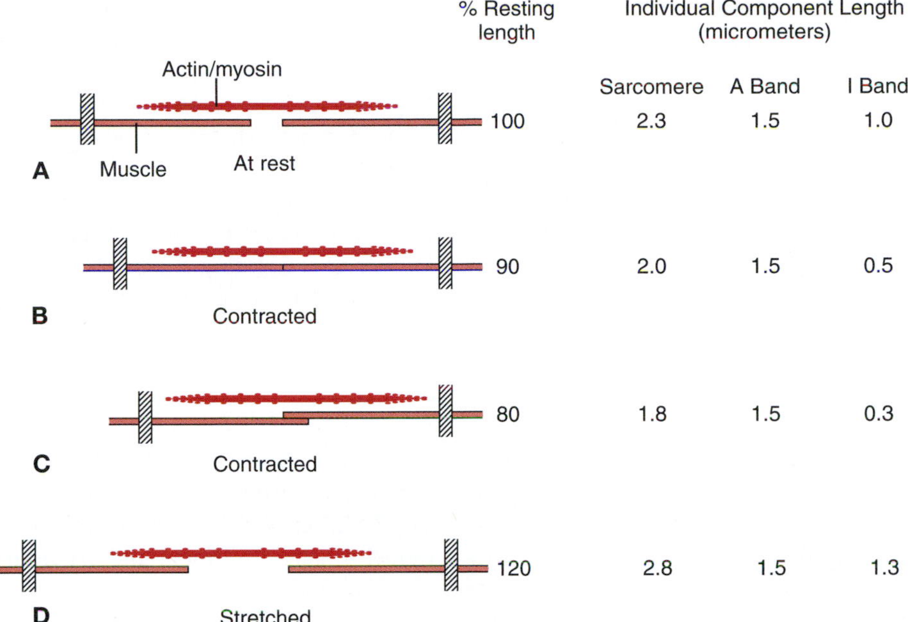

Figure 3.6 The structural basis for changes in muscle length: **A)** A sarcomere at resting length showing changes; **B, C)** in arrangement of filaments under various degrees of contraction; and **D)** when stretched. Relative changes in length of the sarcomere are indicated on the *left*, and the approximate lengths (in micrometers) of the sarcomere, the A-band, and the I-band are listed on the *right*. Note the constancy of the A-band length. (Adapted from Schottelius, BA, and Schottelius, DD: *Textbook of Physiology*, ed 17. St. Louis: CV Mosby, 1973, p 87.)

rigid insoluble chain. Tropomyosin is about 40 nm long. These straight molecules are arranged along the actin filament so one tropomyosin is coupled with approximately six actin molecules (Fig. 3.5F). Troponin is a regulatory protein that is bound to a specific region of the tropomyosin filament. This arrangement provides one troponin globule per 40 nm of tropomyosin filament. Regulatory proteins, such as troponin, impact the interactions between an actin filament and its adjacent myosin filaments. An important function of troponin is based on its enormous avidity for calcium ions (Ca^{++}), a property that is important in activating the contractile process. This arrangement of actin, tropomyosin, and troponin forms the actin filaments in the sarcomere. In simple terms, the functional purpose of actin is to provide a binding site for the myosin during a muscle contraction.

Myosin filaments (Fig. 3.5G) are thicker than actin filaments and are composed of myosin molecules (Fig. 3.5H). Myosin consists of polypeptide chains, one pair of heavy chains and two pairs of lighter chains, which are coiled together into one large chain (Fig. 3.5G-I). Myosin molecules form a rod about 1.6 μm long and 1.5–2.0 nm in diameter, about 1/10,000 of the diameter of a hair from your head. The end of each heavy chain has a globular structure that forms two "heads" of myosin. These heads look similar to the distal end of a hockey stick (Fig. 3.5). These globular heads are at the end of an "arm" portion that is "hinged" to the myosin. These "hinges" allow the arms to project out laterally from the myosin filament and move during muscle activation. These heads are called **crossbridges** because they bridge the thick filaments to the thin filaments during muscle activity (Fig. 3.8). Crossbridges are not present at the central portion of the myosin filament, and the crossbridges on the two halves of the myosin project in opposite directions. These crossbridges align in groups of three called "crowns." Each consecutive crown is positioned such that it is rotated on the myosin from the previous crown. This arrangement provides crossbridges for each actin that is adjacent to the myosin. There are about 300 to 400 crossbridges on a 1.6 μm-long myosin filament.[7] Myosin exhibits enzyme-like qualities capable of splitting adenosine triphosphate (ATP) into adenosine diphosphate (ADP) and phosphate (PO_4) plus energy. The significance of this reaction is discussed in the section dealing with the energetics of muscle contraction.

Muscle Contraction and Relaxation

Investigators using light and electron microscopy have observed relaxed and contracted states of muscle tissue. The length of each serially repeating sarcomere unit is approximately 2.5 μm when the muscle is relaxed (Fig. 3.6A). The length of each sarcomere decreases to about 1.5 μm when the muscle is fully contracted (Fig. 3.6C). In contrast, the sarcomere unit may be increased to about 3.0 μm when the muscle is stretched (Fig. 3.6D).

As mentioned, a sarcomere is secured at each of its ends by a Z-line (Figs. 3.5D and 3.7). Widths of individual A-bands do not change during contraction. However, the I-band where only actin filaments are seen does become narrower, and the H-zone, where only myosin filaments are seen within the A-band, is obliterated. These observations demonstrate that the free ends of the actin filaments slide toward each other into the central H-zone of the A-bands when muscles contract. As the actin filaments move toward each other, the Z-lines are pulled closer together so that the I-bands shorten (Fig. 3.6A, B, C). Although the amount of shortening of each sarcomere unit is small (0.5–1.0 μm) the shortening of several thousands of these sarcomere units linked in series produces a noticeable reduction in the entire muscle's overall length. For example, a muscle fiber 10 cm in length, like the biceps brachii muscle, has approximately 40,000 sarcomere units lined up end to end.* If each of these 40,000 sarcomere units shortened by 1 μm, the ends of the entire muscle fiber would move 40,000 μm (or 4 cm) closer together. Thus, an overall shortening of 40% of the length of the muscle occurs.

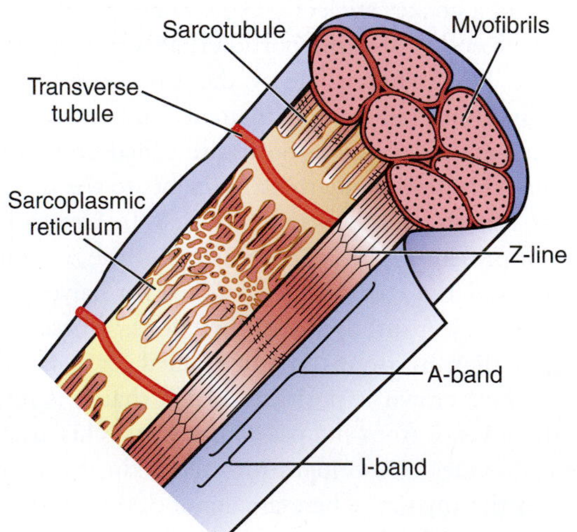

Figure 3.7 Endoplasmic reticulum of the skeletal muscle fiber. Sketch of the fine structure of part of a muscle fiber based on an electron micrograph. The cell membrane invaginates at the level of each Z-line, sending transverse tubules across the interior of the fiber. Between the Z-lines and parallel to the myofibrils runs the sarcoplasmic reticulum, of which saclike enlargements (the terminal cisternae) adjoin the transverse tubules.

This concept of actin and myosin filaments sliding past each other to produce muscle contraction is known as the **sliding filament model** of muscle contraction.[8, 9] The specific way in which actin filaments are drawn past myosin filaments to develop muscle tension and muscular shortening is complex. Simply summarized, however, the myosin's heads attach to and pull on the actin causing the actin filament to slide over the myosin into the H-zone to shorten the sarcomere during muscle contraction (Fig. 3.5 E, Fig. 3.8). Let us delve deeper into the sliding filament model to gain additional understanding of how muscles contract.

Myoneural Junction: Transmission of Impulses from Nerves to Skeletal Muscle Fibers

The nervous system regulates the activity of muscle fibers by sending control signals in the form of action potentials. Conversion of a nerve impulse to a muscle impulse, however, occurs through a complex process. The nerve fiber branches at its end to form a motor end plate, which adheres tightly to surface of the muscle fiber but does not penetrate the muscle fiber membrane (Fig. 3.2). This connection is a type of synapse referred to as the **myoneural** (Gr. *mye,* muscle, plus *neuron,* nerve) **junction,** commonly referred to as the **neuromuscular junction.** The motor neuron end plate contains mitochondria that synthesize a neurotransmitter, acetylcholine. Molecules of acetylcholine are stored in small vesicles located in the presynaptic ending of motor neurons. The arrival of a nerve impulse at the myoneural junction causes release of acetylcholine from some of the vesicles. When freed from storage in the vesicles, acetylcholine diffuses rapidly across the short distance between the motor end plate and muscle fiber membrane. Acetylcholine then interacts with receptor sites on the muscle fiber membrane. The interaction increases the permeability of the muscle cell membrane to ions in the fluid bathing the junction. Movement of these ions into the muscle cell depolarizes the muscle fiber (postjunctional) membrane and triggers a muscle action potential that moves along the muscle fiber by an

*1 cm = 10^4 μm = 10,000 μm; thus, the 10 cm muscle fiber = 100,000 μm in length. 100,000 μm divided by 2.5 μm per sarcomere = 40,000 sarcomere units.

electrochemical mechanism similar to that of a nerve impulse (Fig. 3.4).

After causing increased permeability at the postjunctional membrane, acetylcholine is rapidly inactivated by an enzyme, cholinesterase. Cholinesterase is present in the fluid bathing the synaptic space and immediately splits acetylcholine when it comes in contact with it. The very short time that acetylcholine remains in contact with the muscle fiber membrane, about 2 msec, is usually sufficient to excite the muscle fiber, and yet the rapid inactivation of acetylcholine by cholinesterase prevents re-excitation after the muscle fiber repolarizes.

Conduction of Muscle Impulses to the Interior of the Muscle Fiber: Endoplasmic Reticulum

Change in electrical potential in the immediate vicinity of actin and myosin filaments triggers a process that leads to shortening of each sarcomere. The interior of a muscle fiber contains two interlaced systems of tubes that play an important role in excitation of and contraction of muscle fibers (Fig. 3.7). One system, the **transverse tubular system (T-system),** runs perpendicular to the myofibrils and speeds the transmission of a muscle action potential to all portions of the muscle fiber. The other system, the **sarcoplasmic reticulum (SR),** is found deep to the sarcolemma, running parallel and superficial to the myofibril. The sarcoplasmic reticulum stores and releases calcium ions during the contractile process. The two systems, the transverse tubular system and the sarcoplasmic reticulum, together comprise the **endoplasmic reticulum** (Fig. 3.7).

Excitation-Contraction Coupling

Energy must be supplied to myofilaments to cause movement of the actin filaments toward the center of the A-bands. Energy for this purpose is available from adenosine triphosphate (ATP) molecules, which are coupled to myosin crossbridges. The energy is provided when myosin acts as a **catalyst** to split molecules of ATP into adenosine diphosphate (ADP) and inorganic phosphate (P_i). Calcium stimulates the myosin to split ATP. This process is called myosin **ATPase activity.** The following section describes how this process works.

Sliding Filament Model of Muscle Contraction

A sequential series of events explains how sliding filaments develop tension and shorten (Fig. 3.8). Projections of **crossbridges** are located on the myosin myofilaments. At rest, the crossbridges between myosin and actin myofilaments lie perpendicular to the myosin filaments and are prevented by regulatory mechanisms from making contact with the actin filaments (Fig. 3.8A). Also, at rest, calcium is stored in the SR, and the ATP molecules are coupled near the end of each crossbridge (Fig. 3.8A). Potential reactive sites on actin myofilaments are covered by troponin and, therefore, are not available to the myosin crossbridges.

When a pulse of depolarization descends the T-tubules, quantities of calcium are released from storage sites in the SR. Some of the calcium ions interact with troponin, causing a deformation in the shape of

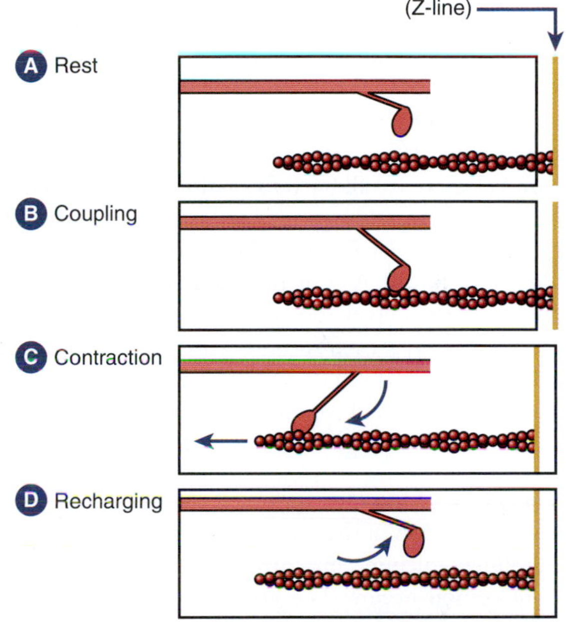

Figure 3.8 The hypothesized sequential series of reactions between active sites on actin and myosin filaments that pull the actin filament along the myosin filament to produce shortening of the sarcomere. The recovery process is also illustrated. Many repetitions of the cycle at a large percentage of the active sites are needed to produce a strong contraction. **A)** Rest. Crossbridges project from a myosin myofilament but are not coupled with an actin myofilament. Adenosine triphosphate (ATP) is attached near the head of the crossbridge; troponin covers the active sites on the actin myofilament; calcium ions are stored in the sarcoplasmic reticulum. **B)** Coupling. Arrival of the muscle action potential depolarizes the sarcolemma and T-tubules; calcium ions are released and react with troponin; change in the shape of the troponin-calcium complex uncovers active sites on actin; a crossbridge couples with an adjacent active site, thereby linking myosin and actin myofilaments. **C)** Contraction. Linkage of a crossbridge and an active site triggers adenosine triphosphatase (ATPase) activity of myosin; ATP splits to adenosine disphosphate (ADP) + PO_4 + energy; the reaction produces a transient flexion of the crossbridge; the actin myofilament is pulled a short distance along the myosin myofilament; Z-lines are moved closer together. **D)** Recharging. The crossbridge uncouples from the active site and retracts; ATP is replaced on the crossbridge. The recoupling, flexion, uncoupling, retraction, and recharging processes are repeated hundreds of times per second.

the troponin molecule (Fig. 3.8B). The changes in shape caused by the interaction of calcium with troponin uncover an active site on the thin actin filament that electrostatically attracts the myosin crossbridge. So, in the presence of calcium, myosin and actin are attracted to each other and a globular head of a myosin filament and an active site on an actin filament forms an actomyosin crossbridge. The actomyosin crossbridge, in turn, triggers the ATPase activity of myosin to cause ATP to split into ADP plus phosphate and produce energy. This chemical energy is converted into mechanical energy by the muscle cell to produce motion. Mechanically, this ATP hydrolysis (split into ADP and P_i) produces transient "flexion" of the crossbridge (Fig. 3.8C), which pulls the actin filament a short distance. Once this motion occurs, the ADP and P_i are released to allow reformation of ATP which binds once again to myosin. In the presence of ATP, the myosin's affinity for actin diminishes and linkage is broken (Fig. 3.8D). A cycle of coupling, flexion, uncoupling, retraction, recharging, and recoupling repeats hundreds of times each second as long as calcium and ATP are present. If either calcium is removed from the myoplasm or the ATP supply is exhausted, the cycle of actomyosin crossbridge formation and release ceases.

Muscle Relaxation

As depolarization of the muscle fiber ends (5–10 msec), intracellular calcium concentration drops very quickly, and relaxation occurs. The rapid drop in intracellular calcium results from an active "pumping" of calcium ions from the region of the myofilaments back into the SR storage sites. Active transport of calcium against a concentration gradient continues until the concentration of calcium remaining in the intracellular fluid bathing the myofilaments reaches a very low resting-condition level. Removal of calcium ions from the vicinity of the actin filaments results in the troponin returning to its original shape, covering the active sites on the actin filament; thus, the actin and myosin filaments return to their "resting," relaxed state. In effect, an insufficient concentration of intracellular calcium ceases actin and myosin myofilament interaction.

Muscle Fiber Types

To most efficiently perform various functions, different types of skeletal muscle fiber exist. Early research of muscle fibers classified an entire muscle as either fast or slow, based on speeds of shortening.[10, 11] With more recent investigations, an expansion in identification of main fiber types has evolved to include two types: type I and type II, with a further subdivision of type II into type IIa, and type IIb.[10, 11] Some investigators have described a more detailed breakdown of fiber types,[11-14] but, for the purpose of this text, only the two main types of muscle fibers are discussed. Each type of fiber has different properties. Most skeletal muscles contain a mixture of both types, with the proportion of one type more predominant than the other type in a muscle. More importantly, the functional unit of muscle contraction, the **motor unit**, which includes the alpha motor nerve and all of the muscle fibers that it innervates, can be classified based on contractile speed, as detailed below.[10, 15, 16]

The **type I** muscle fiber appears dark (like the dark meat of a domestic chicken*) because it contains large numbers of mitochondria and a high concentration of myoglobin. Myoglobin is muscle hemoglobin that stores oxygen. Type I also is referred to as **slow-twitch, tonic**, or **slow oxidative (SO)**, because biochemically, these fibers depend on aerobic or oxidative energy metabolism.[11, 12, 18]

The **type II** muscle fiber appears paler (like the white meat of a domestic chicken*) because it contains fewer mitochondria and only small amounts of myoglobin. Type II, further subdivided into IIa and IIb, are fiber

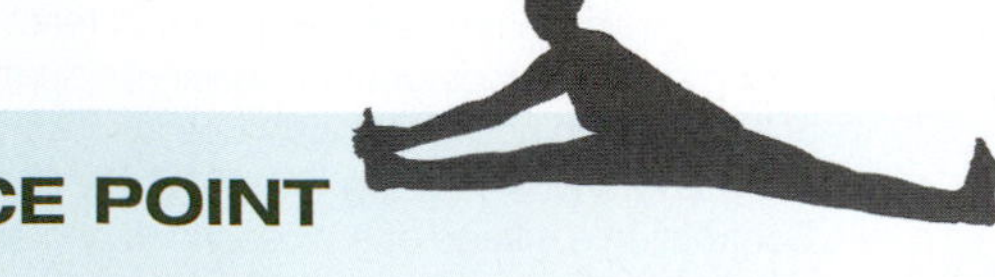

PRACTICE POINT

Live muscle has a continual availability of ATP for muscle activity. Rigor mortis is a condition caused by a lack of ATP with an arrest of the actomyosin crossbridge cycle with attachment of the two myofilaments in the presence of calcium. Since there is no ATP, the actin and myosin filaments remain attached until muscle tissue begins decomposing. Rigor mortis is a condition that occurs around 3 hours after death and remains to some degree for up to 72 hours.

* A different situation exists in birds that predominantly fly.

types that are fast-twitch in their contractile speed but which rely on glycolytic (anaerobic) processes and oxidative (aerobic) metabolic processes. Type II muscle fibers, also termed **fast-twitch, phasic,** or **fast glycolytic (FG)** or **fast oxidative glycolytic (FOG)**, are larger in diameter than type I muscle fibers. Type IIa are the fast oxidative glycolytic and type IIb are the fast glycolytic. Type IIa fibers may seem like a "transition" fiber type between the slow oxidative type I and the fast glycolytic type IIb since it possesses characteristics of each. Type IIb fibers develop a greater contraction force and complete a single twitch in a significantly shorter time than type I muscle fibers. Type IIb fibers, however, fatigue more quickly than type I fibers. Type I fibers are innervated by small diameter axons of the motor nerve and are recruited first in a muscle contraction. On the other hand, type IIb fibers are innervated by larger diameter motor axons and are recruited after type I and type IIa fibers.[17] Table 3–2 summarizes the characteristics of each fiber type.

All human muscles contain various proportions of these different types of muscle fibers. Postural muscles such as the soleus and erector spinae, which are vital for stabilizing the body in positions such as standing for long periods of time, are largely composed of type I fibers, whereas muscles involved in large or quick bursts of activity, such as the biceps brachii, are composed largely of type IIb fibers. Some investigators suggest that the proportions of fast-twitch and slow-twitch muscle fibers in a particular muscle can vary from subject to subject.[20-23] Despite subject-to-subject variation, the proportion of slow-twitch (type I) fibers is high in postural control muscles such as the human soleus muscle in the leg (as great as 85% of the fibers) and low in quick-moving, refined movement muscles such as in the orbicularis oculi of the eyeball (10%).[18] Generally, the more type I muscle fibers contained within a muscle, the more it provides postural stability, and the more type IIb fibers contained within a muscle, the more it provides rapid movement over short periods.

Muscle fiber development and adaptation are good examples of how the movement system can change in response to the demands placed upon it. Muscle fibers can adapt to changing demands by changing ratios of fiber types within muscles.[10, 19] For example, type II fibers are predominant at birth, as evidenced by the characteristically quick jerky movements typical of a newborn baby. As the infant develops postural control, an increase in type I fibers occurs. By the time the child is about 2 years old and has upright postural control, balance, and antigravity control, the ratio of type I and II fiber types is similar to the ratio seen in adults.[1, 20] Muscle fiber development and adaptation is also illustrated in children with developmental disabilities such as cerebral palsy, who demonstrate differences in the morphological properties of skeletal muscle.[21] Fiber types change again with aging, resulting in decreases in the total number of both fiber type I and type II fibers and selective atrophy of the type II fibers, and conversion of fiber types.[10, 22-27] These age-associated changes are correlated with some of the declines in motor performance seen in older persons, such as decreased

TABLE 3–2 | CHARACTERISTICS OF SKELETAL MUSCLE FIBERS BASED ON PHYSICAL AND METABOLIC PROPERTIES

Muscle Fiber Type Property	Type I Slow-Twitch SO	Type IIA Intermediate FOG	Type IIB Fast-Twitch FG
Muscle fiber diameter	Small	Intermediate	Large
Color	Red (dark)	Red	White (pale)
Myoglobin content	High	High	Low
Mitochondria	Numerous	Numerous	Few
Oxidative enzymes	High	Intermediate	Low
Glycolytic enzymes	Low	Intermediate	High
Glycogen content	Low	Intermediate	High
Myosin ATPase activity	Low	High	High
Major source of ATP	Oxidative phosphorylation	Oxidative phosphorylation	Glycolysis
Speed of contraction	Slow	Intermediate	Fast
Rate of fatigue	Slow	Intermediate	Fast

SO = slow oxidative; FG = fast glycolytic; FOG = fast oxidative-glycolytic.
Source: Burke, RE and Edgerton, VR. Motor unit properties and selective involvement in movement. *Exer Sport Sci Rev* 3:31, 1975.[107] Adapted with permission.

postural control, coordination and dexterity challenges, along with functional problems such as **hypokinesis** (decreased activity) and frequent falls. There is evidence to indicate that muscle fiber types can change from fast- to slow-twitch fibers with exercise or electrical stimulation.[21, 28] Conversely, muscles that experience disuse demonstrate a transformation in the opposite direction, from slow to fast.[21,28]

This fluctuation of fiber type has implications for rehabilitation, serving as the physiological basis for numerous therapeutic and exercise science intervention programs. Although a fiber-type specification within individuals is thought to be genetically determined, training and rehabilitation can alter contractile and metabolic properties of muscle fibers, allowing for improved responses to functional demands. For example, placing a high metabolic demand on muscle, such as in endurance training, results in an increased oxidative capacity for all muscle fiber types and leads to a conversion from fast glycolytic to fast oxidative glycolytic muscle fibers. In other words, percentages of pure type IIb fibers decrease and the percentages of type IIa fibers increase with endurance training.[12, 34, 35] Researchers have found that the type I fibers become faster and type II fibers convert to slower, more oxidative types with endurance exercise. The converse is also true with type I fibers becoming more plentiful and slower with deconditioning.[29-31]

The Motor Unit

Motor neurons that activate efferent motor responses are located either in the brainstem or in the spinal cord. Those in the brainstem are for the muscles of the face and head, and those in the spinal cord send impulses to the muscles of the neck, trunk, and extremities. Specifically, the motor neurons in the spinal cord are located in the gray matter of the ventral (anterior) horns (Fig. 3.2). Various types of motor neurons exist. The majority, if not all, of the neurons that innervate skeletal muscles are within the A, alpha (α), size classification, and known as **alpha (α) motor neurons**. Motor commands travel from the neuronal cell bodies over peripheral nerve fibers and then across the neuromuscular junction. The number of muscle fibers innervated by a single motor nerve fiber varies from as few as five, as in some of the eye muscles, to as many as 1,000 or more, as in large muscles such as the gastrocnemius. The more control required of a muscle, the fewer muscle fiber to nerve fiber ratios a muscle has. On the other hand, muscles that produce large forces without the need for fine control have much larger ratios of muscle fibers to nerve fibers. The number of motor units and the average number of muscle fibers per motor unit are later summarized in Table 3–3.

As the term "motor unit" implies, all muscle fibers act as one unit, contracting or relaxing nearly simultaneously. Muscle fibers of one motor unit are not adjacent to one another; they are distributed throughout the muscle's length. In addition, if the motor unit's nerve activates its muscle fibers to contract, those fibers will contract maximally. This principle is the **all-or-none law.**

Gradation of Strength of Muscle Contraction

Increased strength of a muscle contraction, as a whole, occurs in three ways and is based on different principles:

- Size principle: The smallest motor units are activated first.
- Recruitment principle: Increasing the number of motor units activated simultaneously increases the overall muscle tension.
- Excitatory input/rate coding principle: Increasing the frequency of stimulation of individual motor units increases the percentage of time that each active muscle fiber develops maximum tension

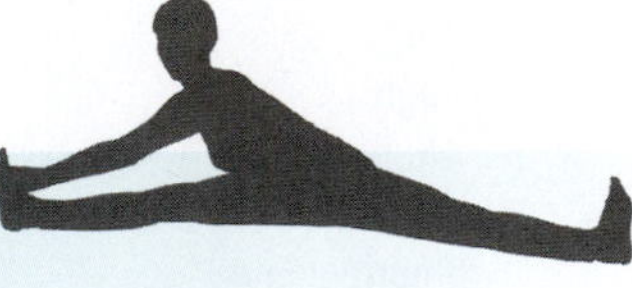

PRACTICE POINT

Changes in fiber type composition may also be at least partially responsible for some of the impairments and disabilities seen in older persons. As the elderly remain active and experience injuries, the clinician must realize that muscle fiber compositions in this age group will require changes in rehabilitation expectations in areas such as maximal strength or balance abilities. Evidence indicates that strength exercises are beneficial for older persons and these individuals will experience the same types of gains as younger individuals, but the maximal level will be lower than younger patients.[32] Additionally, exercise interventions, especially endurance training, can affect muscle fiber types leading to improvements in conditioning, balance, and performance.[33]

The size principle of recruitment describes the fact that the smallest motor neurons are the first to be recruited and the largest motor neurons are recruited last.[38] Small motor neurons participate in most sustained activities because they tend to innervate the slow-twitch, type I muscle fibers that fatigue slowly. When muscle functions require greater strength, the largest fast-twitch and more quickly fatiguing motor units become active. In terms of recruitment order, the smaller motor units are recruited first. Since these smaller motor units have fewer muscle fibers per nerve, more must be recruited to produce force of a specific level. For example, if a small motor unit is able to produce 0.05 kg, it would take 100 small motor units to produce 5 kg of force. On the other hand, the large motor units produce greater force since there are a greater number of muscle fibers in each motor unit. For example, if a large motor unit is able to produce 0.20 kg, 100 large motor units would produce 20 kg of force. Of course, these numbers are exaggerated, but they serve to explain the concept. In summary, a muscle successively fires its small motor units first. Once those units are all recruited, the larger motor units are recruited in order of their size from smallest large unit to the largest large motor unit. In other words, motor units are normally recruited in an orderly pattern with those which produce low force recruited first, followed by higher force-producing units as force requirements increase.[39]

Firing of a single motor unit results in a twitch contraction of the stimulated muscle fibers. With an increase in firing rate, these twitches summate to increase and sustain a force output. An individual increases muscle force by increasing both the number of active motor units and the firing rates of those active motor units.

Joint, Tendon, and Muscle Receptors

Specialized receptors are present in joint structures, tendons, and skeletal muscles. Because these afferent receptors gather information about one's own joints and joint movements, they are called **proprioceptors** (L. *proprio*, one's own, plus *captive*, to receive). These receptors detect changes in tension and position of the structures in which the receptors are situated. A pattern of nerve impulses is generated in the receptor and transmitted to other parts of the nervous system. As a result, moment-to-moment changes in joint angle (position of the joint), speed of joint motion, amount of joint compression or distraction, as well as changes in muscle length, rate of change in muscle length, and force of muscle contraction are relayed to centers in the spinal cord and brain. In the central nervous system, this information is integrated with that coming in from other sensory organs. Additional sensory organs include the eye's retina and the inner ear's vestibular apparatus, both of which provide input on position, balance, and motion. Integrated sensory signals then are used by motor control centers in the brain to automatically adjust the location, type, number, and frequency of motor unit activation so that appropriate muscle tension is developed to perform desired movements.

Joint Receptors

Several different types of sensory receptors are in joint capsules and ligaments. The major anatomic features of various sensory receptors are illustrated in Figure 3.9. Most of these receptors emit several action potentials per second as a "resting" output, so the body always has a sense of position in space. The receptor is stimulated when it is deformed. Depending on the location and magnitude of deforming forces acting on the joint and receptor location, certain receptors are stimulated and discharge a high-frequency burst of nerve impulses when the joint moves. Receptors typically adapt, which means that the frequency of impulses decreases after movement ceases and then transmit a steady train of nerve impulses thereafter. Further movement of the joint may cause one set of receptors to stop discharging impulses and another set to become active. This continual flow of information allows the nervous system to continually appraise joint position and of the rate of joint movement.

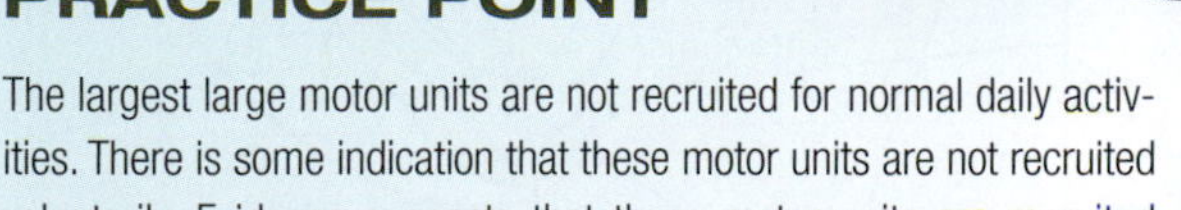

PRACTICE POINT

The largest large motor units are not recruited for normal daily activities. There is some indication that these motor units are not recruited voluntarily. Evidence suggests that these motor units are recruited during times of extreme stress. During these times the autonomic system provides extraordinary functions such as when a nonathletic individual jumps an 8-foot fence to save someone in a house fire.

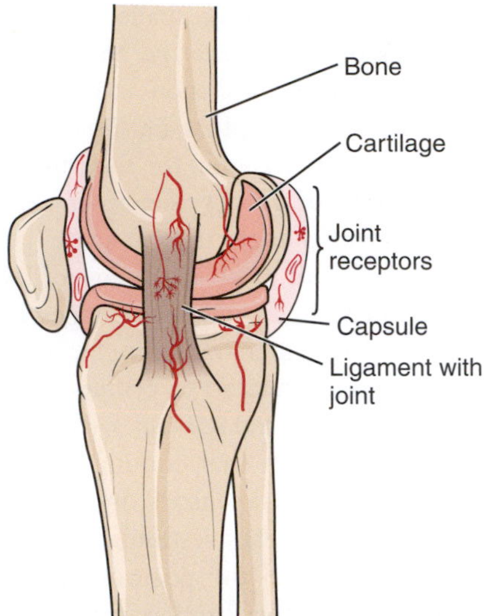

Figure 3.9 Schematic illustration of types of receptors that are usually distinguished in joints. A diagram of the knee joint, showing the distribution of various receptor types in the capsule and ligaments of the joint. The menisci are free from nerve fibers except at their attachment to the fibrous capsule.

Golgi Tendon Organs

Golgi tendon organs (GTOs) lie within muscle tendons near the point of their attachment to the muscle (Fig. 3.10). An average of 10 to 15 muscle fibers is usually connected in direct line with each GTO. Because they are oriented in line (or in series) with the collagen fibers of the tendon and the muscle fibers, the GTO is ideally suited to detect force or tension in either muscle or tendinous collagen fibers but not changes in muscle length.[40] The GTO is stimulated by tension produced within the muscle fibers or the collagenous tendon to which it is attached. Physiologic data indicate that the GTO responds through force-related neural discharge because it is selectively sensitive to the forces produced by in-series muscle fibers. Nerve impulses discharged by the Golgi tendon organ are transmitted over large, rapidly conducting afferent axons (group Ib fibers) to the spinal cord and cerebellum. In turn, several efferent messages are dispatched. These efferent messages go to the agonist (contracting) muscle to inhibit it and to that muscle's antagonist to facilitate it. Inhibiting the agonist limits that muscle's force production to a level that can be tolerated by the tissues being stressed by the contraction. The GTOs thereby mediate nonreciprocal inhibition, or **autogenic inhibition,** referring to this inhibitory input to an agonist muscle (prime mover) and an excitatory message to the antagonist (opposing) muscle.

Muscle Spindles

Skeletal muscles are composed of **extrafusal** (L. *extra,* outside of or in addition, plus *fusus,* spindle) **fibers,** which are "regular" or skeletal muscle fibers. Lying within muscles, parallel to the extrafusal fibers, are unique proprioceptors called **muscle spindles,** so named for their shape. These small but complex organs have multiple functions, both sensory and motor in nature.

Very specialized muscle fibers, called **intrafusal muscle fibers (IFMF),** lie within muscle spindles. Each muscle spindle contains 3 to 10 of these specialized muscle fibers. The intrafusal fibers of the muscle spindle are encapsulated within a connective tissue sheath

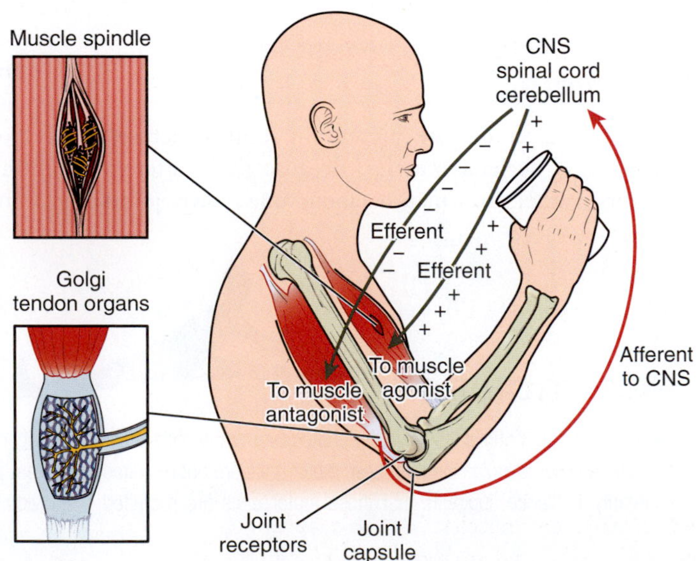

Figure 3.10 A schema to illustrate the anatomic relations among extrafusal muscle fibers, a motor unit, a muscle spindle and a Golgi tendon organ with the attached afferent projection. The force or tension produced by contracting the extrafusal muscle fibers causes the structural fiber network (collagen and elastin) to collapse around the Golgi tendon organ and the muscle spindle to be activated. The muscle spindle activates the agonist while inhibiting the antagonist whereas the Golgi tendon organ does the opposite: inhibits the agonist and activates the antagonist.

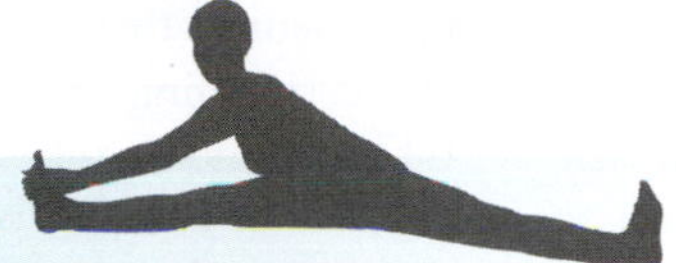

PRACTICE POINT

Autogenic inhibition can be effectively applied to therapeutic stretching techniques, especially in situations in which the patient is extremely anxious about movement due to pain. Stretch the muscle to the end of the range and then ask the client to actively isometrically contract the muscle against your resistance. The muscle will then relax temporarily due to the GTO and stretching into an increased range becomes facilitated. In this technique, called hold-relax, the limb is held by the clinician at the end of the muscle's range of motion (for example, the hamstrings), and the patient is asked to perform an isometric or "holding" contraction at that point in the motion. After the ensuing relaxation of the isometric hold, the limb is then more easily moved into the newly achieved range.[1, 41]

(Fig. 3.11). There are two types of morphological arrangements of the intrafusal fiber nuclei: nuclear bag and nuclear chain fibers. These intrafusal fiber names describe their specific anatomical configuration.[42, 43] The nuclear bag intrafusal muscle fiber has its nuclei grouped in the middle (looks like a bag) of the fiber, whereas the nuclear chain has its nuclei spread along its length, in a chain-like arrangement. Both the nuclear bag and the nuclear chain are surrounded in a spiral fashion by branches of an Ia (also called primary sensory ending) afferent neuron. A secondary neuron ending is formed by group II afferent fibers and found primarily on nuclear chain fibers.[44]

Two types of gamma (γ) axons supply the nuclear fibers with motor innervation. The static gamma motor nerve axons supply the nuclear chain fibers, and the dynamic gamma motor nerve axons supply the nuclear bag fibers. These gamma nerve axons are narrower than the alpha motor axons supplying the extrafusal muscle fibers, so intrafusal muscle fibers respond slower to stimuli than do the extrafusal muscle fibers. However, this unique anatomy illustrates that muscle spindles have both sensory and motor functions.

Focus on the Sensory Function of the Muscle Spindle

As part of the afferent or sensory system, muscle spindles function as a stretch receptor. Muscle spindles send sensory impulses over the Ia and II afferent axons that "inform" other neurons in the spinal cord and brain of their length and, therefore, of the length of the extrafusal muscle and of the rate at which a muscle stretch occurs. This muscle spindle's receptor function transpires because of its parallel alignment with the extrafusal muscle fibers. Therefore, a change in the intrafusal fiber length is associated with a change in the extrafusal fiber's length.

There are varying numbers of muscle spindles located within different muscles. Muscle spindles are present in skeletal muscle and are most numerous in the muscles of

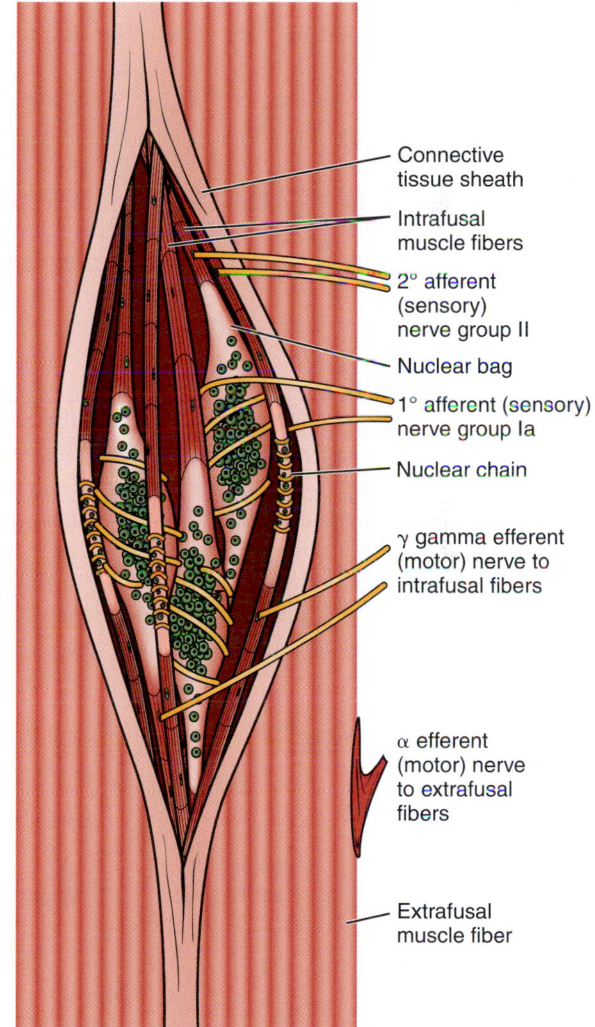

Figure 3.11 The muscle spindle. This diagram shows the anatomic relationships among the major components of a muscle spindle. Although most muscle spindles contain 3 to 10 intrafusal fibers, for simplicity, only 3 sets are shown. Nuclear bag fibers and nuclear chain fibers also are pictured, as well as the afferent and efferent nerve supplies. Extrafusal muscle fibers alongside the muscle spindle and an α motor neuron to the extrafusal fiber also are shown.

the arms and legs (Table 3–3). Muscle spindles are especially abundant in the small muscles of the eye, hand, and foot; all of these muscles have a very high muscle spindle density because of the need for these muscles to be constantly alerted to even small changes.

As a muscle lengthens or shortens, the degree of stretching or relaxation of its intrafusal fibers alters the activity in the Ia and II sensory fibers that innervate them. The Ia afferent fiber detects both the amount of stretch and the velocity of the stretch, thereby exhibiting qualities of both **phasic** (Gr. *Phasis,* an appearance, a distinct stage or phase) and **tonic** (Gr. *tonikos,* continuous tension) activity. On the other hand, the secondary (II) receptor is purely tonic, responding primarily to the amount of stretch. Therefore, the primary and secondary receptors behave differently. As the muscle contracts or stretches to change the length of its extrafusal muscle fibers, its muscle spindles detect this length change and depolarize the Ia afferent sensory nerve wrapped around each muscle spindle. This Ia nerve also has a critical velocity threshold, so it also detects a length change but only if this change exceeds a certain rate or velocity. When this sensory nerve notes a muscle stretch of a sufficient velocity and depolarizes, it sends impulses into the dorsal horn (where all sensory information enters the spinal cord), where it connects with other neurons. Via a monosynaptic reflex, it makes a direct connection to an efferent nerve, an alpha motor neuron (in the anterior horn cell), which then transmits a signal back to the extrafusal muscle fibers in the same muscle as the muscle spindle. This process ceases when the stretch ends. Another pathway the incoming sensory afferent nerve takes is an additional connection through an interneuron (disynaptic) to a different efferent alpha motor neuron that transmits a signal to the antagonist muscle, signaling that muscle to relax.

The monosynaptic component of this example is also known as the deep tendon reflex or **stretch (or myotatic) reflex,** a simple reflex arc mediated at the spinal cord level. Afferent nerves (group Ia) from the primary receptor make an immediate synaptic connection with the motor neurons (A, α motor neurons) that control extrafusal muscle fibers in the same muscle. Therefore, an abrupt stretch of a muscle initiates a burst of impulses from the primary stretch receptor in the muscle spindle, which travels to the spinal cord and excites activity in motor units of the same muscle (Fig. 3.12). We have all experienced this reflex connection when a doctor tests it by tapping a reflex hammer on a muscle tendon. When a muscle shortens, the stretch on the muscle and its muscle spindles is relieved, thereby removing the stretch receptor stimulus.

The neural and muscular structures that participate in the stretch reflex are illustrated using a patellar tendon tap in Figure 3.12. The presence of a reflex contraction in the stretched muscle 100 to 200 msec after tapping the tendon demonstrates an intact circuit. In addition, the briskness and relative amplitude of the reflex contraction reflect the general level of excitability of α motor neurons innervating the stretched muscle.

Focus on the Motor Function of the Muscle Spindle

As mentioned earlier, the cell bodies of the gamma (γ) efferent nerves are located in the ventral or anterior horn of the spinal cord. These gamma cells receive synaptic connections and influences from regions throughout the nervous system including the cortex, cerebellum, and

TABLE 3–3 | NUMBER OF MOTOR UNITS, MOTOR FIBERS, AND MUSCLE SPINDLES PER MOTOR UNIT IN HUMAN MUSCLE

		NUMBER OF MUSCLE FIBERS		NUMBER OF MUSCLE SPINDLES	
Muscle	**Number of Motor Axons**	**Per Muscle × 10^3**	**Average Per Motor Unit**	**Per Muscle**	**Per Motor Unit**
Biceps brachii	774	580	750	320	0.4
Brachioradialis	330	130	390	65	0.2
First dorsal interosseus	119	41	340	34	0.3
First lumbrical	98	10	110	53	0.6
Opponens pollicis	133	79	595	44	0.3
Masseter	1020	1000	980	160	0.2
Temporalis	1150	1500	1300	217	0.2
Gastrocnemius medius	580	1000	1720	80	0.1
Tibialis anterior	445	270	610	284	0.6

Source: Adapted from Buchthal, F, Schmalbruch, H. Motor unit of mammalian muscle. *Physiol Rev* 60:95, 1980.[108]

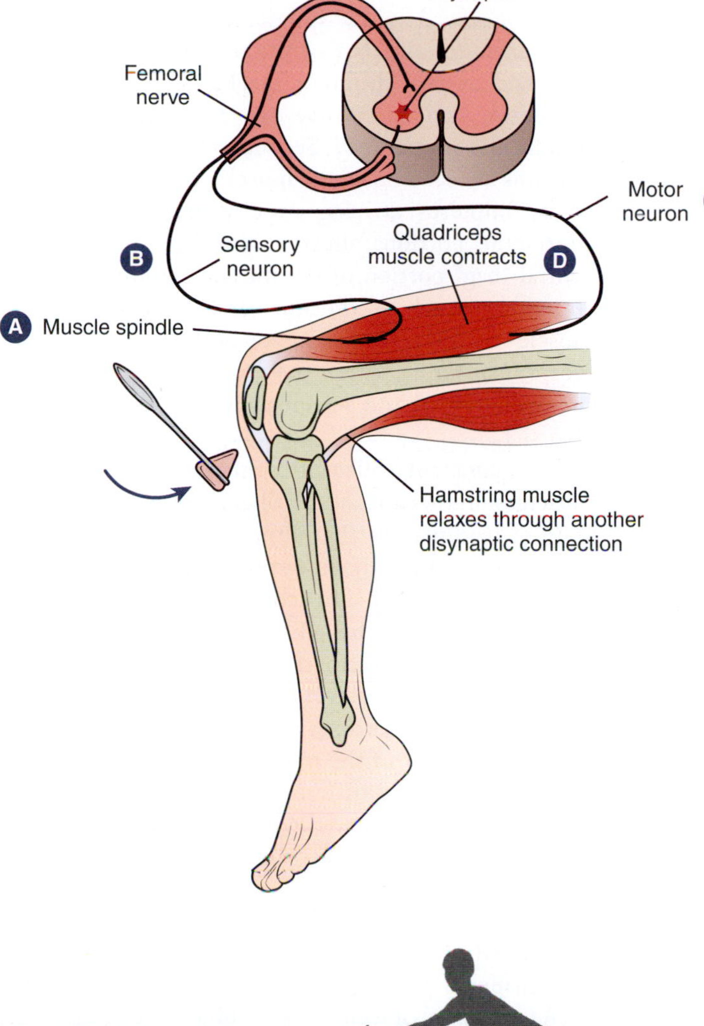

Figure 3.12 The stretch reflex elicited upon a tendon tap. Four fundamental parts of the simple stretch reflex arc are: A) A receptor in the muscle generates nerve impulses in proportion to the degree of deformation; B) An afferent neuron conducts the burst of sensory impulses from the receptor to the spinal cord; C) An efferent neuron conducts motor impulses from the spinal cord to extrafusal muscle fibers; and D) An effector, the muscle, responds to the motor impulses.

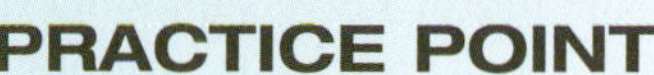

PRACTICE POINT

Active and passive stretching techniques utilize the neuroanatomical connections described above. These connections provide the basis for the rationale behind active stretching, whereby a patient is asked to actively contract a muscle to shut off its opposing muscle so the "shut off" muscle's stretch is more effective. For example, if a patient actively contracts the quadriceps muscles, an induced relaxation of the hamstrings occurs, allowing a more effective stretch of the hamstrings. In addition to the benefits of improved stretching of a tight muscle resulting from this neural reciprocation is the fact that this agonistic muscle contraction with concomitant antagonistic relaxation provides important functional ramifications. This is known as **reciprocal inhibition** and allows for some of the fluidity seen in movement. For example, when the quadriceps is activated to deliver a forceful kick, the hamstrings receive signals to relax during midrange and are activated again at the end of range to slow the motion and prevent injury (Fig. 3.13 and 3.14).

brainstem. The amount of shortening of the contractile portions of the muscle spindle regulates the stretch receptor portion of the muscle spindle. With extrafusal shortening, the length of the spindle is correspondingly adjusted to maintain its sensitivity to additional changes in length or stretch. This relationship is a highly important property of muscle spindles. In essence, as α motor neurons stimulate the contraction of extrafusal fibers, γ motor neurons discharge, causing contraction of the intrafusal (muscle spindle) fibers. The contraction of the intrafusal fibers adjusts the sensitivity range for changing lengths of the muscle.

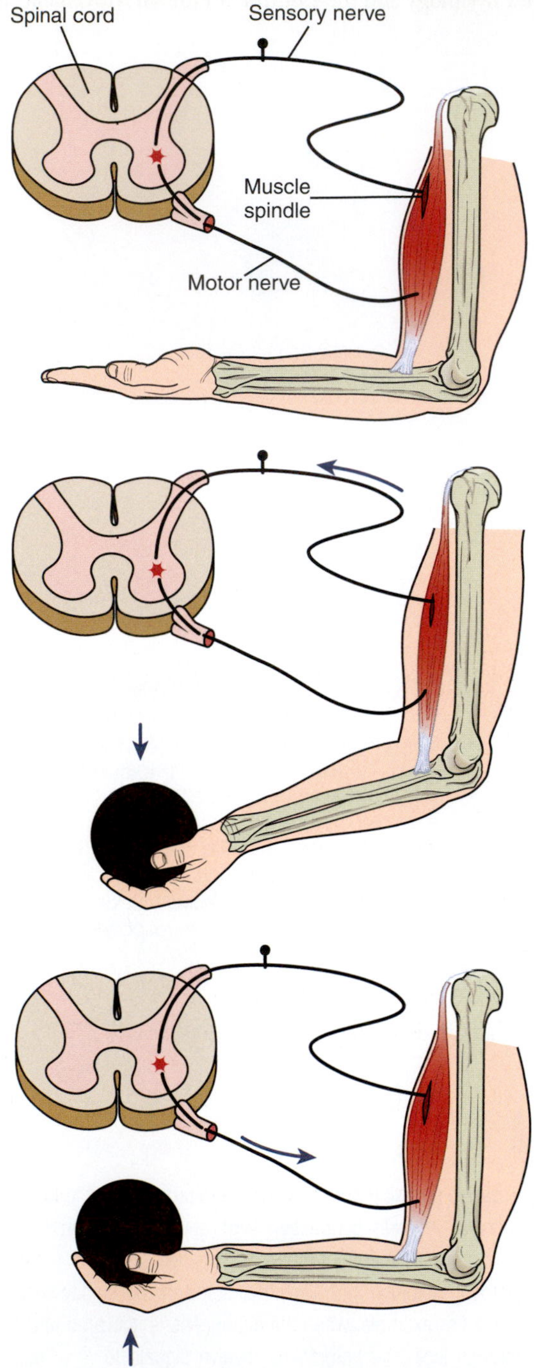

Figure 3.13 Schematic representation of the stretch reflex regulation of muscle length. A muscle is under the influence of the stretch reflex when the muscle is engaged in a steady contraction of a voluntary nature, as when a person's elbow is flexed steadily. A sudden unexpected increase in the load stretches the muscle, causing the sensory ending on the muscle spindle to send nerve impulses to the spinal cord, where the impulses contact a motor nerve cell at the synapse and excite it. As a result, motor impulses are sent back to the muscle, where the impulses cause the muscle to contract. More complicated nerve pathways than the one shown may also be involved in the stretch reflex. Any actual muscle is, of course, supplied with many motor nerve fibers and spindles. In addition, the synaptic connections to even a single motor neuron are multiple.

Gamma motor neurons also are referred to as **fusimotor** (L. *fusus,* a spindle plus *movere,* to move) neurons because the neurons supply motor impulses to the intrafusal muscle spindle fibers. Thus, the middle, noncontractile part of the muscle spindle can be stretched by two different mechanisms. First, when the entire skeletal muscle is stretched, the muscle spindle also is stretched. Second, when the contractile portions at each end of the muscle spindle are activated by impulses arriving over γ motor nerves, the contractile portions shorten, thereby stretching the central "bag" portion of the muscle spindle. In either situation, stretch of the nuclear bag portion of the muscle spindle activates one or both types of sensory receptors residing within the muscle spindle—that is, the primary (Ia) and secondary (II) stretch receptors (Fig. 3.11).

This constant volley of regulatory input onto the muscle spindle's intrafusal fibers sets up a constant state of readiness so that although the muscle is not activated, it is literally on a steady state of alert, ready to act when needed. This constant state of readiness is called **muscle tone,** characterized by an innate amount of muscle stiffness and resting tension. Tone is determined by the level of excitability of the entire pool of motor neurons controlling a muscle, the intrinsic **stiffness** of the muscle itself, and the level of sensitivity of many different reflexes. The contribution of the muscle spindle is only one piece of the puzzle contributing to the phenomenon called muscle tone.

Normal muscles exhibit a firmness to palpation, considered to be typical or "normal" muscle tone. The firmness present in muscles is observed at rest, even in muscles of well-relaxed subjects. The firmness, however, is impaired if the motor nerve supplying the muscle is not intact or the muscle is atrophied. Relaxed muscles exhibit at least a palpable amount of muscle tone, but investigators have failed to detect any muscle action potentials to account for this tone.[45-47] Thus, the tone of relaxed muscles in persons with an intact neuromusculoskeletal system appears to be the result of basic physical properties of muscle, such as elasticity, viscosity, plasticity, and the innate stiffness of the tissue.

Postural tone is a term used to describe the development of muscular tension in specific muscles that maintain body segments in their proper relationships to maintain posture. Postural tone is accompanied by recordable electrical activity from active motor units. Muscles used most often to maintain an erect position of the body are **antigravity muscles.** Muscles of the trunk, flexor muscles of the upper extremities, and extensor muscles of the lower extremities are considered antigravity muscles. Motor centers supply nerve

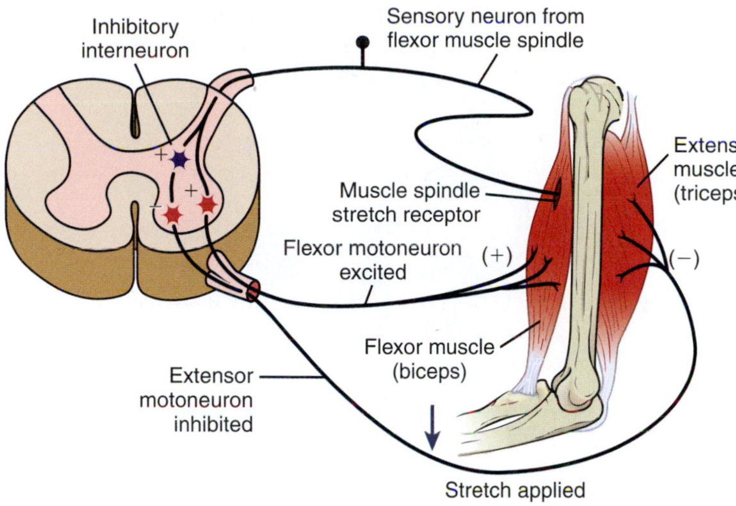

Figure 3.14 Schematic representation of the reciprocal inhibition of motor neurons to the opposing muscle. Impulses from a stretched muscle excite motor units in the same muscle (facilitatory synaptic influence is designated with a plus [+] sign) and inhibit, through an interneuron, motor units in the opposing muscle (inhibitory synaptic influence is designated with a minus [–] sign).

impulses that influence the excitability of lower motor neurons in the spinal cord segments supplying antigravity muscles. These motor centers include the cerebral cortex, basal ganglia, facilitating and inhibiting centers in the midbrain, brainstem reticular formation, and the cerebellum (Fig. 3.15). Postural tone is an automatic (reflexive) phenomenon that is influenced by both afferent impulses from sensory receptors and efferent mechanisms from γ motor neurons.

In functional terms, postural muscle tone in individuals without a pathological condition has been described as "high enough to hold the head, body and extremities against gravity yet low enough to allow for movement."[48] The appropriate amount of muscle tone ensures that the muscle is ready to resist any change in position to maintain posture. In persons with an intact neuromusculoskeletal system, descending motor tracts from the brainstem, particularly from the reticulospinal and vestibulospinal tracts, deliver low frequency trains of impulses to spinal motor neurons, either indirectly through interneurons or directly (Fig. 3.16). Although local postsynaptic depolarizations may not be great enough to provoke complete depolarization and firing of the cell, they maintain the neuron in a slightly oscillating state of high excitability, ready to respond to more concentrated presynaptic input. Muscle tone also ensures that the muscle is ready to contract or relax promptly when appropriate control signals reach the motor neurons. Muscle tone may be influenced by disease or injury affecting various levels of the nervous system resulting in symptoms of insufficient muscle tone (low tone, **hypotonia**) or excessive muscle tone (high tone, **hypertonia**), both to be elaborated upon in later sections of this chapter.

Summary of Muscle Spindle Functions

In essence, muscle spindles function as "thermostats," comparing the length of the muscle spindle with the length of skeletal muscle fibers that surround the muscle spindle (Fig. 3.11 and 3.13). If the length of the surrounding extrafusal muscle fibers is less than that of the muscle spindle, the frequency of muscle spindle's discharged nerve impulses is reduced since they are not being facilitated. However, when the central portion of the muscle spindle is stretched because of γ-efferent activity, its sensory receptors discharge more nerve impulses to excite α motor neurons and activate the extrafusal muscle fibers to contract. The mechanism is particularly important in the regulation and maintenance of postural muscle tone.

Kinesthesia and Proprioception

Under most conditions, a person can be consciously aware of the position of the various parts of his or her body relative to all other parts and whether a particular part is moving or still. This awareness is **kinesthesia** (Gr. *kinen,* to move, plus *aisthesis,* perception) and **position sense**. These two terms are often treated as synonyms and are used frequently to cover all aspects of this awareness, whether static or dynamic. Strictly speaking, however, the term *kinesthesia* regards awareness of dynamic joint motion, and the term *position sense* refers to the awareness of static position. Kinesthetic signals are generated in various sensory receptors residing in muscles, tendons, and joints and respond to body movements and tension within tendons. The impulses produced in the receptors are transmitted predominantly over group II afferent fibers to the spinal cord, the cerebellum, and sensory nuclei. Thus, other sensory and motor centers in the central nervous system are

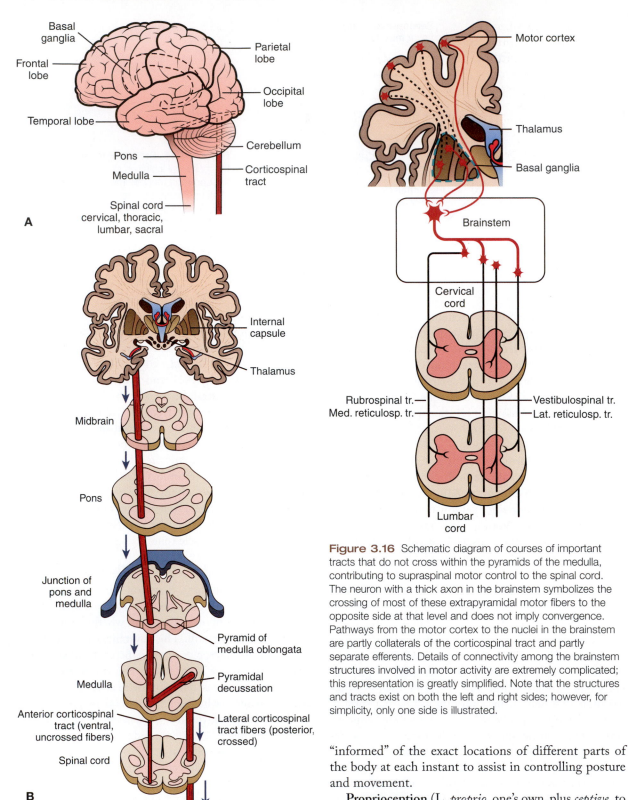

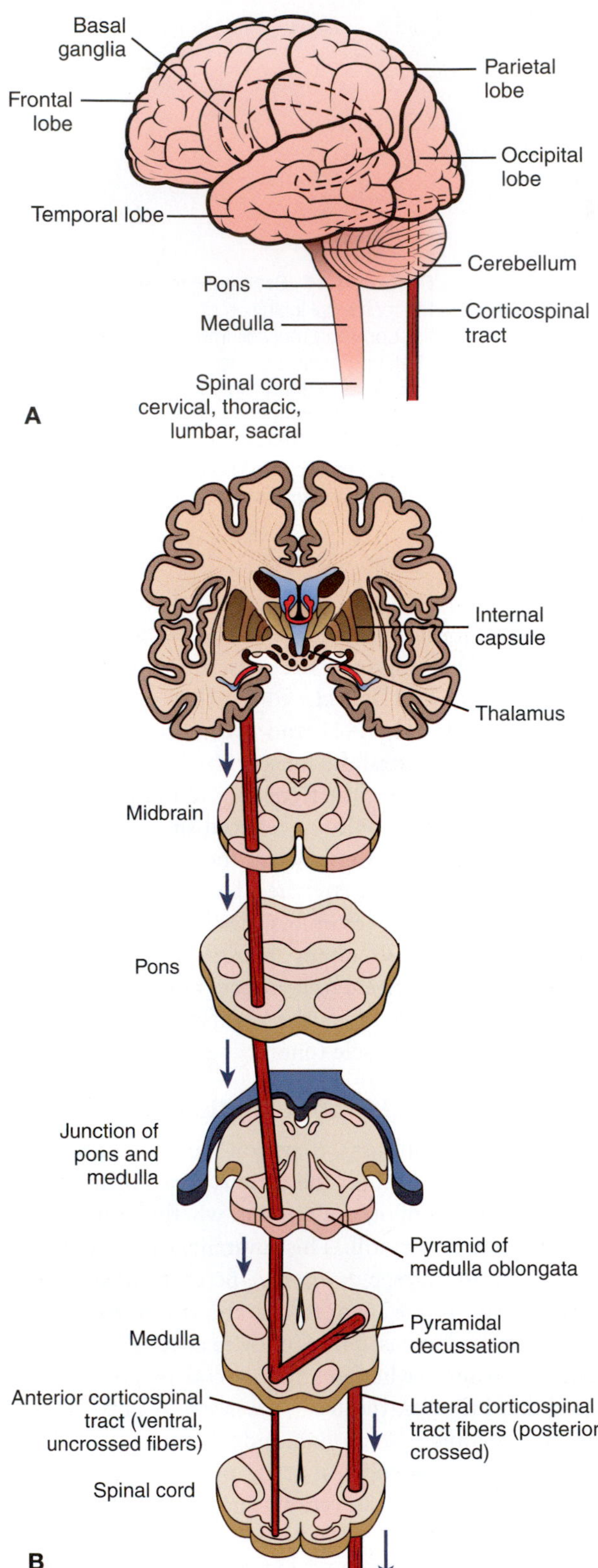

Figure 3.15 A) Central nervous system areas primarily involved in the control of movement; B) shows a cross-sectional view from the internal capsule and thalamus and inferior structures of the midbrain and spinal cord.

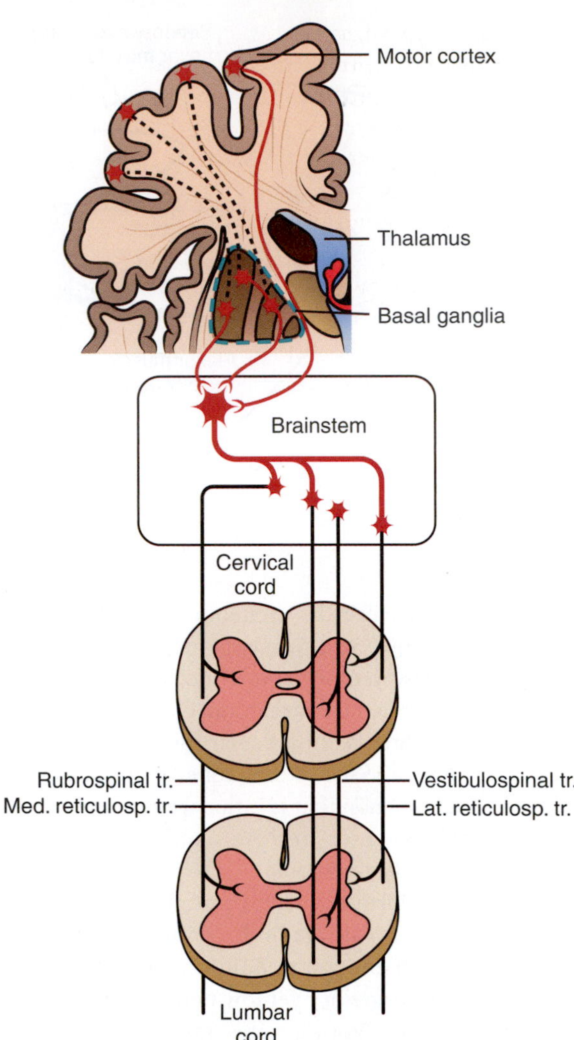

Figure 3.16 Schematic diagram of courses of important tracts that do not cross within the pyramids of the medulla, contributing to supraspinal motor control to the spinal cord. The neuron with a thick axon in the brainstem symbolizes the crossing of most of these extrapyramidal motor fibers to the opposite side at that level and does not imply convergence. Pathways from the motor cortex to the nuclei in the brainstem are partly collaterals of the corticospinal tract and partly separate efferents. Details of connectivity among the brainstem structures involved in motor activity are extremely complicated; this representation is greatly simplified. Note that the structures and tracts exist on both the left and right sides; however, for simplicity, only one side is illustrated.

"informed" of the exact locations of different parts of the body at each instant to assist in controlling posture and movement.

Proprioception (L. *proprio,* one's own, plus *ceptive,* to receive) is a more inclusive term than kinesthesia and refers to the use of sensory input from receptors in muscle spindles, tendons, and joints to discriminate joint position and joint movement, including direction, amplitude, and speed, as well as relative tension within tendons. Proprioceptive impulses are transmitted predominantly over group I afferent fibers and are integrated in various sensorimotor centers to automatically regulate postural muscle adjustments and maintain postural equilibrium.

Several types of **somatosensory** (Gr. *soma,* body, plus L. *sensorius,* pertaining to sensation) inputs also are important in maintaining postural equilibrium. For example, pressure sensations from the soles of the feet provide information about the distribution of load between the two feet and whether the weight is more forward or backward on the feet.

Postural equilibrium is crucial for both static position and dynamic motion. Without it, the body is unable to function. Its importance is underscored by the number of systems the body uses to achieve equilibrium during static and dynamic activities. In addition to proprioceptors and somatosensory receptors, the body uses two additional input mechanisms to aide in equilibrium: the vestibular system and the visual system. The vestibular receptors in the inner ears provide awareness of head orientation and movements. Anyone who has had a middle ear infection can testify to the importance of the vestibular system in balance. Vision of where the body and its segments are relative to the surrounding environment also assist in maintaining equilibrium. In fact, visual input sometimes serves as the primary means of maintaining equilibrium when the proprioception system is impaired. The importance of equilibrium is observed not only during daily activities but also when performing various sports or when assessing impairments of equilibrium and suggesting solutions to balance problems. Even static equilibrium is affected by vision. Try standing on one leg with your eyes open and then with your eyes closed, and you will quickly realize how much you use vision for equilibrium.

Movement or "Motor" Control

When considering the control of movement, we must realize that movement and posture are exceedingly intricate and complex, and may be affected by an abundance of factors. For example, several systems must be intact for appropriate regulation of posture and movement. The neuromuscular systems must be intact, including the muscles that experience excitation or inhibition, muscles spindles, GTOs, neuromuscular junctions, peripheral nerves that innervate the muscles, spinal cord ascending and descending pathways, cortical motor centers, and the interconnections of these systems. The skeletal system, including the bones, ligaments, joints, joint capsules, and joint receptors also must be unimpaired. In addition, the respiratory, cardiovascular, and digestive systems must supply energy sources for muscular contractions and for the maintenance of the neuromusculoskeletal systems. Furthermore, accurate sensory input of the internal and external environments must be provided.

In order to perform skilled motor activities, a highly integrated set of motor commands is required to activate or inhibit several muscles in the proper way and in the proper sequence. We *cannot* view movement simply as the action of the various systems which carry out the movement task; rather, there is a highly complex organization and regulation in play that orchestrates our ability to move. **Motor control** refers to this dynamic regulation of posture and movement. Muscle **synergy** (Gr. *synergia,* together) is a term used to describe functional coordinated muscle activation, such as seen during functional movement when muscles typically work together as a group.[49]

Motor control requires the individual to maintain and change posture, and his or her movement response is based on an interaction between the individual, task, and environment. This interaction utilizes the contributions of many systems to orchestrate coordinated movement. These systems are not arranged in a **hierarchy** (Gr. *hierarchia,* rule or power of the high priest), in which one is more important than the other. Rather, they are a functioning **heterarchy** (Gr. *heteros*, other and *archos*, rule), in which the contributing systems work parallel to each other.[1]

Heterarchy recognizes that different levels of motor control exist and that portions of the nervous system interact with each other. In the heterarchy of motor control, cortical centers interact not only with each other but also with brainstem and spinal regions of the central nervous system, with the peripheral nervous system, and with ascending and descending pathways.[50,51] In this heterarchy, information regarding the environmental milieu both inside and outside the body is provided to the central nervous system, specifically to the cerebral cortex, basal ganglia, and cerebellum, which plan, initiate, execute, coordinate, and regulate movement and posture. These centers also coordinate the timing of specific movements, whether simple or complex, the sequencing and synchronization of movements, as well as the amount of force generated. Which region is considered the "controller" varies, depending on the motor task desired and on the information provided to the central nervous system at a given time. Therefore, no one area is responsible for the control of all movement and posture.[52] The brainstem and spinal cord generate patterns of movement that are referred to as pattern generators, sometimes further clarified as central or stepping pattern generators.[5, 49, 53] Other systems involved in motor control include ascending and descending pathways that provide feedback and feed-forward information.

Interactions within and between the various neural regions provide the most effective and efficient regulation of posture and movement. This model of heterarchy, therefore, considers both the importance of interactions of multiple areas within the CNS and the effect of an individual's ability to anticipate movements and adapt to changes in the environment. Heterarchy suggests that the flow of information is in more than one direction: The interaction occurs within and between levels of the nervous system, the interaction is reciprocal, and the information may be modified as a result of feedback and feed-forward systems.

Movement, therefore, is made possible by the contributions of many systems. Additionally, no system acts in isolation from the others in order to produce movement. In other words, movement emerges through the interaction and self-organization of many subsystems, and a movement behavior is greater than the sum of its individual parts.[54] Absent or disordered movement may result from a problem in the nervous system (either motor or sensory) or skeletal system or due to a difficulty encountered by the moving individual within the environment. In the rehabilitation setting, the patient's movement that a clinician observes is the end result of all of the possibilities and **constraints** (limitations or restrictions) offered by all of the contributing systems. In a simple example, if the gastrocnemius muscle is tight, the patient may stand with hyperextended knees.

Normal movements, therefore, are coordinated not because of muscle activation patterns prescribed only by sensory and motor pathways, but because the strategies of motion emerge from the interaction of the systems working together in this functional heterarchy. It is important to note that included in this complex of interactive systems are subsystems related to the environment and to the task itself. All of these elements are crucially important to movement execution. Our movements are ideally selected, executed, and modified as the best movement choice for a specific task within the environment in which we are moving. Multiple subsystems interact to produce a given motor behavior within a context appropriate for the environment and the task.[55] The interactions between these subsystems within the individual, the requirements of the task, and the unique aspects of the environment all affect the movement outcome.

Motor behaviors are conceived of as functional synergies (groups of muscles working together) rather than specific muscles or individual muscle groups. The human movement system is viewed as tremendously flexible, extremely dynamic, and capable of adapting to changes within the individual, the task, and/or the environment in an effort to produce the most effective movement possible.[1,56]

Dynamic Systems Approach to Understanding Motor Control

It is important to realize that these contributing systems change over time since they are dynamic in nature. A **dynamic action system** is any system that demonstrates change over time.[57] This **dynamical action system model** views movement not as the unfolding of predetermined or prescribed patterns in the CNS, but as emerging from the dynamic cooperation of many subsystems in a task-specific context.[54] The many systems then self-organize to produce movement.[58] Motor behavior emerges from the dynamic cooperation of all subsystems within the context of a specific task including the central nervous system as well as biomechanical, psychological, and social-emotional components.

Movement can then be expressed from among a wide variety of movement combinations, represented by a sum of all the possible degrees of freedom of the total joints involved in a movement. As you remember from Chapter 1, degrees of freedom represent the potential movements possible at specific joints. It is through a wide variety of movement combinations that human movement can be so varied. For example, the shoulder can move within three planes and therefore has three degrees of freedom, the elbow and the forearm each have one, and the wrist has two degrees of freedom. These comprise seven degrees of freedom for the upper extremity, excluding the fingers and thumb. If one was to add all the degrees of freedom available and all of the different directions of muscle pull across those joints, the total number of possible movement combinations is extremely numerous.[59] Every joint contributes its number of degrees of freedom to a movement, so that any functional movement emerges as the sum of all of the possible combinations that can occur. As mentioned, these functional movement synergies are self-assembled according to the interaction between the individual, the task, and the environment.

Motor Control at the Spinal Region

Neural connections within the spinal cord contribute much to the automatic control of movement. Specifically, the spinal region is the site for reflex motions, muscle synergy activations, and central pattern generators. Reflex motion control includes the stretch reflex, reciprocal inhibition, and autogenic inhibition, all described earlier in this chapter. Transmission in local spinal circuits involves very little delay and ensures rapid responses. Interneurons within the spinal cord also link motor neurons into functional groups, or muscle synergies.

Reflexes

Spinal reflexes provide movement that is largely generated as a response to information arising from cutaneous, muscle, and joint receptors. These movements are stereotypical and predictable in nature but can be modified by the central nervous system. For example, arousal or alertness will change a person's response to the stretch reflex.

Pattern Generators

Complex muscle activation patterns that produce purposeful movement through neural connections at a spinal cord level are called **pattern generators.** These flexible networks of interneurons produce stepping and walking patterns that can be modified by cortical commands. Adaptable networks of interneurons in the spinal cord activate the lower motor neurons to elicit an alternating activation of flexor and extensor muscles at the hips, knees, and ankles.[60-63] This mechanism allows for efficiency of movement. These patterns are sensitive to changes in the task and the environment and will adapt body responses to these changes. For example, weight gain concomitant with growth in human infants will change the individual's stepping pattern.[49,64]

Motor Control within the Brainstem

As you recall from anatomy, the brainstem consists of the midbrain, pons, and medulla oblongata (Fig. 3.17). The brainstem contains numerous ascending and descending tracts as well as nuclei. These brainstem elements function as an extremely complex prespinal integrating system. These brainstem efferent tracts are largely responsible for automatic postural control. Most supraspinal postural control and proximal movement are regulated from brainstem centers.[49] Since these neurons are within the central nervous system, they are upper motor neurons. Bundles of axons that originate from neurons within the reticular formation of the brainstem and terminate within the spinal cord form the *reticulospinal tract.* Likewise, bundles of axons originating within the vestibular nuclei and terminating within the spinal cord comprise the *vestibulospinal tract* (Fig. 3.16). The reticulospinal tract provides excitatory input to extensor muscles of the arms and flexor muscles of the legs and trunk. In contrast, the vestibulospinal tract carries excitatory input destined for flexor muscles of the arms and extensor muscles of the legs and trunk.[5] Movement requires sufficient postural support from the limbs and body as a whole. Movement is the end product of a number of control systems that interact extensively together. The postural muscles are chiefly responsible for this control as they respond to efferent input from the reticulospinal tract.

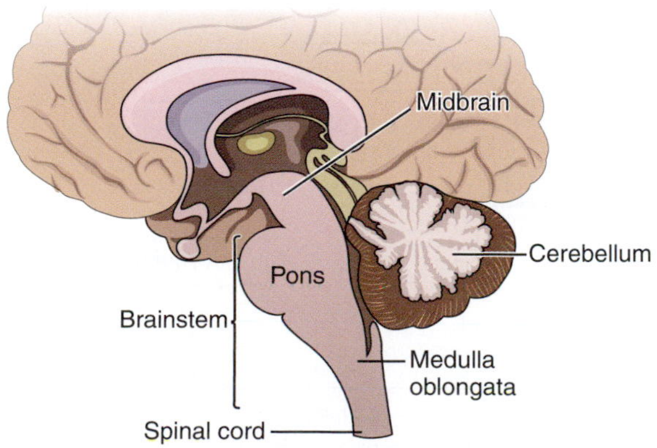

Figure 3.17 Sagittal view illustrating the positions of the main subdivisions of the brainstem.

Cerebral Motor Centers

When considering the motor functions of the nervous system, keep in mind that the motor centers can function appropriately only if an uninterrupted stream of afferent or sensory information about the status of the environment is received from all parts of the body. To emphasize the role of the sense organs in the control of posture and movement, the term *sensorimotor system* is sometimes used to denote the combined afferent and efferent processes required to produce coordinated movement.

Nerve fibers that descend from the motor cortex collectively form the *corticospinal tract* (Figs. 3.2 and 3.15). As the name implies, most of the axons arise from cell bodies in the motor area of the cerebral cortex and route downward in the spinal cord, where synaptic contact is made with motor neurons in the anterior horn gray matter of the spinal cord. The corticospinal tract also is referred to as the **pyramidal tract** because many of the cell bodies located in the motor cortex have a triangular shape and appear as small pyramids when a section of cortex is stained and viewed under a light microscope. Most of the corticospinal axons cross to the opposite side in the brainstem and descend in the lateral corticospinal tract of the spinal cord (Figs. 3.2, 3.15, 3.18). The crossing fibers from the right and left motor cortex also form a pyramid in the brainstem. At the spinal segmental level, axons of the corticospinal tract terminate predominantly on interneurons. The interneurons terminate on α motor neurons. The organization of the corticospinal tract suggests that its design provides precise control of individual muscle groups. Other cortical neurons originating in the same areas of the motor cortex have shorter axons that synapse with second order motor neurons lying in the basal ganglia or brainstem (Fig. 3.18).

Motor Cortex

The frontal lobe is responsible for voluntary control of complex motor activities and cognitive functions, such as judgment, attention, mood, abstract thinking, and aggression. The frontal lobe, frequently referred to as the motor cortex, is further subdivided into the primary motor cortex, the premotor cortex, and the supplementary motor area. All three of these areas have their own somatotopic maps of the body, so that if different cortex areas are stimulated, different muscles and body parts move. However, all three subdivisions offer their own unique yet collaborative contribution to the cerebral control of movement, highlighting once again the beauty of the heterarchical organization of motor control.

The primary motor cortex is responsible for **contralateral** (opposite side of the body) voluntary control of the upper extremity and facial movements. The premotor cortex controls the muscles of the trunk and muscles used in anticipatory postural adjustments, such as required in establishing the correct "postural set" in preparation for standing up from a chair.[1] The supplemental motor cortex controls the initiation of movement, orientation of the head and eyes, and bilateral (involving both body sides) movements.[65,66] The supplemental area also controls the sequencing of movement and plays a role in the pre-programming of movement sequences that are familiar and part of an individual's memory repertoire.[49]

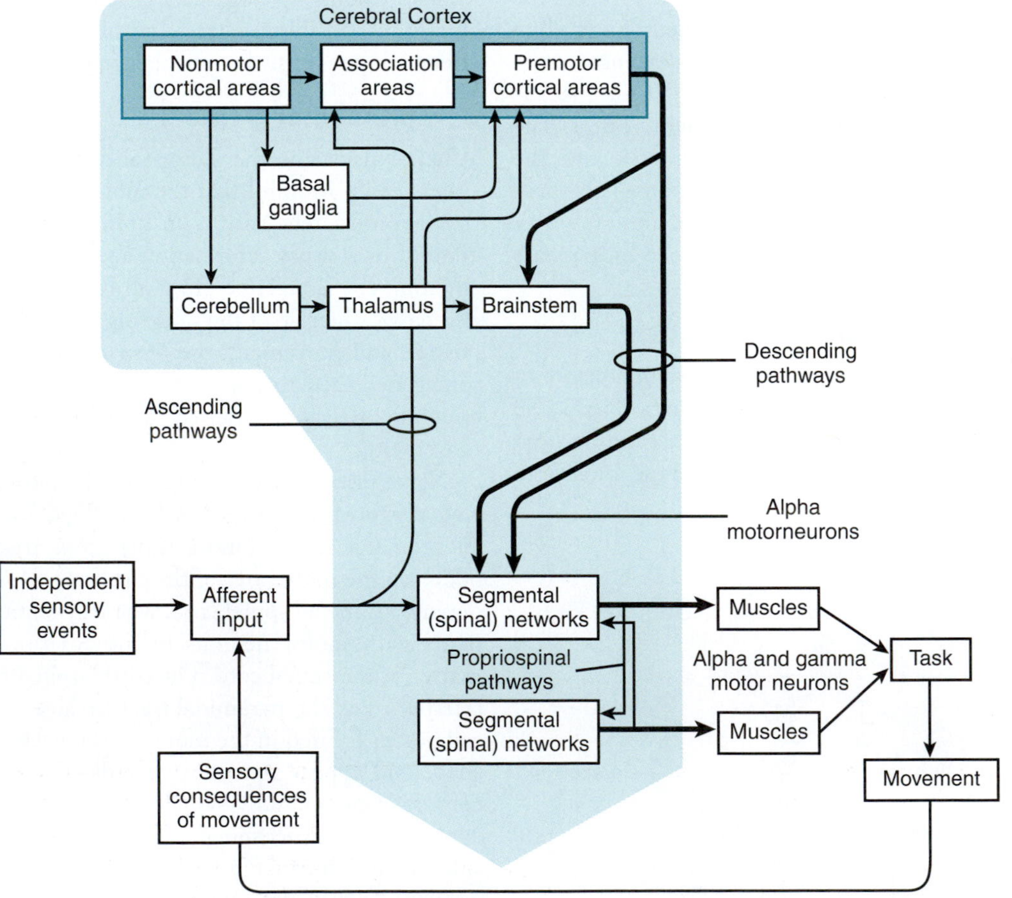

Figure 3.18 Schematic diagram of the course of the lateral and medial corticospinal tracts from the motor cortex to the spinal cord. For simplicity, collaterals to the basal ganglia, the cerebellum, and the motor centers of the brainstem have been omitted. Note that the structures and tracts exist on both the left and right sides; however, only one side is illustrated. For further description, see text.

PRACTICE POINT

Lesions of the primary motor cortex (as seen following a stroke) usually give rise to contralateral weakness or paresis, typically seen as a period of initial **flaccidity**, in which muscle tone is absent. Clinically, this type of damage will produce reduced postural reactions and diminished stretch reflexes in the acute phase. Oftentimes, this event is followed by a slow recovery and eventually overactive neural responses, producing hyperactive stretch reflexes. Recovery is typically gradual but incomplete.

Lesions of the supplemental motor cortex result in complex motor dysfunction, including severe **akinesia** (lack of movement) and difficulty with tasks requiring the cooperative use of both hands. Patients also have difficulty performing self-initiated tasks but are able to benefit from therapeutic approaches that teach them to use additional sensory cues to start a movement.

Lesions of the premotor cortex result in nonspecific motor disturbances or **apraxia**, in which the patient's movements are slow and clumsy with mild proximal weakness and loss of coordination around the proximal joints. Rhythmic movements such as typing or tapping are disrupted, and **perseveration** (stammering or repeating) may occur. Unlike patients with lesions of the supplemental motor cortex, these patients are able to perform self-initiated tasks, but have difficulty with sensory-triggered tasks. Previously acquired sequential tasks deteriorate, even though individual components of the sequenced task can be performed.[1, 67]

Cerebellar lesions cause distinctive motor symptoms. Cerebellar symptomology usually includes balance and coordination deficits. These deficits may produce **ataxia** (wide based movements), intention tremor (tremor accompanying purposeful movement), and **dysmetria** (inability to gauge distance or properly scale the required force in reaching or stepping).[68] Cerebellar damage can cause any number of errors in the kinematic parameters of movement control, including difficulties with timing, accuracy, coordination, and regulation of intensity.[1]

Intermediate Control Centers

The cerebellum and the basal ganglia serve different but related functions in programming cortically initiated movement patterns, and both act as important motor control centers, contributing vital regulatory functions in movement control.

Cerebellum

The cerebellum is interconnected with all levels of the central nervous system and functions as an overall "coordinator" of motor activities. The cerebellum is responsible primarily for programming rapid movements, correcting the course of rapid movements, and correlating posture and movement. The cerebellum regulates balance and coordination. It is responsible for regulating and adjusting the accuracy, intensity, and timing of movement as required by the specific movement task. It sequences the order of muscle firing when a group of muscles work together to perform a complex task such as stepping or reaching.[66] The cerebellar pathways control balance, coordination, and movement accuracy on the **ipsilateral** (same) body side, as opposed to the **contralateral** control feature associated with the cerebral cortex. The cerebellum is often called the "great comparator," because it constantly monitors and compares the movement requested to the actual output, making adjustments as necessary.[1] The cerebellum has the ability to receive sensory feedback from receptors about a movement as the movement is occurring, a property called **reafference.**

Basal Ganglia

At the base of the cerebrum (hence the name "basal") are several nuclei, including the caudate, putamen, globus pallidus, substantia nigra, and subthalamic nuclei. Although all of their functions are unknown, the basal ganglia play a vital role in the regulation of posture and muscle tone. The basal ganglia have no input from the spinal cord, but they do have direct input from the cortex. They have an important role in the control of both automatic and voluntary movement, exerting effects on the motor planning areas of the motor cortex.

The basal ganglia can either inhibit or facilitate cortex output to alter conscious motion. Nuclei of the basal ganglia are particularly significant with respect to the initiation and execution of slow movements (Fig. 3.18).

Integration of Motor Control to Produce Functional Movement

The entire chapter thus far has presented physiological and anatomical information on the integration of the nervous system with the musculoskeletal system to provide motion. Hopefully, you now realize that movement is the result of complex interactions of many systems and subsystems. For example, sensory impulses from muscles are not restricted to influencing only their own motor neurons. Afferent input also spreads through collateral branches of primary sensory neurons and through interneuron circuits to reach the motor neurons of closely related muscles and, to some extent, those of more "distant" muscles. Therefore, stretch or contraction of one muscle affects its own motor neurons most strongly and, to a lesser extent, also affects motor neurons of muscles performing an opposite action. The effect on the muscles that perform the opposite action is to inhibit activity of those muscles (Fig. 3.14). Motor neurons of other muscles that assist in the motion are also affected but to an even lesser extent. The effect on muscles that assist in the movement is to facilitate action. Thus, every primary loop or pathway is part of a larger feedback network serving a group of muscles.

While an immediate response is occurring, the same sensory signals are being transmitted to higher centers by way of collaterals, projection tracts, and secondary relays to widely separated parts of the nervous system for more elaborate analyses of the information. The ascending tracts allow information integration regarding the status of the body and the status of the environment. Many types of receptors in tendons, joints, and skin, as well as from visual, auditory, and vestibular receptors, simultaneously also provide sensory information regarding the body and the environment. Subsequently, motor signals are relayed back to numerous segmental levels to adjust posture and perform other actions.

It is important to recognize that not only is the precise functioning of the musculoskeletal and nervous systems essential for motor control, but cognition also plays an important role. Cognitive factors are necessary to assimilate sensory information, process and integrate the information, and determine appropriate movements and postures at any given instant. Furthermore, memory of movement and the ability to recall movement information are integral components to the regulation of posture and movement. The execution and efficiency of movement are further influenced by factors such as the ability to concentrate; the presence or absence of visual, auditory, mental or emotional distractions; one's level of proficiency; and one's motivation. Likewise, cognitive strategies influence motor control.[70-74]

The more often a motor pattern is learned, the less input from the cortical level is required until the motor pattern becomes subcortical, not requiring conscious thought to produce accuracy. We see this result when we walk. As toddlers, we used our cortex a great deal to provide us with feedback to balance our body weight over our feet, put one foot in front of the other, change the position of our center of mass, and move forward. As we perfected our gait, we were able to walk without conscious correction, relying on our subcortical nervous innervation and corrections to move safely and securely in our environment. **Motor learning** is concerned with how motor skills are acquired and how they are made proficient, transferred, and retained to allow consistent, accurate, and automatic motion. The reader is referred to other sources a complete discussion of motor learning.[75,76]

Health care professionals work to enhance motor control and motor performance in patients as well as healthy individuals engaged in competitive or leisure sports activities and wellness programs. Intervention programs are designed to stretch and strengthen muscles, to increase endurance, to improve balance and

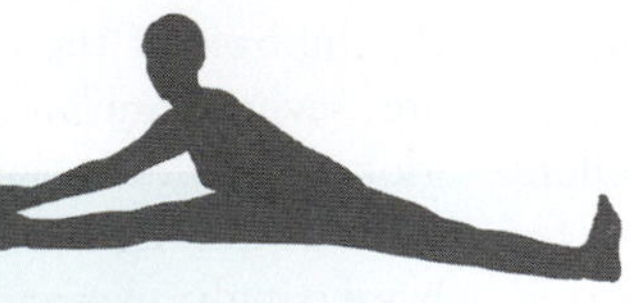

PRACTICE POINT

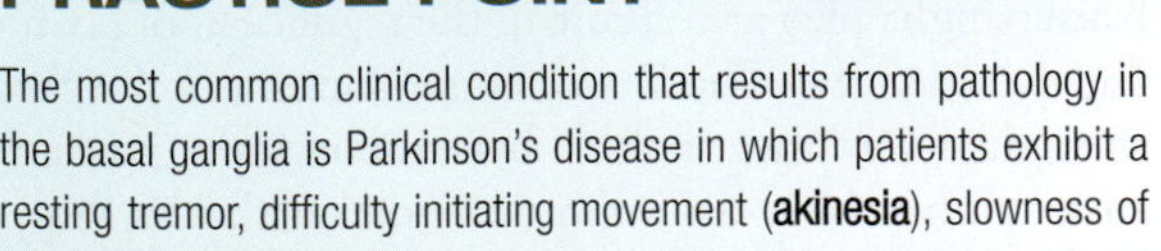

The most common clinical condition that results from pathology in the basal ganglia is Parkinson's disease in which patients exhibit a resting tremor, difficulty initiating movement (**akinesia**), slowness of movement (**bradykinesia**), muscular rigidity, and a stooped posture. This progressive disease, with a mean onset age of 58, is caused by a gradual loss of neurons that produce dopamine (a neurotransmitter) in the basal ganglia.[69]

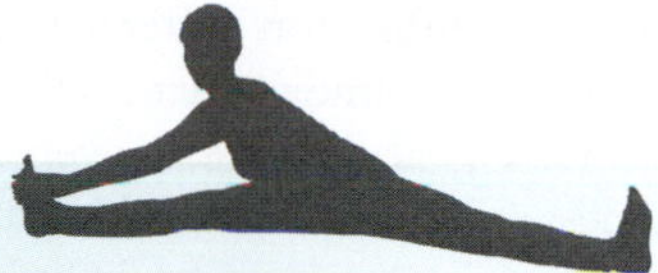

PRACTICE POINT

If we take an example of a motor skill, all of these factors may be more easily appreciated. Kicking a ball towards a target is a complex motor skill. Many cognitive components are first assimilated. The weight of the ball, the distance of the target, the wind speed and direction are all factors that the individual consciously considers before kicking a ball. In the early days of this skill acquisition, the individual also had to rely on his or her coordination and balance input to be able to stand securely on one foot while moving the contralateral leg from hip extension to hip flexion. Additionally, hip abduction to adduction and medial to lateral rotation motions were likely included in the performance. Other joint motions the nervous system had to control included the knee and the ankle. Cocontraction of trunk muscles was necessary for posture control during the kick. Sensory input regarding muscle length, tension, and changes in length as the individual approached the ball were continually being fed, received, and responded to by the neuromuscular system. Once the ball was kicked, the neural system obtained the feedback regarding the performance: Was the ball kicked far enough? Where did the ball land in relation to the target? What part of the foot came in contact with the ball? Where in relation to the body was the foot and leg when contact with the ball was made? The nervous system collects all this data; the subsystems self-organize and alter the next attempt based on this input.

muscle tone, and to improve the ability to regulate posture and movement. These professionals also realize the importance of practice to enhance skill and recognize that more than just the neuromusculoskeletal system must be enhanced to augment performance. It is important to acknowledge that cognitive strategies such as mental practice and imagery, as well as positive self-talk, are important for the client's success.[75-77] Principles of cognition used to enhance motor performance may be applied clinically so that an individual's mindset for rehabilitation is productive to facilitate recovery.

Functional Applications and Clinical Considerations

Neuromuscular impairments encompass a diverse group of problems that constitute a major constraint on functional movement. Impairments of motor control may result from many diseases, injuries, or developmental disabilities and can result from pathology to any part of the movement system. Pathological conditions that affect any part of the neuromuscular system, including motor, sensory, perceptual, and cognitive elements, will result in associated signs, symptoms, and impairments.[78] Other factors may be involved in motor control dysfunction, including the skeletal, cognitive, visual or vestibular systems. Since this chapter deals with movement control and primarily the neuromuscular aspects involved in the control of movement, we will continue to focus on impairments that affect these structures and contribute to alterations in movement.

Impairments are the typical consequences of the disease or pathological process, further defined as the loss or abnormality of function, at the tissue, organ, or system level, resulting in constrained movement. Examples of primary motor impairments include weakness, abnormalities in muscle tone, and motor coordination problems.[1, 68] In addition to primary impairments, secondary impairments also contribute to movement problems. These secondary impairments do not result from the pathology directly, but rather develop as a result of the consequences of the primary impairment and may be preventable. Examples of secondary impairments include loss of range of motion or contracture.[78]

The ability to produce and coordinate an appropriate movement response requires production of muscular force, activation and sustenance of muscle activity, and the coordination and timing of muscle activation patterns. The primary motor system impairments that interfere with functional movement are muscle weakness, abnormalities of muscle tone, and coordination problems.[68]

Muscle Weakness

Muscle weakness is defined as an inability to generate normal levels of muscular force and is a major impairment of motor function in patients with nervous and/or muscular system damage.[68] Lesions within the CNS, PNS, or muscular system can produce weakness. It is important to differentiate the weakness from where in the movement system the damage is located. By definition, damage to the descending motor control systems in the CNS is associated with lesions affecting upper motor neurons, anywhere from the spinal cord superiorly.[68] This damage will produce signs of upper motor neuron (UMN) damage. Upper motor neuron lesions are associated with hypertonicity, or hypotonicity, depending on the site of the lesion and the time of onset (acute vs. chronic). Depending on the extent of the lesion, weakness in the patient with an upper motor neuron lesion can vary in severity from total loss of muscle activity (paralysis or plegia) to a mild or partial loss of muscle activity (paresis).[68] Paresis results from damage to the descending motor pathways, which interferes with the brain's excitatory drive to the motor units, thereby resulting in a loss of descending control of the lower motor neurons.[79] The end result is an inability to recruit and modulate the motor neurons, leading to a loss of movement.

Upper motor neuron lesions are accompanied by secondary abnormal muscle tone and altered motor control.[68, 80] The range of muscle tone abnormalities found within patients who have UMN covers a broad spectrum, ranging from complete flaccidity (loss of tone), to spasticity (hypertonicity).[68] Changes in muscle tone will vary depending on the specific lesion. Following an upper motor neuron lesion, weakness occurs due to loss of motor unit recruitment, changes in recruitment patterns, and changes in firing rates. Additionally, changes occur in the properties of the motor units and in the morphological and mechanical properties of the muscle itself. These secondary changes happen as adaptations to loss of innervation, immobility, and disuse. In upper motor neuron lesions, reduced numbers of motor units and reduced firing rates of motor units have been reported.[14, 81] Within two months of the insult, patients with hemiparesis resulting from a stroke show up to a 50% reduction in motor units on the affected side. Individuals who have had a stroke display atrophy in motor units on the hemiparetic side. The remaining motor units require more time to contract, and they fatigue more rapidly. Altered recruitment and decreased motor unit firing accounts for this apparent weakness.[82] The degree of weakness may differ for different muscle groups. Given that the pyramidal tract is the primary pathway for voluntary goal-directed movement, it has been suggested that interruption of this pathway produces a greater impairment in prime mover muscles.[83] Prolonged paresis, a primary neuromuscular impairment, also produces secondary musculoskeletal impairments. Changes in muscle tissue resulting from damage to upper motor neurons suggest that muscle may not be as "strong" due to changes in the properties of the muscle and the presence of denervated muscle fibers.[82] Specific changes at the motor neuron secondary to the upper motor neuron damage can decrease a patient's ability to produce force.

Muscle weakness most often results from direct injury to the muscle. A wide continuum of injuries, from contusions to ruptures, produce weakness, initially from the injury itself, and secondarily from inactivity and disuse following the injury during the recovery phase. Pain, whether in an injured muscle or in a joint on which the muscle acts, reduces the individual's willingness to move the muscle. When a muscle is not used at its normal functional level, weakness ensues.

Regardless of the underlying etiology or pathology, when a muscle is not used or exercised, muscle weakness and atrophy occur. When a muscle does not function for long periods of time, the quantity of actin and myosin myofilaments in the muscle's fibers actually decrease. This change is reflected in reduced diameters of individual fibers, and diminished overall muscle cross-sectional area.[91] Muscle wasting is due, at least in part, to a decrease in protein synthesis coupled with increased protein degradation; these changes cause alterations in contractile properties and a resultant loss in the muscle's ability to develop and hold tension.[31, 92] In response to decreased use, skeletal muscle also undergoes an adaptive remodeling; this process includes a transition from slow to fast myosin fiber types, a fuel shift toward glycolysis, decreased capacity for fat oxidation, and energy substrate

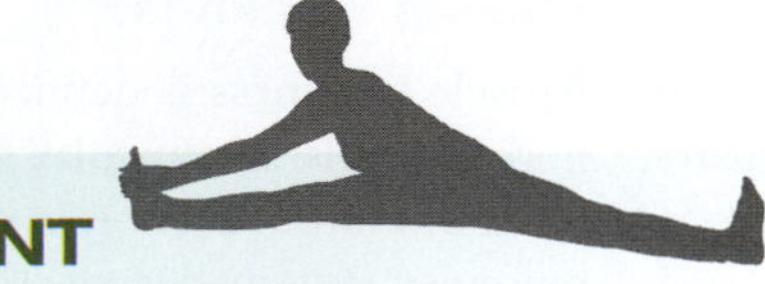

PRACTICE POINT

Clinicians formerly believed that prescribing strength training was not appropriate for patients with UMN pathology. Research has demonstrated that improvements in strength not only contribute to an improvement in functional performance, but that there is also no indication of any associated increase in spasticity.[79-89] Strength training is thought to not only improve voluntary motor control, but it also appears to prevent or slow down some of the mechanical changes and denervation changes seen in muscle tissue following UMN damage.[87, 90] The shift in emphasis to the functional significance of weakness in patients with CNS lesions has led to increased attention on strengthening programs for both adults and children with CNS disorders.

accumulation in the atrophied muscle.[93] A loss of peak muscle force and functional muscle strength results from these changes.[31] **Disuse atrophy** is a term used to specifically describe this atrophy that occurs when a person or limb is immobile, such as during bed rest, or when a limb is restricted in a sling, brace, or cast.[94-96] Current research demonstrates that this disuse atrophy begins within 4 hours of the start of bed rest![97]

Abnormal Muscle Tone

As described briefly earlier, typically muscle tone is characterized by a state of readiness of muscle to perform the task demands to be placed on it. The level of excitability of the pool of motor neurons controlling a muscle, the intrinsic muscle stiffness, the absence of neuropathology, and the level of reflex sensitivity determine this state of readiness. A hallmark of central nervous system pathology is the presence of abnormal muscle tone. Abnormally high (hypertonia) or abnormally low (hypotonia) muscle tone are universally recognized clinical signs of nervous system pathology. Flaccidity and hypotonia are states of muscle hypotonicity, while spasticity and rigidity are states of hypertonicity. Typically, upper motor neuron lesions oftentimes results in hypertonia and lower motor neuron lesions in hypotonia. Terms related to abnormal muscle tone are found in Table 3–4.

Coordination Problems

Coordinated movement involves multiple joints and muscles that are activated at the appropriate time and with the correct amount of force so that smooth, efficient, and accurate movement occurs.[68] The essence of coordinated movement, therefore, is the synergistic organization of multiple muscles for purposeful motion, not just the capacity to fire an isolated muscle contraction. Incoordination can result from pathology in a wide variety of neural structures, including the motor cortex, basal ganglia, and cerebellum. Uncoordinated movement may be displayed through the manifestation of abnormal synergies, inappropriate coactivation patterns, and timing problems.

As mentioned earlier, **synergy** is a group of muscles that often act together as if in a bound unit. Nicolai Bernstein[100] used the term synergy to aptly describe the functional muscle groups that produce motor behavior. Lesions to corticospinal centers can also lead to the ability to recruit only a limited number of muscles controlling a movement. The result is the emergence of mass patterns of movement, referred to as abnormal synergies. Abnormal synergies reflect an inability to move a single joint without simultaneously generating movement in other joints. Abnormal synergies are stereotypical patterns of movement that don't change or adapt to environmental or task demands.[1,68]

Coordination problems can also be manifested as abnormalities with muscle activation patterns and difficulties with muscle sequencing. Inappropriate coactivation of muscles is an example of a sequencing problem. Coactivation, which means that the agonist and antagonist both fire, is normally present in the early stages of learning a skilled movement. Coactivation is commonplace in young children just learning to balance and during early walking patterns. Adults also frequently demonstrate coactivation when attempting to learn a new task. In the neurologically intact adult, coactivation is atypical unless during the early stages of learning a new skill. Coactivation requires unnecessary energy expenditure and results in inefficient movement. Inappropriate coactivation occurs in central nervous system disorders in both children and adults. This inappropriate and ungraded coactivation of agonist and antagonist contributes to functional limitations in force generation. Coactivation has been demonstrated in adults following a stroke and in children with cerebral palsy during walking and the performance of common functional skills.[101,102]

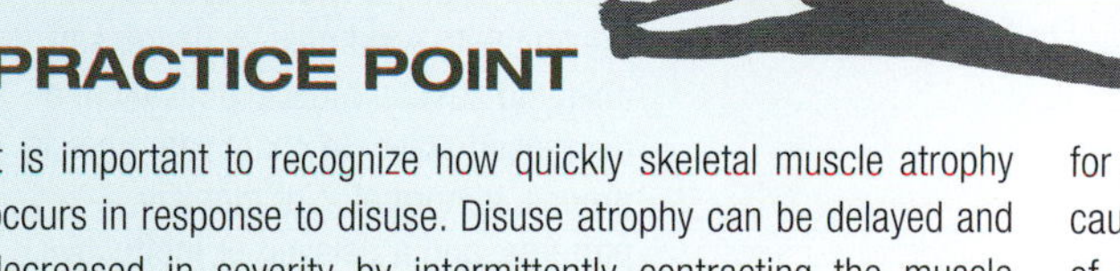

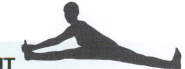

PRACTICE POINT

It is important to recognize how quickly skeletal muscle atrophy occurs in response to disuse. Disuse atrophy can be delayed and decreased in severity by intermittently contracting the muscle isometrically during any period of immobilization or relative inactivity.[98] Exercise and proper nutrition have both resulted in protein synthesis stimulation in muscle and tendon with obvious implications for rehabilitation management.[99] On the other hand, clinicians are cautioned that if atrophy has already occurred, strenuous exercise of atrophied muscle can lead to muscle damage, including sarcolemma disruption and distortion of the myofibrils' contractile components.[97] Prevention with early intervention is truly the best practice.

Uncoordinated movement can also be manifested as an inability to appropriately time the action of muscles, to activate muscles in the appropriate sequence, or to scale or grade the force needed. There can be many facets to timing errors including problems initiating the movement, slowed movement execution, and problems terminating a movement. All of these timing errors have been observed in individuals with neurological damage. Coordination problems, characterized by problems in muscle activation, sequencing, timing, and scaling, can create a tremendous obstacle to efficient functional movement.

Since coordination requires adequate strength and ROM, uncoordinated movement is often characterized by some degree of weakness, fatigue, or instability. Likewise, body segments weakened by injury or disuse may suffer inadequate coordination and sequencing. Even as a patient fatigues during rehabilitation exercises, coordination becomes more difficult. As previously mentioned, muscle recruitment occurs in normal muscles from single joint muscles to multiple joint muscles. Proper muscle sequencing is also important in daily activities, but if correct sequencing is not present, the individual is at risk of injury at the most and inefficient movement at the least. Such consequences place additional stresses on other body segments. For example, studies have demonstrated that muscle recruitment and sequencing vary between back patients and normal groups.[103, 104] It is unclear, however, if the changes in recruitment were the cause of pain or the result of pain. In either situation, an individual is not able to function optimally if proper muscle activation and recruitment sequencing is dysfunctional.

Involuntary Movements

Involuntary movements are a common motor sign of neurological damage and can take many forms. **Dystonia** is a syndrome dominated by sustained muscle contractions, frequently causing abnormal postures, twisting or writhing movements, and repetitive abnormal postures. Dystonic movements usually result from basal ganglia disturbances.[1]

Tremor is defined as a rhythmic, involuntary, oscillatory movement of a body part.[106] A tremor results from damage to the CNS. A **resting tremor** is a tremor occurring in a body part that is not voluntarily activated and is supported against gravity. Resting tremors is a symptom of Parkinson's disease and is secondary to basal ganglia dysfunction. An **intention tremor** occurs when the individual attempts purposeful movement of an extremity. Intention tremors often accompany cerebellar lesions.

Common Pathological Conditions Affecting Movement System Function

The movement system can be impacted by numerous pathological conditions that affect any contributing

TABLE 3–4 | ABNORMAL MUSCLE TONE TERMINOLOGY

Term	Origin of Term	Definition	Clinical Examples
Flaccid	L. *flaccidus,* weak, soft, lax	complete loss of muscle tone	Flaccidity is often seen in the acute stage of injury, immediately following a CNS injury, but it can also be secondary to a lower motor neuron lesion. In patients with flaccidity, deep tendon reflexes (DTRs) are absent.
Hypotonia	Gr. *hypo,* under and *tonos,* tension	reduction in muscle stiffness	Characterized by low muscle tone, weak neck and trunk control, poor muscular co-contraction, and limited stability. Patients with hypotonia present with weakness, a decreased ability to sustain muscle activation, a decreased ability to coactivate muscle groups, abnormal joint mobility patterns, and a delayed or ineffective exhibition of normal postural responses.
Hypertonia	Gr. *hyper,* over, above and *tonus,* tension	excessive muscle tone	See spasticity

TABLE 3–4 | ABNORMAL MUSCLE TONE TERMINOLOGY—cont'd

Term	Origin of Term	Definition	Clinical Examples
Spasticity	Gr. *spastikos,* to tug or draw	motor disorder characterized by a velocity-dependent increase in the stretch reflex with exaggerated tendon jerks, resulting from hyperexcitability	Typically seen as part of the upper motor neuron clinical presentation. As a result, there will be increased alpha motor neuron excitability with a resultant increase in muscle tone and exaggerated stretch reflexes, secondary to this damage in the descending motor systems. Clinically, the term spasticity is used to describe a wide range of abnormal motor behaviors including: 1) Hyperactive stretch reflexes, 2) Abnormal posturing of the limbs, 3) Excessive coactivation of the antagonist muscles, 4) Associated movements, 5) Clonus, and 6) Stereotypical movement synergies
Rigidity	L. *Rigidus,* inflexible, rigid	heightened resistance to passive movement, but independent of the velocity of that stretch or movement.	Rigidity is associated with lesions of the basal ganglia, and appears to be the result of excessive supraspinal drive acting upon a normal spinal reflex mechanism. Rigidity tends to be predominant in the flexor muscles of the trunk and limbs and results in severe functional limitations. There are two types of rigidity, lead pipe and cogwheel. A constant resistance to movement throughout the range characterizes **lead pipe rigidity,** whereas **cogwheel rigidity** is characterized by alternate episodes of resistance and relaxation. Rigidity is frequently associated with lesions of the basal ganglia, commonly seen in Parkinson's disease

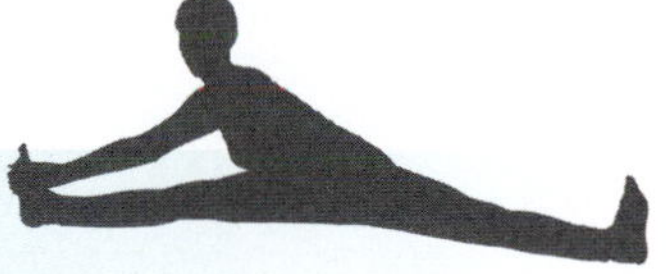

PRACTICE POINT

Because the stretch reflex is velocity dependent, and due to increased muscular stiffness, spasticity limits a patient's ability to move quickly. Regardless of its complex neural basis, it is important to remember that spasticity is simply one of several symptoms of neurological damage and should be treated as it interferes with function. Functional treatment approaches should focus primarily on improving active muscle control in addition to spasticity symptom reduction when it limits movement.

component of the nervous, muscular, or skeletal systems, arising at any phase of the life span. A few commonly encountered pathological conditions with their associated impairments and functional limitations are briefly described in the following section. This section identifies only a few selected conditions to illustrate the functional implications associated with impaired movement.

Peripheral Nerve Injury

Peripheral nerves (Figs. 3.2 and 3.3) may be damaged by disease or trauma. Acute injury includes lacerations or other causes of partial or complete severance of the nerve. Other acute or repetitive injuries may occur from pressure or compression of the peripheral nerve. If the damage is complete, flaccid paralysis of muscle fibers supplied by the damaged lower motor axons will result when the muscles no longer receive efferent signals.

A common peripheral nerve lesion in the upper extremity affects the median nerve. The median nerve is susceptible to damage at the wrist, where it may be compressed within the carpal tunnel. Remember from your study of anatomy that the tendons of the long finger flexors and the median nerve pass under the flexor retinaculum (L. *retinaculum,* a rope or cable). In instances of essential narrowing of the carpal tunnel through anatomical constraints, enlargement of soft tissue structures, or swelling of structures within the tunnel, compression of the median nerve within the carpal tunnel often results in carpal tunnel syndrome. Symptoms associated with the compression of the median nerve include decreased sensation in the area innervated by the nerve, pain and, if the condition progresses, atrophy with weakness of muscles innervated by the median nerve. Peripheral nerves in the more proximal upper extremity also suffer injury secondary to fractures. For example, a fracture of the humerus may cause a lesion of the radial nerve, resulting in weakness or total loss of function of the elbow and wrist extensors. In the lower extremities, the sciatic nerve is a frequent site of pathology.

Peripheral nerve injuries may result in muscular imbalance. Muscle imbalance occurs when one group of muscles is opposed by an impaired muscle group. This condition can then lead to secondary deformities. For example, following a lesion of the ulnar nerve, the individual is predisposed to developing a "claw hand" deformity. In this case, the long flexors and extensors of the fingers are not affected by the ulnar nerve deficiency. Their pull, however, is opposed by nonfunctioning intrinsic muscles in the hand so the balance between the long finger flexors and long finger extensors is lacking. Without occasional movement, adhesions can form between tendons and the sheaths that surround them, as well as between adjacent bundles of muscle fibers. When tissues crossing a joint remain in the same position for prolonged periods, a contracture forms, whereby the tissues adapt to the shortened position and exhibit a decrease from normal joint range of motion. These complications may be prevented by using passive physical activity to maintain full range of movement and increase flow of blood and lymph through the area. Splints also may assist in preventing contractures.

Cerebral Palsy

Cerebral palsy (L. *cerebrum,* brain; *palsy,* paralysis) is a general term used to describe a group of motor disorders that generally result from damage to the developing brain. As one of the most common developmental disabilities, cerebral palsy results from a lesion to the brain during prenatal (L. *prae,* before, plus L. *natal,* birth), perinatal, or early postnatal stages of life. The brain lesion causes a nonprogressive but permanent damage to one or more areas of the brain. Although cerebral palsy is defined as a neurologically static condition, it can be considered orthopedically progressive in nature. Depending on the sites of the neurologic lesion, an individual with cerebral palsy may show a variety of motor or other impairments. Because of the close relationship of motor functions with other neural functions and because of the potential diffuse nature of the lesion, the individual with cerebral palsy also may demonstrate sensory, communicative, perceptual, and/or cognitive impairments.

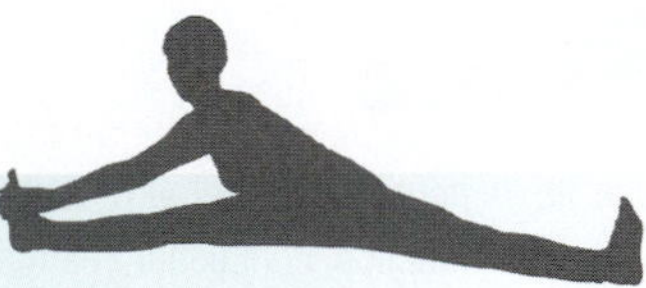

PRACTICE POINT

Loss of sensation can be a more serious problem than loss of muscle strength for a person with a peripheral nerve lesion. Individuals with impaired sensory function may exhibit a loss of awareness of location or position of certain body segments, reduced pressure sensation, deficient temperature detection, and/or loss of pain sensation. If such sensory deficiencies exist, the person may not detect when blood flow is occluded by external pressure or when the part is in contact with excessively hot or cold objects. Various sensory losses place the affected body segment at risk for traumatic injuries, ischemia (Gr. *ischein,* to suppress, plus *haima,* blood), burns, pressure sores, and subsequent infections.

Cerebrovascular Accident

The central nervous system is very vulnerable to reduction of its blood supply. Cerebrovascular accidents (CVAs), or strokes (from the Greek term *streich,* meaning "to strike"), occur when the blood supply to an area in the CNS is disrupted. Residual problems following a stroke vary greatly depending on numerous factors such as the cause of the CVA, the affected CNS area, the extent of the damage, and the functions of the damaged area(s). The clinical deficits may include weakness or paralysis of the muscles of the face, trunk, and/or extremities; impairment of sensation and proprioception; visual deficits; cognitive difficulties; language impairments; and perceptual problems. Impairment of motor and sensory impulse conduction is likely to produce paralysis of muscles on the side contralateral (opposite) to the lesion, causing the clinical presentation referred to as hemiplegia.

Basal Ganglia Disorders

The basal ganglia are generally responsible for the regulation of posture and muscle tone. They convert plans for movement into programs for movement by affecting the motor planning areas of the motor cortex, particularly with respect to the initiation and execution of movements. The most common complex of symptoms resulting from disturbance of basal ganglia connections is Parkinson's disease. Individuals with Parkinson's disease demonstrate movement characterized by slowness of movement; rigidity of facial expressions; decreased or absent communicative gestures; a hesitant, shuffling gait with small steps; and resting tremor of the hands.

Athetosis is another movement disorder involving the basal ganglia. Athetosis, however, results in slow, writhing movements that are exhibited especially in the upper extremities. Basal ganglia disorders also include chorea, a complex disorder in which the individual has involuntary, sudden, nonpurposeful movements.

Cerebellar Disorders

The cerebellum regulates balance and coordination. It is responsible for regulating and adjusting the accuracy, intensity, and timing of movement as required by the specific movement task. It sequences the order of muscle firing when a group of muscles work together to perform a complex task such as ambulation or reaching.[66] The cerebellar pathways control balance, coordination, and movement accuracy on the ipsilateral body side, as opposed to the contralateral-control feature associated with the cerebral cortex. Cerebellar lesions cause distinctive motor symptoms. Cerebellar damage can cause any number of errors in the kinematic parameters of movement control, including difficulties with timing, accuracy, coordination, and regulation of intensity.

Summary

This chapter gave an overview of the human movement system and its main structural components. The anatomy and physiology of muscle tissue was reviewed and an organizational framework for studying the human nervous system was described. Motor control, as a dynamic and heterarchical system controlling functional human movement, was discussed. Movement impairments and their functional consequences were defined and described. Common primary impairments that affect human movement were described. For the purposes of illustration, a few commonly encountered pathological conditions that cause disordered movement were introduced with a focus on the functional consequences to movement.

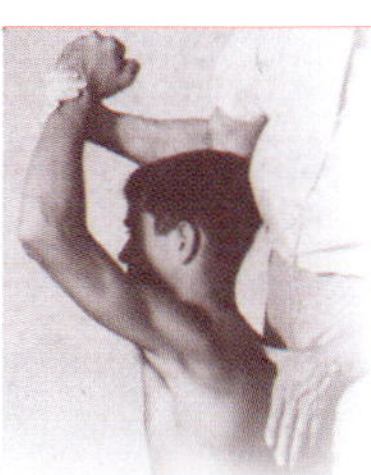

CLINICAL SCENARIO SOLUTION

Joseph has cerebral palsy, and so the weakness that he demonstrates in his lower extremities is caused by a lack of movement control secondary to the developmental nature of that disability. Spasticity is a symptom of upper motor neuron brain damage, secondary to the pathological condition which caused his cerebral palsy. The ulnar nerve injury sustained in Joseph's left upper extremity will result in motor and sensory loss of function to the muscles supplied by the ulnar nerve below the injury, functionally resulting in lost innervation to many of the muscles required for a full grasp. Because the ulnar nerve injury is a lower motor neuron lesion, it will regenerate and function will return over a period of a few months. The transient nature of the ulnar nerve injury is in contrast to the more permanent weakness and overlying spasticity seen in his lower extremities due to the cerebral palsy.

Discussion Questions

1. Think about muscle fiber types in discussing the following: Why is the breast meat of a domestic chicken white as opposed to the breast meat of a pheasant or duck? Along the same lines, why is the leg meat of domestic fowl (chicken and turkeys) dark?
2. What do you think would be the major fiber composition in each of the following muscles, based on their primary function as primarily tonic or phasic: 1) back extensors; 2) biceps brachii; 3) soleus; and 4) finger flexors?
3. What is the overall organization of the nervous system, both anatomically and physiologically?
4. How does the nervous system send signals, utilizing the following physiological processes in order to transduce and communicate a signal: action potential, receptor potential, threshold, excitatory and inhibitory postsynaptic potential, summation?
5. What is motor control? What is the dynamic nature of the systems involved in motor control?

Lab Activities

1. **Stretch Reflex (Materials needed—reflex hammer):**

   Working in pairs, one partner is seated at the edge of a plinth so that the foot is off the ground, hip and knee flexed comfortably. This subject should be sitting and relaxed, with his or her eyes closed. The other partner uses the reflex hammer to elicit the stretch reflex in the quadriceps muscle. Explain Figure 3.12. The most important part of this lesson is for one partner to be able to explain to the other the mechanism involved, including the monosynaptic stretch reflex, reciprocal innervation, and a beginning understanding of the basis for normal muscle tone. Note the length of time between the tap and the response. Observe the "crispness" of the response. Observe variations among different subjects.

2. **Proprioception:**

   One partner is instructed to close his or her eyes. The other partner passively moves the partner's arm into a new position and asks the person to hold it there momentarily. Once the partner has moved the extremity back to a position of rest, the partner whose eyes were closed is instructed to duplicate the arm position that the arm had been placed in by the other partner. Discussion can then follow about the value of proprioception and intact kinesthesia.

References

1. Bertoti DB. *Functional Neurorehabilitation through the Life Span*. Philadelphia: F. A. Davis Company, 2004.
2. *Stedman's Medical Dictionary for the Health Professions and Nursing,* 6 ed. Baltimore: Lippincott, Williams & Wilkins, 2008.
3. Sahrmann S. The Twenty-ninth Mary McMillan Lecture: Moving Precisely? Or Taking the Path of Least Resistance? *Phys Ther* 78(11):1208–1218, 1998.
4. Sahrmann SA. *Diagnosis and treatment of movement impairment syndromes*. St. Louis: Mosby, 2002.
5. Burt AM. *Textbook of Neuroanatomy*. Philadelphia: WB Saunders, 1993.
6. Adal MN, Barker D. Intramuscular diameters of afferent nerve fibres in the rectus femoris muscle of the cat. In Barker D (ed). *Symposium on Muscle Receptors*. Hong Kong: Hong Kong University Press, 1962, p 249.
7. Berne RM, Levy MN. *Physiology*. St. Louis: Mosby, 1998.
8. Hanson J, Huxley HE. Structural basis of the cross-striations in muscle. *Nature* 172:530, 1953.
9. Huxley HE. The mechanism of muscular contraction. *Science* 164:1356, 1969.
10. Scott W, Stevens J, Binder-Macleod S. Human skeletal muscle fiber type classification. *Physical Therapy* 81(11):1810–1816, 2001.
11. Pette D, Peuker H, Staron RS. The impact of biochemical methods for single fibre analysis. *Acta Physio Scand* 166:261–277, 1999.

12. Burke RE. Motor units: Anatomy, physiology and functional organization. In Brooks VS (ed). *Handbook of Physiology, Section I, The Nervous System (Motor Systems)*. Baltimore: Williams & Wilkins, 1981.
13. Staron RS. Human skeletal muscle fiber types: Delineation, development, and distribution. *Can J Appl Physiol* 22:307–327, 1997.
14. MacIntosh B, Gardiner P, McComas AJ. *Skeletal Muscle: Form and Function*. Champaign, IL: Human Kinetics,1996.
15. Burke R. Motor unit types of cat triceps surae muscle. *J Physiol* 193:141–160, 1967.
16. Sieck GC, Prakash YS. Morphological adaptations of neuromuscular junctions depending on fiber type. *Can J Appl Physiol* 22:197–230, 1997.
17. Milner-Brown HS, Stein RB, Yemm R. The orderly recruitment of human motor units during voluntary isometric contractions. *J Physiol* 230:359–370, 1973.
18. Johnson MA, Polgar J, Weightman P. Data on the distribution of fibre types in thirty-six human muscles: An autopsy study. *J Neurol Sci* 18:111, 1973.
19. Glenmark B, Hedberg G, Kaijser L, Jansson E. Muscle strength from adolescence to adulthood—relationship to muscle fibre types. *Europ J Appl Physiology & Occup Physioiology* 68:9–19, 1994.
20. Cech DJ, Martin S. *Functional Movement Development across the Life Span*. Philadelphia: WB Saunders, 2002.
21. Ponten E, Friden J, Thronell LE, Lieber R. Spastic wrist flexors are more severely affected than wrist extensors in children with cerebral palsy. *Devel Med Child Neurol* 47:384–389, 2005.
22. Lee WS, Cheung WH, Qin L, Tang N, Leung KS. Age-associated decrease of type IIA/B human skeletal muscle fibers. *Clin Orthop Related Res* 450:231–237, 2006.
23. Roos MR, Rice CL, Vandervoort AA. Age-related changes in motor-unit function. *Muscle Nerve* 20:679–690, 1997.
24. Lexell J, Taylor CC, Sjostrom M. What is the cause of ageing atrophy? Total number, size, and proportion of different fiber types studied in whole vastus lateralis muscle from 15- to 83-year-old men. *J Neurol Sci* 84:275–294, 1988.
25. Perle SM, Mutell D, Romanelli R. Age-related changes in skeletal muscle strength and modifications through exercise: A literature review. *J Sports Chiropract Rehabil* 1193(97–103):131–132, 1997.
26. Pette D, Staren RS. Mammalian skeletal muscle fiber type transitions. *Int rev Cytol* 170:143–223, 1997.
27. Porter MM, Vandervoort AA, Lexell J. Aging of human muscle: Structure, action, and adaptability. *Scand J Med Sci Sports* 5:129–142, 1995.
28. Ito M, Araki A, Tanaka H, Tasaki T, Cho K, Yamazaki R. Muscle histopatholgy in spastic cerebral palsy. *Brain Dev* 18:299–303, 1996.
29. Larsson L, Li XP, Berg HE, Frontera WR. Effects of removal of weight-bearing function on contractility and myosin isoform composition in single human skeletal muscle cells. *Pflugers Arch* 432:320–328, 1996.
30. Widrick JJ, Trappe SW, Blaser CA, et al. Isometric force and maximal shortening velocity of single muscle fibers from elite master runners. *Am J Physiol* 271(2 pt 1):C666–C675, 1996.
31. Thompson LV. Skeletal muscle adaptations with age, inactivity, and therapeutic exercise. *J orthop sports phys ther* 32(2):44–57, 2002.
32. Frontera W. Aging muscle. *Crit rev phys rehabil med* 18(1):63–93, 2006.
33. Holzer N, Menetrey J. Muscle fiber types and sport medicine: An update in 2005. *Switzerland Journal for Sports Medicine & Sports Trauma* 53:40–44, 2005.
34. Edwards RHT. Human Muscle function and fatigue. In Porter R, Whelan J (eds). *CIBA Foundation Symposium #82 Human Muscle Fatigue: Physiological Mechanisms*. London: Wiley, 1981, p 1.
35. Bennett RL, Knowlton GC. Overwork weakness in partially denervated skeletal muscle. *Clin Orthop* 12:22–29, 1958.
36. Hickok RJ. Physical therapy as related to peripheral nerve lesions. *Phys Ther Rev* 41:113, 1961.
37. Johnson EW, Braddom R. Overwork weakness in facioscapulohumeral muscular dystrophy. *Arch Phys Med Rehabil* 52:333, 1971.
38. Henneman E. Recruitment of motoneurones: The size principle. In Desmedt JE (ed). *Progress in Clinical Neurophysiology,* Vol 9. Basel: S Karger, 1981, p 26.
39. Carr R, Shepherd J. *Neurological Rehabilitation: Optimizing Motor Performance*. Oxford: Butterworth Heinemann., 1998.
40. Macefield VG. Physiological characteristics of low-threshold mechanoreceptors in joints, muscle and skin in human subjects. *Clin and Experimental Pharmacol and Physiol* 32:135–144, 2005.
41. Chalmers G. Re-examination of the possible role of Golgi tendon organs and muscle spindle reflexes in proprioceptive neuromuscular facilitation muscle stretching. *Sports Biomechanics* 3(1):159–183, 2004.
42. Taylor A, Prochazka A. *Muscle Receptors and Movement*. New York: Oxford University Press,1981.

43. Matthews PBC. Proprioceptors and the regulation of movement. In Towe AL, Luschel ES (eds). *Handbook of Behavioral Neurobiology, Vol 5, Motor Coordination*. New York: Plenum Press, 1981, p 93.
44. Palastanga N, Field D, Soames R. *Anatomy and Human Movement*. 4 ed. Boston: Butterworth Heinemann, Elsevier Science, 2004.
45. Clemmesen S. Some studies of muscle tone. *Proc R Soc Med* 44:637–646, 1951.
46. Basmajian JV. Electromyography. *University of Toronto Medical Journal* 30:10–18, 1952.
47. Ralston HJ, Libet B. The question of tonus in skeletal muscle. *Am J Phys Med* 32:85, 1953.
48. DeMauro GJ. Personal Communication, June, 1994.
49. Lundy-Ekman L. *Neuroscience: Fundamentals for Rehabilitation*, 3 ed. St Louis: Saunders Elsevier, 2007.
50. Davis WJ. Organizational concepts in the central motor networks of invertebrates. In Herman RM, Grillner S, Stein PSG, Stuart DG, (eds). *Neural Control of Locomotion: Advances in Behavioral Biology,* Vol 18. New York: Plenum Press, 1976, p 265.
51. Horak FB. Assumptions underlying motor control for neurologic rehabilitation. In Foundation for Physical Therapy: *Contemporary Management of Motor Control Problems: Proceedings of the II STEP Conference*, 1991.
52. Montgomery PC, Connolly BH. *Motor Control and Physical Therapy: Theoretical Framework and Practical Applications*. Hixson, TN: Chattanooga Group, 1991.
53. Grillner S. Control of locomotion in bipeds, tetrapods, and fish. In Brooks VB, (ed). *Handbook of Physiology: The Nervous System*. Bethesda, MD: American Physiological Society, 1981, pp 1179–1236.
54. Thelen E, Kelso S, Fogel A. Self-organizing systems and infant motor development. *Dev Review* 7(1):39–65, 1987.
55. Horak FB. Assumptions underlying motor control for neurologic rehabilitation. Paper presented at Contemporary Management of Motor Control Problems: Proceedings of the II STEP Conference, 1991.
56. Bertoti DB. Functional Neurorehabilitation across the Life Span. Paper presented at Australian Physiotherapy Association, 2007, Cairns, Australia.
57. Heriza C. Motor development: Traditional and contemporary theories. Paper presented at II Step Conference: Contemporary Management of Motor Control Problems, 1991, Alexandria VA.
58. Heriza C. Implications of a dynamical systems approach to understanding infant kicking behaviors. *Phys Ther* 71(3):222–234, 1991.
59. Janeschild ME. Integrating the dynamical systems theory with the neurodevelopmental approach. *Developmental Disabilities, Special Interest Newsletter* 19(1):1–4, 1996.
60. Butt SJ, Lebret J, M. Organization of left-right coordination in the mammalian locomotor network. *Brain Research Reviews* 40(1–3):107–117, 2002.
61. Edgerton VR, Tillakaratne NJ, Bigbee AJ, de Leon RD, Roy RR. Plasticity of the spinal neural circuitry after injury. *Annu Rev Neurosci* 27:145–167, 2004.
62. Lanuza GM, Gosgnach S, Pierani A, Jessell TM, Goulding M. Genetic identification of spinal interneurons that coordinate left-right locomotor activity necessary for walking movements. *Neuron* 42(3):375–386, 2004.
63. Stecina K, Quevedo J, McCrea DA. Parallel reflex pathways from flexor muscle afferents evoking resetting and flexion enhancement during fictive locomotion and scratch in the cat. *J Physiol* 569(1):275–290, 2005.
64. Thelen E, Fisher DM, Ridley-Johnson R. The relationship between physical growth and a newborn reflex. *Infant Behav Dev* 7:479–493, 1984.
65. Morecraft RJ, Van Hoesen G, W. Cortical motor systems. In Fredericks CM, Saladin LK (eds). *Pathophysiology of the Motor Systems: Principles and Clinical Presentations*. Philadelphia: F A Davis Company, 1996, pp 158–180.
66. Martin S, Kessler M. *Neurological intervention for physical therapist assistants*. Philadelphia: W B Saunders, 2000.
67. Cohen H. *Neuroscience for Rehabilitation*, 2 ed. Philadelphia: Lippincott, Williams & Wilkins, 1999.
68. Shumway-Cook A, Woollacott MH. *Motor Control: Translating Research into Clinical Practice*, 3 ed. Philadelphia: Lippincott, Williams & Wilkins, 2007.
69. Jankovic J. Pathophysiology and clinical assessment of motor symptoms in Parkinson's disease. In Koller W (ed). *Handbook of Parkinson's Disease*. New York: Marcel Dekker, 1987, pp 99–126.
70. Nideffer RM. *Athletes Guide to Mental Training*. Champaign, IL: Human Kinetics Publishers, 1985.
71. Nideffer RM. Concentration and attention control training. In Williams JM (ed). *Applied Sports, Personal Growth and Peak Performance*. Mountain View, CA: Bayfield Publishing, 1993, pp 243–261.
72. Schmidt RA. *Motor Control and Learning: A Behavioral Emphasis*. Champaign, IL: Human Kinetics Publishers, 1988.
73. Green LB. Developing self talk to facilitate the use of imagery among athletes. In Sheikh AA, Korn ER (ed). *Imagery in Sports and Physical Performance*. Amityville, NY: Baywood Publishing, 1994, pp 43–57.

74. Green LB. The use of imagery in the rehabilitation of injured athletes. In Sheikh AA, Korn ER (eds). *Imagery in Sports and Physical Performance*. Amityville, NY: Baywood Publishing, 1994, pp 157–174.

75. Schmidt RA, Lee T, D. *Motor Control and Learning: A Behavioral Emphasis*. 6 ed. Champaign, IL: Human Kinetics, 1999.

76. Utley A, Astill S. *Motor Control, Learning and Development*. New York: Taylor & Francis Group, 2008.

77. Feltz D, Landers D. The effects of mental practice on motor skill learning and performance: A meta-analysis. *J Sports Psychol* 5:25, 1983.

78. American Physical Therapy Association. Guide to physical therapist practice, 2 ed. *Physical Therapy* 81(1): S305–S461, 2001.

79. Ghez C. Voluntary Movement. In Kendel E, Schwartz JH, Jessell TM (eds). *Principles of Neuroscience*. 3 ed. New York: Elsevier, 1991, pp 609–625.

80. Fredericks CM, Saladin LK. *Pathophysiology of the Motor Systems: Principles and Clinical Presentations*. Philadelphia: FA Davis Company, 1996.

81. Rosenfalck A, Andreassen S. Impaired regulation of force and firing pattern of single motor units in patients with spasticity. *Journal of Neurology, Neurosurgery, and Psychiatry* 43:907–916, 1980.

82. Craik RL. Abnormalities of motor behavior. Paper presented at Contemporary Management of Motor Control Problems: II Step Conference, 1991, Alexandria, VA.

83. Burke D. Spasticity as an adaptation to pyramidal tract injury In Waxman, SG (ed). *Advances in Neurology: Functional Recovery from Neurological Disease*, 47 ed. New York: Raven Press, 1988, pp 401–423.

84. Andrews AW, Bohannon RW. Distribution of muscle strength impairments following stroke. *Clin and Rehabil* 14: 79–87, 2000.

85. Bohannon RW, Walsh S. Nature, reliability, and predictive value of muscle performance measures in patients with hemisparesis following stroke. *Arch Phys Med Rehabil* 73:721–725, 1992.

86. Bohannon RW. Is the measurement of muscle strength appropriate in patients with brain lesions? A special communication. *Phys Ther* 69(3):225–236, 1989.

87. Light KE. Clients with spasticity: To strengthen or not to strengthen. *Neurology Report* 15(1):19–20, 1996.

88. Nwaobi OM. Voluntary movement impairment in upper motor neuron lesions: Is spasticity the main cause? *The Occup Jl Res* 3(3):132–140, 1983.

89. Bourbonnais D, Vanden Noven S. Weakness in patients with hemiparesis. *AJOT* 43:313–219, 1989.

90. McCartney N, Moroz D, Garner SH, McComas AJ. The effects of strength training with selected neuromuscular disorders. *Medicine and Science in Sports and Exercise* 20(4):362–368, 1998.

91. Symonds BL, James RS, Franklin CE. Getting the jump on skeletal muscle disuse atrophy: Preservation of contractile performance in aestivating *Cyclorana alboguttata*. *Journal of Experimental Biology* 210(5):825–835, 2007.

92. Jackman RW, Kandarian SC. The molecular basis of skeletal muscle atrophy. *American Journal of Physiology: Cell Physiology* 56(4):C834–C843, 2004.

93. Stein TP, Wade CE. Metabolic consequences of muscle disuse atrophy. *Journal of Nutrition* 135(7):1824–1828, 2005.

94. Gutmann E, Hnik P. *The Effect of Use and Disuse on Neuromuscular Functions*. New York: Elsevier, 1963.

95. Browse NL. *The Physiology and Pathology of Bed Rest*. Springfield, IL: Charles C Thomas, 1965.

96. Berg HE, Eiken O, Miklavcic L, Mekjavic IB. Hip, thigh and calf muscle atrophy and bone loss after 5-week bedrest activity. *Eur J Appl Physiol* 99:283–289, 2007.

97. Kasper CE, Talbot LA, Gaines JM. Skeletal muscle damage and recovery. *AACN Clin Issues Adv Pract Acute Crit Care* 13(2):237–247, 2002.

98. Hislop HJ. Response of immobilized muscle to isometric exercise. *J Am Phys Ther Assoc* 44:339, 1964.

99. Rennie MJ. Exercise- and nutrient-controlled mechanisms involved in maintenance of the musculoskeletal mass. *Biochemical Society Symposia* 035(5):1302–1305, 2007.

100. Bernstein N. *The coordination and regulation of movement*. London: Pergamon, 1967.

101. Bertoti D. Cerebral Palsy: Lifespan Management. In *Orthopaedic Interventions for the Pediatric Patient, Orthopaedic Section Home Study Course*. Alexandria: American Physical Therapy Association, 2000.

102. Knutsson E, Richards C. Different types of disturbed motor control in gait of hemiparetic patients. *Brain* 102:405–430, 1979.

103. van Dieën JH, Cholewicki J, Radebold A. Trunk muscle recruitment patterns in patients with low back pain enhance the stability of the lumbar spine. *Spine* 28(8):834–841, 2003.

104. Ng JKF, Richardson CA, Parnianpour M, Kippers V. EMG activity of trunk muscles and torque output during isometric axial rotation exertion: A comparison between back pain patients and matched controls. *Journal of Orthopaedic & Sports Physical Therapy* 20:112–121, 2002.

105. Laufer Y, Ries JD, Leininger PM, Alon G. Quadriceps femoris muscle torques and fatigue generated by neuromuscular electrical stimulation with three different waveforms. *Phys Ther* 81(7):1307–1316, 2001.

106. Deuschl G, Bain P, Brin M. Consensus statement of the Movement Disorder Society on tremor. *Mov Disord.* 1998;13:2-23.

107. Burke RE, Edgerton VR. Motor unit properties and selective involvement in movement. *Exer Sport Sci Rev* 3(31): 31–81, 1975.

108. Buchthal F, Schmalbruch H. Motor unit of mammalian muscle. *Physiol Rev* 60:90–142, 1980.

Muscle Activity and Strength

Greatness lies not in being strong, but in the right use of strength.
—Henry Ward Beecher, 1813–1887
Congregationalist, clergyman, social reformer, abolitionist, and orator

CHAPTER OUTLINE

Learning Outcomes
Clinical Scenario
Introduction
Muscle Activity
Recording Muscle Activity
Muscle Activation
Muscle Anatomic Activity
Muscle Functional Activity
Muscle Characteristics
Viscosity
Elasticity and Extensibility
Stress-Strain
Creep
Muscle Strength
Muscle Size
Fiber Architecture
Passive Components
Length-Tension Relationships and Physiological Length of Muscle
Moment Arm
Speed of Contraction
Active Tension
Age and Gender
Passive Excursion of Muscles
Passive Insufficiency
Tendon Action of Muscle
Active Excursion of Muscles
Active Insufficiency
Leverage and Length-Tension Interactions
Positive and Negative Work
Open Kinetic Chain versus Closed Kinetic Chain

LEARNING OUTCOMES

This chapter discusses muscle structure and activity and factors that produce or affect muscle strength. By the end of this chapter, you should be able to:

- ❑ Explain the differences in various muscle activation methods;
- ❑ Identify the differences in muscle fiber types and their significance in muscle function;
- ❑ Discuss the differences between the types of muscle functions;
- ❑ Provide an explanation of the stress-strain curve and its relevance to stretching tissue;
- ❑ Create two examples of active and passive muscle insufficiency;
- ❑ List and explain the components that determine muscle force;
- ❑ Outline the importance of lever arm length and muscle length in terms of muscle force production;
- ❑ Discuss eccentric muscle force and how it impacts muscle injury.

Factors Affecting Maximum Isometric Muscle Force
Exercise-Induced Muscle Injury
Delayed-Onset Muscle Soreness
Hamstring Strain
Summary
Clinical Scenario Solution
Discussion Questions
Lab Activities
References

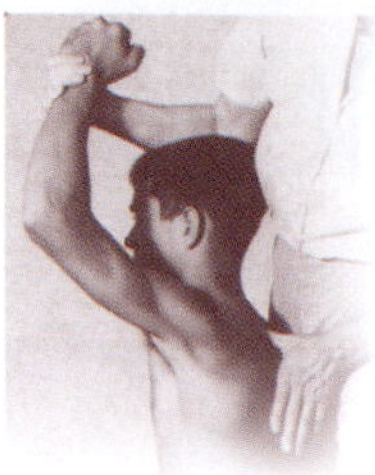

CLINICAL SCENARIO

Two promising track athletes on scholarships at Rochester State University have been in this country for only a couple of weeks. They are both from Ireland and have never experienced workouts as extensive as those that their new coach has been having them perform since they arrived on campus. Both athletes, Owain and Xavier, reported to the injury clinic this morning. They each suffered the same complaints. They had a lot of pain in their hamstrings and calf muscles after their long hill workouts yesterday. They both complained that it was difficult to get out of bed, and the pain in their hamstrings was especially uncomfortable. The clinician who examined each of them found it curious that they both suffered the same symptoms, but she suspected that she knew what the problem was.

Introduction

In the last chapter, we explored the microscopic elements involved in muscle structure and the neural elements that provided muscle activity and responses. This chapter explores the muscles at a macroscopic level. Now that you have an appreciation of the physiological function of the neuromuscular system, we can move on to realize what happens when the factors you learned in the last chapter are put to functional use. This chapter will help you understand how muscles move joints and limbs to produce daily activity and functions without a thought given to their effort. Whereas the last chapter dealt with physiology, this chapter deals with mechanics.

To make muscle mechanics easier to understand, muscle forces are depicted as acting at a single point on the body. This simplification is helpful in demonstrating principles of biomechanics, but it is important to keep in mind that many complex forces impact function. Muscles are not the only force producers affecting motion. Other soft tissues may also transmit forces of muscles through their attachments to fascia, ligaments, cartilage, joint capsules, and tendons of other muscles, as well as to bones. Active and passive structures affecting motion are presented in this chapter.

Muscle Activity

Chapter 3 guided your understanding of the neuromuscular physiology that provides muscle activity via the motor unit. Muscle contraction occurs when several motor units fire asynchronously, and the magnitude of that muscle contraction is dependent upon the number of motor units firing and how often they fire. These factors determine a muscle's activation, but there are other factors that influence how much force, or strength, a muscle ultimately exerts. Before we address the topic of strength, however, we must first identify the types of actions a muscle performs. Along with that information, we must understand how one muscle interacts with other muscles and how it responds to its own functions. This section deals with these topics.

Recording Muscle Activity

Recording muscle output and activity using surface, needle, or indwelling wire electrodes is called electromyography (EMG), (L. *elektra,* lit, brilliant, pertaining to electricity; Gr. *myos,* muscle; and L. *graphicus,* to write). Each pair of electrodes is connected to a "channel" of the recording apparatus (Fig. 4.1). The use of multi-channel instruments allows the contraction and relaxation patterns of several muscles to be recorded simultaneously during a particular movement or joint position. Using EMG, the sequence of activation and relaxation, as well as the relative amount of activity of specific muscles, can be studied as they perform various isolated or coordinated functions. Some of the earliest careful studies of kinesiology using EMG were performed by Inman and co-workers[1] in their analysis of shoulder motions. Reports on the uses and limitations of kinesiologic EMG include those by Clarys[2], Basmajian[3], and Heckathorne and colleagues[4]. Reports

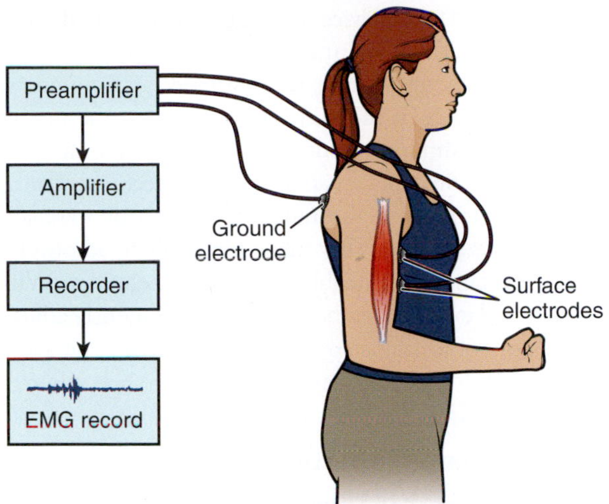

Figure 4.1 Using electromyography to record muscle activity. Electrodes are placed over the muscle to detect changes in electric potential associated with muscle fiber activation. The electrical activity "seen" by the electrodes is greatly amplified by electronic equipment, recorded, and stored for later analysis.

of the use of EMG techniques for kinesiologic studies include those by Ebersole [5], Smidt [6], and Perry.[7] A more detailed discussion of the use and limitations of kinesiologic EMG is presented in Chapter 12.

Muscle Activation

A muscle is able to produce different types of muscle tension, either with or without movement. There are different types of motions that muscle activation produces. This section briefly describes each of them.

Isometric

When a muscle produces force with no apparent change in the joint angle, the activation is **isometric** (Gr. *isos,* equal; *metron,* measure). Isometric activations are also called static, or holding, contractions. During functional activities, isometric activation stabilizes joints. For example, to reach forward with the hand, the scapula must be stabilized against the thorax.

Concentric

A shortening of the muscle is a **concentric activity.** Examples include the quadriceps muscle when an individual rises from a chair or the elbow flexors when an individual lifts a glass of water to her mouth. Concentric motion occurs as the muscle shortens and the muscle's proximal and distal insertion points move closer towards each other. Concentric activity produces acceleration of body segments.

Eccentric

When the muscle lengthens during activation, it is an **eccentric activity.** For example, the quadriceps activates eccentrically when the body moves from standing to sitting, as do the elbow flexors when lowering the glass of water from the mouth to the table. Eccentric motion occurs as the muscle lengthens and the muscle's points of insertion move away from each other. Eccentric motion often occurs against gravity as the muscle controls the speed with which gravity moves the joint. Eccentric activity decelerates body segments and provides shock absorption as when landing from a jump or in walking.

Concentric motion is sometimes also referred to as **positive work** whereas eccentric motion is **negative work.** Positive work is force exerted by the muscle to produce movement of a joint; in other words, the motion is produced *by* the muscle. On the other hand, negative work occurs when an outside force produces joint motion while the muscle controls the rate at which that motion occurs; an external force, often gravity, is responsible for motion that is done *to* the muscle during negative work.

Isotonic

The word **isotonic** is derived from the Greek *isos,* equal, and *tonus,* tension. The term was originally used by muscle physiologists to refer to the contraction of a muscle detached from the body and lifting a load vertically against gravity. The connotation was that shortening of the muscle occurred and the load on the muscle was constant throughout the excursion. Truly

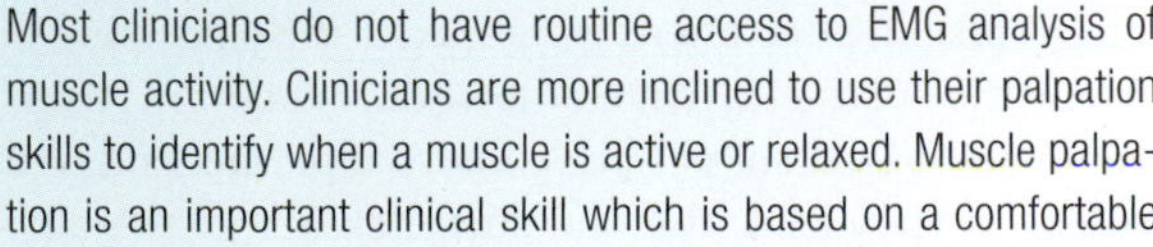

PRACTICE POINT

Most clinicians do not have routine access to EMG analysis of muscle activity. Clinicians are more inclined to use their palpation skills to identify when a muscle is active or relaxed. Muscle palpation is an important clinical skill which is based on a comfortable familiarity of surface anatomy and comprehensive knowledge of three-dimensional anatomy. It is best to palpate a muscle when it is lightly contracting so as to avoid contraction of surrounding muscles.

isotonic contractions seldom, if ever, occur when muscles are acting through the lever systems of the body. Even so, the term is often used, although incorrectly, to refer to a contraction that causes a joint to move through some range of motion, as in flexing the elbow while holding a weight in the hand. Even though the weight remains the same throughout the movement, the tension requirements of the muscle change continuously with changing leverage, and the torque exerted by the weight changes with changing joint angles.

Isometric and 'isotonic' activities are sometimes referred to as "contractions." However, "contraction" means "shortening;" it is not necessarily an accurate term since shortening does not occur in either isometric activation or eccentric activity. Nevertheless, "contraction" is commonly used as a noun with isometric or eccentric as its adjectives.

Isokinetic

An **isokinetic** (Gr. *isos*, equal; *kinetos*, moving) contraction occurs when the rate of movement is constant. In the 1960s, an electromechanical device (an isokinetic dynamometer) was developed that limits the rate of movement of a crank-arm or a pulley to some preset angular velocity regardless of the force exerted by the contracting muscles. In 1967, Hislop and Perrine described the concept and principles of isokinetic exercise.[8] The axis of rotation of the crank arm of the isokinetic device is aligned with the anatomic axis of the moving joint, and the device lever is matched to the skeletal lever (Fig. 4.2). A subject contracts the muscle group being exercised or evaluated, and the device controls the speed of body movement without permitting acceleration to occur. "During isokinetic exercise, the resistance accommodates the external force at the skeletal lever so that the muscle maintains maximum output throughout the full range of motion."[8] A clinician can apply a similar accommodating resistance throughout the range of motion by manually resisting the motion. This manually applied, accommodating resistance is a valuable therapeutic technique. With practice and experience, the clinician continuously adjusts the amount of resistance offered so that the motion speed is essentially constant throughout the range, thereby approaching an isokinetic condition.

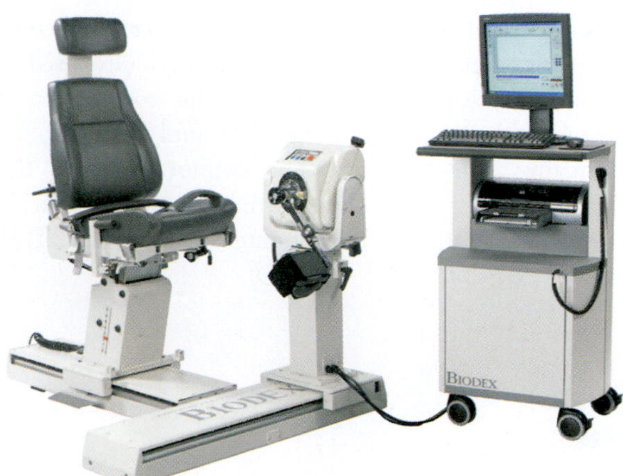

Figure 4.2 An example of an isokinetic exercise and testing unit. Isokinetic dynamometers may be used for testing and exercising muscle groups isokinetically, isometrically, concentrically, or eccentrically. Depending on the specific unit, force or torque exerted by the muscle group is recorded along with joint angles and motion. The computer provides calculations for average peak torque, work, and power.

Muscle Anatomic Activity

Muscle fiber types and muscle attachment sites are presented in this section. They are anatomical designs that influence how a muscle reacts to stimulation and also how a muscle performs during functional activities.

Muscle Attachments

Anatomically, muscles are described by their **proximal attachments** (origin), **distal attachments** (insertion), and **actions** in producing specific joint motions. Although knowledge of the anatomic attachments and actions is essential to the study of kinesiology, it is important to recognize that these factors can predict muscle function when all of the following conditions are present:

(1) The proximal attachment is stabilized;
(2) The distal attachment moves toward the proximal attachment (concentric contraction);
(3) The distal segment moves against gravity or a resistance; and
(4) The muscle acts alone.

Unfortunately, these circumstances rarely occur in normal function.

However, the anatomical attachments and actions of muscles are a good starting point for novice clinicians to begin their understanding of kinesiology. After all, knowing where a muscle's proximal and distal attachments are and understanding the motion a muscle produces is essential to appreciating more complicated muscle functions. Once you know insertions and actions of muscles, you can recall other factors that affect functional application of muscle activity. For example, if the proximal biceps brachii attachment is stabilized, the elbow will flex when the muscle activates; however, when any muscle contracts, it shortens at both ends, so if neither end of the biceps is stabilized, the shoulder flexes and the elbow flexes when the biceps contracts. We can take this notion in another direction to better understand muscle function in a closed chain activity: If the distal segment of a muscle's attachment is stabilized, then the proximal segment is the moving end of the muscle. Since a muscle can produce either a shortening (concentric) or lengthening (eccentric) motion, biceps function changes depending on which type of muscle movement occurs. Therefore, when the proximal end is stabilized and the elbow flexes, the activated biceps produces a concentric force; however, when the elbow extends with gravity, the biceps produce an eccentric force to guide the speed of gravity's pull on the elbow. In fact, gravity is often the force against which muscles act, so eccentric force production of muscles commonly occurs during functional antigravity activity. Most human activity is the result of more than one muscle. Muscles perform functional activity conjointly, either with the assistance of other muscles acting as synergists or with other muscles assisting joint or segmental stabilization.

In summary then, it is necessary to identify a muscle's proximal and distal insertions and its actions, but knowing these factors provides only part of the picture; a true appreciation of how the body produces functional activity production occurs with the realization that movement results from the of modification of these factors: (1) Proximal attachments often move toward fixed distal attachments (closed kinematic chain); (2) Contractions can be concentric, eccentric, or isometric; (3) Movement of the distal segment is often assisted by the force of gravity; and (4) Muscles seldom if ever act alone—they more often act with other muscles.

Since gravity plays a profound role in functional activities, it is interesting to realize that muscles that are named for their function and the joint they cross may not be the muscles that perform the activity. For example, when the hand is placed over the edge of a table with the palm facing the floor and the wrist is slowly flexed, the wrist flexors are inactive; the motion is performed by an eccentric contraction of the wrist extensors. Therefore, an awareness of gravity's influence on motion is vital to understanding functional activity.

Muscle Fiber Types

Chapter 3 described the differences in muscular fiber types. As you recall, there are three types of skeletal muscle fibers. These types may be classified several different ways, according to their metabolic function, structure, chemical composition, or mechanical functions. Two of these fiber types are opposite to one another in most of these categories, and the third one is a blend of the two. Because they may be classified in different ways, they are referred to differently, depending on which classification system is used. Take a quick look at Table 3–2 so you may quickly recall the various classification systems and the characteristics of each fiber type. The major classification system most frequently used identifies the three fiber types as I, IIa and IIb. Types I and IIb are opposite to one another, and type IIa is a blend of the two. It should be kept in mind that these fiber types are on a continuum with type I at one end and type IIb at the other. Type IIa is a meshing of these two types, so some of the type IIa fibers are more similar to type I fiber types whereas others are more similar to type IIb fibers.

Each individual has a combination of these fiber types throughout the body. Some muscles may have more of one fiber type than another and this arrangement varies from one individual to another.[9-10] Although an individual is born with type I and type II fibers, they may change later in life according to the individual's activity and hormone levels.[10] As we age, muscle fibers also change with a reduction in the amount of type II fibers.[11]

To some extent, the type of fibers within a muscle is determined by that muscle's function.[11] Muscles that work against gravity as we sit or stand are called antigravity muscles or postural muscles. Since we may sit or stand for prolonged periods, these muscles contain more slow-twitch or type I muscle fibers. Prolonged standing or sitting requires continual minor adjustments in posture, so these muscles must have fibers that resist fatigue and are able to maintain sustained activity. These muscles include the soleus, peroneals, quadriceps, gluteals, rectus abdominis, upper extremity extensors, erector spinae group, and short cervical flexors. On the other hand, muscles that are used for rapid movement during explosive activities are mobility muscles or nonpostural muscles. These muscles contain more type II muscle fibers.[12] These movement muscles produce force and power rapidly but have low endurance; therefore, they cannot sustain activity for prolonged periods. These muscles include the gastrocnemius, hamstrings, and upper extremity flexors.

Muscle Functional Activity

As has been mentioned, muscles rarely act alone during functional activities. Sometimes a muscle is the primary mover, but at other times, it may assist or oppose an action. Although there are various terms in the literature that describe these functions, three primary terms are used in this text. They are presented here.

Agonist

A muscle that is the principle muscle producing a motion or maintaining a posture is the **agonist** (Gr. *agon*, contest). An agonist actively contracts to produce a concentric, eccentric, or isometric contraction. Agonists are sometimes referred to as prime movers.

Antagonist

An **antagonist** (Gr. *anti*, against) is a muscle or a muscle group that provides the opposite anatomic action of the agonist. During functional activities, the antagonist is usually inactive during the activity so it neither contributes to nor resists the activity, but its passive elongation or shortening allows the desired activity to occur. For example, when a fork is brought to the mouth, the biceps is the agonist providing the movement while the triceps is the antagonist that remains relaxed, passively lengthening to allow the movement to occur.

Synergist

A muscle that contracts at the same time as the agonist is a **synergist** (Gr. *syn*, with, together; *ergon*, work). A muscle may provide synergistic action in different ways. One way is that it may provide identical or nearly identical activity to that of the agonist. An example is the brachioradialis working with the brachialis during elbow flexion.

Another way a synergist may function is to obstruct an unwanted action of the agonist, such as when the wrist extensors prevent wrist flexion when the long finger flexors contract to grasp an object. This type of synergistic activity is a common functional feature of muscles that perform more than one motion. Look at the action of wrist radial deviation as an example. The flexor carpi radialis performs both wrist flexion and radial abduction; similarly, the extensor carpi radialis longus performs both wrist extension and radial abduction. When frontal plane radial abduction occurs, both muscles act synergistically to radially abduct the wrist while the extension and flexion actions of the muscles are neutralized.

Another way synergists act is to stabilize proximal joints for distal joint movement. When synergists act in this manner, they work isometrically at joints that are not being moved by the agonists to stabilize the proximal joint, allowing the desired motion at the more distal segment to occur.

Muscles work more often as synergists than as either agonists or antagonists. When an agonist contracts, its force causes both its proximal and distal attachments to move. To prevent movement of the muscle from both of its attachments and allow the desired movement to occur, one of the muscle's attachment sites must be stabilized; which end—the proximal or distal attachment site—is stabilized depends on the intended activity. Stabilizers are mentioned throughout this text as important factors of joint motion. In fact, without stabilizers, agonistic movement is inefficient and ineffective.

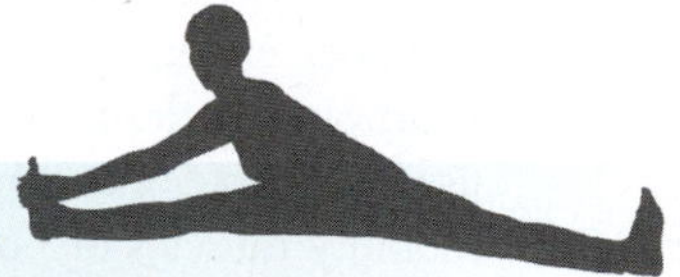

PRACTICE POINT

Some clinicians argue that an antagonist contracts with the agonist to produce a motion such as a squat exercise; however, it has been found that the antagonist's activity is a fraction of the agonist's contraction force.[13-15] In this example, the antagonist (hamstrings) works more as a synergist to the quadriceps, not providing the movement but stabilizing the joint to permit the agonist's desired motion of knee flexion to occur. This rationale makes intuitive sense since if an agonist and an antagonist both contracted with comparable force, movement could not occur. Clinicians desiring to increase strength of the hamstrings would do better to create an exercise that uses the hamstrings as the agonist rather than count on the squat exercise to provide significant strength gains.

Two exercises readily point to the importance of stabilizers during functional movements. One quick exercise is to close the hand into a very firm grip; you are able to palpate tension not only in the finger flexors within the anterior forearm, but also in the posterior forearm, biceps and triceps in the arm, and even the shoulder muscles. These muscles all contract isometrically to stabilize the upper extremity to allow your firm grip to occur. Another exercise example is a sit-up. Lie supine with your lower extremities fully extended and your hands on top of your head. Attempt to do a sit-up and notice that both your trunk and your legs lift off the surface. The hip flexors, like other muscles, contract at both ends, so if one end is not stabilized, both ends of the muscle move. Clinicians must realize how muscle contraction produces either proximal or distal motion so when inadequate stabilization is present during rehabilitation activities, it is easily recognized and corrected. Clinicians must also understand the importance of stabilization during functional activities and appreciate which muscles must function and what their strength requirements are to provide that stabilization.

The relationships of muscles as agonists, antagonists, and synergists are not constant. They vary with the activity, position of the body, and the direction of the resistance which the muscle must overcome. These changing relationships are illustrated in the EMG recordings (Fig. 4.3) of the triceps brachii and the biceps-brachialis muscles during the motions of elbow flexion and extension (Fig. 4.3A1) When the seated subject flexes the elbow to lift a load in the hand, the elbow flexors contract concentrically as agonists (Fig. 4.3A2). The antagonistic extensors are relaxed to elongate and permit elbow flexion motion. As the elbow extends to lower the load to the side, the flexors perform an eccentric activity and are still classified as agonists (Fig. 4.3A3). The extensors remain inactive and are still the antagonists. However, when the subject moves to supine with the shoulder in 90° of flexion and performs the same motions of elbow flexion and extension, the agonist-antagonist relationships are reversed (Fig. 4.3B1). Here, the elbow extensors are the agonists for elbow flexion (eccentric contraction) (Fig. 4.3B2) and for elbow extension (concentric contraction) (Fig. 4.3B3), while the flexors are the antagonists and remain relaxed for both motions.

An interesting switch in the agonistic-antagonistic classification also occurs with these same motions of elbow flexion and extension when the subject is in supine with the arm at the side (Fig. 4.3C1). Now the biceps-brachialis muscles are the agonists for the first part of elbow flexion, but as the elbow passes 90°, the direction of the resistance force changes, and the triceps becomes the agonist (Fig. 4.3C2). The agonist for elbow extension from this position to 90° is the triceps, but once the elbow moves on the other side of to 90°, the elbow flexors (eccentric contraction) control the elbow movement to the start position (Fig. 4.3C3). This change in responsibility changes with gravity's pull on the weight and the relative position of the center of mass to the pull of gravity. Application of manual resistance throughout the motion of flexion (Fig. 4.3D1) and then extension (Fig. 4.3D2) further illustrates the principle that muscles act according to the resistance they meet rather than the motion.

Other examples of the varying relationships among these muscles are shown in Figure 4.4. As seen in this example, the biceps acts as an agonist in supination (along with the supinator), and the triceps acts as a synergist to prevent elbow flexion. When a muscle has multiple functions like the biceps but only one of its motions is desired, the antagonist to the undesired motion is often recruited to serve as a synergist so the undesired motion is prevented from occurring.

Muscle Characteristics

Forces applied to muscles produce stresses to those muscles. A **stress** is a force or load that is applied to a body, segment, or muscle. Stresses may occur as compression, distraction, shear, torsional, bending, twisting, or any combination of these stresses. The muscles and their connective tissue resist these stresses in similar fashion. If they are unable to withstand the stress, injury occurs. Muscle and its surrounding connective tissue possess mechanical and physical properties that provide resistance to stresses. These characteristics are presented in this section. The most important properties are described along with why they are important and how we can use these characteristics to our advantage in exercise and rehabilitation.

Viscosity

Viscosity is the resistance to an external force that causes a permanent deformation. It is a term that is usually applied to fluids. Think of tar versus oil. Although both are viscous, tar has more viscosity than oil. If tar is heated, it becomes less viscous and more easily moldable. Human tissue also has viscosity. Clinicians use the fact that elevating temperature reduces viscosity by applying heat to tissue before stretching it. Lowering tissue temperature, on the other hand, increases the tissue's viscosity. If you have ever been outside without gloves or mittens on a cold day, you know this already because you may recall how stiff your fingers and hands were when you first entered a warm building.

Elasticity and Extensibility

Extensibility and elasticity are closely related. **Extensibility** is the ability to stretch, elongate or expand. **Elasticity** is the ability to succumb to an elongating force and then return to normal length when the force is released. The potential energy that is released by tissue when it is stretched is also the energy that allows tissue to return to its normal length following release of a stretch force. The more elasticity a tissue possesses, the more extensibility, or temporary elongation, it is able to demonstrate. If you take two rubber bands, a thick one and a thin one, and stretch them both with an equal amount of force, you find that the thin one has more elasticity than the thick one; it is able to stretch farther and still return to its normal length when you release the stretch.

Just as elasticity and extensibility are directly related to each other, viscosity is indirectly related to them. The more extensibility a tissue has, the less viscosity it has, and vice versa. Muscle and connective tissue have both properties of viscosity and elasticity and are referred to

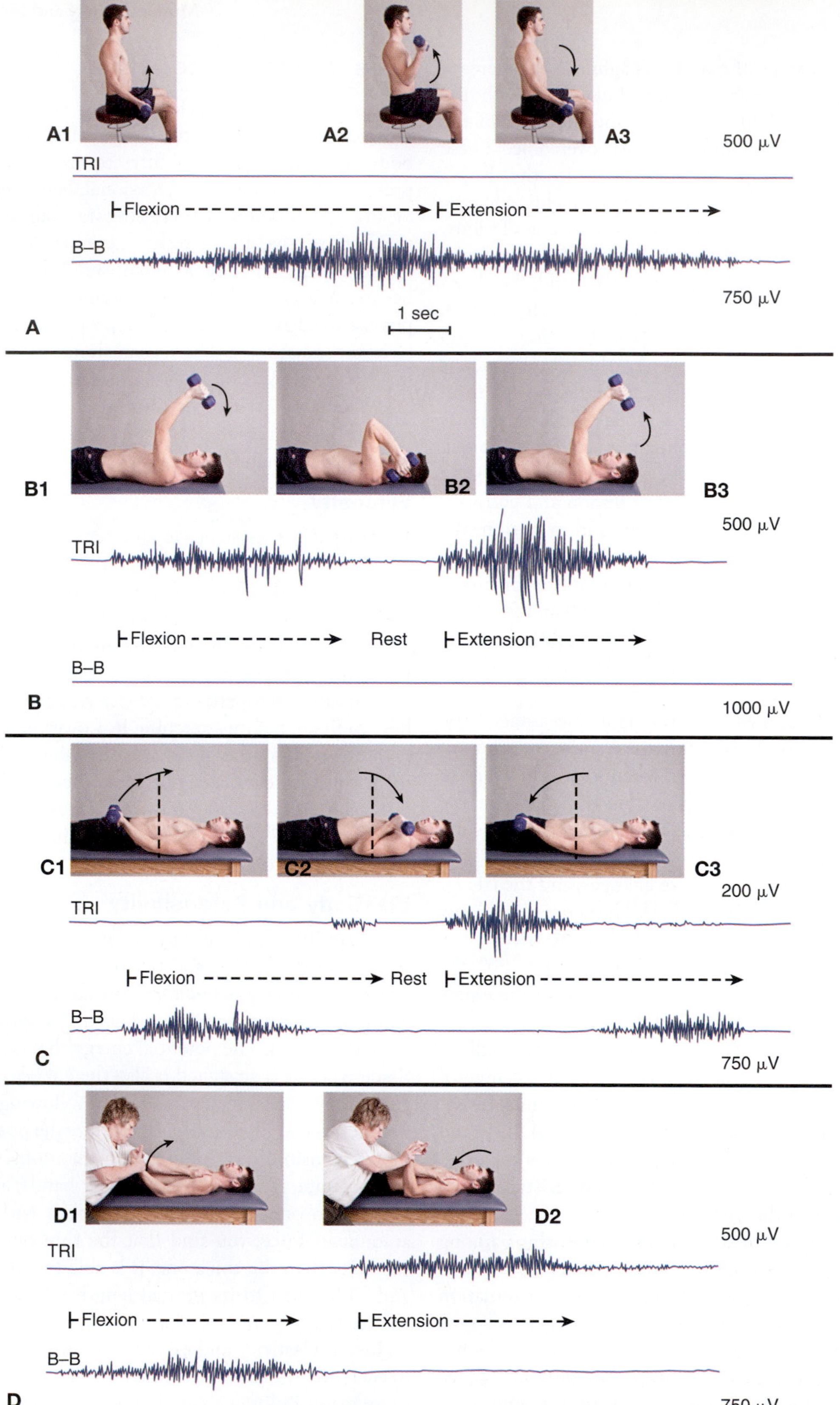

Figure 4.3 EMG activity of the biceps and triceps during elbow flexion and extension changes with changes in body position and the direction of resistive force. **A)** Subject seated with resistance in hand. **B)** Subject supine with resistance in hand. **C)** Subject supine working against manual resistance during concentric muscle activity. Notice in **A** and **B** how the intensity of muscle activity is less during eccentric effort compared to concentric contractions. TRI = triceps. B–B = biceps brachii and brachialis.

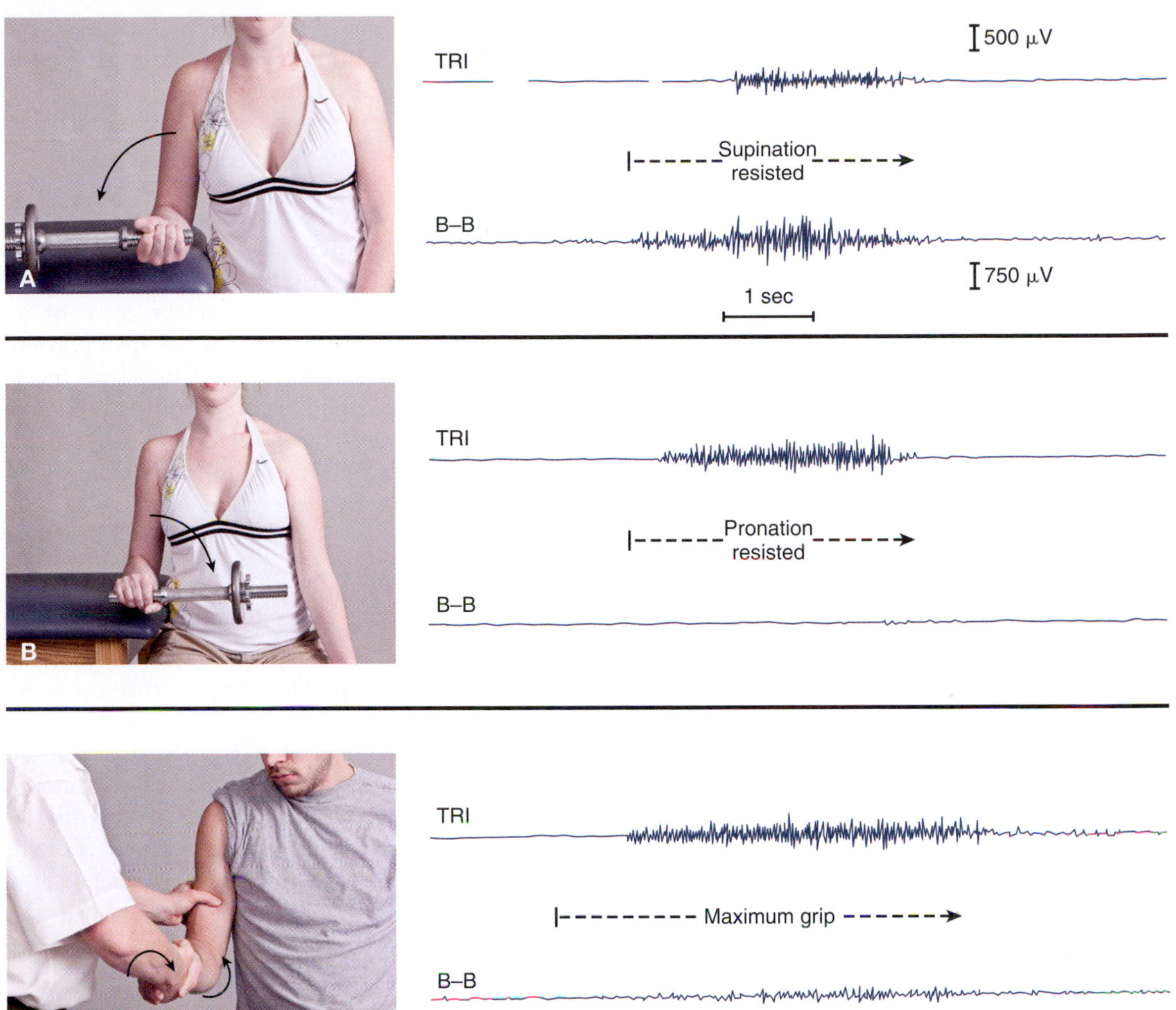

Figure 4.4 Synergistic actions of biceps and triceps during forearm activities. Electromyographic recordings with the subject sitting, the elbow flexed to 90°, and the forearm supported. An isometric contraction at the start of forearm supination requires synergistic activity of the triceps to prevent the biceps from flexing the elbow. TRI = Triceps. B–B = Biceps brachii and brachialis.

as viscoelastic tissue. Tissue that has **viscoelasticity** has the ability to resist changing its shape when a force is applied to it, but if the force is sufficient to cause change, the tissue is unable to return to its original shape. Not only do muscle and connective tissue possess this quality, but all tissues do. In fact, all structures do. Very rigid structures are more viscous and less elastic; very pliable structures are more elastic and less viscous. If you have ever seen an old building with its original windows, it may appear that the window glass looks wavy—the glass has succumbed to the continual pull of gravity and is unable to return to its original clear, see-through structure. This property of viscoelasticity of any structure adheres to the stress-strain principle.

Stress-Strain

As we have mentioned, stress is a force or load that the body or its parts resists. How well those structures are able to resist a stress is dependent upon its ability to deform. This is **strain** of a structure: the amount of deformation it is able to tolerate before it succumbs to the stress. All structures, natural and man-made, have their own specific relationship between stress and strain. This is called the **stress-strain curve** or **stress-strain principle**. Although it varies from one structure to another and from one type of tissue to another, a curve for connective tissue serves to represent a generic stress-strain curve for human tissue (Fig. 4.5). The initial section of the stress-strain curve is the *toe region*. In

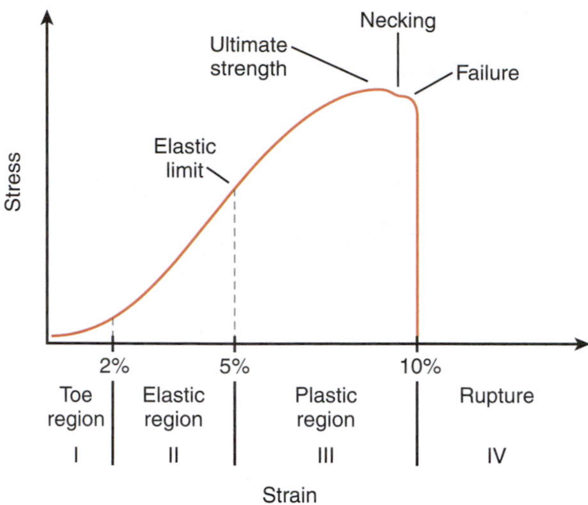

Figure 4.5 Stress-strain curve. Whereas stress is the amount of force applied to a structure, strain is the deformation that occurs with the application of stress. A structure has its own ability to withstand stresses applied to it. This ability is dependent upon the degree of deformation allowed in the toe, elastic, and plastic regions of its stress-strain curve. When the stress applied to a structure moves into the necking range, the next phase is failure of the structure to withstand further stress.

a resting state, tissue has a crimped or wavy appearance. When stress is applied to the tissue, this slack is taken up within the toe region of the stress-strain curve. Once the tissue is elongated to the point at which the slack is taken out of the structure so it becomes taut, the stress force moves the tissue into the *elastic range*. This elastic range is the point at which the tissue's elastic properties are stressed. The tissue strain and the amount of stretch move through a linear relationship when there is a direct relationship between the amount of stress applied to the tissue and the tissue's ability to stretch. If the force or load is released at any time during either of these two ranges, the tissue returns to its normal length. On the other hand, if the force applied continues to increase, the tissue moves from its elastic range into its *plastic range*. In this range, there is microscopic damage to the structure; some of the tissue ruptures because it is unable to withstand this amount of stress. It is at this point that permanent change in the tissue's length occurs. If the force is released at this point, the tissue is elongated compared to what it was prior to the stress application. If the amount of stress continues to increase past the plastic range, the tissue moves into the *necking range*. At this point, more and more microscopic ruptures occur until the tissue becomes macroscopically damaged. It is at this time that the force or load required to create tissue damage is less than previously because the tissue is weakening. If the stress increase continues, immediately before the tissue ruptures entirely, a give in the structure is felt and then the tissue rips apart, moving into the *failure range*. Continuity of the tissue is lost when tissue failure occurs.

Creep

Creep is the elongation of tissue from the application of a low-level load over time. The old glass in the window of the old home that was described earlier underwent deformation by creep. The changes that occur with creep occur in the plastic range of tissue or structures so the changes are permanent. We experience creep on a daily basis. If you measure your height in the morning and then again in the evening, you will discover that you are taller in the morning. The long-term effect of gravity on our tissues causes this height difference by the end of the day. Creep can be either advantageous or deleterious. For example, an individual with a tight Achilles tendon will find it very difficult to effectively stretch such a large, firm structure using a normal short-term stretch. However, using a prolonged stretch of perhaps 10 minutes may produce sufficient creep to increase the flexibility of the Achilles. This is especially true if the prolonged stretch is repetitive.

Muscle Strength

Muscle strength is a general term without a precise definition. Among the many definitions of strength are the

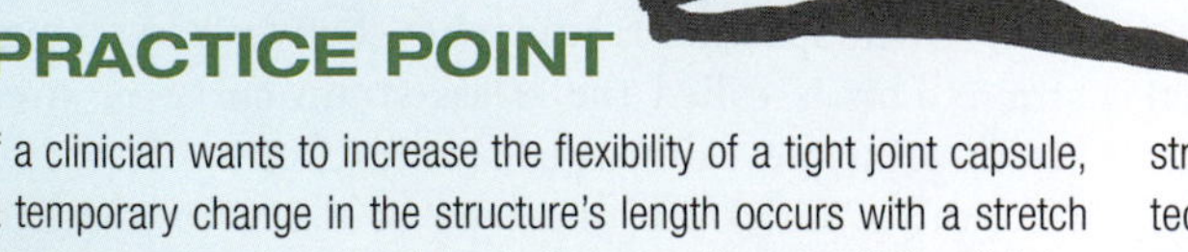

PRACTICE POINT

If a clinician wants to increase the flexibility of a tight joint capsule, a temporary change in the structure's length occurs with a stretch that approaches the capsule's elastic range. However, if the clinician wants to improve range of motion of the joint, the capsule must be stretched into its plastic range. A combination of joint mobilization techniques and stretching exercises must provide this stress to produce a permanent increase in flexibility.

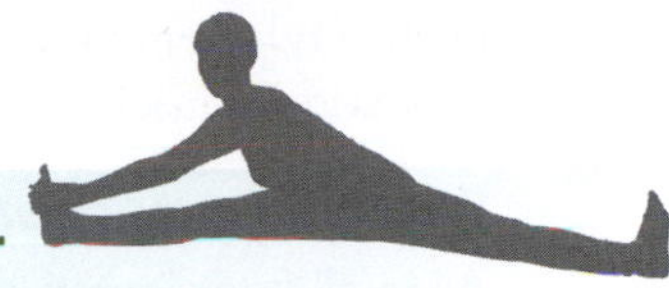

PRACTICE POINT

Creep may also be injurious to the body. If a creep load is more stressful than the tissue is able to tolerate, repetitive bouts applied over time may cause the tissue to become structurally fatigued. Structural fatigue occurs with an accumulation of stress from repeated bouts of application. In bones, we call these **stress fractures**; in tendons, we may refer to it as **tendinopathy.**

state of being strong, the capacity of a muscle to produce force, and the ability of a muscle to generate active tension. How well muscles are able to produce force depends upon a number of factors. In addition to neurologic, metabolic, endocrine, and psychological factors that affect muscle strength, many other factors determine muscle strength.

If bones create levers and joints, muscles provide the forces by which motion occurs in the body. Motion of the body's levers occurs as muscles which cross joints produce force to move those levers. How well this force is produced depends on a number of factors unique to each muscle or muscle group. These factors that influence muscle performance include:

- the muscle's size;
- the architecture of muscle fibers;
- the passive components of the muscle;
- the physiological length of the muscle or length-tension relationship of the muscle;
- the moment arm length of the muscle;
- the speed of muscle contraction;
- the active tension; and
- age and gender

Each of these topics is discussed in this section.

Muscle Size

Muscle size refers to two parameters: length and width. If muscle fibers are placed side by side—as in *parallel* to each other—the muscle's width is greater. On the other hand, if muscle fibers are placed end to end, they are in *series* to each other. As a rule, parallel muscle fibers provide greater force and series muscle fiber arrangements provide greater speed of motion. Given two muscles of the same length, the muscle with a greater width is stronger than one that has a smaller diameter or width. A good rule of thumb to remember is that when there are muscles of variable lengths crossing a joint, the longer muscles provide that segment's mobility whereas the shorter muscles provide its stability. For example, the short multifidus muscles that attach from one spinal segment to the adjacent vertebrae provide spinal stability whereas the longer erector spinae muscles that attach across several spinal segments provide spinal motion.

In terms of cross section, it is well known that larger muscles in normal subjects are stronger than smaller ones. It is also known that muscle size may increase (**hypertrophy**) or decrease (**atrophy**) with exercise or inactivity, respectively. Clinicians are often called upon to measure these changes. However, measurement of actual size and changes in size is difficult. Magnetic resonance imaging (MRI) provides an anatomic cross section of the muscle, so the area of muscle tissue can be measured and small size changes can be detected.[16-17] Muscle biopsies can also measure small size changes.[18] Both of these techniques, however, are expensive, and the biopsy is invasive. Circumferential measurements lack accuracy because they also include skin, fat, fluid, vasculature, and bone and depend on a subjective judgment of the amount of tension on the tape measure.[19] However in spite of their inaccuracy, circumferential measurements are most often used clinically since it is inexpensive and convenient. An important key factor in using circumferential measurements is to be precise and consistent in both the procedure and the recording of the procedure.

Fiber Architecture

All skeletal muscles have the same basic architecture. An entire muscle may be divided into sections called fascicles, or bundles. Within these bundles are numerous muscle fibers. Recall that the number of muscle fibers is one of the factors that determine a muscle's ability to produce force. The more muscle fibers a muscle has, the more force that muscle has the potential to exert.

One skeletal muscle fiber is a single muscle cell which is enclosed by a plasma membrane called the sarcolemma. Each muscle cell contains substances: Some are necessary for cell metabolism and others are the contractile elements of the cell. These contractile structures are myofibrils. There are several myofibrils within each cell. The myofibrils contain protein filaments—actin and myosin. It is at the actin and myosin level that muscle contraction occurs.

Not only is the basic cellular design relevant to strength, but investigators have shown a strong correlation between the physiologic cross-sectional area of a muscle and the maximal force that the muscle can produce.[20] A line that transects each fasciculus at a right angle determines the physiologic cross section of a muscle. Hence, the fiber arrangement of a muscle is fundamental to its strength. By knowing the various fiber arrangements of muscles, we can determine its cross-sectional area and then predict whether the muscle has relatively great or little force production potential.

Muscle fiber arrangement of an entire muscle at the macroscopic level is either **fusiform** (strap) or **pennate** (L. *penna,* feather). In fusiform muscles, the fascicles are parallel and long throughout the muscle. The sartorius is an example of a strap, or fusiform, muscle.[21] These muscles are designed to produce greater shortening distance but less force. Pennate fascicles, on the other hand, attach at oblique angles to a central tendon. There are different pennate designs of muscles, depending upon the number of fiber arrangements within a muscle. Unipennate muscles have one parallel fiber arrangement whereas bipennate muscles have two groups of parallel fibers running to one central tendon. Most muscles in the body are multipennate muscles with more than two pennate groups attaching to more than one centralizing tendon. Pennate fascicles are shorter than fusiform fascicles; they produce greater forces to the sacrifice of speed since their total cross section is larger. Since muscle strength is proportional to the total cross-sectional area of the muscle, strength of pennate muscles is related to the combined cross-sectional size of the pennate muscle. Therefore, total strength of pennate muscles is the sum of the cross-sectional areas of each pennate. The architectural design of most muscles in the body is multipennate.[22] Figure 4.6 demonstrates the various muscle fascicle arrangements.

Passive Components

As in all body structures, muscle is surrounded by connective tissue called **fascia**. Although this connective tissue is composed of various cells and ground substance, its predominant cell type is collagen. Collagen is the protein that forms the majority of the white fibers of fascia. Muscle structural levels from the microscopic fibers to the entire muscle are each encased by a sleeve of fascia; these layers of fascia have different names to identify their structural level. Each muscle cell or fiber is surrounded by a fascial layer called the **endomysium. Perimysium** surrounds groups of muscle fibers or fascicles. The **epimysium** is the fascial layer surrounding the entire muscle. These fascial layers are interconnected with each other as well as with the fascia covering the muscle's tendons. Collectively, these fascial layers form a muscle's **passive elastic component.** The fascia is passive since it is unable to change its length actively but complies with the muscle's change in length. Because the fascial fibers surrounding a muscle are parallel to the muscle fibers, muscle fascia is also known as the muscle's **parallel elastic component.** When a muscle elongates beyond the point at which its slack is removed, the fascia becomes passively stretched as the muscle continues to lengthen. This *parallel* elastic component design is in contrast to the tendon and its fascia that are positioned at either end of the muscle; the tendon and its fascia provide the muscle's **series elastic component.** This name is given to the tendon and its fascia because of their series arrangement with the muscle: tendon–muscle–tendon. This configuration allows the contracting muscle fibers to transfer their forces along the tendon to the bone to produce motion.

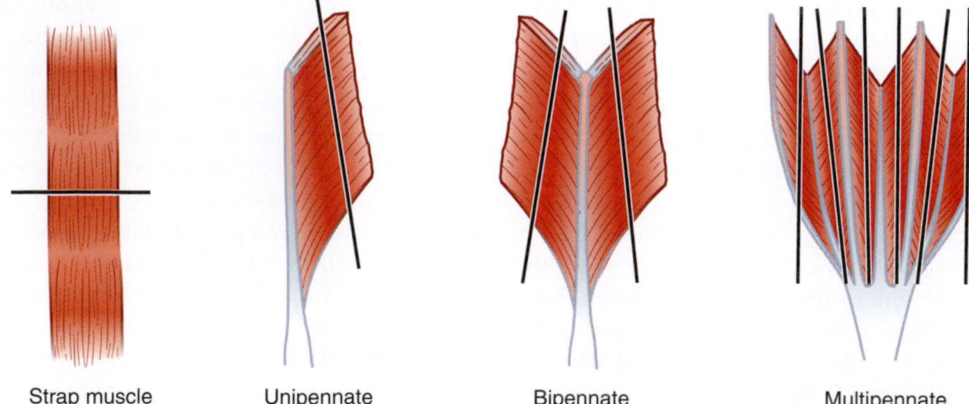

Figure 4.6 Fusiform and pennate muscles with their cross-sections identified. Multipennate muscles have larger cross sections (black lines through the muscle fibers represent cross sections) than unipennate muscles, and the more pennates a muscle has in its fiber arrangement, the greater force it is able to produce.

As mentioned, the parallel elastic component stretches when a muscle lengthens and so, too, does the series elastic component. As the series and parallel elastic components become taut, they provide stiffness to the muscle. Since this increase in the muscle's stiffness occurs because of the muscle's fascia and tendon, it is considered **passive tension** (Fig. 4.7). This passive tension is like stretching a rubber band—as the stretch increases, more tension is produced. When the passive tension is released, a greater rebound response or contraction is produced by the greater tension. This is the length-tension relationship described in the next section.

Length-Tension Relationships and Physiological Length of Muscle

There is a relationship between the amount of tension produced by a muscle and its length. As was just mentioned, passive tissue creates some of that tension as the muscle elongates. Studies have investigated how far a muscle's passive tissue can be stretched before tissue failure occurs: When a sarcomere is stretched to 200% of normal resting length, failure occurs.[23] The **resting length** of a muscle is a position of the muscle in which there is no tension within the muscle. Although this cannot be precisely determined, a muscle's resting length is defined as the length at which the maximum number of actin-myosin crossbridges is available. As a muscle either shortens or lengthens beyond that resting position, its ability to produce force decreases because the number of crossbridges declines when the muscle fiber moves out of its resting length.

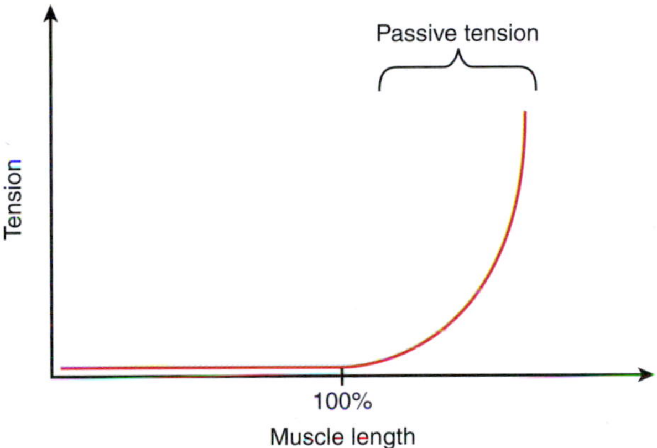

Figure 4.7 Total length-tension relationship curve of a muscle. Passive elastic components provide tension beyond normal resting length whereas active muscle tissue provides tension at less than resting length. Passive tension occurs as the result of stretch.

Active tension declines as the muscle shortens because there are fewer crossbridges available between the actin and myosin fibers. When a sarcomere is at its shortest position, there are no remaining crossbridges available. Likewise, as the muscle lengthens, the actin and myosin fibers move farther apart until crossbridges do not connect between the actin and myosin sufficiently to produce tension. Active tension is responsible for muscle tension during shortening whereas passive tension adds to muscle tension during lengthening. Active muscle tension is graphically presented in Figure 4.8. Together, the active and passive tension elements of a muscle produce the muscle's length-tension relationship as diagrammed in Figure 4.9.

It should be realized that investigations which have provided us with this information on length-tension have been performed in the laboratory with sarcomeres in isolation from the body.[23-25] Isometric resistance applied to these individual fibers in the lab has created the results we all extrapolate to an entire muscle. Unfortunately, the methodology of these investigations makes the findings debatable. These studies investigated individual

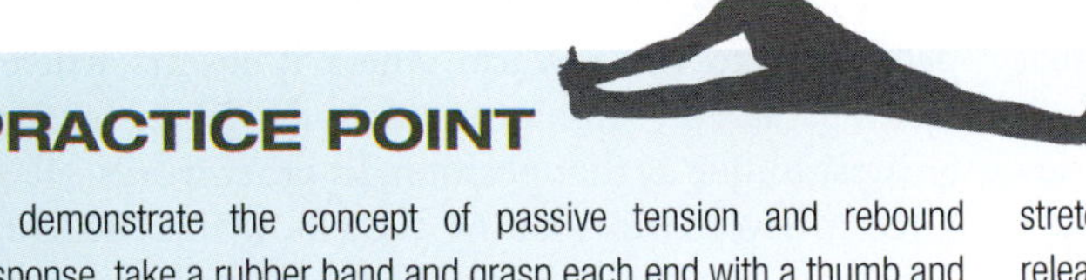

PRACTICE POINT

To demonstrate the concept of passive tension and rebound response, take a rubber band and grasp each end with a thumb and index finger. Pull the band to take up its slack, and then stretch it slightly beyond that point. Release one end of the band and notice how much rebound it provides to the hand that continues to grasp the band. Now, take up the slack of the band and stretch it more but vigorously this time. Release one end again and notice the difference in the rubber band's rebound. One final time, repeat the vigorous stretch on the rubber band, but this time stretch it quickly and release it as soon as you have stretched it out. The passive fascia surrounding our muscles performs the same way: If we stretch the fascia slightly, it has little impact on our muscle's force output, but if we stretch more vigorously and release that stretch quickly, it contributes significantly to the muscle's force. This concept provides rationale for one of the basic theories involving the use of plyometrics in conditioning and reconditioning exercises.

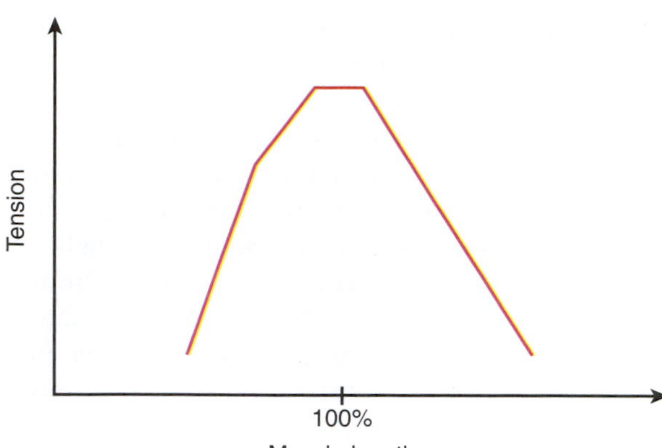

Figure 4.8 Active length-tension curve. Maximal actin-myosin cross bridges occur at the muscle's resting position. As the muscle shortens or lengthens, fewer cross bridges are available.

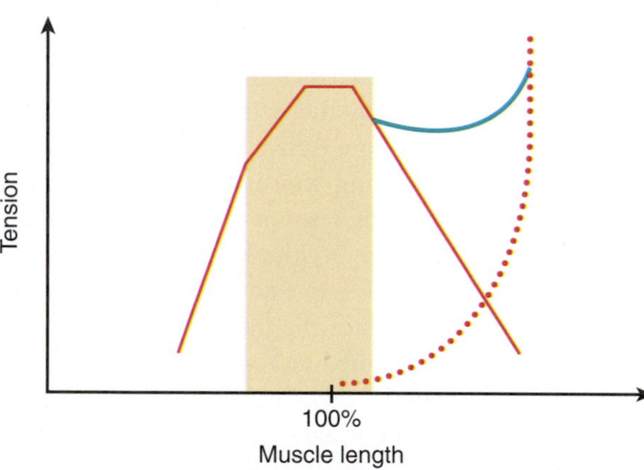

Figure 4.9 Total length-tension relationship curve of muscle. Passive elastic components provide tension beyond normal resting length whereas active muscle tissue provides tension at less than resting length. —— = active length-tension component, ······ = passive elastic length-tension component, —— = resultant combination of passive and active components.

sarcomeres, and this issue raises at least three questions: 1) Since a muscle's sarcomeres are not all the same length, should we expect a variation in responses of sarcomeres at other lengths? 2) Because a sarcomere responds in a specific way, does it necessarily mean that an entire muscle will respond the same way? and 3) Even if we assumed that an entire muscle responds as the sarcomere does, do all muscles respond the same way? Although these length-tension concepts are accurate for sarcomeres in the lab, how reliable they are when discussing entire muscles in the living body is unknown. Unfortunately, we do not yet know the answers to these concerns, so until investigations provide additional knowledge and insight into these issues, most people assume the results of investigations of sarcomere are expandable to entire muscles within the body.

Although resting length cannot be accurately determined *in vivo* (in the body), passive tension is appreciated with a simple exercise. Passively elongate multijoint muscles such as the finger flexors over their full range of motion: Extend the wrist, the metacarpophalangeal joint, and interphalangeal joints through the full range of motion to produce tension in the flexor digitorum superficialis and profundus muscles. You can feel the tension increasing in the muscles as you place them on progressively greater stretch. We will address this factor a little later when we discuss passive insufficiency of muscles.

Although experimental results demonstrating isometric sarcomere length-tension may or may not be applicable to entire muscles, we do know that other experiments investigating whole muscles have provided functional results on length relative to force production. In the normal body, the joints do not permit extreme shortening or lengthening of a muscle. Such safeguards prevent muscles from entering injurious ranges of motion. Early investigations on activity of an entire muscle were generally performed on animals. For example, the gastrocnemius muscle of the frog was used to determine the physiologically functional portion of the length-tension curve.[26] This portion occurs from about 75% to 105% of resting length, a range that is similar to the shaded area in Figure 4.9. More recent investigation of length-tension in humans reveals similar findings.[27]

Moment Arm

As was discussed in Chapter 2, the moment arm of a muscle is the lever arm that produces rotation around a joint. As was also discussed, the muscle's moment arm is the length of a perpendicular line from the joint's axis of motion to the muscle's force vector or line of pull. You may recall from previously presented information that all of the muscle's force rotates the joint (produces torque) when the muscle is aligned perpendicularly to the long axis of the body segment. For example, as we see in Figure 4.10A, the line of pull of the biceps is perpendicular to the forearm where it inserts when the elbow is at 90°; this means that the biceps exerts its greatest torque at that position. In other words, all of its force is devoted to rotating the elbow into flexion. As the elbow changes position, the line of pull of the biceps also changes so it is no longer perpendicular to the forearm; therefore, some of its force is devoted to compressing the joint in positions greater than 90° and to distracting the joint when the elbow is less than 90°. The distraction and compression forces, you recall, are the tangential force of the biceps. You can also observe in Figure 4.10D that the more the elbow moves away

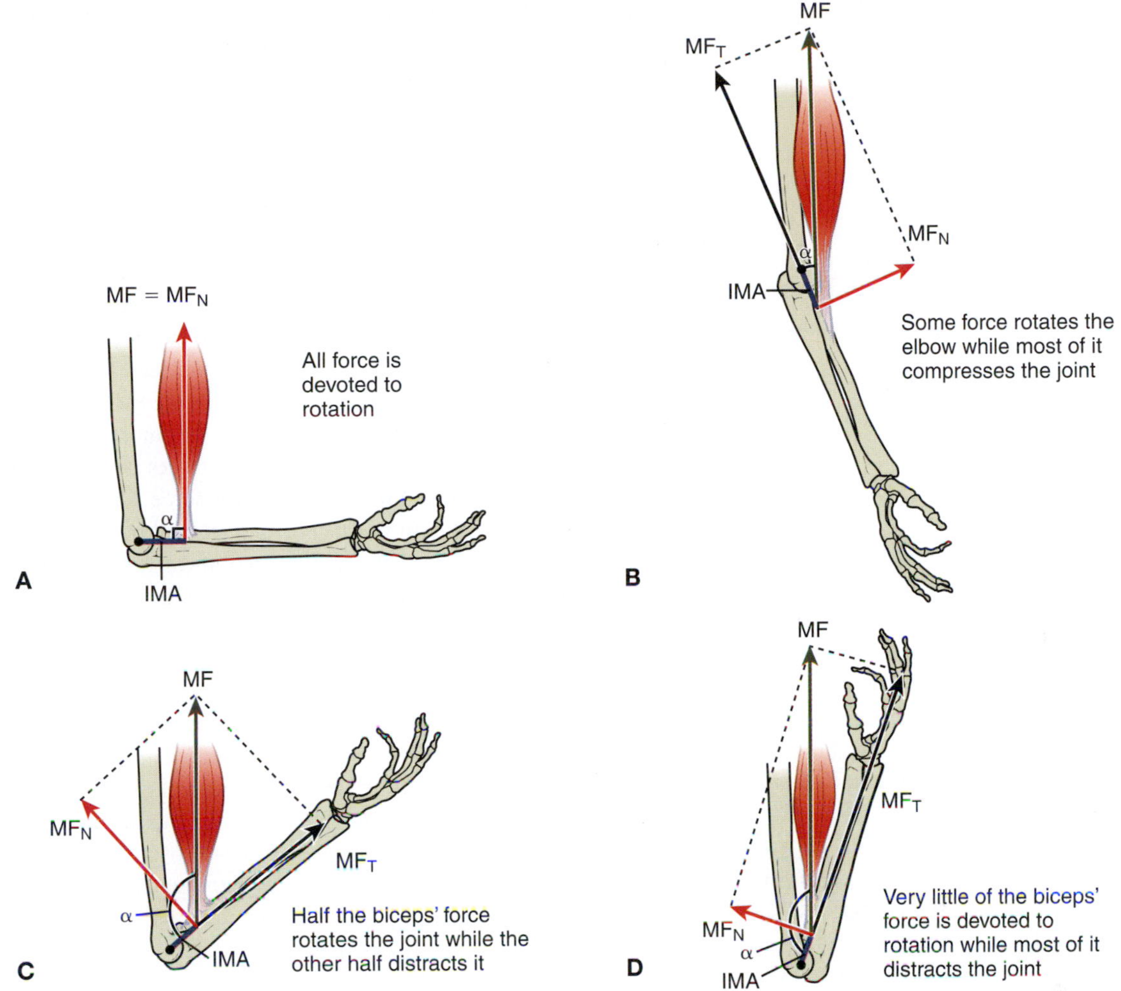

Figure 4.10 A) When the muscle's moment arm is perpendicular to the muscle, all of its force produces joint rotation. B–D) When it is not perpendicular, some of its force is directed to either compression or distraction of the joint and the rest to joint rotation.

from 90°, the less the force of the biceps is devoted to rotation and the greater amount of its force produces either distraction or compression.

Using this elbow example, we see that as the joint moves through its range of motion, muscles producing the movement experience a change in their moment arms, both in length and in the position at which it is relative to the segment. This means that at some points in the range of motion, a muscle generates a large torque (rotational force) and sometimes it produces less torque, depending upon when that muscle's moment arm is perpendicular to its body segment. As we have previously discussed, the muscle's physiological length (length-tension) also influences its strength, or ability to produce force. Although it is likely that the mechanical influence is greater, the physiological and mechanical factors both influence a muscle's ability to produce force *in vivo*. Therefore, they must both be considered when determining the optimal position for a rehabilitative exercise. In addition to these mechanical and physiological influences, the speed of a muscle's contraction also impacts the muscle's ability to produce a force.

Speed of Contraction

Speed is rate of motion. Velocity is rate of motion in a particular direction. The rate of muscle shortening or lengthening substantially affects the force a muscle can develop during activation. The relationship between the maximum force developed by a human muscle and the speed of contraction is shown in Figure 4.11. As the speed of a concentric contraction becomes slower, the muscle's force development increases.[28–29] When there is no motion, this is a maximum isometric contraction, or zero-velocity, contraction. A muscle's decreased ability

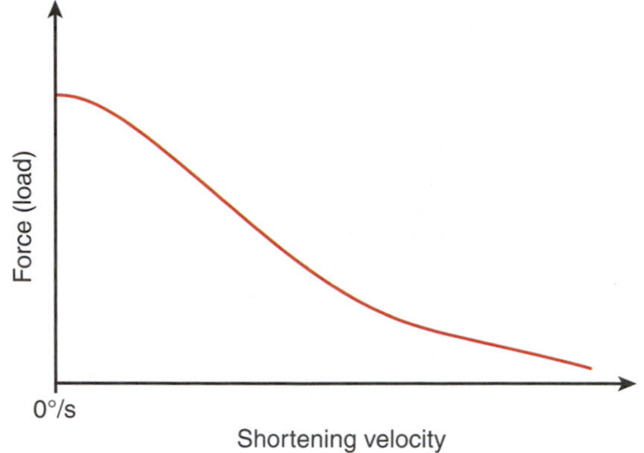

Figure 4.11 Force-velocity during concentric activity. The faster a muscle moves concentrically, the less force it is able to produce.

to produce a contraction force with increasing speed of shortening is based of the number of links between the actin and myosin filaments that can be formed per unit of time (Fig. 4.12). The maximum number of crossbridges that can be formed occurs at slow speeds. The more rapidly the actin and myosin filaments slide past each other, the smaller is the number of links that are formed between the filaments in a unit of time so less force is developed. There is a loose inverse relationship between the muscle's speed of contraction and the amount of force a muscle is able to produce concentrically. It is important to remember that from a clinical perspective, the faster a muscle moves through a range of motion, the less weight it is able to work against, or lift.

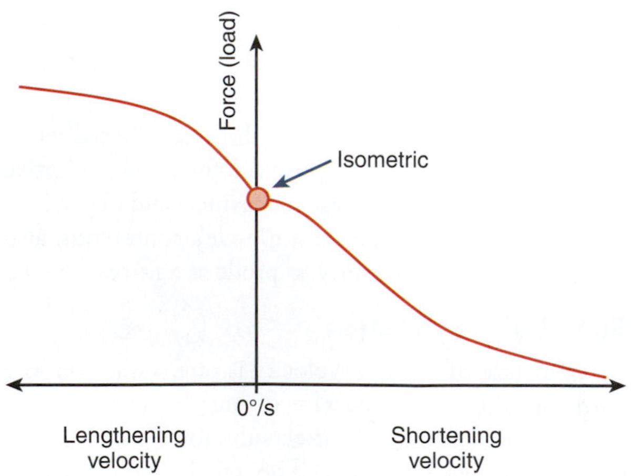

Figure 4.12 The passive length-tension portion of a skeletal muscle's length-tension curve demonstrates the effect of passive tissue tension of a muscle. Passive tension occurs as the result of stretch on parallel and series elastic components when a muscle is elongated. To a point, as a muscle moves faster eccentrically, it produces greater force.

On the other hand, as the muscle lengthens during activity, there is a difference in the relationship between speed of contraction and force production than that which occurs with muscle shortening. As seen in Figure 4.12, muscle strength actually increases as speed increases during eccentric contraction until the speed reaches a point at which the muscle is unable to control the load.

Active Tension

Active tension is the force produced by a muscle. Active tension in a muscle is created by activation of the crossbridges between the actin and myosin elements within muscle fibers. Assuming a normally interacting neuromotor system, active tension is the most important factor in the production of muscle forces used for functional activities. How much active force a muscle contraction is able to produce is determined by the number of motor units that are recruited and the firing rate of the active motor units.[30] Also, the greater the number of muscle fibers activated, the greater the active tension that is produced. The number of muscle fibers within one motor unit varies. There is an inverse relationship between the size of the motor neuron and its excitability; the larger the axon, the less excitable it is.[31]

Not only does the size of the neuron innervating the motor unit matter, but the size of the muscle fiber being innervated is related to the sequential triggering of muscles. Elizabeth Henneman and her associates[32] found a direct relationship between the size of the neuron and the size of the fibers it innervated. In other words, the larger motor units contained the larger neuron and also contained the larger-sized muscle fibers. They concluded that it is reasonable to assume that the smaller muscle fibers, since they are innervated by smaller nerve fibers, are activated before larger muscle fibers.

The type of muscle fiber recruited within a muscle influences the amount of tension produced by a muscle. The type II muscle fibers are facilitated when a rapid or forceful response is required. However, type I muscle fibers are active for postural corrections during prolonged positioning; they frequently fire as needed to make small corrections so a position is maintained in spite of either external factors, such as wind or standing on a boat, or internal factors, such as heart or lung activity, which cause minute changes in the body's position. Once a motor unit receives a stimulus sufficient to cause activation, the muscle fibers within that motor unit contract and immediately relax. If there is a series of stimuli provided to the motor unit, it will produce repeated contractions of the muscle fibers within the motor unit. Fast, repetitive firing will produce repeated contractions at a rate sufficient to cause a sustained contraction of the muscle fibers. The more motor units that are recruited and contract in this manner, the more forceful is the muscle's contraction.

Motor units are recruited in a systematic order.[30, 33–34] Smaller motor units are recruited before larger ones. Smaller motor units usually produce less tension, last a longer time, and require less energy than the larger motor units.[33–34] Recruitment first of smaller motor units and then later of larger motor units, if and when they are needed, assures conservation of energy and efficiency of movement. If greater forces or a higher intensity of activity is required, the larger motor units are recruited to improve the muscle's response to increased or short-term activity demands.

In summary, motor units are recruited in an order according to the size of the motor unit (smaller ones are recruited first), the size of the muscle cells (smaller ones are recruited before larger ones), and the type and speed of conduction of the muscle fibers (slower type I are recruited before faster type II). The smaller motor units are slower to respond but last longer than the larger ones which respond quickly with strong bursts. Therefore, type I motor units are recruited for posture.

As with motor units, some investigators have demonstrated that muscles are also recruited in a systematic manner.[34] Most of the research on this topic has been performed on postural muscles with mixed results. Some researchers find that there is no consistent firing sequence[35–36] whereas others reveal that sequence patterns do exist in muscle firing.[37–38] There seems to be a pattern for some activities but not others and for some muscles but not others. For example, it has been found that an inhibition of erector spinae muscles occurs as an anticipatory adjustment as the person prepares to rise out of a chair.[39] When an individual is in a prone position, Ana Sakamoto and her associates[40] found a consistent sequence of muscle firing starting with the semitendinosus and followed by the contralateral erector spinae, then the ipsilateral erector spinae, and finally the gluteus maximus. Some investigators have found changes in muscle firing sequences with changes in speed of muscle contraction and in subjects with sacroiliac pain or sacrolumbar dysfunction.[36–38, 41–42] Katsuo Fujiwara and associates[35] investigated movement patterns and muscle activity and discovered that although subjects had variable methods of movement patterns and muscle recruitment, each subject performed his or her own pattern consistently over repeated trials. Based on these findings, it may be that, although motor units are systematically recruited, movement patterns rely more on the individual's development of his or her personal strategy. Additional investigations are needed on this topic of movement patterns and muscle recruitment.

Age and Gender

Males are generally stronger than females. In both genders, however, muscle strength increases from birth through adolescence, peaking between the ages of 20 and 30 years, and gradually declining after 30 years of age. For example, the grip strength of the dominant hand of males and females between ages 3 and 90 is plotted in Figure 4.13. As seen in Figure 4.13, the muscle strength of young boys is approximately the same as that of young girls up to the age of puberty. Thereafter, males exhibit a significantly greater grip strength than females, with the greatest differences occurring during middle age (between ages 30 and 50). As individuals age, the number of motor units decline.[43] The greater strength of males appears to be related primarily to the greater muscle mass they develop after puberty. Up to about age 16, the ratio of lean body mass to whole body mass is similar in males and females, as indicated by studies of creatinine excretion and potassium counts. After puberty, however, the muscle mass of males becomes as much as 50% greater than that of females, and the ratio of lean body mass to whole body mass also becomes greater. On the other hand, muscle strength per cross-sectional area of muscle is similar in males and females.[44] The proportion of fast-twitch and slow-twitch muscle fibers in specific muscles is also similar in the two groups.[44]

Although muscle strength is related to age and gender in the population as a whole, many exceptions to the general rule can be found because of two factors: 1) the large variation in the rate at which biologic maturation occurs; and 2) the large variation in individual genetics and specific conditioning levels which are acquired and maintained through proper diet and exercise.[45]

Passive Excursion of Muscles

The paired agonist-antagonist relationship of muscles throughout the body requires that each muscle have the ability to accommodate and change length both passively and actively to permit joint motion. For example, Morrison determined that the hamstrings and quadriceps muscles change their length 3 to 4 inches (8 to 10 cm) during normal walking.[46] The **functional excursion** of a muscle is the distance to which the muscle is capable of shortening after it has been elongated as far as the joint(s) over which it passes allows. Weber[47] investigated the excursions of several muscles and found that these muscles were able to shorten from 34% to 89% of their longest length, with an overall average shortening value

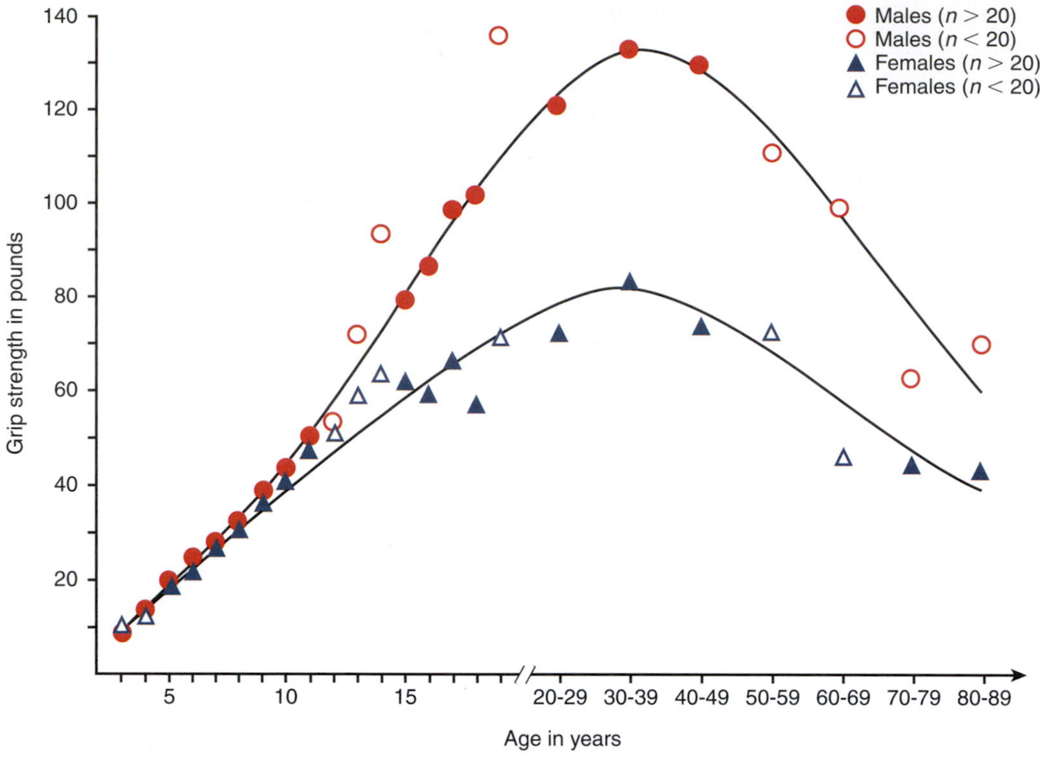

Figure 4.13 Based on data from Komi and Karlsson,[44] the average strength grip of the dominant hand in 537 female and 531 male healthy subjects between 3 and 90 years of age. Until subjects reach puberty, there is essentially no difference in grip strength, but after puberty, significant differences between the sexes are apparent.

of 50%. Muscles that cross more than one joint had the greatest excursion measures. Kaplan[48] and Boyes[49] identified specific measurements of the excursion distances for each muscle of the hand and wrist. Findings by Boyes[49] showed that the flexor digitorum profundus muscle had an excursion of 3 inches (8 cm) when the middle finger and wrist joints were moved from full wrist and finger flexion to full extension. Although there is a large variation from one muscle to another in the ability to shorten, these specific measures are not as important from a clinical perspective as the muscle's ability to function. Since precise measures of shortening are not clinically relevant, clinicians use an average estimate of 70% of a muscle's resting length in discussing an average muscle's ability to shorten.[50] In other words, rather than use precise experimental results that vary from one muscle to another, clinicians generally estimate any muscle's ability to shorten as a maximum of 70% of its resting length.

Passive Insufficiency

When muscles become elongated over two or more joints simultaneously, they may reach the state of **passive insufficiency.** This full elongation of a muscle prevents further shortening by its opposite muscle. This passive insufficiency can be demonstrated with hip flexion in a healthy individual. When the hip is flexed with simultaneous knee extension, the hamstrings is stretched over both of these joints, elongating the hamstrings to its maximum length; the passive stretch of the hamstring to its full length limits the hip flexors' ability to move the hip through its entire range of hip flexion, although the hip flexors have the strength to otherwise perform the full motion. In another example, if the ankle dorsiflexes to 15° when the knee is flexed, it does so freely, but when the knee is extended, the amount of dorsiflexion is reduced because of passive insufficiency of the gastrocnemius muscle which is now stretched over the knee and ankle. Passive insufficiency may occur normally, as demonstrated in these examples. However, passive insufficiency may also occur in pathological conditions. Certain pathologic conditions may cause muscles and tendons to lose their normal range of excursions. Examples of these conditions include muscle tightness, spasticity, scar tissue shortening from trauma or surgery, and adhesion of tendons to their sheaths. Thus, even though an agonist may contract strongly, motion may be significantly limited by passive insufficiency of its antagonist.

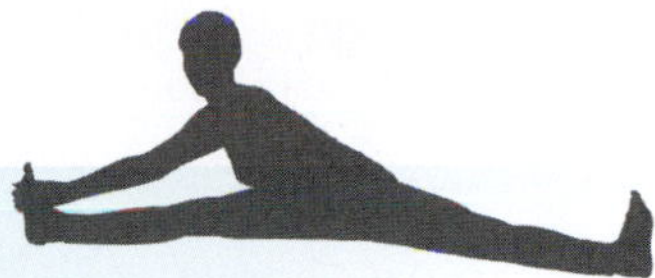

PRACTICE POINT

Passive insufficiency may occur because of either orthopedic restrictions or neurological restrictions. An example of an orthopedically-based restriction is a basketball player who has tight hamstrings. The hip can normally be flexed to 115°-125° when the knee is also flexed; because of normal passive insufficiency of the hamstrings, hip flexion range of motion is limited to 90° with the knee extended. However, if the basketball player has tight hamstrings, his straight-leg raise may be limited even more than normal—perhaps to 60°—since his hamstring length reaches passive insufficiency before that of a normal hamstring (Fig. 4.14).

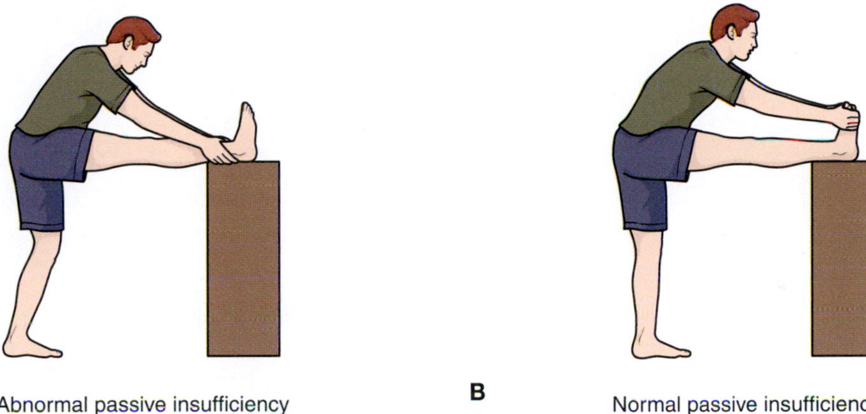

Figure 4.14 Normal passive insufficiency and abnormal passive insufficiency of hamstrings. Passive insufficiency of a muscle will limit its opposing muscle's ability to contract since the lengthening muscle is unable to stretch any farther.

Tendon Action of Muscle

Passive tension of muscles that cross two or more joints may produce passive movements of those joints. This effect is called **tenodesis** (Gr. *tenon,* tendon; *desis,* a binding together) action of muscle. In able-bodied subjects, the effect is seen when the individual flexes and extends the wrist while keeping the hand relaxed. When the wrist flexes, the relaxed fingers extend because of the passive tension of the extensor digitorum, which elongates over the wrist and fingers. When the wrist extends, the fingers passively flex because of the tension of the flexor digitorum profundus and superficialis muscles (Fig. 4.15).

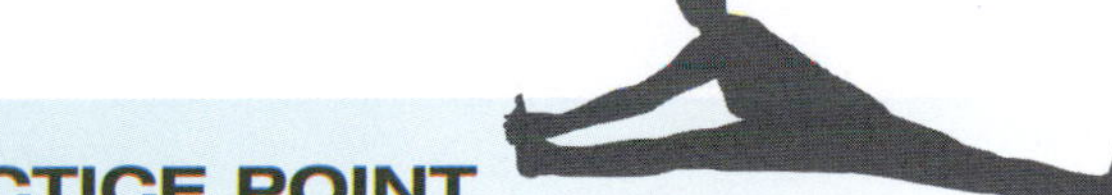

PRACTICE POINT

This tenodesis action is sometimes used functionally by patients with tetraplegia who have motor function loss at a C-6 level.* These individuals are able to contract wrist extensor muscles but have paralysis of finger muscles. When the wrist flexes, the fingers extend by passive insufficiency of the extensors so the hand can be placed over an object. As the individual actively extends the wrist, the passive tension of the finger flexors produces increasing force on the object so it may be picked up and held in the hand. If selective shortening of the long finger flexors has been permitted to occur, several pounds of grasping force can be generated.

* The designation of the level of a spinal cord injury is based on the lowest normally functioning nerve root segment of the spinal cord. If a patient has complete interruption of upper motor neuron connections to lower motor neurons in the seventh cervical segment and below, the patient is classified as having a C-6 level (complete) of motor function. The level of sensory function may also be classified.

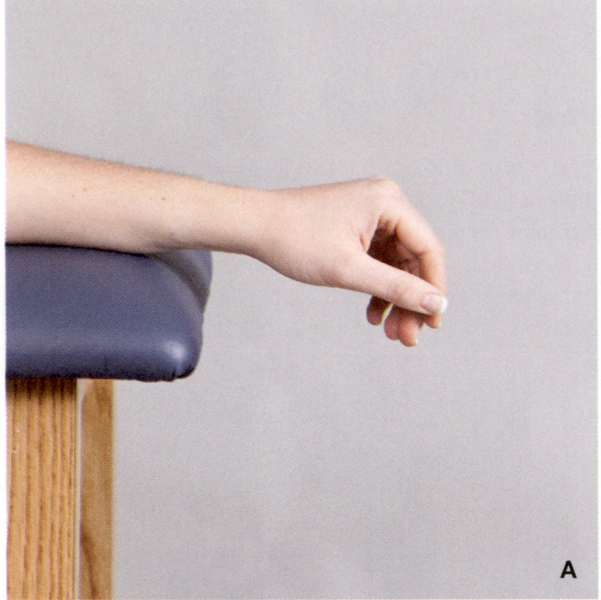

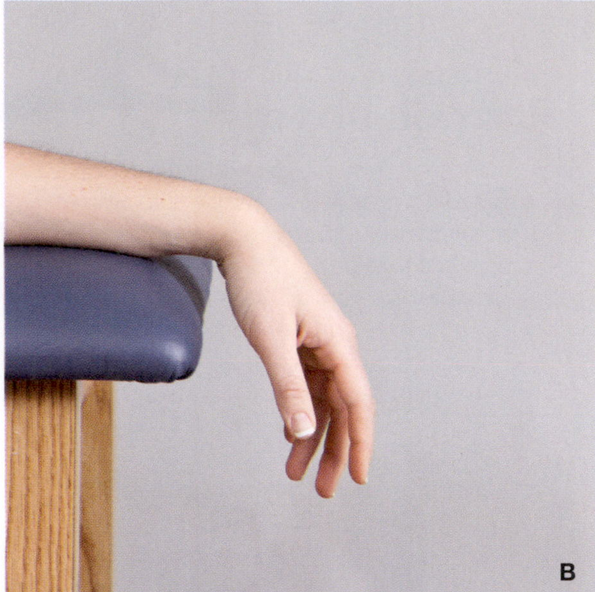

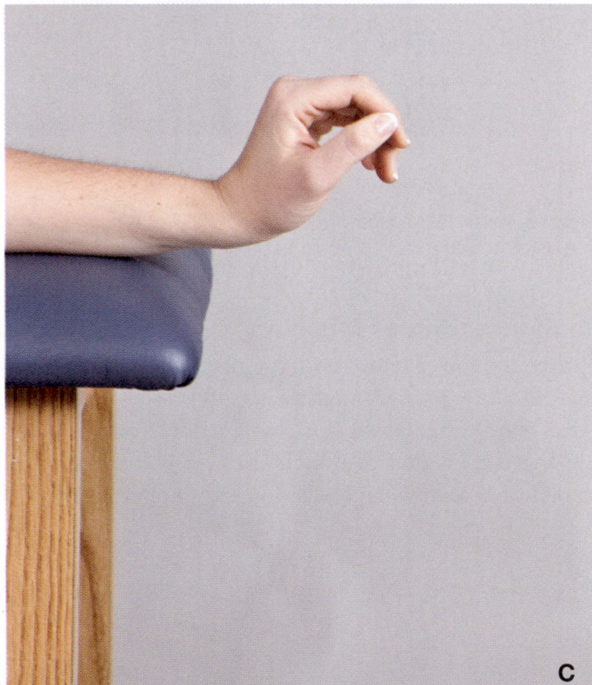

Figure 4.15 Tenodesis occurs in the long finger flexors and extensors with movement of the wrist. **A)** The hand and wrist in a resting position. **B)** As the wrist flexes, the passive insufficiency of the long finger extensors causes the fingers to move into extension. **C)** As the wrist extends, the passive insufficiency of the long finger flexors moves the fingers passively into flexion.

Active Excursion of Muscles

Functional motion involves several muscles working simultaneously to accomplish any given task. Some of these muscles are single-joint muscles whereas others are multijoint muscles. The ability and function of multijoint muscles are impacted by each joint they cross. The performance of these multijoint muscles at one joint is either enhanced or impaired by the position of its other joints. For both multijoint muscles and single-joint muscles, their physiologic length and their mechanical arm length also influence their ability to produce a force. These factors are discussed in this section.

Active Insufficiency

Active insufficiency occurs in multijoint muscles when the muscle is at its shortest length when its ability to produce physiologic force is minimal (Fig. 4.16A).

Recall from a muscle's length-tension relationship that a muscle's optimum strength is at its resting length, and as the muscle shortens, it becomes weaker. Fortunately, the body is designed so that fully shortened, weak positions are avoided in normal activities, especially those which require great force production. Favorable length-tension relationships are usually maintained by movement combinations that cause a muscle to elongate at one joint it crosses while it contracts to produce motion or force at another joint. For example, maximum isometric grip strength is greatest with the wrist in slight extension (Fig. 4.16B), but when the wrist is flexed the grip strength is markedly weakened; finger flexors are lengthened with the wrist in extension so they can provide greater grip strength. On the other hand, when the wrist flexes, the finger flexors shorten at the wrist as well as at the finger digits, causing a weak grip through active insufficiency of the finger flexors (Fig. 4.16A).

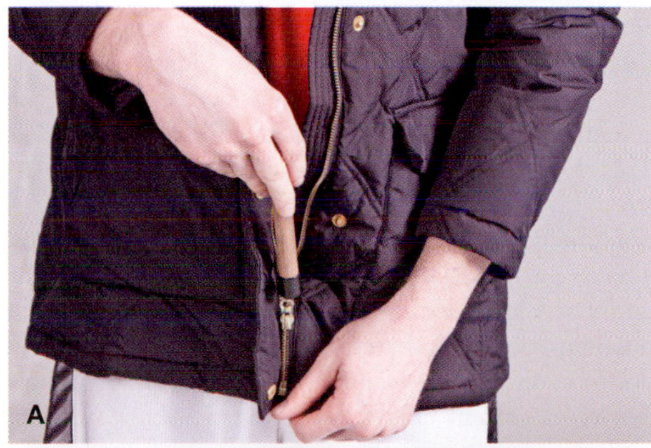

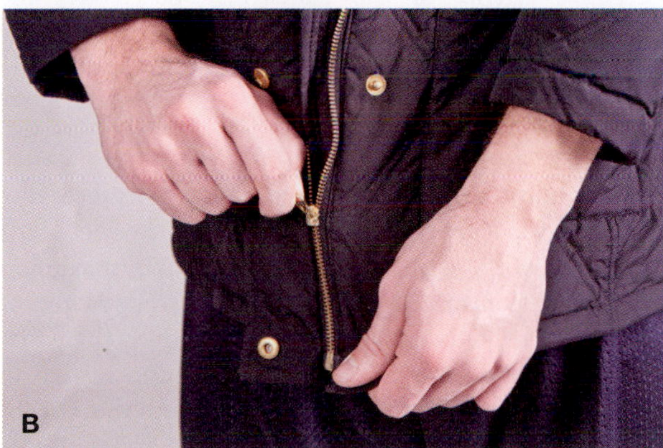

Figure 4.16 Active insufficiency. **A)** When a muscle is at its shortest, its ability to produce tension is at its lowest so finger flexors are unable to provide a strong grip when the wrist is flexed along with the finger flexors. **B)** By lengthening the muscle at another joint the muscle crosses, the muscle's strength is maintained, so if the wrist extends, the finger flexors have enough length to provide a strong grip.

During normal function, however, an antagonistic muscle group (in this example, the wrist extensors) works cooperatively with the agonist multijoint muscle or muscle group (flexor digitorum superficialis and profundus) to create an optimal position and permit functional activity of that multijoint muscle or muscle group at another joint. We call this **optimal sufficiency**—stabilization by antagonists that allows the multijoint agonist to perform the desired function. If optimal sufficiency is not present—antagonists do not stabilize either the proximal or distal joint(s) of the multijoint muscle which is contracting—the multijoint muscle moves all of the joints it crosses, becoming ineffective at any of them. For example, the ineffectual grip produced with the wrist in flexion lacks stabilization of the wrist joint so the long finger flexors shorten at each joint they cross; since the wrist extensors do not provide optimal sufficiency, the long finger flexors become actively insufficient and are unable to provide adequate grasp force. On the other hand, optimal sufficiency of the wrist stabilizers, positioning the wrist in extension, allows the finger flexors to produce the desired function of firmly grasping an object (Fig. 4.16).

Leverage and Length-Tension Interactions

Another unique way the body avoids the weakness caused by active insufficiency is by changes in the mechanical leverage that occurs throughout the joint's range of motion. In the example of the biceps brachii muscle (Fig. 4.17), the physiologic length-tension factor is most favorable when the elbow is in full extension, and the maximum tension that can be produced during muscle contraction decreases as the elbow approaches and passes 90° of flexion. To compensate for this loss in physiologic muscle tension, the muscle's leverage (moment arm length) increases to its maximum at 90°. This increase in moment arm length provides the muscle's greatest mechanically-produced torque at a point in the range of motion which is important for holding heavy objects. In this instance, the torque that the muscle can produce actually increases because of a mechanical change, even though the physiologic muscle tension decreases (Fig. 4.17).

The patella is another example of an increased mechanical force taking over when a muscle's physiologic force declines. Not only does the patella mechanically increase the force arm distance—and, consequently, the torque of the quadriceps muscle group—but as the physiologic length-tension force declines, the force arm distance provided by the patella increases. Kaufer[51] measured a 40% increase in the force arm distance of the quadriceps from 120° of knee flexion to complete

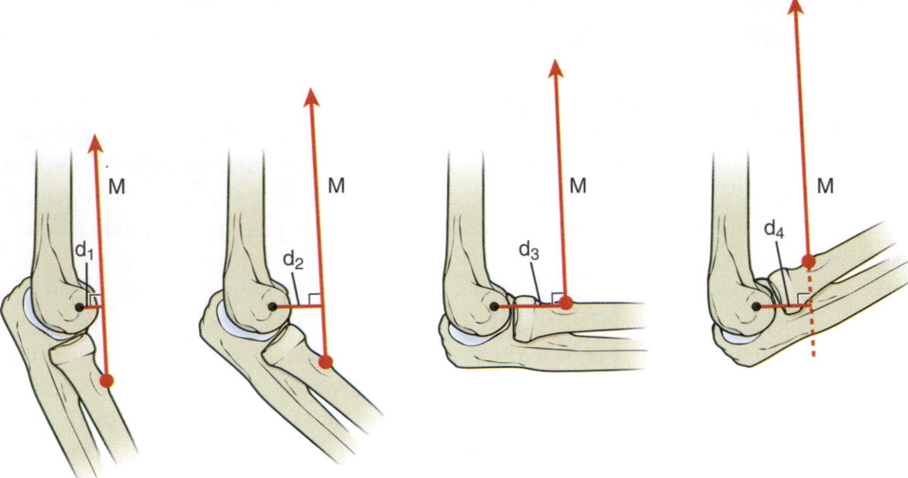

Figure 4.17 Changes in the force arm distance (d) for the biceps brachii muscle in four positions of elbow flexion. The maximum muscle torque occurs at the greatest moment arm distance (when the attachment of the muscle to the bone is perpendicular).

extension (force arm changed from 3.9 cm to 5.8 cm). In the absence of the patella, both the initial force arm distance and the amount of increase with extension were significantly less (force arm changed from 3.5 cm to 4 cm). With creation of a shorter moment arm, strength is undoubtedly affected when the patella is removed. In fact, Gibson and Scott [52] found about a 30% reduction in extension force output in knees whose patella had been removed compared to the contralateral knee.

Positive and Negative Work

When muscles activate, they produce force that results in one of three activities: no motion (isometric); muscle shortening (concentric); or muscle lengthening (eccentric). Although we have addressed these types of activity, we haven't discussed how they are important in functional activities. These types of contractions influence active excursions during all motor functions.

Eccentric Muscle Forces

When a muscle's tension matches the load or resistance against it, an isometric activity of the muscle occurs. However, when the resistance or load increases beyond the force that can be produced by a maximum isometric contraction of the muscle, the muscle can no longer maintain the isometric position. The resistance or load is lowered or decelerated with an eccentric contraction. When the speed of movement is slow, the muscle's ability to resist the force increases up to 50% more than the muscle's ability was in maintaining a maximum isometric contraction (Fig. 4.12). This rapid force increase occurs between ±10% of a muscle's maximum concentric contraction. (For the knee joint, for example, this is approximately a velocity of 30°/sec.) A muscle's force then remains the same as the velocity increases to maximal levels.[50] For practical purposes, the force of an eccentric contraction is independent of velocity.[29, 53] This ability of muscles to withstand higher forces eccentrically is important in deceleration and shock absorption functions, which occur with high-velocity motions. This is an important function of muscles in both the upper and lower extremities. For example, throwing or pitching activities in baseball or softball require forearm deceleration by an eccentric contraction of the elbow flexors to prevent elbow joint injury. During running, eccentric activity of the hamstrings decelerates the swinging leg, and the quadriceps femoris eccentrically contracts to absorb forces of six to seven times the body weight at foot impact.[54]

Energy Expenditure

Higher maximum force production and tolerance during eccentric activities permits managing heavier loads (negative work) than can be lifted with a maximum concentric contraction (positive work). Fewer motor units are activated during an eccentric activity than during a concentric activity. This phenomenon is seen in the EMG recordings of the biceps and the triceps brachii in Figure 4.3A and B. Therefore, for the same force output, energy expenditure (oxygen consumption) is less for an eccentric contraction than it is for a concentric contraction. This reduced energy requirement occurs because of the contributions of the muscle's passive tissue (fascia and tendons) to the muscle's total force output during eccentric activity.

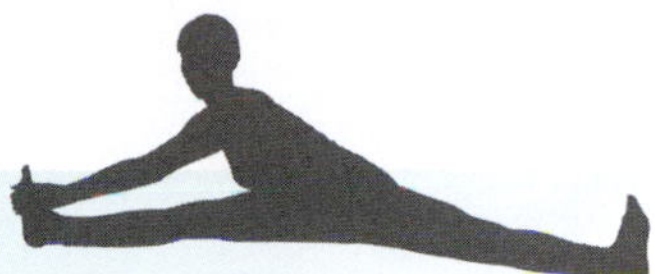

PRACTICE POINT

Because of the excessive forces applied to the body during deceleration activities, clinicians appreciate that it is during this phase of any activity in which most injuries occur. For example, a baseball pitcher will release a pitch with a speed of 7500°/sec at the shoulder.[55] Following release of the ball, the shoulder moves through a bit more than 180° of motion and uses less than 1 second to decelerate to a stop position; substantial eccentric forces place tremendous stresses on the muscles and joints. These stresses become even more significant when the activity is performed repetitively, resulting in accumulative stress injury.

Since eccentric activities are performed with less energy requirements and fewer motor units recruited, if a muscle is very weak, the clinician may assist the patient in a concentric activity and merely guide the patient in an eccentric activity. For example, the patient may require assistance by the clinician to lift the lower extremity during a straight-leg raise exercise against gravity; however, since lowering the extremity to the start position recruits fewer motor units during eccentric muscle activity, the patient may be able to lower the limb without assistance. Such an exercise may assist the patient in facilitating muscle performance in early rehabilitation.

Abbott, Bigland, and Ritchie[56] devised an experiment to measure the relative difference in energy cost of performing positive work (lifting a load a certain distance using a concentric contraction) versus the cost of performing negative work (lowering the load the same distance by means of an eccentric contraction). The results of their experiments showed that with equal loads, the energy cost of positive work was from 2.5 to 6 times greater than the cost of negative work, depending on the rate at which the work was performed. The relative cost of eccentric activity decreased as the rate of motion increased. In other words, less energy is required to lower a given load quickly than to lower it slowly. Most of the energy is used to control the rate at which the object decelerates.

Dick and Cavanagh[57] demonstrated that although negative work (running downhill) required less oxygen consumption than positive work (running on a level surface), there was a gradual increase in oxygen consumption of negative work with time. Oxygen consumption for running at 3.83 M/second at 10 minutes was 33% less for running downhill (10% grade) than for running on a level surface. There was, however, a 10% increase in oxygen consumption in downhill running by 40 minutes, and an increase of only 1.5% in level running. The authors also found that EMG activity of the quadriceps femoris muscle during downhill running increased 23% between 10 and 40 minutes. The increases in oxygen consumption and EMG activity were proposed to be from muscle fiber and connective tissue damage, which is frequently associated with maximum lengthening (eccentric) contractions and additional motor unit recruitment because of fatigue.

In summary, oxygen consumption, a measure of energy requirements for activity, is less during activities such as lifting weights and other short-term muscle functions. On the other hand, if eccentric muscle activity is performed for a prolonged time (more than 10 minutes and less than 40 minutes), then oxygen needs increase. During short-term eccentric activities, passive connective tissue elements utilize their viscoelasticity to provide a portion of the activity force requirement so the muscle works more efficiently.[58] During long-term activities, the reason for additional oxygen is based more on theory. Some theories suggest various reasons for this increased oxygen need: (1) longer activities increase tissue temperature to require additional oxygen uptake;[59] (2) fatigue reduces the efficiency of mitochondria;[60] (3) increased lactate levels requires more oxygen uptake;[61] or (4) more motor units are required because fatigue is occurring in currently recruited fibers, and the breakdown of

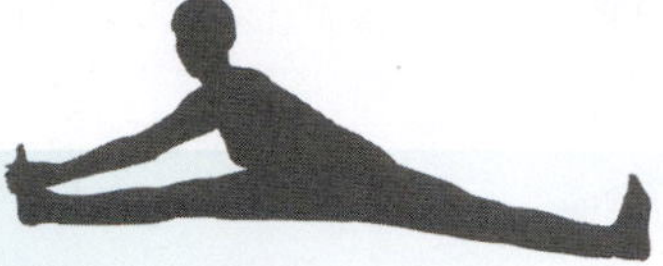

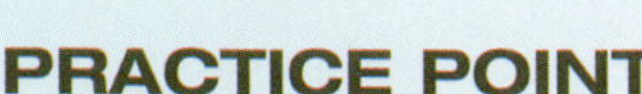

When lifting free weights, it is important to instruct individuals to perform the exercise slowly and in a controlled manner. If a clinician fails to include this factor in the instructions, the individual may lower the weight rapidly to the start position. This rapid movement requires less energy and less muscle activity, so if the intent is to build muscle strength, the eccentric benefit of the exercise is significantly diminished. Additionally, the risk of injury increases since the weight must be controlled at the very end of the motion; the muscle must "put on the brakes" of the movement with a much steeper decline in speed of motion over a much shorter degree of motion.

connective tissue following eccentric activity requires restorative functions which necessitates additional blood flow.[57] It is apparent that we have yet to discover many untold secrets of muscle performance.

Differences in Crossbridge Mechanisms

Since a muscle is able to produce a greater force eccentrically than with either an isometric or a concentric contraction and does so with greater efficiency (requires less energy), regardless of velocity, the crossbridges must somehow provide the mechanism. Since former Soviet Union athletes incorporated plyometric exercises in their conditioning programs and were rewarded with a significant number of gold medals during the 1968 Olympics, heightened interest in eccentric physiology has persisted. Unfortunately, we still have primarily only theories on what happens to produce increased forces with sudden eccentric activity. We know that larger parts of the brain's cortex are involved in eccentric production.[62] We have strong evidence to indicate that when muscle fibers are lengthened during eccentric activity, rather than the ATP mechanisms that provide bonds between actin and myosin during concentric activity, some type of mechanical disruption is used in eccentric activity.[63] Various theories intended to help us understand what happens with crossbridges during the different types of muscle activity include proposals and models set forth by investigators such Sugi and Pollack,[64] Lombardi and Piazzesi,[25] Edman,[65] and Stauber.[66] Of all the developing theories on this topic, it seems that those involving the neural commands appear to be the most promising since neural input influences a number of motor unit factors.[67] Time may eventually reveal the secrets yet to be discovered in the relationship between crossbridges and eccentric forces; until then, we are limited to theory and speculation based on the relatively little we now know about this topic. We do know that crossbridges are active during isometric, concentric, and eccentric activities, but how these crossbridges change in their function and affiliation during these different types of activities is yet to be completely realized.

Elastic Forces of Muscle

During activities such as running and jumping, it has been observed since the time of Marey and Demeny[68] that muscles sometimes behave as if they were capable of storing and transmitting elastic energy. For example, if an individual performs a maximum vertical jump twice in a row, the second jump is always higher; or if a squat jump is preceded by a quick counter stretch of the contracting hip and knee extensor and plantarflexor muscles, the jump is higher.[69-70]

This phenomenon occurs when the muscle performs negative work (eccentric contraction) and the muscle is contracting while being stretched. This activity produces potential energy, and the contracting muscle can store this energy briefly, but the energy is usually dissipated as heat. However, if a maximum concentric contraction of the muscle occurs before the energy dissipates, this stored energy is converted to kinetic energy to increase the force, speed, and power of the contraction beyond that of an isolated maximum concentric contraction.[71] This is the principle behind the incorporation of plyometric exercises into conditioning programs for highly competitive athletes. Activities such as running, in which this type of eccentric-concentric contractions occurs, show a surprising increase in efficiency as speed of the activity increases. For example, in the hopping kangaroo, efficiency increases from 0.23 at 10 km/hour to 0.62 at 27.5 km/hour.[71]

The magnitude of a concentric contraction increases with the intensity of the pre-stretch.[72] Additionally, Aura and Komi[72] also found that EMG activity of the eccentric contraction also increases with the intensity of the pre-stretch but that there is little change in the EMG of the concentric contraction. In other words, the greater force that is produced during the concentric contraction occurs without increased energy expenditure. For this to occur, the time of the eccentric-concentric contraction must be very brief. If the stretch is maintained too long (i.e., more than one second) or the muscle relaxes, the elastic energy dissipates as heat.

Early theories of this enhanced concentric contraction were based on the thought that the elasticity of the connective tissues was the source of improved muscle performance. Currently, the increased force is thought to be due to neural factors including muscle spindles, Golgi tendon organs, and the forces generated by the actin-myosin crossbridges.[70–71, 73] More recent evidence indicates additional reflex mechanisms that occur during rapid exercise and are facilitated by sensory receptors within muscles.[74] These stimulated receptors lie within the primary muscle of the exercise as well as its synergists and antagonists. These muscles are enhanced in their responsibilities through two reflex mechanisms that occur during rapid performance exercises, a length feedback reflex and a force feedback reflex. A **length feedback reflex** is triggered by a muscle when it is stretched and occurs within the same time as the stretch reflex; it not only excites autogenically (itself), but it also excites its synergists while inhibiting its antagonists.[75] This simultaneous excitation of synergists and inhibition of antagonists is thought to improve the muscle's performance. On the other hand, a **force feedback reflex** is an inhibitory neural reflex caused by muscle activity and occurs with activation of the Golgi tendon organ; not as much is known about the impact of this reflex mechanism, but it is thought to play a role in coupling antigravity muscles that cross different joints during sudden movements.[76] It is known that these reflexes rely on length and force for their activation and that they have the potential to improve neuromuscular control.[74]

This enhancement of the maximum concentric contraction is called the *stretch-shortening cycle*.[73, 77–79] The cycle is used to increase maximum concentric contractions and, thereby, performance in many sports activities, such as walking, running, jumping, throwing, gymnastics, skiing, and weight lifting. The stretch-shortening cycle also is used in exercise systems such as Proprioceptive Neuromuscular Facilitation[80–81] and Plyometrics[73, 82–84] to obtain stronger concentric muscle contractions. Although the stretch-shortening cycle is the proper term of a sudden eccentric lengthening followed by a rapid concentric shortening of a muscle or muscle group, this activity is more commonly referred to as plyometric activity.

Because of the short time for coupling of the eccentric-concentric contraction, skill and learning are major aspects in achieving maximum performance with the stretch-shortening cycle. Precise execution of activities and practice allows the individual to experience optimal results of plyometric training.[85]

Open Kinetic Chain versus Closed Kinetic Chain

Open and closed kinetic chain concepts were presented in Chapter 1. As you recall, an open kinetic chain is present when the distal segment of the extremity is free to move while the distal segment is weight-bearing in the closed kinetic chain. Also recall that in an open kinetic chain, each segment of the extremity is free to move, uninfluenced by the other joints or segments. On the other hand, movement of one joint impacts all of the joints of the extremity in closed kinetic chain activities. A common specification for a closed kinetic chain condition is that it is essentially weight-bearing. In contrast, an open kinetic chain condition is a non-weight-bearing position. Although both open and closed chain conditions occur in functional upper and lower extremity activities, the upper extremity is more often used in open kinetic chain activities whereas the lower extremity functions primarily in closed kinetic chain activities. It should be kept in mind that open chain activities often facilitate rapid movements whereas closed chain functions are used to develop force and power. In functional upper extremity open chain activities such as throwing, the proximal portion of the extremity initiates the movement for the distal joints. In closed chain activities, compression of the joints occurs, providing stabilization through joint approximation and coactivation of opposing muscle groups.

However, thinking "outside the box" allows us to approach open and closed kinetic chain concepts from another perspective. Let's use an example to see the relevance of this statement. In standing, the hip is in a closed kinetic chain position. Therefore, if the hip joint angle changes as a result of motion of the femur (e.g. squat), the knee and ankle will also move. On the other hand, if the hip moves from its proximal end, the pelvis rotates, moving the trunk into flexion from the hip. The hip, then, moves in an open kinetic chain manner. Similarly, if an individual lies prone on a table and moves the shoulder from hanging over the side of the table into shoulder hyperextension, he or she is performing an open kinetic chain activity of shoulder extension. However, if the individual is prone on a sled and uses his or her arms to move him or herself on the ground, the activity is still shoulder extension, but it is a closed kinetic chain activity.

As clinicians, we often must take this type of different perspective to alter exercises to accomplish specific goals for an individual. For example, if we want to increase joint stability, a closed kinetic chain activity is used, or perhaps if the individual's weight-bearing is restricted, an open kinetic chain activity is necessary. The important point is to identify the desired goals and understand how the body functions so those goals may be achieved.

Factors Affecting Maximum Isometric Muscle Force

Maximum isometric force at different points in the range of motion were calculated in early studies to identify patterns of muscle groups.[86] Figures 4.18 through 4.21 present this information in simplified form. Such studies have made a valuable contribution to understanding muscle strength characteristics. Inspection of these curves shows that maximum isometric force changes markedly within the range of motion (40 to 80%). As expected, most of the muscles show greater strength when they contract from their elongated position than when they contract from their shortened position. The pronator muscles, for example, show maximum force when the forearm is fully supinated and the least force when the forearm is pronated (Fig. 4.19). This pattern reflects the length-tension effect that we have discussed earlier in this chapter. The decrease in strength of some muscles, such as the forearm pronators and supinators (Fig. 4.19), is linear; in these muscles, the linear decline in strength indicates that the predominant factor determining the muscle's strength is the length-tension curve.

Other muscles, however, rely on moment arm length for strength advantages at other points along the range of motion other than the maximum length of the muscle. For example, Figure 4.21 shows the effect of increasing the force of the knee flexor muscles by flexing the hip to increase the stretch on the hamstring muscles. Curves for the quadriceps femoris muscle (Fig. 4.22) show peak forces in midrange of motion. This is an example of muscles in which the leverage factor is superimposed on the length-tension curve to increase torque in midrange. In this case, there is marked increases in the muscle lever arm length at midrange. As we have mentioned earlier in this chapter, the patella and the shape of the intercondylar groove of the femur increase the moment arm (lever arm) length for the quadriceps femoris muscles at midrange of knee flexion.[87]

Muscles that have this relationship between joint angle and muscle strength are usually muscles that must

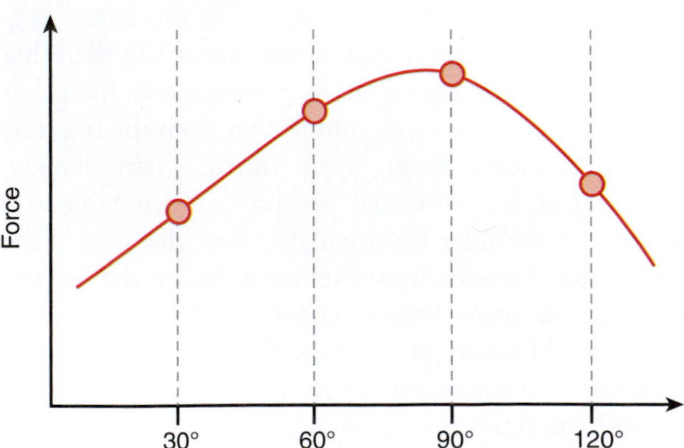

Figure 4.18 Maximum isometric force of elbow flexors (brachialis, biceps brachii, and brachioradialis) in college-aged men. Data of these muscles in college-aged men are based on data from Williams and Stutzman.[86]

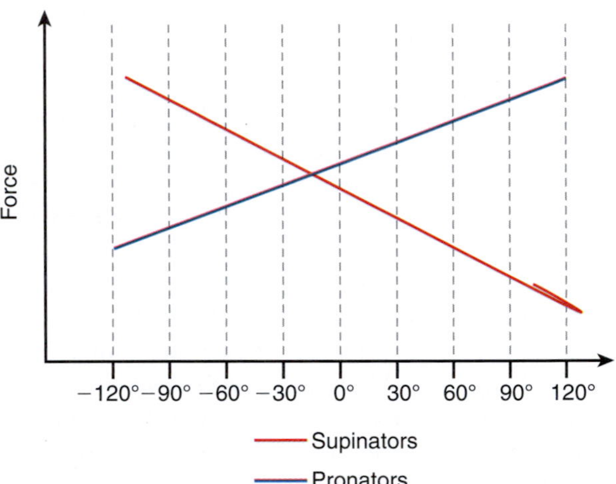

Figure 4.19 Maximum isometric force curves of the pronators (pronator teres and pronator quadratus) and supinators (supinator and biceps brachii).

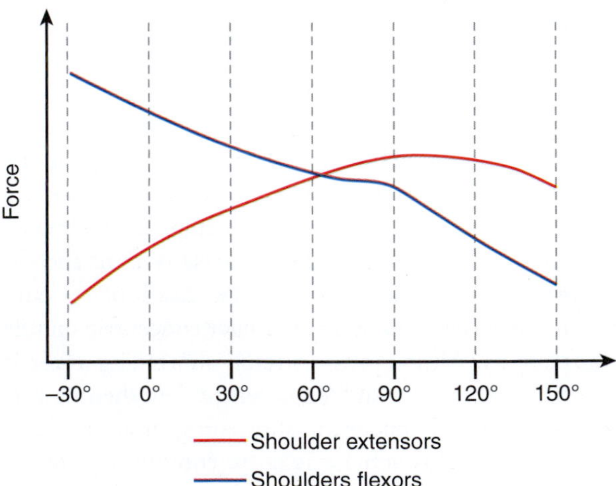

Figure 4.20 Comparison of maximum isometric shoulder flexor muscles (anterior deltoid, coracobrachialis, and biceps brachii) and shoulder extensor muscles (posterior deltoid, teres major, latissimus dorsi, and triceps brachii) based on data from Williams and Stutzman.[86]

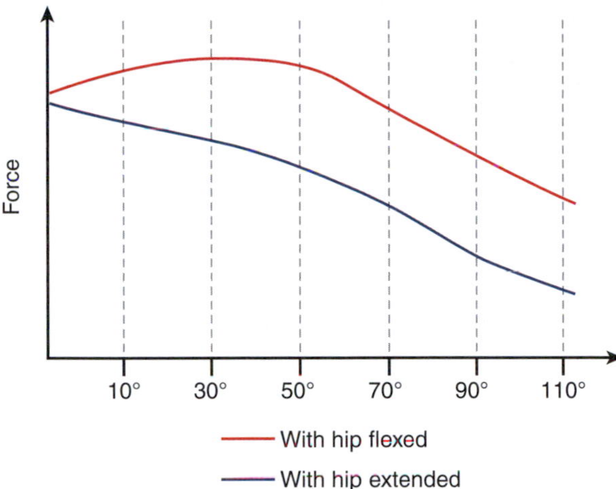

Figure 4.21 Maximum isometric force curves of the knee flexor muscles (semimembranosus, semitendinosus, biceps femoris, and gastrocnemius). Notice that the hip position changes the amount of force available for knee flexion.

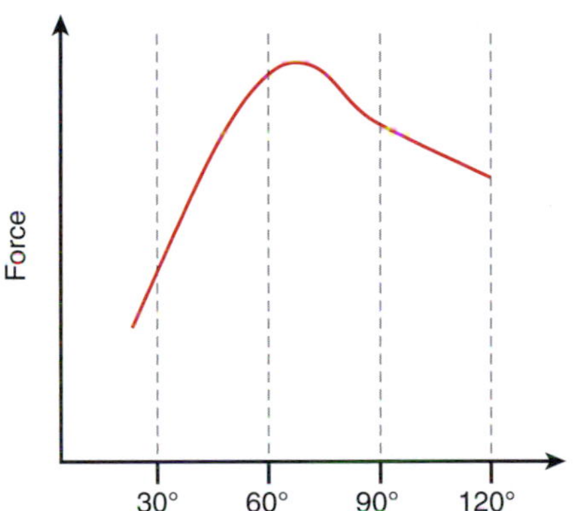

Figure 4.22 Maximum isometric force curves of the knee extensor muscles (quadriceps femoris). Based on data from Williams and Stutzman.[86]

provide large forces during their midranges of motion. For example, great strength of the elbow flexors must be available at a joint angle of 90° of flexion (Fig. 4.18) since that is the angle at which the elbow is positioned for carrying heavy objects. Maximum strength requirement of the knee extensor muscles occurs at 60° of flexion, the position at which great force is needed to elevate the body when a person rises from a chair or climbs stairs.

In Figures 4.19 and 4.20, maximum isometric forces of antagonistic muscle groups are recorded. At one point in the range, one muscle is stronger. At another point, the muscles have equal strength. At the other end of the motion, the antagonistic muscle is stronger. Therefore, when discussing which muscle group is stronger or ratios of strength, be sure to reference a specific point in the range of motion to make your discussion meaningful.

Exercise-Induced Muscle Injury

Muscles are among the most commonly injured orthopedic structures in the body. Injuries to muscles occur as gradual or acute onset injuries. Most muscle injuries, however, occur during eccentric and deceleration activities. Two injuries common in strenuous exercise are attributed to the great forces that occur with maximum eccentric muscle contractions because these contractions can produce up to twice the force of a maximum isometric contraction.

Delayed-Onset Muscle Soreness

One of these common muscle injuries is **delayed-onset muscle soreness (DOMS)**, which begins about 24 hours after the activity and may continue for up to 10 days post-exercise.[88] Other functional signs of DOMS are a decrease in range of motion because of pain and a decrease in maximum concentric and eccentric muscle forces of +50%, depending on the intensity of the exercise.[89–91] Biochemical signs of injury and destruction of muscle contribute to abnormally high levels of creatine kinase (a muscle enzyme) and myoglobin in venous blood, as well as increased plasma concentrations of myosin heavy-chain fragments from slow-twitch muscle fibers.[92,93] Structural damage to the Z-lines with a zigzag appearance and, sometimes, dissolution has been found. (Remember from Chapter 3 that the Z-lines border the ends of the sarcomeres and are a base of attachment of the actin myofilaments.) This alteration of the Z-line changes the alignment of the myofilaments, and, in some cases, the myosin filaments are absent.[90,94] Recovery from the functional and structural injuries of DOMS requires from 5 to 30 days, depending on the severity of the initial exercise. If, after recovery, the eccentric exercise or activity is repeated, it has been found that muscle soreness does not occur, and the muscle adapts to the exercise. Even greater eccentric forces can be made; there are minimal signs of muscle damage, but if injury occurs, recovery is more rapid.[89,92]

Hamstring Strain

A second common type of exercise-induced muscle injury is the muscle strain, and of the muscles strained, hamstrings strains occurs most often, especially in sprinting and jumping activities. This is a sudden and sometimes severe injury, frequently causing the athlete to fall to the ground in agony. In severe injuries, it is a macro-muscle tear of a hamstring with hemorrhage into the muscle. The tear occurs during the late swing phase and early stance phase of running. At this time, the hamstrings are decelerating the forward movement of the thigh and the leg with a maximum eccentric contraction (lengthening) and then instantaneously changing at foot strike (initial contact with the ground) to a maximum concentric (shortening) contraction to accelerate the thigh (hip extension) and prevent knee hyperextension.

Summary

An understanding of the myriad factors involved in the ability of a muscle to generate force and perform a functional movement is crucial for all professionals engaged in rehabilitation or human performance. This chapter described and summarized the key concepts related to muscle activity and strength. Muscle force is produced using isometric, eccentric, or concentric muscle activity. Muscles produce motion as agonists, antagonists, and synergists. A muscle's cross section determines its potential to create force. The larger the cross section, the greater the force a muscle is able to produce. A muscle that is multipennate has the potential to produce more force than a unipennate muscle. All tissue responds to stresses according to the stress-strain curve. If tissue stresses move into the tissue's toe or elastic region, the tissue returns to its normal length, but if the stress occurs in the tissue's plastic range, a permanent deformation occurs. If the stress applied is greater than the plastic range, the tissue fails. Creep is the ability of tissue to change its length with the application of a lower force over a longer time; in this case, tissue length changes occur as the tissue gradually lengthens. Muscle strength is determined by factors such as the muscle's size, fiber architecture, passive and active components, its length-tension relationship, moment arm, the speed of its contraction, and the age and gender of the individual. Active insufficiency and passive insufficiency may prevent a muscle from reaching its maximum strength or length. Optimal sufficiency occurs with the contraction of an antagonist to allow optimal positioning of a multijoint muscle at one of its ends to maximize its function at its other end. Negative work is eccentric activity. Such activity requires less energy expenditure yet provides a greater output of force than positive work, associated with concentric activity. Delayed-onset muscle soreness and hamstring strains are two common injuries that can occur as a result of eccentric muscle activity; described as examples of the application of key concepts to exercise and rehabilitation.

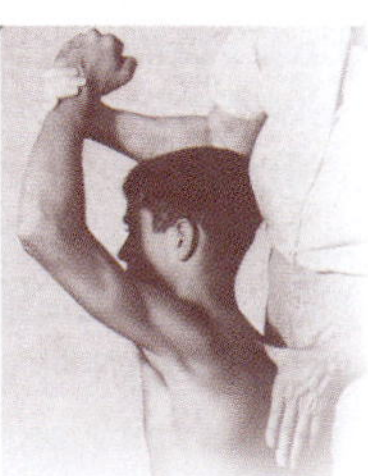

CLINICAL SCENARIO SOLUTION

The clinician correctly assessed Xavier and Owain as having delayed-onset muscle soreness (DOMS) from the previous day's workout. Since they have probably not previously engaged in the eccentric activities that she knows their new coach uses, she suspects that it will be a few days before they feel better, but they should return to their normal activities soon. In the meantime, she suggests light exercise and flexibility exercises to reduce the pain and discomfort they are having. She also explains to them that subsequent workouts will not produce this much pain and discomfort.

Discussion Questions

1. Think about the fiber arrangement of these muscles: biceps brachii, pronator quadratus, gluteus medius, sartorius, and gastrocnemius. Explain how their fiber arrangement is related to their function.
2. Explain how you would identify which muscles are agonists, antagonists, and synergists for an activity such as rising from a chair.
3. Identify the characteristics of the gastrocnemius that affect its ability to resist a stretch and how you would apply a stretch to make a lasting change in its length.
4. How would you position the shoulder to obtain maximal output from the triceps? Explain your answer.
5. Provide three examples of functional activities that include open kinetic chain activities of the lower extremity.
6. Provide three examples of functional activities that include closed kinetic chain activities of the upper extremity.

Lab Activities

1. Take three rubber bands of about the same length and width and loop them on your two index fingers in a parallel arrangement with each other. Pull your index fingers apart, noticing how much force is required to stretch them and how far you can stretch the bands. Now loop one rubber band to another one, and that one to the final one so you have all three attached end to end. Now stretch them and notice how much force is required to stretch them and how far you can stretch the bands. There is a significant difference to the two arrangements of these rubber bands. Now identify as many muscles as you can with a parallel fiber arrangement and those with a series fiber arrangement. How do the functions of the muscles in the parallel fiber group differ from those in the series muscle fiber group?
2. Take a tape measure and measure your lab partner's thigh girth at the following levels: joint margin; 5 cm above the superior patella; 10 cm above the superior patella; 15 cm above the superior patella. Compare the left and right thigh girth measurements. How much difference is there between left and right girth measures? What are you measuring when you measure at each level? If your partner had swelling in the knee, which measurements would be most affected? If your partner had atrophy in the quadriceps, which measurements would be most affected?
3. Place your partner in a supine position with the knee maintained at 30° of flexion. Have your partner perform a maximum isometric contraction of the hamstrings against a dynamometer. Now have your partner positioned leaning on the elbows in about 30° to 45° of hip flexion; once positioned, have your partner once again perform a maximum isometric contraction of the hamstrings. Repeat this procedure with the hip at 90° and at 135° of flexion. Record each maximal isometric measurement and its range of motion on a graph. Explain how the maximal output changes as the length-tension of the muscle changes.
4. Perform a maximum isometric contraction against your partner's manual resistance with your knee positioned at 135°, 90°, 60°, and 0°. In which position did you feel your quadriceps provided the most strength? Where did you feel the weakest? How do you explain the changes in strength as your knee angle changed?
5. Using a grip dynamometer, record your partner's maximum grip strength (dynamometers record maximum contractions within 3 to 4 seconds). Allow 30 to 45 seconds of rest, repeat two times, and record each. Then have your partner perform three 75% maximum contractions (without knowledge of results and with rest periods). Note that the true maximum contractions are not exactly the same but are very close. This is one way to determine if a person has performed a maximum contraction. The 75% contractions are similar to those made by a person who is not motivated or is trying to simulate muscle weakness. There is marked variability to show that this is not a true maximum contraction.
6. Record your partner's maximum grip strength and then repeat the procedure while you hold his or her wrist in wrist flexion. This requires that either you provide sufficient strength to maintain your partner's wrist in flexion while he or she is gripping the dynamometer or that you provide other means to stabilize the wrist in flexion. Note the marked decrease in the strength of grip when the wrist is flexed. Explain why this change in strength occurs.
7. Explain the synergistic motion that results when the extensor carpi radialis and flexor carpi radialis contract simultaneously. Identify two other muscles that work together in such a manner.
8. Lift a 10-lb weight in an elbow curl slowly and lower it slowly. Which motion was easier? Now perform the same motions fast in both directions. Which was easier? Explain why.
9. Perform one open kinetic chain activity with each muscle: biceps, shoulder flexors, and knee extensors. Now perform closed chain activities, one each with each muscle. Explain how each muscle felt during the open and closed kinetic chain exercises.
10. Actively shorten your hamstrings in a prone position and then in a sitting position on the end of a plinth. Which position provided more knee flexion motion? Explain why.

References

1. Inman VT, Saunders JB, Abbott LC. Observations on function of the shoulder joint. *Journal of Bone and Joint Surgery Am* 26:1, 1944.
2. Clark DI, Downing N, Mitchell J, Coulson L, Syzpryt EP, Doherty M. Physiotherapy for anterior knee pain: A randomised controlled trial. *Annals of the Rheumatic Diseases* 59(9):700–704, 2000.
3. Basmajian JV. Cyclobenzaprine hydrochloride effect on skeletal muscle spasm in the lumbar region and neck: Two double-blind controlled clinical and laboratory studies. *Archives of Physical Medicine and Rehabilitation* 59:58–63, 1978.
4. Heckathorne CW, Childress DS. Relationships of the surface electromyogram to the force, length, velocity and contraction rate of the cineplastic human biceps. *American Journal of Physical Medicine* 60(1):1–19, 1981.
5. Ebersole KT, O'Connor KM, Wier AP. Mechanomyographic and electromyographic responses to repeated concentric muscle actions of the quadriceps femoris. *Journal of Electromyography and Kinesiology* 16(2):149–157, 2006.
6. Smidt GL. Hip motion and related factors in walking. *Physical Therapy* 51(1):9–22, 1971.
7. Perry J. *Gait Analysis. Normal and Pathological Function*. Thorofare, NJ: Slack, Inc, 1992.
8. Hislop HJ, Perrine JJ. The isokinetic concept of exercise. *Physical Therapy* 47:114, 1967.
9. Pette D, Peuker H, Staron RS. The impact of biomechanical methods for single fibre analysis. *Acta Physiologica Scandinavica* 166:261–277, 1999.
10. Staron RS. Human skeletal muscle fiber types: Delineation, development, and distribution. *Canadian Journal of Applied Physiology* 22(4):302–327, 1997.
11. Thompson LV. Skeletal muscle adaptations with age, inactivity, and therapeutic exercise. *Journal of Orthopaedic and Sports Physical Therapy* 32(2):44–57, 2002.
12. Garrett WE, Califf JC, Bassett FH. Histochemical correlates of hamstring injuries. *American Journal of Sports Medicine* 12(2):98–103, 1984.
13. Gryzlo SM, Patek RM, Pink M, Perry J. Electromyographic analysis of knee rehabilitation exercises. *J orthop sport phys ther* 20(1):36–43, 1994.
14. Qi Z. Influence of knee joint position on co-contractions of agonist and antagonist muscles during maximal voluntary isometric contractions: Electromyography and Cybex measurement. *Journal of Physical Therapy Sciences* 19:125–130, 2007.
15. Wilk K, Escamilla R, Fleisig G, Barrentine S, Andrews J, Boyd M. A comparison of tibiofemoral joint forces and electromyographic activity during open and closed kinetic chain exercises. *American Journal of Sports Medicine* 24(4):518–527, 1996.
16. Fiatarone MA, Marks EC, Ryan ND, Meredith CN, Lipsitz LA, Evans WJ. High-intensity strength training in nonagenarians. *JAMA* 263(22):3029–3034, 1990.
17. Frontera WR, Meredith CN, O'Reilly KP, Knuttgen HG, Evans WJ. Strength conditioning in older men: Skeletal muscle hypertrophy and improved function. *Journal of Applied Physiology* 64(3):1038–1044, 1988.
18. Leivseth G, Reikerås O. Changes in muscle fiber cross-sectional area and concentrations of Na, K-ATPase in deltoid muscle in patients with impingement syndrome of the shoulder. *Journal of Orthopaedic and Sports Physical Therapy* 19(3):146–149, 1994.
19. Maylia E, Fairclough JA, Nokes LDM, Jones MD. Can thigh girth be measured accurately? *Journal of Sport Rehabilitation* 8(1):43–49, 1999.
20. Folland JP, Williams AG. The adaptations to strength training: Morphological and neurological contributions to increased strength. *Sports Medicine* 37(2):145–168, 2007.
21. Gans C, DeVries F. Functional bases of fiber length and angulation in muscle. *Journal of Morphology* 192(1):63–85, 1987.
22. Lieber R, Fridén J. Clinical significance of skeletal muscle architecture. *Clin Orthop* 383:140–151, 2001.
23. Ramsey RW, Street SF. Isometric length-tension diagram of isolated skeletal muscle fibers of frog. *J Cell Comp Physiol* 15:11, 1940.
24. Bagni MA, Cecchi G, Colomo F, Poggesi C. Tension and stiffness of frog muscle fibres at full filament overlap. *Journal of Muscle Research and Cell Motility* 11(5):371–377, 1990.
25. Lombardi V, Piazzesi G. The contractile response during steady lengthening of stimulated frog muscle fibres. *Journal of Physiology* 431:141–171, 1990.
26. Beck O. Die gesamte kraftkurve des tetanisierten froschgatrocnemius und ihr physiologisch ausgenutzter anteil. *Pfluegers Arch Ges Physiol* 193:495, 1921–1922.
27. Lieber RL, Loren GJ, Fridén J. In vivo measurement of human wrist extensor muscle sarcomere length changes. *Journal of Neurophysiology* 71(3):874–881, 1994.

28. Lord SF, Clark RD, Webster OW. Visual acuity and contrast sensitivity in relation to falls in an elderly population. *Age and Aging* 20:175, 1991.

29. Westring SH, Seger JY, Karlson E, Ekblom B. Eccentric and concentric torque-velocity characteristics of the quadriceps femoris in man. *European Journal of Applied Physiology and Occupational Physiology* 58(1–2):100–104, 1988.

30. Adam A, DeLuca CJ. Recruitment order of motor units in human vastus lateralis muscle is maintained during fatiguing contractions. *Journal of Neurophysiology* 90(5):2919–2927, 2003.

31. Henneman E. Recruitment of motorneurones: The size principle. In Desmedt JE (ed). *Progress in Clinical Neurophysiology.* Vol 9. Basel: S. Karger, 1981, p 26.

32. Henneman E, Somjen G, Carpenter DO. Functional significance of cell size in spinal motoneurons. *Journal of Neurophysiology* 28:560–580, 1965.

33. Henneman E, Somjen G, Carpenter DO. Excitability and inhibitability of motoneurons of different sizes. *Journal of Neurophysiology* 28:599–620, 1965.

34. Milner-Brown HS, Stein RB, Yemm R. The orderly recruitment of human motor units during voluntary isometric contractions. *Journal of Physiology* 230:359–370, 1973.

35. Fujiwara K, Maeda K, Kunita K, Tomita H. Postural movement pattern and muscle action sequence associated with self-paced bilateral arm flexion during standing. *Perceptual and Motor Skills* 104(1):327–334, 2007.

36. Pierce MN, Lee WA. Muscle firing order during active prone hip extension. *Journal of Orthopaedic and Sports Physical Therapy* 12(1):2–9, 1990.

37. Hungerford B, Gilleard W, Hodges P. Evidence of altered lumbopelvic muscle recruitment in the presence of sacroiliac joint pain. *Spine* 28(14):1593–1600, 2003.

38. Rogers MW, Pai YC. Dynamic transitions in stance support accompanying leg flexion movements in man. *Experimental Brain Research* 81(2):398–402, 1990.

39. Cheynel N, Mourey F, Peschaud F, Durand-Fontanier S, Didler JP, Trouilloud P. Standing-up/sitting-down movement: Electromyographic analysis of four muscles of lower limb and the erector spinae muscle: study of anticipatory postural adjustments. *Morphologie* 86:23–26, 2002.

40. Sakamoto ACL, Teixeira-Salmela LF, de Paula-Goulart FR, de Morais Faria CDC, Guimaraes CQ. Muscular activation patterns during active prone hip extension exercises. *Journal of Electromyography and Kinesiology* 19(1):105–112, 2009.

41. Miller JP, Croce RV, Hutchins R. Reciprocal coactivation patterns of the medial and lateral quadriceps and hamstrings during slow, medium and high speed isokinetic movements. *Journal of Electromyography and Kinesiology* 10(4):233–239, 2000.

42. O'Sullivan PB, Beales DJ, Beetham JA, et al. Altered motor control strategies in subjects with sacroiliac joint pain during the active straight-leg-raise test. *Spine* 27(1):E1–8, 2002.

43. McNeil CJ, Doherty TJ, Stashuk DW, Rice CL. Motor unit number estimates in the tibialis anterior muscle of young, old, and very old men. *Muscle & Nerve* 31:461–467, 2005.

44. Komi PV, Karlsson J. Physical performance, skeletal muscle enzyme activities and fibre types in monozygous and dizygous twins of both sexes. *Acta Physiologica Scandinavica. Supplementum* 462:1–28, 1979.

45. Frontera W. Aging muscle. *Crit rev phys rehabil med* 18(1):63–93, 2006.

46. Morrison JB. The mechanics of the knee joint in relation to normal walking. *Journal of Biomechanics* 3(1):51–61, 1970.

47. Weber EF. *Ueber die Langeverhaltnisse der Muskeln im Allgemeinen*. Leipzig: Verh Kgl Sach Ges d Wiss, 1851.

48. Kaplan EB. *Functional and Surgical Anatomy of the Hand*. Philadelphia: JB Lippincott, 1965.

49. Boyes JH. *Bunnell's surgery of the hand*. Philadelphia: Lippincott, 1970.

50. Lieber RL, Bodine-Fowler SC. Skeletal muscle mechanics: Implications for rehabilitation. *Physical Therapy* 73(12):844–856, 1993.

51. Kaufer H. Mechanical function of the patella. *Journal of Bone and Joint Surgery Am* 53(8):1551–1560, 1971.

52. Gibson JNA, Scott M. Long-term effects of patellectomy on quadriceps and hamstring isokinetic function. *Physiotherapy* 77(10):711–714, 1991.

53. Griffin JW, Tooms RE, vander Zwaag RV, Bertorini TE, O'Toole ML. Eccentric muscle performance of elbow and knee muscle groups in untrained men and women. *Medicine & Science in Sports & Exercise* 25(8):936–944, 1993.

54. Stanton P, Purdam C. Hamstring injuries in sprinting: The role of eccentric exercise. *Journal of Orthopaedic and Sports Physical Therapy* 10(9):343–349, 1989.

55. Pappas AM, Zawacki RM, Sullivan TJ. Biomechanics of baseball pitching, a preliminary report. *American Journal of Sports Medicine* 13:216–222, 1985.

56. Abbott BC, Bigland B, Ritchie JM. The physiological cost of negative work. *J Physiol* 117:380–390, 1952.

57. Dick RW, Cavanagh PR. An explanation of the upward drift in oxygen uptake during prolonged sub-maximal downhill running. *Medicine & Science in Sports & Exercise* 19(3):310–317, 1987.

58. Dean E. Physiology and therapeutic implications of negative work: A review. *Physical Therapy* 68:233–237, 1988.

59. Ferguson RA, Ball D, Sargeant AJ. Effect of muscle temperature on rate of oxygen uptake during exercise in humans at different contraction frequencies. *Journal of Experimental Biology* 205:981–987, 2002.

60. Whipp BJ, Rossiter HB, Ward SA. Exertional oxygen uptake kinetics: A stamen of stamina? *Biochemical Society Transactions* 30(2):237–247, 2002.

61. Roston WL, Whipp BJ, Davis JA, Cunningham DA, Effros R, M., Wasserman K. Oxygen uptake kinetics and lactate concentration during exercise in humans. *American Review of Respiratory Disease* 135(5):1080–1084, 1987.

62. Fang Y, Siemionow V, Sahgal V, Xiong F, Yue GH. Distinct brain activation patterns for human maximal voluntary eccentric and concentric muscle actions. *Brain Research* 1023(2):200–212, 2004.

63. Flitney FW, Hirst DG. Crossbridge detachment and sarcomere "give" during stretch of active frog's muscle. *Journal of Physiology* 276:449–465, 1978.

64. Sugi H, Pollack GH. *Mechanism of Myofilament Sliding in Muscle Contraction. Advances in Experimental Medicine and Biology,* Vol 332. New York: Plenum Press, 1993.

65. Edman KA. Mechanism underlying double-hyperbolic force-velocity relation in vertebrate skeletal muscle. *Advances in Experimental Medicine and Biology* 332:667–676, 1993.

66. Stauber WT. Eccentric action of muscles: physiology, injury, and adaptation. *Exercise and Sport Sciences Reviews* 17:157–185, 1989.

67. Enoka RM. Eccentric contractions require unique activation strategies by the nervous system. *Journal of Applied Physiology* 81(6):2339–2346, 1996.

68. Marey EJ, Demeny G. Etude experimentale de la locomotion humaine. *Comptes Rendus Hebdomadoires des Seances de l'Academie des Sciences* 105:544, 1887.

69. Häkkinen K, Komi PV, Kauhanen H. Electromyographic and force characteristics of leg extensor muscles of elite weight lifters during isometric, concentric and various stretch-shortening cycle exercises. *International Journal of Sports Medicine* 7(3):144–151, 1986.

70. Komi PV. Physiological and biomechanical correlates of muscle function: Effects of muscle structure and stretch-shortening cycle on force and speed. *Exercise and Sport Sciences Reviews* 12:81–121, 1984.

71. Cavagna GA. Storage and utilization of elastic energy in skeletal muscle. *Exercise and Sport Sciences Reviews* 5:89–129, 1977.

72. Aura O, Komi PV. Effects of prestretch intensity on mechanical efficiency of positive work and on elastic behavior of skeletal muscle in stretch-shortening cycle exercise. *Int J Sports Med* 7:137–143, 1986.

73. Wilk KE, Voight ML, Keirns MA, Gambetta V, Andrews JR, Dillman CJ. Stretch-shortening drills for the upper extremities: Theory and clinical application. *Journal of Orthopaedic and Sports Physical Therapy* 17(5):225–239, 1993.

74. Chmielewski T, Kauffman D, Myer GD, Tillman SM. Plyometric Exercise in the Rehabilitation of Athletes: Physiological Responses and Clinical Application. *J orthop sport phys ther* 36(5):308–319, 2006.

75. Burkholder TJ, Nichols TR. The mechanical action of proprioceptive length feedback in a model of cat hindlimb. *Motor Control* 4(2):201–220, 2000.

76. Nichols TR. Receptor mechanisms underlying heterogenic reflexes among the triceps surae muscles of the cat. *Journal of Neurophysiology* 81(2):467–478, 1999.

77. Helgeson K, Gajdosik RL. The stretch-shortening cycle of the quadriceps femoris muscle group measured by isokinetic dynamometry. *Journal of Orthopaedic and Sports Physical Therapy* 17(1):17–23, 1993.

78. Koutedakis Y. Muscle elasticity-plyometrics: Some physiological and practical considerations. *J applied res coach athl* 4:35–49, 1989.

79. Witvrouw E, Mahieu N, Roosen P, McNair P. The role of stretching in tendon injuries. *Br J Sport Med* 41(4):224–226, 2007.

80. Lundin P. A review of plyometric training. *Strength Condit* 7:69–74, 1985.

81. Voss DE, Ionta MK, Myers BJ. *Proprioceptive Neuromuscular Facilitation*, 3 ed. Philadelphia: Harper & Row, 1985.

82. Allerheiligen B, Rogers R. Plyometrics program design. *Strength and Conditioning* 17:26–31, 1995.

83. Pretz R. Plyometric exercises for overhead-throwing athletes. *Strength condit* 28(1):36–42, 2006.

84. Wilt F. Plyometrics. What it is—How it works. *Athletic Journal* 55:76–79, 1975.

85. Chu D. *Jumping into plyometrics*, 2nd ed. Champaign, IL: Human Kinetics, 1998.

86. Williams M, Stutzman L. Strength variation through the range of joint motion. *Physical Therapy Review* 39(3):145–152, 1959.

87. Smidt GL. Biomechanical analysis of knee flexion and extension. *Journal of Biomechanics* 6(1):79–92, 1973.

88. Dutto DJ, Braun WA. DOMS-associated changes in ankle and knee joint dynamics during running. *Medicine & Science in Sport & Exercise* 36(4):560–566, 2004.

89. Clarkson PM, Tremblay I. Exercise-induced muscle damage, repair and adaptation in humans. *Journal of Applied Physiology* 65(1):1–6, 1988.

90. Faulkner JA, Brooks SV, Opiteck JA. Injury to skeletal muscle fibers during contractions: Conditions of occurrence and prevention. *Physical Therapy* 73(12):911–921, 1993.

91. Rodenburg JB, Bär PR, DeBoer RW. Relations between muscle soreness and biochemical and functional outcomes of eccentric exercise. *Journal of Applied Physiology* 74(6):2976–2983, 1993.

92. Golden CL, Dudley GA. Strength after bouts of eccentric or concentric actions. *Medicine & Science in Sports & Exercise* 24(8):926–933, 1992.

93. Mair J, Koller A, Artner-Dworzak E, et al. Effects of exercise on plasma myosin heavy chain fragments and MRI of skeletal muscle. *Journal of Applied Physiology* 72(2):656–663, 1992.

94. Fridén J, Lieber RL. Structural and mechanical basis of exercise-induced muscle injury. *Medicine & Science in Sports & Exercise* 24(5):521–530, 1992.

INTRODUCTION TO

Unit 2: Upper Quarter

This unit investigates each upper extremity and axial skeleton body segment from a clinical kinesiological perspective. Anatomy is summarized in tables with the body of each chapter presenting information on the unique joint, arthrokinematics, osteokinematics, and clinical functions of each segment.

Chapter 5 presents the shoulder complex. The shoulder complex includes the scapulothoracic, sternoclavicular, acromioclavicular, and glenohumeral joints. The relationship between these structures is discussed, and the muscles are presented along with their functions for each joint. Additionally, how these joints interact with each other to produce smooth, effective shoulder movement is presented.

Chapter 6 addresses the elbow and forearm joints. The discussion includes the interaction between the muscles functioning at both of these joints and how they affect each other. The importance of synergistic functions of the elbow and forearm muscle groups is discussed.

Chapter 7 presents the wrist and hand, a complex structure. The multiple joints and muscles providing optimal performance of the hand and how the hand's unique functions are accomplished are discussed in this chapter. The various types of power and prehension grips are presented along with pathologies in these grips that occur with muscle or neural injuries.

Chapter 8 investigates the axial skeleton. The spine from the cervical region to the sacroiliac joint is presented along with information on the temporomandibular joint. The axial skeleton is a complex segment of the body that often determines the quality of activity possible in the extremities, so the relationship between the spine and extremities is presented along with elements of trunk stabilization and balance.

Shoulder Complex

"Every generation stands on the shoulders of the generation that came before. Jealously guard the values and principles of our heritage. They did not come easy."

—Ronald Reagan, 1911–2004, 40th President of the United States

CHAPTER OUTLINE

Learning Outcomes
Clinical Scenario
Introduction
Bones
Manubrium
Clavicle
Scapula
Humerus
Joints
Definition of Shoulder Girdle Movements
Sternoclavicular Joint
Acromioclavicular Joint
Scapulothoracic Joint
Glenohumeral Joint
Resting and Close-Packed Positions of the Shoulder Complex Joints
The Bicipital Groove
Scapulohumeral Rhythm
Muscles of the Shoulder Complex
Scapular Stabilizer Muscles of the Shoulder Complex
Glenohumeral Stabilizing Muscles of the Shoulder
Large Muscle Movers of the Shoulder
Function of Muscles of the Shoulder Complex
Passive and Dynamic Stabilization of the Glenohumeral Joint
Synergistic Muscle Actions
Muscle Forces and Moment (Lever) Arm Lengths
Muscle Activity during Functional Motions
Functional Deficiency Applications
Summary

LEARNING OUTCOMES

This chapter investigates the shoulder complex. By the completion of this chapter, you should be able to:

- ❑ Identify the bones, joints, and muscles of the shoulder complex;
- ❑ Discuss the relationship between each of the joints that determine scapular motion;
- ❑ Explain the relationship between movements of the scapulothoracic and glenohumeral joints and their inter-reliability;
- ❑ List muscles that stabilize the scapulothoracic joint and the glenohumeral joint;
- ❑ Discuss the influence of gravity and body position in determining muscles acting on the shoulder complex during functional motions;
- ❑ Name muscle groups that function to position and move the shoulder complex in specific functional activities.

CHAPTER OUTLINE

Clinical Scenario Solution
Discussion Questions
Lab Activities
References

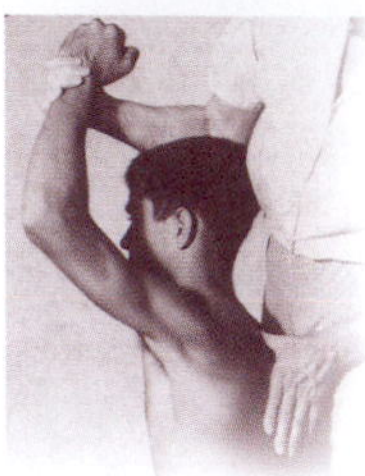

CLINICAL SCENARIO

Ella, the clinician, is in the middle of examining Tyler, her first patient for the day. Because of the history she has taken, Ella knows that Tyler's right dominant shoulder became injured while he was working. He is a house painter who has spent the last month painting ceilings in a very large mansion. His right shoulder is painful in the area just above the glenohumeral joint, especially when he raises his arm above his head. The pain has increased so much that it now bothers him when he reaches up to comb his hair or pulls his wallet out of his back pocket. Ella knows that she must examine all of the shoulder muscles, especially those that function to move and position his arm over his head. She also realizes that in order to do the appropriate muscle tests she must first know what each of those muscles do and the best position in which to test them. As Ella begins her manual muscle tests on Tyler, she is thinking of each of these muscles and the positions she must put Tyler in to obtain the most accurate results.

Introduction

The shoulder region is a complex of 20 muscles, three bony articulations, and three soft tissue moving surfaces (functional joints) that permit the greatest mobility of any joint area found in the body. The primary purpose of the shoulder is to put the hand in a position for function. The shoulder is able to place the hand in about 16,000 different positions,[1] thereby allowing the hand to produce myriad functions that we usually take for granted. The shoulder complex not only provides a wide range of positions for hand placement, but it also stabilizes the upper extremity for hand motions, lifts and pushes objects, elevates the body, assists with forced respiratory inspirations and expirations, and even bears weight when walking with crutches or performing handstands. Mobility, however, is at the expense of structural stability. The only bony attachment of the upper extremity to the trunk is at the sternoclavicular joint. Thus, support and stabilization of the shoulder are primarily dependent on muscles and ligaments. Muscles acting on this complex structure do not act alone but rather in concert with other muscles to provide for its smooth function. If ligaments become disrupted or muscles are unable to provide their normal function, normal motion within the shoulder complex is lost and the upper limb's efficiency is hampered.

When we speak of the shoulder complex, we include all of the structures that provide upper limb movement at this most proximal upper extremity segment. The bony structures of the shoulder complex include the sternum, clavicle, scapula, and humerus; the joints make up the connections between each of these bones; and the soft tissue connection between the scapula and the thorax. When we discuss the shoulder joint, reference is made to only the glenohumeral joint: the humerus and scapula as they form the shoulder joint and the soft tissue structures that surround this joint. However, care must be made to use the correct terminology since the "shoulder joint" is only one element of the shoulder complex. Each of the elements included in the shoulder complex are presented and discussed in this chapter.

Bones

The entire shoulder complex is held to the **axial skeleton** by a combination of the bony attachment between the sternum (manubrium) and clavicle and the muscles originating from the axial skeleton and attaching to the bony shoulder complex structures. The bones connecting the shoulder complex to the axial skeleton are the manubrium (of the axial skeleton) and the clavicle (of the shoulder complex). The manubrium with the left and right clavicles and scapulae form an incomplete girdle (Fig. 5.1). It is incomplete since a true girdle completely surrounds a structure, and the shoulder girdle does not have a bony connection posteriorly; in spite of this technicality, however, the structure is often referred to as the **shoulder girdle**.

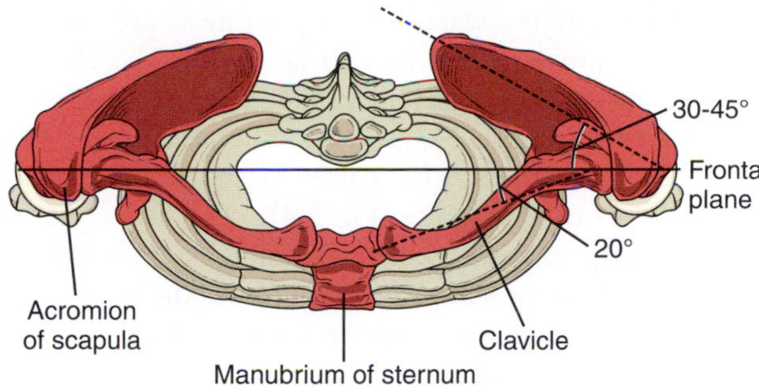

Figure 5.1 Superior view of the shoulder girdle. Notice the angles of the scapula and clavicle from the frontal plane.

Manubrium

The manubrium (L. manubrium, handle) is the most cephalic aspect of the sternum and the site at which the left and right clavicles secure the upper extremities to the axial skeleton. The superior aspect of the manubrium contains a shallow depression for the medial clavicular attachments. Sitting between these two clavicular facets is the sternal or jugular notch, a prominent concavity that is easily palpated. On the lateral aspects of the manubrium immediately adjacent and inferior to the clavicular facets are the slightly concave facets for attachment of the first ribs.

Clavicle

From a superior to inferior view, the clavicle (L. *clavicula,* diminutive of *clavus,* key) is S-shaped, like a crank, with its forward convexity at its sternal end to clear the brachial plexus and upper extremity vascular bundle and its forward concavity at the humeral end. In the anatomical position, the long axis of the clavicle is slightly above the horizontal plane, resting 20° to the frontal plane. The medial end of the clavicle is prominent where it articulates with the manubrium. It has a costal facet inferiorly that articulates with the first rib. Just lateral and posterior to this costal facet is the costal tuberosity, the attachment site for the costoclavicular ligament. Beginning at its medial aspect, the clavicle may be palpated laterally along its crank-like curve to its acromial end (Fig. 5.2). The clavicle begins as a round bone at its sternal end and transitions at about two-thirds of its length to a flatter bone, so it has a broad, flat oval expansion by the time it reaches its lateral end where it articulates with the scapula's acromion process. The acromial end of the clavicle, like the sternal end, is enlarged and is palpated as a protuberance.

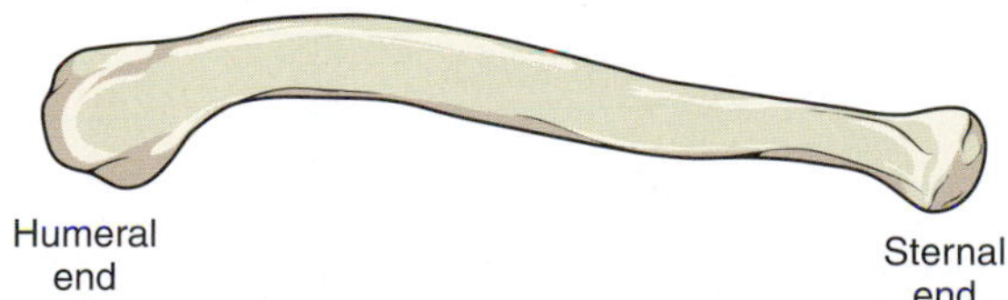

Figure 5.2 A left clavicle with its rounded medial end and flat lateral end.

Animals that stand and run in a quadruped position, such as horses and dogs, do not have clavicles, and their scapulae are on the lateral surfaces of the thorax. On the other hand, bipedal humans have a strong, well-developed clavicle that acts as a lateral strut to the scapula and the humerus. This increases glenohumeral mobility to permit greater motion in reaching and climbing activities.[2]

Scapula

The scapula (L. *scapula,* shoulder blade) is a flat, triangular-shaped bone with three sides and three angles that sits against the posterior thorax. In an anatomical resting position, its medial vertebral border is approximately 5 to 6 centimeters, or two to three finger-widths, from the thoracic spinous processes and between thoracic levels 2 (T2) and 7 (T7). It has a dual function: to provide a place for muscles controlling the glenohumeral joint to venture from and to provide a stable base from which the glenohumeral joint can function. It works intimately with the clavicle to provide the glenohumeral joint more motion so the hand can be placed in more positions.

The inferior angle of the scapula where the vertebral border and lateral border meet is palpated by following the vertebral border distally. The lateral axillary border angles upward and laterally from the inferior angle toward the glenoid fossa. The glenoid fossa is the superior lateral aspect of the scapula that forms the concave portion of the glenohumeral joint. The superior border is difficult to palpate but lies essentially parallel to the spine of the scapula. The scapular spine lies on the posterior scapula and divides the scapula into two fossae, the supraspinatus fossa and the infraspinatus fossa. The spine of the scapula can be palpated from its root on the medial vertebral border at T3 to its lateral end where it becomes the acromion process (Gr. *acron,* tip; *omox,* shoulder) of the scapula. As it traverses laterally and slightly upward along the posterior scapula, the scapular spine transitions from a flat prominence on the vertebral border to become more prominent dorsally in its middle and then becomes larger at its lateral end. The lateral acromion end hooks slightly forward and superiorly to meet the clavicle. The acromion process sits over the glenohumeral joint to protect it from overhead forces applied down toward the shoulder. At its lateral end, the acromion process is broad and extends like an easily palpated shelf over the shoulder joint. The acromion's free edge may be felt at its very anterior aspect. Its junction with the clavicle (acromioclavicular joint) is somewhat protected since it is covered by the acromioclavicular ligament. In most individuals, two bony enlargements can be differentiated in this region—one is the acromion and the other is the clavicle with a slight depression between them. This depression is the acromioclavicular (AC) joint itself and is palpated between the two bone ends (Fig. 5.3).

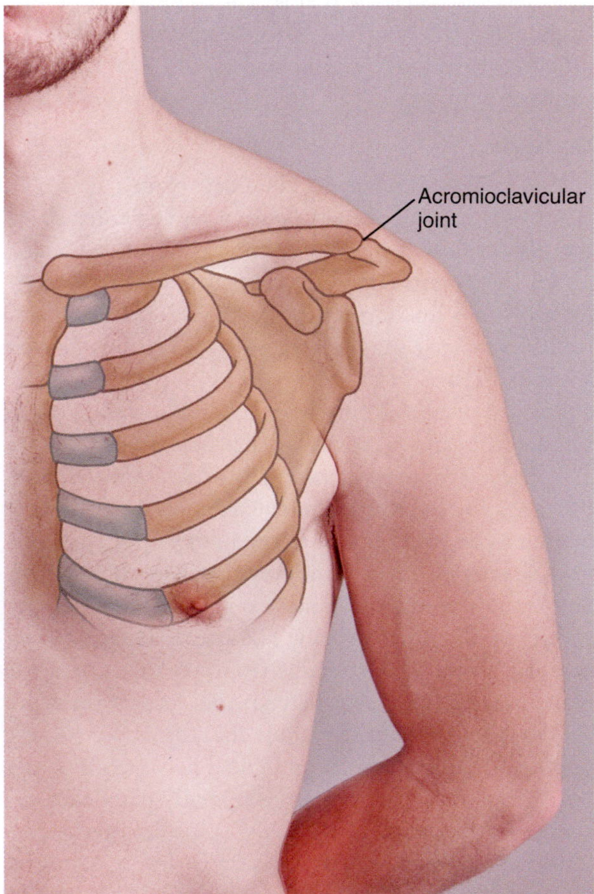

Figure 5.3 This view of the anterior left shoulder reveals the distal end of the clavicle as the more proximal "bump" on the top of the shoulder that is separated from the more lateral "bump," the acromion, by the slight depression between them which is the acromioclavicular joint.

Anteriorly, the scapula has a prominent process: the coracoid process. This process sits below the clavicle and is medial to the glenoid fossa. It protrudes anteriorly from the scapula and is a site of multiple ligament and muscle attachments. Its name means "crow's beak" because of its appearance (Fig. 5.4).

To palpate the scapular structures, it is easiest to identify the acromion process and follow the bony ridge posteriorly along the scapular spine as it goes transversely across the scapula to the scapula's vertebral border where it flattens out to form a smooth, triangular-shaped area. The supraspinatus fossa, above the scapular spine, and the infraspinatus fossa, below the scapular spine, can be readily identified; because both are filled with muscles, their depths cannot be fully appreciated, particularly the supraspinatus fossa. The vertebral and axillary borders of the scapula are easily palpable when the scapular muscles are relaxed. As previously mentioned, the inferior angle of the scapula is the lowest part of the scapula where the vertebral and axillary borders join. Also previously mentioned, the superior angle of the scapula is more difficult to palpate because it is well covered by muscles. Anteriorly, just medial to the anterior roundness of the anterior deltoid over the glenohumeral joint and about one thumb's width below the inferior clavicle, the coracoid process is a small, round protuberance that is located with deep palpation. Even in normal individuals, the coracoid process is usually tender to deep palpation.

The glenoid fossa, or cavity, (Gr. *glene,* socket) of the scapula is the most lateral aspect of the scapula. It is the

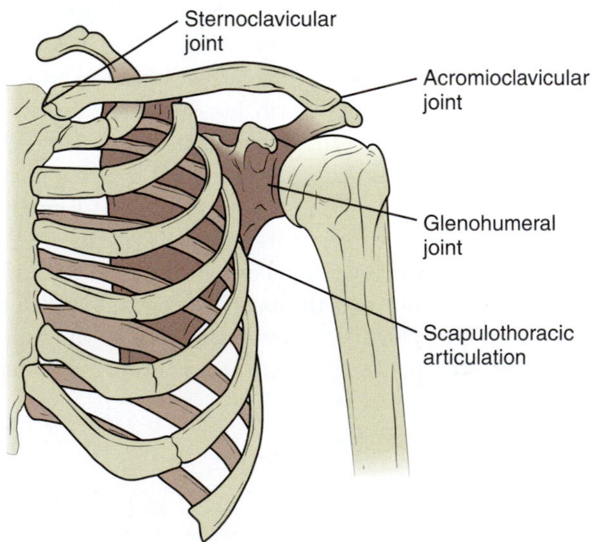

Figure 5.4 Joints of the shoulder complex. Note that the distal acromion forms a "crow's beak" at it protrudes anteriorly from the scapula.

concave portion of the glenohumeral joint that receives the convex portion of the joint, the humeral head. The glenoid fossa is a shallow socket that has two tubercles. The supraglenoid tubercle on the superior rim of the fossa serves as the attachment site for the long head of the biceps. The other tubercle, the infraglenoid tubercle on the inferior rim, is the site of attachment of the long head of the triceps. The glenoid fossa and its tubercles cannot be palpated because of the ligaments, capsule, and muscles covering them. The glenoid labrum, a dense fibrous connective tissue rim that surrounds the glenoid fossa,[3, 4] expands the depth of the glenoid fossa to increase joint congruence and assist in stress reduction by increasing the area of joint surface contact. The glenoid labrum adds about 50% more surface area to the depth and curve of the glenoid fossa. The labrum attaches securely to the inferior glenoid. It attaches more loosely to the superior glenoid where the long head of the biceps tendon anchors itself on the most superior aspect of the glenoid. The alignment of the glenoid fossa is tilted approximately 5° upward relative to the scapula's vertebral border (Fig. 5.5A). The fossa is narrower at its superior aspect and broadens slightly towards its inferior border to take on a teardrop, or pear-shaped, appearance (Fig. 5.5B). The importance of this configuration will become apparent when we discuss glenohumeral motions.

The scapula lies on the posterior ribs and conforms to the upper thorax when in its resting position; therefore, it does not lie in a pure frontal plane. Rather, it is rotated on its transverse axis approximately 30° to 45° so the glenoid fossa is tilted anterior to the frontal (coronal) plane. This position is the **plane of the scapula** or the scapular plane. Because of the position of the upper thorax and ribs, the scapula sits tipped in the sagittal plane approximately 10° to 20° so the superior aspect of the scapula lies more anterior than its inferior angle (Fig. 5.1).

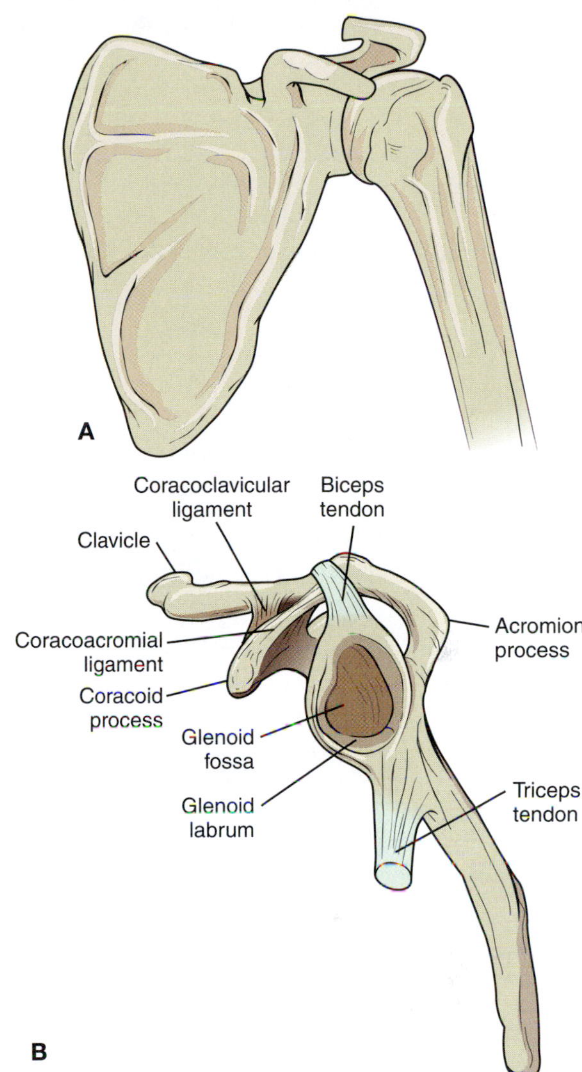

Figure 5.5 Glenoid fossa. A) There is about a 5° tilt of fossa relative to the scapula's vertebral border. B) The glenoid fossa has a pear shape with a narrower superior portion and a broader inferior aspect.

Humerus

The head of the humerus is the convex segment that interfaces with the concave glenoid fossa to form the glenohumeral joint. The head is one-third to one-half of a sphere and is positioned medially and superiorly in the frontal plane and rotated posteriorly in the transverse plane to meet the glenoid fossa that usually faces a slightly lateral, superior, and anterior direction. The humeral head is adjacent to a short humeral neck, the anatomic neck, which connects to the shaft of the humerus. In the frontal plane, the humeral head is angled at 135° to the long axis of the humeral shaft. This angle is referred to as the **angle of inclination**. The humeral head also has an **angle of torsion** relative to the shaft of the humerus. The resting position of the humeral head in posterior rotation relative to the distal condyles of the humerus allows the head to be aligned in the scapular plane while maintaining proper elbow joint alignment; this relative position of posterior rotation is called **retroversion** (L. *retro,* backward; *verto,* to turn) and is usually 30°. Figure 5.6 shows both the angle of inclination and the angle of torsion of the humeral head relative to the shaft humerus.

The greater and lesser tubercles are located on the neck of the humerus adjacent to the humeral head. The greater tubercle sits lateral to the lesser tubercle and is a

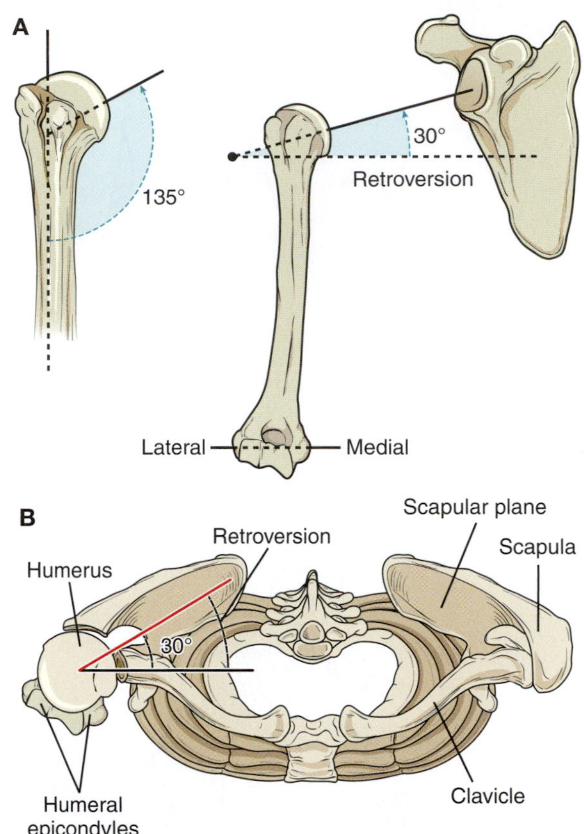

Figure 5.6 Humeral position. **A)** In the frontal plane, the humeral head is angled relative to the long axis of the humeral shaft to create an angle of inclination. **B)** In the transverse plane, the humeral head is rotated slightly posterior relative to the distal condyles of the humerus. This is the angle of torsion, or retroversion, and allows the humeral head to align with the glenoid fossa while maintaining the elbow and hand in a functional position.

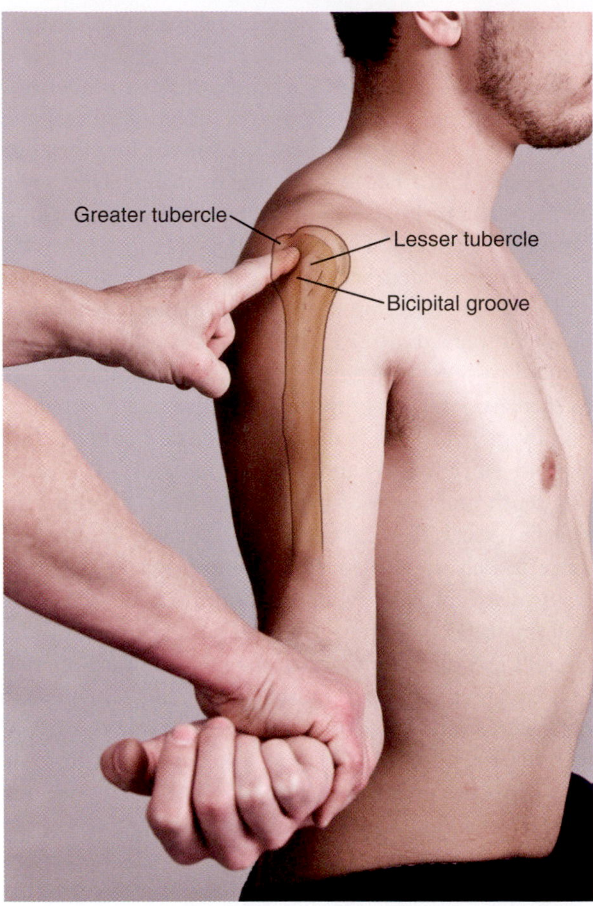

Figure 5.7 Palpation of the greater and lesser tubercles and the bicipital groove. These structures lie directly inferior and slightly posterior to the acromion when the shoulder is in lateral rotation.

large round protuberance. The lesser tubercle is smaller and sharper and lies more medially. Separating the two tubercles is an indentation, the bicipital groove (intertubercular groove), through which the long head of the biceps runs from its proximal insertion on the supraglenoid tubercle. The surgical neck of the humerus is a circumferential area on the proximal humerus. This region is distal to the bicipital groove and called the "surgical neck" because it is a common site for humeral fractures, especially in the elderly, when a fall occurs and the individual lands on an outstretched arm.

If the humerus is laterally rotated while the arm is hanging at the side, the greater tubercle of the humerus may be palpated slightly posterior and just inferior to the acromion process (Fig. 5.7). In full medial rotation, this tubercle is no longer palpable because it disappears under the deltoid muscle. The greater tubercle has three facets, serving as points of attachment for muscles, but these facets cannot be distinguished by palpation. With the humerus in full lateral rotation, the lesser tubercle is just medial to the greater tubercle. The indentation of the bicipital groove is between the two tubercles; because of its location, this groove is also referred to as the intertubercular groove. In full shoulder lateral rotation, the bicipital groove is directly in line with the acromion process. All three of these structures can be palpated in most individuals.

Joints

The bones of the shoulder complex join at three synovial joints: (1) the clavicle articulates with the manubrium of the sternum at the sternoclavicular (SC) joint; (2) the clavicle and the scapula join at the acromioclavicular (AC) joint; and (3) the humerus articulates with the scapula at the glenohumeral (GH) joint. During movements of the shoulder complex, the scapula also slides on the thorax; this connection is the scapulothoracic (ST) joint, although it is not a joint in the technical sense of the word.

Definition of Shoulder Girdle Movements

Before we can discuss all the joints of the shoulder complex in detail, we should identify the motions of these joints. Some of these motions are unique to the shoulder girdle and, therefore, need to be defined. As mentioned, "shoulder girdle" is a term that refers to the scapula, clavicle, and manubrium (Fig. 5.1). The special motions of the scapula that occur as a result of scapulothoracic, acromioclavicular, and sternoclavicular joint motions are illustrated in Figure 5.8. Scapulothoracic motions are the result of sternoclavicular and acromioclavicular joint movements. In essence, there is coupling between the motions of the clavicle and the scapula. In

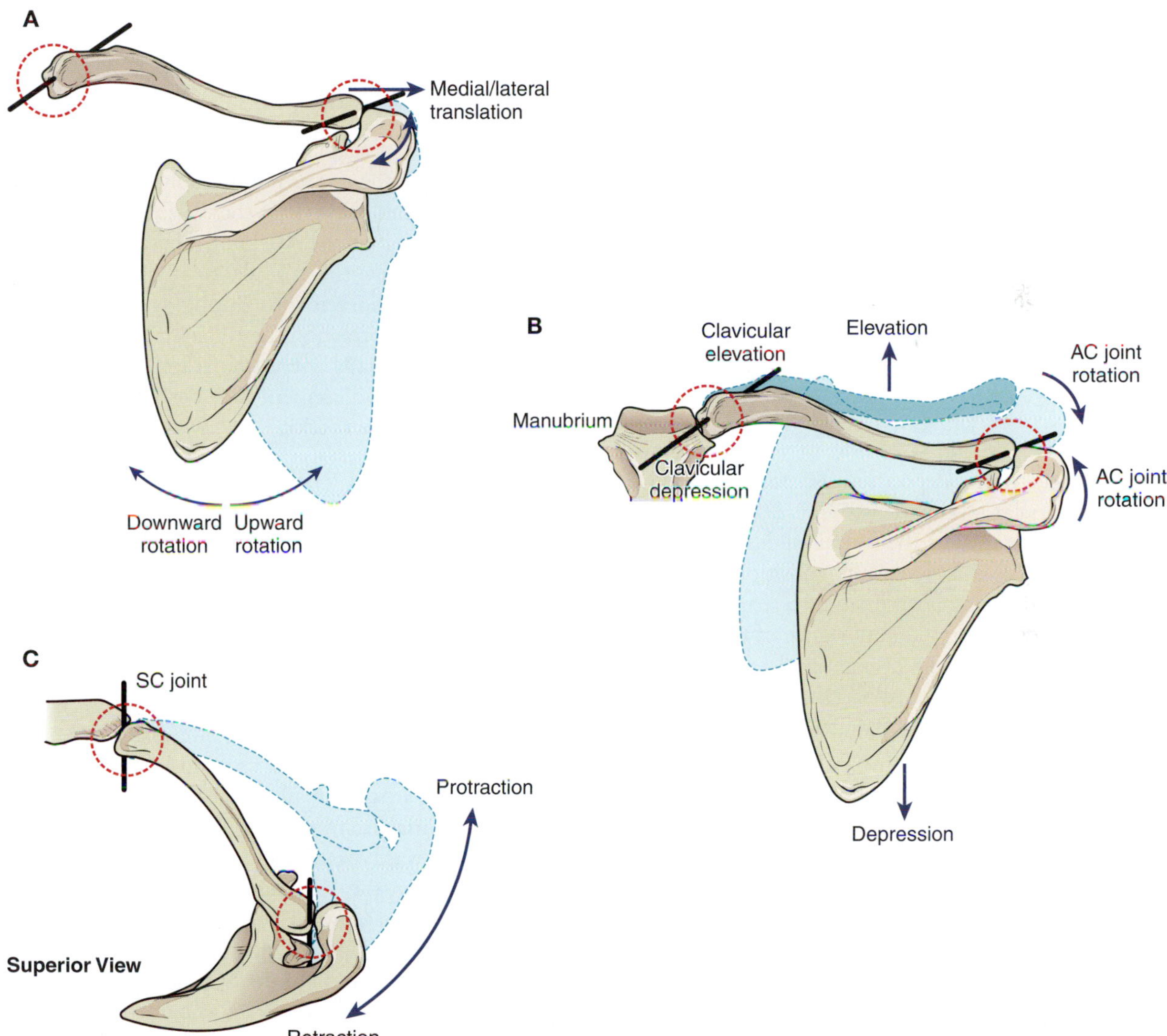

Figure 5.8 Scapula motion is the result of the SC and AC joints working together to produce scapulothoracic movement. The SC joint moves the scapula in position and the AC joint provides an adjustment to achieve the final desired position. First and second motions identified for a joint correlate with the corresponding first and second motions of the other joints, respectively. Corresponding first motions are underlined for each joint. **A)** AP axis motion of **elevation** or depression at SC joint and **upward rotation** or downward rotation adjustment at AC joint produce **upward rotation** or downward rotation of the scapula on the thorax. **B)** AP axis motion of **elevation** or depression at the SC joint and **downward** or upward rotation adjustment at the AC joint produce **elevation** or depression of the scapula on the thorax. **C)** Vertical axis motion of **protraction** or retraction at SC joint and **anterior rotation** or posterior rotation adjustment in the horizontal plane at the AC joint produce **protraction** or retraction of the scapula on the thorax.

other words, motions at the AC and SC joints produce movement of the scapula on the thorax. Therefore, if there are deficiencies that restrict movement of any of these three joints, the other two are also affected. Of the two clavicular joints, the sternoclavicular joint is responsible for the majority of the scapula's movement whereas the acromioclavicular joint provides minimal movement and acts more as a fine tuner of scapula motion than a producer of its motion.[5, 6] Think of the SC joint as the major transporter and the AC joint as the scapula's position modifier for each scapular motion (Fig. 5.8). The terms in this section identify and describe motions unique to the scapula and these joints.

Shoulder Girdle Elevation

Elevation is a motion primarily used to describe the scapula. In elevation, the scapula slides upward on the thorax relative to its resting position (Fig. 5.9A). Shrugging the shoulders produces this motion. In order for scapular elevation to occur, there must also be elevation of the clavicle at the sternoclavicular joint. Because of this SC motion, the distal end of the clavicle and the acromion process move superiorly (toward the ear) approximately 60°.[7]

Shoulder Girdle Depression

As with elevation, depression is used primarily to describe scapular motion. It is the reverse movement of elevation. In depression, the scapula slides downward on the thorax relative to its resting position (Fig. 5.9B). From a seated resting position, only 5° to 10° of depression occurs. However, the importance of the movement is in stabilization of the scapula and elevation of the body during upper extremity weight-bearing as in gymnastic maneuvers on the parallel bars, walking with crutches, or wheelchair transfers for individuals with a disability such as paraplegia. From a position of maximum elevation, the movement of shoulder depression can elevate the trunk 4 to 6 inches (10 to 15 cm).

During elevation and depression motions, there are slight changes in the amount of scapular tilting and rotation. Downward rotation of the lateral scapula and slight anterior medial tilting of the superior scapula accompany elevation, and upward rotation of the lateral scapula with slight posterior and lateral tilting of the superior scapula occur with depression. These minor adjustments allow the scapula to stay in contact with the thorax throughout each motion.

Shoulder Girdle Protraction

Although the scapula is generally thought of as the foundation of motion during protraction, both the scapula and clavicle play important roles in producing this motion. During protraction, the lateral end of the clavicle and the scapula move anteriorly around the rib cage, with the medial border of the scapula moving away from the midline 5 to 6 inches (13 to 15 cm). This motion is also referred to as abduction of the scapula (Fig. 5.9C).

Shoulder Girdle Retraction

Retraction is the opposite motion of protraction. In retraction, the lateral end of the clavicle and the scapula move posteriorly, and the medial border of the scapula approaches the midline (Fig. 5.9D). This motion is also called scapular adduction. At the sternoclavicular joint, the total range for protraction and retraction is approximately 25°.[7]

The motions of scapular protraction and retraction must also include the concurrent motions of protraction and retraction of the clavicle at the SC joint and medial and lateral rotation at the AC joint. These SC and AC joint motions allow the scapula to maintain contact along the upper thoracic ribs during protraction and retraction. With protraction the AC joint makes a slight adjustment to medially rotate the scapula, and during retraction, the AC adjustment includes lateral rotation of the scapula on the thorax.

Shoulder Girdle Upward Rotation

Upward rotation is a scapular motion in which the glenoid fossa moves to face superiorly and the inferior angle of the scapula slides laterally and anteriorly on the thorax (Fig. 5.9). Maximum range of upward rotation occurs with the full shoulder (glenohumeral) flexion.

Shoulder Girdle Downward Rotation

Downward rotation is a scapular motion in which the glenoid fossa moves to face inferiorly (Fig. 5.9). Complete range of downward rotation occurs when the hand is placed in the small of the back or when the shoulder is in maximum extension.

Scapular upward rotation and downward rotation are named relative to the movement of the glenoid fossa. The total range of upward and downward rotation is approximately 60°. Upward rotation of the scapula is accompanied by elevation of the SC and AC joints, and scapular downward rotation is accompanied by depression of these joints. Both upward and downward rotations occur about an anterior-posterior axis through the scapula.

Scapular Tilting

Scapular tilting accompanies glenohumeral motions.[8, 9] Tilting is also referred to as tipping or rotation. In addition to scapular upward and downward rotation, the scapula undergoes both anterior-posterior tilting and

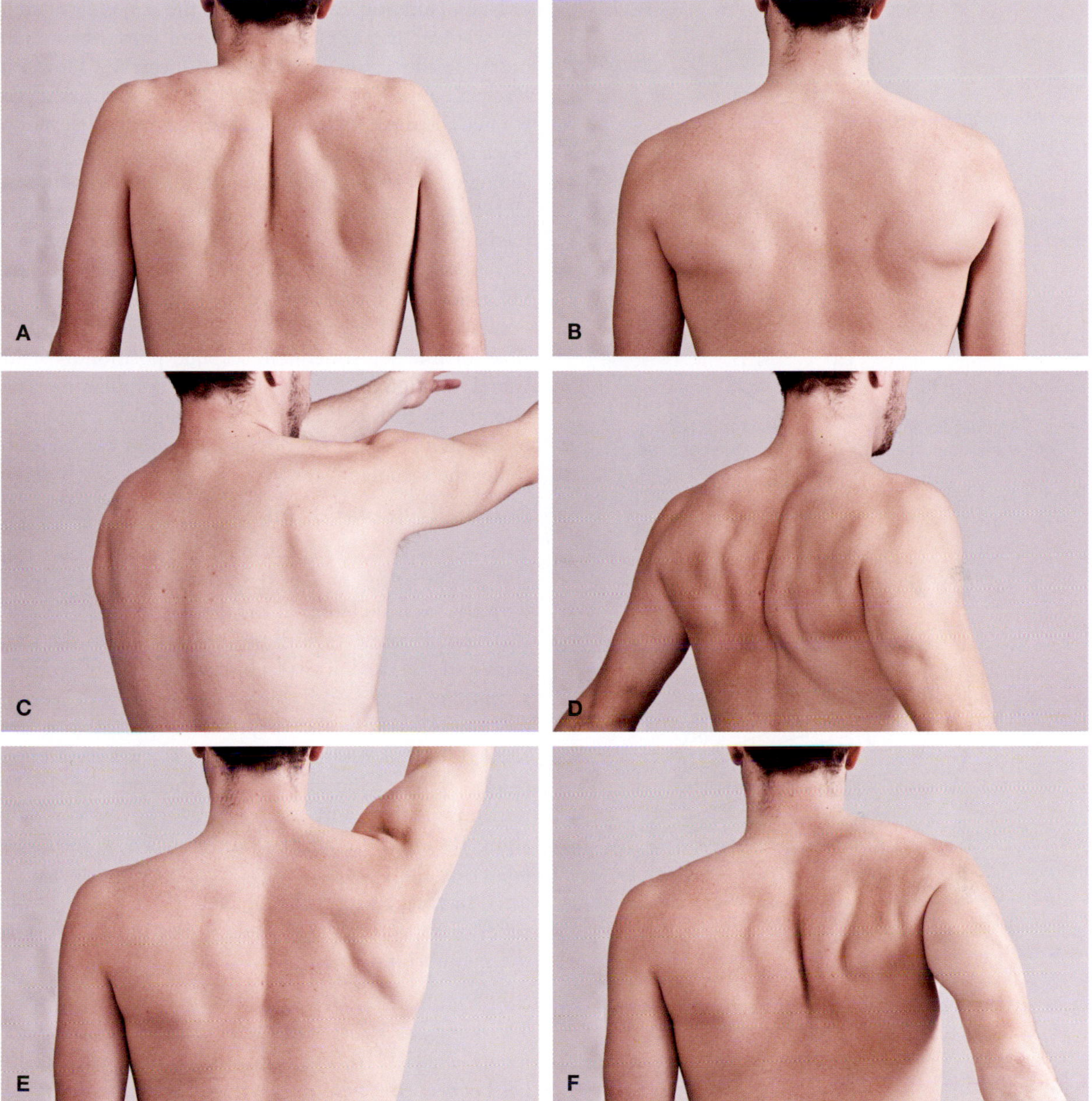

Figure 5.9 Motions of the scapula. A. Elevation B. Depression C. Protraction D. Retraction E. Upward rotation F. Downward rotation

medial-lateral tilting. Differences in scapular tilting have been noted in pathological conditions, muscle imbalances, or poor posture when compared to normal subjects.[8, 9]

Anterior-Posterior Tilting of the Scapula

Anterior and posterior tilting is rotation of the scapula along a near medial-lateral axis.[10-13] The direction of scapular anterior-posterior tilting is identified according to the direction of movement of the superior scapula. Anterior tilting occurs when the superior border of the scapula tilts forward with its inferior angle moving away from the thorax. Anterior tilting of the scapula occurs when the humerus is positioned behind the back and the hand is lifted away from the back (Fig. 5.10). Posterior tilting will occur as the scapula returns to the resting position from an anteriorly tilted position. From a resting position or anatomical position, the scapula will posteriorly tilt as the humerus is elevated during shoulder flexion and abduction. Posterior tilting is

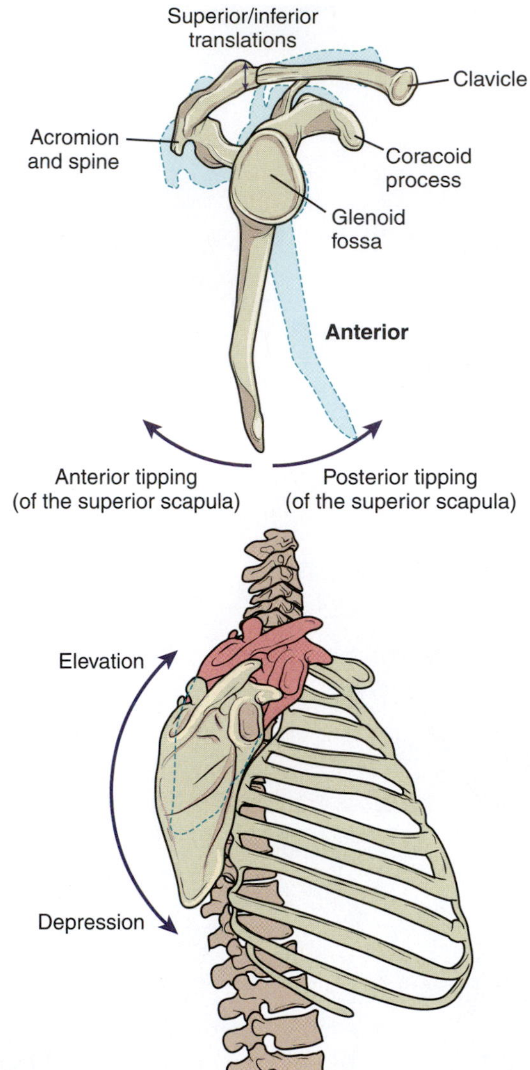

Figure 5.10 Anterior and posterior tipping of the scapula is identified according to the direction in which the superior scapula moves. Anterior tilting occurs when the superior border of the scapula tilts forward with its inferior angle moving away from the thorax, and posterior tilting occurs when the superior border tilts backward. As demonstrated in the image, when the scapula elevates on the ribs, it also tilts anteriorly.

accompanied by posterior rotation of the clavicle at the SC and AC joints.[14]

Medial-Lateral Tilting of the Scapula

Medial tilting and lateral tilting are rotation around a vertical axis. Tilting around the vertical axis occurs at the acromioclavicular joint.[15] Medial tilting causes the glenoid fossa of the scapula to face more anteriorly whereas lateral tilting causes the glenoid to face more laterally. Medial tilting and lateral tilting are sometimes referred to as internal, or medial, rotation and external, or lateral, rotation, respectively. As the arm is elevated in the scapular plane, a combination of upward rotation, posterior tilting and lateral tilting occurs.[13] However, Rachael Teece and her associates[15] found that the scapula tilted medially in the lower degrees of elevation. If we consider the shape of the scapula and the forward sliding of the scapula on the thorax during glenohumeral elevation, it makes intuitive sense that the scapula medially rotates during the first half of glenohumeral elevation. On the other hand, since Philip McClure and his associates[13] found most of the scapula's lateral tilting occurs above 90°—perhaps since the AC joint is responsible for fine adjustments in scapular positioning—this lateral rotation is the result of the scapular muscles' attempt to further maintain the scapula's conformity to the thorax as the sternoclavicular joint continues to rotate the scapula upward.

Sternoclavicular Joint

The sternoclavicular (SC) joint is the only joint that acts as a strut to connect the upper extremity directly with the axial skeleton; at this joint, the medial end of the clavicle connects with the manubrium of the sternum and the medial first rib. Because the SC joint is a complex sellar (saddle) joint, it has three degrees of motion: elevation and depression, protraction and retraction, and rotation. This joint can vary significantly from one individual to another, but the clavicle portion of the joint is generally convex vertically along its longitudinal axis, and concave anterior-to-posterior along its transverse axis, with the manubrium's surface reciprocally shaped (Fig. 5.11A). The superior aspect of the clavicle is not in contact with the manubrium.

Sternoclavicular Joint Ligaments

The joint has a disc and three strong stabilizing ligaments (Fig. 5.11B). The fibrocartilaginous articular disc lies between the two joint surfaces, attaching inferiorly near the lateral aspect of the clavicular facet on the sternum's manubrium. Superiorly, it attaches to the clavicular head and interclavicular ligament. The outer rim of the disc attaches to the inner surface of the joint's capsule. This arrangement divides the joint into two separate synovial cavities. This arrangement allows motion to take place both between the clavicle and the disc and between the disc and the sternum. The disc serves as a hinge for motion. The disc attachments add stability to the joint and reduce the risk of the clavicle sliding over the manubrium. The disc also increases stability by increasing congruency between the joint surfaces and provides reduced joint stresses by improving shock absorbency.

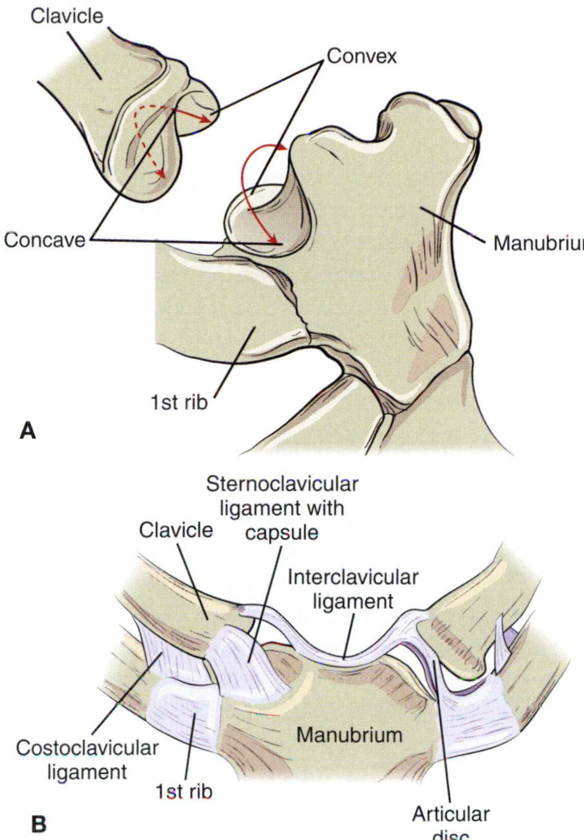

Figure 5.11 Sternoclavicular joint. **A)** The clavicle portion is convex vertically along its longitudinal axis and concave anterior-to-posterior along its transverse axis whereas the manubrium's surface is reciprocally shaped. **B)** A disc lies between the two joint surfaces.

The ligaments surrounding and supporting the joint include the anterior and posterior sternoclavicular ligaments that blend with the joint capsule to protect against anterior and posterior joint stresses. The third ligament, the superior sternoclavicular ligament, traverses over the superior aspect of the jugular notch to form the interclavicular ligament; this ligament prevents upward clavicular displacement at the SC joint. Although the bony articulations appear small, these ligamentous attachments are sufficiently strong that when sufficient stresses are applied, the clavicle usually fractures before the joint dislocates. The ligament attaching the clavicle to the first rib is the costoclavicular ligament. This ligament lies outside the articular capsule and has two heads that cross each other so the anterior fibers on the first rib lie in a superior and lateral direction while the posterior fibers traverse and angle from the first rib to the clavicle in a superior and medial direction (Fig. 5.12A). The costoclavicular ligament restricts clavicular elevation, rotation, and medial and lateral movements. The joint capsule and ligaments are further reinforced by the proximal tendinous attachments of the sternocleidomastoid muscles (Fig. 5.12B).

The shoulder girdle and the entire upper extremity are suspended from the axial skeleton by muscles, ligaments, and fascia. The position of this hanging structure is determined partly by the action of gravity and partly by the clavicle, which restricts shoulder girdle movements in all directions, particularly in a forward direction.

Sternoclavicular Joint Kinematics

Although the clavicle's axes of motions lie slightly oblique to the cardinal planes of movement, sternoclavicular motions are close enough to the cardinal planes so that they are classified and discussed in cardinal plane terms (Fig. 5.13). As mentioned, the sternoclavicular joint's osteokinematic motion occurs within three degrees of freedom: elevation and depression, retraction and protraction, and rotation.

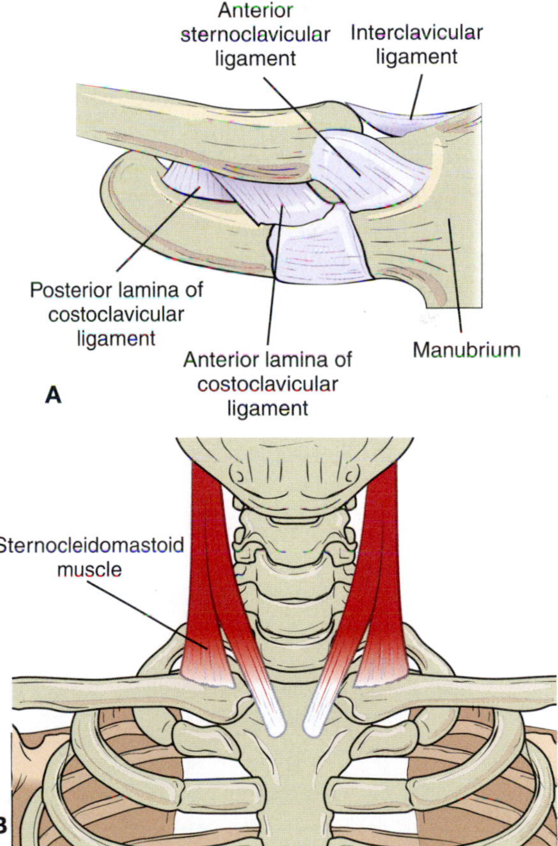

Figure 5.12 Anterior SC joint. **A)** The costoclavicular ligament restricts motion of the clavicle in elevation, rotation, and medial and lateral movements. **B)** The sternocleidomastoid muscle's tendon also provides some reinforcement to the sternoclavicular joint.

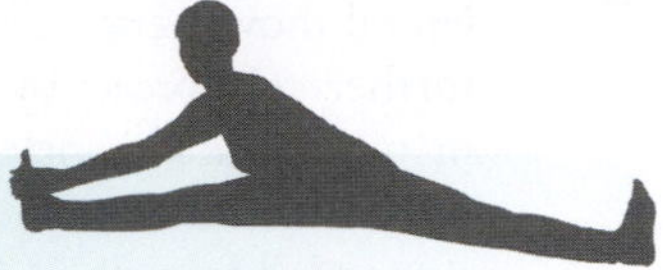

PRACTICE POINT

Cases of an absent clavicle have been reported in the medical literature—these individuals were able to move their shoulders so far forward that the tips of the shoulders almost met in front of the body. With complete surgical removal of the clavicle, Michael Lewis and associates[16] found shoulder joint ranges of motion to be the same as those on the uninvolved side. The maximum isokinetic torques for shoulder extension, medial rotation, and lateral rotation were also the same. The shoulder flexors, abductors, and adductors on the involved side, however, had a 50% loss of isokinetic torque.

Sternoclavicular elevation and depression occur in a frontal plane around an anterior-posterior axis. The A-P axis pierces the sternal end of the clavicle and takes a backward-downward course (Fig. 5.13). Movement about this axis takes place between the sternal end of the clavicle and the articular disc. Because of the slight obliquity of this axis, shoulder girdle elevation occurs in an upward-backward direction, and depression occurs in a forward-downward direction. Elevation of the sternoclavicular joint is 30° to 45°,[4, 17] with most of the motion occurring in the first 90° of shoulder elevation. Elevation of the SC joint is limited by the costoclavicular ligament and the subclavian muscle. From the resting position, the SC joint can be depressed 5° to 10° until the clavicle is stopped by the interclavicular ligament, superior capsule, and first rib.

The joint between the articular disc and the sternum is involved mainly in retraction-protraction of the shoulder girdle. These motions take place in a plane parallel to the transverse plane about a nearly vertical axis. This axis pierces the manubrium close to the SC joint (Fig. 5.13). From the resting position, protraction of the sternoclavicular joint is 15° to 30° and retraction is 15° to 30°.[4, 18] The posterior sternoclavicular ligament and the costoclavicular ligament limit protraction, and the anterior sternoclavicular ligament limits retraction.[19] Scapular retraction and protraction accompany retraction and protraction of the clavicle, respectively. Since these clavicular movements occur in an anterior-posterior direction along a vertical axis, the moving surface is the concave clavicular joint surface.

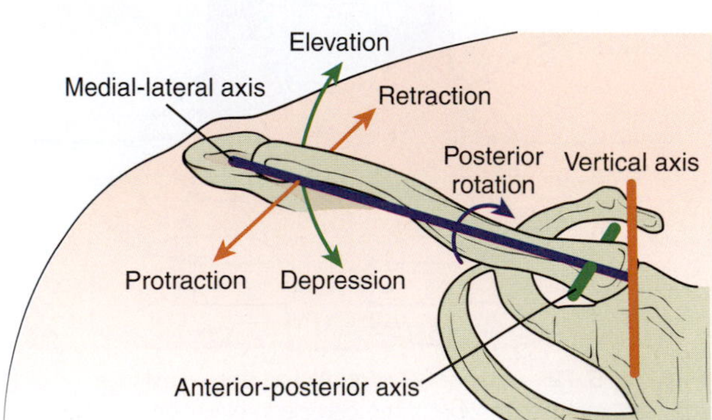

Figure 5.13 Three motions of the clavicle include elevation and depression on an anterior-posterior axis, protraction and retraction on a vertical axis, and rotation on a medial-lateral axis.

In addition to elevation-depression and protraction-retraction, the clavicle also posteriorly rotates at the sternoclavicular joint approximately 40° to 50° around its long axis.[17, 20] This motion is upward rotation or backward rotation. Anterior rotation is limited to returning to the resting position. This transverse rotation occurs after the shoulder joint has been elevated to 90° when the SC joint starts to reach its maximum elevation. This transverse rotation is essential for full, normal upward rotation of the scapula and full shoulder elevation. If rotation of the clavicle is prevented, elevation of the arm is limited to 110°.[17]

This posterior rotation occurs along a medial-lateral axis that runs between the sternoclavicular and acromioclavicular joints. Posterior rotation is a passive motion of the clavicle and is caused by the tightening of the acromioclavicular ligaments—the trapezoid and the conoid (Fig. 5.14)—which are attached to the inferior surface of the clavicle and at right angles to each other. As the conoid ligament becomes taut, its attachment on the clavicle becomes an axis for the upward rotation which is occurring at the sternoclavicular joint. Because of the clavicle's S-shape, the acromial end becomes higher. The clavicle's unique shape provides additional elevation and upward rotation of the scapula than would be possible if the bone was straight (Fig. 5.15). The trapezoid and conoid ligaments also function to limit separation of the clavicle from the scapula.

Sternoclavicular Joint Arthrokinematics

Arthrokinematic motion during elevation includes a superior roll of the clavicle with a concomitant inferior slide of the convex clavicle on the concave sternum

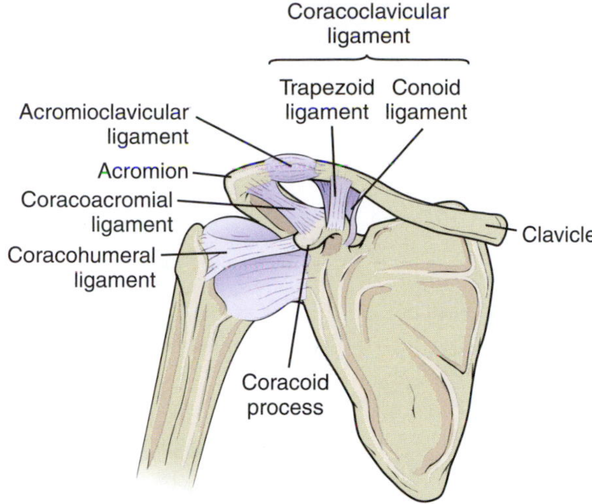

Figure 5.14 Acromioclavicular joint with its ligaments. The trapezoid and the conoid ligaments on the inferior aspect provide significant stability to this joint.

(Fig. 5.16A). During depression, the clavicle rolls inferiorly and slides superiorly on the sternum (Fig. 5.16B). During protraction and retraction, the moving clavicle's surface is concave; therefore, in arthrokinematic terms, as the clavicle rolls anteriorly in protraction, it also slides anteriorly; conversely, as it moves in retraction, the clavicle rolls and slides posteriorly (Fig. 5.16C). During rotation, the axis of motion is a medial-lateral axis with spin of the clavicular head occurring about the articular disc.

Acromioclavicular Joint

The acromioclavicular (AC) joint is a plane synovial joint with three degrees of freedom involving the medial margin of the acromion and the lateral end of the clavicle (Fig. 5.17). The acromial end faces medially and slightly superiorly while the clavicular end faces laterally and slightly inferiorly to form a wedge-like surface. In a

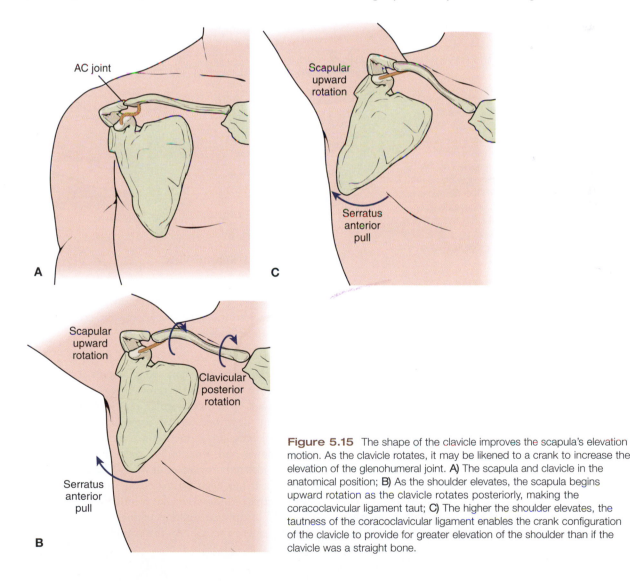

Figure 5.15 The shape of the clavicle improves the scapula's elevation motion. As the clavicle rotates, it may be likened to a crank to increase the elevation of the glenohumeral joint. **A)** The scapula and clavicle in the anatomical position; **B)** As the shoulder elevates, the scapula begins upward rotation as the clavicle rotates posteriorly, making the coracoclavicular ligament taut; **C)** The higher the shoulder elevates, the tautness of the coracoclavicular ligament enables the crank configuration of the clavicle to provide for greater elevation of the shoulder than if the clavicle was a straight bone.

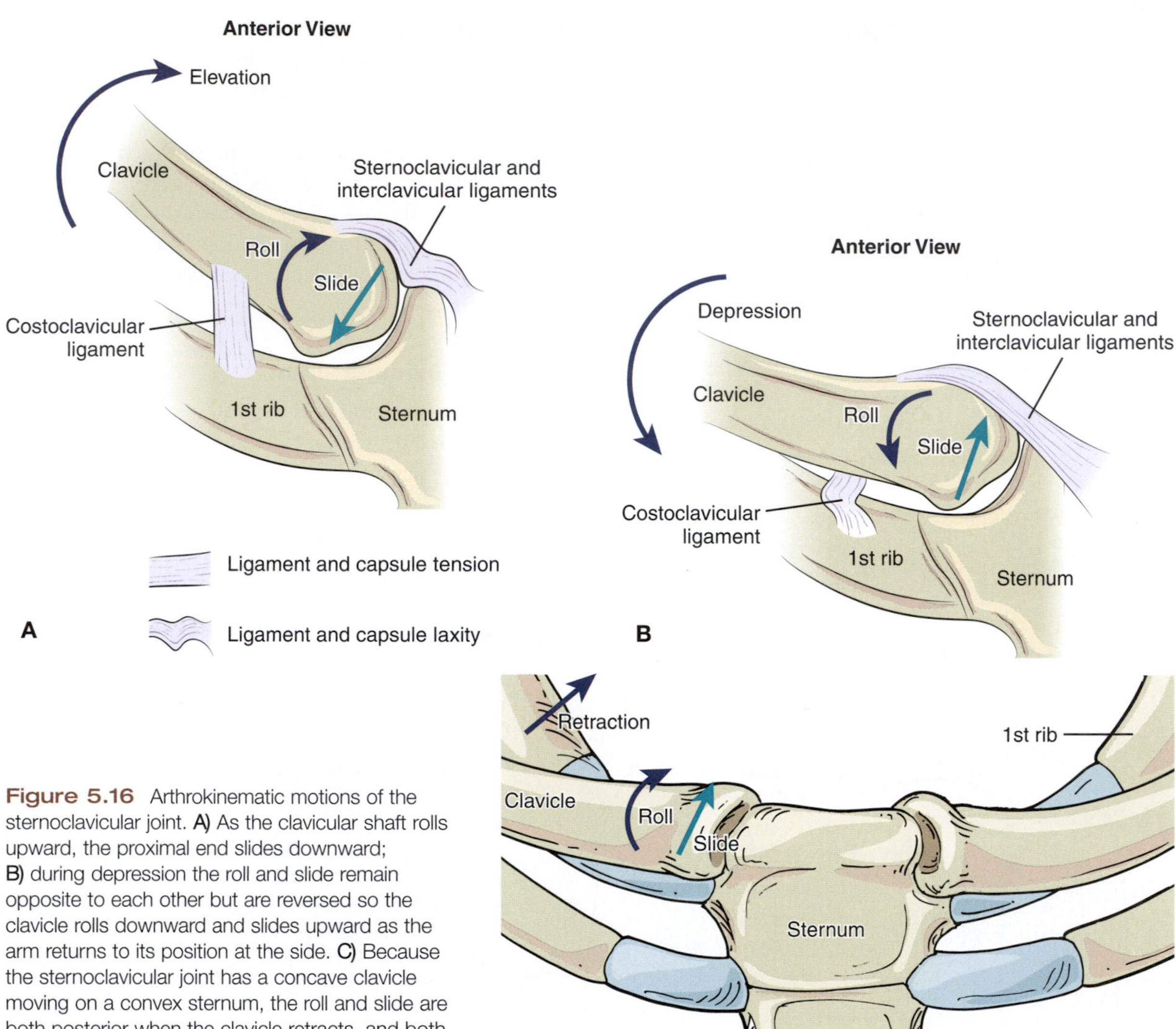

Figure 5.16 Arthrokinematic motions of the sternoclavicular joint. A) As the clavicular shaft rolls upward, the proximal end slides downward; B) during depression the roll and slide remain opposite to each other but are reversed so the clavicle rolls downward and slides upward as the arm returns to its position at the side. C) Because the sternoclavicular joint has a concave clavicle moving on a convex sternum, the roll and slide are both posterior when the clavicle retracts, and both roll and slide move in an anterior direction when the clavicle protracts.

study of dissected cadavers, there was only about 10% of the shoulders examined presented with complete articular discs, but most often only partial discs were present.[21] It was concluded that the incomplete discs were secondary to disc wear and fragmentation. Although there is considerable variation in the convexity or concavity of the joint's surfaces, they are most often flat, so roll and slide arthrokinematics do not occur at this joint. The articular surfaces of this joint are unusual in that they are lined with fibrocartilage, not articular cartilage as is the case with most synovial joints.

Acromioclavicular Joint Ligaments

Superior and inferior acromioclavicular ligaments reinforce the joint capsule (Fig. 5.14). This joint binds the scapula with the clavicle so the two structures have similar motions; at the same time, individual accommodation of each of the bones occurs so subtle movements of each of these bones can transpire.

Acromioclavicular Joint Kinematics

Since the AC joint is a plane synovial joint, it has three axes and three degrees of freedom. As was mentioned in the discussion of sternoclavicular joint motions, the AC motions are described as the scapular movements of elevation-depression, abduction-adduction, and upward rotation-downward rotation as seen in Figure 5.13. Although isolated movement of the AC joint is difficult to identify, it has been estimated that during full arm elevation, the acromioclavicular joint contributes about 20° to 30° of upward rotation of the scapula along an anterior-posterior axis.[17] As the scapula moves on the

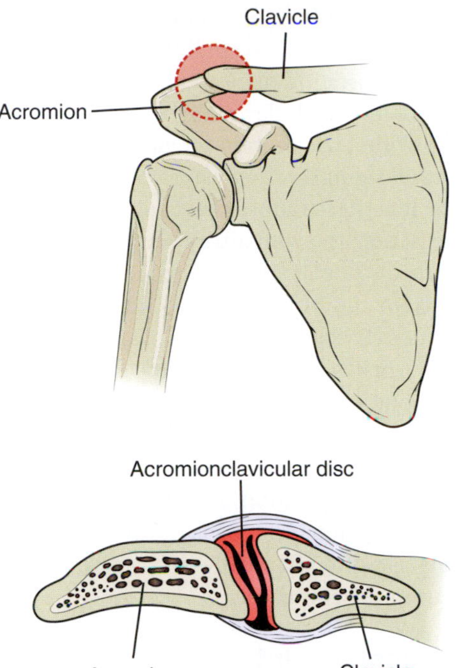

Figure 5.17 Acromioclavicular joint. The acromion end of this joint faces medially and slightly superiorly whereas the clavicular end faces laterally and slightly inferiorly to form a wedge-like surface with relatively flat interfaces with each other.

thorax, the primary function at the AC joint is to allow the scapula to maintain contact with the thorax throughout its movement by providing slight adjustments in the scapular motions provided via the sternoclavicular joint. Acromioclavicular joint motions are limited by two strong ligamentous pairs: the anterior and posterior ligaments of the joint and the more medially located coracoclavicular ligaments, the conoid and the trapezoid (Fig. 5.14).

Whereas the sternoclavicular joint provides for extensive clavicular motion and guides the general path of the scapula, the acromioclavicular joint motions are more subtle and provide for key but small adjustments of the scapula to allow continuity between the scapula and thorax during scapular movements (Fig. 5.8). Small rotational movements of the AC joint on a vertical axis in the horizontal plane will facilitate minor adjustments in the scapula's medial border to move either toward or away from the posterior thoracic ribs. Along a medial-lateral axis, minor sagittal plane motions at the AC joint will cause the superior border of the scapula to tilt downward and the inferior border to tilt away from the posterior ribs. Acromioclavicular joint motions also keep the glenoid fossa aligned with the humeral head during glenohumeral elevation.

Scapulothoracic Joint

As previously mentioned, this is not a true joint. Because there are no bony articulations, the moving surfaces are called a false joint, a pseudo joint, or a functional joint. Separating the scapula from the thorax are soft tissue structures, including a large subscapular bursa. The serratus anterior muscle attaches to the medial border of the scapula and passes under the scapula to attach on the anterolateral border of the first nine ribs. A large amount of motion occurs between the fascia of the muscle and the fascia of the thorax.

Scapulothoracic Joint Function

Normal function of the scapulothoracic joint is essential for the mobility and stability of the upper extremity. Motion of the scapulothoracic joint provides a movable base for the humerus and thereby provides several important functions. These scapulothoracic functions include:

(1) Increasing the range of motion of the shoulder to provide greater reach;
(2) Maintaining favorable length-tension relationships for the deltoid muscle to function above 90° of glenohumeral elevation to allow better shoulder joint stability throughout a greater motion;
(3) Providing glenohumeral stability through maintained glenoid and humeral head alignment for work in the overhead position;
(4) Providing for injury prevention through shock absorption of forces applied to the outstretched arm; and
(5) Permitting elevation of the body in activities such as walking with crutches or performing seated push-ups during transfers by persons with a disability such as paraplegia.

Scapulothoracic Kinematics

There is an intimate relationship between the quantity and quality of motion available in the scapulothoracic joint and the motions of the sternoclavicular and acromioclavicular joints. As previously mentioned, scapulothoracic motion is a direct result of motion within the acromioclavicular and sternoclavicular joints. The combined effect of AC and SC joint motions provides scapulothoracic movement so that its glenoid fossa may face forward, upward, or downward, as the need may be, while its anterior surface remains close to the thorax. In full arm elevation (flexion or abduction), the scapula rotates upward 60°. Because of the intimate attachment of the scapula to the clavicle, the scapula's motion results directly from movement of the joints at either end of the clavicle. Hence, the sum of the ranges of motion at the sternoclavicular and acromioclavicular joints equals the range of motion of the scapula.

Scapular Elevation and Depression

Scapular elevation is the result of the large motion of elevation at the SC joint and lesser motion at the AC joint. The SC joint accounts for the majority of motion, but subtle AC joint motions during scapular movement allows the scapula to maintain contact on the thorax throughout its ranges of movement (Fig. 5.8B). Additionally, slight downward AC motion during scapular elevation on the thorax allows the scapula to maintain a near-vertical position throughout elevation. Without this fine AC motion, the scapula would take an upward and lateral path, moving the scapula's inferior angle laterally on the thorax as the clavicle's distal end elevates higher than its medial aspect. Scapular depression involves the reverse joint motions. Degrees of motion in these scapular movements are estimated to be up to 10 cm in elevation and 2 cm in depression.[7, 22]

Scapular Protraction and Retraction

During scapular protraction, both the SC and AC joints work together to move the scapula around the thoracic cage along a vertical axis in a horizontal plane (Fig. 5.8C). The SC and AC joints also compensate for each other if motion loss at one of them restricts the amount of scapular protraction on the thorax so forward reach is minimally affected. In normal function, the forward movement of the scapula occurs at the SC joint and the adjustment to maintain the scapula on the ribs occurs at the AC joint. Scapular retraction involves the reverse SC and AC joint motions. Scapular motion ranges have been reported up to 10 cm in protraction and 5 cm in retraction.

Scapular Upward Rotation and Downward Rotation

Upward rotation of the scapulothoracic joint occurs on an anterior-posterior axis and provides 60° of total shoulder or humeral elevation. Therefore, this important scapulothoracic motion provides the glenohumeral joint with a significantly greater ability to position the hand for function in more positions, especially in overhead activities. As with other scapulothoracic movements, this scapular motion requires the combined activity from the SC and AC joints. As the SC joint elevates the clavicle to raise the scapula, the AC joint upwardly rotates the scapula to complete scapular upward rotation and simultaneously maintain the scapula on the thorax. The AC and SC motions are reversed for downward rotation and occur from an upwardly rotated position until the arm returns to the anatomical position. The plane of these motions during functional elevation is usually in the scapular plane but can occur in the frontal plane.

Glenohumeral Joint

The glenohumeral joint is often what is referred to when the "shoulder" is discussed. However, it is only one of the joints of the entire shoulder complex. If the glenohumeral joint is discussed by itself, the more preferred name is "shoulder joint" rather than simply "shoulder" since "shoulder" is not a definitive term and may also include the sternoclavicular, acromioclavicular, and scapulothoracic joints in addition to the glenohumeral joint.

Type of Joint

The glenohumeral (GH) joint, a ball-and-socket, spheroid, or universal joint, has three degrees of freedom, but the joint has little bony stability. The convex head of the humerus rests on the small, shallow,

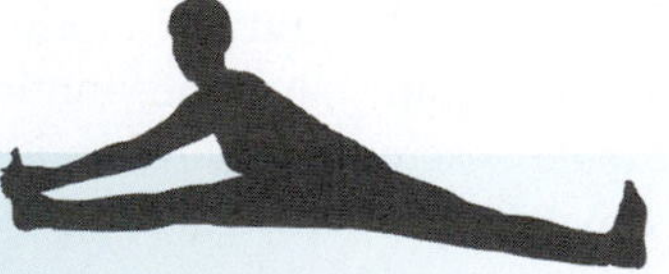

PRACTICE POINT

Total arm elevation is 180°. Since 60° of that motion is provided by the scapulothoracic joint, then 120° actually occurs in the glenohumeral joint itself. These numbers provide the shoulder complex with a 2:1 ratio of glenohumeral motion to scapulothoracic motion. However, this ratio is not maintained throughout the entire movement from start to finish but is variable throughout the motion. Investigators have found that scapular motion occurs most readily during the middle ranges of elevation.[13, 23] It is speculated that the scapular muscles work to "set" the scapula as the glenohumeral joint begins its movements. Clinicians must remember this concept when rehabilitating individuals with shoulder injuries. It is important to begin rehabilitation exercises in the lower one-third of shoulder elevation before allowing the patient to move the arm into higher elevations; this procedure allows the scapular muscles to gain strength sufficiently to stabilize the scapula before increased stresses are applied to them in higher levels of shoulder positions.

inclined concavity of the glenoid fossa (Fig. 5.4). The humeral head is more than twice the size of the glenoid fossa with only a fraction of its surface in contact with the glenoid fossa. In the resting position, the glenoid lies in the scapular plane in an anterior and lateral position (Fig. 5.1, 5.4). Although there is considerable variability, the glenoid is also commonly slightly upwardly rotated. Correspondingly, the humeral head faces a posterior, medial, and superior direction in the scapular plane. Surrounding the rim of the glenoid is a cartilaginous labrum, or lip. A loose and thin fibrous capsule covers the joint from the neck of the glenoid to the anatomic neck of the humerus (Fig. 5.18A). The capsule's inner wall is lined with a synovial membrane. This capsule has a surface area twice that of the humeral head and, in the normal subject, permits injection of 10 to 15 mL of fluid.[2] There is an area of redundancy in the inferior capsule to allow humeral head mobility during shoulder elevation. This redundancy is the axillary pouch. The importance of this axillary pouch is discussed further in glenohumeral kinematics.

Capsular Reinforcement

Since there is great disparity between the size of the humeral head and its glenoid fossa, the bony arrangement is unable to provide joint stability; therefore, the joint must rely on surrounding soft tissue supports for its stability. Ligaments and tendons blend with and reinforce the glenohumeral joint capsule for added stability. The coracohumeral ligament crosses from the coracoid process of the scapula to the greater and lesser tubercles of the humerus, where it forms a tunnel for the tendon of the long head of the biceps brachii (Fig. 5.18B). The superior, middle, and inferior glenohumeral ligaments (called capsular ligaments in Fig. 5.18B) arise from the glenoid and its labrum, form capsular thickenings, and attach to the humeral neck and lesser tubercle. There is a weakness in the capsule between the superior and middle glenohumeral ligaments. This weak capsular region is the foramen of Weitbrecht, a frequent site of anterior dislocations of the joint (Fig. 5.18B). The coracohumeral, superior glenohumeral, and middle glenohumeral ligaments support the dependent (hanging down) arm and limit

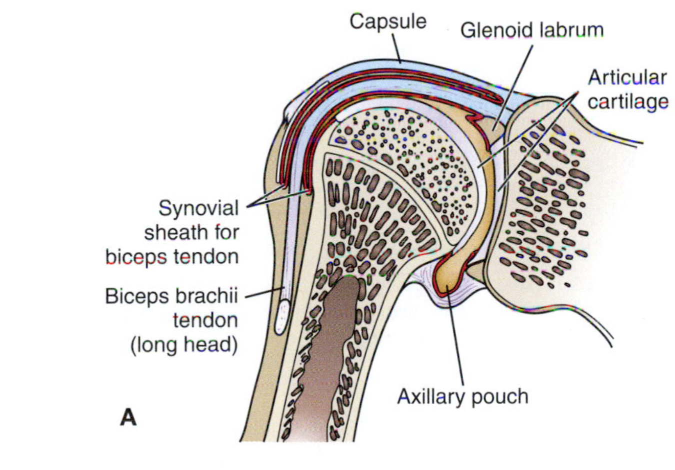

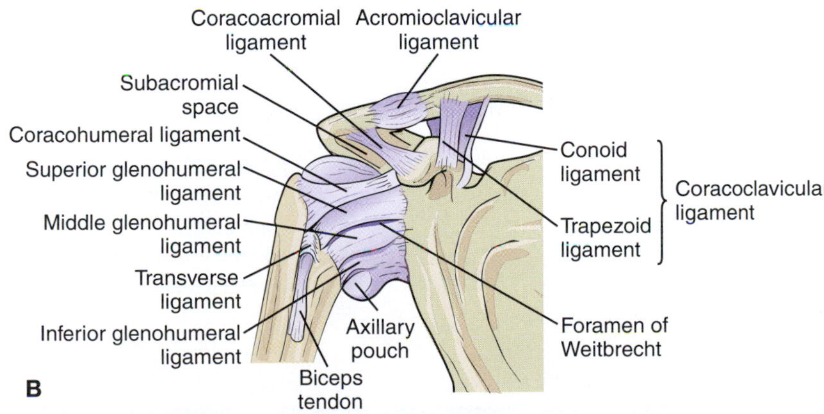

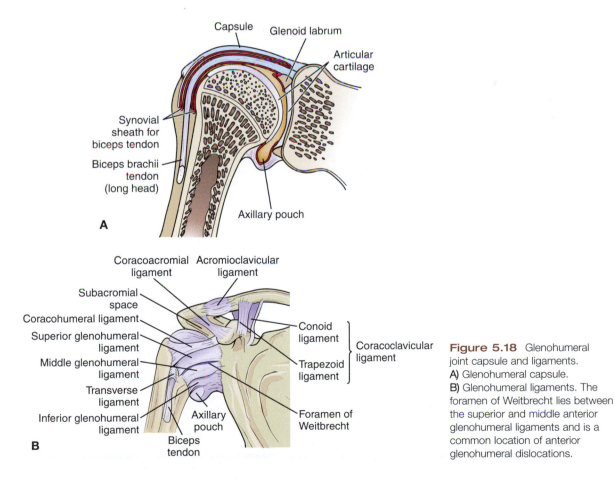

Figure 5.18 Glenohumeral joint capsule and ligaments. A) Glenohumeral capsule. B) Glenohumeral ligaments. The foramen of Weitbrecht lies between the superior and middle anterior glenohumeral ligaments and is a common location of anterior glenohumeral dislocations.

lateral rotation in the lower ranges of abduction.[24] The inferior glenohumeral ligament forms a hammock-like sling with anterior and posterior bands around the lower portion of the humeral head and is part of the axillary pouch. O'Brien and associates[2] consider this ligament the main stabilizer of the abducted shoulder. In the abducted position, different parts of the ligament tighten to limit medial and lateral rotation. Table 5–1 provides specific origin and insertion sites, and the protections each of these ligaments provide the glenohumeral joint.

It is believed that the coracohumeral ligament's most important function is to serve as the primary force against gravity's downward pull on the joint in a resting position.[25-27] There is some indication that the ligament may also assist in protection against superior humeral head translation when the rotator cuff fails to provide this protection.[28] The ligament also limits lateral rotation with the arm resting at the side.

The deep muscles of the shoulder also provide intimate reinforcement of the joint capsule by the attachments of their tendons. Anteriorly, the tendon of the long head of the biceps brachii arises from the supraglenoid tuberosity and the glenoid labrum. The tendon arches over the head of the humerus under the joint capsule to exit and descend in the bicipital (intertubercular) groove of the humerus (Fig. 5.18). Although the bicipital tendon is within the joint capsule, the tendon is covered by reflection of the synovial membrane, so the tendon is not exposed to the synovial fluid of the joint cavity. Thus, the tendon is considered to be

TABLE 5–1 | GLENOHUMERAL JOINT LIGAMENTS

Ligament	Proximal attachment	Distal attachment	Position of greatest joint protection	Joint protections provided
Superior glenohumeral ligament	Near supraglenoid tubercle anterior to attachment site of long head of biceps tendon	Anatomic neck above the lesser tubercle	With arm at the side	Protects against inferior and anterior displacement with the arm at the side
Middle glenohumeral ligament	Anterior glenoid rim at its middle and superior aspects	Broad attachment to anterior aspect of anatomic neck	With the arm at the side and lower levels (up to about 45°) of abduction	Provides anterior stability from 0°–45° abduction Limits anterior translation and lateral rotation of the humeral head
Inferior glenohumeral ligament	Forms a hammock-like sling in the inferior capsule from the anterior-inferior and posterior-inferior glenoid	Anterior, inferior, and posterior bands attach to corresponding areas of anatomic neck	Higher levels of abduction (above 45°), with or without rotation	All limit inferior translation of humeral head. Anterior fibers limit anterior humeral head translation during abduction and lateral rotation. Posterior fibers limit posterior humeral head translation during abduction and medial rotation. Inferior pouch limits abduction at 90° and provides AP stability in abduction.
Coracohumeral ligament	Lateral border of the coracoid process	Two bands (long head of the biceps tendon tunnels under): Anterior aspect of greater tubercle and edge of supraspinatus tendon; second band inserts on subscapularis and lesser tubercle	With arm at the side	Protects against lateral rotation with the arm adducted. Protects against inferior translation of the dependent arm and superior translation of a shoulder with a weak rotator cuff

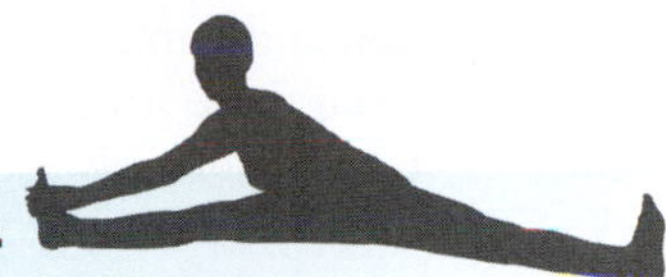

PRACTICE POINT

There is greater lateral rotation of the glenohumeral joint when the arm is elevated than when it is at the side. The reason for this is that when the arm is at the side, the coracohumeral and anterior glenohumeral ligaments are taut and limit lateral rotation. When the arm is elevated to 90°, however, these two ligaments are lax and allow greater lateral rotation of the glenohumeral joint. When examining a patient, the clinician should record the position in which lateral rotation is measured since these two different positions will likely produce two different results.

intra-articular but extrasynovial. Strong contraction of the biceps brachii muscle, as when the elbow is flexed and a weight is held in the hand, produces depression force on the head of the humerus.[29] The forces causing that effect are similar in action to forces that restrain the pull on a rope by "snubbing" the rope around a pole or tree. Such depression of the head of the humerus prevents elevation of the head, which might otherwise cause impingement injuries to suprahumeral soft tissues positioned between the humeral head and the rigid acromial structures.

Posteriorly, the long head of the triceps brachii has a broad proximal attachment on the infraglenoid tubercle of the scapula. This tendon blends with and becomes part of the posterior capsule.

The tendons of four short rotator cuff muscles that produce medial and lateral rotation of the glenohumeral joint blend with the capsule and form their distal attachments on the tubercles of the humerus. Anteriorly, the subscapularis attaches by a broad tendon to the lesser tubercle of the humerus. This tendon covers the head of the humerus below 90° of abduction and is considered by Jobe[30] to be a passive stabilizer to prevent anterior subluxation of the humerus. The lower part of the capsule and the subscapularis are the primary structures limiting lateral rotation.[31] Superiorly, the supraspinatus muscle attaches to the greater tubercle of the humerus, and posteriorly, the infraspinatus and the teres minor blend with the capsule to attach lower on the greater tubercle. These two tendons were found by Ovesen and Nielsen[31] to be the major structures limiting medial rotation in the first half of abduction. These rotator cuff tendons can be injured when they make contact and move against the acromion, the coracoid process, or the strong connecting coracoacromial ligament under the coracoacromial arch (Fig. 5.14). Injuries to these tendons often occur with elevation activities of the arm, such as working overhead or in throwing sports.

Coracoacromial Arch

The coracoacromial ligament runs from the anterior acromion and the lateral coracoid process to form the coracoacromial arch. This osteoligamentous arch is the roof of the glenohumeral joint. The area between the arch and the superior humeral head is called the subacromial space. The subacromial space contains important soft tissue shoulder structures. These structures include the supraspinatus muscle and tendon, long head of the biceps tendon, subacromial bursa, and superior capsule. The coracoacromial arch protects the soft tissue structures from superior blows directed downward and protects the glenohumeral joint from superior dislocations.

The subacromial space is approximately one centimeter wide, about the width of a pencil. This is a narrow space that limits the room available for the soft tissue structures during shoulder motion and in pathological conditions. The space narrows to approximately half of its normal width as the arm is elevated[32] If pathologies exist in the soft tissue or bony structures or in the shoulder's biomechanics, this space may become even narrower, threatening soft tissue injury. Glenohumeral kinematics and pathological movements are discussed later in this chapter.

Motions of the glenohumeral joint impact the positional relationship between the head of the humerus and the arch formed by the neck of the scapula, the acromion process, the rigid coracoacromial ligament, and the coracoid process. This area has been named the **supraspinatus outlet** by Neer and Poppen.[33] This region is essentially the area under the coracoacromial arch. The clinical importance of this area is the propensity for compression and injury of the soft tissues that lie between the rigid structures: the rotator cuff (especially the supraspinatus), the tendon of the long head of the biceps brachii, the capsule, the capsular ligaments, and the subdeltoid and subacromial bursae. During normal shoulder elevation, the downward line of pull of the rotator cuff along with depression of the humeral head by the supraspinatus and long head of the biceps tendons depress the humeral head as the arm is elevated by the supraspinatus and deltoid. In cases of shoulder impingement, the deltoid's line of pull for humeral elevation lies directly superior to the joint's axis of motion and is not adequately opposed by the rotator cuff and biceps, so the humerus moves vertically, striking the acromion. Unfortunately, there is no space for error in the supraspinatus outlet, and impingement injuries occur when the subacromial space diminishes. This space can be narrowed either by structural or biomechanical causes. Structural causes include a reduction of the available space by an enlarged tendon, hooked or angled acromion, or other space-infringing object.[34] Biomechanical causes include changes in the position of the glenohumeral joint during motion that may be the result of muscle imbalances,[35] improper muscle firing sequences,[36] muscle fatigue,[37] poor posture,[9] or uncontrollable forces.[38] Microtrauma and repetitive stress injuries are common; for example, 50% to 60% of all problems in competitive swimmers are from microtrauma to soft tissue structures.[39] People with poliomyelitis and paraplegia who perform repetitive activities such as walking with crutches, propelling manual wheelchairs, or seated push-ups to transfer the body have an extraordinarily high incidence of shoulder pain and rotator cuff tears.[40, 41] Bayley and associates,[40] Smith,[42] and Neer[29] consider the most frequent cause of injuries to be narrowing of the supraspinatus outlet, which may be congenital or caused by inflammation, scarring, or the development of bone spurs. Attrition (wearing down) of the capsular structures has a high incidence in cadaver dissections and has been documented with aging by Brewer[43] and Ferrari.[44]

Bursae

There are several bursae within the shoulder joint area. A bursa reduces friction between two structures, so it is not surprising to realize that with the close proximity of so many soft tissue and bony structures within the shoulder complex, there are several bursae in the area as well. Although there are eight bursae within the shoulder area, some of them actually extend from the synovial lining of the capsule or are continuous with each other. The two most important are the subacromial bursa and the subdeltoid bursa. The subacromial bursa is located between the supraspinatus tendon and the coracoacromial arch; it serves to protect the supraspinatus tendon and allow for smooth tendon movement during shoulder motion.[45] The subdeltoid bursa is continuous with the subacromial bursa and is located between the deltoid muscle and the supraspinatus tendon and humeral head (Fig. 5.19) to reduce friction between these structures.

Bursae normally have a very small amount of fluid within them. If they become irritated and inflamed, however, the amount of fluid increases. Within the subacromial region, this volumetric increase can become problematic since the space is limited, and an increase in bursa fluid will further limit available space. Inflamed glenohumeral bursae are usually not primary conditions but secondary conditions that are brought on by other existing injuries. For example, initial injuries in the subacromial space usually affect the tendons, especially the supraspinatus tendon; as the condition continues, secondary bursae inflammation occurs with continued narrowing of the space and impingement of the soft tissue structures lying within it.

Glenohumeral Joint Kinematics

The glenohumeral joint's three degrees of motion include flexion-extension, abduction-adduction, and medial rotation-lateral rotation. Glenohumeral joint motions without scapular motions are presented here.

Abduction and adduction occur in a frontal plane around an anterior-posterior axis. As the humerus moves into abduction, the humeral head glides inferiorly into the deeper aspect of the glenoid fossa. Dynamic stability of the glenohumeral joint is vital for these motions to occur. Dynamic stability during motion results from a coordinated and well-timed effort of the rotator cuff and deltoid muscles. This is discussed in more detail when muscles and muscle activity are presented later in this chapter.

The amount of abduction possible depends on rotation at the glenohumeral joint. When the joint is in full medial rotation, active abduction is limited to approximately 60°, because the greater tubercle is in alignment

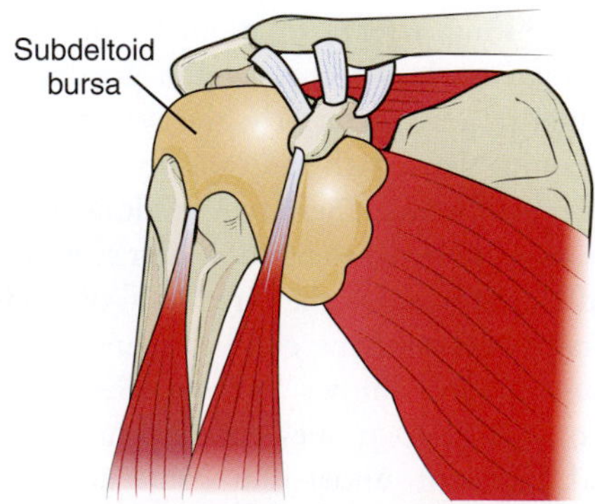

Figure 5.19 Because of the close proximity of so many soft tissue and bony structures within the shoulder complex, there are several bursae in the area.

with and strikes the acromion process and the acromioclavicular ligament. With 90° of lateral rotation, the greater tubercle rotates behind the acromion so active abduction increases to approximately 90°, where it becomes limited by active insufficiency of the deltoid muscle. Abduction can be continued passively to 120°, where it is then limited by tension of the inferior glenohumeral ligament. In full shoulder abduction, Murray[46] measured an average of 124° of glenohumeral motion (Table 5–2).

Medial and lateral glenohumeral rotations take place about a vertical axis through the head and shaft of the humerus in the horizontal plane. Rotation at the glenohumeral joint is isolated from supination and pronation of the forearm by flexion of the elbow to 90°. If the arm is at the side of the body, lateral rotation causes the medial epicondyle of the humerus to move anteriorly whereas medial rotation causes the medial condyle to move posteriorly. The amount of rotation changes with elevation of the arm. Approximately 160° of total rotation is present when the arm is abducted at 90°[47] and is reduced to about 90° because of the twisting and tightening of the coracohumeral and glenohumeral ligaments when the arm is fully elevated. When the glenohumeral joint is positioned in 90° of shoulder abduction with 90° of elbow flexion,[48] the normal range of motion for lateral rotation is approximately 90° and for medial rotation, approximately 70° (Table 5–2). Brown and associates[49] found 136° of lateral rotation in major league baseball pitchers; Chang, Buschbacher, and Edlich[50] found 78° in power lifters.

Elevation of the glenohumeral joint includes either flexion or abduction. Flexion and extension occur in the sagittal plane around a medial-lateral axis. Flexion motion of the glenohumeral joint is up to 120°.[51] Full flexion to 180° is possible because of the motion provided by scapulothoracic joint. As the shoulder reaches its terminal degrees in flexion, the inferior glenohumeral capsule tightens posteriorly.[52] This posterior capsule tightness may cause a slight forward and nearly imperceptible medially rotated translation of the humerus on the glenoid. When the arm is at the side and then passes behind the body, the

TABLE 5–2 | AVERAGE SHOULDER RANGE OF MOTION IN NORMAL SUBJECTS (DEGREES)

Author	Boone & Azen [53]		Murray et al [46]		Brown Chang, et al [49]	Buschbacher & Edlich [50]	
SUBJECTS	109 M		20 M 20 F		41 M*	10 M 10 M†	
Age (yrs)	2–19	19–54	25–66		27 ± 4.2	21 – 35	
Flexion	168	165	167	171	163	171	157
Abduction	185	183	178	179	168	—	—
Extension	67	57	56	59	76	55	42
Lateral rotation	108	100	88	97	136	82	78
Medial rotation	71	67	54‡	54‡	84	83	56
Glenohumeral abduction	—	—	122	126	99	—	—

NOTE: Notice the tendency for more flexibility in the younger males (Boone and Azen) and in the females versus the males (Murray et al), the decreased flexibility of the power lifters versus normal controls (Chang, Buschbacher, and Edlich), and the marked amount of lateral rotation in the baseball players (Brown et al).
*Major league baseball players.
†Power lifters matched to non-power lifters.
‡The goniometric positions were described as standard, except that the scapula was stabilized.

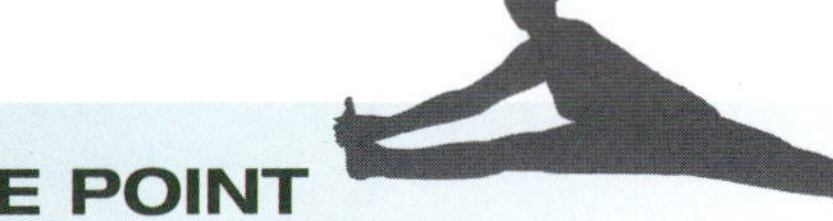

PRACTICE POINT

When tested, individuals generally want to perform their best. When clinicians examine an individual's range of motion, they must be watchful for substitutions the individual may unintentionally use to provide an optimum result. For example, if the clinician has the individual laterally rotate the glenohumeral joint, the individual may inadvertently retract the scapula in an attempt to demonstrate as much glenohumeral lateral rotation as possible. Likewise, scapular protraction may occur with movement into end-range medial rotation. Clinicians must be aware of these possible substitutions and prevent them from occurring if accurate measurements are to be obtained.

terminal extension motion is sometimes called hyperextension. The range of hyperextension is 40° to 60° and is limited by the superior and middle glenohumeral ligaments.[51] As the glenohumeral joint reaches terminal extension motion, the anterior capsule becomes slightly tight to cause an anterior tilt of the scapula. This scapular tilt may increase the extension reach of the arm. Just as tautness of the capsule causes medial rotation in terminal flexion, capsular tautness in terminal shoulder extension produces slight lateral rotation.

Normal range of shoulder flexion or abduction is conventionally reported as 180°, but when carefully measured to eliminate trunk motions, the mean angle is close to 170°[53-55] (see Table 1–2). This amount of elevation is the compilation of motion at both the glenohumeral and scapulothoracic joints, with the scapular movements accompanied by motions at the sternoclavicular and acromioclavicular joints. Ninety degrees to 110° of motion occur at the glenohumeral joint, and an additional 60° to 70° occur at the sternoclavicular and acromioclavicular joints. Although not technically part of shoulder elevation, additional overhead reach may result from trunk movement with lateral flexion in shoulder abduction or with trunk extension in shoulder flexion. Achievement of the maximum glenohumeral elevation range requires lateral rotation of the glenohumeral joint in abduction; for flexion, medial rotation and posterior tilting of the scapula are required.[10, 13] Additionally, upward rotation of the scapula is required for full arm elevation in either flexion or abduction.

Two other planar motions occur at the glenohumeral joint. They are horizontal abduction (horizontal extension) and horizontal adduction (horizontal flexion). These motions occur from a starting position of 90° of abduction. Horizontal abduction is a posterior motion from this position, and horizontal adduction is an anterior motion of the arm across the body. These motions occur around a vertical axis in a horizontal plane with the arm elevated to 90°.

All normal limitations of motion on the glenohumeral joint are due to ligamentous and passive muscle tightening. Thus, the end feels are all firm. Even when the greater tubercle of the humerus strikes on the acromion process, the end feel is firm because of the soft tissues lying between the two bony structures.

Glenohumeral Arthrokinematic Motions

Arthrokinematic motion of the shoulder joint during flexion and extension consists of the humeral head spinning in the glenoid fossa. Neither roll nor slide occurs in the joint during these motions. However, as the shoulder reaches higher levels of flexion elevation, an anterior slide of the humeral head on the glenoid occurs, and during end phases of hyperextension, a posterior slide of the humeral head occurs. During abduction, the humeral head rolls superiorly as it slides inferiorly (Fig. 5.20A). Since the humeral head is so much larger than the glenoid fossa, its slide in direction opposite to the motion allows the humeral head to stay within its socket with minimal translation. If the slide did not accompany the roll as it does, the humeral head would translate or move out of the upper glenoid rim when the arm was raised. The inferior slide also limits the humeral head from jamming into the upper part of the glenohumeral joint, thereby averting impingement of the humeral head against the soft tissue structures under the coracoacromial arch. During adduction, the humeral head moves in opposite motions to produce a downward roll and upward slide. Arthrokinematics for lateral rotation has the humeral head rolling posteriorly and sliding anteriorly on the glenoid fossa (Fig. 5.20B).

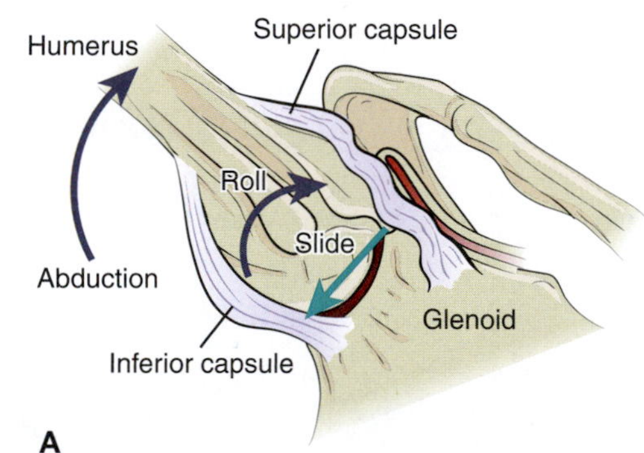

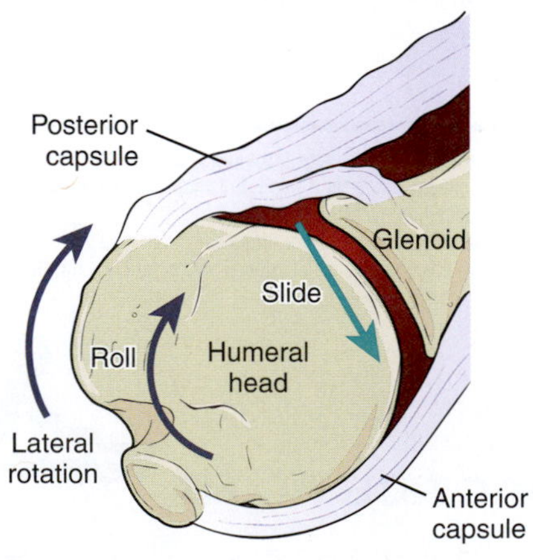

Figure 5.20 Arthrokinematics of the shoulder joint during **A)** abduction and **B)** lateral rotation occur with the roll in the opposite direction as the slide since the convex humeral head moves within the concave glenoid fossa.

Humeral head roll and slide are the reverse for medial rotation of the glenohumeral joint: The roll is anterior and the slide is posterior.

Shoulder Abduction in the Plane of the Scapula (Scaption)

Scapular plane glenohumeral abduction occurs 30° to 40° anterior to the frontal plane. **Scaption** is the term coined by Perry[56] to define this plane of motion. This position is recommended for examination of glenohumeral elevation because the capsule is in a loose-packed position, and there is less likelihood of impingement on the coracoacromial structures.[56] Thus, it is important to specify the plane of abduction used during your examination because the ranges of motion vary slightly and the torque of the lateral rotators is greater in the scapular plane than in the frontal plane.[57] Most functional shoulder abduction motions in daily and sports activities actually occur in the scapular plane, not the frontal plane.

Resting and Close-Packed Positions of the Shoulder Complex Joints

With the glenohumeral joint capsule being twice as large as the joint, there is considerable laxity in the normal capsule. The loose capsule of the glenohumeral joint normally permits 1 to 2 cm of joint play motions in distal and lateral distraction of the humeral head on the glenoid as well as anterior and posterior translatory glides.[58] The resting position of the glenohumeral joint is in about 20° to 30° of horizontal abduction and 55° of flexion.[58] The close-packed position of the glenohumeral joint occurs in full abduction with full lateral rotation; in this position, the capsular structures twist tightly around the joint and the joint surfaces are most congruent. This is a common position of the shoulder in people who sleep on their backs and is frequently a source of shoulder pain and injury. The sternoclavicular joint's close-packed position occurs when the arm is fully elevated whereas the close-packed position of the acromioclavicular joint occurs when the arm is abducted to 90°.[58]

The Bicipital Groove

The tendon of the long head of the biceps brachii attaches to the supraglenoid tubercle of the scapula and arches over the head of the humerus to descend in the intertubercular groove of the humerus (Fig. 5.18). The tendon is retained in the groove by the coracohumeral ligament and by the transverse humeral ligament, which bridges the groove from the lesser to the greater tubercle. During motions of the shoulder, the head of the humerus slides on the undersurface of the tendon so the bone moves under the tendon. A fixed point on the groove moves along 1.5 inches of tendon during full arm elevation.[59] When the glenohumeral joint is in full lateral rotation, the proximal and distal attachments of the tendon are in a straight line with each other, but in all other positions of rotation, the bicipital tendon is bent around the medial wall of the groove.[56] Thus, the bicipital tendon is subject to not only wear and injury with time, but to impingement injuries as well.

Scapulohumeral Rhythm

Joints of the shoulder complex rarely work alone. Rather, they move together to provide greater motion of the shoulder than any one of them could by itself. For each glenohumeral motion, there are important companion motions of the shoulder girdle, ensuring that the scapula is placed accurately on the thorax with the glenoid fossa appropriately partnered with the humeral head so that upper extremity function is optimized. Table 5–3 lists these companion motions. Shoulder elevation occurs in a precisely coordinated series of synchronous motions termed **scapulohumeral rhythm.** The classic work by Inman and associates[17] demonstrated that both the scapular and humeral segments participate throughout the motion. They found that the early phase of abduction was individually variable. This

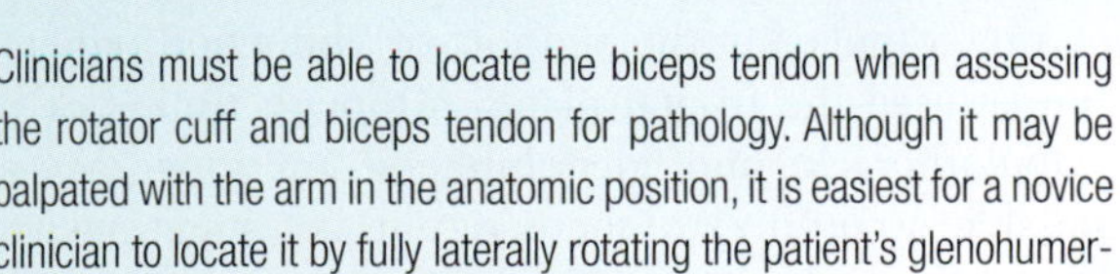

PRACTICE POINT

Clinicians must be able to locate the biceps tendon when assessing the rotator cuff and biceps tendon for pathology. Although it may be palpated with the arm in the anatomic position, it is easiest for a novice clinician to locate it by fully laterally rotating the patient's glenohumeral joint. With the shoulder in this position, the clinician identifies and palpates the lateral end of the acromion process. The bicipital groove is immediately inferior to the tip of the acromion. The clinician should be able to palpate the biceps tendon within the groove as well as the greater and lesser tubercles on either side of the bicipital groove as they form the lateral and medial walls of the groove, respectively.

TABLE 5-3 | COMPANION MOTIONS OF THE SHOULDER GIRDLE AND GLENOHUMERAL JOINTS

Glenohumeral Motion	Scapulothoracic Motion	Sternoclavicular Motion	Acromioclavicular Motion
Flexion	**Traditional View** Upward rotation, elevation, and protraction **Tri-planar motion** Upward rotation, posterior tilting Medial tilting initially followed by lateral tilting in higher ranges of flexion	Elevation Posterior rotation Protraction	Upward rotation Horizontal & sagittal plane rotational adjustments
Extension	**Traditional View** Downward rotation, depression, and retraction **Tri-planar motion** Downward rotation, anterior tilting Reverse of all tri-planar motion occurring in flexion	Depression Anterior rotation Retraction	Downward rotation Horizontal & sagittal plane rotational adjustments
Abduction	**Traditional View** Upward rotation, elevation, and protraction **Tri-planar motion** Upward rotation, posterior tilting Medial tilting initially followed by lateral tilting in higher ranges of abduction	Elevation Posterior rotation Retraction	Upward rotation Horizontal & sagittal plane rotational adjustments
Adduction	**Traditional View** Downward rotation, depression, and retraction **Tri-planar motion** Downward rotation, anterior tilting Lateral tilting initially followed by medial tilting when returning to anatomic position	Depression Anterior rotation Protraction	Downward rotation Horizontal & sagittal plane rotational adjustments
Lateral rotation	Retraction	*Retraction (speculation at this time)*	*Undocumented at this time*
Medial rotation	Protraction	*Protraction (speculation at this time)*	*Undocumented at this time*
Horizontal abduction	Retraction	*Retraction (speculation at this time)*	*Undocumented at this time*
Horizontal adduction	Protraction	*Protraction (speculation at this time)*	*Undocumented at this time*

early stage of motion was termed the "setting phase." After about 30° of abduction, a 2:1 ratio occurred: For every 2° of glenohumeral motion, 1° occurred at the scapulothoracic joint. Other investigations have found that the motions are not as linear as this 2:1 ratio implies and that there is variation in patterns. The most common pattern, found by Bagg and Forrest,[60] showed greater glenohumeral motion at the beginning and end of the range and more scapular motion between 80° and 140° of abduction. The average ratio of glenohumeral to scapulothoracic joint motions was 1.25:1, which is the same as the mean values obtained by Poppen and Walker.[61] Both of these investigations used the plane of the scapula for the motion of abduction, whereas Inman used the frontal plane. Although timing of the scapulothoracic and glenohumeral motions may be variable according to these recent investigations, the case still remains that 60° of elevation is attributed to the scapulothoracic joint and 120° is attributed to the glenohumeral joint. If normal scapular rotation occurs throughout elevation, when the arm is in full elevation, the inferior angle of the scapula lies directly inferior to the axilla and is in line with the mid-axillary line.

As the scapula rotates during scapulohumeral motion, the axis of rotation of the scapula migrates from the medial root of the spine of the scapula to the region of the acromioclavicular joint during elevation.[60] This large movement of the axis causes marked changes in the force arms of the trapezius and the serratus anterior, which is considered later with the discussion of factors determining scapular rotation.

Mention should be made that early investigations of the shoulder complex used a two-dimensional view of motions, but more recent research inquiries have available technology the early investigators did not have. The use of three-dimensional tools provides new degrees of accuracy and additional information that allows results to identify previously immeasurable motions. For example, it has only been in the past few years that scapular tilting has been identified, and its importance is now recognized not only in identifying normal kinesiological function but also in finding causes of pathological function of the shoulder complex.[6, 15, 62, 63] Because of the new perspectives we are gaining in understanding shoulder girdle motion, Table 5–3 information is divided into traditional (two-dimensional) and triplanar motions. The most recent investigations using three-dimensional analysis provides us with more detailed understandings of all motions occurring in these complex and interrelated structures.

Muscles of the Shoulder Complex

The shoulder is unique in that its stability during motion occurs not only from ligaments that restrict terminal motions, but also from muscles that simultaneously provide motion to the same joints they are stabilizing. Although other joints also rely on muscles for stabilization, very few use the same muscles that are stabilizing to also serve as movers at the same time. The muscles of the shoulder girdle also participate significantly in skilled movements of the upper extremity, such as writing, and are essential in activities requiring pulling, pushing, and throwing, to mention only a few of the important activities of the upper extremity.

The shoulder region muscles are divided into three groups for study: 1) scapular stabilizers of the shoulder complex; 2) glenohumeral stabilizers of the shoulder complex; and 3) large movers of the shoulder. See Tables 5–3 through 5–5 for these muscle groups and their muscle descriptions along with methods to palpate them. Some additional highlights and unique features of each of the muscles are provided below.

Scapular Stabilizer Muscles of the Shoulder Complex

These muscles are primarily responsible for movement and stabilization of the scapula during glenohumeral joint motion. They each originate on the thorax and end on the scapula (Table 5–4).

Serratus Anterior

Serratus anterior (L. *serra,* saw) is one of the most important muscles of the shoulder girdle. Since it is the primary scapular protractor, without it, the arm cannot be raised overhead. It is called the "saw muscle" because of its serrated-looking insertions on the ribs and thorax. The lowest four or five slips of this muscle interdigitate with the external oblique abdominal muscle. It lies close to the thorax and passes underneath the scapula to its distal attachment. The lowest five digitations is the strongest portion of the muscle.

On well-developed individuals, the lower digitations may be seen and palpated near their proximal attachment on the ribs when the arm is overhead (Fig. 5.21). When the serratus anterior is paralyzed or weak and forward reaching is attempted (Fig. 5.22), a typical "winging" of the medial border of the scapula is seen as the scapula fails to protract or slide forward on the rib cage or to remain in contact with it.[64]

Trapezius

The trapezius is a superficial muscle of the neck and upper back and is accessible for observation and palpation in its entirety (Fig. 5.23). Because of its shape, it has been called the "shawl" muscle. Early anatomists named it "musculus cucullaris" (shaped like a monk's hood). The present name refers to its geometric shape. From a widespread origin, the muscle fibers converge to its distal attachments. Scapular upward rotation and protraction occur together during glenohumeral flexion. As the axis for scapular rotation moves from the root of the scapular spine to the acromion process during upward rotation, the moment arm for the lower trapezius becomes larger for upward rotation.[60]

In full abduction with scapular retraction, all parts of the trapezius are recruited: retraction of the shoulder girdle by the entire muscle and upward rotation of the scapula by the upper and lower portions of the muscle. Although the upper and lower trapezius work together to perform scapular upward rotation, their fiber arrangement also allows them to perform contradicting motions; the upper trapezius produces scapular elevation whereas the lower trapezius produces scapular depression.

Dysfunction of the muscle results in an inability to achieve full scapular upward rotation. In complete trapezius

(text continues on page 190)

TABLE 5–4 | SCAPULAR STABILIZING MUSCLES OF THE SHOULDER GIRDLE

Scapular Muscles

Group	Muscle	Proximal Insertion	Distal Insertion	Innervation	Action	Palpation/ Inspection
Muscles from Trunk to Shoulder Girdle	Serratus anterior 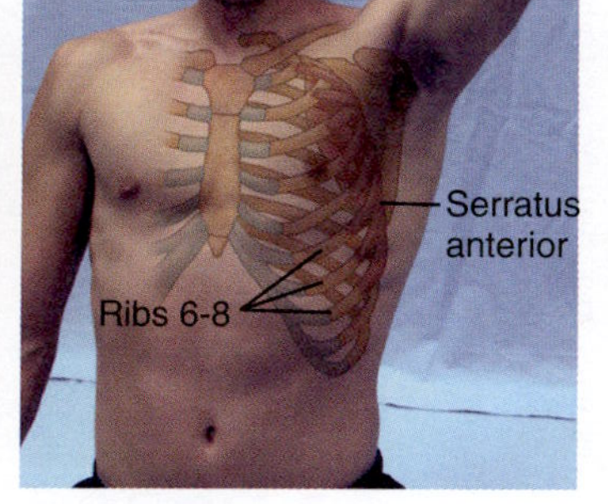	Anterior and superior aspects of ribs #1-9	Anterior surface of vertebral border of scapula	Long thoracic nerve	Protracts and upwardly rotates the scapula	Although the upper portions of the muscle is covered by the pectoral muscles, its lower digitations may be palpated distal to the axilla, close to the ribs posterior to the pectoralis major. With the arm in about 135° in the scapular plane, palpation may be possible of these lower digitations as the subject protracts the scapula.
	Trapezius	Occipital bone, ligamentum nuchae, and spinous processes from C_7-T_{12}	On the acromial end of the clavicle, the acromion, and the spine of the scapula. The fibers of the upper portion course downward and laterally, those of the middle portion more horizontally, and those of the lower portion obliquely upward	Spinal accessory nerve (C_3-C_4 and spinal portion of cranial nerve XI).	The **upper trapezius** performs elevation and upward rotation of the scapula, as well as extension, lateral flexion, and contralateral rotation of the neck; the **lower trapezius** performs upward rotation, adduction, and depression of the scapula; the **middle trapezius** performs upward rotation and adduction of the scapula.	The entire muscle can be observed during shoulder abduction with shoulder girdle retraction. If the trunk is simultaneously inclined forward or the subject lies prone, the muscle has to act against the force of gravity to hold the shoulders back, and the intensity of the contraction increases.

Muscles from Trunk to Shoulder Girdle	Rhomboids Major & Minor 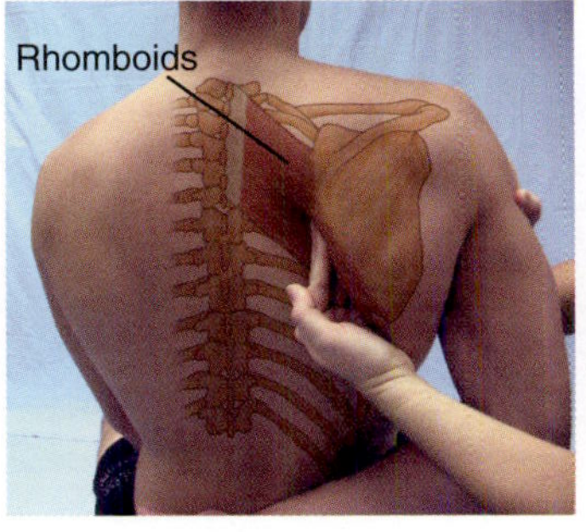	Ligamentum nuchae and spinous processes of the lowest two cervical and the upper four thoracic vertebrae.	Medial border of scapula	Dorsal scapular nerve ("the nerve to the rhomboids," C_4-C_5).	The oblique direction of the muscles indicates that they serve to elevate as well as to retract the scapula. The rhomboid major also has the important function of downward rotation of the scapula since it attaches to the inferior angle of the scapula. Downward rotation, adduction, and elevation of the scapula	Because the rhomboids are covered by the trapezius, they are best palpated when the trapezius is relaxed. The subject's hand is placed in the small of the back. The investigator places the palpating fingers underneath the medial border of the scapula, which can be done without causing discomfort to the subject, provided that the muscles in this region are relaxed (Fig. 5.24). If the subject raises the hand just off the small of the back, the rhomboid major contracts vigorously as a downward rotator of the scapula and pushes the palpating fingers out from underneath the medial border of the scapula. If the lower trapezius is not too bulky, the direction of the contracting fibers of the rhomboids may be seen under the skin. In the case of trapezius paralysis, the course of the rhomboids is easier to observe.

continued

TABLE 5–4 | SCAPULAR STABILIZING MUSCLES OF THE SHOULDER GIRDLE—cont'd

Scapular Muscles

Group	Muscle	Proximal Insertion	Distal Insertion	Innervation	Action	Palpation/ Inspection
Muscles from Trunk to Shoulder Girdle	Pectoralis Minor	By four tendomuscular slips from the second to the fifth ribs	The muscular slips converge into the coracoid process of the scapula	Medial pectoral nerve (C_7-T_1)	Depression and anterior tilt of the scapula as well as elevation of ribs 2 to 5.	The forearm is placed in the small of the back. In this position, the pectoralis major is relaxed, a prerequisite for palpation of the pectoralis minor. The examiner places one finger just below the coracoid process of the scapula, as seen in Figure 5.25, pressing down gently to let the finger sink in as far as possible. In this position, the finger lies across the tendon of the pectoralis minor, the muscle of which is relaxed as long as the forearm rests in the small of the back. When the subject raises the forearm off the back, the pectoralis minor contracts, and its tendon becomes tense under the palpating fingers. The muscle can also be palpated in its important function of shoulder depression (trunk elevation). The palpating fingers should be placed distal to the coracoid process, and the subject (sitting on a table) should be asked to push down on the table with the hands as if to elevate the body (actual trunk elevation or sitting push-up will cause other muscles to contract and obscure palpation of the muscle).

Muscles from Trunk to Shoulder Girdle	Levator Scapulae 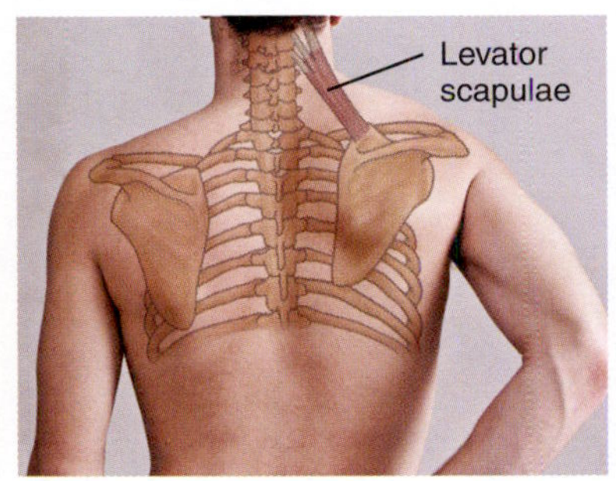	Transverse processes of the upper cervical vertebrae	Medial border of the scapula, above the spine, near the superior angle.	Dorsal scapular nerve (C_3-C_5).	Elevation and downward rotation of the scapula as well as lateral flexion and ipsilateral rotation of the cervical spine.	The levator is difficult to isolate and palpate. To bring out levator action with a minimum of trapezius participation, the subject places the forearm in the small of the back, then shrugs the shoulder. The levator may then be palpated in the neck region, anterior to the trapezius but posterior to the sternocleidomastoid muscle. A comparatively isolated action of the levator may be obtained if the shrug is made briefly and quickly and in a short range. If much effort is exerted in raising the shoulder and if the elevated position is maintained, the trapezius will contract in spite of the above precautions.

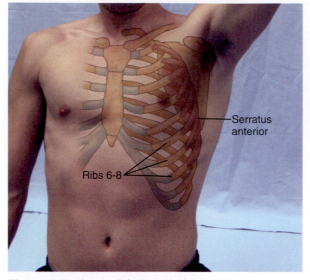

Figure 5.21 Lower digitations of the serratus anterior near their origins on the ribs. The upper portion of the muscle is covered by the pectoralis major.

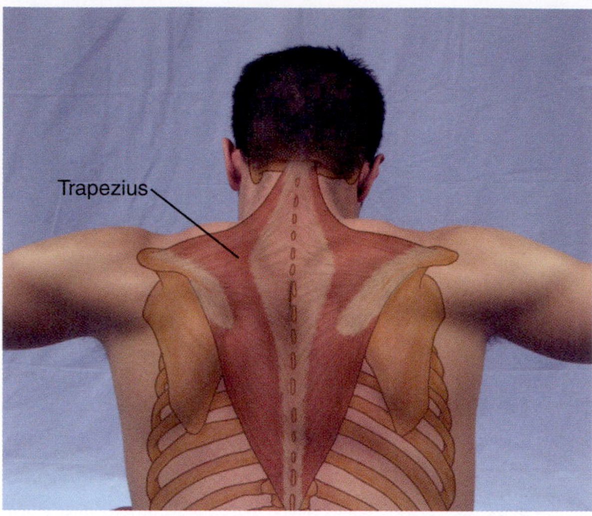

Figure 5.23 All portions of the trapezius in contraction. For strong action of this muscle, the subject inclines the trunk forward. Note also the contraction of the posterior deltoid, infraspinatus, and teres minor.

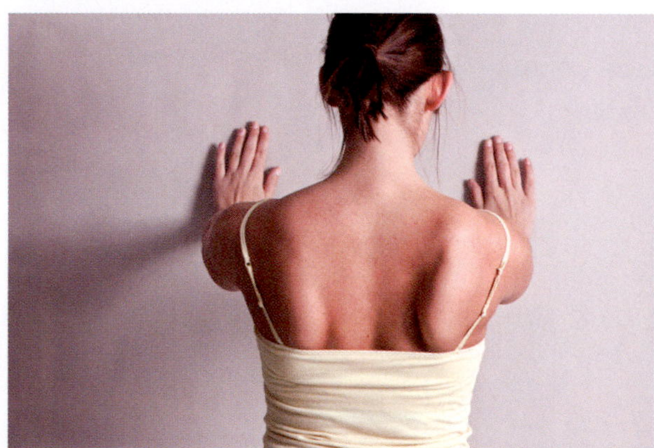

Figure 5.22 Dysfunction of the serratus anterior produces winging of the scapula's medial border.

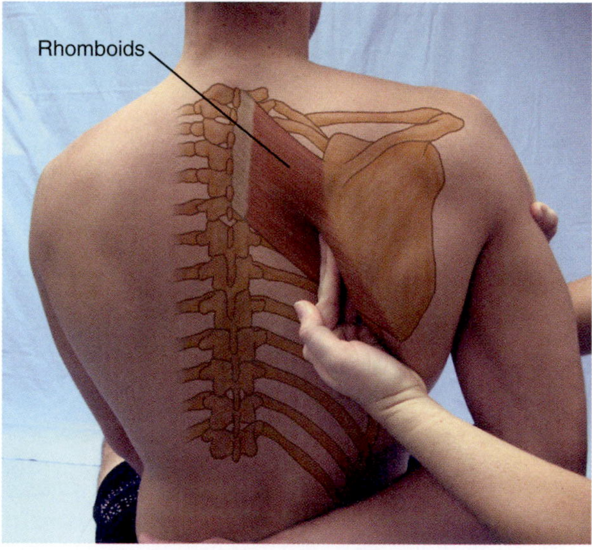

Figure 5.24 Rhomboids. Palpation of the rhomboids. When the trapezius and rhomboids are relaxed, the examiner's finger may be placed under the medial border of the scapula. As the subject raises the hand off the back, contraction of the rhomboid major is observed. Note also the contraction of the teres major.

paralysis, elevation is limited to 120° since elevation is the result motion only at the glenohumeral joint.

Rhomboid Major and Minor

The rhomboids (Gr. *rhombos,* parallelogram-shaped) that connect the scapula with the vertebral column lie under the trapezius. The more cranial portion is known as rhomboid minor; the larger, more caudal portion is the rhomboid major (Fig. 5.24). The rhomboids are made up of parallel fibers, the direction of which is almost perpendicular to those of the lower trapezius.

Weakness or loss of rhomboids function will cause the scapula to assume a protracted position on the thorax. Posterior observation of such a patient reveals a scapula positioned farther laterally from the thoracic spinous processes than the normal 6 cm from the thoracic spinous processes.

Pectoralis Minor

The pectoralis minor (L. *pectus,* breast bone, chest) is located anteriorly on the upper chest, entirely covered by the pectoralis major (Fig. 5.25). The muscle spans from proximal to distal insertions to give the muscle a triangular shape. Weakness of this muscle results in reduced strength during scapular depression and downward rotation of the scapula against resistance.

Levator Scapulae

The levator scapulae, as its name indicates, is an elevator of the scapula, an action it shares with the upper trapezius and with the rhomboids. The levator is difficult to palpate since it is covered by the upper trapezius, and its upper portion is also covered by the sternocleidomastoid muscle (Fig. 5.26). Note that the line of action of the upper trapezius produces elevation and upward rotation of the scapula, whereas the levator—at least in a certain range—has a downward rotary action on the scapula. Therefore, the levator muscle is more likely a scapular elevator when elevation occurs with the scapula in a downward rotation position, as in shrugging the shoulder when the hand is behind the body. Deficiencies in this muscle produce a reduced ability to elevate and downwardly rotate the scapula.

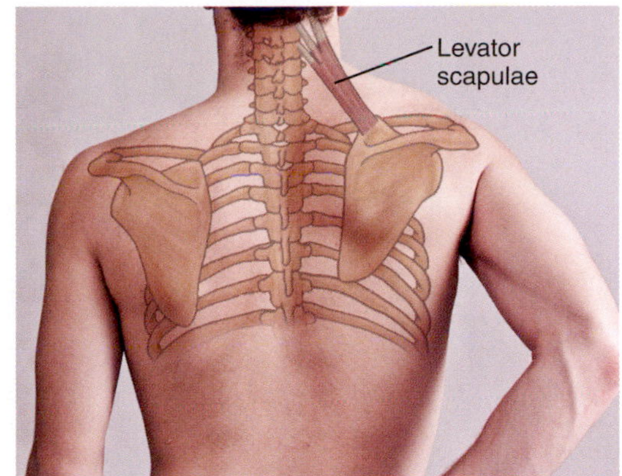

Figure 5.26 Levator scapulae palpation. With the forearm in the small of the back, the subject lightly shrugs the shoulders while the examiner palpates the muscle in the neck.

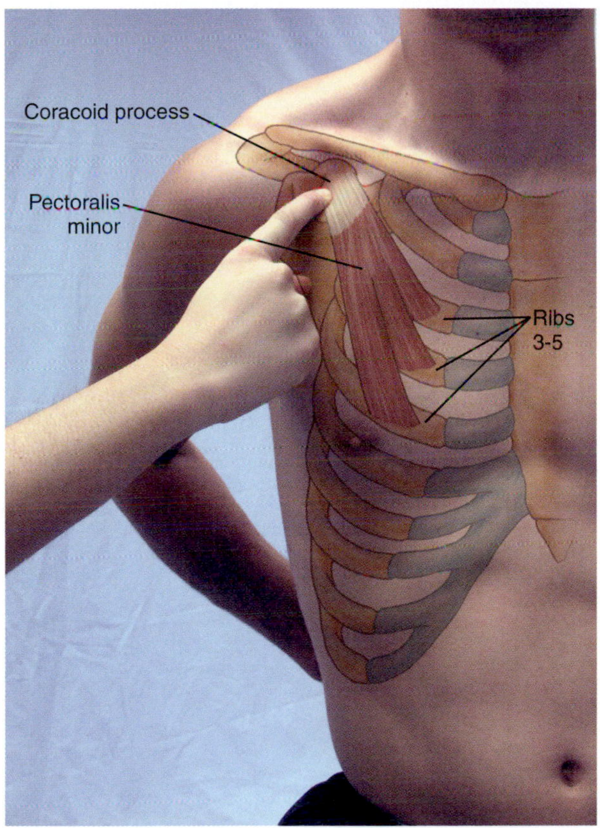

Figure 5.25 Palpation of the pectoralis minor. With the subject's hand resting in the lumbar region of the back, both the pectoralis major and minor are relaxed. The tendon of the pectoralis minor is palpated at the inferior aspect of the coracoid process when the subject raises the hand off the back.

Glenohumeral Stabilizing Muscles of the Shoulder

These muscles include the rotator cuff group (Table 5–5). The rotator cuff muscles provide glenohumeral stability as well as glenohumeral motion. Weakness or dysfunction of any of these muscles will result in reduction of the motion the specific muscle provides as well as a significant decrease in glenohumeral joint stability during shoulder activities. Since they offer some stability to the glenohumeral joint, the biceps and triceps are also included in this group of glenohumeral stabilizers.

The four rotator cuff muscles are sometimes referred to as the "SITS" muscles. This label refers to the order in which they attach to the humerus and their arrangement around the glenohumeral joint. Figure 5.27 demonstrates their arrangement on the humerus as they form the rotator cuff.

Supraspinatus

As its name indicates, the supraspinatus muscle is located above the spine of the scapula. It is hidden by the trapezius and the deltoid; the trapezius covers its muscular portion and the deltoid lies over its tendon. Note that the deepest portion of the supraspinatus lies too deep in the supraspinous fossa to be palpated, but the more superficial fibers of the supraspinatus may be felt through the trapezius. In addition to the method of palpation provided in Table 5–5, the muscle may also be palpated with the subject seated. In this position, first identify the spine of the scapula and place your palpating fingers on the muscle immediately cranial to the scapular spine (they should be moved along the

(text continues on page 195)

TABLE 5-5 | GLENOHUMERAL STABILIZER MUSCLES OF THE SHOULDER GIRDLE

Group	Muscle	Proximal insertion	Distal insertion	Innervation	Action	Palpation
Glenohumeral stabilizers: rotator cuff	Supraspinatus	Supraspinous fossa of the scapula, which it completely fills	Muscles fibers converge toward the tip of the shoulder to form a short tendon that inserts on the uppermost facet of the greater tubercle of the humerus	Suprascapular nerve (C_5-C_6).	Abduction of the glenohumeral joint.	With the subject prone and the arm hanging over the edge of the table, the scapula moves anteriorly around the rib cage by the weight of the arm and is already partially upwardly rotated. When abduction is carried out in this position, a contraction of the supraspinatus may be felt in the supraspinatus fossa with little or no interference by the trapezius. The supraspinatus also may be palpated when the subject lifts a heavy object with the trunk inclined forward. As the weight of the object exerts its downward traction, the supraspinatus becomes tense, apparently for the purpose of preventing excessive separation of the glenohumeral joint.
Glenohumeral stabilizers: rotator cuff	Infraspinatus	Infraspinous fossa	Greater tubercle of the humerus, into its middle facet	Suprascapular nerve (C_5-C_6).	Lateral rotation and adduction of the glenohumeral joint.	To have as large parts of the muscle as possible available for palpation, the arm must be away from the body and the posterior deltoid must be relaxed. This is accomplished if the subject lies prone or stands with the trunk inclined forward and if the arm hangs vertically. The margin of the posterior deltoid is first identified. The palpating fingers are placed below the deltoid on the scapula, near its lateral margin. While the subject maintains the arm in a vertical position, the subject laterally rotates the shoulder by turning the palm forward. The infraspinatus and teres minor then rise under the palpating fingers, Lateral rotation in this position requires only a mild contraction of these muscles, and consequently they do not show beneath the skin in the illustration.

Glenohumeral stabilizers: rotator cuff	Teres Minor	Cephalic aspect of the lateral border of the scapula	Greater tubercle of the humerus, into its lower (posterior) facet	axillary nerve (C_5-C_6).	Lateral rotation and adduction of the glenohumeral joint.	The same procedure for palpation of the infraspinatus will locate the teres minor, but the teres minor is palpated lateral to the infraspinatus and spine of the scapula.
Glenohumeral stabilizers: rotator cuff	Subscapularis	Costal surface of scapula	Broad tendinous insertion on the lesser tubercle of the humerus and shaft distal to the tubercle.	Subscapular nerves (C_5-C_6).	Medial rotation of the glenohumeral joint.	If the trunk is inclined forward so that the scapula slides forward on the rib cage by the weight of the hanging arm, a portion of this muscle may be palpated. The fingers are placed in the axilla anterior to the latissimus dorsi and, with gentle pressure, are moved in the direction of the costal surface of the scapula. With the arm hanging vertically, the subject medially rotates the shoulder by turning the palm posteriorly. The firm, round belly of the subscapularis can then be felt rising under the palpating fingers. If a person wishes to feel the muscle on himself or herself, the thumb is used for palpation. As far as can be ascertained by palpation, the size of the muscle varies considerably from person to person.

continued

TABLE 5-5 | GLENOHUMERAL STABILIZER MUSCLES OF THE SHOULDER GIRDLE—cont'd

Group	Muscle	Proximal insertion	Distal insertion	Innervation	Action	Palpation
GHJ movers from scapula	Teres Major Teres major	Inferior angle of the scapula	Strong, broad tendinous attachment on the crest of the lesser tubercle of the humerus	Subscapular nerves (C_5-C_6).	Medial rotation, adduction, and extension of the glenohumeral joint.	The belly of the muscle can be palpated on the inferior aspect of the axillary border of the scapula when the subject is prone on a table with the arm hanging over the side. If the relaxed subject inwardly rotates the glenohumeral joint, the teres major rises under the palpating fingers. If at the same time other fingers are placed higher on the axillary border and the subject is asked to laterally rotate, the teres minor is felt to contract as the teres major relaxes.
	Coracobrachialis 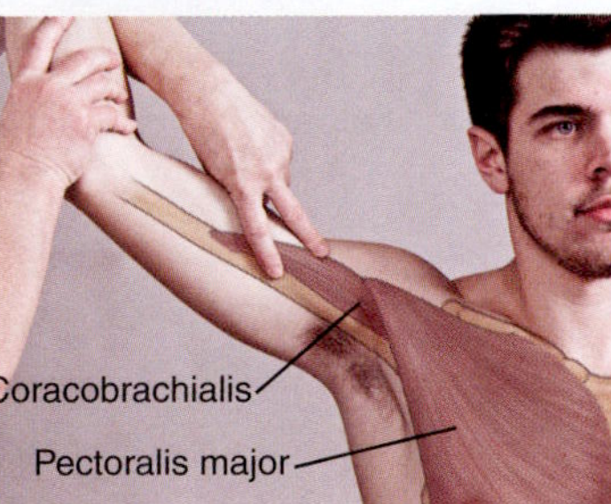 	Coracoid process of scapula	Medial surface of humerus, about halfway down the shaft of the humerus	Musculocutaneous nerve (C_6-C_7).	Flexion and adduction of the glenohumeral joint.	The coracobrachialis may be palpated in the distal portion of the axillary region if the arm is elevated above the horizontal, as seen in Figure 5.31. It emerges from underneath the inferior border of the pectoralis major where it lies medial to, and parallel with, the tendon of the short head of the biceps. The biceps is first identified by supination of the forearm; the palpating fingers then follow the short head of the biceps proximally until the muscle tapers off, and this is the height best suited for palpation of the coracobrachialis. In the illustration, the subject is bringing the arm in a direction toward the head.

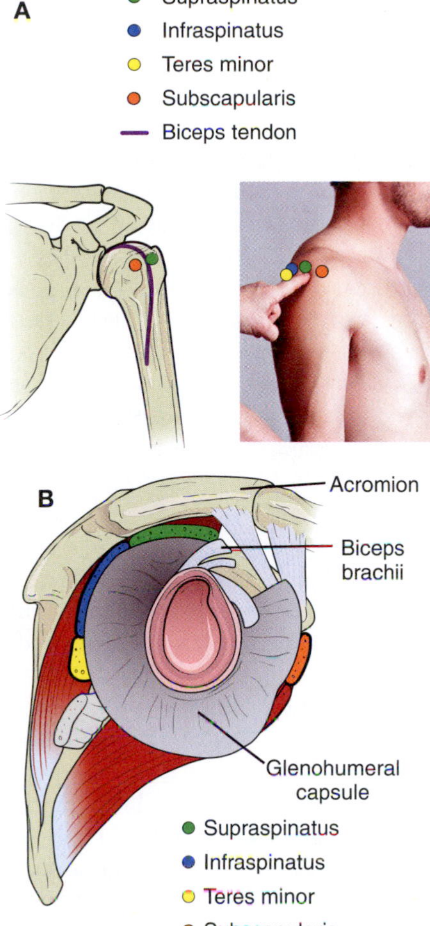

Figure 5.27 SITS tendon arrangement on the humerus. A) Drawing is of a left shoulder and the photo is of a right shoulder. From anterior to posterior, the rotator cuff tendon insertions on the greater tubercle include the supraspinatus, infraspinatus, and teres minor. The rotator cuff tendon inserting on the lesser tubercle is the subscapularis. B) Drawing is of a right shoulder with the humerus removed. With the humerus removed, the arrangement of the rotator cuff muscles around the glenoid fossa appears as a cuff surrounding the glenohumeral joint.

scapular spine until the best spot for palpation is located). A quick active abduction movement in an early, short range of abduction motion is performed by the subject as the clinician palpates a momentary contraction of the muscle. In wider ranges of abduction, the supraspinatus is more difficult to palpate because the trapezius becomes increasingly tense and it is then not easy to distinguish one muscle from the other.

The supraspinatus is capable of performing the total motion of abduction without the assistance of the deltoid. This has been demonstrated in persons with paralysis of the deltoid muscle in both poliomyelitis and axillary nerve block. Howell and associates[65] found the supraspinatus is able to abduct the humerus against resistance and to contribute approximately 50% of normal maximum isokinetic torque. Additionally, however, Howell and associates[65] proposed that the supraspinatus may contribute to 12% of abduction torque at and above 120° of motion.

Infraspinatus and Teres Minor

Although the infraspinatus and teres minor are supplied by two different nerves, they are described together here because they are closely related in location and action (Fig. 5.28). The infraspinatus lies closest to the spine of the scapula and occupies most of the infraspinatus fossa. The teres minor (L. *teretis,* round and long) is attached to the lateral border of the scapula. The tendons of both muscles are adherent to and blend with the capsule.

The largest parts of the infraspinatus and the teres minor are superficial and may be palpated; however, some portions are covered by the trapezius and the posterior deltoid.

The distal attachments of these muscles can be palpated on the greater tubercle of the head of the humerus just distal and anterior to the acromion if the glenohumeral joint is passively hyperextended and the deltoid muscle is relaxed. If pathology is present, palpation of these structures may produce complaints of pain or discomfort.

Subscapularis

The subscapularis is located on the anterior scapula (Fig. 5.29). The muscle's tendon passes over the anterior aspect of the capsule of the glenohumeral joint. Depending on the arm position, the subscapularis can flex, extend, adduct, or abduct the glenohumeral joint in addition to its primary medial rotation function. Other subscapularis functions are dependent upon its moment arm and are, therefore, related to the glenohumeral position. When the arm is overhead, the subscapularis is able to assist with extension. There is also evidence that it may work to adduct when the shoulder is medially rotated and abduct when the shoulder is laterally rotated.[66, 67] The subscapularis has a cross section nearly equal that of the middle deltoid, which indicates that the muscle is of considerable size.[68]

Biceps Brachii and Triceps Brachii

The biceps and triceps muscles do not belong to the rotator cuff; however, the two heads of the biceps and the long head of the triceps cross the shoulder joint and, therefore, act on it. The long and short biceps heads attach to the supraglenoid tubercle and to the coracoid process, respectively, whereas the triceps attaches to the infraglenoid tubercle. At the shoulder, the biceps serves

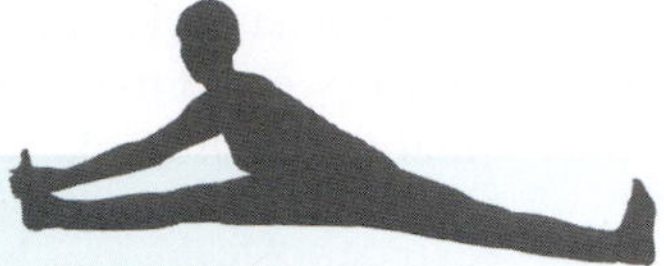

PRACTICE POINT

The distal attachment of the supraspinatus, infraspinatus, and teres minor blend into the glenohumeral joint's capsule and is a frequent site of injury and cause of shoulder pain. To locate and palpate these insertion sites, the clinician should first passively hyperextend the shoulder and assure that the deltoid muscle is relaxed. By placing the clinician's hand in the small of the patient's back and hooking the patient's arm behind his or her arm, this hyperextended position of the patient's arm can be easily achieved. Once the clinician identifies the bicipital groove, the greater tubercle is located immediately adjacent and lateral to the groove. The greater tubercle is the insertion site for the supraspinatus, infraspinatus, and teres minor and is located and forms the lateral ridge of the groove whereas the lesser tubercle where the subscapularis tendon attaches forms the medial ridge of the groove. Although the clinician is unable to delineate the tendons from one another, those on the greater tubercle are arranged in sequence with the supraspinatus most adjacent to the bicipital groove and the teres minor farthest from the groove, so the location of the patient's complaint of pain to palpation as well as other components of the examination provide the clinician with the identity of the specific structure of injury or pain.

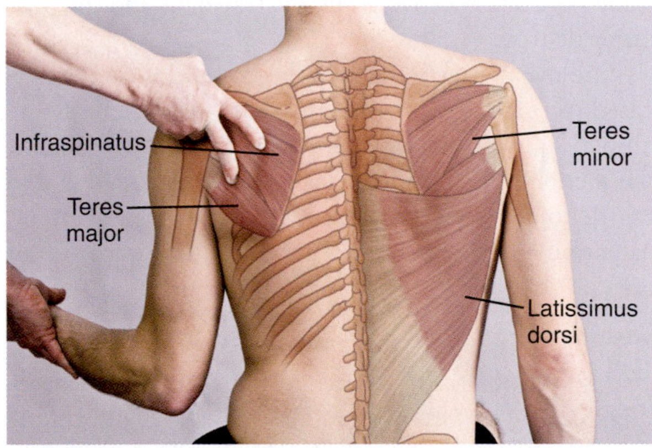

Figure 5.28 Infraspinatus and teres minor may be located near the lateral border of the scapula when the shoulder is laterally rotated. Vertical position of the arm allows activation of these two muscles in a rather isolated fashion.

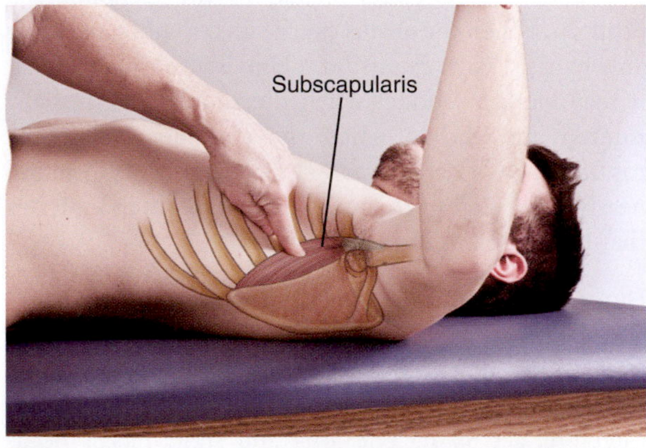

Figure 5.29 The subscapularis is palpated in medial rotation of the shoulder. The palpating fingers are placed in the axilla and are moved in a direction toward the costal surface of the scapula.

as a glenohumeral joint flexor and an abductor, and the triceps is an extensor and an adductor of the glenohumeral joint. These two muscles are described in detail in Chapter 6.

The long head of the biceps is also important in stabilizing the humeral head in the glenoid during glenohumeral motion. When stimulated, the biceps tendon pushes the humeral head into the lower portion of the glenoid to reduce stress on the joint.[69] However, it must be kept in mind that since the long head of the biceps crosses both the shoulder and elbow joints, its influence on one joint is dependent upon its position at the other.[70] Itoi and colleagues[71] demonstrated that both the long and short heads of the biceps added to shoulder stability when the shoulder was in abduction and lateral rotation. They also concluded from their investigation that as the joint's stability provided by other structures decreased, such as with a tear in the anterior capsule, the biceps' role increased. It is agreed upon by several investigators that the biceps is an important stabilizing structure for the glenohumeral joint during elevation, especially if there is injury to other stabilizing structures.[71-73]

When the deltoid and the supraspinatus are paralyzed, the long head of the biceps is capable of substituting as an arm elevator. The biceps is able to provide this motion when the glenohumeral joint is in lateral rotation, slightly anterior to the frontal plane and without resistance or a tool in the hand. This motion is useful for placement of the hand over the head, but the long head of the biceps is not strong enough to lift objects or to perform work in this position.

The long head of the triceps also lends stability to the glenohumeral joint during elevation activities. As the humerus moves into abduction, the triceps' long head helps to steady the humeral head in the glenoid.[74] During weight-bearing activities, the triceps also provides stabilization of the glenohumeral joint; Marisa Pontillo and associates[75] found that as upper extremity weight-bearing activities became more difficult, the triceps becomes more active as a shoulder stabilizer.

Large Muscle Movers of the Shoulder

These muscles have their proximal attachments on the trunk and their distal attachments on the humerus, having little or no attachment to the scapula (Table 5–6). They act on the humerus as primary movers, but through their connection to the humerus, they may also indirectly affect the position of the entire shoulder girdle. Because of their attachments, these muscles each perform multiple actions at the shoulder joint.

Deltoid

The deltoid (Gr. *delta*, the letter Δ; *eidos*, resemblance) is a large, superficial muscle consisting of three parts: anterior, middle, and posterior. The muscle covers the glenohumeral joint on all sides except in the inferior axillary region and comprises 40% of the mass of the scapulohumeral muscles.[2] The muscle is covered by skin only, so it is easy to observe and palpate in its entirety. The characteristic roundness of the normal shoulder is due to the deltoid muscle (Fig. 5.30). All parts of the deltoid are described in Table 5–6.

The three portions of the deltoid should be observed in action while horizontal abduction and adduction are performed and in pulling and pushing activities. Although all three heads of the deltoid work together to produce abduction as a common motion, similar to the upper and lower trapezius, the anterior and posterior portions of the deltoid also act antagonistically to each other; the anterior deltoid produces horizontal flexion (horizontal adduction) whereas the posterior deltoid produces horizontal extension (horizontal abduction). Similarly, the anterior deltoid contributes to medial rotation whereas the posterior deltoid laterally rotates the humerus.

In normal abduction, the supraspinatus initiates motion. However, in persons with supraspinatus paralysis or debilitating injury, the deltoid is able to abduct the humerus throughout the range of motion if the other functioning rotator cuff muscles are able to counteract the deltoid's translatory force. Even though deltoid-only abduction occurs, it is produced with less than normal strength. Howell and associates[65] found an approximately 50% reduction in maximum isokinetic abduction torque with nerve blocks to the suprascapular nerve. After recovery from surgical removal of the deltoid muscle (because of soft tissue tumors), Markhede, Monastyrski, and Stener[76] documented a loss of 5° to 15° of active abduction and a decrease in maximum isometric torques of only 30% to 40%. In the resting position with the arm at the side, the deltoid's angle of pull tends to primarily elevate the humeral head towards the coracoacromial arch with essentially no lever arm for rotation. As the arm continues into higher degrees of abduction, however, the middle deltoid's translatory moment arm decreases, and its rotary moment arm increases starting at about 50° and becomes larger than that of the supraspinatus above 50°.[77] This change in moment arms allows the deltoid to work synergistically with the rotator cuff to be a prime mover in shoulder elevation after the initial ranges of motion. In summary, the deltoid does not rotate the glenohumeral joint into abduction until the higher levels of abduction motion unless the supraspinatus is unable to perform its duties; in these cases, the deltoid may be able to initiate abduction provided the other rotator cuff muscles are intact to counterbalance the deltoid's strong initial translatory force.

Latissimus Dorsi

The name latissimus dorsi is derived from the Latin *latus,* meaning broad. This muscle is the broadest muscle of the low back and the lateral thoracic region. It lies superficially, except for a small segment that is covered by the lower trapezius.

The largest part of this muscle is thin and sheet-like on the posterior thorax, which makes it difficult to distinguish from the fascia and the deeper muscles of the back. The latissimus forms the posterior fold of the axilla. Its shoulder functions commonly relate with those of the teres major and the long head of the triceps (Fig. 5.28).

If the arms are stabilized, as in pushing down on crutch handles or in a seated press down, the distal attachment aids to lift the pelvis. In crutch walking, the latissimus dorsi activity allows the foot to clear the ground, and during a seated press down, the hips lift off the surface. This function is of particular importance to someone with paraplegia whose lower extremity muscles, including the hip-hikers (quadratus lumborum and lateral abdominals), are paralyzed because of a spinal cord injury. By placing the hands on the armrests of the wheelchair, the person can perform a seated push-up and decrease pressure from sitting on the buttocks and minimize the likelihood of developing pressure sores. Additionally, this muscle serves a vital function for gymnasts, wrestlers, divers, and other athletes who must support their body weight with their upper extremities.

TABLE 5–6 | LARGE MUSCLE MOVERS OF THE SHOULDER

Group	Muscle	Proximal insertion	Distal insertion	Innervation	Action	Palpation
Large muscle movers of the shoulder	Deltoid	The acromial end of the clavicle, the acromion process, and the spine of the scapula	The three portions converge on the deltoid tuberosity, a rather rough area about halfway down the shaft of the humerus	Axillary nerve (C_5-C_6).	Abduction of the glenohumeral joint. Anterior deltoid performs flexion and horizontal adduction of the glenohumeral joint. Posterior deltoid performs extension and horizontal abduction of the glenohumeral joint.	The **anterior deltoid** may be observed and palpated when the arm is held in a horizontal position. Note that its inferior border lies close to the upper portion of the pectoralis major. The anterior deltoid contracts strongly when horizontal adduction is resisted. The **middle deltoid** has the best anatomic position for abduction and is seen contracting whenever this movement is carried out or the abducted position is maintained. The **posterior deltoid** contracts strongly when the shoulder is hyperextended against resistance, or resistance is given to horizontal abduction. The inferior border of the posterior portion of the deltoid has a close relation to the long head of the triceps and to the teres muscles. The patient (postpoliomyelitis) had extensive paralysis of the shoulder muscles, including the middle and anterior portions of the deltoid, while the posterior portion was more or less preserved.

Large muscle movers of the shoulder	Latissimus dorsi	Spinous processes of the thoracic vertebrae from T-6 downward, dorsolumbar fascia, crest of ilium (posterior portion), and the lowest ribs, here interdigitating with the external oblique abdominal muscle. The fibers converge toward the axilla, some fibers passing over or near the inferior angle of the scapula, often adhering to it.	The tendon courses in the axilla and attaches to the crest of the lesser tubercle of the humerus, proximal to that of the teres major.	Thoracodorsal nerve (C_6-C_8).	Medial rotation, extension and adduction of the glenohumeral joint, scapular depression, elevation of pelvis.	Laterally, in the axillary line and where the fibers converge, the muscle has considerable bulk, and here it is easy to observe and palpate. The latissimus and the teres major contract when adduction or extension of the shoulder is resisted, as seen in the illustration, in which the subject is pressing down on the examiner's shoulder.
	Pectoralis major	Inferior & medial clavicle; costocartilages of ribs #2-6 & body of sternum	Crest of the greater tubercle of the humerus	Medial and lateral pectoral nerves ($C_5 - T_1$)	Glenohumeral adduction, horizontal adduction, and medial rotation. clavicular head flexes the glenohumeral joint. Sternocostal head extends the glenohumeral joint from fully flexed position.	Being superficial and of considerable bulk, the muscle is easily observed and palpated along its origin along the sternum or distal to the clavicle. The entire muscle contracts when horizontal adduction is resisted, as in pressing the palms together in front of the body.

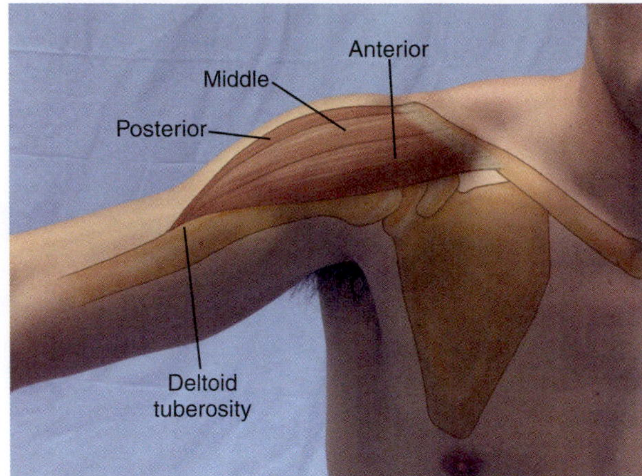

Figure 5.30 Deltoid. The clinician grasps around the anterior portion of the deltoid, separating it from the middle deltoid and from the pectoralis major.

Teres Major

The teres major lies distal to the teres minor on the lateral scapula border (Fig. 5.28). It is round like the minor, but larger. The muscular portion of the teres major is well accessible to palpation, but the tendon of its distal attachment is not. The teres major acts in most pulling activities when the shoulder is extended or adducted against resistance. Its function is closely aligned with that of the latissimus dorsi.

Pectoralis Major

Its name (L. *pectus*, breastbone, chest) indicates that the pectoralis major is a large muscle of the chest. It has an extensive origin but does not cover nearly as large an area as the latissimus dorsi. The muscle is described as consisting of two parts: the clavicular and sternocostal. This delineation into two segments is based on its muscle fiber directions and functions. Their fiber arrangements and sites of proximal attachments allow these two heads to work independently of one another during shoulder flexion and extension.[74] Because of its wide origin with a convergence of its fibers toward the axilla, the muscle takes the shape of a fan. The manner in which the muscle fibers approach their distal attachment should be noted—the tendon appears to be twisted around itself, so that the uppermost fibers attach lowest on the crest and the lower fibers attach more proximally.

Coracobrachialis

The name of this muscle identifies its proximal and distal insertions. Parts of this muscle are covered by the deltoid, pectoralis major, and biceps brachii (Fig. 5.31). It is considered a mover of the glenohumeral joint rather than a stabilizer since its line of pull is sufficiently distant from the joint's axis of motion.

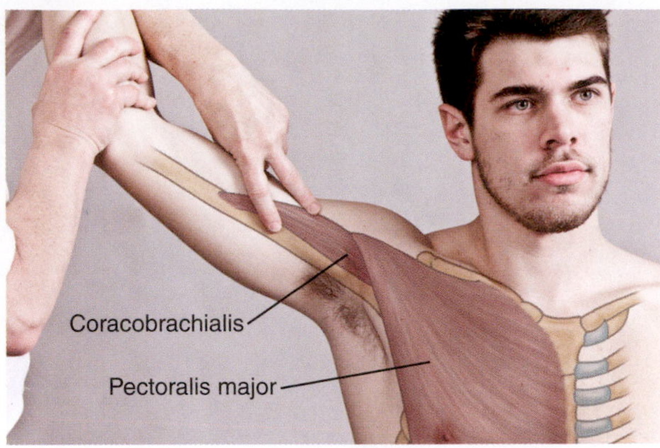

Figure 5.31 Identification of coracobrachialis. This muscle emerges from under the inferior border of the pectoralis major, where it lies close to the tendon of the short head of the biceps.

Function of Muscles of the Shoulder Complex

As has been mentioned, each of the joints within the shoulder complex provides important contributions to overall upper extremity movement. Clinicians must understand how these segments interact to provide smooth function of the shoulder complex and entire upper extremity in order to properly examine and assess patients prior to providing correct treatment to resolve those conditions. This section of the chapter presents information relevant to the functions of these segments. Some synergistic movements are also described. However, the last unit of this text presents information on integrated motions for proper execution of numerous activities including sports and recreational activities, activities of daily living, functional work activities, and gait. Information in this section provides a basic comprehension of how the shoulder complex works, so when you study these later chapters, the information in them can be more fully appreciated.

Passive and Dynamic Stabilization of the Glenohumeral Joint

As with any synovial joint, the joints of the shoulder complex rely on a combination of passive and dynamic elements for their stabilization. The passive elements include the capsule and ligaments whereas the muscles are the dynamic elements. The sternoclavicular and acromioclavicular joints rely primarily on passive restraints whereas the glenohumeral and scapulothoracic joints look to their muscles for stability. Some texts refer to the passive stabilizers as "static" stabilizers;

however, static implies that these structures do not change, but these structures do change as the joint moves. For example, as the clavicle rotates upwardly, the coracoclavicular ligament becomes progressively taut until it reaches a level of tension that prevents further clavicular rotation. Therefore, rather than call these structures "static," we prefer to identify them as passive stabilizers since their motions occur passively.

Passive Stabilization

Motions at the sternoclavicular and acromioclavicular joints are limited by strong ligamentous attachments and, to a lesser degree, by bony configuration. On the other hand, the glenohumeral and scapulothoracic joints have little ligamentous or bony stability. As previously mentioned, these latter two joints attach to the body via muscles, and the glenohumeral joint has the additional supporting advantage of a loose joint capsule which is reinforced by ligaments.

Normally, there is no contraction of muscles of the shoulder girdle during relaxed sitting or standing, giving rise to the question of what structures prevent the humerus from subluxating when the person is upright. The clavicle and scapula rest on the thorax. The head of the humerus is maintained in the glenoid fossa by the horizontal coracohumeral and superior glenohumeral ligaments and by negative atmospheric pressure within the capsule. In fresh cadavers, Kumar and Balasubramaniam[78] found that subluxation of the humeral head occurred only after puncture of the capsule when the atmospheric pressure variant was eliminated.

Dynamic Stabilization

Low-level continuous activity of the upper trapezius frequently occurs during sitting and standing, but when attention is called to this activity, most subjects can relax the muscle easily. The trapezius activity is probably related to head posture because the upper fibers are neck extensors as well as scapula elevators; continuous muscle activity of these neck muscles is a common source of tension and neck pain in people who work at a desk or who have poor posture. Upper trapezius pathology also affects the shoulder complex; it has long been noted that trapezius paralysis is accompanied by scapular dropping and downward rotation.[64] This evidence leads to the conclusion that maintenance of the normal resting position of the scapula may be from passive fascial forces produced by the 15 muscles that have attachments on the scapula as well as from the support of the rib cage.

Rotator Cuff Stabilization

It was once thought that, when a person is carrying a heavy load such as a briefcase in the hand, contraction of the deltoid, biceps, or triceps brachii muscles with their vertical action lines kept the humeral head apposed to the glenoid cavity. These muscles, however, have been found to be electromyographically silent even with loads of 25 lb in the hand.[79, 80] Instead, EMG activity has been found in the horizontally directed rotator cuff muscles—the supraspinatus, infraspinatus, and teres minor. Contraction of these muscles holds the humeral head tightly against the glenoid to prevent subluxation when carrying a weight in the hand. Although these rotator cuff muscles produce motion of the glenohumeral joint, their most important and primary function is to provide stability to the joint by compressing the humeral head into the glenoid fossa. During elevation of the glenohumeral joint, these rotator cuff muscles create dynamic stabilization of the joint as the humerus moves into flexion or abduction. During elevation, the rotator cuff secures and protects the joint and its surrounding soft tissue structures by not only pulling the humerus to the glenoid, but it also moves the humeral head into the lower portion of the glenoid fossa where it is able to sit more securely against a larger surface of the glenoid, thereby allowing sufficient space under the coracoacromial arch for the soft tissues positioned between the arch and glenohumeral joint.

Biceps Brachii

The tendon of the long head of the biceps brachii courses over the humeral head and descends in the intertubercular groove. In the tendon, tension is produced when the muscle contracts to compress the humeral head against the glenoid cavity. This force is similar to pulling a rope around a post. Thus, the biceps aids in preventing subluxation of the glenohumeral joint when the elbow flexes with a weight in the hand.

The Deltoid and Rotator Cuff

In the evolution of primate and human development, the deltoid muscle increases its relative size markedly with the upright position.[2] In humans, the muscle is prominent and surrounds the glenohumeral joint on three sides. Attention has been focused on the deltoid in its function as an abductor of the glenohumeral joint. The deltoid, however, has a small rotary component to its muscle force vector (Fig. 5.32A). In the early part of elevation, the major force of the deltoid is directed vertically, producing a shear of the humeral head in the glenoid, causing the humeral head to move upward to hit the coracoacromial arch. However, this movement is prevented by the horizontal and downward pulls of the rotator cuff muscles (Fig. 5.32B). As mentioned earlier,

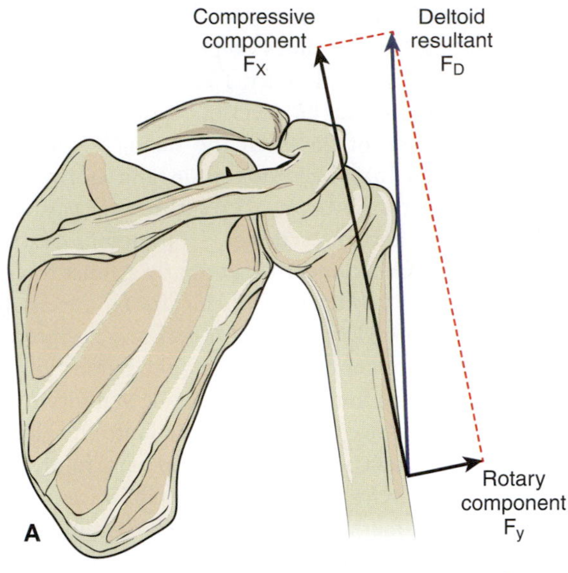

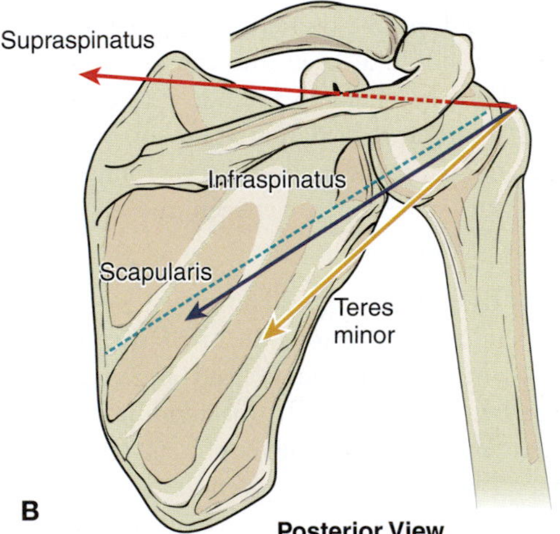

Figure 5.32 Rotary forces in glenohumeral abduction. **A)** The deltoid's vector forces. The deltoid has a very small rotary component when the arm is at the side. **B)** The horizontal and downward pull of the rotator cuff muscles prevents the deltoid from pulling the humerus into the coracoacromial arch.

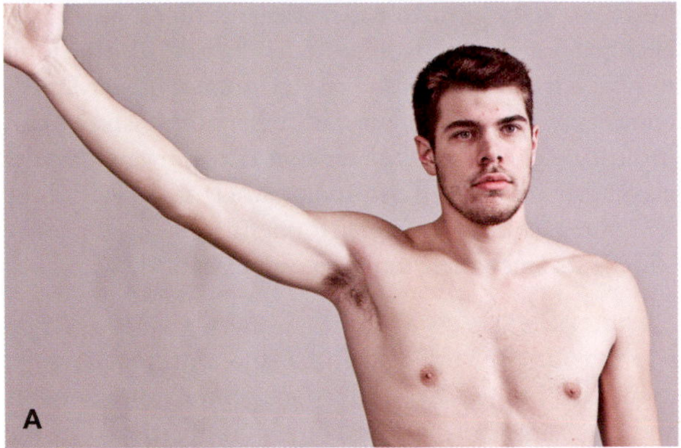

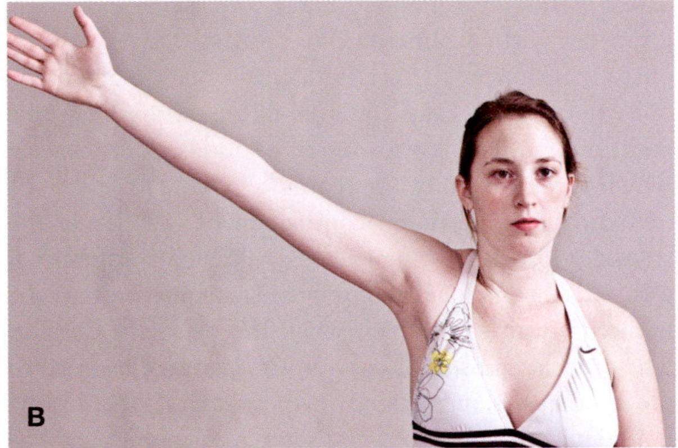

Figure 5.33 Shoulder elevation in the scapular plane. **A)** Normal elevation with properly functioning muscles. **B)** Elevation with inadequate rotator cuff strength to maintain the humerus in the lower glenoid fossa is revealed by the humeral head's inability to maintain its proper position in the lower portion of the glenoid fossa so the shoulder appears to have a slight shrug as the arm elevates.

the inferior glenoid surface is larger than its superior aspect. When the arm elevates, the rotator cuff pulls the humerus into this larger inferior area. This action accomplishes two important factors: 1) the surface of contact between the glenoid and humeral head is greater, providing more joint stability; and 2) with the humeral head depressed in the socket, the subacromial soft tissue structures have optimal room and less risk of impingement. Figures 5.33A and 5.33B demonstrate a visualization of the difference between when the rotator cuff does not provide a downward pressure of the humeral head in the glenoid fossa during elevation (Fig. 5.33B) and when the muscles perform the task adequately (Fig. 5.33A). Some consider the posterior deltoid itself to be an adductor or to cause joint compression in the early part of the motion and have found lines of force inferior or very close to the axis of motion.[81, 82] As elevation progresses, the lever arms for abduction increase, but most of the force generated by the deltoid is directed into the stabilizing component, which compresses the head of the humerus against the glenoid. When the arm is fully elevated, the deltoid and the horizontal forces of the rotator cuff muscles provide stability for the glenohumeral joint. In full shoulder elevation, as in an overhead press (open chain) or standing on the hands (closed chain), the protracted and upwardly rotated scapula is positioned so that it forms a platform for the head of the humerus. In turn, the serratus anterior and the trapezius muscles stabilize the scapula in this position. Therefore, the scapular stability provided by its upward rotators allows the glenoid to be stable in overhead motions. At the same time, the humeral head is held in a secure position within the glenohumeral joint during overhead activities by the rotator cuff muscles (Fig. 5.34). If either the scapular rotators or the rotator cuff fails in its duty to provide scapular or glenohumeral stability, respectively, injury will occur to the glenohumeral structures. A fateful but common pathological combination of scapular rotator muscle imbalances (e.g., when the upper trapezius overpowers the lower trapezius) with weakness of the rotator cuff muscles causes a predictable effect. These two deficiencies—either by themselves or in combination with each other—result in subacromial impingement during elevation: 1) the deltoid overpowers the rotator cuff to pull the humeral head into the superior aspect of the glenoid socket; and 2) the scapula shrugs upward rather than rotating upward (Fig. 5.35).

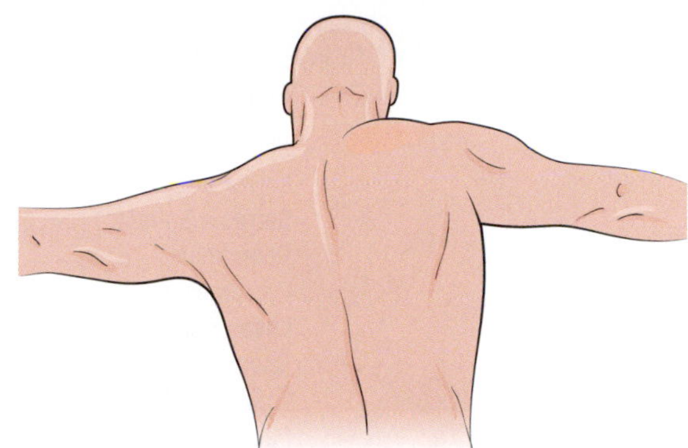

Figure 5.35 With lower trapezius and serratus anterior weakness, the upper trapezius overpowers these scapular upward rotators to cause the scapula to elevate rather than rotate, leading to glenohumeral impingement.

Synergistic Muscle Actions

Individual muscles and parts of the same muscle in the shoulder girdle have multiple anatomic actions because of the number of joints, the large ranges of motion, and the absence of structural stability. Likewise, it is rare in the shoulder complex that only one muscle performs any one action. In fact, many muscles work during any shoulder motion. For example, elevation of the arm can activate 11 of the 17 major muscles of the shoulder girdle. Sometimes the muscles work synergistically to produce a desired motion, and at other times, they are antagonistic to each other. For example, elevation of the scapula occurs with activity from the upper trapezius and levator scapulae with the opposite motion, depression, the result of lower trapezius and pectoralis minor contraction. On the other hand, upward rotation is the result of cooperative efforts from the serratus anterior, upper trapezius, and lower trapezius whereas the pectoralis minor, levator scapulae, and rhomboids produce downward rotation. Table 5–7 shows how muscles moving the scapula change from synergists to antagonists, sometimes working with one muscle and other times working against the same muscle, depending upon the motion produced.

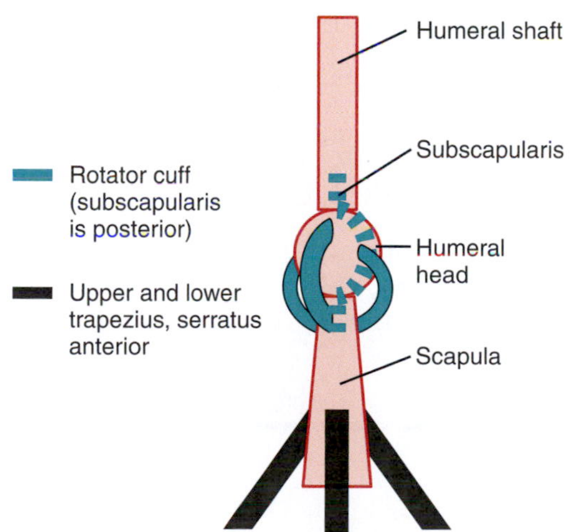

Figure 5.34 Schematic of the stabilization provided in overhead activities by the scapular upward rotators and rotator cuff. The scapular rotators stabilize the scapula so it serves as a stable platform from which the rotator cuff muscles function during glenohumeral motion.

When synergistic muscles produce rotation, they are referred to as a force couple. A **force couple** is defined in mechanical terms as two forces whose points of application occur on opposite sides of an axis and in opposite directions to produce rotation of the body. Because they are on opposite sides of an axis, when they work by themselves, they produce a motion that is opposite to the synergist. However, when they work together, these muscles produce rotation. There are several force couples in the shoulder complex. Such synergy occurs during elevation of the arm. During elevation, there are two primary force couples acting on the shoulder complex: One acts on the glenohumeral joint and the other acts on the scapulothoracic joint. The scapulothoracic force couple includes the upper and lower trapezius and the serratus anterior combining forces to produce upward rotation of the scapula (Fig. 5.36). The glenohumeral force couple consists of the deltoid and the rotator cuff—the deltoid and supraspinatus contract together to produce elevation (abduction or flexion) at the glenohumeral

TABLE 5-7 | ANTAGONISTS AND SYNERGISTS OF THE SCAPULA AND HUMERUS

Scapular Motion	**Synergists**	**Antagonists**
Upward rotation	Upper trapezius Lower trapezius Serratus anterior	Rhomboids Pectoralis minor Levator scapulae
Downward rotation	Rhomboids Pectoralis minor Levator scapulae	Upper trapezius Lower trapezius Serratus anterior
Retraction	Rhomboids Trapezius	Pectoralis minor Serratus anterior
Protraction	Pectoralis minor Serratus anterior	Rhomboids Trapezius
Elevation	Upper trapezius Rhomboids Levator scapulae	Pectoralis minor Lower trapezius Lower serratus anterior
Depression	Pectoralis minor Lower trapezius Lower serratus anterior	Upper trapezius Rhomboids Levator scapulae
Glenohumeral Motion	**Synergists**	**Antagonists**
Flexion	Pectoralis major (clavicular head) Coracobrachialis Biceps brachii	Latissimus dorsi Teres major Triceps brachii (long head) Pectoralis major (costosternal head)
Extension	Latissimus dorsi Teres major Triceps brachii (long head) Pectoralis major (costosternal head)	Pectoralis major (clavicular head) Coracobrachialis Biceps brachii
Abduction	Deltoid Supraspinatus Biceps brachii (long head)	Pectoralis major Latissimus dorsi Teres major Triceps brachii (long head)
Adduction	Pectoralis major Latissimus dorsi Teres major Triceps brachii (long head)	Deltoid Supraspinatus Biceps brachii (long head)
Lateral rotation	Infraspinatus Teres minor Posterior deltoid	Subscapularis Teres major Pectoralis major Latissimus dorsi Anterior deltoid
Medial rotation	Subscapularis Teres major Pectoralis major Latissimus dorsi Anterior deltoid	Infraspinatus Teres minor Posterior deltoid

joint while the infraspinatus, teres minor, and subscapularis work to pull the humeral head down into the lower part of the socket as the deltoid elevates the humerus, thereby producing rotation of the joint. Another force couple of the scapulothoracic joint includes the rhomboids, levator scapulae, and pectoralis minor producing downward rotation of the scapula on the thorax (Fig. 5.37).

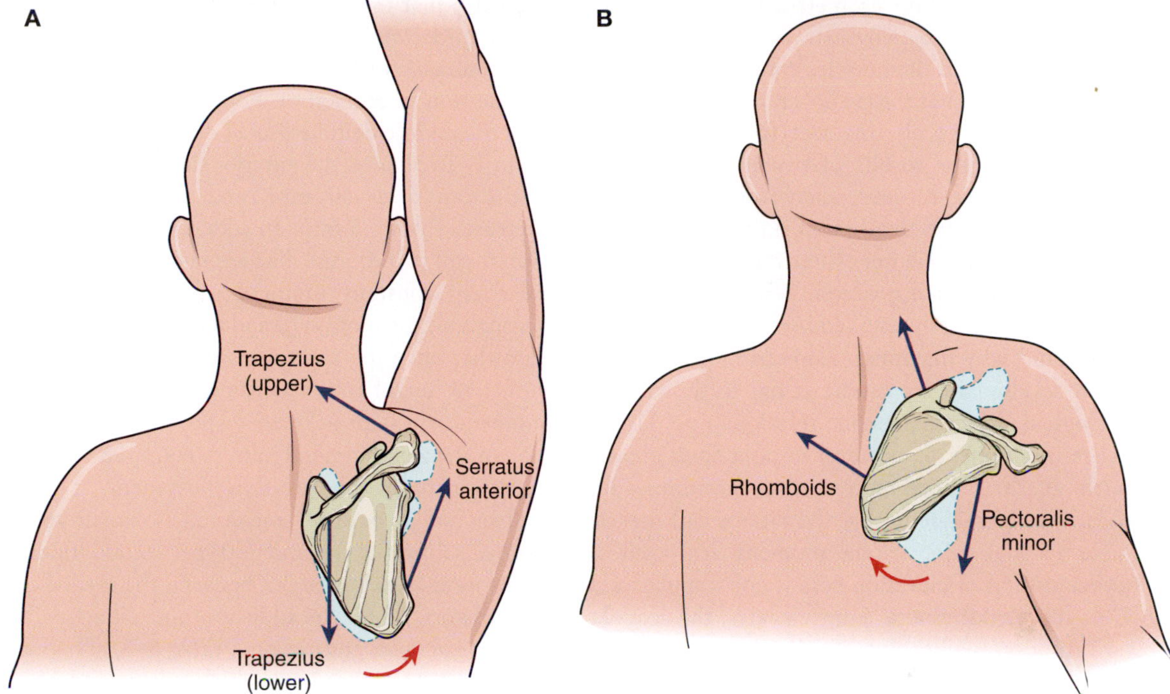

Figure 5.36 Force couple of the scapulothoracic joint. A) Upward rotators include the upper trapezius, lower trapezius, and serratus anterior. B) Downward rotators include the levator scapulae, rhomboids, and pectoralis minor.

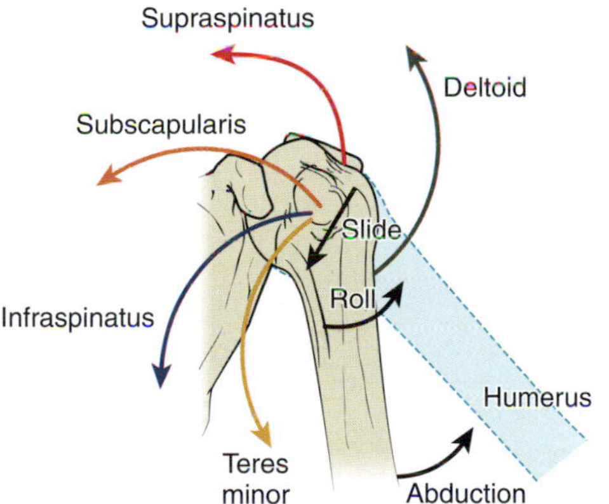

Figure 5.37 Force couple of the glenohumeral joint. The rotator cuff and deltoid work together to produce rotation of the humerus in the glenoid.

Muscle Forces and Moment (Lever) Arm Lengths

Large forces are generated by the shoulder when an implement or tool such as a hammer or tennis racquet is added to the hand. These implements extend the resistance arm length; however, the muscle's force arm lengths do not change. Although the resistance arms may be measured in meters or feet, depending on the length of the implement, the muscle's force arms are measured in fractions of centimeters or inches. Therefore, in order to overcome the greater resistance, the muscles must produce a much greater force to perform the desired activity. This point will become a bit clearer when you do the lab activities at the end of this chapter.

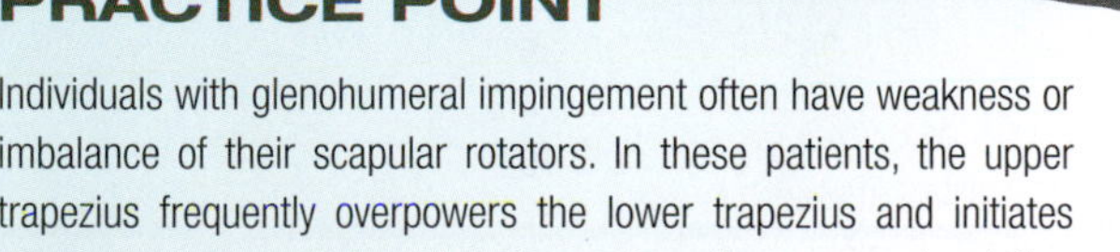

PRACTICE POINT

Individuals with glenohumeral impingement often have weakness or imbalance of their scapular rotators. In these patients, the upper trapezius frequently overpowers the lower trapezius and initiates movement so scapular elevation rather than upward rotation becomes the primary scapular motion. Such movement elevates the humeral head towards the coracoacromial arch, impinging the rotator cuff tendons and other soft tissues between the arch and the humeral head (Fig. 5.35). Clinicians must be able to identify when this occurs, strengthen the weak scapular rotators, and correct their timing sequence to relieve impingement symptoms.

Studies of maximum isometric torque measurements in the shoulder demonstrate that the greatest strength occurs when the muscles contract in the elongated position and that torque decreases as the muscles shorten.[46, 83] (We recall this fact from Chapter 2.) Table 5–8 shows the results of two investigations of maximum isometric torques taken from normal subjects.[46, 83] When more than one position is tested, the resulting torques are higher when the muscle is contracted in the elongated position. When we remember the concepts that were presented in Chapter 4, it is easy to understand why maximum isometric torque is produced in an elongated position. It has to do with the physiological length-tension relationship. Muscle fibers are in an optimal position to offer their greatest strength at their maximum resting positions. The shoulder is very unique in that the rotator cuff muscles are able to maintain a long moment arm over an extended motion of elevation because of scapular rotation. As the glenohumeral joint elevates, the scapula's upward rotation maintains a steady relative position of the rotator cuff to the humerus, so its length-tension relationship remains essentially unchanged over a large range of elevation. This scapular motion allows the rotator cuff to maintain a high level of force output through a greater range of shoulder elevation.[77] In the first 30° to 60° of abduction, the leverage for the supraspinatus is greater than that of the deltoid, which indicates that the supraspinatus provides a major force in the initiation of shoulder abduction.

Moment arm lengths for the deltoid increase with the motion of abduction. Poppen and Walker[82] found that the middle deltoid almost doubled its moment arm from 17 to 30 mm, the anterior deltoid increased eightfold from 5 to 40 mm, and the posterior deltoid increased from −5 mm (an adduction or joint compression force) to +20 mm. The supraspinatus maintained a relatively constant moment arm of about 20 mm throughout the motion of abduction. These results indicate that once the supraspinatus elevates the arm to a sufficient height (60° according to Liu[77]), the deltoid's moment arm is positioned to provide additional rotation of the glenohumeral joint to continue and assist the supraspinatus in the elevation movement.

Ivey and associates[84] measured isokinetic torques in normal subjects at 60° and 180° per second. Peak torque ratios were found to be 3:2 between the medial and lateral rotators, 2:1 for the adductors and abductors, and 5:4 for the extensors and flexors (Table 5–8). There was no significant difference between dominant and nondominant sides. The angle at which the peak torque occurred was constant for the same person but had a wide variation among individuals. Isokinetic studies on athletes engaged in throwing sports show slightly different ratios, particularly at high speeds, and some significant differences between dominant and nondominant sides.[49, 85]

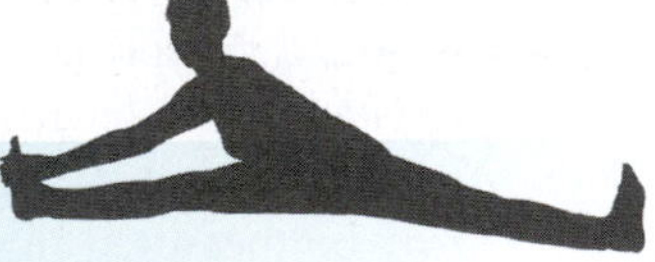

PRACTICE POINT

Another cause of glenohumeral impingement is weakness in the rotator cuff, especially the supraspinatus. In these cases, the deltoid initiates glenohumeral elevation and pushes the humeral head towards the coracoacromial arch, narrowing the subacromial space. If the rotator cuff is weak, clinicians must identify this deficiency and improve its strength before the patient is permitted shoulder elevation above 60°.

TABLE 5–8 | AVERAGE MAXIMUM ISOMETRIC TORQUE IN NORMAL SUBJECTS (FT-LB)*

	Shoulder Abduction			Shoulder Flexion		
Joint position	0°	45°	90°	0°	45°	90°
Subjects and age						
36 Males † (X̄ = 25.8 yr)	53	43°	42°	69°	59°	55°
20 Males ‡ (X̄ = 31 yr)	—	45°	—	76°	41°	—
20 Males ‡ (X̄ = 62 yr)	—	31°	—	62°	35°	—
20 Females ‡ (X̄ = 29 yr)	—	20°	—	37°	24°	—
20 Females ‡ (X̄ = 62 yr)	—	16°	—	28°	16°	—

*Maximum isometric torques from two studies that used similar methods have been converted from Newton-meters and kilograms-centimeters to foot-pounds. One foot-pound of resistance is the application of 1-lb force just above the elbow.

† Otis et al (1990).

‡ Murray et al (1985).

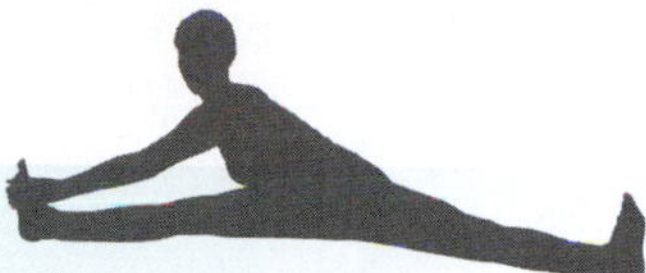

PRACTICE POINT

It matters whether a clinician is treating a throwing athlete or a non-throwing athlete or a non-athlete. Non-athletic populations and patients not involved in throwing sports are expected to have comparable left to right strengths in the upper extremities whereas throwing athletes should have greater strength in the dominant extremity. Differences in these expectations directly impact treatment goals and plans.

Muscle Activity during Functional Motions

Functionally, which muscles perform a desired motion is dependent upon a number of factors. These factors include the position of the body and the limb in relation to gravity, the amount of resistance applied to the limb, and the velocity of motion required. In essence, these factors are the primary determinants, rather than the anatomic motions, as to which muscles are recruited. For example, reaching overhead in a standing or sitting position (a flexion-abduction-upward rotation movement) requires concentric contraction of the anterior deltoid, pectoralis major (clavicular head), coracobrachialis, biceps brachii, and the rotator cuff muscles at the glenohumeral joint as well as the trapezius and serratus anterior muscles at the scapulothoracic joint. When the arm is returned to the side in the same sitting or standing position, the motion is antagonistic (extension-adduction-downward rotation), but the muscles providing the movement are not the antagonistic muscles. In this example, the muscles that moved the arm overhead now lower the arm against gravity with eccentric activity. On the other hand, if we provide manual resistance against the return motion from an overhead position, this time the antagonistic muscles—posterior deltoid, pectoralis major (sternal head), triceps brachii (long head), latissimus dorsi, teres major, levator scapulae, and rhomboids—push against the force to return the arm to the side. If we position the body in supine and have the subject now move the arm overhead, the first half of the motion is provided by concentric movement of the flexors, abductors, and upward rotators, but once the arm passes 90° of elevation, the antagonistic muscles perform eccentrically to control the final half of the motion. On the return motion in supine, the reverse is true: The antagonistic muscles perform the motion concentrically until the arm returns to 90°, at which point the flexors, abductors, and upward rotators return the arm to the side using eccentric activity. Therefore, knowledge of the relationship between muscle actions and body positions relative to gravity is essential in the analysis of muscular requirements during functional activities. The best way to start understanding muscle function during functional activities is to become acquainted with the muscles' anatomic actions first, then advance to the effect of other determinants influencing muscle recruitment. A summary classification of muscles according to their anatomic actions at the shoulder joints is in Table 5–7.

In forceful movements, all muscles in the upper extremity may contract, making it difficult to analyze the muscle activity. They may contract to produce or restrain the motion, to hold the desired position, to counteract an undesired motion of another active muscle, or to stabilize the scapula or glenohumeral joint. The rotator cuff muscles are almost always active in shoulder motions in order to provide glenohumeral stabilization, even if the muscles are not called upon to move the glenohumeral joint. Likewise, the scapular rotators activate to stabilize the scapula on the thorax during glenohumeral activity so that a stable base for the shoulder joint is provided. In the following analyses of muscle activity, it is helpful to have a subject perform the activity with a minimum of resistance so that the prime movers can more easily be identified visually and by palpation.

Placing the Hand behind the Head

Placing the hand behind the head, as in combing one's hair, requires the following shoulder complex motions: sternoclavicular joint elevation to about 18°, retraction of 38°, and posterior rotation of approximately 40°; scapular elevation, upward rotation, and protraction; and glenohumeral joint elevation to about 100° to 120° along with full lateral rotation.[86] Shoulder complex muscles producing these motions in the standing position are: the trapezius and serratus anterior acting as a force couple at the scapula; the deltoid and supraspinatus providing the force couple at the glenohumeral joint; and the infraspinatus and teres minor providing lateral rotation. The contractions of the muscles are concentric except for the eccentric contraction of the trapezius during scapular protraction and for the posterior parts of the deltoid, which lengthen during

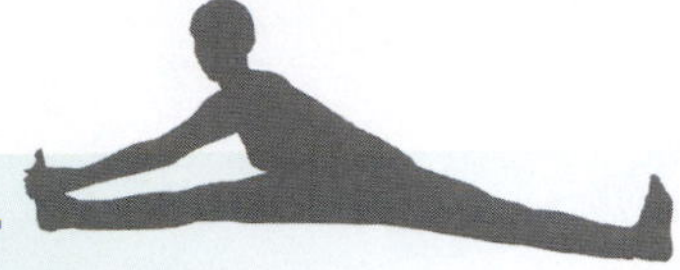

PRACTICE POINT

When a clinician wishes to isolate a muscle or tendon from other surrounding structures, he or she should first place the palpating fingers over the muscle or tendon to be palpated and then instruct the patient to provide a light contraction of the muscle. A mild contraction allows minimal activity sufficient for palpation of the muscle or tendon without excitation of surrounding dynamic structures.

movement from 0° to 60° and then shorten as elevation continues. When the extremity is returned to the side, the motions reverse to include sternoclavicular depression, protraction, and anterior rotation along with depression, downward rotation, and retraction of the scapula with glenohumeral adduction, extension, and medial rotation. However, the primary muscles controlling this motion are the same as with elevation. The type of contraction of these muscles changes to eccentric to control lowering of the arm against gravity.

Pulling

If we examine another functional motion such as pulling, muscle activity changes. When pulling an object, the shoulder's motion is adduction-extension, similar to lowering the arm after combing hair, but now the motion occurs against an external resistance. Examples of this situation include pulling down on a window to close it or an exercise using an overhead bar. With the hands in place on the bar connected to the overhead pulley, the pulling motion is open chain and includes similar joint motions as those just presented in lowering the arm after combing the hair. These joint motions include: elbow flexion; sternoclavicular depression and posterior rotation; scapular retraction, downward rotation, and depression; and glenohumeral adduction, extension, and rotation. However, glenohumeral rotation in this example changes depending on how the hands are placed; if the hands are placed close together, medial rotation occurs, but if the hands are widely separated, the motion is lateral rotation. In this activity, the muscles working include the glenohumeral adductors and extensors (latissimus dorsi, pectoralis major, long head of the triceps brachii, and posterior deltoid) and scapular downward rotators and depressors (pectoralis minor and rhomboids). They are all working concentrically to overcome the resistance.

When the overhead bar is fixed and the person performs a chin-up to lift the body weight, closed-chain motion occurs. The joint motions that occur during this activity include glenohumeral joint adduction, extension, and medial rotation along with scapular retraction, downward rotation, and depression. Concentric muscle activity of the muscles providing these joint motions occurs in pulling on the overhead bar to lift the body up. This example is similar to the pulling activity in the previous paragraph. In both of these motions, the muscle activity is the same except that in the first instance, the bar moves down while the body stays stationary, whereas in the second example, the body moves up while the bar remains stationary. When the person lowers the body from the chin-up position, eccentric contractions of the same muscle groups that lifted the body upward occur (glenohumeral extensors and adductors, and the scapular downward rotators and depressors). As these muscles work eccentrically, they control the rate and motion of lowering the body by flexing and abducting the glenohumeral joint and upwardly rotating, protracting, and elevating the scapula. In daily functional motions and sports activities, the muscle activity in a chin-up is similar to a gymnast on the rings moving into an iron cross from an arm hang. The muscles used are also similar to those needed in a pull-up when patients grasp overhead bed trapezes to lift their body weight for transfers and bedpan use.

Functional Deficiency Applications

At the glenohumeral joint, there are three to five muscles that can perform each motion (Table 5–7). Thus, weakness from an injury or paralysis of an individual muscle will cause functional deficits from loss of strength during a motion, but the arm and hand often can still be placed in desired positions through reliance on other muscles that also perform the motion.

On the other hand, the scapular muscles often perform very specific actions; therefore, a deficiency of a single muscle can seriously compromise use of the hand and arm. Although there is more than one scapular muscle performing any one scapular motion, these muscles must work in concert together to produce the motion correctly; if one is deficient, the motion usually does not occur as it should. Kibler[87] originally named this principle "scapular dyskinesis" to define an abnormal position and pattern of motion of the scapula. Although there are many factors that could lead to scapular dyskinesis, Kibler indicated that scapular dyskinesis may lead to many conditions such as subacromial impingement, glenohumeral instability, and Superior Labrum Anterior to Posterior (SLAP) lesions.

In normal subjects standing in the erect position with the arms at the sides, the medial border of the scapula is nearly parallel to the vertebral column. When the arm is raised overhead, the scapula rotates upward and simultaneously protracts on the rib cage, so that the medial border of the scapula assumes an oblique position, and its inferior angle lies approximately in line with the axilla yet remains in contact with the thorax. The serratus anterior, upper trapezius, and lower trapezius work together to produce this movement and simultaneously fixate the scapula in any partially upward rotated position. With dysfunction of the serratus anterior, the scapula is not held against the rib cage and the medial border is winged (Fig. 5.22). Scapulohumeral rhythm is abnormal with a dysfunctional serratus anterior, so the person is unable to fully elevate the arm normally. To compensate, some people with a serratus anterior deficiency will combine trapezius activity with a lateral trunk shift to position the hand overhead. In addition to the inability to elevate the shoulder for hand placement, the person with serratus anterior paralysis is unable to push on doors or drawers because without stabilization of the scapula by the serratus anterior, pressure on the extended hand causes the scapula to move posteriorly. This would be an example of scapular dyskinesis.

Isolated paralysis of the trapezius muscle can occur if the spinal accessory nerve is severed during radial neck dissection surgery for complete removal of lymph nodes in people with cancer of the head and neck. Although the trapezius is electromyographically inactive in the erect posture, clinicians have long noted that the resting posture of the scapula in the presence of paralysis of the trapezius is that of downward rotation, protraction, and depression.[64, 88] This dropped position is best attributed to loss of passive tension of the trapezius. The downward rotation position of the scapula in turn places the glenohumeral joint in a position of abduction, with forces on the humeral head promoting subluxation and pain in the sternoclavicular joint (Fig. 5.38). Functionally, people with excessive trapezius weakness have difficulty retracting the scapula, but usually they can partially elevate the arm by using the levator scapulae, the serratus anterior, the deltoid, and the pectoralis major.

Paralysis of both the trapezius and the serratus destroys scapular stability and its ability to upwardly rotate; since upward scapular rotation accounts for 60° of total glenohumeral elevation, and the arm cannot be elevated greater than 120°. If the scapula cannot be stabilized on the thorax, the rotator cuff's moment arm cannot be maintained, so its strength is diminished. If this happens, then the deltoid cannot achieve an appropriate position that will allow it to elevate the arm.

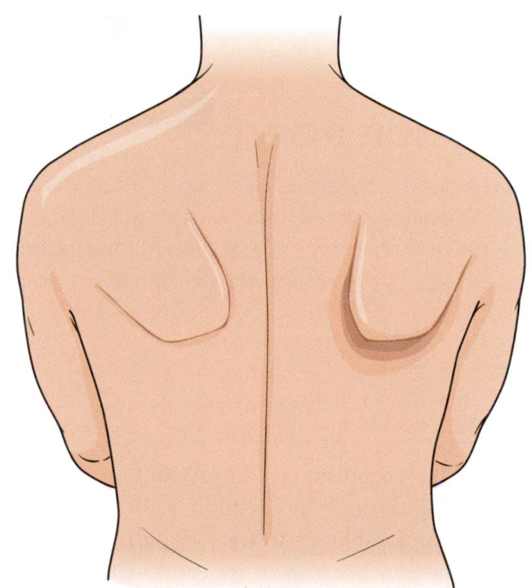

Figure 5.38 Weakness in the trapezius causes instability of the scapula with positioning in downward rotation and protraction.

Scapular stability, as has been mentioned, is crucial for efficient activity of the glenohumeral joint. The most important scapular stabilization occurs during glenohumeral elevation activities when the scapula is also simultaneously rotating upward and moving anteriorly and laterally on the thorax as it is providing glenohumeral stability. These scapular motions are the primary responsibility of the serratus anterior, upper trapezius, and lower trapezius. As has been discussed, weakness or paralysis of these muscles significantly impairs glenohumeral motion, but imbalance of these muscles' strength can also lead to injury within the glenohumeral joint. For example, in a shoulder with a strong upper trapezius and a proportionately weaker lower trapezius and/or serratus anterior, the scapula glides superiorly prior to rotating upward during glenohumeral elevation. This activity causes the humeral head to move into the upper portion of the glenoid fossa. If there is rotator cuff weakness in addition to this muscle imbalance, this upward migration of the humeral head becomes even more significant. As has been mentioned, the result is an impingement of those soft tissue structures beneath the subacromial arch.

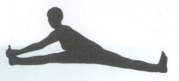

PRACTICE POINT

When investigating shoulder complex injuries, it is as vital for the clinician to examine scapular rotator strength as it is to evaluate rotator cuff strength. Many clinicians attend to the rotator cuff to the exclusion of the scapular rotators, but both are intimately connected to the health and stability of the glenohumeral joint. Therefore, the clinician must examine the scapular rotators for their ability, function, and performance during both isolated and functional activities.

Summary

The shoulder complex is comprised of four joints: three real joints and one pseudo joint. The glenohumeral joint is able to move through its extensive ranges of motion because of its construction and the contributions of the other joints within the shoulder complex. Although the acromioclavicular joint does not often succumb to injury because of its stability, it is not as secure as the sternoclavicular joint, which rarely is injured secondary to its strong ligamentous support. The good news is that the glenohumeral joint has more motion available to it than any other joint of the body; the bad news is that its mobility and lax ligamentous support make it susceptible to injury. The rotator cuff provides active support to stabilize the humerus in the glenoid fossa. Although the scapula is not secured directly to the thorax by a bony joint, the scapulothoracic joint is positioned and moved by its dynamic stabilizers—the trapezius, rhomboids, levator scapulae, pectoralis minor, and serratus anterior. These muscles form force couples to provide rotation of the scapula, just as the rotator cuff forms a force couple with the deltoid to rotate the humerus in the glenoid during arm elevation. Through these scapular muscles, the scapula provides a stable base from which the humerus moves and performs functional activities. Just as the scapular stabilizers hold the scapula in position for the glenohumeral joint, the rotator cuff holds the humerus in position to allow performance of upper extremity functions. As the glenohumeral joint moves into flexion or abduction, the scapula and humerus each move throughout elevation to provide maximal reach. This relationship between scapula and humerus movement is called scapulohumeral rhythm, an important ratio of movement between the two segments, which is overall a 1:2 ratio between the scapula and humerus movements. Larger muscles such as the deltoid, pectoralis major, latissimus dorsi, and teres major are considered the movers of the shoulder joint and provide the power for forceful shoulder movements. If any of these muscles fail to function as they should, injury to the shoulder is likely. Which muscles function during shoulder complex movements is dependent upon the shoulder's position relative to gravity and the presence of external forces and how they are applied.

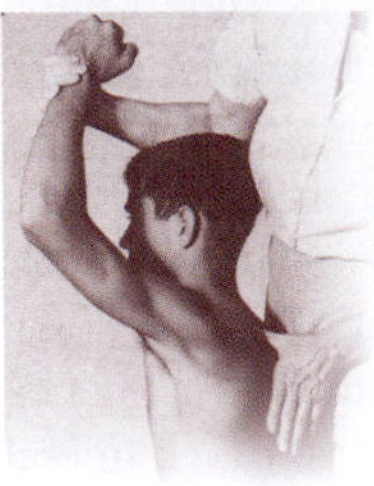

CLINICAL SCENARIO SOLUTION

As she expected, Ella found mild weakness in the rotator cuff and even more weakness in the scapular stabilizers during her examination of Tyler's shoulder complex. Fortunately, he has full range of motion in the region, but she knows that it is weakness of these crucial muscles that has lead to Tyler's present complaints of shoulder pain. She explains to him how the weakness in these two groups is causing the pain and impingement he is suffering in the glenohumeral joint. She assures him that with proper a proper rehabilitation program, he will be able to resume his full work responsibilities.

Discussion Questions

1. Explain the motions at the sternoclavicular joint and acromioclavicular joint, and identify the role they play in scapular motion.
2. Define scapulohumeral rhythm and explain its significance.
3. Illustrate how weakness in the muscles stabilizing the scapula may result in impingement of the glenohumeral joint.
4. Describe the roles of the deltoid and rotator cuff during glenohumeral elevation.
5. Identify the shoulder complex muscles that perform an activity such as a push-up, moving into the elbow extended position, explaining their actions; then identify the muscles required to return to the start position with the elbows flexed.
6. Explain how you can differentiate between palpation of the upper trapezius and the levator scapulae, and know which muscle you are palpating with confidence.

Lab Activities

1. On the bones, identify the following parts and bony landmarks. Determine which ones are palpable on a human subject, and identify these on a partner. (Wear appropriate attire for this unit to permit exposure of the shoulder and shoulder girdle.)

Scapula

acromion process
spine
coracoid process
supraspinous fossa
infraspinous fossa
glenoid cavity
superior angle
inferior angle
medial border
axillary border
supraglenoid tubercle
infraglenoid tubercle

Humerus

head
neck
greater tubercle
lesser tubercle
bicipital (intertubercular) groove
deltoid tuberosity

Sternum

manubrium body
xiphoid process
jugular (sternal) notch
facet for clavicle

Clavicle

trapezoid line
conoid tubercle
articulating surfaces of sternal and acromial ends

2. Locate the sternoclavicular, acromioclavicular, and glenohumeral joints on the bones or skeleton, and perform all movements that are possible at these joints. Identify axes about which each movement occurs.
3. Passively move your partner's shoulder through its range of flexion and hyperextension; medial and lateral rotation (shoulder abducted to 90° and elbow flexed to 90° to rule out supination and pronation); and abduction (laterally rotate at 90° of abduction) to reach maximum range of motion. State the approximate range of motion and the end feels for each.
4. With your partner in prone, passively move the scapula through its normal ranges of elevation and depression, protraction and retraction, and upward and downward rotation.
5. With a skin pen, mark the following landmarks on your partner (in a sitting position):
   a. The two angles of the scapula
   b. The three borders of the scapula
   c. The spine, acromion process, and glenoid fossa
   d. Spinous processes of C-7 and T-12
   e. Outline the clavicle

6. Use the marked side for reference and have your partner perform motions of abduction, flexion, medial rotation (place hand behind back), and lateral rotation (place hand behind neck). Observe the motions from anterior and posterior views and palpate the motions of both the scapula and the humerus when the shoulder is at the side (0°) and when the shoulder is at 45°, 90°, 135°, and 180° of abduction.
7. On the bones, identify the muscles and the attachments for these muscles connecting the:
   a. Shoulder girdle with trunk
   b. Scapula and humerus
   c. Trunk and humerus

   Note particularly the:
   a. Lines of action
   b. Muscles with extensive proximal attachments and, hence, the multiple actions
   c. Movements these muscles can perform
8. Identify the muscles that:
   a. Flex the shoulder
   b. Extend the shoulder
   c. Abduct the shoulder
   d. Adduct the shoulder
   e. Medially and laterally rotate the shoulder
   f. Elevate the shoulder girdle
   g. Depress the shoulder girdle
   h. Protract the shoulder girdle
   i. Retract the shoulder girdle
   j. Upwardly rotate the scapula
   k. Downwardly rotate the scapula
9. Palpate and obtain isolated contractions of the muscles as described in the text and in Tables 5–4, 5–5, and 5–6.
10. Place your hand firmly against the lateral border of your partner's scapula; stabilize the scapula so it cannot move. Instruct your partner to slowly abduct the arm while you continue to stabilize the scapula. Note the amount of elevation motion present. Now, have your partner forward flex the shoulder while you continue to stabilize the scapula and note the motion at its end range. Finally, repeat both motions and allow the scapula to move freely. Compare the quantity and quality of both motions in both conditions. Explain your findings.
11. With your partner in the supine position, place palpating fingers on the biceps and triceps; have your partner raise the arm overhead and then return the arm to the start position at his or her side Note which muscles were active and when they were active throughout the motion. Now, place palpating fingers on the costosternal and clavicular heads of the pectoralis major and have your partner repeat the motion while you note which muscles were active and when they were active throughout the motion. Explain what you palpated through these two movements.
12. Repeat the palpation and movements in #11, but this time offer resistance to movement in both elevation and returning the arm to the side. Explain the differences in your palpation between this activity and what you palpated during the activity in #11.
13. Functional analysis of the shoulder complex in any three of the activities listed below. Perform the analysis by palpating muscles at rest and during activity and observing motions and muscles on a partner or a member of a small group. The analysis should include:
   1) The name of the motion at each joint area;
   2) The primary muscle group(s) responsible for the motion or for maintaining a position; and
   3) The type of contraction that occurs (eccentric, concentric, or isometric).

Difficult activities should be modified so that injury or exhaustion does not occur with the repetitions required; for example, push-ups should be done from the knees (modified) instead of the toes (regular), and chin-ups should be done with partial support of the feet on the floor (modified).

a. Seated push-up in a wheelchair (or arm chair) or standing push-up in parallel bars.

b. Have the person perform a seated or standing push-up; when in the highest position, keep the elbows straight and lower the body by permitting the scapula to elevate. Measure how many inches the body can be elevated by scapular elevation and depression alone.

c. Modified push-ups. How does muscle activity in these push-ups differ from push-ups in the seated or standing position?

d. Chin-ups from the erect position (modified).

e. Pull-ups from a supine position (as in a bed with an overhead trapeze bar).

f. Push forward on an object such as a table or door.

g. Pull back on an object such as a table or door.

h. Reach overhead to grasp a pulley or an open window; then pull down.

i. Lift a backpack or purse from the floor; then lower it back to the floor.

j. Walking with crutches, nonweight-bearing one leg.

k. Propelling a manual wheelchair.

Sports activities such as swimming, throwing, or tennis or playing musical instruments such as violin, cello, flute, and so on.

14. Compare your partner's ability to provide resistance against you in elbow flexion when your shoulder is elevated to 90° in the sagittal plane to your partner's ability to provide resistance in elbow flexion when his or her shoulder is hyperextended 10° to 20°. Which position provides the greater force output by your partner? Explain why this occurs.

References

1. Perry J. Normal upper extremity kinesiology. *Physical Therapy* 58:265–278, 1978.
2. O'Brien SJ, Arnoczky SP, Warren RF, et al. Developmental anatomy of the shoulder and anatomy of the glenohumeral joint. In Rockwood CA, Matsen FA (eds): *The Shoulder*, *Vol I*. Philadelphia: WB Saunders, 1990.
3. Moseley HF. Recurrent dislocation of the shoulder. *Postgraduate Medicine* 31:23–29, 1962.
4. Moseley HF. The clavicle: Its anatomy and function. *Clinical Orthopaedics Related Research* 58:17–27, 1968.
5. Goldstein B. Shoulder anatomy and biomechanics. *Physical Medicine and Rehabilitation Clinics of North America* 15(2):313–349, 2004.
6. Ludewig PM, Behrens SA, Meyer SM, Spoden SM, Wilson LA. Three-dimensional clavicular motion during arm elevation: Reliability and descriptive data. *Journal of Orthopaedic and Sports Physical Therapy* 43(3):140–149, 2004.
7. Kapandji IA. *The Physiology of the Joints, Vol 1, Upper Limb*, ed 5. Edinburgh: Churchill Livingstone, 1982.
8. Finley MA, Lee RY. Effect of sitting posture on three-dimensional scapular kinematics measured by skin-mounted electromagnetic tracking sensors. *Archives of Physical Medicine and Rehabilitation* 84(4):563–568, 2003.
9. Lewis JS, Green A, Wright C. Subacromial impingement syndrome: The role of posture and muscle imbalance. *Journal of Shoulder and Elbow Surgery* 14(4):385–392, 2005.
10. Blakely RL, Palmer ML. Analysis of rotation accompanying shoulder flexion. *Physical Therapy* 64(8):1214–1216, 1984.
11. Ludewig PM, Cook TM, Nawoczenski DA. Three-dimensional scapular orientation and muscle activity at selected positions of humeral elevation. *Journal of Orthopaedic and Sports Physical Therapy* 24(2):57–65, 1996.
12. Lukasiewicz AC, Michener LA, Pratt N, Sennett BJ, McClure PW. Comparison of three-dimensional scapular position and orientation between subjects with and without shoulder impingement. *Journal of Orthopaedic and Sports Physical Therapy* 29(10):574–586, 1999.
13. McClure PW, Michener LA, Sennett BJ, Karduna AR. Direct three-dimensional measurement of scapular kinematics during dynamic movements in vivo. *Journal of Shoulder and Elbow Surgery* 10(3):269–277, 2001.
14. Ludewig PM, Phadke V, Braman JP, Hassett DR, Cieminski CJ, LaPrade RF. Motion of the shoulder complex during multiplanar humeral elevation. *Journal of Bone and Joint Surgery* 91A(2):378–389, 2009.

15. Teece RM, Lunden JB, Lloyd AS, Kaiser AP, Cieminski CJ, Ludewig PM. Three-dimensional acromioclavicular joint motions during elevation of the arm. *Journal of Orthopaedic and Sports Physical Therapy* 38(4):181–190, 2008.

16. Lewis MM, Ballet FL, Kroll PG, Bloom N. En bloc clavicular resection: Operative procedure and postoperative testing of function. Case reports. *Clinical Orthopaedics and Related Research* 193:214–220, 1985.

17. Inman VT, Saunders JB, Abbott LC. Observations on the function of the shoulder joint. *Journal of Bone and Joint Surgery Am* 26:1–30, 1944.

18. Conway A, Malone TR, Conway P. Patellar alignment/tracking alteration: Effect on force output and perceived pain. *Isokinetics and Exercise Science* 2:9–17, 1992.

19. Peat M. Functional anatomy of the shoulder complex. *Physical Therapy* 66(12):1855–1865, 1986.

20. Van der Helm FC, Pronk GM. Three-dimensional recording and description of motions of the shoulder mechanism. *Journal of Biomechanical Engineering* 117(1):27–40, 1995.

21. DePalma AF. Degenerative changes in sternoclavicular and acromioclavicular joints in various decades. Springfield, IL: C.C. Thomas, 1957.

22. Kelley MJ. Anatomic and biomechanical rationale for rehabilitation of the athlete's shoulder. *Journal of Sport Rehabilitation* 4:122–154, 1995.

23. Scibek JS, Mell AG, Downie BK, Carpenter JE, Hughes RE. Shoulder kinematics in patients with full-thickness rotator cuff tears after a subacromial injection. *Journal of Shoulder and Elbow Surgery* 17(1):172–181, 2008.

24. Ferrari DA. Capsular ligaments of the shoulder. *American Journal of Sports Medicine* 18(1):20–24, 1990.

25. Curl LA, Warren RF. Glenohumeral joint stability: Selective cutting studies on the static capsular restraints. *Clinical Orthopaedics and Related Research* 333:54–65, 1996.

26. Hawkins RJ, Schutte JP, Janda DH, Huckell GH. Translation of the glenohumeral joint with the patient under anesthesia. *Journal of Shoulder and Elbow Surgery* 5(4):286–292, 1996.

27. Itoi E, Berglund LJ, Grabowski JJ, Naggar L, Morrey BF, An KN. Superior-inferior stability of the shoulder: Role of the coracohumeral ligament and the rotator interval capsule. *Mayo Clinic Proceedings* 73(6):508–515, 1998.

28. Soslowsky LJ, Carpenter JE, Bucchieri JS, Flatow EL. Biomechanics of the rotator cuff. *Orthopedic Clinics of North America* 28(1):17–30, 1997.

29. Neer CS. *Shoulder Reconstruction*. Philadelphia: WB Saunders, 1990.

30. Jobe CM. Gross anatomy of the shoulder. In Rockwood CA, Matsen FA (eds): *The Shoulder, Vol 1*. Philadelphia: WB Saunders, 1990.

31. Ovesen J, Nielsen S. Stability of the shoulder joint: Cadaver study of stabilizing structures. *Acta Orthopaedica Scandinavica* 56(2):149–151, 1985.

32. Flatow EL, Duralde XA, Nicholson GP, Pollock RG, Bigliani LU. Arthroscopic resection of the distal clavicle with a superior approach. *Journal of Shoulder and Elbow Surgery* 4(1 Pt 1):41–50, 1995.

33. Neer CS, Poppen NK. Supraspinatus outlet. *Orthopaedic Trans* 11:234, 1987.

34. Woodward TW, Best TM. The painful shoulder: Part II. Acute and chronic disorders. *American Family Physician* 61(11):3291–3300, 2000.

35. Cools A, Witvrouw E, Mahieu N, Danneels L. Isokinetic scapular muscle performance in overhead athletes with and without impingement symptoms. *Journal of Athletic Training* 40(2):104–110, 2005.

36. Cools AM, Witvrouw EE, De Clercq GA, et al. Scapular muscle recruitment pattern: Electromyographic response of the trapezius muscle to sudden shoulder movement before and after a fatiguing exercise. *Journal of Orthopaedic and Sports Physical Therapy* 32(5):221–229, 2004.

37. Ebaugh DD, Karduna AR, McClure PW. Scapulothoracic and glenohumeral kinematics following an external rotation fatigue protocol. *Journal of Orthopaedic and Sports Physical Therapy* 36(8):557–571, 2006.

38. Bradley JP, Laudner KG, Lephart SM, Myers JB, Pasquale MR. Scapular dysfunction in throwers with pathologic internal impingement. *Journal of Orthopaedic and Sports Physical Therapy* 36(7):485–494, 2006.

39. Reid DC, Saboe L, Burham R. Current research in selected shoulder problems. In Donatelli R (ed): *Physical Therapy of the Shoulder*, New York: Churchill Livingstone, 1987.

40. Bayley JC, Cochran TP, Sledge CG. The weight-bearing shoulder: The impingement syndrome in paraplegics. *Journal of Bone and Joint Surgery Am* 69(5):676–678, 1987.

41. Davis JL, Growney ES. Three-dimensional kinematics of the shoulder complex during wheelchair propulsion: a technical report. *Journal of Rehabilitation Research and Development* 35(1):61–72, 1998.

42. Smith LK. Poliomyelitis and the post-polio syndrome. In Umphred DA (ed): *Neurological Rehabilitation*, ed 2, St Louis: CV Mosby, 1990.

43. Brewer BJ. Aging of the rotator cuff. *American Journal of Sports Medicine* 7(2):102–110, 1979.

44. Ferrari DA. Capsular ligaments of the shoulder: Anatomical and functional study of the anterior superior capsule. *American Journal of Sports Medicine* 18(1):20–24, 1990.

45. Birnbaum K, Prescher A, Heller KD. Anatomic and functional aspects of the kinetics of the shoulder joint capsule and the subacromial bursa. *Surgical and Radiologic Anatomy* 21(1):41–45, 1998.

46. Murray MP, Gore DR, Gardner GM, Mollinger LA. Shoulder motion and muscle strength of normal men and women in two age groups. *Clinical Orthopaedics and Related Research* 192:268–273, 1985.

47. Bechtol CO. Biomechanics of the shoulder. *Clinical Orthopaedics and Related Research* 146:37–41, 1980.

48. Norkin C, White D. *Measurement of Joint Motion: A Guide to Goniometry*, ed 2. Philadelphia: FA Davis, 1995.

49. Brown LP, Niehues SL, Harrah A, Yavorsky P, Hirshman HP. Upper extremity range of motion and isokinetic strength of the internal and external shoulder rotators in major league baseball players. *American Journal of Sports Medicine* 16(6):577–585, 1988.

50. Chang DE, Buschbacher LP, Edlich RF. Limited joint mobility in power lifters. *American Journal of Sports Medicine* 16:280–284, 1988.

51. Hislop HJ, Montgomery P. *Daniels and Worthingham's Muscle Testing: Techniques of manual examination*, ed 7. Philadelphia: WB Saunders, 2002.

52. Morrey BF, An K. Biomechanics of the shoulder. In Rockwood CA, Matsen FA (eds): *The Shoulder, Vol 1*. Philadelphia: WB Saunders, 1990.

53. Boone DC, Azen SP. Normal range of motion of joints in male subjects. *Journal of Bone and Joint Surgery Am* 61(5):756–759, 1979.

54. Doody SG, Freedman L, Waterland JC. Shoulder movements during abduction in the scapular plane. *Archives of Physical Medicine and Rehabilitation* 51(10):595–604, 1970.

55. Freedman L, Munro RR. Abduction of the arm in the scapular plane: Scapular and glenohumeral movements. A roentgenographic study. *Journal of Bone and Joint Surgery Am* 48(8):1503–1510, 1966.

56. Perry J. Biomechanics of the shoulder. In Rowe C (ed): *The Shoulder*. New York: Churchill Livingstone, 1988.

57. Greenfield B, Donatelli R, Wooden MJ, Wilkes J. Isokinetic evaluation of shoulder rotational strength between the plane of the scapula and the frontal plane. *American Journal of Sports Medicine* 18(2):124–128, 1990.

58. Kaltenborn FM. *Mobilization of the Extremity Joints*. Oslo: Olaf Norlis Bokhandel,1980.

59. Burkhead WZ. The biceps tendon. In Rockwood CA, Matsen FA (eds): *The Shoulder, Vol 2*. Philadelphia: WB Saunders, 1990.

60. Bagg SD, Forrest WJ. A biomechanical analysis of scapular rotation during arm abduction in the scapular plane. *American Journal of Physical Medicine* 67:238–245, 1988.

61. Poppen NK, Walker PS. Normal and abnormal motion of the shoulder. *Journal of Bone and Joint Surgery Am* 58(2):195–201, 1976.

62. Ludewig PM, Reynolds JF. The association of scapular kinematics and glenohumeral joint pathologies. *Journal of Orthopaedic and Sports Physical Therapy* 39(2):90–104, 2009.

63. Meyer KE, Saether EE, Soiney EK, Shebeck MS, Paddock KL, Ludewig PM. Three-dimensional scapular kinematics during the throwing motion. *Journal of Applied Biomechanics* 24(1):24–34, 2008.

64. Brunnstrom S. Muscle testing around the shoulder girdle. *Journal of Bone and Joint Surgery Am* 23:263–272, 1941.

65. Howell SM, Imobersteg AM, Seger DH, Marone PJ. Clarification of the role of the supraspinatus in shoulder function. *Journal of Bone and Joint Surgery Am* 68(3):398–404, 1986.

66. Hughes RE, Niebur G, Liu J, An KN. Comparison of two methods for computing abduction moment arms of the rotator cuff. *Journal of Biomechanics* 31(2):157–160, 1998.

67. Kuechle DK, Newman SR, Itoi E, Morrey BF, An KN. Shoulder muscle moment arms during horizontal flexion and elevation. *Journal of Shoulder Elbow Surgery* 6(5):429–439, 1997.

68. Lehmkuhl LD, Smith LK. *Brunnstrom's Clinical Kinesiology,* ed 4. Philadelphia: FA Davis, 1983.

69. Andrews JR, Carson WGJ, McLeod WD. Glenoid labrum tears related to the long head of the biceps. *American Journal of Sports Medicine* 13(5):337–341, 1985.

70. Furlani J. Electromyographic study of the m. biceps brachii in movements at the glenohumeral joint. *Acta Anatomica* 96(2):270–284, 1976.

71. Itoi E, Kuechle DK, Newman SR, Morrey BF, An KN. Stabilising function of the biceps in stable and unstable shoulders. *Journal of Bone and Joint Surgery Br* 75(4):546–550, 1993.

72. Karistinos A, Paulos LE. Anatomy and function of the tendon of the long head of the biceps muscle. *Operative Techniques in Sports Medicine* 15(1):2–6, 2007.

73. Schultz JS. Clinical evaluation of the shoulder. *Physician Medicine and Rehabilitation Clinics of North America* 15(2):351–371, 2004.

74. Moore K. *Clinically Oriented Anatomy*. Baltimore: Williams & Wilkins, 2004.

75. Pontillo M, Orishimo KF, Kremenic IJ, McHugh MP, Mullaney MJ, Tyler T. Shoulder musculature activity and stabilization during upper extremity weight-bearing activities. *North American Journal of Sports Physical Therapy* 2(2):90–96, 2007.

76. Markhede G, Monastyrski J, Stener B. Shoulder function after deltoid muscle removal. *Acta Orthopaedica Scandinavica* 56(3):242–244, 1985.

77. Liu J, Hughes RE, Smutz WP, Niebur G, Nan-An K. Roles of deltoid and rotator cuff muscles in shoulder elevation. *Clinical Biomechanics* 12(1):32–38, 1997.

78. Kumar VP, Balasubramaniam P. The role of atmospheric pressure in stabilising the shoulder: An experimental study. *Journal of Bone and Joint Surgery Br* 67(5):719–721, 1985.

79. Basmajian JV. *Muscles Alive: Their Function Revealed by Electromyography*, ed 4. Baltimore: Williams & Wilkins, 1978.

80. Berne RM, Levy MN. *Physiology*. St. Louis: Mosby, 1998.

81. Duca CJ, Forrest W. Force analysis of individual muscles acting simultaneously on the shoulder joint during isometric abduction. *Journal of Biomechanics* 6:385–393, 1973.

82. Poppen NK, Walker PS. Forces at the glenohumeral joint in abduction. *Clinical Orthopaedics and Related Research* 135:165–170, 1978.

83. Otis JC, Warren RF, Backus SI, Santer TJ, Mabrey JD. Torque production in the shoulder of the normal young adult male. *American Journal of Sports Medicine* 18(2):119–123, 1990.

84. Ivey FM, Jr., Calhoun JH, Rusche K, Bierschenk J. Isokinetic testing of shoulder strength: Normal values. *Archives of Physical Medicine and Rehabilitation* 66(6):384–386, 1985.

85. Hinton RY. Isokinetic evaluation of shoulder rotational strength in high school baseball pitchers. *American Journal of Sports Medicine* 16(3):274–279, 1988.

86. Veeger HE, Magermans DJ, Nagels J, Chadwick EK, Van der Helm FC. A kinematical analysis of the shoulder after arthroplasty during a hair combing task. *Clinical Biomechanics* 21(Suppl 1):S39–44, 2006.

87. Kibler W, McMullen J. Scapular dyskinesis and its relation to shoulder pain. *Journal of the American Academy of Orthopaedic Surgeons* 11(2):142–151, 2003.

88. Herring D, King AI, Connelly M. New rehabilitation concepts in management of radical neck dissection syndrome: A clinical report. *Physical Therapy* 67(7):1095–1099, 1987.

Elbow and Forearm Complex

CHAPTER OUTLINE

Learning Outcomes
Clinical Scenario
Introduction
Bones
Humerus
Ulna
Radius
Joints
Humeroulnar and Humeroradial Joints
Radioulnar Articulations
Muscles
Elbow Flexors
Elbow Extensors
Forearm Supinators
Forearm Pronators
Functional Movement and the Muscles of the Elbow/Forearm Region
Muscles as Agonists, Antagonists, and/or Synergists
Selection of Muscles in Functional Movement: Synergistic Contractions
One-Joint and Multijoint Muscles of the Elbow and Forearm
Typical Elbow and Forearm Muscular Function: Summary and Comparisons
Closed Kinematic Chain Motion at the Elbow Complex
Analyses of Muscle Activity during Common Functional Movements
Placing the Hand behind the Head
Pulling

LEARNING OUTCOMES

This chapter investigates the elbow and forearm complex. By the end of this chapter, you should be able to:

- ❑ Identify the bones, joints, soft tissue, and muscles of the elbow/forearm complex;
- ❑ Discuss the relationship between the elbow and radioulnar joints and their contribution to functional movement;
- ❑ List muscles that are prime movers in elbow flexion, elbow extension, forearm pronation and forearm supination;
- ❑ Discuss the influence of gravity and body position in determining muscles acting on the elbow/forearm complex during functional motions;
- ❑ Name muscle groups that function to position and move the elbow and forearm in specific functional activities;
- ❑ Describe commonly encountered movement disorders of the elbow complex and their functional consequences.

CHAPTER OUTLINE

Summary
Clinical Scenario Solution
Discussion Questions
Lab Activities
References

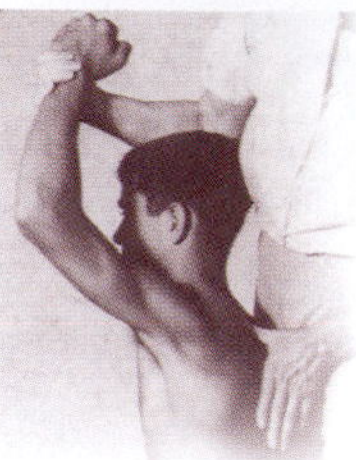

CLINICAL SCENARIO

Bethany has just met her new patient, Chris. Chris is a manager of a prosperous shoe store and presents with weakness in his grip and pain and swelling over the medial surface of his elbow, especially when he flexes his wrist. However, his chief complaint and concern is not the pain at the elbow but rather his weakened grasp, which is interfering with his ability to maintain the quickly changing stockroom. He complains of frequent incidences of what he calls "having the dropsies." Bethany knows that she must examine both his elbow and wrist area to identify the source of his pain and weakness. She needs to pinpoint the area of tenderness and make some recommendations to manage the pain and swelling. She must also test all of the muscles that are attached in the painful area and primarily involved in grasp. As Bethany begins her assessment and manual muscle tests on Chris, she is thinking of each of these muscles and their functions, and she is concerned about how she can convince this high-energy workaholic to limit his activity in order to rest the area.

Introduction

The elbow region is a complex structure that includes three individual joints that are surrounded by only one capsule. The first two joints are the humeroulnar and humeroradial joints; these articulations are what we typically think of as the "elbow." Another joint, the proximal radioulnar articulation, is the third joint of the elbow complex. Even though this joint lies within the elbow capsule, it is technically not part of the elbow joint; it is where forearm rotation occurs and is not involved in movement at the elbow. Although motion occurs and an articulation exists between the humerus and radius, most of the contact and osteokinematic elbow motion comes from the humeroulnar rather than from the humeroradial articulation. These two articulations (humeroulnar and humeroradial) act as one joint, creating a modified uniaxial hinge joint with one degree of freedom. This uniaxial joint's motions include elbow flexion and extension in the sagittal plane around a medial-lateral axis. Since the uniaxial elbow joint moves in only the sagittal plane, the uniaxial proximal radioulnar joint also offers only one degree of freedom. The proximal radioulnar joint also has one degree of freedom, but its motion occurs in the transverse plane around a vertical axis. The radioulnar joint provides forearm supination and pronation. The elbow and radioulnar joints are each uniaxial, but because they work together in different planes, they collectively offer a variety of functional movements.

The combined two degrees of freedom offered by these elbow and forearm joints provide numerous hand placement possibilities by rotating the forearm and lengthening or shortening the distance between the hand and the shoulder. Although this mobility is vital for hand positioning and function in the open chain, equally important is the elbow's ability to provide stability during closed chain activities such as pull-ups, push-ups, and while using assistive devices during ambulation. The elbow's anatomy provides this significant stability because of its bony congruency.

In addition to this bony congruency, several muscles crossing the elbow complex also provide stability and functional mobility. There are five main muscles of the elbow complex, two extensors and three flexors. Additionally, the radioulnar joint's motion is supplied with contributions from four primary muscles, a pair of supinators and a pair of pronators.

Other structures are important to the stability and function of the elbow complex. Ligaments provide vital stability to these joints. Branches of the brachial plexus innervate elbow and forearm muscles; these branches include predominantly the musculocutaneous, radial, and median nerves, arising from C5 through C7.

Pathological conditions affecting the elbow and forearm region are common and lead to varying degrees of functional impairment. As with any other region of the body, specific pathological conditions affect various tissues and can include acute injuries such as bony fracture, muscular strain, ligamentous sprain, distraction injuries of the bony partners, or chronic injuries including overuse or repetitive microtrauma. Because of its location as the middle link in the upper extremity, the elbow complex is prone to distraction injuries and to a whole series of either acute or chronic processes involving its muscles, tendons, ligaments, and peripheral nerves.[1,2]

Bones

The elbow complex possesses one of the more congruent joint designs of the body. Bones in the elbow region possess notches, ridges, and grooves that fit like jigsaw puzzle pieces, creating both stability and function (Fig. 6.1).

Humerus

The proximal articulating bone of the elbow joint is the humerus, a long bone with several distinct markings on its distal end, some of which are palpable. The most distinct palpable bony landmarks are the epicondyles. The epicondyles are prominences immediately proximal to the distal condyles of the humerus. They are the most easily identifiable landmarks in this region. When the shoulder is laterally rotated, the **medial epicondyle** lies closest to the trunk; the less prominent **lateral epicondyle** lies on the lateral side of the humerus, farthest from the trunk. When the humerus is medially rotated, however, the medial epicondyle points posteriorly, and the lateral epicondyle points anteriorly. In anatomical position, it is easy to locate the large and prominent medial epicondyle. The medial epicondyle serves as the proximal attachment site for a primary forearm pronator (pronator teres), for a major stabilizing ligament (the ulnar collateral ligament), and for most of the wrist and finger flexor muscles. The lateral epicondyle, although less prominent, is easily located by positioning the elbow at 90 ° of flexion with the forearm in midposition as if to shake someone's hand; as the body leans laterally towards an adjacent wall (on the flexed elbow side), the knobby bony landmark that makes contact with the wall is the lateral epicondyle. The lateral epicondyle serves as the attachment for many of the wrist and finger/thumb extensors and the forearm supinator. Superior to the lateral epicondyle is the **lateral supracondylar ridge**, a landmark that is palpable between the lateral head of the triceps posteriorly and the brachioradialis muscle anteriorly.

The distal humerus that forms the proximal portion of the elbow joint has two prominences, the medial **trochlea** and the lateral **capitulum.** The trochlea articulates with the ulna and the capitulum articulates with the radius (Fig. 6.1). The hourglass-shaped trochlea is large and comprised of two portions that are separated by the **trochlear groove.** The capitulum is almost spheroid in shape. Between the lateral spheroid-shaped capitulum and medial hourglass-shaped trochlea is the

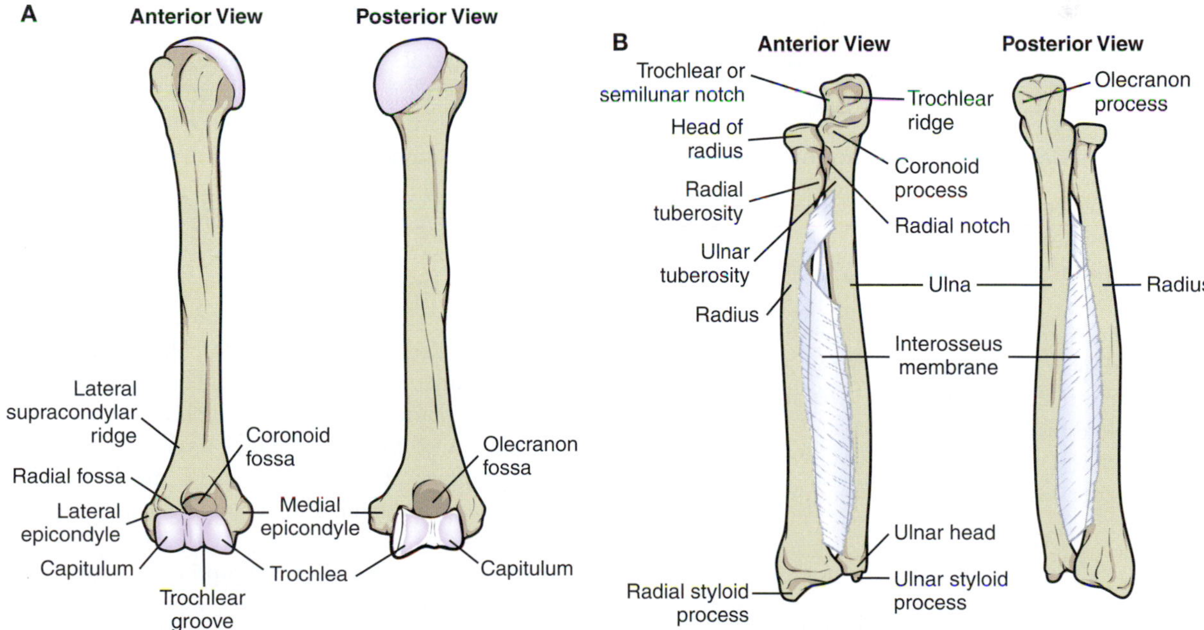

Figure 6.1 Anterior and posterior view of humerus, radius, and ulna highlighting bony characteristics. **A)** Humerus: anterior and posterior view. **B)** Ulna and radius: anterior and posterior view,

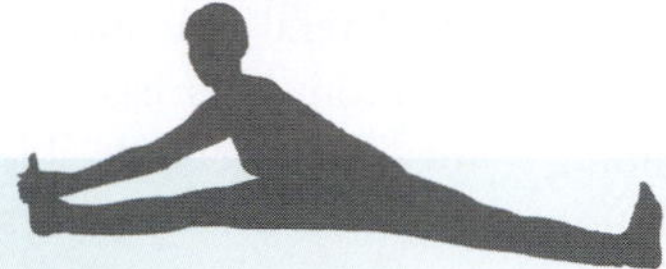

PRACTICE POINT

Because of multiple tendinous attachments to both the medial and lateral epicondyle, the epicondyles are frequent sites of pain due to either acute injury or chronic overuse. As mentioned, many of the wrist extensors have their proximal attachments on the lateral epicondyle, whereas the wrist flexors attach to the medial epicondyle. With chronic overuse, degenerative tissue changes may occur within the tendon at its attachment onto the epicondyle, leading to a condition known as epicondylopathy. Lateral epicondylopathy is commonly called "tennis elbow" because of its prevalence among people who play racquet sports. With the advent of occupations which require extended periods of work at a computer, this condition is now commonly seen in groups such as computer workers. Clinically, lateral epicondylopathy is characterized by pain that is usually exacerbated with resisted wrist extension. Medial epicondylopathy, commonly called "golfer's elbow," also results from overuse pathomechanics of the structures attached to the medial epicondyle. In preadolescents, we see a medial epicondylar condition known as "Little League elbow." This condition is a complex of symptoms sustained by the skeletally immature, resulting from repetitive overload trauma and/or abnormal pathomechanics such as excessive compressive or valgus forces. Little League elbow begins as a stress of the **apophyseal plate** and may progress to apophysitis,[3] secondary ossification changes, vascular disruption or irritation of any of the supporting structures.[1, 4] Elbow pain, swelling and loss of full extension motion are signs and symptoms of this syndrome. Regardless of the age group with which we work, clinicians are reminded that one of our most important roles as health care professionals with any of these conditions is the important role we play in assessing the patient's pathomechanics and teaching effective ways to change deleterious movement habits to help prevent reoccurrence.

capitulotrochlear groove. The radial head slides within this groove when the elbow flexes. Superior to the trochlea on the anterior humerus is the **coronoid fossa;** when the elbow fully flexes, the ulna's coronoid process moves into this fossa. Similarly, superior to the capitulum is the **radial fossa,** The radial fossa houses the radial head at the end of elbow flexion. The posterior aspect of the distal humerus has a pronounced **olecranon fossa,** providing a deep and stable articulating surface for the superior ulna when the elbow is in full extension (Fig. 6.1).

Distinctive Bony Features of the Distal Humerus

- Medial epicondyle
- Lateral epicondyle
- Lateral supracondylar ridge
- Trochlea
- Trochlear groove
- Capitulum
- Capitulotrochlear groove
- Coronoid fossa
- Radial fossa
- Olecranon fossa

Ulna

The ulna is the more integral articulating bony partner with the humerus at the elbow, forming the humeroulnar joint. Located on the medial forearm in the anatomical position, the ulna plays a very prominent role at the elbow but provides minimal function at the wrist. The **olecranon process** is the distinctive posterior prominence of the superior ulna and is the most posterior portion of the elbow when the joint is flexed. The dorsal margin of the ulna may be palpated along its entire length from the olecranon process to the styloid process of the ulna at the wrist. Medial to the olecranon process is a groove between it and the medial epicondyle; this groove houses the ulnar nerve, which is palpated as a round cord within the groove.

The concave ulnar **trochlear notch** articulates with the more proximal humeral trochlea to form the medial elbow joint. Shaped like a half-moon, this ulnar articulation is also known as the **semilunar notch.** This large articulating ulnar surface is divided in the center by a prominent **trochlear or longitudinal ridge** that articulates with the trochlear groove of its humeral companion. During elbow flexion and extension, the ulna's trochlear ridge glides within the humerus' trochlear groove. The anterior surface of the ulna is marked by a distinctive, sharp, medial superior process called the **coronoid process.** When the elbow flexes, this ulnar process moves to fit snugly into the **coronoid fossa** of the humerus, providing stability in that position. Inferior to the coronoid process is the **ulnar tuberosity,** an attachment site for a primary elbow flexor muscle, the brachialis. On the lateral aspect of the proximal ulna, distal to the trochlear notch is the slightly concave **radial notch.** This radial notch articulates with the radius to form the proximal radioulnar joint (Fig. 6.1).

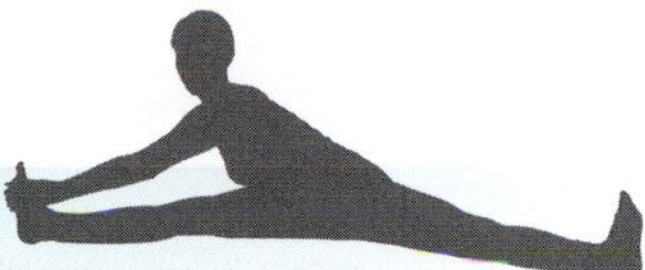

PRACTICE POINT

Because it is so superficial as it passes the medial epicondyle, the ulnar nerve is susceptible to injury. Ulnar nerve injury produces pain over the medial elbow with tingling or pain radiating down the forearm and into the little finger. Friction across the nerve within the ulnar groove produces a prickling sensation in the little finger; hence, this location of the ulnar nerve is popularly known as the "funny bone."

Distinctive Bony Features of the Proximal Ulna

- Olecranon process
- Coronoid process
- Trochlear or semilunar notch
- Trochlear or longitudinal ridge
- Ulnar tuberosity
- Radial notch

Radius

Although the radius contributes to proximal forearm function, it plays a more important role at the distal radioulnar joint and at the wrist. At the proximal end, the **head of the radius** is located just distal to the humeral lateral condyle. The superior surface of the radial head has a deep concave **fovea,** which articulates with the round convex head of the humeral capitulum to form the humeroradial joint. With the elbow in full extension, the roundness of the radial head, which forms the convex portion of the proximal radioulnar joint, may be palpated distal to the lateral epicondyle when the radius rolls under the skin during pronation and supination. During elbow flexion, the radial head slides within the capitulotrochlear groove until it nestles within the radial fossa of the humerus at the end of flexion. Just distal to the radial head on the anterior **radial neck** is the **radial tuberosity**. The radial tuberosity is the attachment site for the biceps brachii (Fig. 6.1).

Distinctive Bony Features of the Proximal Radius

- Radial head
- Fovea of radius
- Radial neck
- Radial tuberosity

Joints

Three joints are within the elbow joint capsule. These joints include the elbow and proximal forearm joints. The elbow joints include the humeroulnar and humeroradial joints whereas the proximal forearm joint is the proximal radioulnar joint.

Humeroulnar and Humeroradial Joints

The primary articulating segments at the elbow joint are the humerus and ulna. Although the radius moving on the humerus offers important companion motion, it does not contribute substantially to the elbow joint's function. As mentioned earlier, the elbow is an uniaxial hinge joint (ginglymus type), permitting one degree of freedom of motion: flexion and extension in the sagittal plane around the frontal axis (Fig. 6.2). The joint has ulnotrochlear and radiocapitular components that work in unison in flexion and extension. The strong structural stability of the joint is derived from both the bony configuration and the strong collateral ligaments (Fig. 6.3). Although the capsule surrounding all of the joints is reinforced by these collateral ligaments, it is thin and loose, especially posteriorly, with many folds to allow for the joint's significant motion. A large, olecranon bursa is located in the olecranon fossa, buffering the locking of the elbow when it moves into full extension.

Osteokinematics

The axis for elbow flexion-extension is medial-lateral (x-axis) and runs through the centers of the trochlea and capitulum and then near the lateral epicondyle (Fig. 6.2A). Because the trochlea is more distal than the capitulum, the line drawn through them is off from horizontal, creating the carrying angle at the elbow. This angle is discussed in more depth later in this chapter. The approximate location of this axis is located by placing fingers on the elbow slightly distal to the lateral and medial epicondyles and imagining a line connecting the two fingers. If the line were horizontal, the elbow's function would be akin to a rigid hinge, similar to that of a door. Since the elbow's

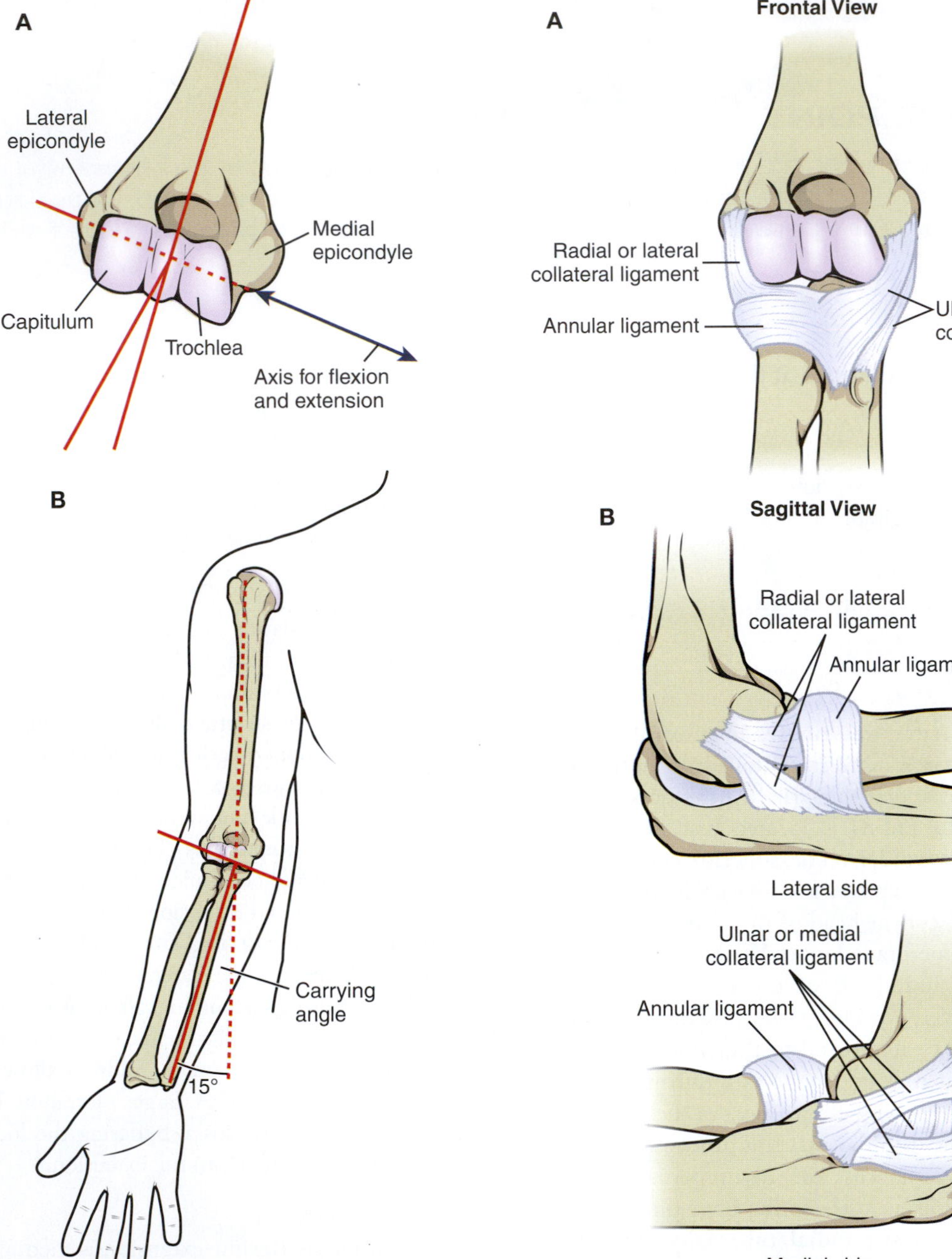

Figure 6.2 A) Axis for flexion and extension of the elbow courses through the trochlea and capitulum (one degree of freedom of motion). B) Carrying angle of the elbow when the extremity is in the anatomic position.

Figure 6.3 A) Frontal plane and B) sagittal plane views of the elbow illustrate the strong bony and ligamentous stability of the joint. Note the following ligaments: medial collateral, lateral collateral, and annular.

axis of motion is a few degrees off of the horizontal, the elbow has variability in excursion; this alignment provides a better joint and the elbow is best referred to as a "loose" hinge joint. Such a design allows for smooth instantaneous elbow flexion within multiple forearm positions so functional motion is easily performed.[5] A few degrees of medial and lateral rotation occur at the extremes of flexion and extension in this "loose" hinge joint.[6] Additionally, the distal end of the humerus lies in 30° of anterior rotation with respect to the humeral shaft, and the proximal ulna is rotated about 30° posteriorly in relation to the ulnar shaft. This matching relationship provides the 145° range in flexion as well as the stability of the joint in full extension.[7,8]

Elbow joint range of motion is variable. Although typical passive range of elbow flexion motion averages 145°, normal variability ranges from 120° to 160°.[7,9,10] Active flexion range of motion is less when the forearm is not in full supination.[11] Flexion motion is usually stopped by contact between the forearm and arm muscles with a soft end feel. In heavily muscled and obese persons, the flexion range can be reduced so significantly that the individual may not be able to place the fingers on the shoulder. At the other extreme, people with little soft tissue may have a hard end feel with bone contact of the ulnar coronoid process into the humeral coronoid fossa. We seldom use our full range of elbow motion; research indicates that most activities of daily living occur within an arc of elbow motion between 30° and 130°.[6]

Elbow extension has a hard end feel with contact between the ulna's olecranon process and the humeral olecranon fossa. Average extension motion is 0° with only a few degrees of normal variation. Outside of the normal spectrum, there may be people who are heavily muscled or have tight ligaments and lack a few degrees of elbow extension and others with a lighter structure or joint laxity with 5° or more of normal hyperextension.

Arthrokinematics

Accessory or component motions of the elbow are small compared to the motions possible in the shoulder, wrist, and fingers. Great joint stability is provided by the corrugated fit of the trochlea and capitulum of the humerus with the matching surfaces of the ulna and radius as well as to the strong medial and lateral collateral ligaments (Fig. 6.3). Slight distraction of the flexed elbow joint occurs if the distal humerus is stabilized and a traction force is applied to the proximal forearm. Some anteroposterior joint play occurs with the elbow placed in flexion and a posterior force is applied to the anterior surface of the proximal forearm. Minimal mediolateral joint play movements are also present. Remember from Chapter 1 that normal accessory motions requires muscle relaxation because any muscle contraction causes joint compression and restricts accessory motions. The close-packed position of the humeroulnar joint is full extension whereas the humeroradial joint's close-packed position is 90° of flexion with 5° of supination, and the radioulnar joint close-packed position is either full supination or full pronation. As with the close-packed positions, the resting positions of the elbow complex is different for each specific joint: the humeroulnar joint's resting position is 70° elbow flexion with 10° forearm supination; the humeroradial joint's resting position is full elbow extension with full forearm supination; and the resting

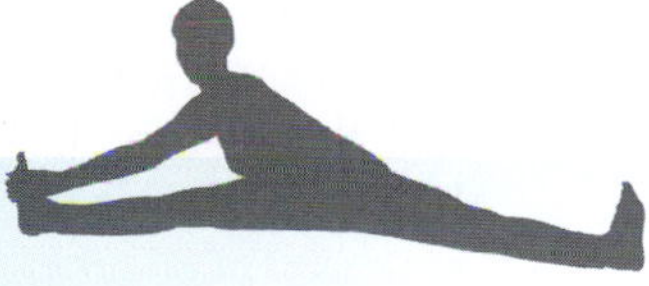

PRACTICE POINT

Although the elbow is classified as a uniaxial ginglymus joint, it really is more accurately described as a **modified hinge joint** because the axis for motion is outside the pure sagittal plane. This slight rotation or "extra-sagittal" motion that occurs in the elbow is a key factor that bioengineers must consider in their prosthetic designs of a mechanical joint. Although advances continue, a mechanical joint for use either in prosthetic design or total elbow joint replacements does not yet duplicate the biomechanical sophistication of the natural anatomical design.

A few degrees of elbow hyperextension can be of great functional use to individuals with spinal cord injuries who have paralysis of their triceps brachii muscles. These individuals cannot actively extend their elbows to push doors open or perform a push-up in a seated position to either relieve pressure or transfer out of a chair. With a few degrees of elbow hyperextension, they can use gravity and leverage to mechanically lock their elbows to push light objects or perform a seated push-up to lift their buttocks out of a chair for either pressure relief or sliding transfers.

position of the radioulnar joint is 70° elbow flexion with 35° forearm supination.[12]

Humeroulnar Arthrokinematics

Humeroulnar motion occurs between the concave ulnar trochlear notch and the convex humeral trochlea. During flexion, the ulnar trochlear notch rolls and glides in the same direction anteriorly over the humeral trochlear groove until the end of flexion when the coronoid process of the ulna reaches the coronoid fossa of the humerus. During extension, the trochlear notch rolls and glides in the same direction posteriorly over the trochlea. Smooth mobility and maximum stability is served well by the reciprocal concave-convex relationship between the trochlea and ulna, guiding the motion between flexion and extension similar to a train staying on its track.[12]

Full flexion motion requires normal length of the posterior capsule and skin, the elbow's extensor muscles, the ulnar nerve, and the posterior fibers of the medial collateral ligament. Contrarily, full extension motion requires normal length of the anterior capsule and skin, the elbow's flexor muscles, and the anterior fibers of the medial collateral ligament.

Humeroradial Arthrokinematics

Functional movement at the primary humeroulnar joint as described above is complemented by the motions between the humerus and radius. The concave proximal radial surface rolls and glides over the convex rounded capitulum of the distal lateral humerus in the same direction; therefore, the radius moves anteriorly during flexion and posteriorly during extension.

In full extension, there is no contact between the radius and humerus, but during flexion the deep fovea atop the head of the radius is pulled against the rounded capitulum of the humerus and the radial head slides in the capitulotrochlear grove until full flexion occurs when the head settles snuggly into the radial fossa of the humerus.

Carrying Angle

Since the joint axis is not perpendicular to the shaft of the humerus, the forearm alignment angles laterally in relation to the shaft of the humerus in the anatomical position. This angulation creates the **cubital angle**, commonly called the **carrying angle** (Fig. 6.2B). The biomechanical term for this angulation is **cubital valgus** (L., turned outward). This angle is approximately 15°, but it varies with a greater angle usually in women than in men.[13] Studies measuring the carrying angle cite mean values from 5° to 19° with males measured between 11° and 14°[10,11] and females between 13° and 16° and mean differences between men and women at 0° to 6°.[14–16] The variations in these values are attributed to the different methods of measurement and differences in population characteristics such as age, sex, body weight, and body build.[17]

Although cubital valgus angles up to about 15° are normal, excessive cubital valgus can be present secondary to injury or abnormal pathomechanics. Medial deviation, **cubitus varus** (L., turned inward), is considered pathological; this biomechanical change is usually due to a distal humeral fracture sustained during childhood. Cubital varus, or a carrying angle, less than the normal 5° to 15° of valgus is sometimes called a **gunstock deformity.**[3]

Functionally, the carrying angle results from a combination of glenohumeral lateral rotation, elbow extension, and forearm supination; all of these positions are present in the anatomical position.[17] The carrying angle is so named because it is believed to maintain objects that are carried in the hand away from the body. However, the natural and common way of carrying an object in the hand is with the forearm in some degree of pronation; in such a position, the carrying angle is obliterated. To date, no clear function for the carrying angle has been described, although it has been proposed to make hand-to-mouth motions more biomechanically efficient and effective. Kinematic studies on cadavers have demonstrated that flexion and extension at the elbow executed with the forearm in supination follows a consistent motion path and a gradual decrease in carrying angle occurs during progressive flexion.[18] This finding could support the notion that the carrying angle and the humeroulnar joint function best as a "loose" hinge subservient to functional purposeful movement.

Soft Tissue of the Humeroulnar and Humeroradial Articulations

As mentioned, the capsule contains many folds. You can imagine the importance of these folds during elbow motion, especially during elbow flexion when the posterior capsule unfolds as the joint moves farther into flexion. The capsule attaches posteriorly to the humerus above the olecranon fossa and to the trochlea. Anteriorly, the capsule attaches above the radial and coronoid fossa, and distally, it attaches medially to the ulna's coronoid process and laterally to the annular ligament. Although it is able to unfold to permit joint motion, capsular strength is reinforced by ligaments. The capsule attaches to and blends with both the medial collateral and annular ligaments to provide increased stability to the elbow complex. See Table 6–1 for a list of all ligaments, attachments, and functional description.

(text continues on page 228)

TABLE 6–1 | ELBOW AND FOREARM LIGAMENTS

Joint	Ligament	Proximal Attachment	Distal Attachment	Motions it Limits
Elbow joint: Humeroulnar radial articulation	Medial (ulnar) collateral ligament (MCL)	Medial epicondyle of humerus	Coronoid process and olecranon process of ulna	Excessive valgus stress that would force forearm laterally; anterior fibers also limit extension whereas posterior fibers limit flexion; prevents subluxation at humeroulnar articulation.

continued

TABLE 6–1 | ELBOW AND FOREARM LIGAMENTS—cont'd

Joint	Ligament	Proximal Attachment	Distal Attachment	Motions it Limits
Elbow joint: humeroradial articulation	Lateral (radial) collateral ligament (LCL)	Lateral epicondyle of humerus	Blends into annular ligament and attaches to olecranon process of ulna	Excessive varus stress that would force forearm medially; by attaching to ulna, prevents subluxation of humeroulnar articulation by securing humerus to ulna; stabilizes radial head and humeroradial articulation.
Proximal radioulnar joint	Annular ligament (see Frontal View image on page 225)	Anterior and posterior aspects of radial notch of ulna; encircles radial head	Anterior and posterior aspects of radial notch of ulna; encircles radial head	Maintains integrity of radioulnar articulation; prevents proximal radioulnar dislocation; prevents excessive radial distraction
Proximal radioulnar joint	Oblique cord	On ventral forearm, inferior aspect of radial notch of ulna	below radial tuberosity	Fibers run perpendicular to interosseous membrane to offer major stabilization to proximal radioulnar connection
Proximal radioulnar joint	Quadrate ligament	Inferior to radial notch of ulna	Medial surface of neck of radius	Limits spinning of radial head; maintains radial head up against ulnar radial notch; reinforces joint capsule

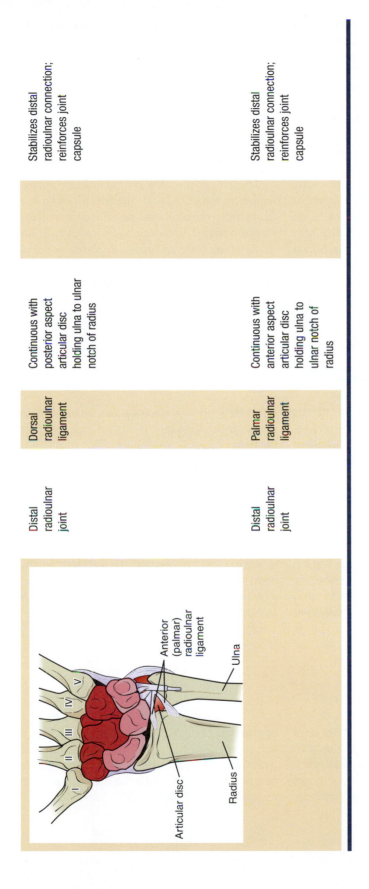

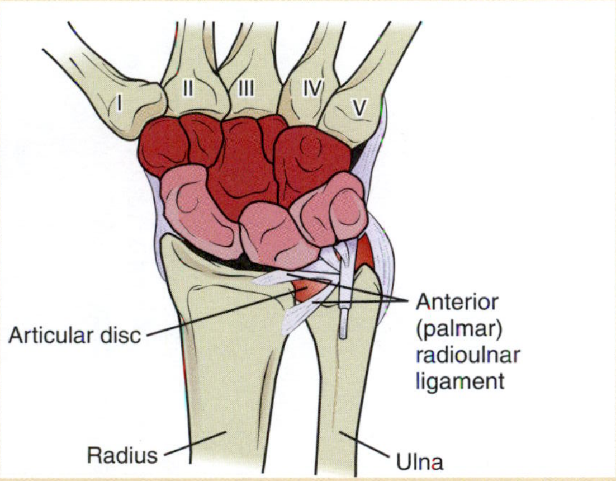	Distal radioulnar joint	Dorsal radioulnar ligament	Continuous with posterior aspect articular disc holding ulna to ulnar notch of radius		Stabilizes distal radioulnar connection; reinforces joint capsule
	Distal radioulnar joint	Palmar radioulnar ligament	Continuous with anterior aspect articular disc holding ulna to ulnar notch of radius		Stabilizes distal radioulnar connection; reinforces joint capsule

Since the primary motions at the humeroulnar joint are flexion and extension, the primary reinforcing ligaments are specialized thickenings of the capsule—the medial (ulnar) and lateral (radial) collateral ligaments. These two ligaments stabilize the capsule medially and laterally, respectively, to offer stability in the frontal plane. Medially, the **medial (ulnar) collateral ligament (MCL)** is quite large and comprised of three distinct parts: anterior, posterior, and transverse. The MCL extends from the medial epicondyle of the humerus to the ulna's coronoid process anteriorly and olecranon process posteriorly (Fig. 6.3). It stabilizes the elbow against excessive valgus forces to restrict the forearm from excessive lateral displacement on the arm. The MCL is the primary stabilizer of the elbow; damage to it may result in an unstable elbow joint.

The **lateral (radial) collateral ligament (LCL)** on the lateral elbow is a fan-shaped structure. Like the MCL, the LCL also has three parts; these segments extend from the humeral lateral epicondyle to the annular ligament surrounding the radial head and to the ulna's olecranon process (Fig. 6.3). This ligament stabilizes the elbow against excessive varus forces, prevents humeroulnar subluxation, stabilizes the humeroradial joint, and assists the annular ligament in stabilizing the radial head against the ulna (Fig. 6.3).

The elbow complex contains seven bursae. Three bursae are associated with the triceps, and a large bursa lies between the olecranon and the olecranon fossa (olecranon bursa). The olecranon bursa is vitally important in absorbing force and reducing shock occurring when the elbow extends forcefully, compressing the olecranon process into the humeral olecranon fossa.

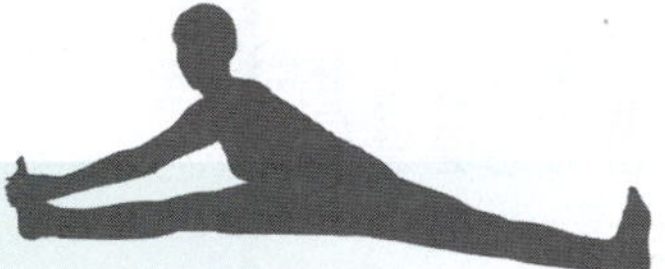

PRACTICE POINT

Since it is a primary stabilizer against valgus stress, the MCL is at risk for injury either from sudden traumatic valgus force or repetitive valgus forces as seen during some sports activities such as pitching a baseball, throwing a javelin, or spiking a volleyball. This is particularly true when side arm throws are used or when pathomechanical techniques at the shoulder increase valgus stresses at the elbow.

Elbow dislocation can occur when excessive force is sustained with the elbow "unpacked," as in slight flexion, causing the proximal ulna to dislocate posterior to the distal humerus. Since the brachial artery is located in the cubital fossa, it is also susceptible to trauma during dislocations. Damage to the brachial artery during a dislocation can result in a clinical presentation known as Volkmann's ischemia, which results in a loss of blood supply to the forearm muscles. If this clinical situation progresses, a Volkmann's ischemic contracture results due to necrosis of the forearm muscles that are dependent on the brachial artery for their blood supply.[19]

Olecranon bursitis can result from chronic overuse with the elbow slamming forcefully into extension or from a fall onto the tip of the olecranon producing swelling or bleeding into the bursal space. Usually painless, bursitis is often seen in football players and wrestlers because of combinations of both repetitive friction and direct trauma.[3] Olecranon bursitis may also present as part of a clinical picture associated with either concomitant lateral or medial epicondylopathy.[2, 20] Considerable swelling is readily apparent. After ruling out olecranon fracture, the bursitis responds to anti-inflammatory medications, compression, rest, and modalities.

Radioulnar Articulations

The radioulnar articulations include a proximal, or superior, component that lies within the elbow joint capsule and a distal, or inferior, component that is just proximal to the wrist. Motions of these joints include forearm supination and pronation. During these forearm motions, the radius pivots around a stationary ulna. These two joints act together to produce one degree of freedom: forearm pronation and supination in the transverse plane around a vertical axis in the anatomical position. In supination, the ulna and radius lie parallel to each other, whereas in pronation the radius crosses over the ulna (Fig. 6.4). During radioulnar motion, the radius pivots around the stationary ulna; this is an important point to remember when studying the prime movers of this joint because if a muscle attaches only to the ulna, it cannot perform supination or pronation. This concept is illustrated by palpating your olecranon while pronating and supinating the forearm and noting that the olecranon (a prominence of the ulna) does not move. As we will see when studying the wrist, the hand is attached to the radius at the radiocarpal articulation and follows the movement of the radius so that the palm turns up during supination and down during pronation. This is a relevant point to remember: the hand and wrist connect only to the radius and the ulna is stationary. A stable ulna is vitally important because it forms a rigid base, or bony lever, from which the forearm and wrist can function.

Radioulnar Joint Kinematics

The axis of motion of the radioulnar articulation occurs as a line from the center of the head of the radius through the center of the ulnar styloid process as shown in Figure 6.5. The proximal axis of rotation is in the head of the radius.[12, 18, 21] The ulnar styloid process is the distal axis of rotation.

The combined range of motion of both radioulnar joints is 150° to 180°.[9, 11, 12] With the forearm in mid-position as the thumb points to the ceiling, there may be up to 90° in supination and 90° in pronation; however, most people have only about 80° of pronation. In supination, the end feel at the proximal radioulnar joint is firm secondary to the tautness of the stretched ligaments, interosseous membrane, and both pronator muscles. In pronation, the end feel may be either hard if the radius and ulna come in contact with each other or firm because of stretch to the radioulnar joints' soft tissue capsules and the interosseous membrane between the two bones.[22] When range of pronation-supination motion is examined, the elbow should be flexed to 90° and in contact with the side of the body. This position

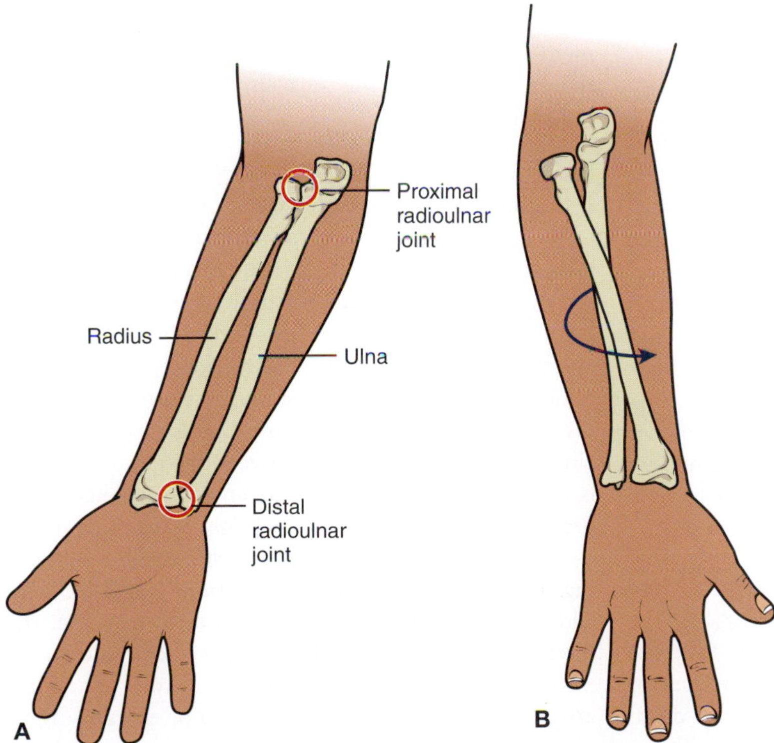

Figure 6.4 Note the positions of the radius and ulna. **A)** Parallel to each other in supination. **B)** The radius crosses over the ulna during pronation.

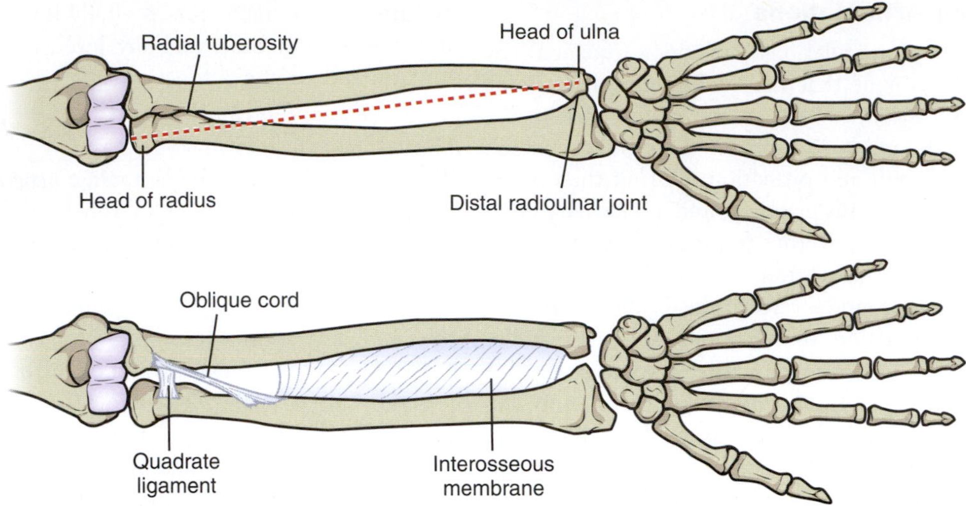

Figure 6.5 Axis for pronation and supination of the forearm courses through the head of the radius proximally and the head of the ulna distally (one degree of freedom of motion). Note also the ligaments at the proximal r-u joint—quadrate ligament and oblique cord, as well as the interosseous membrane.

prevents the shoulder from substituting for forearm movement. The entire range of pronation motion, starting from the fully supinated position, is slightly less than 180° (average is 170°). If pronation and supination occur with the elbow extended, medial and lateral shoulder rotation also occur simultaneously; in this case, the palm of the hand can be turned through almost a full circle or approximately 360°.

Arthrokinematics of the Proximal Radioulnar Joint

The proximal radioulnar joint is classified as a trochoid or pivot joint. The articular surfaces of this joint include the convex radial head and the slightly concave radial notch of the ulna. The annular ligament surrounds the radial head. During supination and pronation, the convex radial head spins within a contiguous fibro-osseous articular surface formed by the annular ligament and the concave radial notch of the ulna. The **annular ligament (L.,** *annulus;* ring) forms most of the articulating ring around the head of the radius, and the smaller radial notch of the ulna completes the articular ring formation. The radial head's motion is restricted to only rotation by this firm ring (Fig. 6.3).

Arthrokinematics of the Distal Radioulnar Joint

Whenever pronation and supination occurs at the proximal radioulnar joint, the distal, or inferior, radioulnar joint also moves. The articular surfaces of this distal joint include the ulnar notch of the distal radius, the rounded head of the ulna and an articular disc. Since the articular surface (ulnar notch) of the distal radius is concave, the radius slides around the ulnar convex head and rolls in the same direction as it slides. For example, when the forearm pronates (from a fully supinated position), the radius crosses over the ulna to roll anteriorly while it also slides anteriorly; motion and sliding is reversed during supination movement (Fig. 6.4). An articular disc, interposed between the distal ulna and the adjacent carpal bones, follows radial motion.

Soft Tissue of the Radioulnar Joint Complex

In contrast to the humeroulnar joint which derives most of its stability from its bony structure, the radioulnar joints are dependent on soft tissue for stability. Soft tissue stability at the proximal radioulnar joint is provided by the annular ligament and reinforced by the LCL, the oblique cord, and the quadrate ligament. The distal radioulnar joint stability is derived from the articular disc and the dorsal and palmar radioulnar ligaments. A close anatomic relationship between the radius and ulna is enhanced by the presence of an **interosseous membrane** located between the two bones. This thick membrane reinforces both radioulnar joints without restricting pronation or supination motions (Fig. 6.5). In addition to serving as a muscle attachment site, the interosseous membrane also absorbs shock and transmits force along the kinetic chain to protect the forearm bones from injury during times of excessive force application as when a person falls and lands on an outstretched arm.

The annular ligament has firm, fibrous connections to the ulna, attaching to it on either side of the radial notch, anchoring firmly around the radial head and neck. Attaching to the anterior and posterior aspects of the ulnar radial notch, this ring encircles the head of the radius forming a circle within which the radial head can pivot, or rotate. The underside of the annular ligament adjacent to the radial head is lined with cartilage to reduce friction and provide smooth pivoting of the radial head during forearm motion. As previously discussed, the lateral collateral ligament (LCL) blends into the annular ligament and offers additional stability for the proximal radioulnar joint. The **quadrate ligament** is quite short but strong, arising from the ulna just inferior to the radial notch and attaching to the medial surface of the radial neck. The quadrate ligament reinforces the joint capsule and maintains a close relationship of the radial head against the ulnar radial notch, thereby limiting spinning of the radial head (Fig. 6.5). The strong anterior portion of the quadrate ligament is a major stabilizer of the proximal radioulnar joint during full supination, whereas the weaker posterior component stabilizes full pronation.[20, 23] The **oblique cord** is a flat band of fascia on the ventral forearm running from the inferior aspect of the ulna's radial notch to just below the ulna's radial tuberosity. Its fibers run perpendicular to those of the interosseous membrane and become taut in full supination, providing additional stability to the radioulnar connection[20] (Fig. 6.5).

As mentioned, the distal ulna is attached to an articular disc. This disc is known as the **triangular fibrocartilage,** because of its shape and strong fibrous structure. The triangular fibrocartilage is part of the triangular fibrocartilage complex (TFCC) at the wrist and has two articular surfaces: the proximal surface and the distal surface. The proximal surface articulates with the ulnar head at the distal radioulnar joint and the distal surface articulates with the carpal bones as part of the radiocarpal joint. The disc's superior and inferior surfaces are concave, but the proximal surface is comparatively more concave to better accommodate the rounded head of the ulna. The TFCC provides some stability to the distal

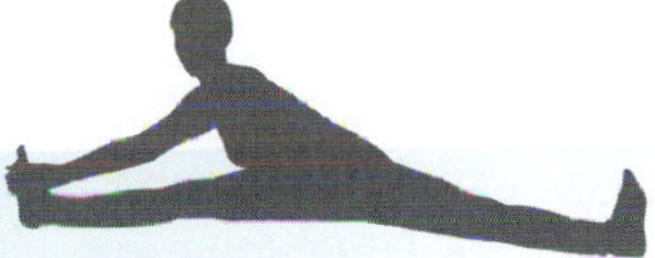

PRACTICE POINT

The anatomical structure of the interosseous membrane is an interesting example of how our bodies are engineered to minimize injury risk. As you have seen in this discussion of the elbow and forearm complex, the ulna is the larger and more dominant of the two at its proximal end, serving as the primary connection with the humerus, whereas the radius is the dominant and larger bone at the wrist where it serves as the primary connecting bone. The strong collagen fibers of the interosseous membrane run in a diagonal, medial-and-distal direction from the radius to the ulna; this design creates an anatomical *bridge* so that the some of the forces can be efficiently transmitted from the radius through the membrane to the ulna and then dissipated to the larger humerus above the elbow. Therefore, when you fall on an outstretched hand, some of the forces are transmitted from the distal radius to the interosseous membrane rather than risking certain injury by being entirely absorbed along the radius. Likewise, it is easier for waiters to carry heavy trays with the elbow flexed and the tray overhead because the tray's weight can be transmitted from the radius to the ulna, distributing the force over a larger area of the extremity.

As the middle link in the upper extremity chain, the elbow and forearm are occasionally at risk for distraction injury from excessive pulling forces. This is especially true for children and adolescents because of normal ligament laxity and the number of ossification centers in the elbow region. A common distraction injury, identified over 100 years ago as "nursemaid's elbow," is a condition whereby the radial head is pulled away from or even subluxed from within the annular ligament.[24] This syndrome, accurately described as "pulled elbow syndrome," occurs in young children aged 5 and younger. It occurs when the child is lifted by his or her hands or forearms, as in lifting the child up from the floor or swinging the child around by their arms during play. Parents should be cautioned not to pull their child in this manner.

radioulnar joint and is described in more detail in Chapter 7. Continuous with the anterior and posterior portions of the disc are the **anterior (palmar)** and **posterior (dorsal) radioulnar ligaments**; they blend into the taut joint capsule and hold the ulna against the ulnar notch of the radius (see Fig. 7.5).

Muscles

The muscles of the elbow and forearm complex include flexor and extensor muscles of the humeroulnar and humeroradial joints and supinator and pronator muscles of the forearm. Some muscles have duplicate functions and the remaining muscles act on only one joint. When studying the actions and functions of the muscles in this region, it is important to remember that a muscle can only act on a joint if it crosses it and can only move a bone to which it attaches. For example, the biceps brachii crosses the shoulder and the humeroulnar joint and attaches to the radius; since it crosses three joints, it is able to flex the shoulder, flex the elbow, and supinate the radius. On the other hand, the brachialis attaches to the humerus proximally and the ulna distally, crossing only the elbow; therefore, the brachialis can only perform elbow flexion. This section addresses the *primary* actions of the muscles of the elbow and forearm complex. See Table 6–2 for detailed information about these muscles. For a general overview, see Table 6–3 for a list of muscles that are primarily responsible for *typical* muscle actions at the elbow and forearm complex. The muscles are summarized according to their anatomic actions.

Elbow Flexors

The primary muscles that flex the elbow include the brachialis, biceps brachii, and brachioradialis. The pronator teres assists to a limited degree; since its primary responsibility is in forearm pronation, it is presented with that group of muscles. Of the primary elbow flexors, both the biceps brachii and brachioradialis also influence forearm motion. There are other muscles which cross the humeroulnar joint but have weak leverage at the elbow and are primarily active at their distal insertions in the wrist and hand. These muscles include the flexor carpi radialis longus, flexor carpi ulnaris, flexor digitorum superficialis, and palmaris longus. These muscles are discussed in the next chapter.

Brachialis

The brachialis (Fig. 6.6), located deep to the prominent biceps brachii, attaches only to the ulna acting across the humeroulnar joint and, therefore, will always be recruited in elbow flexion regardless of forearm position. It is the only one-joint elbow flexor muscle, unaffected by shoulder or forearm position. The brachialis is known as the "workhorse" of the elbow because it has a large work capacity due to a large cross section area, is the largest of all of the elbow flexors, and it crosses only the humeroulnar joint. It is recruited in all tasks requiring elbow flexion. This muscle is also very efficient for achieving mobility at the humeroulnar joint because its insertion is close to the joint axis, exerting its greatest moment arm of force at around 90° to 100° of elbow flexion.[12, 25, 26] The muscle belly of the brachialis is located in the distal half of the arm and is largely covered by the biceps.

Biceps Brachii

As its name implies, the biceps brachii (Fig. 6.7) is a fusiform-shaped muscle with two heads located on the anterior arm. The biceps brachii originates from the scapula and attaches below the elbow joint so it has no direct connection with the humerus and can be passively moved about easily. As the long tendon of biceps courses within the glenohumeral joint capsule under the subacromial arch, traveling then within the intertubercular or bicipital groove of the humerus, it is at risk for entrapment and subsequent pathology. The short head attaches to the scapula's coracoid process. The two heads have separate bellies in the proximal arm but fuse to form one belly in the midarm. The muscle fibers

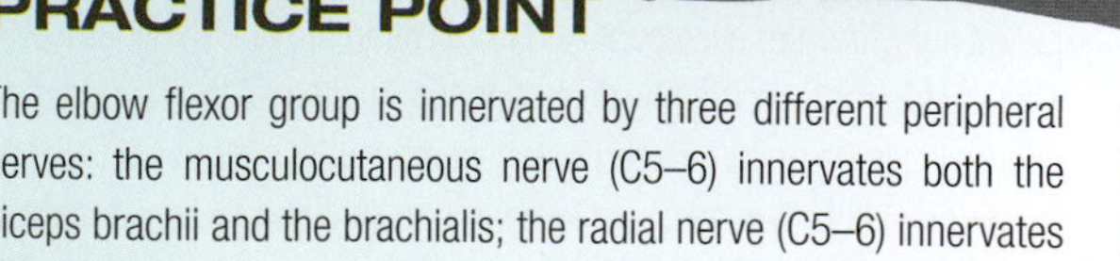

PRACTICE POINT

The elbow flexor group is innervated by three different peripheral nerves: the musculocutaneous nerve (C5–6) innervates both the biceps brachii and the brachialis; the radial nerve (C5–6) innervates the brachioradialis; and the median nerve (C6–7) innervates the pronator teres. This innervation design is a sharp contrast to the single primary elbow extensor—the triceps brachii—served solely by the radial nerve. This innervation pattern allows an individual to perform functional activities such as bringing objects closer to the trunk or performing hand-to-mouth functions even if the individual suffers a peripheral nerve or spinal cord injury.

(text continues on page 239)

TABLE 6–2 | MUSCLES OF THE ELBOW/FOREARM COMPLEX

Group	Muscle	Proximal attachment	Distal attachment	Nerve	Action	Palpation
Elbow Flexors	Brachialis 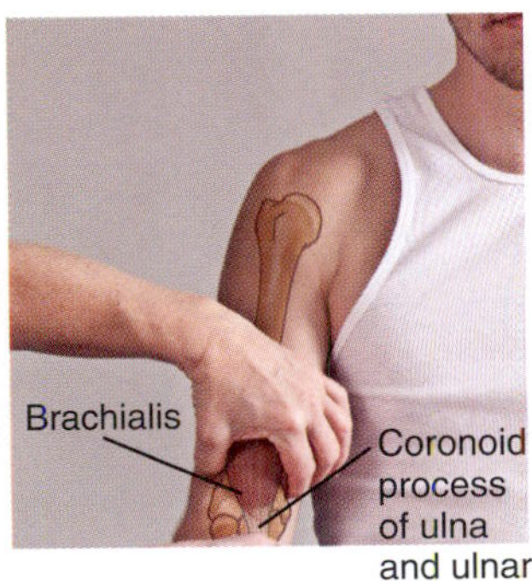	Midway on anterior aspect of shaft of the humerus	Coronoid process of the ulna and ulnar tuberosity	Musculocutaneous (C_5–C_6)	Flexion of the humeroulnar joint	The palpating fingers are placed laterally and medially to the biceps, an inch or two higher than the grasp seen in Figure 6.6. The subject's forearm is pronated, which ensures relaxation of the biceps. The elbow is flexed with as little effort as possible, so that the contraction of the brachialis may be felt. Under these conditions, the brachialis flexes the elbow with little or no participation by the biceps. Once the palpating fingers are properly placed, a quick flexion in small range may be performed, resulting in stronger contraction of the brachialis.
	Biceps Brachii 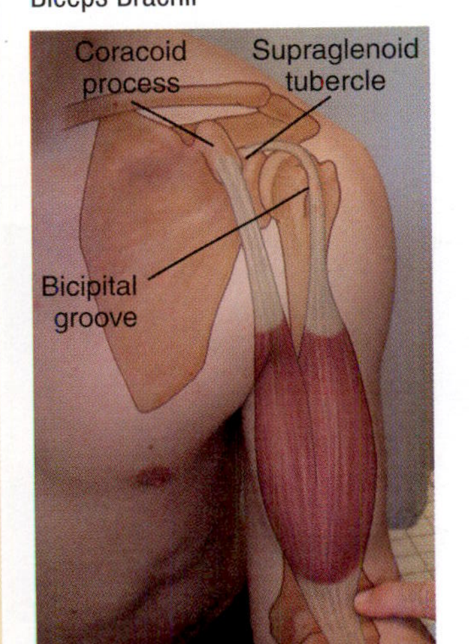	Two heads originate from above the glenohumeral joint: Long head: supraglenoid tubercle of the scapula, the tendon coursing within the capsule of the glenohumeral joint and in the intertubercular (bicipital) groove of the humerus. Short head: coracoid process of the scapula.	Tuberosity of the radius spreading out to form part of the bicipital aponeurosis	Musculocutaneous (C_5–C_6).	Flexion at the glenohumeral joint, flexion of the elbow joint, supination of the radioulnar joint.	The biceps and its tendons are palpated with the muscle relaxed, as when the forearm rests on the table or in the lap. It is then possible to grasp around the muscle, lift it from underlying structures, and move it from side to side, a maneuver that is useful in separating it from the deeply located brachialis muscle. The contour of the biceps is easily identified by resisting elbow flexion; to the layman "making a muscle" means tightening the biceps. The tendon of the biceps is best identified in the "fold" of the elbow when the forearm is supinated. The examiner's finger indicates the location of that part of the tendon that dips into the antecubital fossa on its way to the tuberosity of the radius.

continued

TABLE 6–2 | MUSCLES OF THE ELBOW/FOREARM COMPLEX—cont'd

Group	Muscle	Proximal attachment	Distal attachment	Nerve	Action	Palpation
Elbow Flexors	Brachioradialis	Lateral supracondylar ridge of the humerus	Styloid process of the radius	Radial nerve (C_5–C_6).	Flexion of the elbow joint, supination and pronation of radioulnar joint from midposition. The brachioradialis will pronate or supinate the forearm to neutral against heavy resistance.[33]	The brachioradialis is best observed and palpated when resistance is given to flexion of the elbow while the elbow angle is about 90° and the forearm is in midposition between pronation and supination. Note the tendon of brachioradialis as it bowstrings across the elbow and the belly becomes prominent in the forearm. Figure 6.8 shows the contour of this muscle and one can derive its relation to the extensor carpi radialis longus and brevis. The brachioradialis is superficial and is readily palpated along most of its course. Above the elbow, it lies between the triceps and the brachialis. At and below the elbow, the brachioradialis forms the lateral border of the antecubital fossa. Its muscular part may be followed halfway down the forearm, but its point of distal attachment is less readily palpated because its tendon attachment is flat and partially covered by tendons of muscles passing over the wrist to the hand. These tendons are held down by ligamentous structures that cross obliquely from the ulnar to the radial side of the wrist. When the muscle contracts, its upper portion rises from the underlying structures so that its perpendicular distance to the elbow joint increases, increasing the moment arm, which enhances its function.

	Muscle	Proximal attachment	Distal attachment	Innervation	Action	Palpation
	Pronator teres 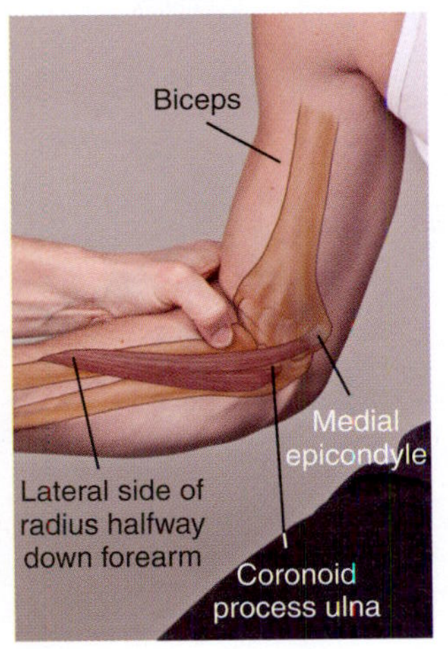	Humeral head: Medial epicondyle of humerus; Ulnar head: coronoid process of the ulna. The muscle fibers cross obliquely from medial to lateral on the anterior aspect of the forearm.	Lateral side of the radius about halfway down the forearm	Median nerve (C_6–C_7).	Pronation at the radioulnar joint, and weak elbow flexor	The muscle is superficial and may be palpated in the fold of the elbow and below, forming the medial margin of the antecubital fossa. Its fibers are easily identified in this region when the forearm is pronated while the elbow is flexed or semiflexed during resistance to elbow flexion. The subject's thumb grasps around the edge of the pronator teres. If, from the position shown, the forearm is further pronated or resistance is given to pronation or flexion, the muscle hardens markedly. The pronator teres lies close to the flexor carpi radialis, and both these muscles are covered by the bicipital aponeurosis. More distally, as it crosses over toward the radial side, the pronator teres is covered by the brachioradialis, and if the pronator teres is to be palpated close to its distal attachment, the brachioradialis must be relaxed, accomplished by resting the forearm in the lap or on the table. The forearm is then pronated, which activates the pronator while the brachioradialis remains essentially relaxed. The movement of pronation should be performed with little effort, or additional muscles in the region become tense.

continued

TABLE 6–2 | MUSCLES OF THE ELBOW/FOREARM COMPLEX—cont'd

Group	Muscle	Proximal attachment	Distal attachment	Nerve	Action	Palpation
Elbow Extensors	Triceps brachii 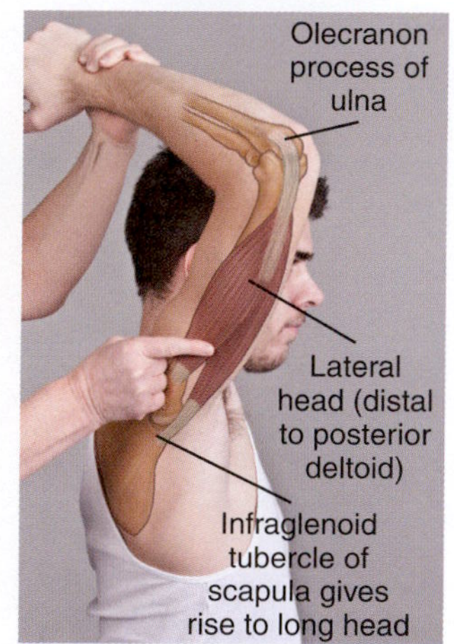 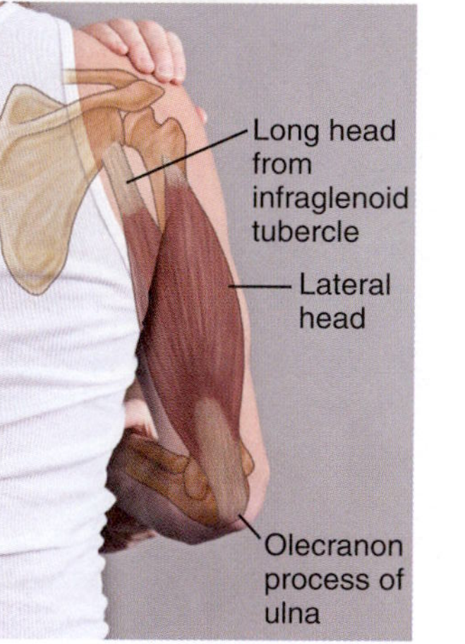 	By three heads: Long head: infraglenoid tubercle of the scapula by a broad tendon closely related to the shoulder joint capsule; Medial head: distal portion of the posterior humerus (fleshy); Lateral head: postero-lateral aspect of the humerus, inferior to the greater tubercle.	Three heads join to form a sturdy broad tendon, attaches to the olecranon process of the ulna and that also sends an expansion spreading out over the anconeus muscle into the dorsal fascia of the forearm	Radial nerve (C_7–C_8).	Extension at the glenohumeral joint and extension at the humeroulnar joint.	The long head is identified proximally as it emerges from underneath the lowest fibers of the posterior deltoid. (Fig. 6-10A) It may be followed distally halfway down the arm. The muscular portion of the lateral head, which is the strongest of the three heads, is palpated distal to the posterior deltoid. The long head and the lateral head join the common tendon of insertion from opposite sides, much as the two heads of the gastrocnemius approach the Achilles tendon. Note in the illustration the flat area between the lateral and the long heads (Fig. 6.10B). This is the broad superficial portion of the triceps tendon into which the two heads insert, partially from underneath and partially from the sides. The medial head is covered, in part, by the long head and is best palpated in its distal portion, near the medial epicondyle. For palpation of the medial head, it is suggested that the dorsum of the wrist be placed on the edge of a table and pressure be applied in a downward direction, the table supplying resistance to elbow extension. The medial head may then be felt contracting.

Elbow Extensors	Anconeus	Region of the lateral epicondyle of the humerus	Proximal ulna, into and inferior to the olecranon process	Radial nerve (C_7–C_8).	Extension at the humeroulnar joint	If one fingertip is placed on the lateral epicondyle and one on the olecranon process, the muscular portion of the anconeus is palpated distally at a point that forms a triangle with the other two points. Although it lies near to the extensor carpi ulnaris, each muscle may be easily differentiated by keeping in mind that the direction of the two muscles differs and that the anconeus lies more proximally and is very short, whereas the extensor carpi ulnaris runs down the forearm.
Forearm Supination	Supinator	Lateral epicondyle of the humerus and adjacent areas of the ulna	Anterior and lateral surfaces of the proximal part of the radius	Radial nerve (C_5–C_6).	Supination at the radioulnar joint	A fairly short, flat, triangular muscle, which winds around the proximal portion of the radius close to the bone. The area where the supinator, although deeply located, may be palpated is shown in Figure 6.11. The fingertips are pushing the muscles of the radial group in a radial direction so that there is no interference with palpation. The best position for palpation is to sit with the pronated forearm resting in the lap and to grasp the radial muscle group from the radial side, pulling it out of the way as much as possible. As the forearm is supinated slowly through short range to avoid activating the biceps, the supinator may be felt under the palpating fingers.

continued

TABLE 6–2 | MUSCLES OF THE ELBOW/FOREARM COMPLEX—cont'd

Group	Muscle	Proximal attachment	Distal attachment	Nerve	Action	Palpation
Forearm Pronation	Pronator Quadratus 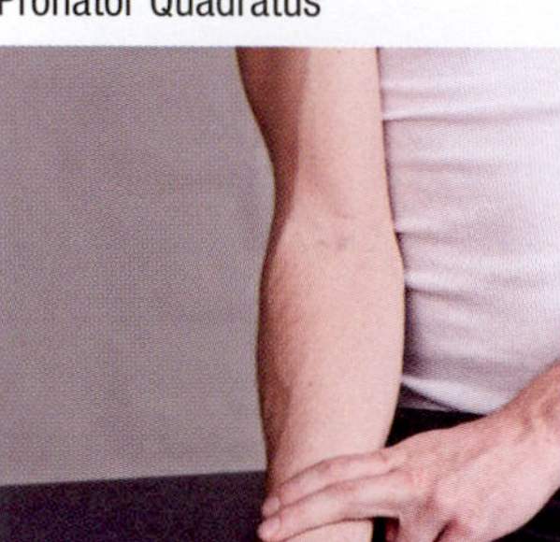	Distal one-fourth of the ulna; anterior surface	Distal one-fourth of the radius; anterior surface	Median nerve (C_8–T_1)	Pronation at the radioulnar joint	Pronator quadratus crosses diagonally over ulna and radius near wrist lying over the bones and against the interosseous membrane. Palpation: impossible because the muscle is covered by the tendons of the wrist and fingers. The approximate length and direction of the muscle fibers are indicated in Fig. 6.12.

TABLE 6–3 | PRIME MOVERS AT THE ELBOW COMPLEX (SUMMARIZED BY ANATOMIC ACTIONS)

Humeroulnar Joint	
Flexion	Brachialis Biceps Brachii • especially in forearm supination Brachioradialis • especially with forearm in midposition
Extension	Triceps Brachii
Radioulnar Joint	
Supination	Supinator • especially in elbow extension Biceps Brachii • especially in elbow flexion
Pronation	Pronator Teres Pronator Quadratus

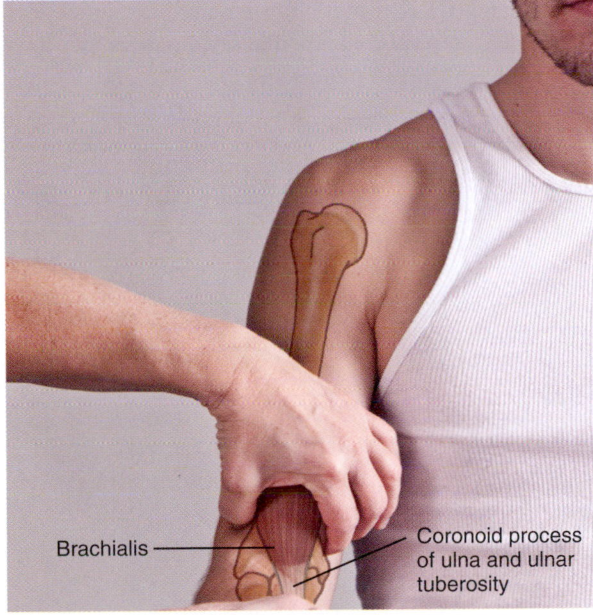

Figure 6.6 Brachialis. Model demonstrates location of brachialis muscle and the artwork overlay draws attention to the attachments and line of muscle pull.

belonging to the short head make up the medial portion of the common belly whereas those of the long head make up the lateral portion.

Functionally, the biceps is selectively recruited when the task requires elbow flexion with forearm supination

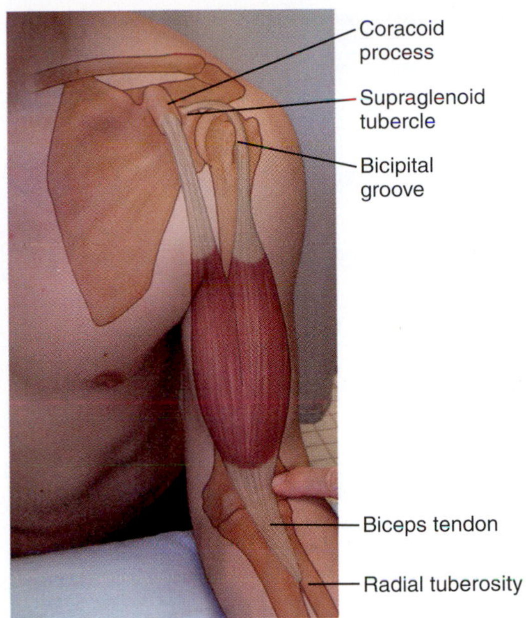

Figure 6.7 Biceps Brachii. The characteristic contour of the biceps is brought out by flexion of the elbow and movement into supination of the forearm. The examiner points out the prominent tendon of biceps in the "fold" of the elbow. Model demonstrates location of biceps brachii muscle and the artwork overlay draws attention to the attachments and line of muscle pull.

such as in carrying a loaded tray or bringing a spoon to the mouth. The muscle has a large cross section and has its the greatest moment arm at 90° to 110° of flexion.[12,25,26] Beyond 100° of flexion or when the elbow is close to full extension, the contractile force becomes more translatory. This translatory force provides joint compression to add stability to the elbow.

Brachioradialis

The brachioradialis (Fig. 6.8) is the longest of the elbow flexors and is the only primary elbow flexor whose belly lies in the forearm. This muscle is a strong contributor to elbow flexion and has a limited role in forearm pronation and supination. Because of its attachment site on the radius, it may contribute to pronation or supination. Although it has a relatively small cross section, it exerts peak force at 100° to 120° of elbow flexion.[12,25,26] Since it inserts far distally from the humeroulnar joint axis, some of its force compresses the joint to provide additional stability to the joint. Figure 6.8 shows the contour of this muscle. When the muscle contracts, its upper portion rises from the underlying structures so its perpendicular distance to the elbow joint increases, increasing its moment arm to add more leverage to its function.

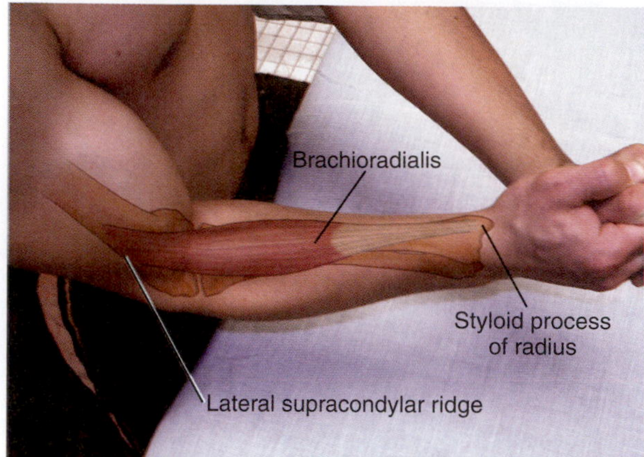

Figure 6.8 Brachioradialis. A contraction of the brachioradialis is demonstrated by resistance to flexion of the elbow with the forearm in midposition between pronation and supination.

Pronator Teres

The pronator teres (Fig. 6.9) is a weak elbow flexor, predominantly contributing to flexion when the forearm is pronated. Since its main action is forearm pronation, this muscle will be described in detail with the forearm muscles.

Elbow Extensors

The principal extensor of the elbow is the triceps brachii. The small anconeus adds only minimally to the total strength of elbow extension.

Triceps Brachii

The triceps brachii, so named because it has three heads, makes up the entire muscle mass on the posterior aspect of the arm (Fig. 6.10). The lateral head is the most muscular portion and strongest of the three heads; it is easily identifiable, distal to the posterior deltoid (Fig. 6.10B). Because the triceps only attaches to the ulna, this muscle extends the elbow regardless of forearm position. Its greatest extension force is exerted in midrange at 70° to 90° of elbow flexion.[27–29] The triceps acts concentrically to extend the elbow, eccentrically as a major elbow stabilizer during elbow flexion, and as a powerful stabilizer of the upper extremity during any functional closed-chain activity.

Anconeus

The anconeus is a small muscle located deep, adjacent to the joint, blending close to the fibers of the humeroulnar joint capsule (Fig. 6.10C). It contracts during elbow extension to tighten the loose posterior elbow capsule, perhaps helping to prevent pinching of the capsule folds as the olecranon locks into the olecranon fossa. It is an accessory muscle for elbow extension. It provides only 10% to 15% of required extensor force, although it is important in that it initiates most low-load elbow extension motions.[30, 31]

Forearm Supinators

Forearm supinators include primarily the biceps brachii and supinator. The brachioradialis may assist

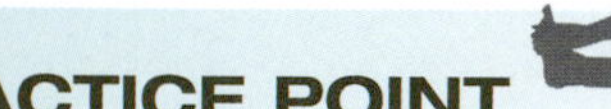

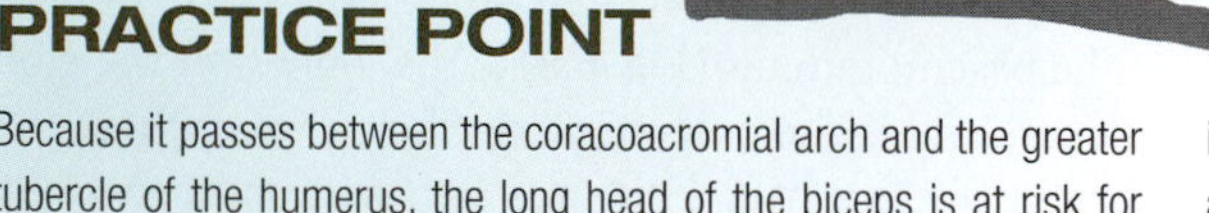

PRACTICE POINT

Because it passes between the coracoacromial arch and the greater tubercle of the humerus, the long head of the biceps is at risk for impingement and is a frequent site of pathology and functional impairment. Chronic irritation from impingement results in pain radiating into the middle aspect of the arm, tenderness over the bicipital grove, and weakness of elbow flexion force.

Since the musculocutaneous nerve innervates both the brachialis and the biceps brachii muscles, injury to this nerve results in loss of these flexor muscles. If the biceps brachii and the brachialis are paralyzed, weak elbow flexion is achieved through function of the brachioradialis with assistance from the pronator teres, extensor carpi radialis longus, and extensor carpi radialis brevis. Although the elbow flexion leverage of these muscles is poor with the elbow in extension, in cases of impairment the entire upper extremity swings to utilize momentum to start elbow flexion movement. Once the elbow swings to 90°, the forearm muscles are in a better position of leverage to provide functional elbow motion, so the hand may be positioned for use and light objects may be lifted.

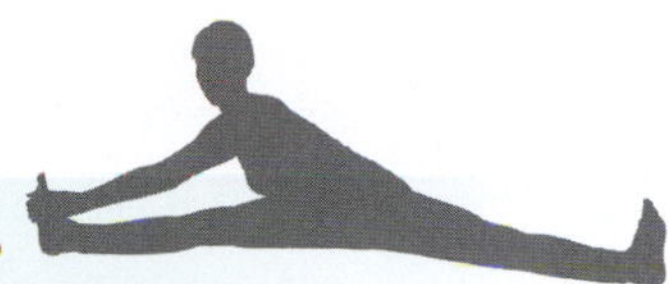

PRACTICE POINT

Paralysis of the triceps brachii occurs with a radial nerve injury or a spinal cord injury affecting C7. Since the entire posterior compartment of the elbow and forearm is innervated by the radial nerve, injury to that nerve can have devastating consequences. A seated individual with a C7 spinal cord injury performs elbow flexion and extension by performing concentric and eccentric contractions of the biceps and brachialis muscles. This is a frequently used function that is required for activities such as cutting food, performing a push-up, or pushing open a door.

to a limited degree. The supinator is able to supply adequate force when supination occurs slowly, when the resistance is light, or when the elbow is extended. As a supinator, the biceps is a powerful participator but supinates best when the elbow is flexed. Therefore, the biceps supinates when the elbow is in a flexed position or when the motion occurs against a heavy resistance. The brachioradialis aids supination from pronation to midposition with the elbow in flexion, but its action is quite weak.[32] Several muscles of the wrist and hand complex, including the abductor pollicis longus, extensor pollicis brevis, and extensor

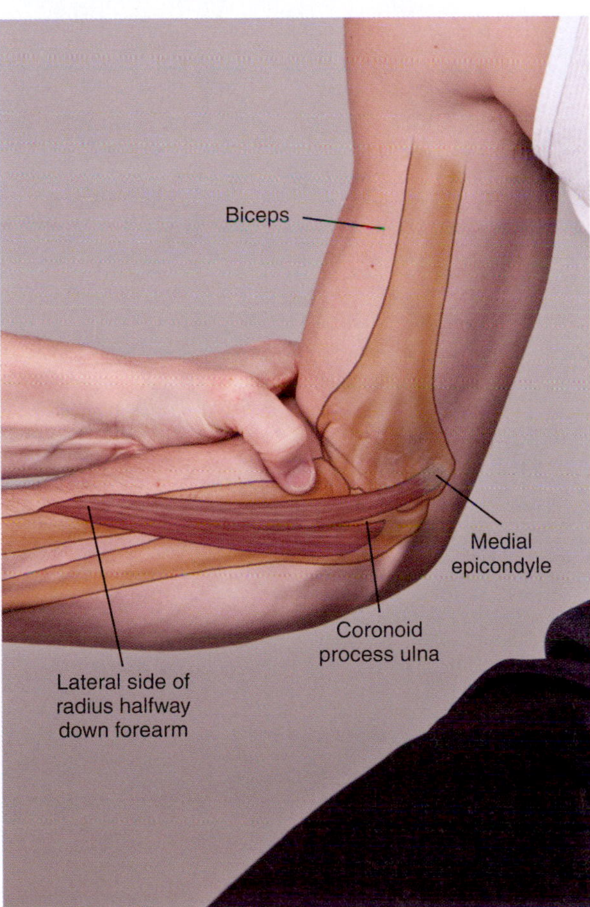

Figure 6.9 Pronator teres. Model demonstrates location of pronator teres muscle and the artwork overlay draws attention to the attachments and line of muscle pull.

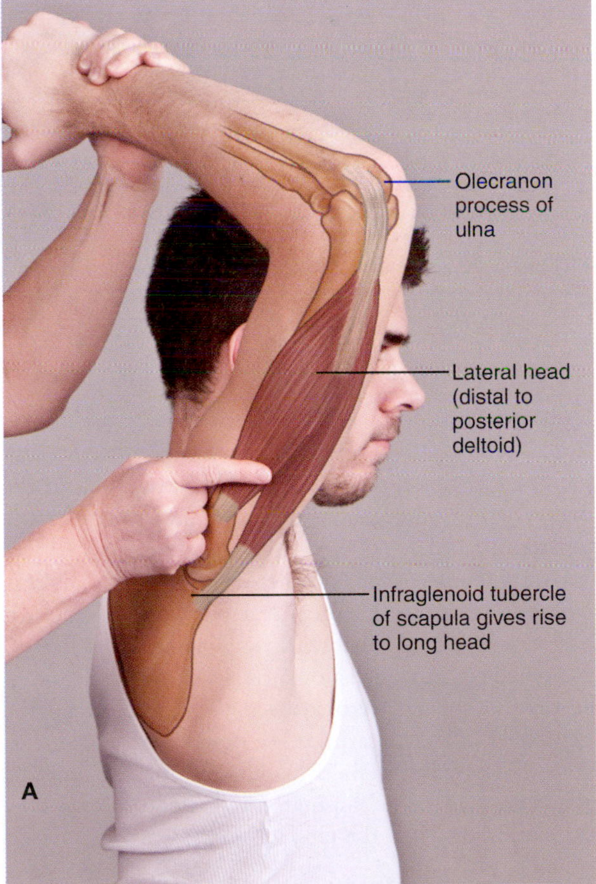

Figure 6.10 Triceps brachii and anconeus. Elbow extension is resisted. **A)** Triceps brachii is demonstrated by the examiner's resistance to extension of the elbow. The long head of the triceps is responsible for the contour at the lower margin of the arm. Note its relation to teres major and the latissimus near the axilla.

continued

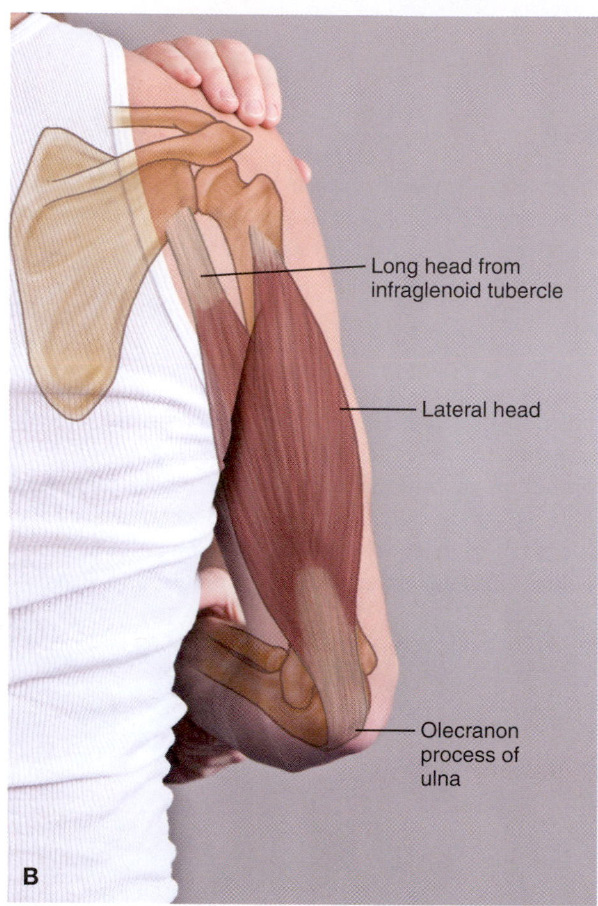

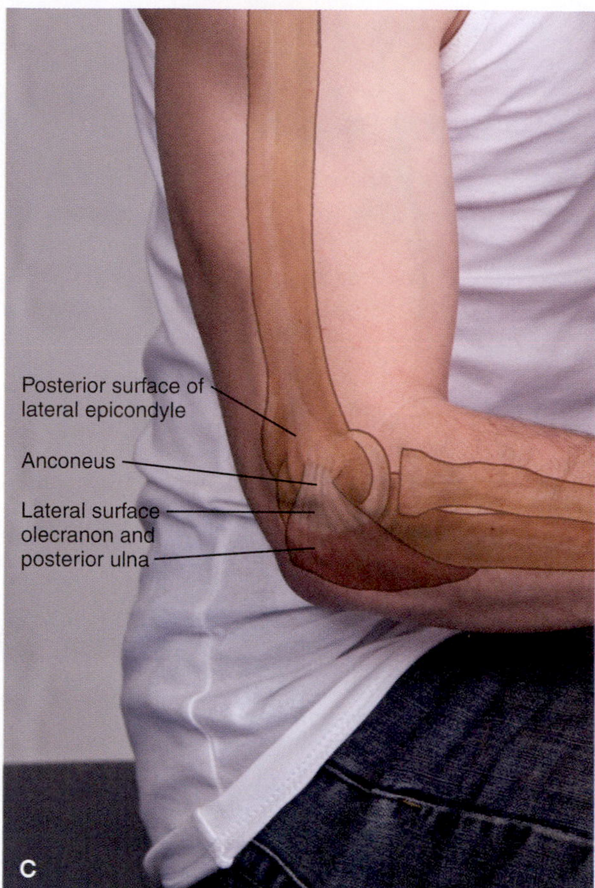

Figure 6.10 B) The lateral head appears separated from the deltoid by a groove. The distal flat area between the lateral and the long heads identifies the broad common tendon of attachment. C) The short, triangular-shaped anconeus lies close to the tip of the elbow and near the upper portion of extensor carpi ulnaris.

indicis may also act as weak contributors to supination, but since their role here is minimal, they are not included in this discussion. They are presented in the next chapter since their primary role occurs at the wrist and hand.

Aptly named, the **supinator** is the only muscle whose sole action is forearm supination. As such, it is always recruited for forearm supination, regardless of the speed or load. The supinator is a deep muscle located on the dorsal interosseous membrane between the two bones of the forearm. It is covered by the anconeus, the extensor carpi radialis longus, and the brachioradialis (Fig. 6.11). The supinator acts alone during slow supination or when the elbow is extended.

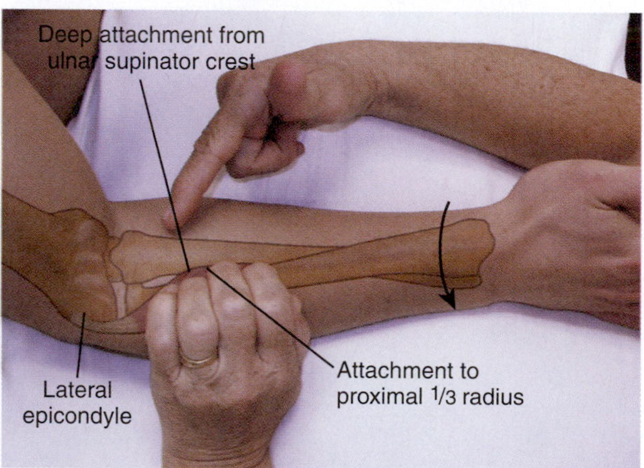

Figure 6.11 Supinator. Examiner points out identification of the location of the supinator muscle, best identified if the forearm is slowly supinated from pronation with the elbow extended in an effort to reduce activation of the biceps. The artwork overlay draws attention to the attachments and line of muscle pull.

Forearm Pronators

The muscles that are primarily responsible for pronating the forearm are named by their prime action and include the pronator teres and pronator quadratus. Pronators originate on the stable ulna and attach to the radius, pulling the radius around the stationary ulna. During forearm pronation, the pronator teres and pronator quadratus act as synergists to pronate the radius over the ulna at the proximal and distal radioulnar joints respectively. The brachioradialis will pronate the forearm from a supinated position to midposition in the face of heavy resistance, especially when the elbow is flexed.[33] The flexor carpi radialis, palmaris longus, and extensor carpi radialis longus are all muscles of the wrist and hand that have the capability for pronation but have poor leverage for pronation and contribute little force. They will be discussed in Chapter 7.

Pronator Teres

Named by its function and shape (cordlike, from the Latin *teres),* the pronator teres is primarily a forearm pronator. The bulk of the pronator teres muscle is located below the elbow. It runs rather close to the axis of the elbow joint so that it has a poor moment arm for elbow flexion; this muscle supplies added force to elbow flexion only when there is a significant resistance or a heavy load.[12] Because of its proximity to the joint, the pronator teres exerts some of its force to stabilize the proximal radioulnar joint and works synergistically with the pronator quadratus to rotate or pivot the radius around the ulna during pronation. The muscle is superficial and its fibers run obliquely—medially to laterally—on the anterior forearm (Fig. 6.9).

Pronator Quadratus

By virtue of its location near the wrist at the distal or inferior radioulnar joint, the deeply situated pronator quadratus (named for its function and shape) crosses transversely over the ulna and the radius in the distal anterior forearm (Fig. 6.12). This one-joint muscle performs forearm pronation regardless of elbow position. Since it is located close to the joint, this muscle also acts as a dynamic stabilizer of the distal radioulnar joint.[27,34]

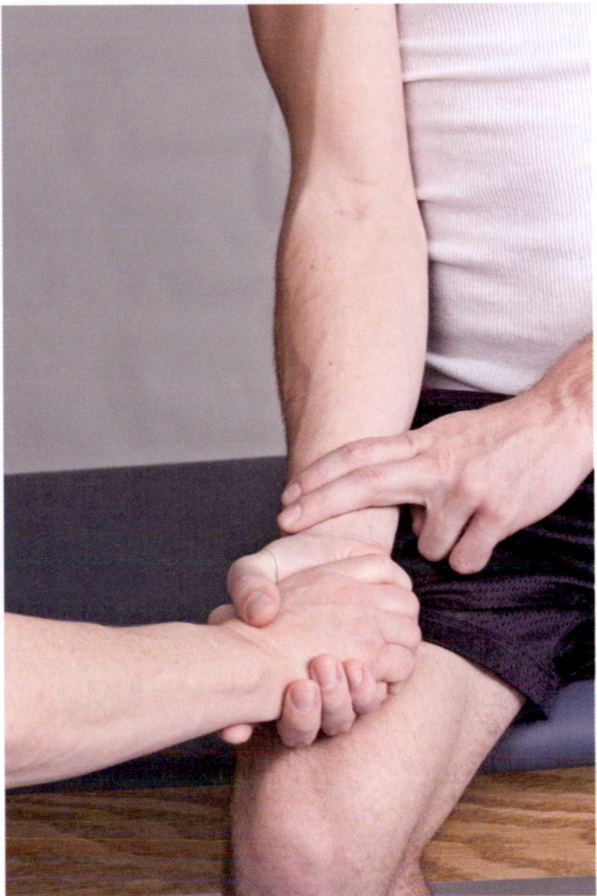

Figure 6.12 Pronator quadratus. The model demonstrates the line of action of the deeply situated pronator quadratus.

Functional Movement and the Muscles of the Elbow/Forearm Region

Since you are now familiar with the primary anatomic actions of the muscles in this region, you can identify how these muscles work together to perform functional activity. Recall from Chapter 4 that a given muscle can contribute to the motion in multiple ways: as an

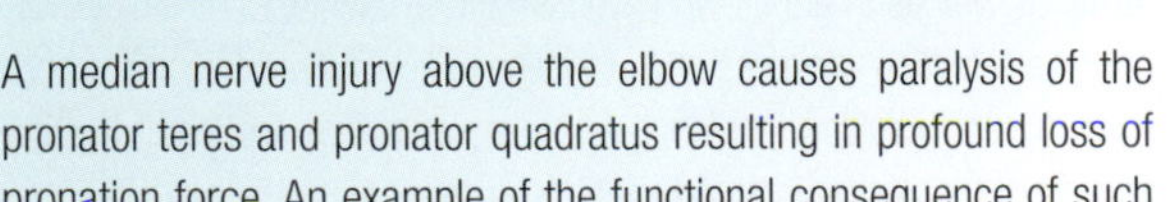

PRACTICE POINT

A median nerve injury above the elbow causes paralysis of the pronator teres and pronator quadratus resulting in profound loss of pronation force. An example of the functional consequence of such an injury is the inability to produce sufficient force to turn a key counterclockwise or hold a glass and keep it from tipping.

agonist, antagonist, synergist, stabilizer, or neutralizer to provide the desired functional action. This section presents examples of ways in which the elbow and forearm muscles work synchronously to provide us with a wide variety of movement to accomplish functional tasks.

Muscles as Agonists, Antagonists, and/or Synergists

Muscle function is first learned by studying the primary motion of muscles when they act as an agonist in a concentric contraction. During such activities, a muscle's proximal attachment is stabilized by other muscles or body weight while the distal attachment moves in open kinematic chain motions (see Fig. 4.3). As discussed in Chapter 4, functional movement occurs because of multiple muscles acting synergistically to accomplish a task. Muscles rarely act in total isolation. At times, the task requires active recruitment of several muscles that perform the same action, such as recruiting all elbow flexors to lift a heavy load. However, a heavier load will also require the synergistic recruitment of additional muscles, including forearm, wrist, and shoulder muscles, during resisted elbow and forearm movement.

Selection of Muscles in Functional Movement: Synergistic Contractions

Some muscle pairs, such as the triceps and the anconeus in elbow extension, coactivate regardless of demand, but typically, activation of synergists depends on the specific needs for a functional movement. Synergistic activation of muscles is affected by the demands of the task, the force required, the direction of the load or stress, and the type of muscle contraction (eccentric, concentric, or isometric).[35] For example, although the biceps and triceps may act antagonistically in flexion or extension, they are more likely to act as synergists, as when a forceful grip is made (see Fig. 4.4C). These muscles cocontract to stabilize the elbow during wrist and finger movement. Turning a doorknob is another example of biceps and triceps synergistic actions. During these activities, the triceps stabilize the elbow and prevent elbow flexion by the biceps as the forearm supinates (see Fig. 4.4A).

Recall from Chapter 4 that the number of muscles involved in synchronous movement is largely determined by the effort required to perform a particular task; if great resistance is encountered, more muscles are recruited, not only at the joint or joints where the movements take place, but also at joints far away from the actual action. The importance of this concept at the elbow and forearm appears when we make a tight fist: Both elbow flexors and extensors contract to stabilize the elbow. These synergistic contractions are automatic and cannot be voluntarily inhibited. By stabilizing the elbow, these muscles provide a firm base for the proximal attachments of the finger and wrist muscles from which they can then function to produce the desired activity. Without this stabilization, a significant amount of finger and wrist muscle force must be diverted to control their proximal position, so their ability to provide appropriate distal function is diminished. Palpation of the shoulder during a strong grip activity also demonstrates the need to maintain stabilization of even more proximal segments along the kinetic chain. With very demanding hand and wrist activities such as opening a stuck container lid, the trunk, lower limbs, and even facial muscles may participate in synergistic action as the individual makes a supreme effort to open the container.

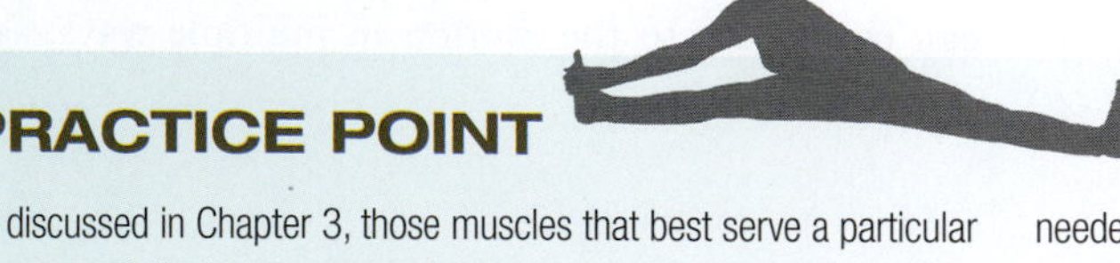

PRACTICE POINT

As discussed in Chapter 3, those muscles that best serve a particular purpose with the least amount of energy expenditure are the ones typically selected by the nervous system to perform the task. The greatest energy conservation during functional movements, however, is achieved best by highly skilled individuals. Movements of unskilled individuals waste energy because muscles not necessarily needed for the movement are "coactivated" and contract along with those needed. Unnecessary coactivation is normally present in the early stages of learning a skilled movement. Such activation is commonplace in young children just learning to balance and during early walking patterns, as well as in adults who are learning a new task. As skill develops, the selection improves and gradation of contraction becomes more finely tuned, resulting in smoother movements that are less fatiguing and, from the aesthetic standpoint, more pleasing to the eye.

One-Joint and Multijoint Muscles of the Elbow and Forearm

As was mentioned in Chapter 4, the single-joint muscles are recruited before the multijoint muscles. Since the brachialis is a one-joint muscle, it abides by this law of nature and is the muscle of choice for elbow flexion if neither supination nor pronation is desired. Indeed, the brachialis is recruited in all tasks requiring elbow flexion.[31] The body desires efficiency by design and function; it is inefficient to use the biceps brachii if the task simply requires elbow flexion or an isometric contraction with a low load because supination would have to be neutralized by the pronators so additional muscles would have to be recruited for simple elbow flexion.

Many elbow and forearm muscles act over more than one joint, and they are the ones usually selected for a task which simultaneously involves those joints. For example, the biceps brachii is the natural selection when elbow flexion and forearm supination occur simultaneously. Ordinarily, for light tasks, the nervous system typically recruits one muscle to perform the job of two when such a muscle is available and strong enough. In cases in which injury prevents a multijoint muscle from acting as it should, single-joint muscles are recruited in their place. For example, if a musculocutaneous nerve injury prevents the biceps from functioning, the brachioradialis and supinator are recruited to perform simultaneous elbow flexion and supination.

When a muscle crosses more than one joint, the muscle has an effect on each joint it crosses, and likewise, the muscle is also influenced by the position at those joints. As we have mentioned, the biceps brachii is a three-joint muscle whereas the long head of the triceps brachii and the pronator teres are two-joint muscles. As you remember from Chapter 4, when a muscle contracts to its shortest length, the muscle is at a weakened length since it is at its minimum on the length-tension curve; when this occurs in multijoint muscles, it is called active insufficiency. Therefore, the biceps is at its point of active insufficiency with full shoulder flexion, elbow flexion, and supination with the palm touching the back of the shoulder. Testing the maximum force of supination in this position compared to when the arm is at the side and the elbow is in 90° of flexion demonstrates the marked loss of biceps force. Active insufficiency of the long head of the triceps occurs at end-range shoulder and elbow extension. The pronator teres is actively insufficient with the elbow in flexion and pronation.

Most functional motions avoid active insufficiency and provide optimal muscle length for optimal sufficiency. For example, the biceps elongates when the shoulder is extended or hyperextended, so it maintains a favorable tension when the elbow flexes through a large range of motion with the arm at the side. This combination—elbow flexion and shoulder extension—occurs naturally in "pulling" activities. On the other hand, the long head of the triceps elongates when the shoulder flexes, so elbow extension combines with shoulder flexion to maintain effective triceps forces. This mechanism is used advantageously in "pushing" activities. The flexion and extension combinations are used alternately in the performance of many functional activities, such as sanding, polishing, using a vacuum cleaner, sawing wood, throwing a ball, archery, and bowling.

Typical Elbow and Forearm Muscular Function: Summary and Comparisons

Recent EMG studies indicate that, as would be expected, there are considerable variations of muscle action

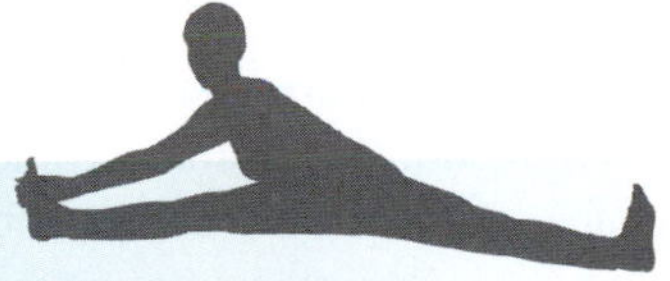

PRACTICE POINT

The maximum length position of the biceps brachii is shoulder hyperextension, elbow extension, and pronation. This position is used in an examination to determine if a multijoint muscle is abnormally shortened or if the muscle or its attachments have been injured. In cases of multijoint muscle tightness or injury, individual passive joint motions are usually within normal ranges. However, when the multijoint muscle is passively elongated to its full end range, the muscle's deficiency becomes apparent. If the muscle is restricted, the last motion attempted will be abnormally limited with a firm end feel. If the muscle is injured, pain occurs before the last joint motion is completed and the end feel is called "empty" since an end feel is not achieved. Since the long head of the triceps and the pronator teres are also multijoint muscles, this same type of test may be used to identify restricted motion or injury of these muscles as well.

among individuals, both in the selection of muscles and in the sequence of recruitment of elbow and forearm muscles. Based on the current literature, the functional patterns presented here are most typical of elbow and forearm function.

Elbow Flexion

Throughout elbow and forearm motions, the moment arm and the length of functioning muscles change, making some muscles more effective than others at specific points within the range of motion. We know that elbow strength peaks at around the midpoint of elbow flexion, between 90° and 120°.[12, 25, 26] As we have already discussed, the biceps brachii and the brachialis are best suited to generate large amounts of elbow force, whereas the brachioradialis is most active under certain conditions, and the pronator teres is a rather weak flexor. Because the biceps and brachialis have the largest moment arms, they provide strength and power for the elbow. On the other hand, the brachioradialis has a short moment arm and provides a large compression force to offer the elbow stability.

The brachialis is the least controversial of the flexors of the elbow. As mentioned, it is uninfluenced by the position of the forearm. Early and still undisputed studies by Basmajian and Latif[36] show that the brachialis is always active as an elbow flexor with or without a load and whether the motion is rapid or slow.

Although the brachioradialis is an elbow flexor, its role as a forearm supinator and pronator is more controversial. Early anatomists called it the *supinator longus*. Fick[37] states that mechanically, the brachioradialis is capable of performing a limited range of supination from the fully pronated position. Beevor first considered the brachioradialis to be a pure flexor of the elbow; his early observations have been substantiated by later EMG studies.[36, 38] Individuals with paralysis of the biceps, supinator, and pronators but who possess a strong brachioradialis cannot generate pronation or supination force. Functionally, these patients have difficulty maintaining a glass of water in an upright position to avoid spilling. Based on these findings, the brachioradialis may be considered a pure flexor of the elbow when the forearm is in midposition.

An isolated, unopposed contraction of the biceps produces simultaneous shoulder flexion, elbow flexion, and forearm supination. During functional motion, undesired biceps movements are prevented by synergistic contraction of other muscles or by gravity. The EMG studies cited previously show that the biceps plays little or no part in slow flexion of the elbow when the forearm is pronated, even when a 2 pound load is lifted or lowered. With the forearm supinated, however, the biceps acts in elbow flexion both with and without a load, in slow as well as in fast movements, regardless of whether the motion is concentric or eccentric. With increasing speed and increasing load, the biceps also acts when the forearm is pronated. Studies indicate that when a significant load is lifted, the biceps is always recruited, regardless of forearm position.[39]

Supination and Pronation

Supination and pronation are frequently used motions of the forearm. Each has muscles that are uniaxial and multiaxial. Unique considerations of supination are covered first, followed by those of pronation.

Comparison of actions of the biceps brachii and the supinator in supination

As mentioned earlier in this chapter, the biceps brachii acts most effectively as a supinator when the elbow is at about 90° of flexion. In this position, the muscle's tendon is at a right angle to the long axis of the radius, so its largest moment arm for supination occurs here. As the elbow extends and the moment arm diminishes, the effectiveness of the biceps as a supinator lessens. Recall that the effectiveness of the supinator muscle is not influenced by the elbow angle. At 90°, the biceps is almost four times as effective as the supinator in performing supination.[37] When the elbow is extended and supinated, however, the effectiveness of the biceps is only twice that of the supinator.[37]

The ability of the supinator to perform supination without the aid of the biceps has been verified by Basmajian and Latif.[36] In most subjects, no electromyographic activity registered in either head of the biceps during forearm supination while the elbow was in extension. But if resistance was applied to supination, the biceps became active. In conclusion, the supinator works alone during most low-power functional tasks.

Comparison of actions of the pronator teres and the pronator quadratus in pronation

The pronator teres is the strongest pronator. Because it is superficial, its contraction can be palpated. On the other hand, the role played by the pronator quadratus is difficult to assess because it cannot be palpated, although it is consistently active in all pronation movements, regardless of power demands or elbow position.[40] Since the pronator teres is an elbow flexor, its ability to pronate is determined somewhat by the elbow position. The cross section of the pronator quadratus is almost two-thirds the size of the pronator teres and compares favorably with the supinator. However, the shortening distance of the pronator quadratus is small. Based on its size and position, we can conclude that the pronator quadratus pronates the forearm unaided by other muscles during slow pronation, without resistance, and without active elbow flexion.

Extension: Comparison of action of the triceps and the anconeus

The triceps has a cross section about five times as large as the anconeus and a shortening range about twice that of the anconeus.[37, 41] The fascia over the triceps tendon also extends over the anconeus, illustrating the very close synergistic relationship between these two muscles. In addition, the anconeus has a close relation to the elbow joint and the proximal radioulnar joint. Both muscles contribute to the protection of these joints. They also provide dynamic elbow extension. Since it is a one-joint muscle, it is not surprising that the anconeus is typically the first muscle recruited to initiate elbow extension; the anconeus may also have sufficient strength to maintain low force levels. As force requirements increase, the medial head of the triceps is recruited first. The medial head strength is usually sufficient to handle typical demands.[42] With higher force demands, the lateral and then the long head of the triceps are recruited.[43]

Closed Kinematic Chain Motion at the Elbow Complex

Although most skilled functional upper extremity movements are in the open kinematic chain (OKC), it is important to recognize the importance of stability of this middle upper-extremity link when the extremity works in a closed kinematic chain (CKC). Although the bony configuration and joint's ligaments provide most of the elbow's stability in full extension, the demand for stability transfers to the joint's flexor and extensor muscles when the elbow is even slightly flexed; these muscle groups cocontract to provide this stability in a CKC activity.

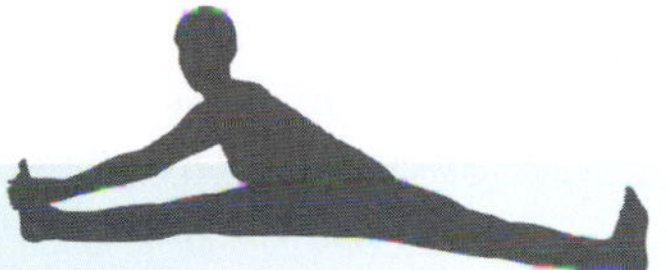

PRACTICE POINT

Because the supinator's sole action is supination and it is a one-joint muscle, it is logical to conclude that the supinator is called upon to contract when supination without elbow flexion is desired and when motion occurs slowly and without resistance. Clinically, this assumption may be confirmed as follows: Have your partner sit with the forearm resting in his or her lap. Place your palpating fingers on the tendon of the biceps at the elbow. If supination is performed slowly and the forearm remains in the lap, the tendon of the biceps remains relaxed since the movement is performed by the supinator.[32] As the speed of motion increases, the biceps brachii is recruited; you can easily palpate the biceps tendon working immediately when a quick supination is performed. This test is useful when working with clients with radial nerve injuries to determine when regeneration of the nerve has progressed to the supinator. As long as the supinator is denervated, a slow supination of the forearm recruits the biceps tendon in place of the supinator. When the supinator has been reinnervated, the normal preferential recruitment order is restored. In other cases, this testing procedure can be useful to isolate the supinator, although in individuals without pathology, no information about the strength of the supinator is obtained.

Even though the pectoralis major does not cross the elbow, this muscle is able to cause elbow extension in closed chain motion as it adducts the shoulder. This function is extremely useful to persons with spinal cord lesions who have paralysis of the triceps brachii (C_7–C_8) but retain innervation of the pectoralis major (C_5–C_7). With the hand anchored, the pectoralis major pulls the shoulder across the body. As the shoulder moves medially, the forearm rolls into supination and the elbow locks in extension. Functional tasks such as moving the body in a sliding board transfer is accomplished by anchoring the hand on the sliding board, then contracting the pectoralis major to pull on the humerus forward to extend the elbow; aligning the elbow anterior to the wrist and shoulder places the extremity's line of force posterior to the elbow joint, thereby passively locking it in extension.

Analyses of Muscle Activity during Common Functional Movements

Like the shoulder, the elbow's purpose is to position the hand for functional activities. However, unlike the shoulder, the elbow also determines the relative position of the hand to the body, bringing the hand either closer to the body or moving it farther away from the body. Additionally, the forearm moves the hand in degrees of pronation and supination so the hand may be positioned for specific functions, such as supination to bring a spoon to the mouth, neutral to grasp a glass of liquid without spilling it, or pronation to use a toothbrush. In Chapter 5, muscle activity during the commonly observed functional motions of placing the hand behind the head and pulling were briefly kinematically analyzed. Now that we have added another link in the upper extremity chain, the following section describes the kinematic analysis of those same functional activities with a focus on the muscular contributions from the elbow and forearm complex. A key factor to consider for the elbow and forearm is how far away from the body the upper extremity needs to move to produce the desired function. As the middle link in the chain, the elbow complex provides the amount of reach outward away from the body or pulling inward toward the body that is required for the upper extremity to accomplish its task.

Do not forget that gravity is a factor in determining which muscles function. For example, elbow extension performed with the assist of gravity is performed by the elbow flexors acting as decelerators to control the speed of elbow extension; the triceps is not involved. On the other hand, if elbow extension occurs against gravity, the triceps perform the movement, acting as accelerators to concentrically extend the elbow.

Placing the Hand behind the Head

In Chapter 5, the first functional movement example discussed placing the hand behind the head, as in combing one's hair. In addition to the shoulder motions you already know occur, the elbow flexes and the forearm pronates. Since there is some resistance of the hair to the comb moving through it, the elbow and forearm muscles providing these actions include the biceps brachii and brachialis, contracting to flex the elbow against this resistance as the hand holding the comb moves down the head. The pronator teres and pronator quadratus cocontract to hold the forearm in full pronation and the comb in the desired position. Prior to the movement of the comb through the hair, the elbow flexes to position the comb on the head after the shoulder is elevated; as the elbow flexes to lower the comb, the triceps eccentrically contract to place the comb.

Pulling

Pulling may occur in either OKC or CKC. Muscle activity and requirements may change as these conditions change. Let's look at closed-chain motion first since, as you remember from Chapter 1, closed-chain motions are somewhat more consistent and, therefore, easier to visualize. As with the example in Chapter 5, closed-chain motion occurs during a chin-up on a fixed overhead bar. Elbow flexion and forearm supination occur during a chin-up. The brachialis (the "workhorse") and the biceps brachii provide the primary muscular elbow force, flexing the elbow concentrically to lift the body weight. The supinator and biceps provide the sustained supination forearm force. On the return from the full chin-up position, the biceps and brachialis continue working, now acting eccentrically to control the rate at which gravity exerts its downward pull. This is a good example of muscular function switching from concentric to eccentric because of the influence gravity has on the body.

In the open chain, things can become more complex because the arm and forearm are freer to move in space so there is a possibility of more variation in motion and function. Let's look at the example in Chapter 5 of an overhead exercise pulley used in a pulldown exercise. There are a variety of ways such an exercise device may be manipulated: 1) It may be pulled toward you with palms up so that the hands move down to the chin (Fig. 6.13A); 2) it may be pulled down behind the back with palms in a down position (Fig. 6.13B); or it may be pulled down in front of the body until the hands are at hip level. (Fig. 6.13C2) In all of these examples, the elbow starts in extension reaching overhead for the bar, and in the first two the elbow ends in flexion. In the third example, the elbow moves into flexion during the first half of the activity (Fig. 6.13C1) but then moves back into extension by the end of the motion (Fig. 6.13C2). The brachialis, brachioradialis, and biceps brachii provide elbow flexion force, and the biceps also works with the supinator to provide forearm supination in the first example. In the second case, the same elbow flexors function to flex the elbow, but the biceps is not contributing as much with the forearm in pronation. Additionally, the pronators are now working to maintain the forearm position through the activity as the bar is brought behind the head. In the final example, the forearm remains pronated, so the pronator quadratus and teres work to hold this position while the elbow flexors and extensors become involved at different points within the activity. The elbow flexors are involved as they are in the second example to flex the elbow as the bar moves down to the chest, but once the bar is moved to the point that the elbow is at 90° of flexion and then continues to move into extension, the triceps take over the movement as the motion converts from a pull to a push; the triceps, with assistance from the anconeus, extends the elbow against the external force until the end position is reached (Fig. 6.13C2).

Summary

This chapter describes the kinesiological principles related to functional motion at the elbow complex. The elbow complex includes the humeroulnar, humeroradial, and the proximal radioulnar joints. Anatomy review and guides to palpation are described and displayed in table format with special factors of each segment presented within the text. The focus of the chapter is functional relationships between and among the different joints and primary muscles providing elbow and forearm motions. Functional movement of this region is optimized by a supportive and synergistic relationship between the joints and the muscles of the elbow and forearm. Contributions to muscular function from the primary muscles at this region are discussed. Common functional movements are described and kinematically analyzed. Pathological conditions are included as an illustration of the functional consequences encountered when the mechanics of this area are compromised.

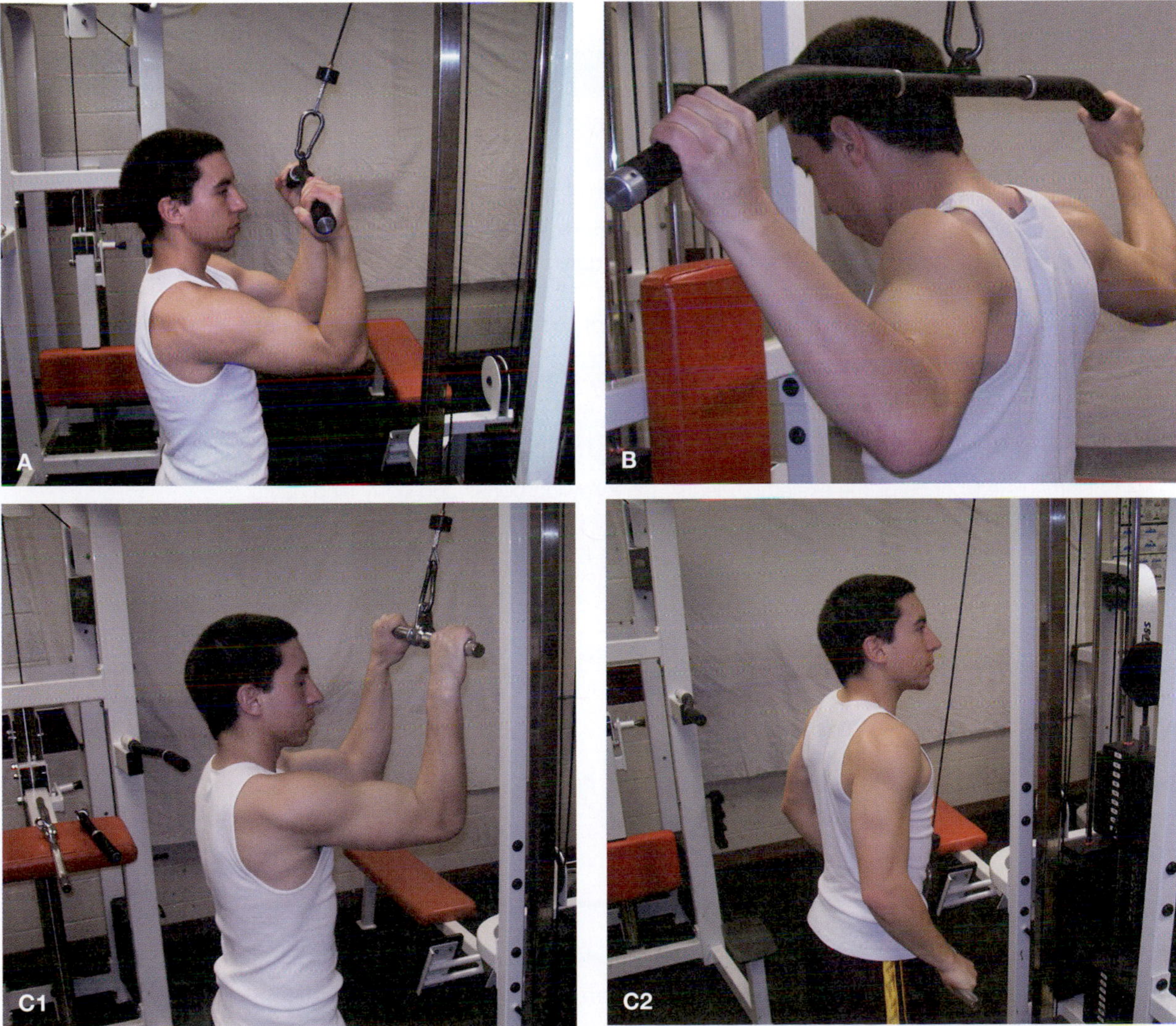

Figure 6.13 Model demonstrates performing the action of pulling on an overhead bar. **A)** The model pulls the bar down in front of the chin with elbow flexion forearm supination. **B)** The model pulls the overhead bar with the forearm pronated with the bar going behind the head. **C)** The model pulls the bar down in front of the body, engaging the biceps in the first half of the motion (C1). When the elbow extends beyond 90°, note the activation of the triceps contracting to push the bar down (C2).

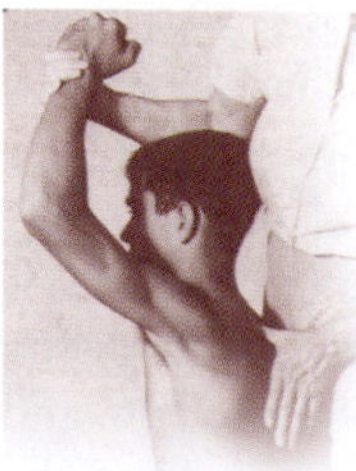

CLINICAL SCENARIO SOLUTION

Through obtaining a history from Chris and palpating his elbow, Bethany was able to identify that Chris's pain was at the medial epicondyle, the point of attachment for many of the wrist and finger flexors. This explained why the pain at the elbow resulted in a functional consequence at the hand—a weakened grasp—and hence, Chris's complaint of "the dropsies." In her examination, Bethany noted pain and tenderness over the medial epicondyle, and this pain was exacerbated not by elbow joint motion but rather by resisted wrist flexion. Intervention was first directed to resting the area and treating the acute symptoms at the medial epicondyle. Chris's wrist was placed in a resting splint with his wrist in neutral so that he would not aggravate the injury by using his wrist flexors. Most importantly, Bethany gave Chris some instruction on the pathomechanics of his injury and offered movement suggestions which could prevent this injury from recurring. After the symptoms subsided, intervention included strengthening of the wrist and finger flexor muscles.

Discussion Questions

1. How does the structural anatomy at the humeroulnar and humeroradial articulations contribute to both stability as well as mobility at this region?
2. What do *you* think is the functional purpose of the carrying angle?
3. What are the varying contributions from the five primary muscles at this region to the accomplishment of the following common activities: pulling a hat down onto your head; opening and closing a window; pushing a shopping cart; or tossing a Frisbee? How are the muscles functioning—as agonists, antagonists, and/or synergists? What types of contractions (concentric, eccentric, and isometric) are involved?

Lab Activities

1. On disarticulated bones or the skeleton, identify the following bones and bony landmarks.

Humerus

shaft
medial epicondyle
lateral epicondyle
lateral supracondylar ridge
trochlea
capitulum
trochlear groove
capitulotrochlear groove
olecranon fossa
radial fossa
coronoid fossa

Ulna

shaft
olecranon process
coronoid process
trochlear or semilunar notch
trochlear (longitudinal) ridge
ulnar tuberosity
head
radial notch
styloid process

Radius

shaft
head
fovea
neck
tuberosity of radius
styloid process

2. Which of these bony landmarks can you palpate? Locate these on yourself and then on a partner.
3. Using the skeleton or disarticulated bony model, perform the following motions with the skeleton; also, perform the motions yourself. Identify and examine bony surfaces where the movements of elbow flexion, elbow extension, pronation, and supination take place. Move the radius on the ulna by turning the palm of the hand up into supination and then by turning it down into pronation. Note that when the palm turns up in supination, the radius and ulna are parallel; when the palm turns down in pronation, these bones are crossed—that is, the radius rotates and crosses over the ulna.

4. Perform the following elbow and forearm movements on yourself and then observe as a partner performs them:
   a. Flex and extend the elbow first with the forearm supinated, then with the forearm pronated.
   b. Pronate and supinate the forearm while palpating the head of the radius. As you do this, hold your upper arm against the side of your body, maintain your wrist in one position, and maintain your elbow flexed at a right angle. Note that isolated forearm movement occurs for approximately 180° of total motion.
   c. Pronate both forearms as described. Now extend your elbows, lift your arms to shoulder height, and continue to turn the palms of your hands in the direction of pronation and then supination as far as they will move. Note the increased movement that results from shoulder rotation (approximately 360°). Now isolate the forearm movement by again flexing the elbow and holding the upper arm against the side of the body. Which forearm and shoulder movements occur synchronously?
5. On the skeleton, on yourself, and on a partner, identify and visualize the axes for elbow flexion and extension and for forearm pronation and supination. Identify and palpate bony landmarks to locate these axes.
6. Using a universal goniometer, measure the carrying angle of various members of the class as each member stands in anatomical position. Note any trends related to body build or gender and discuss.
7. Using an anatomy text, this text, a skeleton, a partner and Table 6–2, determine points of attachment for and palpate the following muscles:
   a. biceps brachii
   b. brachioradialis
   c. brachialis
   d. pronator teres
   e. triceps brachii
   f. anconeus
   g. supinator
   h. pronator quadratus

   Especially note the action line of each muscle and the axes each one crosses; from these observations, determine the movements each can perform. A helpful method to facilitate such observations is to cut lengths of adhesive tape or elastic bands to reach from one attachment of the muscle to the other. Tape these pieces onto the skeleton from the point of proximal attachment to the point of distal attachment.
8. List muscles that:
   a. Flex the elbow
   b. Extend the elbow
   c. Pronate the forearm
   d. Supinate the forearm
9. Perform elbow flexion with the forearm in supination, pronation and midposition. Palpate the muscles that participate in each motion and discuss with a partner the varying contributions of the individual muscles.
10. Perform the same action as above and, in order to integrate knowledge gained from the previous chapter on the shoulder region, palpate and name the muscles required for scapular and glenohumeral stabilization in order to perform this movement function.
11. End feels: Perform slow passive motion to the end of the range of motion of elbow flexion, extension, pronation, and supination on your partner. Describe the end feels and the tissues that limit the motion.
12. Perform a kinematic analysis of the elbow and shoulder for the following functional activities:
    a. Opening a door by turning the doorknob;
    b. Reaching overhead to grasp onto and then pull a window shade down;
    c. Serving a volleyball;
    d. Rolling out piecrust or cookie dough;
    e. Doing jumping jacks.

13. Active insufficiency of the biceps brachii: Test your partner's strength of supination with the arm at the side and the elbow in 90° of flexion and then when the biceps brachii is in its shortest position of shoulder flexion, elbow flexion, and supination.

14. Muscle excursion: Measure the excursion of the biceps brachii from its shortest length (full shoulder flexion, elbow flexion, and supination) to its longest length (shoulder hyperextension, elbow extension, and pronation) on an articulated skeleton or on your partner. Measure the excursion of the brachialis from its shortest length (full flexion) to its longest length (full extension). Compare the two muscles and discuss the functional implications.

References

1. Andrews JR, Whiteside JR. Common elbow problems in the athlete. *Journal of Orthopaedic and Sports Physical Therapy* 17:289–295, 1993.
2. Noteboom T, Cruver R, Keller J, Kellogg B, Nitz AJ. Tennis elbow: A review. *Journal of Orthopaedic and Sports Physical Therapy* 19:357–366, 1994.
3. Schultz SJ, Houglum PA, Perrin DH. *Examination of Musculoskeletal Injuries*, ed 3. Champaign, IL: Human Kinetics, 2010.
4. Shaughnessy WJ. Osteochonditis dissecans. In Morrey BF (ed): *The Elbow and its Disorders*, 3 ed. Philadelphia: WB Saunders Company, 2000, pp 255–260.
5. Ericson A, Arndt A, Stark A, et al. Variation in the position and orientation of the elbow flexion axis. *Journal of Bone and Joint Surgery Br* 85:538, 2003.
6. Morrey BF, Askew L, J, An K, N, Chao EY. A biomechanical study of normal elbow motion. *Journal of Bone and Joint Surgery* 63A:872–877, 1981.
7. Kapandji IA. *The Physiology of the Joints,* Vol 1, Upper Limb, ed.5. Edinburgh: Churchill Livingstone, 1982.
8. Stroyan M, Wilk KE. The functional anatomy of the elbow complex. *Journal of Orthopaedic and Sports Physical Therapy* 17:279–288, 1993.
9. American Academy of Orthopaedic Surgeons. *Joint Motion: Method of Measuring and Recording*. Chicago: American Academy of Orthopaedic Surgeons, 1965.
10. Greene WB, Heckman JDE. *The Clinical Measurement of Joint Motion*. Rosemont, IL: American Academy of Orthopaedic Surgeons, 1994.
11. Levangie PK, Norton CC. *Joint Structure & Function: A Comprehensive Analysis*, ed 4. Philadelphia: FA Davis, 2005.
12. Oatis CA. *Kinesiology: The Mechanics & Pathomechanics of Human Movement*, ed 2. Philadelphia: Lippincott, Williams & Wilkins, 2008.
13. Stokdijk M, Meskers C, G, M, Veeger H, E, J, deBoer Y, Rozing P. Determination of the optimal elbow axis for evaluation of placement of prosthesis. *Clinical Biomechanics* 14:177–184, 1999.
14. Atkinson WB, Elftman H. The carrying angle of the human arm as a secondary sex character. *Anatomical Record* 91:49–52, 1945.
15. Steel FL, Tomlinson JD. The 'carrying angle' in man. *Journal of Anatomy* 92:315, 1958.
16. Beals RD. The normal carrying angle of the elbow: A radiographic study of 422 patients. *Clinical Orthopaedics* 119:194–196, 1976.
17. VanRoy P, Baeyans D, Fauvart R, Lanssiers R, Clarijs JP. Arthrokinematics of the elbow: Study of the carrying angle. *Ergonomics* 48:1645–1656, 2005.
18. Chao EY, Morrey BF. Three-dimensional rotation of the elbow. *Journal of Biomechanics* 11:57–73, 1978.
19. Lippert L. *Clinical Kinesiology and Anatomy*, ed 4. Philadelphia: FA Davis, 2006.
20. Morrey BF. *The Elbow and its Disorders*, ed 3. Philadelphia: FA Davis, 2000.
21. Youm Y, Dryer RF, Thambyrajah K, Flatt A, Sprague B. Biomechanical analysis of forearm pronation-supination and elbow flexion-extension. *Journal of Biomechanics* 12:245–255, 1979.
22. Starkey C, Ryan J. *Orthopedic & Athletic Injury Evaluation Handbook*. Philadelphia: F A Davis, 2003.
23. Spinner M, Kaplan E, B. The quadrate ligament of the elbow: Its relationship to the stability of the proximal radio-ulnar joint. *Acta Orthopaedica Scandinavica* 41(6):632–647, 1970.
24. Letts RM. Dislocations of the child's elbow. In Morrey BF, editor: *The Elbow and its Disorders*. Philadelphia: WB Saunders Company, 2000, pp 261–286.

25. Pigeon P, Yahia L, Feldman AJ. Moment arm and lengths of human upper limb muscles as functions of joint angles. *Journal of Biomechanics* 29:1365–1370, 1996.
26. Murray WM, Delp SL, Buchanan TS. Variation of muscle moment arms with elbow and forearm position. *Journal of Biomechanics* 28:513–525, 1995.
27. Askew LJ, An KN, Morrey BF, Chao EYS. Isometric elbow strength in normal individuals. *Clinical Orthopaedics* 222:261–266, 1987.
28. Currier DP. Maximal isometric tension of the elbow extensors at varied positions. Part I: Assessment by cable tensiometer. *Physical Therapy* 52:1043–1049, 1972.
29. Knapik JJ, Wright JE, Mawdsley RH, Braun J. Isometric, isotonic, and isokinetic torque variations in four muscle groups through a range of joint motion. *Physical Therapy* 63:938–947, 1983.
30. LeBozec S, Maton B, Cnockaert JC. The synergy of elbow extensor muscles during static work in man. *European Journal of Applied Physiology* 43:57–68, 1980.
31. Zhang LQ, Nuber GW. Moment distribution among human elbow extensor muscles during isometric and submaximal extension. *Journal of Biomechanics* 33:145, 2000.
32. Naito A, Sun YJ, Yajiima M. Electromyographic study of the flexors and extensors in a motion of forearm pronation/supination while maintaining elbow flexion in humans. *Tohoku Journal of Experimental Medicine* 186:267, 1998.
33. Basmajian JV, DeLuca CJ. *Muscles Alive: Their Functions Revealed by Electromyography,* ed 5. Baltimore: Williams & Wilkins, 1985.
34. Stuart PR. Pronator quadratus revisited. *Journal of Hand Surgery* 21B:714–722, 1996.
35. Prodoehl J, Gottleib GL, Corocs DM. The neural control of single degree of freedom elbow movement: Effect of starting position. *Experimental Brain Research* 153(1):7–15, 2003.
36. Basmajian JV, Latif A. Integrated actions and functions of the chief flexors of the elbow: A detailed electromyographic analysis. *Journal of Bone and Joint Surgery* 39:1106–1118, 1957.
37. Fick R. *Anatomie und Mechanik der Gelenke: Teil III, Spezielle Gelenk und Muskel Mechanik*. Jena, Germany: Fisher, 1911.
38. Beevor C. *Croonian Lectures on Muscular Movement: Guarantors of Brain*. New York: MacMillan, 1903.
39. Kasprisin JE, Grabiner MD. Joint angle-dependence of elbow flexor activation levels during isometric and isokinetic maximum voluntary contractions. *Clinical Biomechanics (Bristol, Avon)* 15:743, 2000.
40. Basmajian JV, Travill A. Electromyography of the pronator muscles of the forearm. *Anatomical Record* 139:45–49, 1961.
41. Lehmkuhl LD, Smith LK. *Brunnstrom's Clinical Kinesiology*, ed 4. Philadelphia: FA Davis, 1983.
42. Travill AA. Electromyographic study of the extensor apparatus. *Anatomical Record* 144:373–376, 1962.
43. Neumann DA. *Kinesiology of the Musculoskeletal System: Foundations for Physical Rehabilitation*. St. Louis: Mosby, 2002.

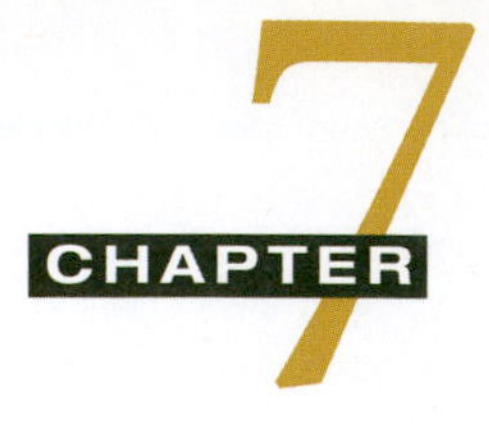

Wrist and Hand

Ingrid Provident, EdD, OTR/L, and Peggy A. Houglum, PhD, PT, ATC

"Take your life in your own hands, and what happens? A terrible thing: no one to blame."
—Erika Jong, Author and educator

CHAPTER OUTLINE

Learning Outcomes
Clinical Scenario
Introduction
Bones
Wrist
Hand
Phalanges
Joints
Wrist
Hand
Fingers and Thumb
Soft Tissue Supporting Structures
Muscles
Muscles Acting on the Wrist
Muscles Acting on the Digits
Extensor Mechanism
Motions
Motions of the Wrist
Motions of the Fingers
Functional Movements of the Wrist and Hand
Types of Grasp
Strength of Grip
Grasping
Intrinsic-Plus and Intrinsic-Minus Positions
Abduction and Adduction of Digits 2 to 5
Balanced Forces
Fingers
Thumb
Synergic Action of Wrist Muscles in Movements of the Thumb and Little Finger

LEARNING OUTCOMES

This chapter investigates the wrist and hand. By the end of this chapter, you should be able to:

- ❑ Identify the bones, joints, soft tissue, and muscles of the wrist and hand;
- ❑ List muscles that are prime movers in wrist flexion, extension, radial, and ulnar deviation and intricate hand movements;
- ❑ Name muscle groups that function to position and move the wrist and hand in specific functional motions;
- ❑ Identify the nerves that innervate the main muscles of the wrist and hand;
- ❑ Describe commonly encountered movement disorders of the wrist/hand and their functional consequences;
- ❑ Identify normal grasping patterns of the hand and their importance in functional activities.

Peripheral Nerves of the Wrist and Hand
Peripheral Nerve Innervations
Peripheral Nerve Injuries
Summary
Clinical Scenario Solution
Discussion Questions
Lab Activities
References

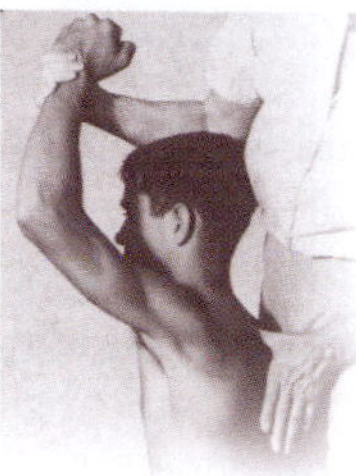

CLINICAL SCENARIO

Lori is a hairdresser who has been trying to build her business and clientele. She has noticed most recently that she is experiencing numbness in her hands, and she is frequently dropping the combs and brushes she uses. At night, she experiences pain and tingling which radiate up to her fingertips, and the pain often wakes her up at night. Lori loves her work and is proud of her new shop. She is concerned that if she goes to her physician, she will need surgery and will be forced to take time off from work.

Introduction

Several bones, joints, muscles, tendons, nerves, and blood vessels make up the hand. The hand is a predominant part of the body, serving many purposes. As such, it is a very versatile body segment, adapting to the many demands placed upon it. As with the shoulder and elbow, the wrist positions the hand and provides a stable platform from which the hand functions, but unlike the shoulder and elbow, the wrist is responsible for finely tuned hand positioning as well as more global positioning. The hand contains the palm and fingers. These structures are both sturdy and mobile. The fingers are sometimes referred to as digits and are named for either their position or their purpose:

- Thumb comes from the Latin word *pollex*, which is the medical term for the thumb: pollicis. It is our first digit or number one (#1) digit.
- The second digit, sometimes referred to as the "first finger" is also called the index finger, pointer finger, or forefinger. "Index finger" was perhaps attached to this #2 digit because it is often used to point, and pointing is a method of making things clearer; making things clearer is the purpose of an index.
- The third digit is also the middle finger or second finger. It is usually the longest finger of the hand.
- The fourth digit is commonly referred to as the ring finger or third finger. Sometime around the fifth century, it was believed that this finger contained a "vein of love" that flowed directly to the heart, so people started wearing wedding rings on this finger.
- The fifth digit, or fourth finger, is the smallest finger. For this reason, it is often referred to as the "pinky" or "little" finger.

Whereas the first two digits are used for dexterous or fine manipulations of objects, the last three provide the hand with gross or strength manipulations.

The hand is a complex, multipurpose organ. As a prehensile organ (L., *prehensus,* to seize), the hand can grasp with forces exceeding 100 lb (445 N or 45 kg) as well as hold and manipulate a delicate thread. Its complex structure allows it to conform around objects of all sizes and shapes; for example, the hand is able to conform around an egg so well that squeezing a raw egg will not break it since the pressure is so well distributed by the conforming ability of the hand. In addition to these functions, the hand can be used for pushing and pulling, and can even provide locomotion using crutches or wheelchairs. As a sense organ for touch, the hand is an extension of the brain to provide information about the environment. The hand is also an important organ for expression and nonverbal communication. How important the hand is to humans is demonstrated by the mere fact that the reason we have a shoulder, elbow, and wrist is to position the hand so it can performs its functions.

Hand placement and stabilization depend on the trunk, shoulder, elbow, and wrist. With the multiple degrees of freedom allowed by the upper extremity, the versatility of hand placement is inconceivably high.

Bones

Within the compact structure of the wrist and hand are 29 bones and even more ligaments and tendons.

This section presents the bones of the wrist and hand; the following sections discuss ligaments and muscles.

Wrist

Although the primary forearm bone for the elbow joint is the ulna, the primary forearm bone of the wrist is the radius. There are two proximal carpal bones that interact with the radius to form the wrist joint.

Distal Ulna

Unlike the radius, the ulna is not in direct contact with the carpal bones. A fibrocartilaginous disc separates the ulna from the carpal bones. In spite of this separation, the distal portion of the ulna is an important part of the wrist. The distal ulna has three parts: the **ulnar styloid process**, the **fovea,** and the pole. The ulnar styloid process is a bony projection, easily palpated with the forearm pronated, on the ulnar side of the wrist. The fovea is a depression at the base of this styloid process and provides attachment for the fibrocartilaginous disc. The pole is a concave articular surface allowing ulnar articulation with the fibrocartilaginous disc.

Distal Radius

The distal end of the radius has several surfaces that are important for proper wrist function. The dorsal surface has a palpable tubercle that is known as the **tubercle of the radius, Lister's tubercle,** or **dorsal tubercle.** It lies about one-third of the wrist's width from the radial styloid process and has grooves on either side of it that serve as a pulley for the extensor pollicis longus tendon on the ulnar side and the extensor digitorum and extensor indicis tendons on the radial side as they pass adjacent to the tubercle. The dorsal tubercle's pulley function serves to redirect the pull of the extensor pollicis longus. On the radial surface of the radius is a distal projection called the **radial styloid process.** This process extends somewhat more distally than the corresponding ulnar styloid process. The ulnar and radial styloid processes serve as attachment sites for the ulnar and radial carpal collateral ligaments, respectively.

On the ulnar (lateral) aspect of the distal radius is the articulating surface for the distal radioulnar joint, commonly called the **ulnar notch** or **sigmoid notch**. The distal surface of the radius makes up the proximal joint surface of the wrist and articulates with the scaphoid and lunate carpal bones.

Carpal Bones

There are eight carpal bones which are more or less cuboid-shaped in the wrist. They have articulating surfaces on their proximal, distal, medial, and lateral aspects with roughened surfaces on their volar and dorsal sides that provide attachment sites for the wrist ligaments. The sole exception is the pisiform bone, which has only one articulating surface. These eight carpal bones are arranged in two rows: The proximal row of carpal bones contains, laterally to medially, the scaphoid, lunate, triquetrum, and pisiform; the distal row contains, laterally to medially, the trapezium, trapezoid, capitate, and hamate (Fig. 7.1B).

Occupying a central position at the wrist (in line with the middle finger), the **capitate bone** (os magnum) is best approached from the dorsum, where a slight depression indicates its location (Fig. 7.2A). The axis of motion for ulnar and radial deviation goes through this bone in a dorsopalmar direction (Fig. 7.2B).

The scaphoid (formerly known as the navicular) bone is palpated distally to the styloid process of the radius (Fig. 7.1B). Ulnar abduction of the wrist causes the bone to become prominent to the palpating fingers, whereas radial abduction causes the bone to recede. The scaphoid bone and the trapezium make up the floor of the "anatomic snuff box" (fovea radialis), the depression seen between the tendons of the thumb extensor muscles (extensor pollicis longus and brevis) when these muscles are tensed (Fig. 7.3). Based on its appearance, the scaphoid seems to extend across both rows of carpal bones, giving the impression that the proximal row curves around the capitate. However, it should be remembered that the scaphoid belongs to the proximal row and the trapezium is in the distal row of carpal bones between the scaphoid and first metacarpal.

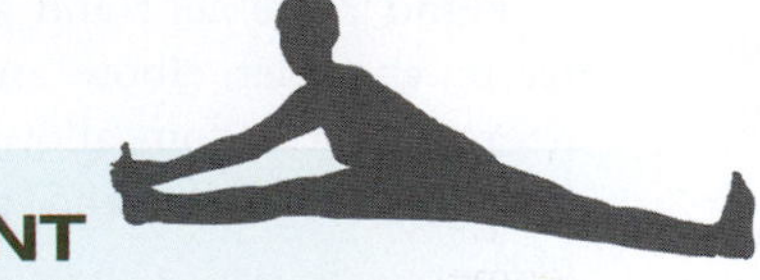

PRACTICE POINT

It can be difficult for the novice to remember these carpal bones, but it is necessary for clinicians to remember their arrangement and position. A simple mnemonic is frequently used to more easily remember the carpal bones. A mnemonic (nee MON ic) is a formula or system that is used to "jog" the memory. In the case of the carpal bones, the mnemonic is: **S**he **L**ooks **T**oo **P**retty, **T**ry **T**o **C**atch **H**er.

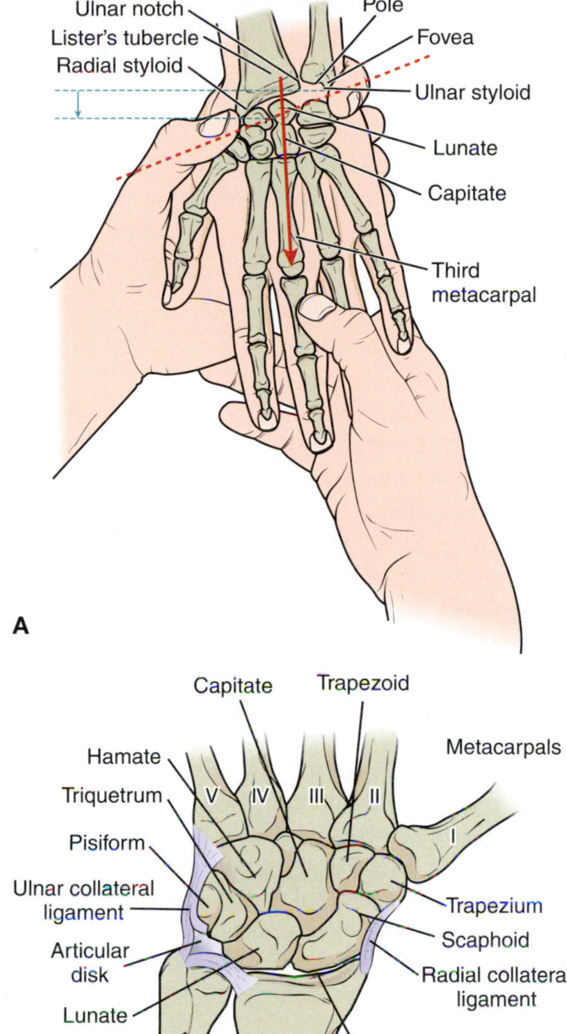

Figure 7.1 Bony landmarks on the wrist. **A)** A dorsal view of the wrist and hand. The approximate location of the axis for radiocarpal flexion and extension is a line connecting the tips of the palpating thumb and forefinger of the palpating hand with a horizontal line between the distal radial and ulnar styloid processes. **B)** A ventral view of the wrist and hand showing the articulating surfaces and some of the ligaments of the wrist and hand. The midcarpal joint is formed by the distal articulating surfaces of the proximal row of carpals and the proximal articulating surfaces of the distal row. The proximal carpal row from lateral to medial wrist is the scaphoid, lunate, triquetrum, and pisiform; the distal row from lateral to medial wrist includes the trapezium, trapezoid, capitate, and hamate.

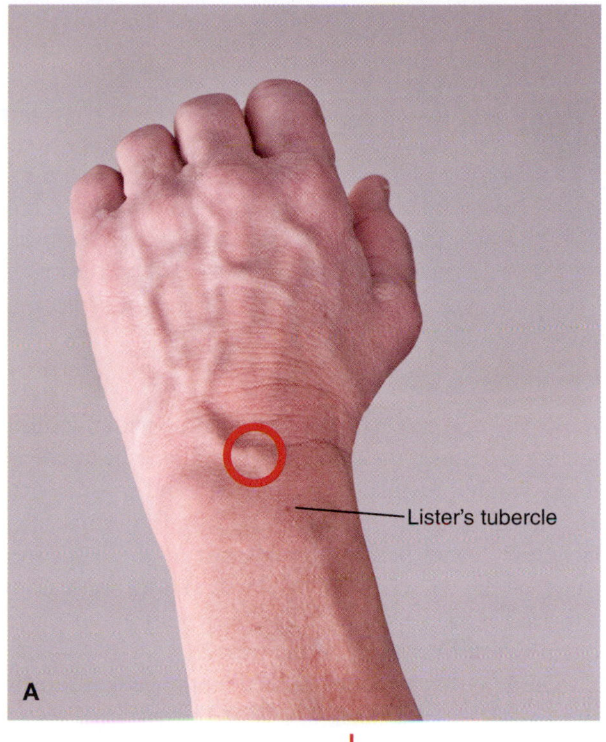

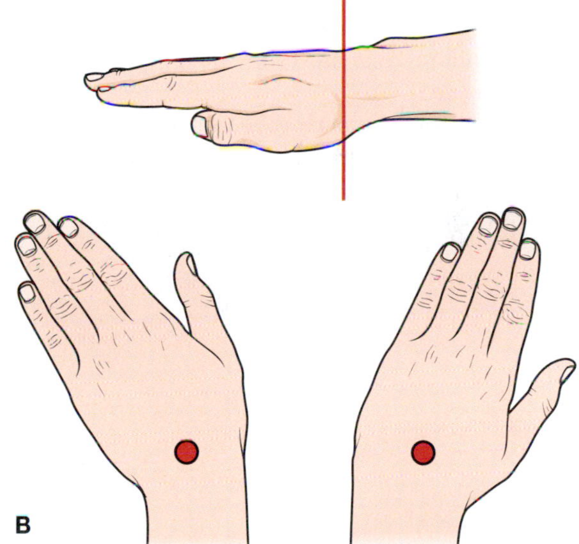

Figure 7.2 **A)** Photo image of the depression overlaying the capitate bone of the wrist. **B)** The axis of motion for ulnar and radial deviation goes through the capitate in a dorsal-to-palmar direction.

The trapezium (formerly known as the greater multangular) is palpated proximally to the first carpometacarpal (CMC) joint of the thumb and distal to the identified scaphoid by passively flexing and extending the thumb to identify the joint margin (Fig. 7.3).

The lunate is palpated more easily if the capitate bone is located first. The capitate is palpated as the

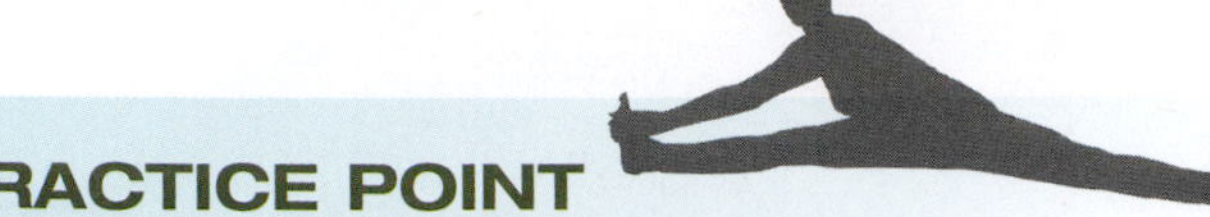

PRACTICE POINT

The scaphoid is the most commonly fractured bone of the wrist. The common mechanism of injury is a fall on an outstretched arm with the forearm pronated. Because it has a poor vascular supply, a fracture of this bone frequently does not heal, becoming a nonunion fracture. Since it is often difficult to diagnose a scaphoid fracture, it is prudent to treat any injury to this region as a fracture until such a diagnosis is ruled out. Conservative treatment is not successful if it is a nonunion fracture. Persistent pain in the anatomic snuff box is a leading complaint for these fractures.

proximal bone making up the articulation with the third metacarpal. Once the capitate is identified, the lunate is immediately proximal to the capitate and in line with and distal to Lister's tubercle (Fig. 7.2). In normal subjects, the lunate becomes prominent to the palpating finger as the wrist is passively flexed and recedes as the wrist is passively extended. The lunate is the most frequently dislocated bone in the wrist.[1]

The pea-shaped bone palpated on the palmar side of the wrist near the ulnar border is the pisiform bone. This bone can be grasped and moved from side to side. Serving as the point of attachment for the flexor carpi ulnaris tendon, this moveable bone qualifies as a sesamoid bone.[1]

The trapezoid (formerly called the lesser multangular), the triquetrum (formerly called the triangular), and the hamate bones seen in Figure 7.1B are more difficult to distinguish directly by palpation. However, they can be palpated and identified using their relationships to the other carpal bones and bony structures that are more easily palpated. The hamate is located by palpating its hook. This protuberance lies at a 45° angle into the palm from the pisiform; lay the base of your thumb's distal phalanx over the pisiform so the tip of your thumb points toward the first web space between the thumb and index finger. The tip of your thumb should then be on the hook of the hamate. With deep palpation, you should be able to identify the hook protuberance; it may be tender to palpation. The triquetrum is under the pisiform and best palpated on the dorsal wrist with the wrist in radial abduction. It is palpated as a bony prominence just distal to the ulnar styloid process. The trapezoid is the most difficult carpal bone to palpate. It lies distal to the scaphoid, medial to the trapezium, and lateral to the capitate.

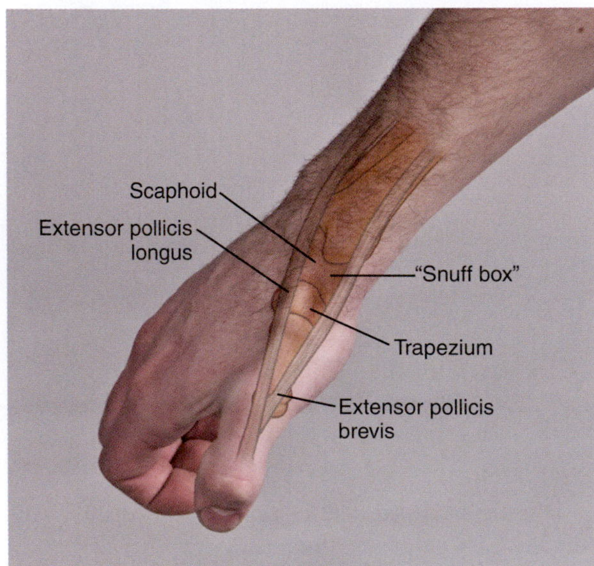

Figure 7.3 The floor of the anatomical snuff box comprises the scaphoid proximally and the trapezium distally. The anatomical snuff box is bordered medially by the extensors pollicis longus and laterally by the extensor pollicis brevis and abductor pollicis longus.

Hand

Distal to the carpal bones are the metacarpals and phalanges. These bones comprise the hand. The phalanges make up the digits. The metacarpals and digits are identified numerically, laterally to medially (from the anatomical position), one through five.

Metacarpals

Each of the five metacarpals has a base that articulates proximally with one or more carpal bones and with its adjacent metacarpals (Fig. 7.1B), a shaft that is slightly curved with a palmar concavity, and a head that articulates with the base of a proximal phalanx. Each metacarpal can be palpated throughout its length on the dorsum of the hand. A tubercle at the medial base of the fifth metacarpal serves as the distal attachment site for the extensor carpi ulnaris; it may be palpated on the hand's dorsolateral aspect just distal to the hamate. At the base of the second metacarpal bone (dorsally), an eminence may be felt that serves as the distal attachment site for the extensor carpi radialis longus. The palmar surface of the base of the second metacarpal also has a rough area, which serves as the attachment site for the flexor carpi radialis, but this lies in a position that is too deep for palpation. The head of each metacarpal bone is a biconvex articular surface that becomes part of the metacarpophalangeal (MCP) joint and that may, in part, be palpated when the joint is flexed.

Phalanges

The two phalanges of the thumb and the three phalanges of each of the other digits may be palpated without difficulty. To differentiate the phalanges of the thumb, the terms proximal and distal are used; proximal, middle, and distal are terms used to identify the three phalanges of each finger. The base of each proximal phalanges is biconcave and has a smaller articular surface than the metacarpal head. The distal phalangeal heads are bicondylar with an intercondylar depression. These surfaces can be palpated at the distal end of the phalanges when the proximal interphalangeal joints are flexed. The middle phalanges and the base of the distal phalanges have articulating surfaces similar to the proximal phalanges.

Joints

With so many bones in the wrist and hand complex, there are also several joints formed by adjacent bones. Because they are synovial joints, ligaments and capsules secure and stabilize them. As with many other body segments, the ligaments in the wrist and hand are usually named for the bones they connect.

Wrist

The wrist joints provide both wide mobility of the hand and great structural stability in the wrist, which allows the hand an extensive degree of function. Although the wrist is often collectively classified as an ellipsoidal joint with two degrees of freedom, it is in reality a highly complex area of 15 bones, 17 joints, and an extensive ligament system.

Radiocarpal Joint

The radiocarpal joint is formed by the biconcave distal end of the radius and the biconvex proximal articulating surfaces of the scaphoid and lunate bones (Fig. 7.4). A triangular fibrocartilaginous disc attaches to the distal end of the radius and the styloid process of the ulna proximally while the apex of the disc attaches to the triquetrum distally (Fig. 7.5). The disc binds the radius and ulna together and separates the distal radioulnar joint and the ulna from the radiocarpal joint. Part of the wrist motions of flexion (volar flexion), extension (hyperextension), radial deviation, and ulnar deviation occurs at the radiocarpal joint.

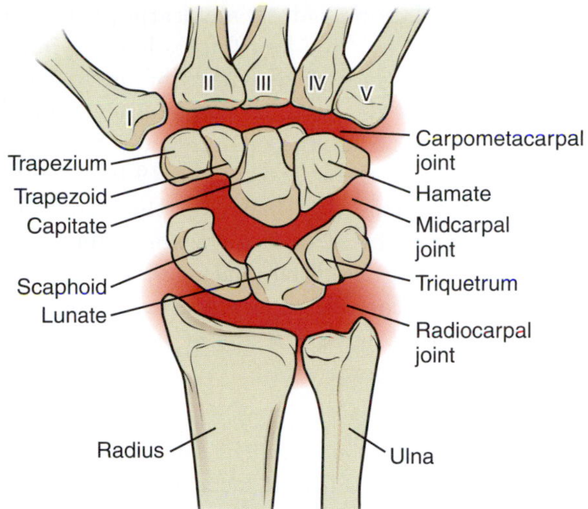

Figure 7.4 Radiocarpal, intercarpal, and carpometacarpal joint surfaces.

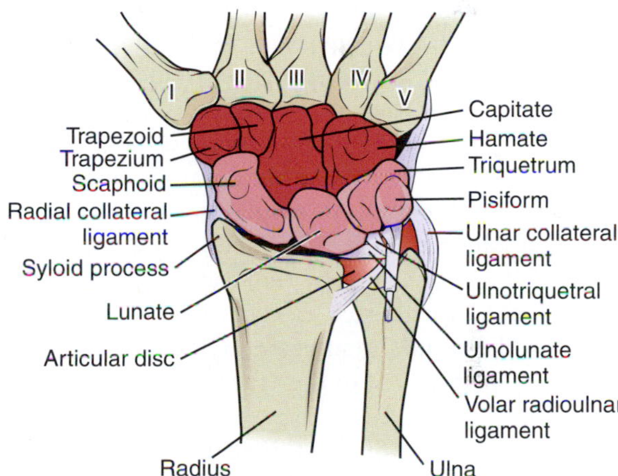

Figure 7.5 A triangular, fibrocartilaginous disc attaches to the distal end of the radius and the styloid process of the ulna while the apex of the disc attaches to the triquetrum.

Midcarpal Joint

The midcarpal joint is formed by the proximal and distal carpal rows. The scaphoid articulates with the trapezium, trapezoid, and capitate; the lunate articulates with the capitate; and the triquetrum articulates with the hamate (Fig. 7.4). The wrist motions of flexion, extension, and radial and ulnar deviation also take place at this joint.

Hand

The hand consists of five digits (four fingers and one thumb). Each digit includes the carpometacarpal

(CMC) articulation and a metacarpophalangeal (MCP) joint. Each of the four fingers has two interphalangeal (IP) joints whereas the thumb has only one. The digits of the hand are commonly numbered with the thumb as 1 and the small finger as 5. As previously mentioned, there are a total of 19 bones distal to the carpal bones that make up the hand: five metacarpal bones, five proximal phalanges, four middle phalanges and five distal phalanges. The palm of the hand has a concave appearance even when the hand is fully open due to the arches produced by the carpal bones and ligaments.

Carpometacarpal Joints

The bases of the second through fourth metacarpals articulate with their adjacent metacarpals. They also articulate with the distal row of carpal bones, forming carpometacarpal (CMC) joints. A common joint cavity exists between these four carpals, the CMC articulations, and into the intermetacarpal joints. The motion in the second CMC joint is minimal and even less in the third CMC joint whereas the fourth CMC joint has 10° to 15° of dorsovolar movement, and the fifth CMC joint is the most flexible with 25° to 30° of motion.[2] Because the third CMC joint is least mobile, it is the central pillar of the hand around which the rest of the hand rotates. Although movements at each individual joint are small, their motions are important for hand function and are the reason the hand is able to function with such an extensive change in the shape of the hand's transverse arch from the one extreme of a closed fist to the other extreme of a fully open hand (Fig. 7.6).

The CMC joint of the thumb is formed by the trapezium and the base of the first metacarpal; the surfaces of both of these bones are both convex and concave and form a saddle joint (Fig. 7.7). The joint capsule is thick but loose, and the metacarpal can be distracted up to 3 mm from the trapezium. Thumb motions include abduction and adduction (in a plane at a right angle to the palm (Fig. 7.8A); flexion and extension (in a plane parallel to the palm (Fig. 7.8B); and **opposition,** a rotation of the first metacarpal on the trapezium to place the pad of the thumb opposite the pads of the fingers (Fig. 7.8C). **Reposition** is the reverse of opposition.

Fingers and Thumb

The fingers and thumb joints include the MCP joints and the interphalangeal joints of the five digits. Each of these joints has a convex proximal surface that articulates with a concave distal surface (Fig. 7.9).

Metacarpophalangeal Joints

The metacarpophalangeal (MCP) joints of the fingers are of the condyloid type with two degrees of freedom. Motions of flexion, extension, abduction, and adduction occur at the MCP joints of the digits. The rounded surfaces of the heads of the metacarpals articulate with the more shallow concave surfaces on the bases of the proximal phalanges. Approximately three-quarters of the circumference of the metacarpal heads are covered with articular cartilage, which extends onto the volar surface. The articular surfaces of the base of the phalanges are extended by fibrocartilaginous volar plates (Fig. 7.10). As the joint flexes, the volar plate slides proximally under the metacarpal with a folding of its membranous part. This mechanism provides a

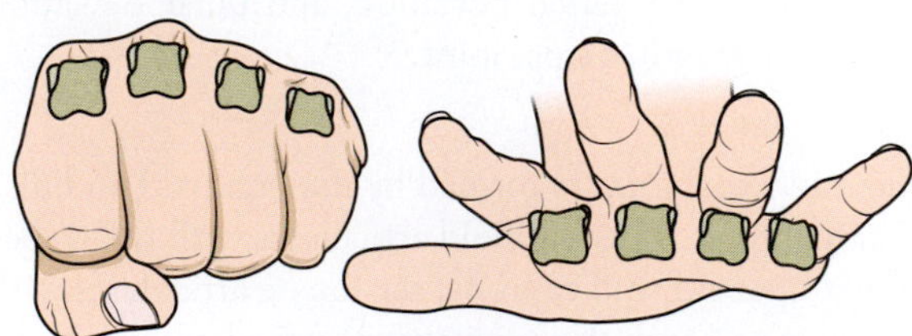

Figure 7.6 The flexible transverse arch of the hand showing the position of the metacarpal heads when **A)** making a fist and **B)** opening the hand. The third carpometacarpal joint is stable whereas the second, fourth, and fifth joints provide increasing mobility, Thus, as the extended hand is opened, the span of the fingers increases to surround the objects, and as the hand is closed, the fingers are approximated to increase the force of the grip.

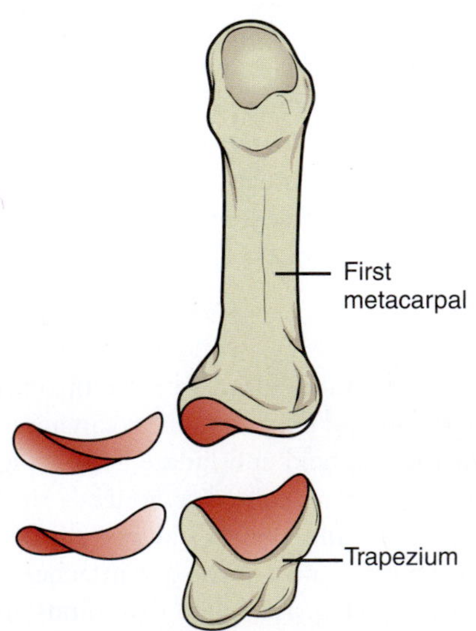

Figure 7.7 The first carpometacarpal joint is formed by the triquetrum and first metacarpal. Each bone surface is convex and concave, forming a saddle joint.

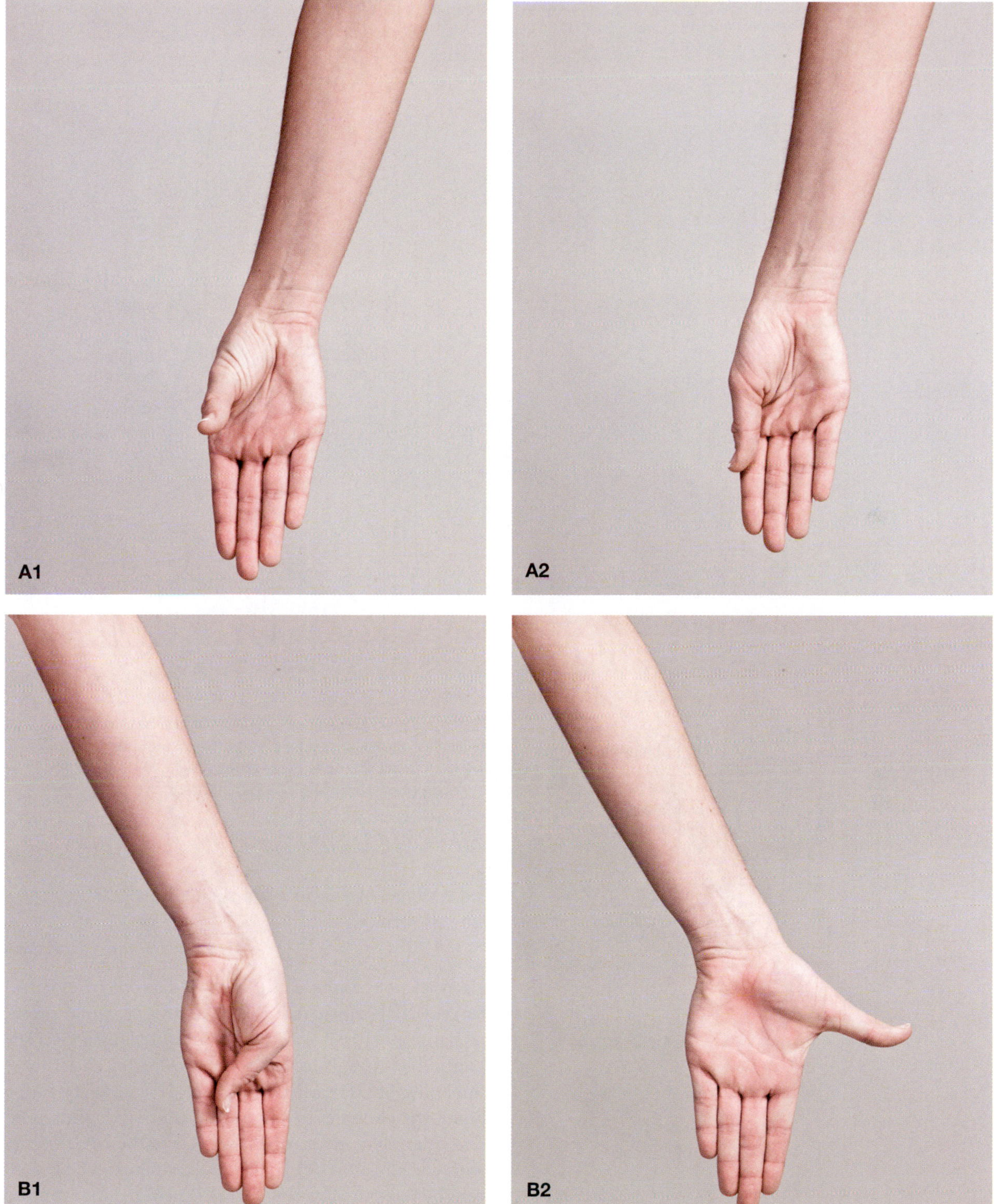

Figure 7.8 Motions of the thumb at the CMC joint. **A1)** Abduction; **A2)** Adduction; **B1)** Flexion; **B2)** Extension;

continued

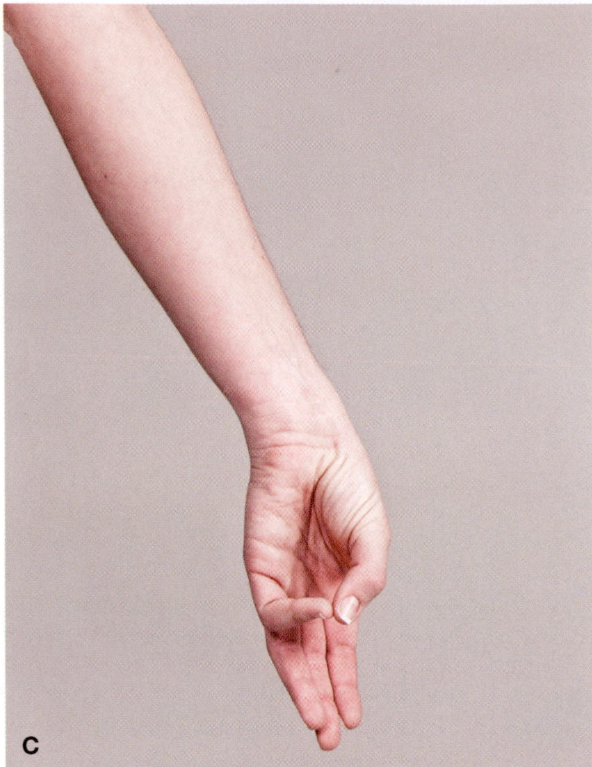

Figure 7.8—cont'd C) Opposition.

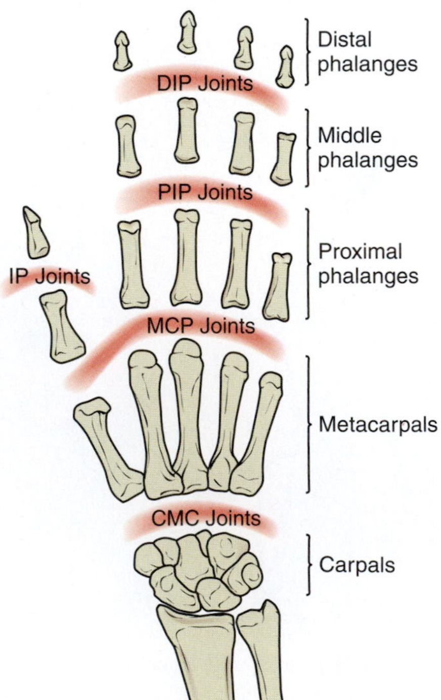

Figure 7.9 Each of the surfaces of the metacarpophalangeal and interphalangeal joints has a convex proximal surface which articulates with a concave distal surface.

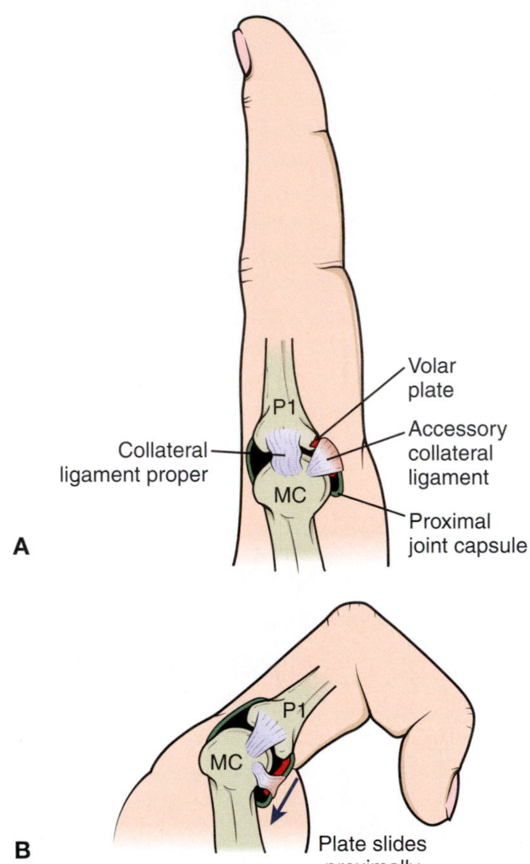

Figure 7.10 The articular surfaces of the base of the phalanges are extended by fibrocartilaginous volar plates. As the joint flexes, the volar plate slides proximally under the metacarpal with a folding of the membranous part.

large range of motion for a small articulating phalangeal surface.

Interphalangeal Joints

Each of the digits 2 through 5 has two interphalangeal (IP) joints, referred to as the proximal interphalangeal (PIP) and distal interphalangeal (DIP) joints. The thumb has only two phalanges and, therefore, only one IP joint. All of the IP joints are hinge joints with one degree of freedom. The IP joints possess volar plate mechanisms similar to the MCP joints with the addition of check rein ligaments, which prevent hyperextension (Fig. 7.11). These ligaments cross the joints on the volar surface on either side of the flexor tendon sheath.

Soft Tissue Supporting Structures

Ligaments throughout the wrist and hand provide support of the joints. These ligaments function to stabilize

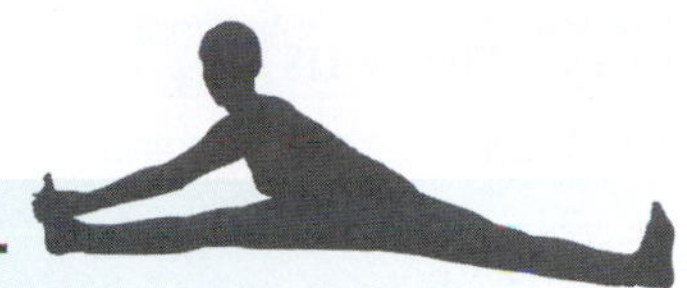

PRACTICE POINT

Finger sprains more often occur at the PIP joint than at the DIP joint. Commonly referred to as a "jammed finger," a severe sprain may cause dysfunction of the hand. Sprains of collateral ligaments and the surrounding joint capsule may lead to degenerative joint changes if not properly treated. Additionally, adjacent lateral bands of the extensor tendon or the oblique retinacular ligament may become adherent in any collateral ligament sprain if edema or prolonged immobilization follows an injury. If the lateral bands do become adherent, the oblique retinacular ligament must be stretched to regain mobility. To stretch the oblique retinacular ligament, place it on maximum stretch by holding the PIP joint in full extension and having the patient actively flex the DIP joint. If active motion is not possible, the DIP joint should be flexed passively in a gentle manner. This motion is performed slowly and does not go beyond the point of pain.

joints, permit and guide motion of bones, limit joint motion, transmit forces from the hand to the forearm, and prevent dislocation of carpal bones with movement.

Ligaments of the Wrist

Ligaments cover the volar, dorsal, radial, and ulnar areas of the wrist. The complexity of these ligaments is illustrated in Table 7–1. In the classification system used in this table, extrinsic ligaments connect the radius, ulna, or metacarpals to the carpal bones; intrinsic ligaments run between the carpal bones only. Short, strong ligaments bind the distal row of carpal bones to each other (intrinsic, short, interossei) and to the bases of the metacarpals (extrinsic, distal, CMC ligaments) (Fig. 7.12). The distal row of the carpal bones and the second to fourth metacarpals form a fixed unit or block without appreciable motion. Intrinsic, intermediate-length ligaments that permit more motion connect the carpal bones where most of individual carpal movements occur—the triquetrum, lunate, scaphoid, and trapezium.

The two rows of carpals are joined to each other and to the radius and the ulnar fibrocartilaginous disc by medial and lateral collateral ligaments and strong oblique V-shaped ligaments. The extrinsic ligaments extend from the radius and ulna to converge on the capitate and the lunate (Fig. 7.4). The intrinsic V-shaped

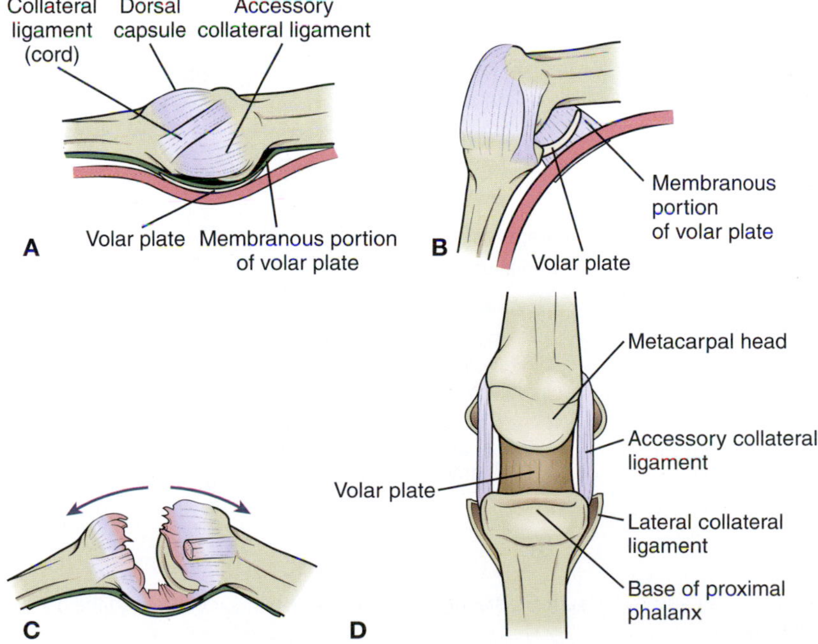

Figure 7.11 Lateral views of the capsular and ligamentous structures of the metacarpophalangeal joint are seen in **A**) and **B**). Note the relationships of the volar plate, articulating surfaces, capsule, and collateral ligaments in extension **A**) and in flexion **B**). In **C**) and **D**), the capsule and ligaments have been cut to show the volar plate.

TABLE 7–1 | CLASSIFICATION OF LIGAMENTS OF THE WRIST*

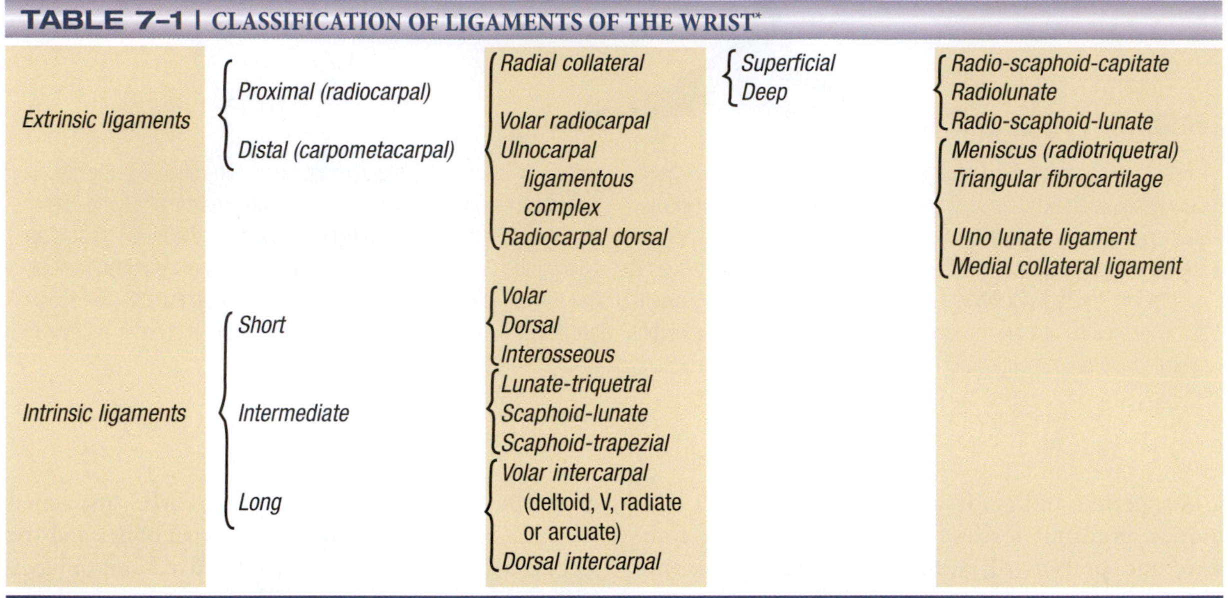

Extrinsic ligaments	*Proximal (radiocarpal)*	*Radial collateral*		
		Volar radiocarpal	*Superficial* *Deep*	*Radio-scaphoid-capitate* *Radiolunate* *Radio-scaphoid-lunate*
		Ulnocarpal ligamentous complex		*Meniscus (radiotriquetral)* *Triangular fibrocartilage* *Ulno lunate ligament* *Medial collateral ligament*
		Radiocarpal dorsal		
	Distal (carpometacarpal)			
Intrinsic ligaments	*Short*	*Volar* *Dorsal* *Interosseous*		
	Intermediate	*Lunate-triquetral* *Scaphoid-lunate* *Scaphoid-trapezial*		
	Long	*Volar intercarpal* (deltoid, V, radiate or arcuate) *Dorsal intercarpal*		

*Extrinsic ligaments are those that connect carpal bones to the radius, ulna, or metacarpals. Intrinsic ligaments attach between the carpal bones only.
Source: Adapted with permission from Taleisnik, J: Ligaments of the carpus. In Razemon, JP and Fisk, GR (eds): *The Wrist.* Edinburgh: Churchill Livingstone, 1988, p 17.

ligament attaches to the triquetrum and the scaphoid and converges on the capitate. There are no ligamentous connections between the capitate and lunate. Thus, considerable movement is allowed, including 2 to 3 mm of distraction.

Included in the extra-articular ligamentous structures of the wrist are the flexor and extensor retinacula (L. *halter*), which contain the tendons going to the fingers. Part of the flexor retinaculum includes the transverse carpal ligament. This ligament is 1 to 2 mm thick and 2 to 3 cm wide, attaching to the hook of the hamate and pisiform bones ulnarly and coursing to the radial side, where it attaches to the trapezium and the scaphoid. These attachments create the transverse

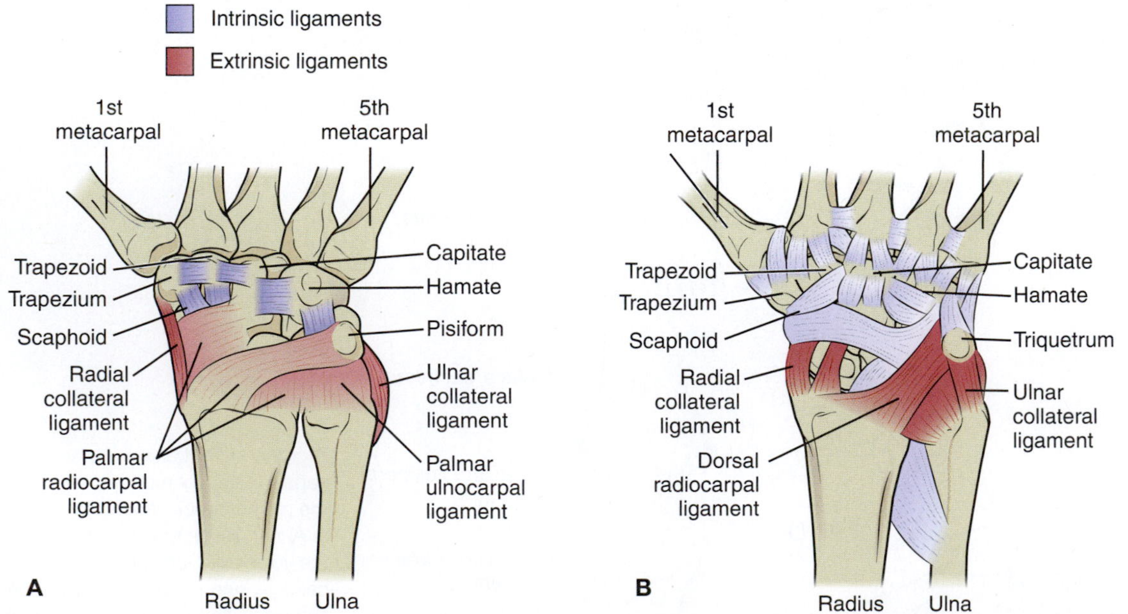

Figure 7.12 Intrinsic and extrinsic ligaments of the carpals provide support, stability, and transmission of forces through the hand. **A)** Anterior view, left hand. **B)** Posterior view, right hand.

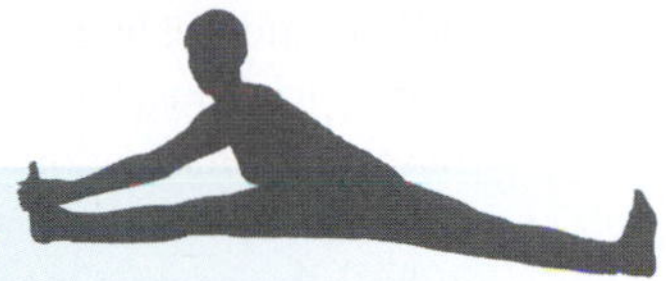

PRACTICE POINT

The fibrocartilaginous disc is part of the triangular fibrocartilage complex (TFCC). It sits between the medial proximal carpal row and distal ulna and serves to cushion the wrist against compressive forces and augment the wrist joint. When a waiter carries a tray overhead with the elbow flexed and hand flat, the TFCC assists in transmitting the weight force of the load to the forearm. The TFCC is commonly injured by either falling on an outstretched arm with the forearm in supination or by a sudden hyperextension force applied to the wrist. Pain is located over the ulnar wrist. Pain occurs with ranges of motion of the wrist and forearm, especially forearm motions. Gripping is painful. A painful crepitus or clicking of the wrist during wrist motions is also common.

carpal arch and form a tunnel through which the median nerve and the tendons of the flexor pollicis longus, flexor digitorum superficialis, and flexor digitorum profundus travel to the hand (Fig. 7.13). Repetitive or acute trauma, swelling, or other factors that encroach to narrow the space in this area can cause carpal tunnel syndrome, producing compression of the median nerve, which may result in pain, loss of sensation, and weakness of the thenar muscles.

Ligaments of the Hand and Fingers

Collateral ligaments of the hand and fingers are strong and run along the sides of the joints. Accessory collateral ligaments control movement of the volar plate, and the metacarpal pulley for the long flexor tendons blends with these structures.

Medial and lateral collateral ligaments attach from the heads of the metacarpals to the bases of the phalanges (Fig. 7.14). There is a longer distance between the points of attachment of these ligaments when the joints are flexed than when they are extended. Thus, abduction and adduction can occur when the joints are extended. When the MCP joints are flexed to 90° the collateral ligaments become taut so abduction cannot be performed. This is functionally important because in flexion MCP joints are mechanically stabilized for gripping.

The deep transverse metacarpal ligament attaches to the volar plate and runs between the metacarpal heads to connect the adjacent sides of the metacarpals 2 through 5. The ligament permits a flexible metacarpal arch and limits the spread of the bones.

In the thumb, two sesamoid bones are attached to the volar plate on its palmar surface. One is ulnarly located in the tendinous attachments of the adductor pollicis and first dorsal interosseous, and the other is radially located at the flexor pollicis brevis and abductor pollicis brevis attachments. The sesamoid bones have medial and lateral ligaments at the metacarpals as well as several ligaments joining the structure to the base of the phalanx.[3] The sesamoid mechanism produces a dynamic rotation of the thumb segment for precision of the pinch.

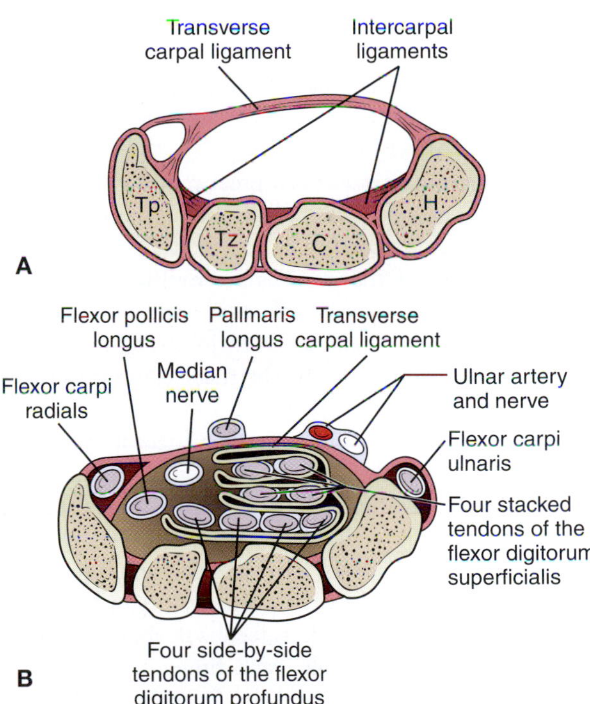

Figure 7.13 The intercarpal ligaments form the floor of the carpal tunnel. The transverse carpal ligament is 1 to 2 mm thick and 2 to 3 cm wide, attaching to the hook of the hamate and pisiform bones and coursing to the radial side, where it attaches to the trapezium and the scaphoid. These attachments maintain the transverse carpal arch and form the carpal tunnel. **A)** The carpal tunnel without its contents. **B)** The carpal tunnel with the median nerve and the tendons of the flexor pollicis longus, flexor digitorum superficialis, and flexor digitorum profundus on their way to the hand.

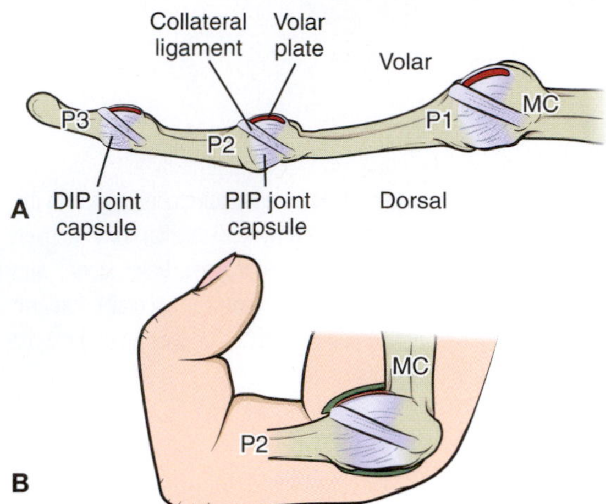

Figure 7.14 Ligaments supporting the IP joints. **A)** In full extension, the distance between the ligament's attachment points is shorter than when the joint is **B)** in flexion.

Muscles

Function of the hand is complex and difficult to understand for many reasons:

- The hand is a compact, multipurpose organ with interdependency of structures in which injury to one may affect many others.
- The hand possesses both great mobility and great stability and can shift from one to the other in a fraction of a second.
- Almost all of the muscles are multiarticular and, therefore, can have an effect on each joint crossed. Some cross as many as seven joints, so to prevent an undesired motion by the muscle, other muscles must contract.
- The hand has many automatic, neurophysiologic synergies, which are so strongly linked that a person cannot willfully separate them. For example, when making a fist, the wrist extensors contract forcefully and cannot be voluntarily inhibited.
- The hand is a wonderful sensory organ that provides us with tremendous feedback about our environment. For example, each finger tip has about 100 sensory endings and the fingertips and hands are among the most sensitive parts of the body.

Basic to the understanding of muscle function is knowledge of the anatomic actions of each muscle. This information is used to determine what happens if a muscle shortens completely or elongates passively and to isolate muscles for examination and assessment of their individual strength. As is true of any other body segment, wrist and hand muscles should be studied on the skeleton, the cadaver, and the living subject, considering: (1) over which joints each muscle passes; (2) the line of action of the muscle and its tendon; (3) the distance of the muscle to the axis of joint motion at various positions of the joint; and (4) the relative length of the muscle.

Muscles Acting on the Wrist

Most wrist muscles have more than one function. Depending on their location, they will either flex or extend the wrist as well as either radially or ulnarly abduct (deviate) the wrist. These muscles also serve as important wrist stabilizers during finger and hand motions. Specific anatomic information of the extrinsic muscles of the wrist and hand is in Table 7–2.

Wrist Extensors

The proximal attachments of the wrist extensors have a common tendon attachment at the lateral humeral epicondyle, with the extensor carpi radialis longus also attaching higher onto the lateral supracondylar ridge. With the elbow extended, the line of action of these muscles crosses on or slightly posterior to the axis of the elbow. After 15° of elbow flexion, their line of pull moves anterior to the axis, so the wrist extensors also become elbow flexors. The higher attachment of the extensor carpi radialis longus provides good lever arm distance from the elbow axis when the elbow is flexed to 90°. This muscle is often used to flex the elbow if the brachialis and biceps are paralyzed.

The primary muscles that extend the wrist are the extensor carpi radialis longus, the extensor carpi radialis brevis, and the extensor carpi ulnaris. If the wrist is extended with the fist closed, the tendon of the extensor carpi radialis longus becomes prominent and is easily observed (Fig. 7.15A). The tendon of the extensor of the index finger crosses over the extensor carpi radialis brevis, making identification of the muscle by palpation somewhat difficult.

The tendon of the extensor carpi ulnaris becomes prominent if the wrist is extended and even more prominent if the wrist is simultaneously abducted ulnarly (Fig. 7.15B). The muscular portion of the extensor carpi ulnaris is best palpated about 2 inches (5 cm) below the lateral epicondyle of the humerus, where it lies between the anconeus and the extensor digitorum. From this point on, it may be followed distally along the dorsoulnar aspect of the forearm in a direction toward the head of the ulna.

The extensor digitorum participates in extension of the wrist only when the fingers are simultaneously extended; in fact, the finger extensors then appear to take over the task of wrist extension altogether. The extensor digitorum is described in the digit muscle section of this chapter.

(text continues on page 274)

TABLE 7–2 | EXTRINSIC MUSCLES OF THE WRIST AND HAND

Muscle group	Muscle	Proximal Attachment	Distal Attachment	Innervation	Action	Palpation
Wrist extensors	Extensor carpi radialis longus	Lateral supracondylar ridge of the distal humerus	Base of the second metacarpal	Radial nerve C6–7	Extends and radially deviates the wrist	The tendon lies on the radial side of the capitate bone but on the ulnar side of the tubercle of the radius and courses toward the base of the metacarpal bone of the index finger, to which it is attached.
Wrist extensors	Extensor carpi radialis brevis	Lateral epicondyle of humerus	Base of third metacarpal	Radial nerve, deep branch C7–8	Extends the wrist	Its tendon can usually be felt rising if the thumb is moved in a palmar direction, perpendicular to the palm of the hand.

continued

TABLE 7-2 | EXTRINSIC MUSCLES OF THE WRIST AND HAND—cont'd

Muscle group	Muscle	Proximal Attachment	Distal Attachment	Innervation	Action	Palpation
Wrist extensors	Extensor carpi ulnaris	Common extensor tendon and proximal three-fourths of dorsal ulna	Base of fifth metacarpal	Posterior interosseous (deep radial) C7–8	Extends and ulnarly deviates the wrist	Muscular portion is palpated about 2 inches (5 cm) distal to the lateral epicondyle of the humerus where the muscle lies between the anconeus and extensor digitorum. It may be followed distally to its insertion and abducted.
Wrist flexors	Palmaris longus	Common flexor tendon	Palmar aponeurosis	Median nerve C7–8	Flexes wrist	The tendon is easily identified by touching the tips of the thumb and little finger together and flexing the wrist. The middle prominent tendon at the wrist is the palmaris longus.

Wrist flexors	Flexor carpi radialis 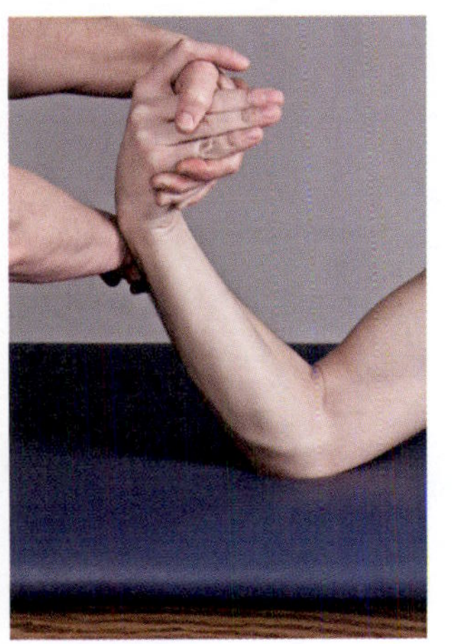	Medial humeral epicondyle	Base of second metacarpal	Median nerve C6–7	Flexes wrist and radially deviates wrist	With the wrist flexed and the tips of the first and fifth digits touching, the tendon is located laterally to the palmaris longus tendon at the wrist. It cannot be followed to its distal attachment on the base of the second metacarpal bone.
Wrist flexors	Flexor carpi ulnaris 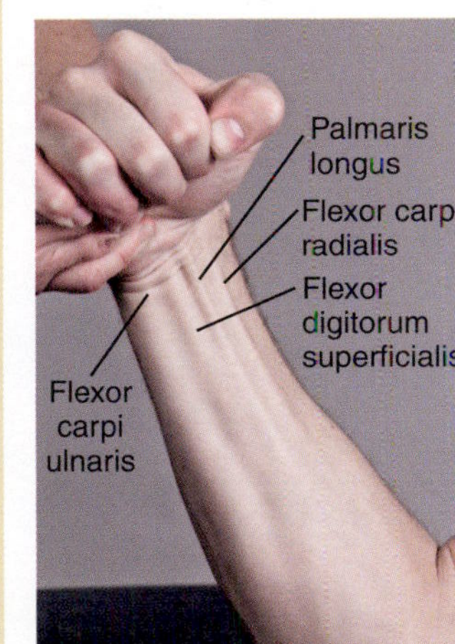	Common flexor tendon	Pisiform bone	Ulnar nerve C7–8	Flexes and ulnarly deviates the wrist	This tendon lies medial to the palmaris longus and may be palpated between the styloid process of the ulna and the pisiform bone, to which it is attached.

continued

TABLE 7–2 | EXTRINSIC MUSCLES OF THE WRIST AND HAND—cont'd

Muscle group	Muscle	Proximal Attachment	Distal Attachment	Innervation	Action	Palpation
Extrinsic finger extensors	Extensor digitorum	Lateral humeral epicondyle	Base of each phalanx of digits #2–5	Posterior interosseous nerve (deep radial branch) C7–8	Extends digits #2–5 at MP joints and assists in extending IP joints and wrist	The four tendons are palpated between the carpals and MCP joints when the MCP and IP joints are actively moved into extension.
Extrinsic finger extensors	Extensor indicis	Proximal part of the lower one-third of the ulna and interosseous membrane	Base of the proximal phalanx of #2 digit	Posterior interosseous nerve C7–8	Extends index (#2) finger. Assists in wrist extension	With the fingers in extension, palpate the index finger's extensor digitorum tendon. Immediately adjacent to this tendon, the extensor indicis is palpated as only the #2 digit is actively flexed and extended.

Extrinsic finger extensors	Extensor digiti minimi 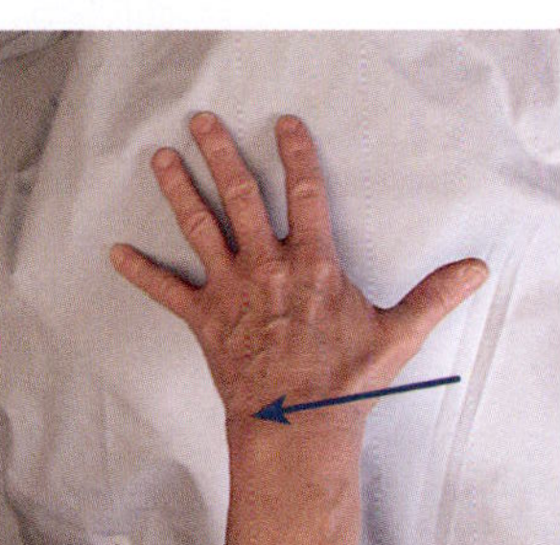	Lateral humeral epicondyle	Base of proximal phalanx and dorsal expansion of #5 digit	Posterior interosseous nerve C7–8	Extends MCP and IP joints of #5 digit	With the hand very gently pushing down on a table top so as to prevent extensor digitorum facilitation, raise only the little finger into extension. The tendon is palpated just lateral and distal to the ulnar styloid process.
Extrinsic flexor muscles	Flexor digitorum superficialis 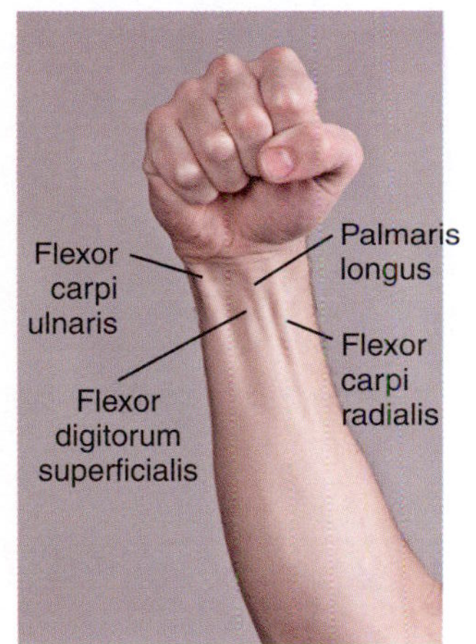	1. Common flexor tendon on medial humeral epicondyle. 2. Medial side of coronoid process of ulna. 3. Oblique line of radius	Medial and lateral aspects of middle phalanx of #2–5	Median nerve C7–8, T1	Flexes MCP and PIP joints of #2–5	If the fist is tightly closed and wrist flexion is simultaneously resisted, one or more tendons of the flexor digitorum superficialis become prominent in the space between the palmaris longus and the flexor carpi ulnaris.

continued

TABLE 7-2 | EXTRINSIC MUSCLES OF THE WRIST AND HAND—cont'd

Muscle group	Muscle	Proximal Attachment	Distal Attachment	Innervation	Action	Palpation
Extrinsic flexor muscles	Flexor digitorum profundus	Proximal two-thirds of anterior surface of ulna and adjacent interosseous membrane	Bases of distal phalanx of #2–5 digits	Median branch of ulnar nerve to medial FDP and radial branch of median nerve to lateral FDP	Flexes DIP joints of #2–5 and assists with flexion of PIP, MCP, and wrist	Because this muscle is deep, it is difficult to palpate. If the PIP is stabilized with a palpating finger on the distal aspect of the middle phalanx, the FDP may be palpated as the distal phalanx is actively flexed.
Extrinsic thumb muscles	Extensor pollicis longus	Middle posterior one-third of ulna and interosseous membrane	Base of distal phalanx of #1	Posterior interosseous nerve C7–8	Extends distal phalanx of #1 and assists with extension of IP and MCP of #1	This tendon forms the ulnar border of the anatomical snuff box and may be palpated when the thumb is actively extended.

Extrinsic thumb muscles	Extensor pollicis brevis 	Posterior radius and interosseous membrane	Base of proximal phalanx of #1	Posterior interosseous nerve C7–8	Extends MCP joint and proximal phalanx of #1	This tendon along with the abductor pollicis longus tendon form the radial border of the anatomical snuff box. If the thumb is extended without abduction, the tendon may be differentiated from the abductor pollicis longus.
Extrinsic thumb muscles	Flexor pollicis longus	Middle one-third of anterior radius and interosseous membrane	Distal phalanx of #1	Anterior interosseous nerve aspect of median nerve C7–8	Flexes phalanx, MCP, and CMC joints of #1	The tendon may be palpated in the anterior mid-section of the proximal phalanx as the thumb is actively flexed.

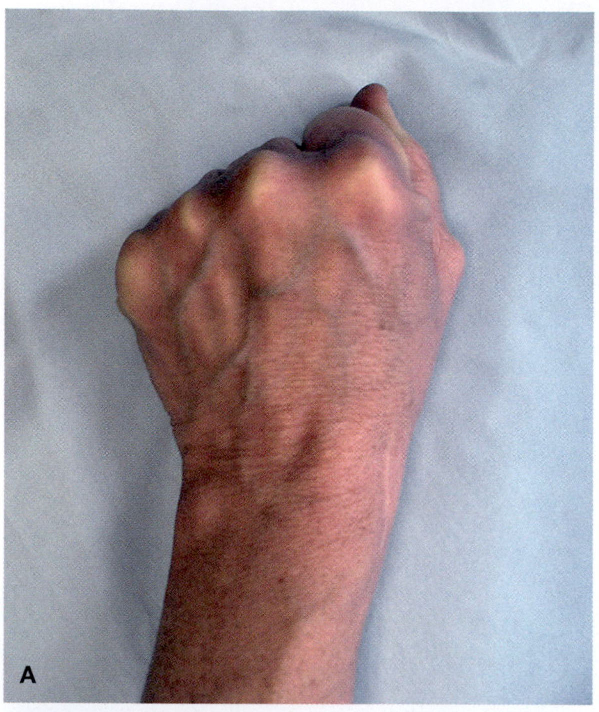

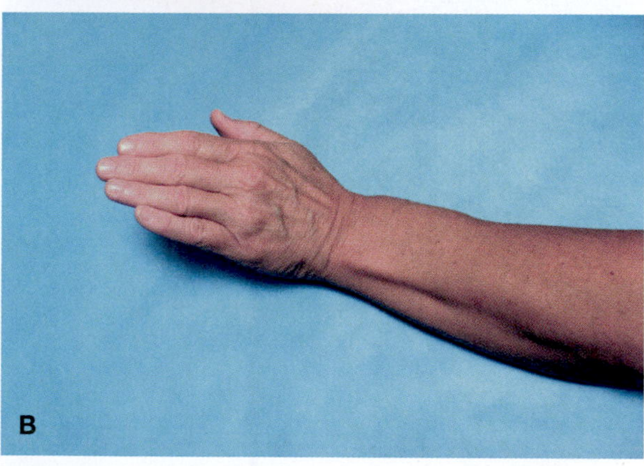

Figure 7.15 A) The tendon of the extensor carpi radialis longus is evident at the base of the second metacarpal when the fist is closed. B) The tendon of the extensor carpi ulnaris becomes prominent at the wrist during wrist extension with simultaneous ulnar deviation.

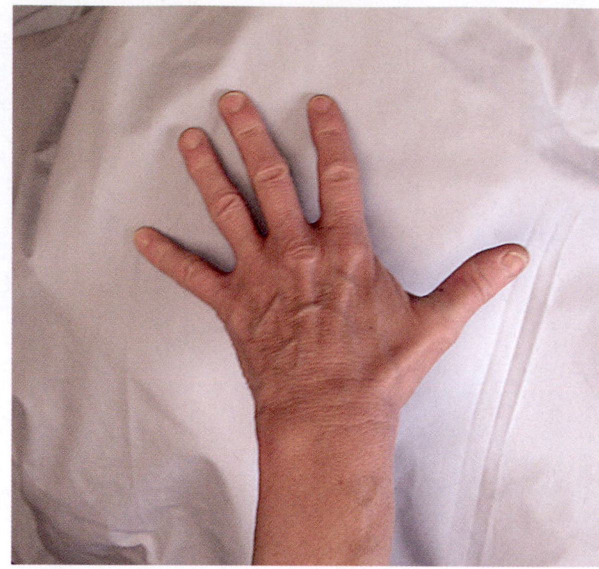

Figure 7.16 When the fingers are extended, the extensor digitorum takes over the task of extending the wrist and the extensor carpi radialis longus tendon becomes less prominent.

Wrist Flexors

Part of the proximal attachment of the wrist flexors is the common flexor tendon at the medial humeral epicondyle. With the elbow in the anatomical position and in flexion, these muscles lie on the anterior side of the elbow axis. Their leverage for elbow flexion is not as good as that of the wrist extensors, but their maximum elongation occurs when the wrist and elbow are extended.

The primary muscles involved in wrist flexion are the flexor carpi radialis, flexor carpi ulnaris, palmaris longus, flexor digitorum superficialis, flexor digitorum profundus, flexor pollicis longus, and abductor pollicis longus. The three wrist flexor tendons become prominent when resistance is provided against wrist flexion (Fig. 7.17). The most centrally located tendon is that of the palmaris longus; it varies in size in different

PRACTICE POINT

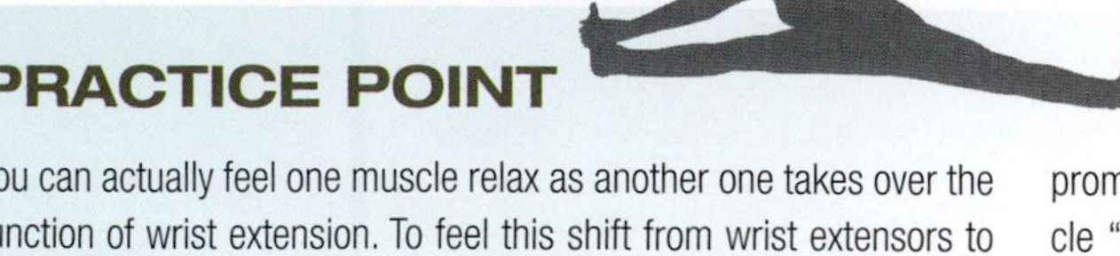

You can actually feel one muscle relax as another one takes over the function of wrist extension. To feel this shift from wrist extensors to finger extensors, extend the wrist with the fist closed, and palpate the prominent tendon of extensor carpi radialis longus at the base of the second metacarpal (Fig. 7.15A). While maintaining the wrist in this position, the fingers are extended. It is then noted that the prominent tendon being palpated "disappears," a sign that the muscle "lets go," or diminishes, its contraction. At the same time, the tendons of the extensor digitorum can be seen and palpated on the dorsum of the hand (Fig. 7.16). This shift in tendon function is regulated automatically.

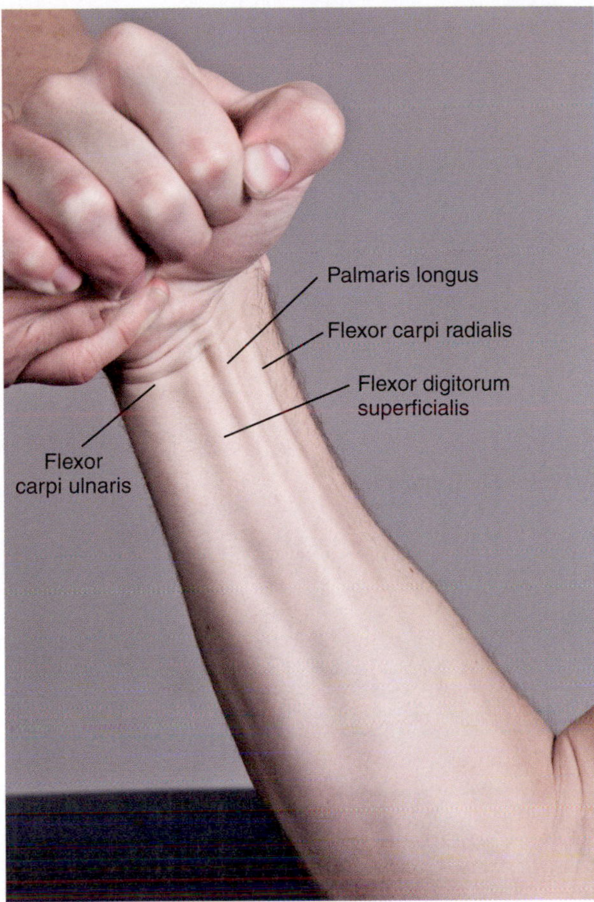

Figure 7.17 Resistance to wrist flexion applied in the palm of the hand brings out tendons of the wrist flexors.

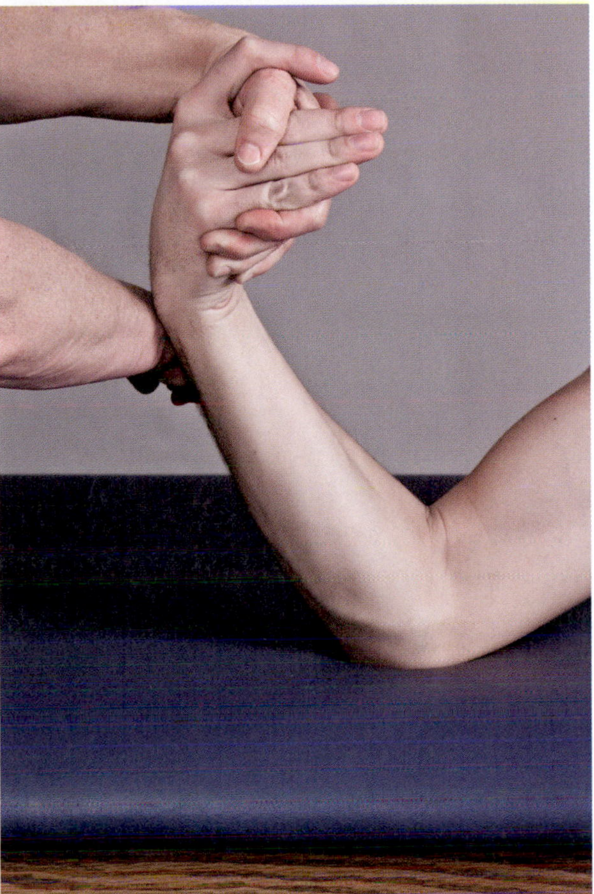

Figure 7.18 Palpation of the flexor carpi ulnaris proximal to the pisiform bone when ulnar deviation is resisted.

individuals, or it may be missing altogether. Radial to it, the strong tendon of the flexor carpi radialis is identified. This tendon lies in a superficial position in the distal forearm, is held down by the transverse carpal ligament at the wrist, and disappears into a groove in the trapezium bone. The flexor carpi ulnaris tendon lies close to the ulnar border of the forearm (Fig. 7.18). Muscle bellies of the wrist flexors may be palpated as indicated in Figure 7.19.

If the fist is tightly closed and wrist flexion is simultaneously resisted, one or more tendons of the flexor digitorum superficialis become prominent in the space between the palmaris longus and the flexor carpi ulnaris (Fig. 7.20). The tendon of the fourth digit appears to rise to the surface. In individuals lacking the palmaris longus, a more complete display of the tendons of the long finger flexors may be observed if flexion of the wrist is resisted and the subject then flexes one finger after the other or flexes all fingers simultaneously.

Radial and Ulnar Motions

The palmaris longus and the extensor carpi radialis brevis are centrally located at the wrist. In contrast to these two muscles, the other wrist flexors and extensors are situated either toward the radial or toward the ulnar side of the wrist; with this arrangement, they are capable of producing wrist movements from side to side as well as flexion and extension. In the anatomical position, these side-to-side movements of the wrist occur in the frontal plane on an anterior-posterior axis. Wrist movement of the hand away from the side of the body is called radial deviation or radial abduction. Wrist movement of the hand towards the side of the body is known as ulnar deviation or ulnar abduction.

When two muscles that normally oppose each other during flexion and extension motions work together, radial deviation or ulnar deviation occur. For example, ulnar deviation of the wrist occurs when the extensor carpi ulnaris and flexor carpi ulnaris contract together.

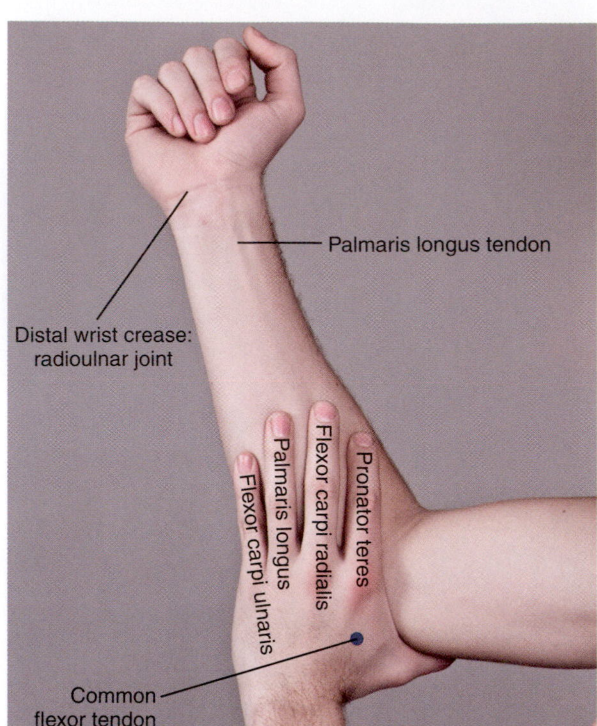

Figure 7.19 The wrist flexor muscles may be located with the palpating hand on the forearm in a manner that places the first web space around the medial epicondyle. The muscle bellies are then identified in the forearm in order of their arrangement as shown.

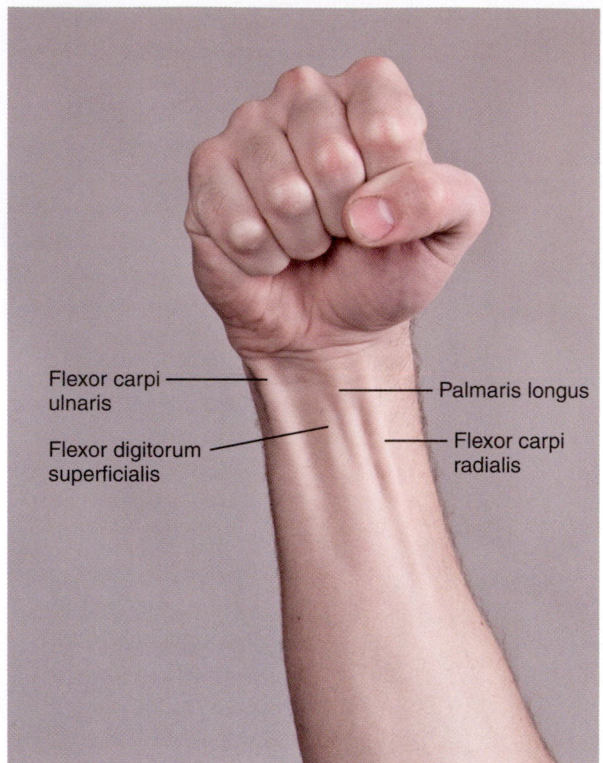

Figure 7.20 When a tight fist is made and wrist flexion is resisted, four tendons are visible. Moving from the ulnar to the radial side of the wrist, the sequence of tendons includes first the flexor carpi ulnaris; next, the flexor digitorum superficialis; then, the prominent palmaris longus; and the flexor carpi radialis on the farthest radial aspect.

Likewise, the extensor carpi radialis longus and the flexor carpi radialis produce radial deviation. When additional force is required for radial deviation, the abductor pollicis longus and the extensor pollicis brevis are able to assist these radial deviators. Since these two thumb muscles have a favorable line of action for performing radial deviation, they are able to assist regardless of the position of the thumb, whether flexed, extended, abducted, or adducted.

By now, you may have realized that the wrist muscles may act as either synergists or antagonists. For instance, in flexion and extension of the wrist, the flexor carpi ulnaris and the extensor carpi ulnaris are antagonists, but in ulnar deviation of the wrist these two muscles act as synergists.

Muscles Acting on the Digits

Normal hand function depends on the teamwork of the many muscles of the digits. These muscles are divided into two basic groups: (1) extrinsic muscles with proximal attachments in the forearm or humerus and distal attachments in the hand; and (2) intrinsic muscles with both proximal and distal attachments existing within the hand. Muscles of each of these groups include:

Extrinsic Muscles	Intrinsic Muscles
Dorsal muscles	**Mid-Palm muscles**
Extensor digitorum	Four lumbricals
Extensor indicis	Three palmar interossei
Extensor digiti minimi	Four dorsal interossei
Extensor pollicis longus	**Thenar muscles**
Extensor pollicis brevis	Opponens pollicis
Abductor pollicis longus	Abductor pollicis brevis
Ventral muscles	Adductor pollicis
Flexor digitorum superficialis	Flexor pollicis brevis
Flexor digitorum profundus	**Hypothenar muscles**
	Opponens digiti minimi
Flexor pollicis longus	Abductor digiti minimi
	Flexor digiti minimi brevis

Extrinsic Muscles

Because extrinsic muscles of the fingers have their proximal attachments in the forearm or on the humerus, they also affect the wrist when they contract. The main function of the extrinsic muscles is to provide strength and gross motor control in hand function. See Table 7–2 for details of these muscles. Since these muscles have long tendons, they are collectively referred to as long finger extensors and long finger flexors.

Long Finger Extensors

The extensor retinaculum at the wrist holds the extensor tendons in place and prevents bowstringing of the tendons during wrist and finger motions. The retinaculum forms six osseofibrous tunnels through which the nine extensor tendons travel to the hand. As they travel under the retinaculum, these tendons are each surrounded with their own synovial sheath that ends in the region of the carpometacarpal joints. The osseofibrous tunnels through which these tendons pass are numbered 1 through 6 from the lateral to medial wrist and serve to anatomically divide the extensor tendons into functional groups. Tunnel 1 includes tendons of the abductor pollicis longus and extensor pollicis brevis; tunnel 2 contains the extensor carpi radialis longus and extensor carpi radialis brevis; tunnel 3 has only the extensor pollicis longus; tunnel 4 encloses the tendons of the extensor digitorum and extensor indicis; tunnel 5 contains the extensor digiti minimi; and tunnel 6 has the extensor carpi ulnaris (Fig. 7.21).

The extensor digitorum muscle is located on the posterior forearm and inserts distally on digits 2 through 5. The extensor digitorum is the only muscle that extends all four fingers. The extensor digiti minimi is a long narrow muscle located on the posterior forearm and functions to extend all the joints of the little finger. The extensor indicis is a fairly small and narrow muscle located on the posterior forearm and acts as the main extensor of the index finger at the metacarpophalangeal joint.

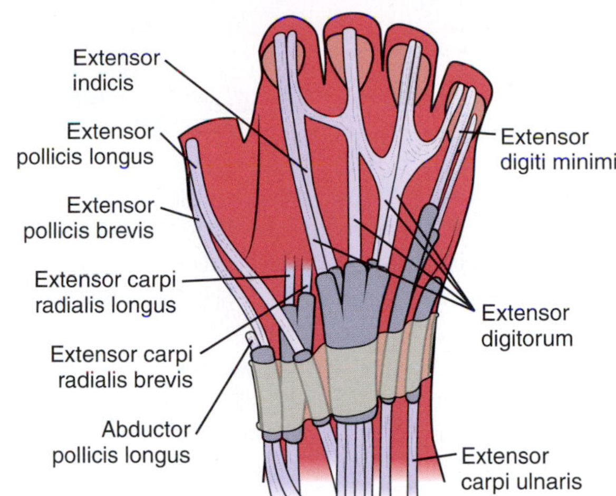

Figure 7.21 Dorsal compartments formed by extensor retinaculum create six tunnels through which the long extensor tendons travel to the wrist and hand. Notice the juncturae tendinae interconnecting the extensor digitorum communis tendons.

Long Finger Flexors

Unlike the extrinsic extensor digitorum, there are two extrinsic flexors on the anterior forearm for digits 2 through 5: the flexor digitorum superficialis and flexor digitorum profundus. The flexor digitorum superficialis muscle has a large muscle belly proximally that divides into a superficial and a deep muscle belly more distally in the forearm; its two superficial tendons attach to digits 3 and 4 whereas the two deep tendons attach to digits 2 and 5. Right before each of these tendons attach, their ends split to insert on either side of the middle phalanges of their respective digits. The flexor digitorum profundus is located on the ulnar aspect of the anterior forearm and has one muscle belly that divides into four tendons; each tendon lies under its respective superficialis tendon in the hand and digits until they become more superficial when they each emerge through the split of their digit's flexor digitorum superficialis to attach at the distal phalanges of the fingers. The flexor digitorum profundus tendon that attaches to the second digit often separates from the muscle belly earlier than the other tendons in the distal forearm.[4] The median nerve innervates the muscle's lateral aspect whose tendons flex digits 2 and 3 whereas the ulnar nerve supplies innervation to the medial aspect of the muscle whose tendons insert onto digits 4 and 5. The flexor digitorum profundus works synergistically with the flexor digitorum superficialis to flex the fingers.

Thumb Muscles

As with the other digits, the thumb has both intrinsic and extrinsic muscles. The extrinsic muscles of the thumb include the flexor pollicis longus, extensor pollicis longus and brevis, and abductor pollicis longus. The intrinsic muscles are the adductor pollicis, flexor pollicis brevis, abductor pollicis brevis, and opponens pollicis. In addition, the lateral head of the first dorsal interosseous attaches to the shaft of the first metacarpal. As with most muscles, the thumb muscles have been named after motions they produce. Because of the large range of motion of the thumb as well as multiple attachments of the intrinsic muscles,

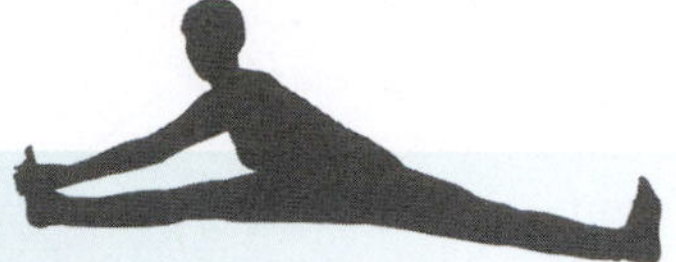

PRACTICE POINT

It may be difficult to determine if the flexor digitorum profundus is functioning or if its lack of function is masked by function of the flexor digitorum superficialis. Isolation of the flexor digitorum profundus may be performed by passively maintaining the metacarpophalangeal and proximal interphalangeal joints in extension and having the patient actively flex the distal phalanx as shown in Figure 7.22.

On the other hand, clinical isolation of the flexor digitorum superficialis may be made with one of two simple techniques—one is an active technique and the other uses passive assistance. The active method uses active flexion of the proximal IP joint while the distal IP joint is maintained in extension (Fig. 7.23A). The other method of isolating the FDS is to passively maintain all MCP and IP joints in extension except for one digit; in this position, the patient actively flexes the fingers as shown in Figure 7.23B. The finger will flex at the PIP joint while the DIP joint flexor is completely relaxed since the flexor digitorum profundus is passively restricted from flexing the fingers. This technique works because the flexor digitorum profundus has only one muscle belly and four tendons: If one or more of its tendons are restricted from functioning, then the other tendons will also be unable to function.

additional motions occur; this can sometimes be confusing since the muscle's name may not reflect these motions. Visualizing a muscle's anatomy relative to an axis of motion may reduce this confusion.

Thumb Flexors

The flexor pollicis longus is a small muscle located on the anterior forearm. The muscle is the primary thumb flexor and is the only flexor of the IP joint. It also contributes to MCP, CMC, and wrist joint flexion as well as adduction from the abducted position.

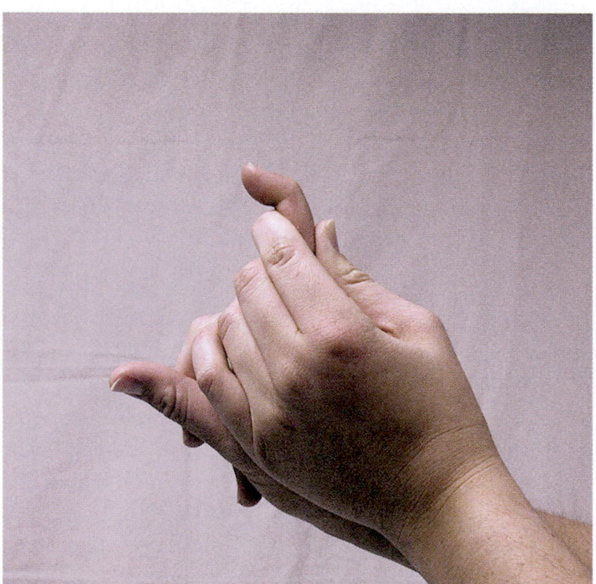

Figure 7.22 Flexor digitorum profundus can be isolated when the MCP and IP joints are held in extension and the individual flexes the DIP joint.

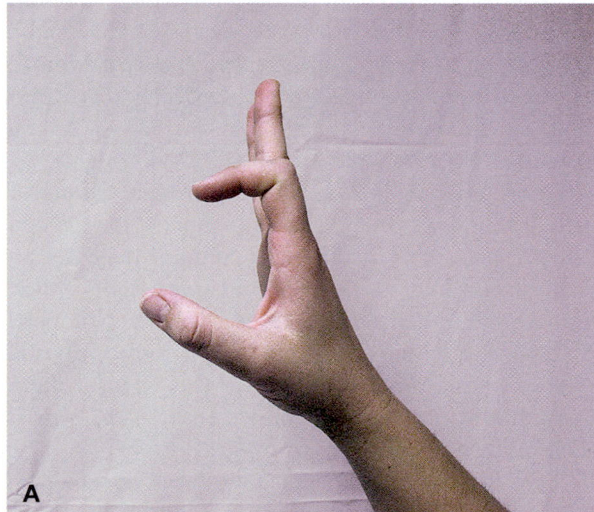

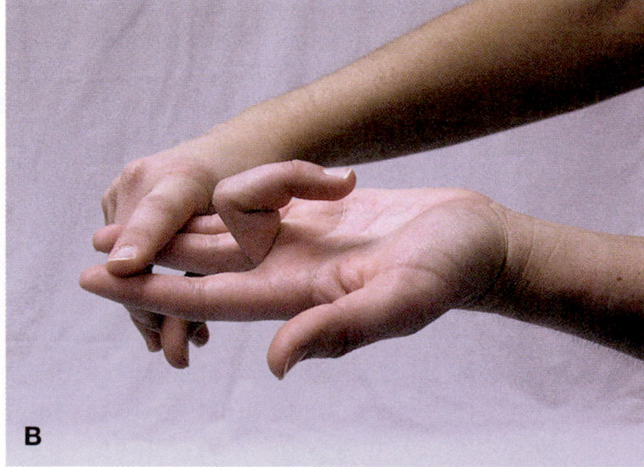

Figure 7.23 Isolation of flexor digitorum superficialis (FDS). **A)** Isolated action of the FDS of the index finger by flexing only the PIP joint. **B)** Method for testing individual FDS muscles by holding all other fingers in extension. In this position, slight pressure on the distal aspect of the flexed digit will prevent function of its FDS.

Thumb Extensors

The two main muscles that extend the thumb are the extensor pollicis longus and the extensor pollicis brevis. These muscles work together as the primary thumb extenders: The extensor pollicis longus inserts on the distal phalanx of the thumb and the extensor pollicis brevis inserts on the base of the proximal phalanx (Fig. 7.3). The abductor and flexor brevis have attachments into the dorsal hood and also can extend the IP joint.

Thumb Abductors

The abductor pollicis longus is a small muscle located on the posterior aspect of the forearm and hand (Fig. 7.24A). It is the main agonist in thumb abduction.

Intrinsic Muscles

Whereas the extrinsic muscles are the muscles that provide strength in hand movement, the intrinsic muscles are responsible for the hand's fine motor movements. The coordinated movements of the long finger flexors and extensors working with the intrinsic muscles are integral to the complexity and function of the human hand. The intrinsic muscles are relatively small and are grouped by their position within the hand. The *thenar* muscle group is located at the base of the thumb, the *hypothenar* group is located at the base of the fifth finger, and the deep muscle group is located in the palm of the hand. These intrinsic muscles are listed in Table 7–3.

Thenar Muscle Group

The thenar muscles function at the thumb. Three muscles make up the thenar mass of the hand: the flexor pollicis brevis, the abductor pollicis brevis, and the opponens pollicis. The abductor pollicis brevis is the most superficial of the three and attaches to the anterolateral side of the proximal phalanx and abducts the thumb (Fig. 7.24B). The flexor pollicis brevis inserts on the proximal phalanx of the thumb and flexes the CMC and MCP joint (Fig. 7.24C). Finally, the opponens pollicis attaches to the lateral and palmar areas of the first metacarpal and works to oppose the thumb. The opponens pollicis muscle is located in the thenar eminence just ulnar to the abductor pollicis brevis. Once the abductor pollicis brevis is located, move the palpating finger just medial to it and have the individual move the thumb into opposition (Fig. 7.25). The flexor pollicis brevis, abductor pollicis brevis, and opponens pollicis all participate in movements of unresisted opposition, MCP flexion, and CMC abduction.

Hypothenar Muscle Group

The hypothenar group of muscles consists of three muscles that lie in the ulnar palm between the wrist and base of the little finger. These muscles are the flexor digiti minimi, abductor digiti minimi, and the opponens digiti minimi (Table 7–3). These muscles

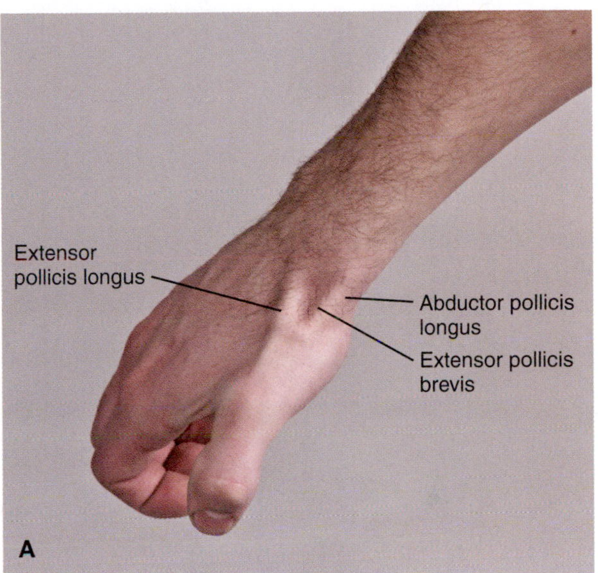

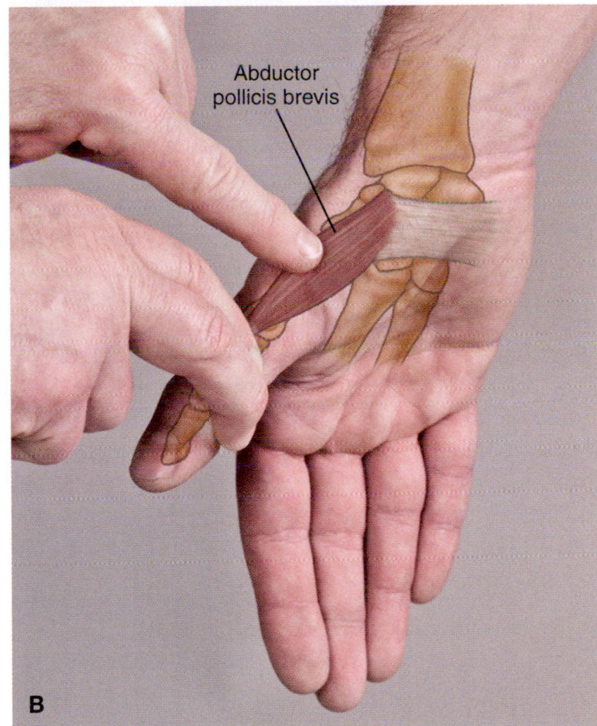

Figure 7.24 A) The extensor pollicis longus on the ulnar aspect and the abductor pollicis longus with the extensor pollicis brevis on the radial aspect form the tendinous borders of the anatomical snuff box. B) Abductor pollicis brevis is located on the anterolateral aspect of the first metacarpal. Place a palpating finger over the region and then instruct the individual to actively abduct the thumb allows the muscle to be readily palpated.

continued

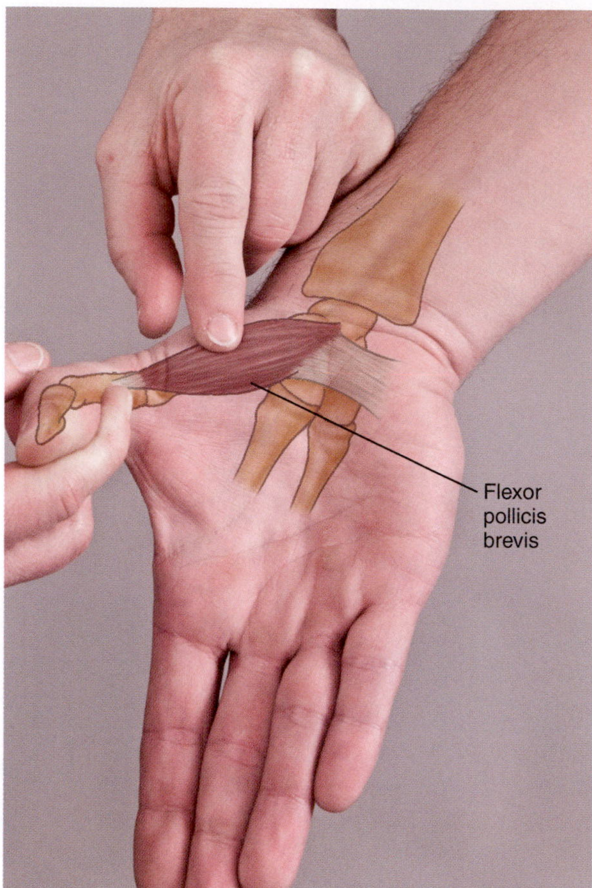

Figure 7.24—cont'd C) Flexor pollicis brevis is slightly ulnar to the abductor pollicis brevis and may be palpated when flexion of the thumb is resisted.

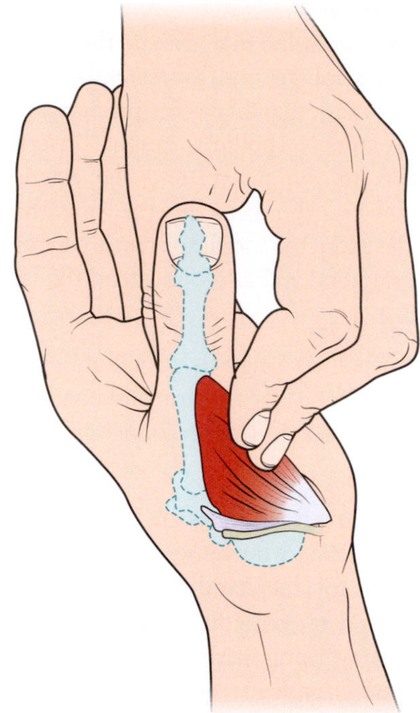

Figure 7.25 Opponens pollicis muscle is located in the thenar eminence just ulnarly to the abductor pollicis brevis. Once the abductor pollicis brevis located, move the palpating finger just medial to it and have the individual move the thumb into opposition.

all act on the little finger. The proximal and distal insertion alignment of the flexor digiti minimi allows it to flex the fifth metacarpophalangeal joint. The abductor digiti minimi abducts the fifth finger's metacarpophalangeal joint. The opponens digiti minimi is the deepest of the three hypothenar muscles. As its name implies, it opposes the fifth finger; it is able to do so because of its slightly angular alignment and medial insertion.

Deep Muscle (Midpalm) Group

This muscle group lies between the thenar and hypothenar eminences and is situated, as the name implies, in the palm of the hand. The muscles in this area include the interossei, lumbricals, and adductor pollicis. The interossei muscles are a group of three palmar and four dorsal muscles that originate in the metacarpal region of the hand and insert at the base of the proximal phalanges. The palmar interossei muscles are responsible for the adduction of the MCP joint of digits 2 to 5 (Fig. 7.26A), whereas the dorsal interossei abduct the digits (Fig. 7.26B). To make the palmar interossei and dorsal interossei function easier to remember, they are sometimes referred to as PAD and DAB muscles, respectively.

The lumbricals are the only muscles that have no bony attachment. Their proximal and distal insertions are on the tendons of other muscles: Their proximal insertions are on the tendons of the flexor digitorum profundus, and their distal insertions are on the tendons of the extensor digitorum. Because of this unique arrangement, these intrinsic muscles flex the MCP joints and extend the IP joints of digits 2 through 5 (Fig. 7.27).

The final midpalm muscle is the adductor pollicis muscle. This muscle is responsible for thumb adduction and has a broad origin ranging from the capitate, the second, and the third metacarpals (Fig. 7.28).

Extensor Mechanism

The hand's extensor mechanism is a complex interaction of the three vital movement groups of the hand: the intrinsic muscles, long finger extensors, and—indirectly through their connection to the intrinsics—the long

(text continues on page 285)

TABLE 7-3 | INTRINSIC MUSCLES OF THE WRIST AND HAND

Muscle group	Muscle	Proximal insertion	Distal insertion	Innervation	Action	Palpation
Thenar muscles	Abductor pollicis brevis	Flexor retinaculum and scaphoid and trapezium tubercles	Base of #1 proximal phalanx, lateral aspect	Median nerve C8–T1	Abducts #1. Assists with opposition	Place a palpating finger over the anterolateral #1 metacarpal and instruct the individual to actively abduct the thumb allows the muscle to be readily palpated.
Thenar muscles	**Opponens pollicis**	Flexor retinaculum and scaphoid and trapezium tubercles	All along the lateral aspect of #1 metacarpal	Median nerve, C8–T1	Flexes, abducts, and medially rotates #1 metacarpal to face the palm and touch #5 finger	The opponens pollicis lies deep to the abductor pollicis brevis and flexor pollicis brevis. Since all three thenar muscles activate during opposition motion, it is difficult to palpate.

continued

TABLE 7–3 | INTRINSIC MUSCLES OF THE WRIST AND HAND—cont'd

Muscle group	Muscle	Proximal insertion	Distal insertion	Innervation	Action	Palpation
Thenar muscles	Flexor pollicis brevis	Flexor retinaculum and scaphoid and trapezium tubercles	Base of #1 proximal phalanx, lateral aspect	Median nerve, C8–T1	Flexes #1	It lies over the opponens pollicis and may be palpated during very light flexion of #1 MCP.
Hypothenar muscles	Abductor digiti minimi	Pisiform	Medial aspect of #5 proximal phalanx	Ulnar nerve, deep branch C8–T1	Abducts #5	With light palpation of medial #5 metacarpal, the muscle is palpated with active abduction.
Hypothenar muscles	Flexor digiti minimi	Hamate and flexor retinaculum	Medial aspect of #5 proximal phalanx	Ulnar nerve, deep branch C8–T1	Flexes MCP and PIP of #5	The FDM is palpated in the hypothenar eminence just lateral to the abductor digiti minimi against light resistance to #5 flexion.
Hypothenar muscles	Opponens digiti minimi	Hamate and flexor retinaculum	Medial border of #5 metacarpal	Ulnar nerve, deep branch C8–T1	Flexes, abducts, and medially rotates #5 metacarpal to face and touch #1	It lies deep to the flexor digiti minimi, just ulnar to the abductor pollicis brevis. Once the

						abductor pollicis brevis is located, move the palpating finger just medial to it and have the individual move the thumb into opposition.
Deep intrinsic (midpalm) muscles	Adductor pollicis 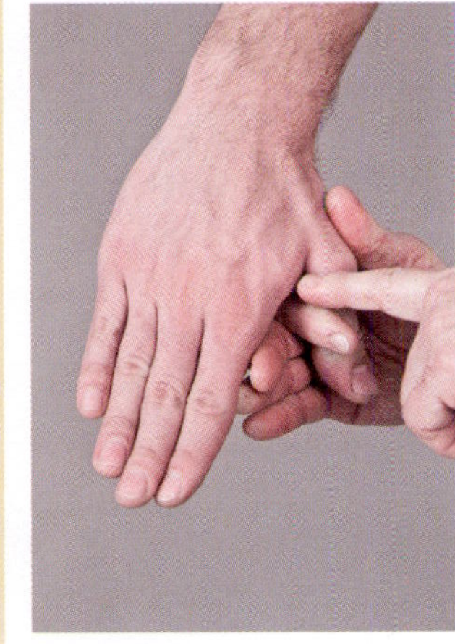	**Transverse head:** anterior aspect of #3 metacarpal. **Oblique head:** #2 & 3 metacarpal bases, capitates	Anteromedial base of #1 proximal phalanx	Ulnar nerve, deep branch C8–T1	Adducts #1 toward palm	This muscle is not in the thenar eminence. It is palpated in the #1–2 web space during #1 adduction against light resistance.
Deep intrinsic (midpalm) muscles 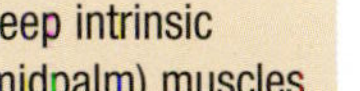	Lumbricals 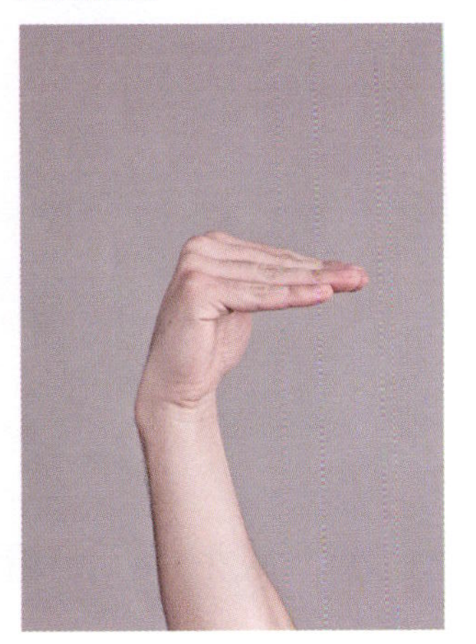	**#1–2:** Lateral 2 FDP tendons **#3–4:** Medial 3 FDP tendons	Lateral aspects of extensor expansions of #2–5 fingers	#1-2: Median nerve C8–T1	Flex MCP joints and extend IP joints	The muscle bellies are located on the radial side of the tendons of the long finger flexors. Identification of the lumbricals is difficult because these muscles are small and covered with fascia and skin.

continued

TABLE 7–3 | INTRINSIC MUSCLES OF THE WRIST AND HAND—cont'd

Muscle group	Muscle	Proximal insertion	Distal insertion	Innervation	Action	Palpation
Deep intrinsic (midpalm) muscles	Interossei	**Dorsal (#1–4):** Adjacent sides of 2 MC	Both: extensor expansions Dorsal (#1–4): bases of proximal phalanges of #2–4 fingers.	Ulnar nerve, deep branch C8–T1	Dorsal: Abducts fingers toward hand midline.	The muscular portion of #1 is palpated in the #1–2 web space with resistance to abduction of #2 digit; #2–4 dorsal interossei are difficult to palpate between MC bones. Resistance with a rubber band around the fingers in various combinations in finger abduction allows palpation. It may be easier to palpate the interossei with the digits in MCP and IP extension: palpate between the metacarpal bones while the fingers are actively abducted and adducted.
Deep intrinsic (midpalm) muscles		**Palmar (#1–3):** Anterior surface of #2, 4 & 5 metacarpals	Palmar (#1–3): bases of proximal phalanges of #2, 4, & 5 fingers		Palmar: Abducts fingers toward hand midline. Both: Flex MCP joints and extend IP joints of #2–4 fingers. Their available force for MCP flexion is greater than that of the lumbricals but over less range; primarily at 90 degrees flexion for a strong grip.	

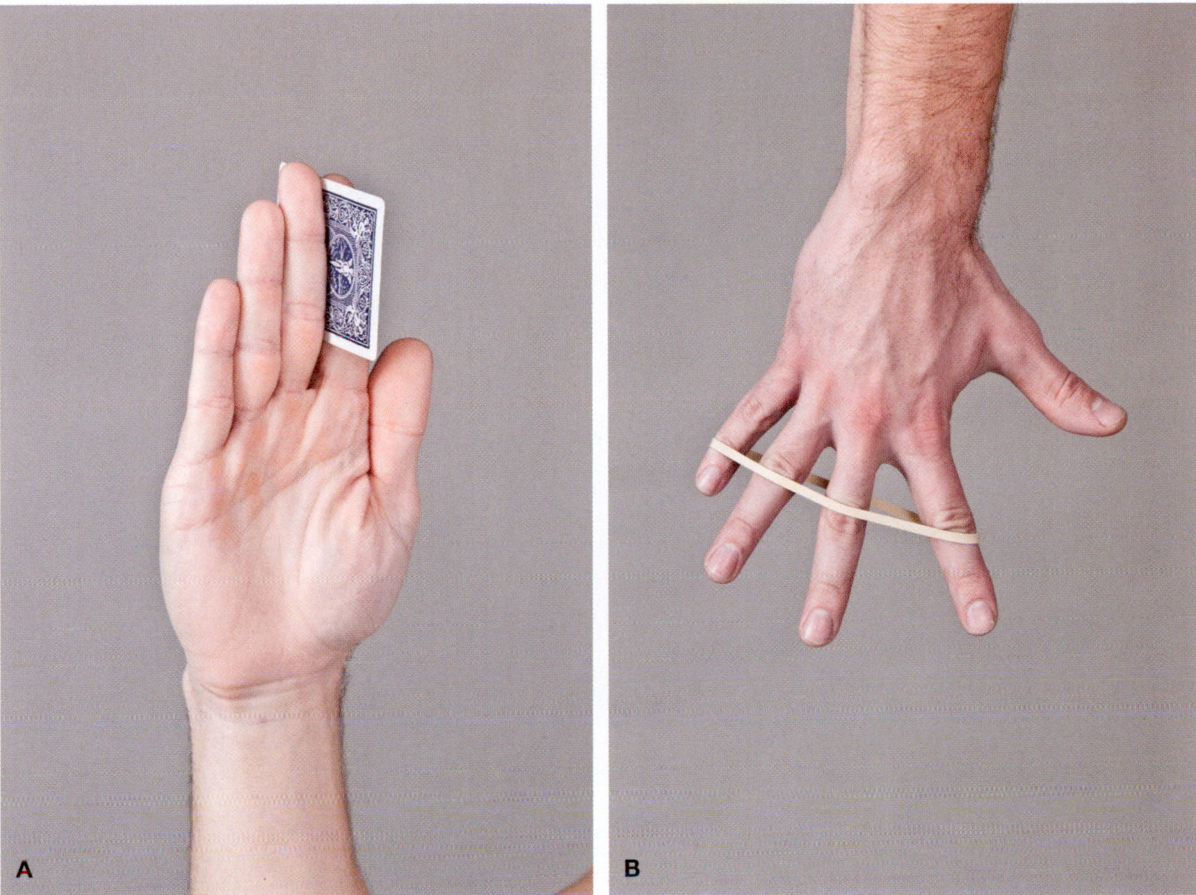

Figure 7.26 A) Palmar interossei adduct the fingers. B) Dorsal interossei abduct the fingers. With the MCPs in flexion and the IPs in extension, palpate between the MC bones as the fingers are actively abducted and adducted.

finger flexors. For the hand to function as it should, all three elements must provide their specific contributions. The extensor mechanism is also known as the extensor hood mechanism, extensor expansion, apparatus, aponeurosis, retinaculum, dorsal hood, or hood.

As shown in Figure 7.29, the digital tendons of the extrinsic extensor muscles and almost all of the intrinsic muscles terminate in the extensor mechanism. (Exceptions are the palmaris brevis, the opponens pollicis, and the opponens, abductor, and flexor digiti minimi muscles.) The extensor mechanism is made up of a tendinous system composed of the distal tendons of attachment of the extensor muscles, lumbricals, interossei, and thenar and hypothenar muscles and a retinacular system of fasciae and ligaments to retain and stabilize the tendons and the skin. The purpose of the assembly is to extend the digits in different positions of finger flexion. Another purpose is to provide shortcuts for the extensor tendons across the joints and to permit the digits full flexion. The extensor tendons must cover a longer distance from maximum extension to full flexion. This distance is about 25 mm and can be measured in the normal subject by placing a string over the dorsum of a finger and marking the change in length from full extension to end flexion.

Tendinous System

Proximally to the metacarpophalangeal joints, the extensor digitorum tendons are joined by three obliquely arranged fascial bands. The long extensor digitorum tendons then cross their respective MCP joint and, from the undersurface, extend a lax tendon, which inserts into the MCP joint capsule and the base of the proximal phalanx.[5] Over the proximal phalanx, the extensor tendon divides into three flat tendon bands: one central band that inserts into the base of the middle phalanx, and two lateral bands that course on either side to the PIP joint and continue on to

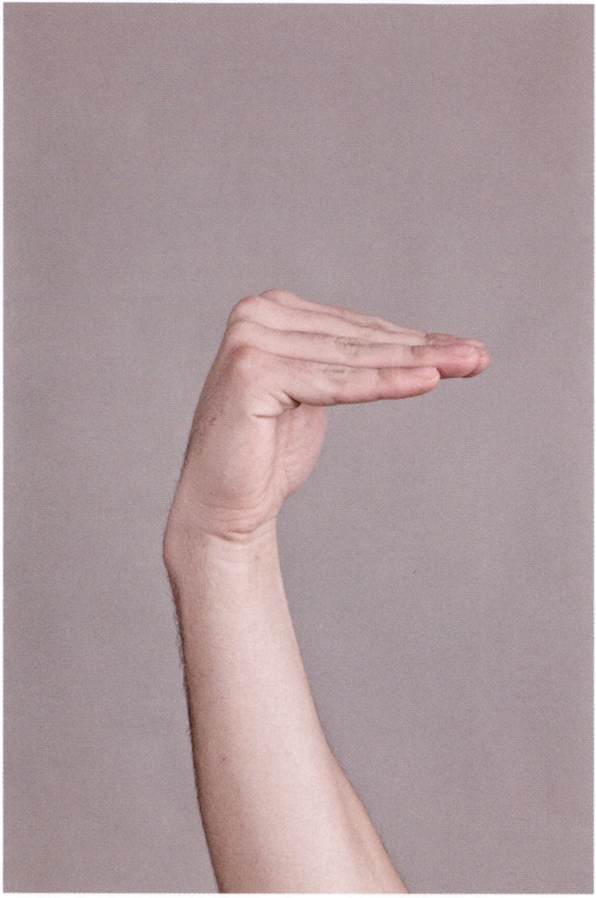

Figure 7.27 Muscular portions of the lumbricals are located on the radial side of the long finger flexor tendons and occasionally may be palpated when the MCPs move into flexion with the IPs in extension; palpate between the MC bones as the fingers are actively abducted and adducted.

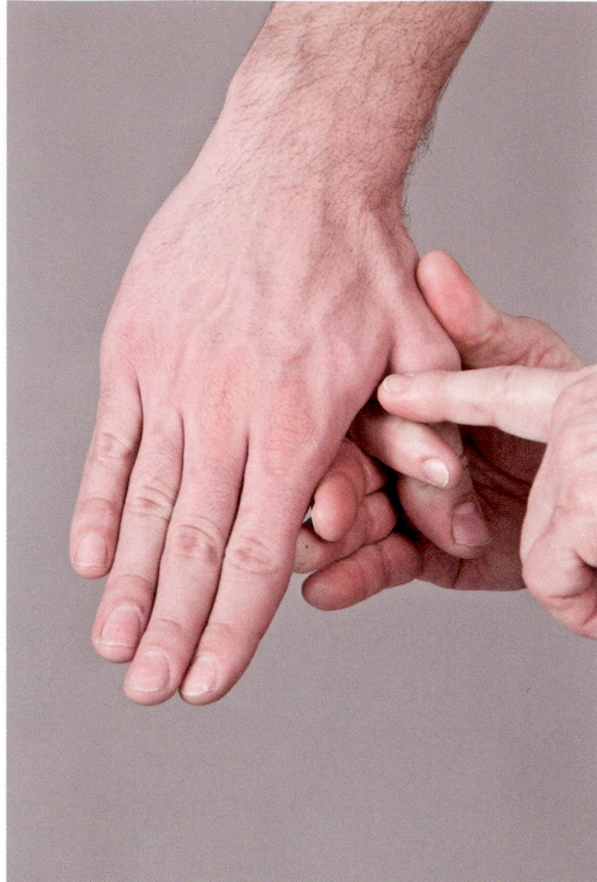

Figure 7.28 Adductor pollicis is seen in the first web space when resistance is offered to adduction of the thumb. The pollicis is not considered part of the thenar eminence, although it is an intrinsic thumb muscle. It lies deep to the thenar muscle group.

rejoin over the middle phalanx and finally insert into the base of the distal phalanx. These bands form the extensor expansions or extensor hoods (dorsal hoods) of the digits. An aponeurosis is formed from each of these bands and covers the dorsum and medial and lateral sides of each digit's metacarpal and proximal phalanx. The extensor expansion includes a middle band that inserts at the base of the middle phalanx and two lateral bands that insert at the base of the distal phalanx.

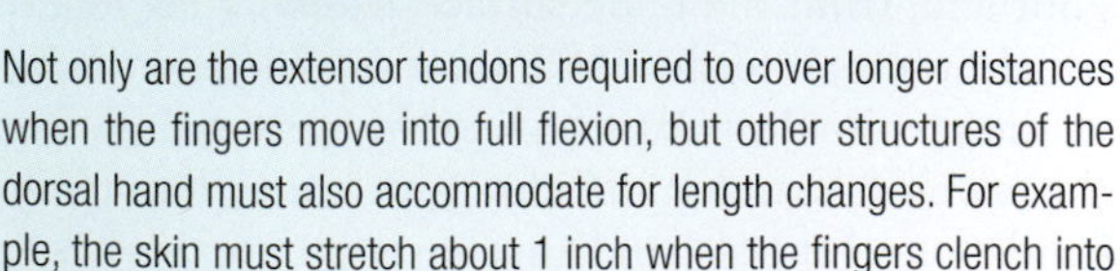

PRACTICE POINT

Not only are the extensor tendons required to cover longer distances when the fingers move into full flexion, but other structures of the dorsal hand must also accommodate for length changes. For example, the skin must stretch about 1 inch when the fingers clench into a fist. Some of this expansion is possible because of the wrinkles around the posterior MCP and IP joints we see when the fingers are in full extension. If an injury such as a severe laceration or burn occurs to the dorsum of the hand, the clinician must restore flexibility of the skin and other affected dorsal soft tissues if full finger flexion function is to be restored.

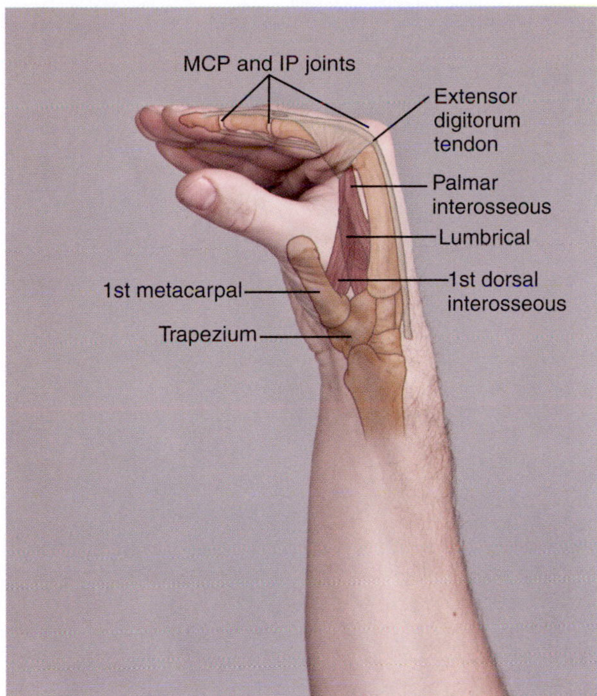

Figure 7.29 Extensor mechanism of the hand. The extensor mechanism is made up of several structures including the distal tendinous attachments of the extensor muscles; insertion of intrinsic muscles such as the lumbricals, interossei, and thenar and hypothenar muscles; and a retinacular system of fasciae and ligaments.

Interossei muscles have several terminal tendons on the sides of each finger (Figs. 7.26 and 7.27). These include insertions into the base of the proximal phalanges, attachments to the volar plate, insertions to the expansion of the lateral bands, and tendons at the base of the middle phalanx. The terminal attachments of the lumbricals pass on the radial side of the MCP joints and volar to the tendons of the interossei. The distal lumbrical tendons insert into and help form the lateral bands of each digit. Thus, for each finger, the motor input into the lateral bands, which extend the PIP and DIP joints, is provided by at least four muscles: the long extensor, two interossei, and a lumbrical.

The tendon of the extensor indicis parallels the extensor digitorum on the ulnar side of the finger. The extensor indicis has a separate muscle belly in the forearm and provides independent movement of the index finger even when the other fingers are flexed. Therefore, the extensor indicis allows us to point the index finger while the other fingers are flexed. The extensor digiti minimi usually divides into two tendons in the area of the dorsal hood and is the primary long extensor of the little finger. According to Brand,[6] the extensor digitorum tendon to the fifth digit is usually small and inadequate to extend the finger. The abductor digiti minimi inserts into the dorsal hood and the lateral bands of the extensor mechanism, as do the interossei.

The thumb has a similar extensor mechanism as the other digits. The extensor mechanism of the thumb includes the extensor pollicis longus along with intrinsic tendinous insertions of the adductor pollicis, flexor pollicis brevis, and abductor pollicis brevis.

Retinacular System

The retinacular system influences both the flexors and extensors of the fingers. The complex fascial and ligamentous parts of the retinacular system enclose, compartmentalize, and restrain the joints and tendons as well as the nerves, blood vessels, and skin.

Extensor Hood

On the extensor surface, the retinacular system includes a fibrous band connecting the proximal phalanx and distal sheath that covers the proximal and distal interphalangeal joints and middle phalanx. It continues to

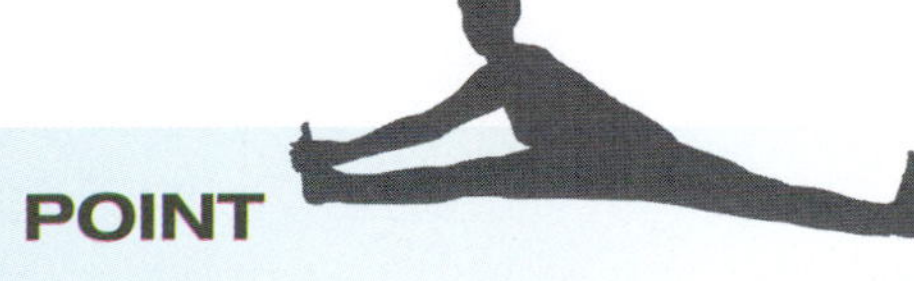

PRACTICE POINT

During sports activities such as baseball and volleyball, the extensor digitorum is occasionally injured when the ball impacts the end of a digit. The compression force of the ball on the finger tip causes a sudden flexion of the DIP joint, resulting in rupture of the extensor tendon's attachment on the distal phalanx. Because the distal phalanx is unable to extend with the rest of the digit and takes on the appearance of a mallet, this injury is commonly referred to as a mallet finger. Such an injury is not usually surgically repaired unless there is a fracture associated with the tendon avulsion. The common treatment is application of a dorsal extension splint of the DIP to allow scar tissue formation and the tendon ends to heal. The splint is worn continuously for about six weeks.

the distal phalanx where it merges with the extensor expansion. This fibrous visor-like hood or dorsal expansion encircles the MCP joints and retains the tendons crossing the joint.

Attachments of the dorsal hood are on the palmar sides at the junction of the volar plate and the transverse intermetacarpal ligament. Distally, the extensor hood and tendons are difficult to distinguish. When the fingers are flexed, the extensor hood is pulled distally so that the hood lies over the proximal phalange rather than over the MCP joint. At the level of the PIP joint, the retinacular system joins and restrains the tendinous system, capsular structures, and skin. During finger flexion, for example, the lateral bands must move volarly on the PIP joint to permit the motion, but to effectively extend the IP joints, the tendons must move dorsally. It is the purpose of the fascia and ligaments of the retinacular system to control and to limit these motions.

Flexor Pulleys

The retinacular system is also connected to the flexor compartment. The flexor digitorum superficialis and profundus tendons are enclosed in synovial-lined tunnels, which are maintained against the palmar surfaces of the phalanges by pulleys. Annular (L., ring) pulleys attach to the shafts of the proximal and distal phalanges and to the sides of the volar plates of the MCP, PIP, and DIP joints at the junctions with the extensor hood and the retinaculum. Cruciate pulleys attach on the shafts of the phalanges and cross to form distal attachments on the volar plates of the PIP and DIP joints.[7] Much like the loops for the line on a fishing pole, these pulleys prevent bowstringing of the long flexor tendons during flexor activities. Severance of a pulley causes loss of finger motion.[8] These pulleys are illustrated in Figure 7.30 and demonstrate their supporting function to the flexor digitorum profundus tendon.

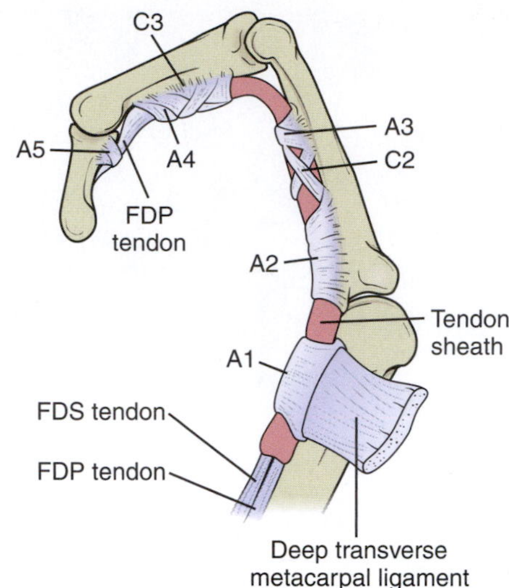

Figure 7.30 Annular rings and pulleys of the flexor tendons of the fingers maintain these tendons in their positions adjacent to the fingers during flexion motion.

Motions

The wrist and metacarpophalangeal joints move in two planes whereas the interphalangeal joints move in one plane. Although some individuals refer to a circumduction movement of the wrist, this movement is actually a combination of its motion in the frontal and sagittal planes of motion.

Motions of the Wrist

As with other joints, the wrist has osteokinematic motions and arthrokinematic motions. Both types of motions must be present in order to have full function of the wrist and hand.

Osteokinematic Wrist Motions

Motions of the wrist occur at the radiocarpal and the midcarpal joints. According to Kapandji,[3] the midcarpal joint is responsible for one-half of the motion of radial

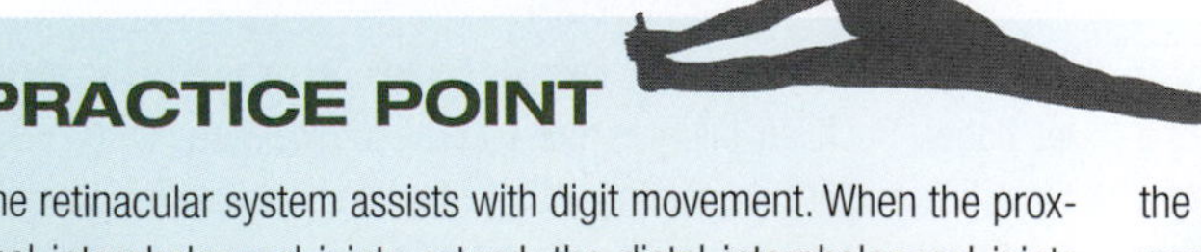

PRACTICE POINT

The retinacular system assists with digit movement. When the proximal interphalangeal joints extend, the distal interphalangeal joints also move into extension. When the distal interphalangeal joints initiate finger flexion, the proximal interphalangeal joints also flex as the retinacular ligament becomes taut. Such an anatomical arrangement provides some biomechanical assist in finger motion when isolated muscle injuries of either the long finger extensor or flexor muscles occurs.

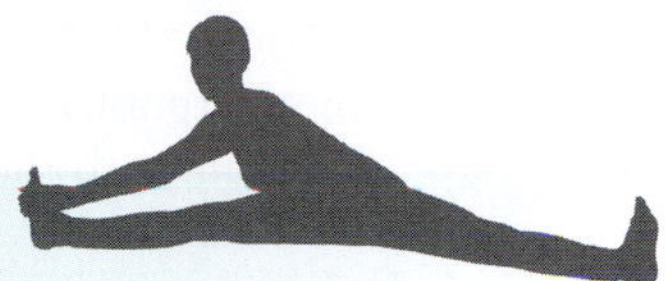

PRACTICE POINT

The retinacular system can be compared to an interconnecting structure that encircles the digit and creates balanced forces. Destruction of a ligament by injury or disease such as rheumatoid arthritis can cause disruption of the balanced forces and movement of tendons to abnormal positions, which create further deforming forces. For example, destruction of the capsule and collateral ligaments of the MCP (Fig. 7.31) can cause bowstringing of the flexor tendons.

deviation and for one-third of the range of ulnar deviation with the remaining motion occurring at the radiocarpal joint. These motions occur around an axis through the head of the capitate (Fig. 7.32). The normal end feel for radial deviation is usually hard from contact of the scaphoid on the styloid process of the radius. Ulnar deviation provides more motion and has a firm end feel caused by tension on the radial collateral ligament.

When the wrist goes through flexion, Kapandji[3] states that there are 50° of motion at the radiocarpal joint and 35° at the midcarpal joint. When the wrist moves into full extension, these values reverse with 35° occurring at the radiocarpal and 50° at the midcarpal joint. Overall, total wrist flexion and extension occurs because of equal contributions from the radiocarpal and midcarpal joints. The axes of motion for both flexion-extension and radial-ulnar deviation both go through the capitate. However, the flexion-extension axis migrates distally from full flexion to extension (Fig. 7.33). The migration is caused by complex movements of the lunate and scaphoid, which include rotational and translatory motions with change in their effective height. These complex motions are compensatory in order to maintain tension of the ligaments at all times.[9]

Full wrist extension requires slight spreading of the distal radius and ulna. If these bones are grasped and held together firmly, the subject is unable to completely extend the wrist.

Arthrokinematic Wrist Motions

In arthrokinematic terms, the radiocarpal and ulnocarpal joints consist of a concave radius and ulna and a convex carpal row (Fig. 7.4). Therefore, maintaining the proximal segment's position, the roll and glide of the distal segment occur opposite to one another; with a dorsal roll, the glide is anterior or palmar, and with a palmar or anterior roll, the glide occurs dorsally. The same is true for the midcarpal joint.

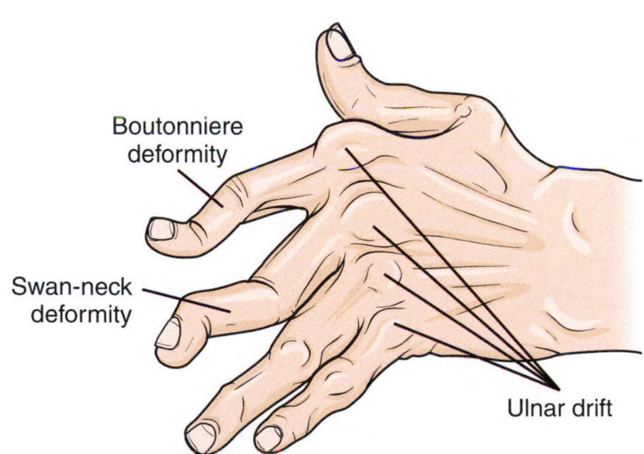

Figure 7.31 Bowstringing of flexor tendons. The passive tension created by the long finger tendons on the MCP joint is normally resisted in a hand with normal ligaments. If the hand has degenerative changes in the joints, ligamentous structures become weakened and unable to resist these normal forces. Over time, the deteriorated capsule and ligaments succumb to the bowstringing force.

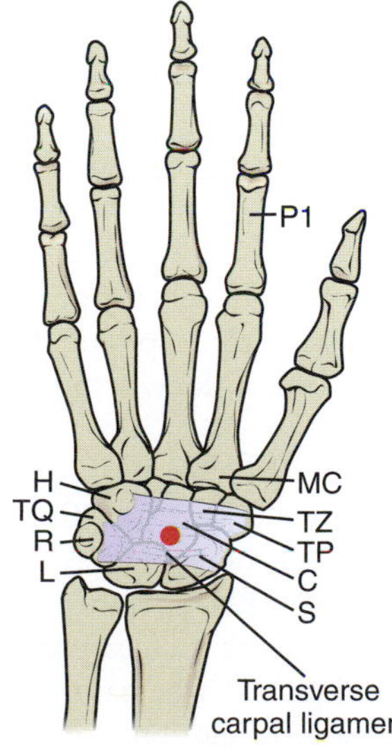

Figure 7.32 Axis for radial-ulnar flexion runs through the head of the capitate.

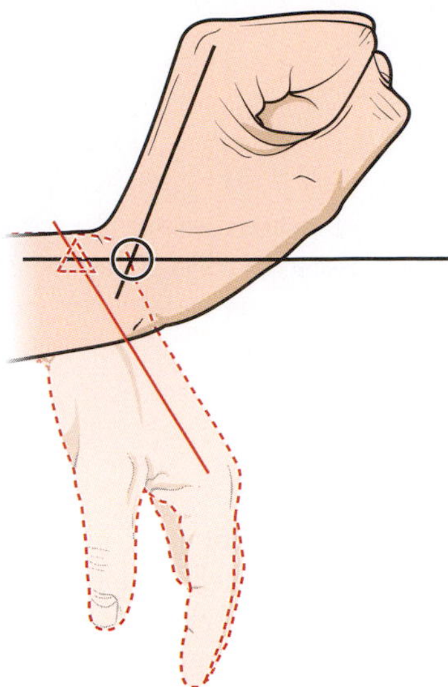

Figure 7.33 Axis for flexion-extension changes in positions of flexion and extension because of the complex movements of the lunate and scaphoid during these motions.

When the forearm and hand are relaxed with the wrist in a neutral position, the wrist is unstable and permits a considerable amount of passive joint play movement. If the clinician stabilizes the patient's distal radius and ulna with one hand and places his or her other hand around the proximal carpal row, the patient's carpals can be moved with ease in dorsal, volar, medial, and lateral translatory glides and distracted several millimeters. Similar movements with less motion occur with hand placement on either side of the midcarpal joint. In addition, each metacarpal bone can be passively moved relative to its neighbors. For example, the capitate can be stabilized on its dorsal and volar surfaces by the examiner's left thumb and forefinger; an individual carpal such as the trapezoid, scaphoid, lunate, or hamate can be grasped between the examiner's right thumb and forefinger and moved on the capitate; however, the roll and glide are variable for each of the individual joints these bones form with the capitate. The most stable (close-packed) position of the wrist is in full extension.

Motions of the Fingers

Metacarpophalangeal joints of the fingers and thumb are different from each other. The MCP joints of the fingers are also different from the interphalangeal joints of the fingers. The finger's metacarpophalangeal joints have two degrees of motion whereas the interphalangeal joints have one degree of motion.

Osteokinematic Motions of the Fingers

The metacarpophalangeal joints have approximately 90° of flexion, with the index finger having slightly less and the middle, ring, and little fingers having successively more range. The end feel may be hard with contact of the phalanx on the metacarpal or firm from capsular limitation. Hyperextension is variable depending on ligamentous structure. Some people may be able to extend the MCP joints to only 0° whereas others with ligamentous laxity may be able to actively hyperextend up to 45°. Passively, some can hyperextend to 90°. The normal end feel is firm from limitation by the volar plate and capsule.

When the MCP joint is extended, its collateral ligaments are slack and permit about 20° of abduction and, if adjacent fingers are moved away, about 20° of adduction. In 90° of flexion, the collateral ligaments are taut and abduction or adduction is limited to a few degrees at best. This is the close-packed position of the joint.

The MCP joint of the thumb is usually described as a hinge joint. It has less motion than the MCP joints of the fingers. Flexion motion ranges from 45° to 60°, and hyperextension is normally from 0° to 20°. In full flexion and extension, ligaments tighten and there is little abduction or adduction. In semi-flexion, 5° to 10° of side-to-side motion can occur plus a dynamic rotation of the phalanx produced by contraction of the muscles to the medial or the lateral sesamoid bone. These small motions provide a precise fit of the thumb around objects for grasping.

Proximal and distal IP joints are hinge joints with one degree of freedom. The bicondylar heads of the phalanges and the greater tension of the collateral ligaments prohibit abduction and adduction motions of these joints. Flexion of the PIP joints is about 120°. The DIP has slightly less than 90° of flexion. Extension of the PIP and DIP joints is to 0° except in individuals with ligamentous laxity, in which some hyperextension is seen. Hyperextension of the thumb IP joint may be 5° to 10° and can be considerably more when performed passively, as when applying weight to the joint's palmar surface (Fig. 7.34).

Arthrokinematic Motions of the Fingers

During flexion and extension of the metacarpophalangeal and interphalangeal joints, the arthrokinematic roll and slide are in the same direction since the proximal aspects of these joints are convex and the distal aspects are concave. For example, when the phalanx rolls in a palmar direction during flexion, slide within the joint also occurs in a palmar direction.

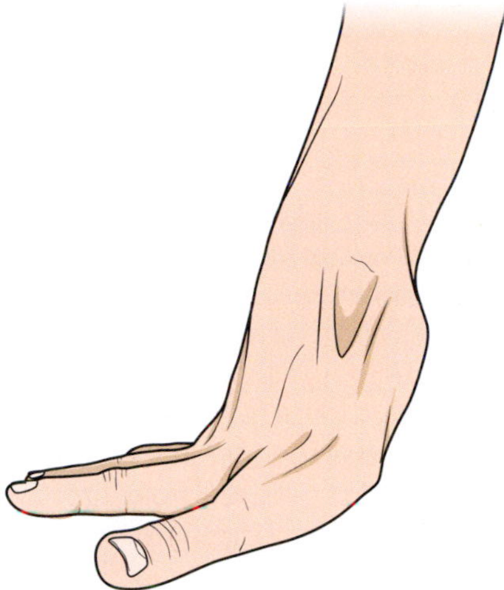

Figure 7.34 Hyperextension of the MCP and IP joints occurs with laxity of the capsule and ligaments surrounding the joints.

Arthrokinematic motion in abduction and adduction movements of the MCP joints also have roll and slide occurring in the same direction. The resting position for all of the MCP and IP the joints is the same—20° of flexion. The close-packed position for the thumb's MCP and IP joints is full extension, and for each of the joints of digits 2 through 5, the close-packed position is full flexion.

Large joint play movements are possible when a person is relaxed and the capsules of the MCP joints are loose with the joints in their resting positions. When the examiner stabilizes the metacarpal with one hand and grasps the proximal phalanx with the other hand, accessory motions of anterior-posterior glides, lateral glides, rotation, and distraction can be made between the metacarpal head and base of the phalanx. Similar accessory motions—but with smaller excursions—are found in the IP joints.

Functional Movements of the Wrist and Hand

Wrist and hand function depends on the close interaction of the extrinsic extensors, extrinsic flexors, and intrinsic muscles. If any of these three groups are unable to function normally, normal hand function is also lost. A careful balance of these three structures is required for the hand and finger's daily activities. Additionally, just as the scapula must be stable on the thorax for the glenohumeral joint to function properly, so too, the wrist must be stable for the digits to function as they should.

Types of Grasp

The hand makes the rest of the upper extremity limb purposeful. The primary function of the shoulder and elbow is to position the hand for function. The hand is used to either serve as a transmitter of force or as a mobile device. As a force transmitter, it is used as a fist, palm, or hook. As a mobile device—its most common function—it is used to manipulate objects, perceive the environment, or express the individual's thoughts or emotions. The hand is used in a multitude of postures and movements that in most cases involve both the thumb and the other digits. Of all the positions and functions for which the hand is used, it is frequently used to grasp objects. Napier[10] describes two types of grasps of the human hand: the "power grip" (7-35A) and the "precision grip" (Fig. 7.35B). The power grip incorporates the entire hand and is used for gross activities to grasp an object rather than to manipulate it. The power grip involves holding an object between the partially flexed fingers and the palm while the thumb usually applies counterpressure to maintain and stabilize the object within the hand; there is only one power grip in which the thumb is not required to participate, the hook grip (Fig. 7.36A1). Table 7–4 describes each of the power grips (See Fig 7.36A, 1–3). In the precision grip, an object is pinched between the flexor surfaces of one or more fingers and the opposing thumb. The precision grip is used when accuracy and refinement of touch are needed to manipulate or use an object (Fig. 7.36B, 1–3). Table 7–5 describes each of the precision grips and Figure 7.37 is a concept map of the power and precision grips. The thumb postures differ in the two types of grips. In the power grips, the thumb is in adduction or opposition, and it reinforces the pressure of the fingers to stabilize the object in the hand. In precision grips, the thumb is abducted and is usually positioned to oppose the pulp of the fingers. Napier[10] states that the nature of the task to be performed determines the grip to be used and that these two types of grips incorporate the whole range of prehensile activity in the human hand.

The names used to identify the various grips imply that hand posture is conditioned by the shape of the object being held. These terms are commonly used in rehabilitation although the general terms, power grip and precision grip, are quite universally accepted.

Schlesinger,[11] in investigating designs for terminal devices for artificial arms, studied the versatility of the human hand in grasping and holding objects of various sizes and shapes. He distinguished among 12 different types of prehension; 7 are divided into power and precision

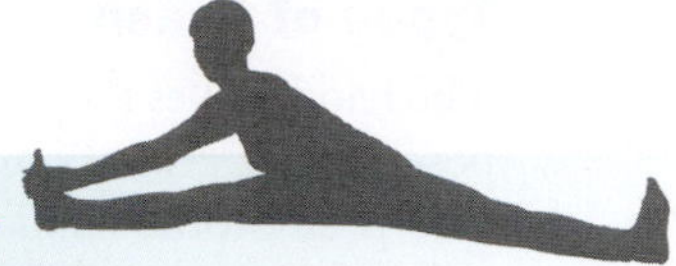

PRACTICE POINT

Individuals with spinal cord injuries who lack function in their finger flexors are still able to grasp objects such as drinking glasses and other items for functional use. **Tenodesis** is utilized to provide a grasping mechanism (Fig. 4.15). Tenodesis is joint movement that occurs because passive tension is applied to a tendon. For example, a person with a C6 tetraplegia lacks innervation to the long finger flexor and extensor muscles to make a fist but does have innervation to perform wrist extension. When the wrist is actively extended, passive tension is placed on the finger flexor tendons because of the length-tension relationship. Extending the wrist shortens the flexor tendons (FDP) to produce finger flexion. Likewise, allowing gravity to flex the wrist will shorten the extensor digitorum so the fingers extend. This is easily seen on yourself when you maintain relaxed fingers as you actively extend and flex your wrist. Clinicians who treat individuals with tetraplegia rely on this technique to grasp objects and encourage the patient's extrinsic finger muscles to shorten so tension of these muscles may occur during wrist motion, providing the individual with a grasp and release mechanism of the hand.

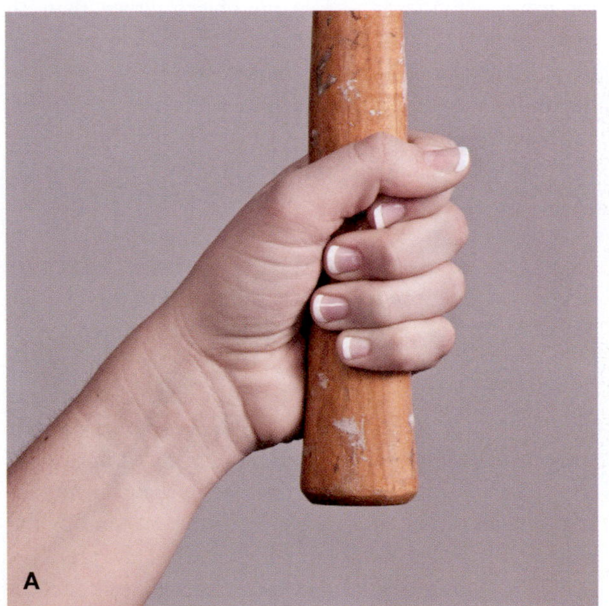

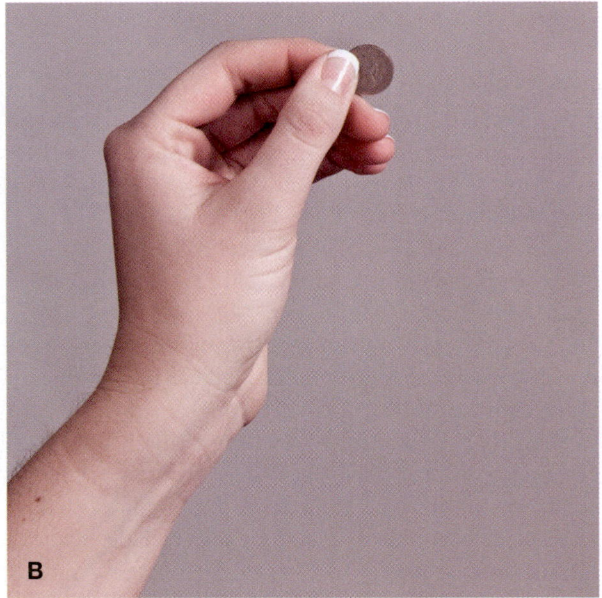

Figure 7.35 Types of grips. **A)** Power grips usually involve all of the fingers and the thumb and provide for strength in grasping activities. **B)** Precision grips usually involve the thumb with the index or the index and middle fingers and are used when a fine grasp is required to manipulate small objects.

grips and described in Tables 7–4 and 7–5, respectively. Schlesinger also points out that some of these prehension types may be compared to simple tools, such as a hook (hook grasp), pincers (tip-to-tip prehension), and pliers (palmar prehension). Palmar prehension is no longer used in the terms presented by Schlesinger; this grip with the thumb pad opposing the index and middle digits is now called "three-jaw chuck" or "three-prong chuck".

Keller, Taylor, and Zahm, as cited by Taylor and Schwarz,[12] investigated the frequency of three types of common prehension patterns in picking up objects and holding them for use. Their findings were as follows:

	Palmar (3-Prong chuck)	Tip	Lateral
Pick up	50%	17%	33%
Hold for use	88%	2%	10%

This study showed that palmar, or three-prong chuck, prehension is by far the most commonly used type for both picking up and holding small objects. An adaptation of this grasp was subsequently used in the design of terminal devices for artificial arms.

Three-prong chuck and tip prehension grips both require that the thumb and fingers be opposed to each other. The awareness that these grips are frequently used in daily activities points to the importance of opposition of the thumb in the human hand. Individuals who have lost their ability to oppose the thumb but who are capable of adducting it, however, may use lateral prehension for grasping and holding small objects. Lateral prehension makes use of pressure of the thumb against the radial side of the index finger, which is held in a semi-flexed position. This is the prehension pattern of choice for patients with upper motor neuron lesions for whom contact on the palmar surface of the fingers increases spasticity of the finger flexors, which is frequently the case. Such patients may be able to release an object held with lateral prehension, whereas an object that touches the palm of the hand may be very difficult to release because of the spasticity.

Strength of Grip

Swanson, Matev, and deGroot[13] studied normal grip and pinch strength to establish a baseline for evaluation of the disabled hand. Strength measurements were taken on 50 normal males and 50 females, ranging in

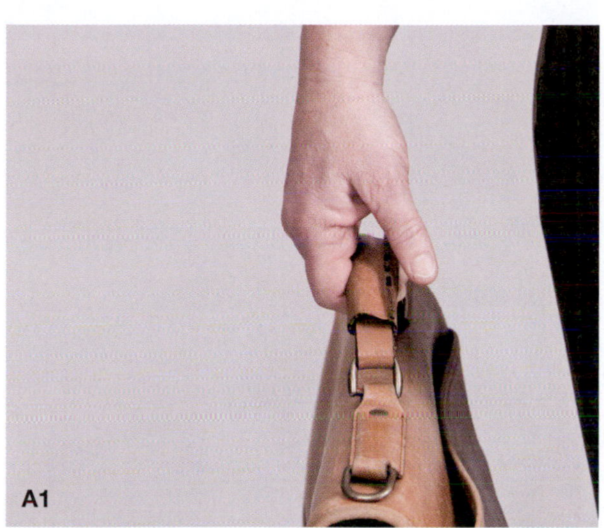

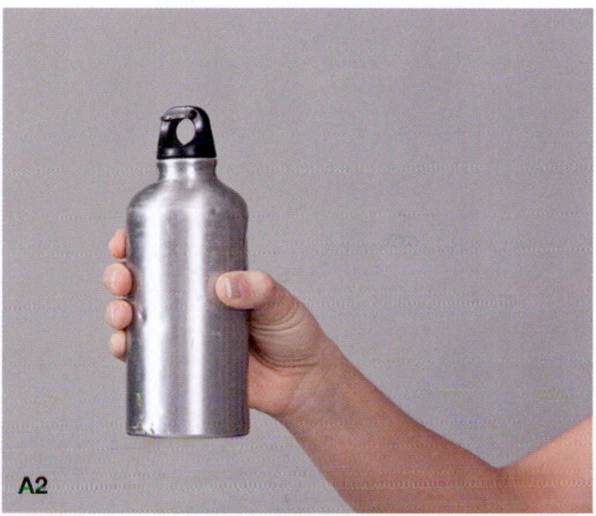

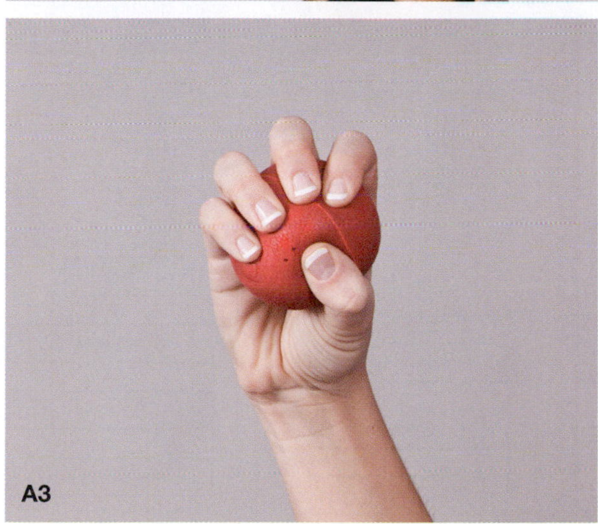

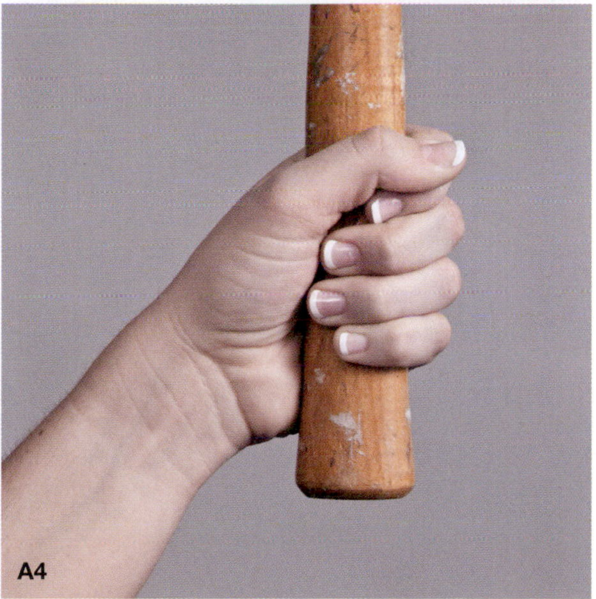

Figure 7.36 A) Power grips: A1) Hook grip is the only power grip that does not require use of the thumb; A2) Cylindrical grip is used to make a firm grasp around a cylindrical object such as a large canister or bottle; A3) A spherical grasp is used to conform around balls or other sphere-shaped objects; A4) A fist grip is similar to the cylinder grip but the hand encloses securely around a small object so the thumb is often in contact with other digits such as when grasping a hammer, shovel, or broom.

continued

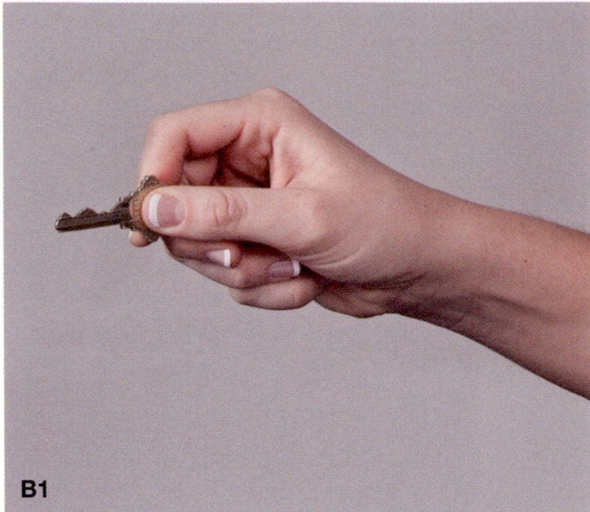

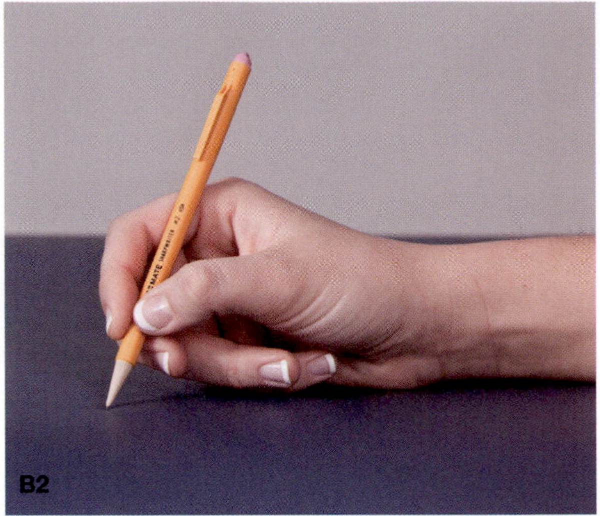

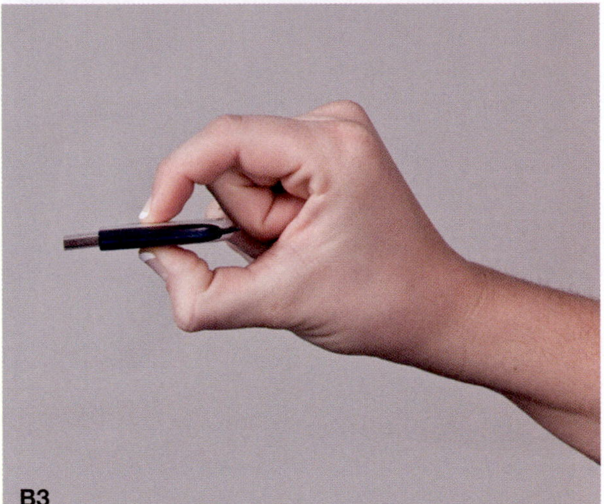

Figure 7.36—cont'd Precision grips: **B1)** Lateral Pinch is also referred to as the key pinch and places the pad of the thumb along the lateral aspect of the index finger; **B2)** Three-jaw chuck or three-prong chuck rotates the thumb so it may be used with digits #2 and 3; **B3)** The tip-to-tip pinch positions the thumb and index finger pads facing each other.

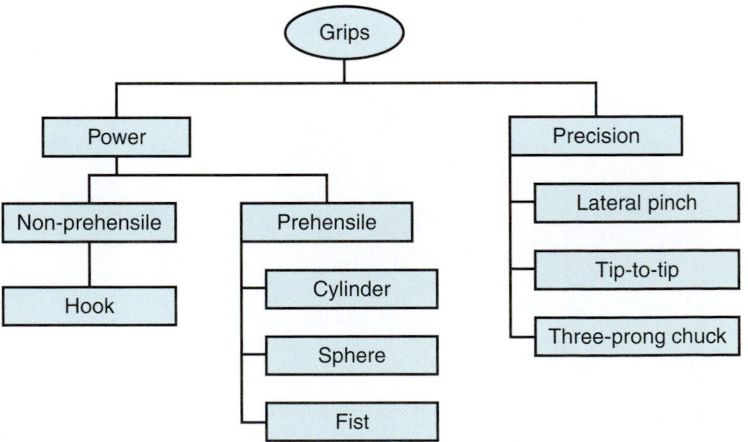

Figure 7.37 Concept map of the various hand grips.

age from 17 to 60 years. Some of the mean values (expressed in pounds) are as follows:

	Age	Male	Female
Grip (major hand)	20	100	53
	20–30	107	54
	30–40	109	68
	40–50	108	52
	50–60	101	49
Chuck pinch (dominant hand)	17–60	17	11
Lateral pinch (dominant hand)	17–60	17	11

In addition to providing some normal values useful for making comparisons, this study found only a 4% to 9% decrease between the dominant and nondominant hands, which substantiates the 6% difference found by Toews.[14] Others have found that the difference between dominant and nondominant grip strength is about 10% with the dominant hand providing the stronger grip.[15, 16] This strength difference is referred to by some as the "10% rule."[17] Other investigators have disputed the 10% rule. Alfred Swanson and associates[13] found that 29% of the subjects had the same or greater grip strength in the nondominant hand. Still, other investigators have found no conflicting differences between dominant and nondominant grip in their studies.[18, 19] The vast differences in these and other studies may reflect the differences in the populations studied and the testing methods used by these studies.

Grasping

When the fist closes, the fingers fold into the palm of the hand or close around an object by the action of the long finger flexors (profundus and superficialis). This long tendon action is probably aided by some of the intrinsic muscles of the hand. Because these long finger flexors have proximal attachments in the forearm and their tendons pass on the flexor side of the wrist, these muscles—if unopposed—would cause the wrist to flex during grasp. Such action is prevented by the stabilizing action of the wrist extensors. The strength of contraction exerted by the wrist extensors is in direct proportion to the effort of the grip: the harder the grip, the stronger the contraction of the wrist extensors.

Role of the Wrist Extensors in Grasping

If the wrist flexes during finger flexion, the grip is markedly weakened (Fig. 7.38); in fact, it then becomes almost impossible to close the fist completely (Fig. 7.39A). This difficulty arises partly because the finger extension apparatus may not permit further elongation (passive insufficiency) and partly because of the significant shortening that occurs in the finger flexors, which weakens their ability to produce effective tension (active insufficiency).

Note that normal wrist movements are in a direction opposite to the finger motions, so that an alternate elongation of the finger extensors and the finger flexors over the wrist is obtained (Fig.7.39B). Such elongation adds to the efficiency of these muscles in extending and flexing the fingers, promoting optimal sufficiency.

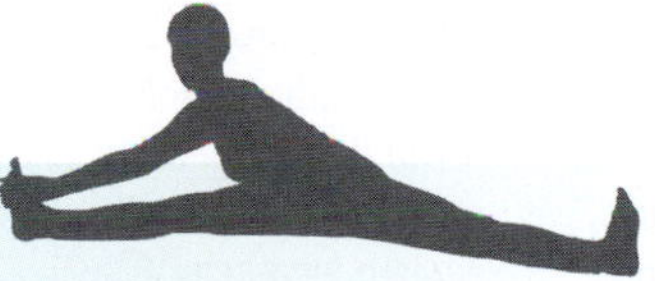

PRACTICE POINT

With such a conflict in research results, the clinician may be easily confused as to whether findings during a patient's examination of grip strength are significant or not. Perhaps the best advice a clinician should heed is that if a *noticeable functional difference* exists in the grip strength of the patient's two hands, it is important to suspect pathology and provide appropriate rehabilitation based on the examination findings.

To determine forces of grip and pinch that should be provided in artificial hands, Keller and associates, as cited by Klopsteg and Wilson,[20] measured the minimum prehension forces required in the manipulation of common objects and other activities of everyday life. They found, for example, that pulling on a sock required a 7.7-lb force, whereas manipulation of a screw cap like that found on a toothpaste tube required a 2.5-lb force, and holding a soup spoon, a 1.6-lb force. Prehension forces available in the natural hand as shown by the Swanson study[13] are considerably greater than the forces that are actually required for most everyday activities.

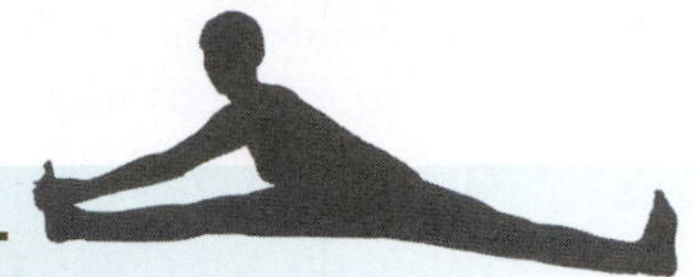

PRACTICE POINT

Just as the wrist extensors influence grasping activity, the wrist flexors influence finger extension. The long finger extensors begin in the dorsal forearm and pass over the wrist and MCP joints. If these muscles contracted in an isolated fashion, they would extend not only the joints of the fingers but also the wrist. To prevent them from moving the wrist, the wrist flexors contract synergistically, keeping the wrist in a neutral position or flexing it. The association between finger extensors and wrist flexors is strong, and it takes a concentrated effort to interrupt the linkage. If full finger extension motion is alternated with full finger flexion motion in rapid succession, you can see that the wrist and fingers are both in constant motion: wrist flexion accompanies finger extension; wrist extension occurs when the fist closes completely. These combinations are automatic in the normal hand, and the less attention the performer pays to the details of the performance, the more obvious they are. Injured wrists that are splinted in flexion often lose this relationship so when the splint is removed, the wrist extensors and finger flexors do not work in concert with each other to provide optimal grasping. Clinicians must correct this asynchrony for proper grasping to be restored.

TABLE 7–4 | POWER GRIPS

Grip	Purpose	Finger Contribution	Thumb Contribution	Examples of uses
Hook grip 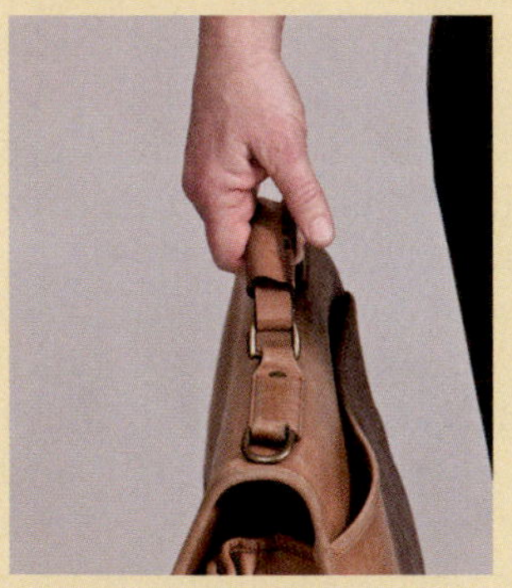	The finger digits provide this grip. Used primarily to support or carry an object.	The fingers and palm are the primary contributors. Primary function occurs from the flexor digitorum superficialis primarily and the profundus secondarily with the IP joints in flexion, especially the PIP joints.	Thumb does not contribute to this grip. It is usually held in extension, away from the hand.	Carrying a suitcase or briefcase. Weight lifters may use a hook grip to lift a barbell off the floor.
Cylinder grip  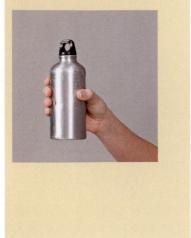	Grasp objects that are cylindrical in shape and large enough that the thumb does not touch the fingers. The fingers and palm are on one side of the object and the thumb is placed on the opposite side to secure the object to the palm.	Primarily flexion of the IP and MCP joints with activity from the flexor digitorum profundus. The flexor digitorum superficialis assists when increased forces are required. Interossei muscles flex the MCP joints and move the MCP joints in an ulnar direction. This ulnar deviation is counteracted by radial collateral	Thumb position varies. Most often, it flexes and adducts, acting as a vice to secure the object to the fingers and palm. Rotation to provide opposition at the CMC joint occurs but depends on the width of the grip.	Holding a beverage container or a telephone receiver incorporates the cylinder grip.

TABLE 7–4 | POWER GRIPS—cont'd

Grip	Purpose	Finger Contribution	Thumb Contribution	Examples of uses
		ligaments of the MCP joints. The fingers usually lie adjacent and parallel to each other and in contact with the adjacent fingers.		
Spherical grip 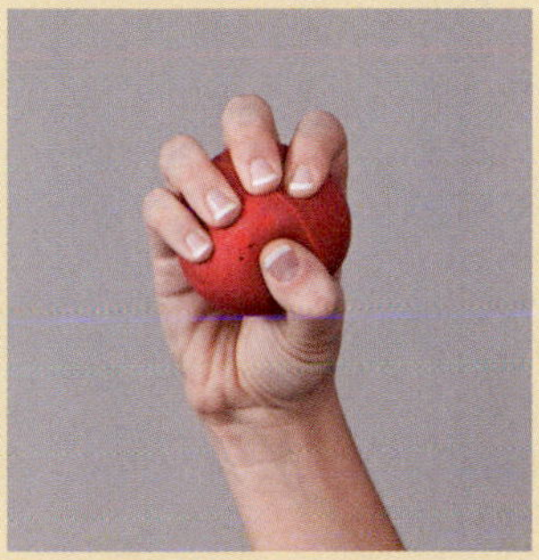	Grasp round objects. Fingers are spread apart more than in the cylinder grip, so interossei muscles work more in this grip. The grasp is adjusted so the size and shape of the spherical object.	MCP joints are abducted and partially flexed. The abductor and adductor interossei co-contract to stabilize the MCP joints. Both extrinsic flexor muscles work to flex the fingers. The extensor digitorum contracts to counteract the flexor force and control release of the object.	The thumb position varies according to the size and weight of the object. The thumb opposes the other fingers and is flexed at the MCP joint and may be flexed at the IP joint. The adductor pollicis and other thenar muscles are active.	Holding a ball or an apple.
Fist grip 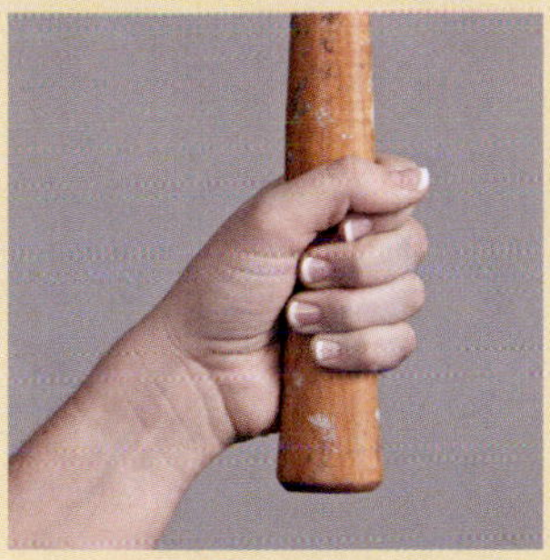	Also known as a digital palmar prehension pattern, the palm and fingers flex around the object and the thumb wraps around from the other direction to enclose the object. Objects grasped using this grip are not usually large since the thumb closes over the object and is often in contact with the other digits as the hand wraps around the object.	All three joints of the digits are flexed. The digits are usually parallel to one another, similar to the cylinder grip. Firm grasping is provided by the FDP and FDS.	The thumb is held either in adduction against the object or in opposition to the fingers that are flexed around the object. As with the cylinder grip, the thumb is used to provide a counterforce against the finger flexors to maintain the object in the hand.	This grip is used for powerful grasps of objects. Grasping a broom handle, baseball bat, hammer, or rake are examples.

TABLE 7-5 | PRECISION GRIPS

Grip	Description	Finger Function	Thumb Function	Examples of uses
Lateral pinch grip 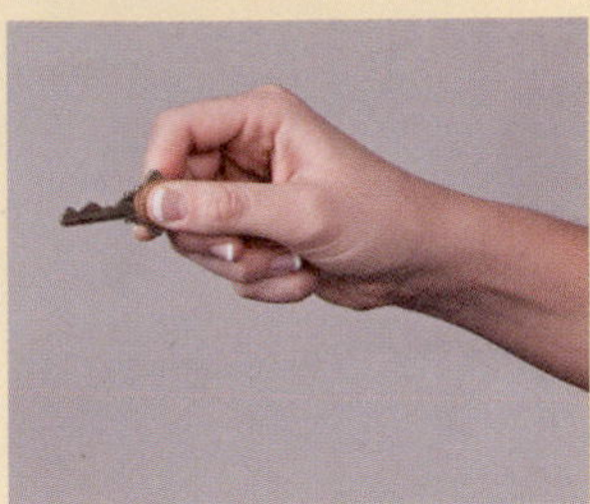	Also called a key grip. This is the least precise of the precision grips. A small object is placed between the index finger and thumb so it may be manipulated or used.	The index finger is abducted at the MCP joint and partially flexed at the MCP and IP joints. Muscles used include the FDP, FDS, and first dorsal interossei.	The thumb is adducted and the IP joint is flexed. Muscles performing these tasks include the FPL, FPB, and adductor pollicis.	Placing a key in the ignition, grasping papers.
Three-prong chuck 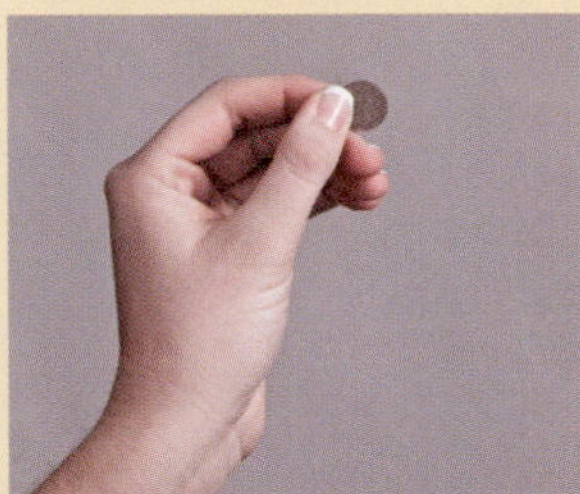 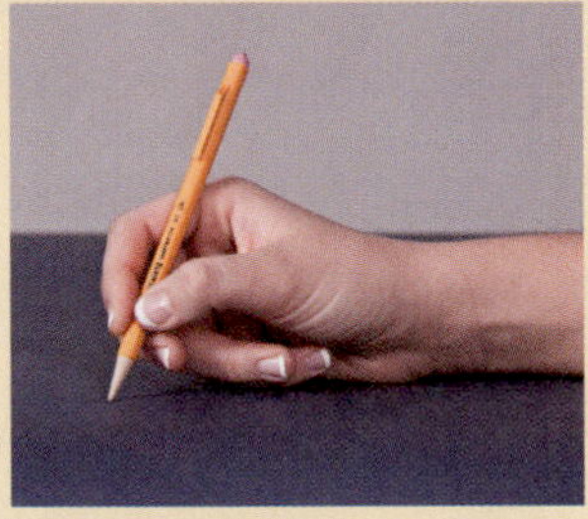	This is also known as pad-to-pad prehension grip and was originally identified as a palmar prehension grip. The pads of distal #2–3 digits contact the pad of the distal thumb for the purpose of picking up or grasping objects.	Fingers are in flexion at the MCP and PIP joints. There may also be some flexion of the DIP joints. The FDS performs the task if the DIP is in extension, but if the DIP is partially flexed, the FDP is also activated. During manipulation of the object, the interossei work to provide MCP joint abduction and adduction. Other fingers not involved in the grip are usually held in variable degrees of flexion so as to not obstruct the desired activity.	The thumb is positioned in opposition, flexion at the MCP and IP joints and adduction at the CMC joint. Muscles providing these positions include the adductor pollicis working with the FPB to stabilize the first metacarpal while the FPL flexes the thumb joints.	Grasping a coin, using a writing utensil such as a pen or pencil.
Tip-to-tip grip 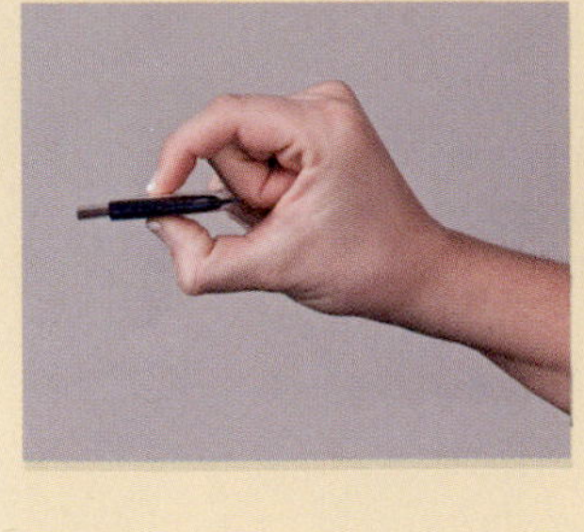	This grip is also known as the tip prehension grip. The thumb faces one of the fingers. Most often, the index finger is used in this grip. This grip is used to pick up or manipulate small objects.	The finger used is position in flexion at all three of its joints. Some lateral movement of the MCP joint towards the ulnar side occurs to allow the finger to meet the thumb with the finger tip facing a radial direction.	The thumb is in opposition with flexion at the MCP and IP joints. The thumb is also adducted so its tip is in alignment with the opposing finger's tip. In addition to the	Picking up a small object such as a pin, bead, or strand of hair.

TABLE 7–5 | PRECISION GRIPS—cont'd

Grip	Description	Finger Function	Thumb Function	Examples of uses
		Finger muscle activity is similar to that seen with the three-prong chuck grip but the FDP plays a greater role since DIP flexion is consistent with this grip although it is not in the three-prong chuck grip.	muscles used in the three-prong chuck, the FPL plays a more important role in this grip.	

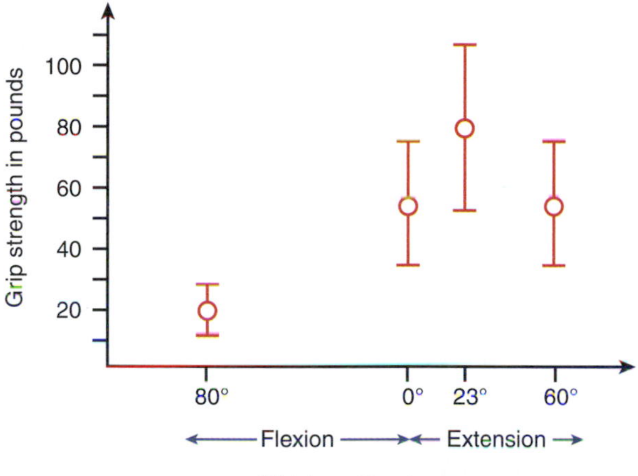

Figure 7.38 Maximum isometric grip strength in four different positions of the wrist.

When the fingers grasp an object, the wrist flexor and extensor muscles co-contract.[21] This co-contraction stabilizes the wrist to allow accurate finger and hand function.[22] Optimal wrist position during grip activities is 20° to 35° of extension with slight ulnar deviation;[3] this is known as the functional position of the wrist since, in this position, all of the wrist muscles have some tension and the finger flexors are placed on some stretch at the wrist to improve their power in grasping. In this functional position, the finger joints are all in slight flexion and the thumb is in slight flexion and opposition. Therefore, if an individual is to have a strong grip, he or she must have good wrist stabilization strength. Long finger tendons also assist in stabilizing the wrist.[22] Accurate finger movement is dependent upon the cooperative activity of the wrist stabilizers,

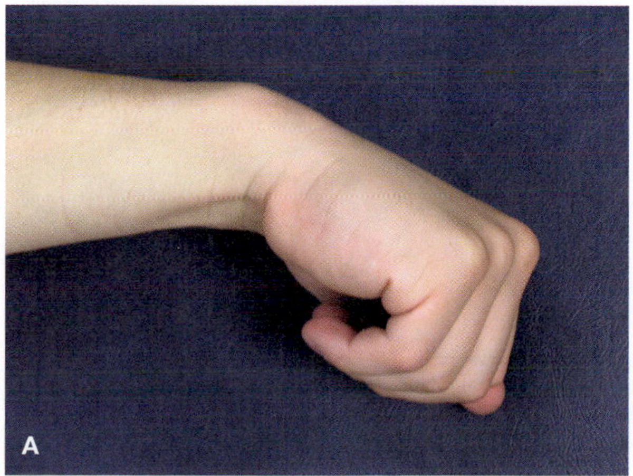

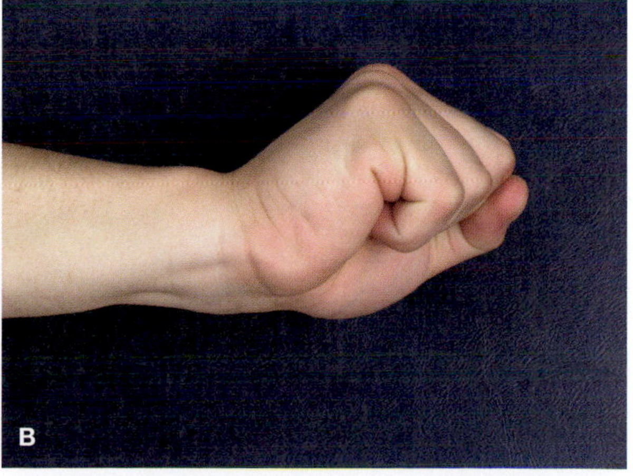

Figure 7.39 Fist strength relative to wrist position. **A)** With the fingers and wrist flexed, grip strength is reduced because of passive insufficiency of the finger extensors. **B)** When the wrist is extended, full grip strength may be achieved since the long finger flexors have adequate length to allow full finger flexion.

finger muscles, and sensory feedback of the cutaneous receptors.[23]

Role of the Long Finger Flexors in Grasping

Flexor digitorum superficialis and profundus flex the IP joints of the second through fifth digits. Because the tendons of these muscles pass on the palmar side of the wrist and the MCP joints, they also tend to flex these joints. In using the hand for grasping, flexion of the MCP joints is necessary for the hand to assume the shape of the object grasped or to properly shape the hand for its desired use. Although, as we have discussed, the ability of the long finger flexors to flex the wrist is counteracted by the synergistic wrist extensor activity, the long finger flexors are vital to our ability to grasp. A brief recollection of the anatomy of these tendons will assist in further understanding their functions.

Attaching to the sides of the middle phalanx, the flexor digitorum superficialis flexes the proximal IP joint. After perforating the superficialis tendon, the flexor digitorum profundus tendon attaches to the base of the distal phalanx and flexes the distal as well as the proximal IP joint. The profundus is the only muscle capable of flexing the distal joint.

In the motion of closing a normally functioning hand, flexion is almost simultaneous at all of the digital joints. The IP joints initiate the motion, and the PIP has the greatest amount of motion. This mechanism permits the pads of the fingers to contact and feel the object to be grasped. The only muscle that shows EMG activity during easy, unresisted motion is the flexor digitorum profundus.[24, 25] MCP flexion is attributed to passive tension of the lateral bands and the tendons of the intrinsic muscles.[5, 26, 27] Contraction of the flexor digitorum profundus exerts traction on the proximal attachment of the lumbrical, and the simultaneous flexion of the IP joints places the intrinsic muscles on a stretch distally, thus producing MCP flexion. The existence of passive tension can be seen in the semi-flexed position of the fingers in the resting hand. This same position is seen in astronauts sleeping in space, where no gravitational force acts on the hand.

When the wrist extends, the length-tension relationship of the flexor digitorum profundus allows sufficient tension development by this muscle to close the fist. With progressive flexion of the wrist, however, the length-tension relationship of the profundus diminishes, so the flexor digitorum superficialis is recruited to aid in fist closure. Forceful closure of the hand or power grip elicits high-level activity of the flexor digitorum superficialis, the interossei, and the flexor digitorum profundus.

Role of the Intrinsic Muscles in Grasping

The location of the dorsal interosseous muscles, with the MCP joints extended, positions these muscles in neutral with respect to flexion and extension of the MCP joints. In other words, they would not affect MCP flexion and extension motions. However, the pathway of palmar interossei and the lumbrical muscles is on the palmar side of the axis for flexion-extension of the MCP joints, so they are mechanically aligned to flex these joints. The mechanical leverage of the lumbrical muscles for flexion is more favorable than that of the palmar interossei since the lumbricals, course is on the palmar aspect and the palmar interossei are on the dorsal side of the transverse metacarpal ligament. As mentioned previously, none of the intrinsic muscles show EMG activity with easy or light-resisted closure of the fingers. Their role in MCP flexion is thought to be from passive stretch.

When a lumbrical is stimulated by a high-intensity electric current, the result is strong extension of the IP joints and flexion of the MCP joint to about 80°. However, when a low current is used (minimal to produce response) the IP joints extend, but the MCP joint flexes very little or not at all.[24] This suggests that the leverage of a lumbrical muscle for extension of the IP joints is far better than its leverage for flexion of the MCP joint.

PRACTICE POINT

Part of the rehabilitation program for finger and hand injuries should always include wrist and forearm strengthening exercises. Since the wrist flexors and extensors play an important role in stabilization of the wrist, their stabilization provides a stable base from which the fingers and hand function. Without a stable wrist, finger function is inefficient and deficient.

TABLE 7–6 | MUSCLES INVOLVED IN MOVEMENT OF THE WRIST AND HAND

Movement	Major Muscles	Movement	Major Muscles
Wrist Flexion	Flexor carpi radialis Flexor carpi ulnaris Palmaris longus Flexor digitorum superficialis Flexor digitorum profundus Flexor pollicis longus Abductor pollicis longus	Finger Extensors	Extensor digitorum Interossei Lumbricals Extensor digiti minimi Extensor indicus
Wrist Extension	Extensor carpi radialis longus Extensor carpi radialis brevis Extensor carpi ulnaris Extensor digiti minimi Extensor digitorum	Thumb Flexion	Flexor pollicis longus Flexor pollicis brevis Abductor pollicis brevis Adductor pollicis Opponens pollicis Dorsal interossei
Wrist Radial Deviation	Flexor carpi radialis Extensor carpi radialis longus Abductor pollicis longus Extensor pollicis brevis Extensor pollicis longus	Thumb Extension	Abductor pollicis longus Extensor pollicis longus Extensor pollicis brevis
Wrist Ulnar Deviation	Flexor carpi ulnaris Extensor carpi ulnaris Extensor indicis	Finger Abduction	Abductor digiti minimi Dorsal interossei Extensor digiti minimi
Finger Flexion	Flexor digitorum profundus Interossei Flexor digiti minimi brevis Abductor digiti minimi Flexor digitorum superficialis Flexor pollicis longus Abductor pollicis Flexor pollicis brevis Abductor pollicis brevis	Finger Adduction	Opponens digiti minimi Extensor indicis Palmar interossei
		Thumb Abduction	Abductor pollicis brevis Abductor pollicis longus Opponens pollicis
		Thumb Adduction	Flexor pollicis brevis Adductor pollicis Extensor pollicis longus Flexor pollicis longus

Finger flexion pulls the extensor hood distally over the proximal phalange, and the tendons of the interossei cross the MCP joint on the volar side with considerable distance from the joint center. In pinching, grasping, and power grip, the interossei have high levels of activity.[28] This muscle contraction serves to rotate the fingers to fit the surface of the object, strengthen the grip, stabilize the proximal phalanges against the metacarpal head, and stabilize the extensor tendons on the dorsum of the MCP joints through attachments to the extensor hood.

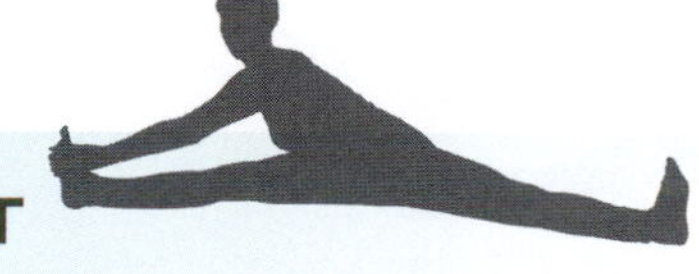

PRACTICE POINT

Individuals with long-standing paralysis of the intrinsic muscles, even though the flexor digitorum profundus and superficialis are intact, have an ineffective grasp. Such an individual is still capable of making a fist, but the IP joints flex first and the MCP joints flex a significant fraction of a second later. Without functioning intrinsic muscles, some difficulty arises when the subject attempts an activity that requires quick closure of the hand, as in catching a ball. Disturbance of the normal extrinsic/intrinsic muscle balance eventually results in a "claw" posture of the hand. Changes in capsules and ligaments as well as atrophy and loss of elastic properties of the intrinsic muscles eventually develop in these individuals.

Although the lumbricals cross the MCP joint at a distance farther from the joint center than do the interossei, the lumbricals are electrically silent in MCP flexion unless the IP joints are extended. The lumbricals do not participate in grip and rarely contract synchronously with the flexor digitorum profundus.

Intrinsic-Plus and Intrinsic-Minus Positions

The motion of MCP flexion with IP extension produces major EMG activity in the intrinsic muscles and slight variable activity in the extrinsic muscles (Fig. 7.40A). This position of the digits is called the "intrinsic-plus" hand position. It is also the position in which the interossei and lumbricals assume their shortest length. The hand assumes this position with contracture of the intrinsic muscles as is often found in rheumatoid arthritis. Normal length of the intrinsic muscles permit full passive flexion of the DIPs and the PIPs followed by hyperextension of the MCP joints. This position is known as the "intrinsic-minus" hand position. (Fig. 7.40B) An intrinsic-minus hand has paralysis of the interossei and lumbrical muscles. The resting posture of this hand is referred to as a "claw hand," with the MCP joints in slight hyperextension and the IP joints in partial flexion. As mentioned previously, none of the intrinsic muscles show EMG activity with easy or lightly resisted closure of the fingers because their role in MCP flexion is likely the result of a passive stretch.

Abduction and Adduction of Digits 2 to 5

Movements away from the midline of the hand are called abduction; movements toward the midline are called adduction. The midline is a longitudinal line through the center of the forearm and hand and through the middle finger; thus, when the fingers spread apart they are abducted, and when they lie close together they are adducted. The third finger, being in the midline, abducts in both directions and does not adduct.

Relationship of MCP Abduction and Adduction to Flexion and Extension

Abduction and adduction movements are unrestricted when the MCP joints are extended because the collateral ligaments are loose; when the MCP joints flex, the fingers automatically adduct, and the range of abduction becomes extremely limited or is absent since the collateral ligaments tighten. The natural tendency is to abduct the fingers as they extend; it may be said that extension and abduction belong together, as do flexion and adduction. If the fist is closed and opened in rapid succession, this pattern becomes obvious: The fingers abduct as they extend and adduct as they flex. In slower motions, and with some concentration, it is entirely possible to keep the fingers adducted as they extend. The extension-abduction combination appears to be part of a mass movement that is considerably easier to execute than other combinations.

When the fingers are flexed one at a time, they point toward the base of the thumb (Fig. 7.41). The literature often states that the point of convergence is on the scaphoid. Fess,[29] however, found more variability among hands and even some variation between dominant and nondominant hands. Knowledge of this motion is of particular importance in applying stretching techniques to fingers that have limited range of motion.

Muscles Acting in Abduction of the Fingers

The four dorsal interossei are responsible for abduction of the second and fourth fingers and for abduction of the third finger. The fifth finger has its own abductor—the abductor digiti minimi—located on the ulnar border of the hand; it is part of the hypothenar muscle group.

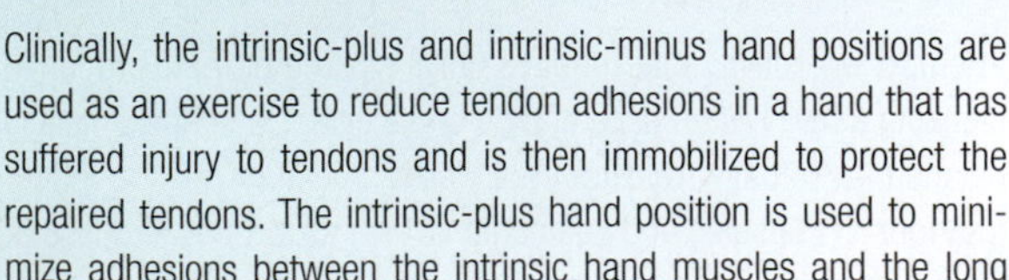

PRACTICE POINT

Clinically, the intrinsic-plus and intrinsic-minus hand positions are used as an exercise to reduce tendon adhesions in a hand that has suffered injury to tendons and is then immobilized to protect the repaired tendons. The intrinsic-plus hand position is used to minimize adhesions between the intrinsic hand muscles and the long extensor tendons: The hand is moved from MCP and IP extension to MCP flexion and IP extension and back to the start position. The intrinsic-minus hand position is used to minimize adhesions between the flexor digitorum superficialis and flexor digitorum profundus: The fingers begin in full extension at the MCP and IP joints and, while maintaining MCP extension or hyperextension, move the IPs into full flexion before returning to the start position.

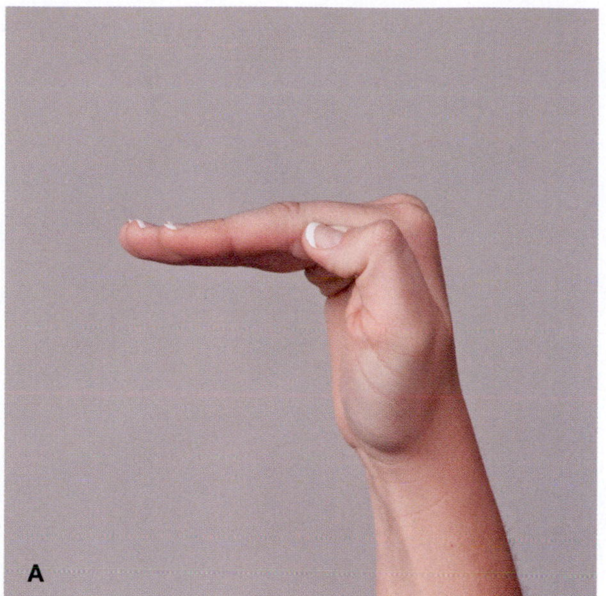

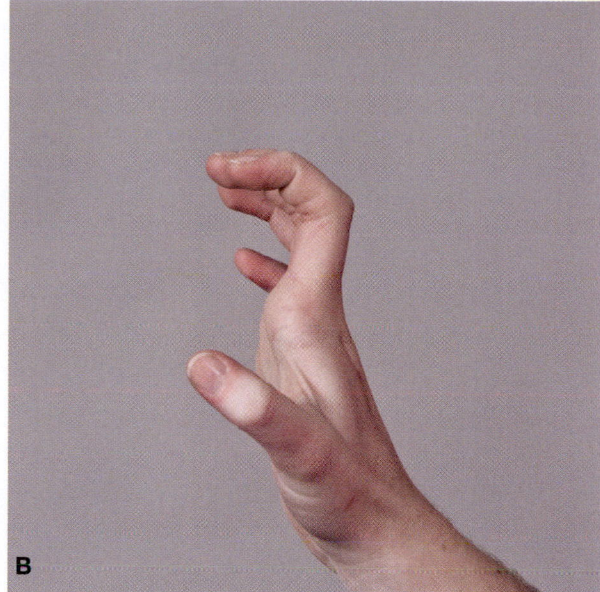

Figure 7.40 A) Flexion of the MCP joints and extension of the IP joints is the "intrinsic-plus" hand position. B) Flexion of the IP joints and hyperextension of the MCP joints is an "intrinsic-minus" hand.

The extensor digiti minimi, with its proximal attachment proximal to the wrist, has its distal attachment at the base of the proximal phalanx in such a manner that it is able to both extend and abduct the little finger. This muscle receives its innervation from the radial nerve. The ability of this muscle to abduct the little finger (in a small range) is clearly seen in cases of ulnar nerve paralysis when the hypothenar muscle group is paralyzed. The little finger then tends to maintain a somewhat abducted position, and the individual is unable to adduct it.

Muscles Acting in Adduction of the Fingers

The palmar interossei are responsible for adduction of the index, ring, and little fingers. These muscles, unlike the dorsal interossei, have only a single proximal attachment to the metacarpal bone of the digits that they serve. The palmar interossei may be tested by manual resistance to adduction of each finger separately or by squeezing three small objects between the fingers. If a piece of paper is slipped between two adjacent fingers and the patient is asked to hold on to it, one palmar and one dorsal interosseous muscle are tested simultaneously (Fig. 7.26A).

Some anatomists identify the deep portion of the flexor pollicis brevis (innervated by the ulnar nerve), or of a division of the adductor pollicis, as the first palmar interosseous muscle. In that case, the index finger is served by the second, the ring finger by the third, and the little finger by the fourth palmar interosseus.

Opposition of the Little Finger

The opponens digiti minimi, aided by the flexor digiti minimi, is responsible for the motion referred to as opposition of the fifth finger. Although the muscle is well aligned to perform the action, the movement is not nearly as well developed as is opposition of the thumb. When both thumb and little finger move toward each other in opposition, "cupping" of the hand results; that is, the hand narrows considerably from side to side.

Balanced Forces

Normal hand function is dependent upon not only balanced mechanics but also balanced forces in the hand. Balanced forces must exist between the muscles acting on the wrist and hand as well as between the muscles and outside forces. The sheer number of these muscles acting on the wrist and hand (Table 7–6) reveals the complexity involved in balancing forces for hand function. Imbalances between either of these groups result in reduced function, inefficient function, or deformity.

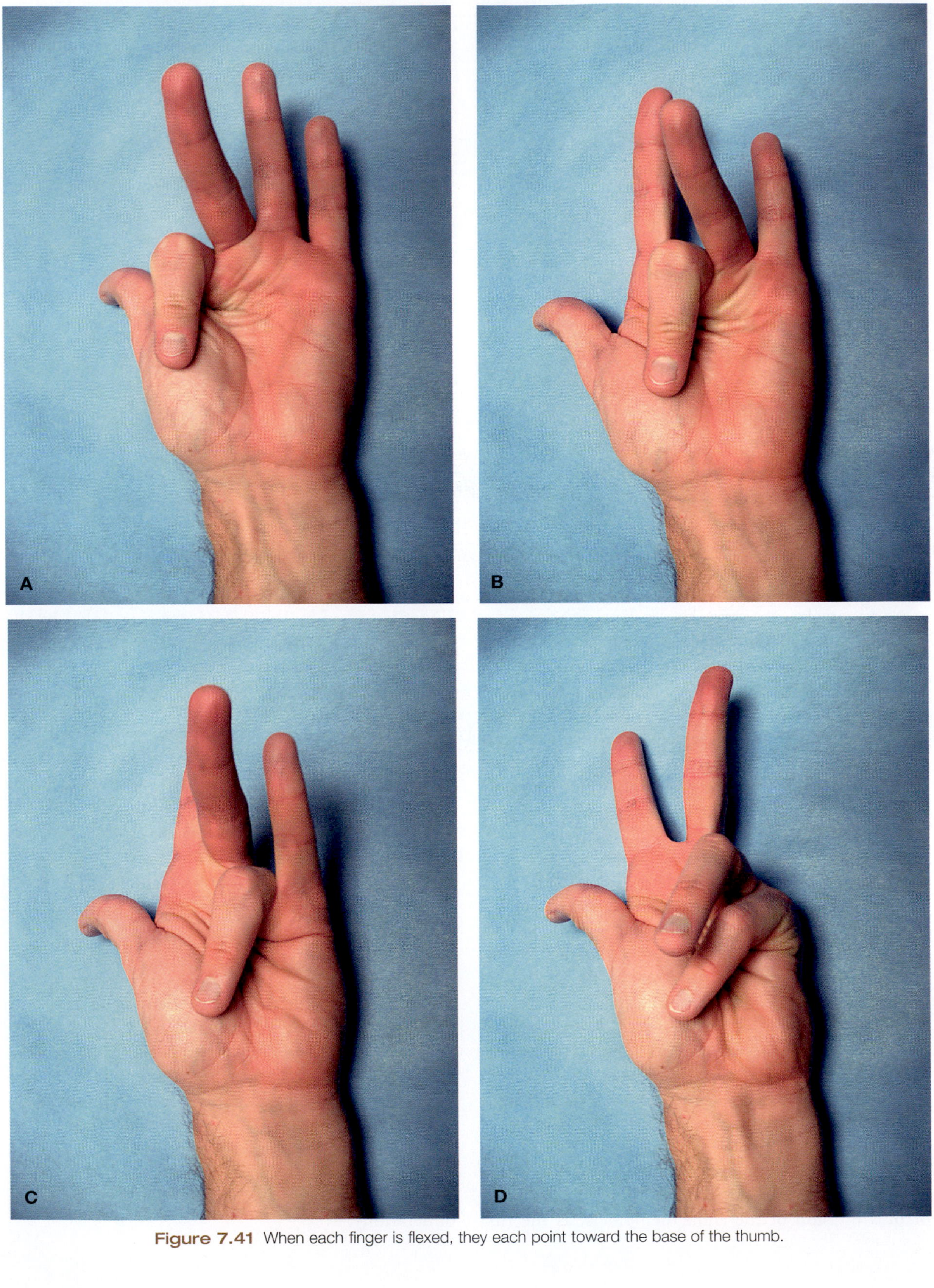

A

B

C

D

Figure 7.41 When each finger is flexed, they each point toward the base of the thumb.

Fingers

A way to appreciate the vast complexity of muscle function of the hand is to imagine a 4-lb force applied to the tip of the index finger as may occur when pressing down on a table with the finger tip. If the torque created by the applied force is not balanced by an equal muscle torque at the DIP, PIP, MCP, and wrist joints, the joints will all hyperextend.

From a clinical perspective, it is sufficient to appreciate that finger force applications are complex and require balance of forces of the flexor extrinsics, extensor extrinsics, and intrinsic muscles accompanied by adequate wrist control for optimal function. Beyond this level of appreciation, additional details are complex and involve specific biomechanical applications. Since the focus of this text is clinical applications, they are not addressed here. Individuals interested in these specific calculations are encouraged to investigate biomechanical-based texts.

Thumb

Thumb mobility provides the thumb with unique responsibilities that make the thumb vital to hand function. Its position relative to the other digits, its mobility and length, and its sensory nerve endings make it vital to overall hand performance. The sensory receptors in the thumb, index, and middle fingers allow the hand to function as a sensory organ. In fact, many hand functions, such as determining the grip force to use and the size of the grip, is based on sensory input. The thumb is used in all precision grips and all but one of the power grips. It has been determined that the thumb is responsible for 50% of the hand's function,[30] so if thumb function is lost, half of the hand's ability to perform its normal functions is also lost.

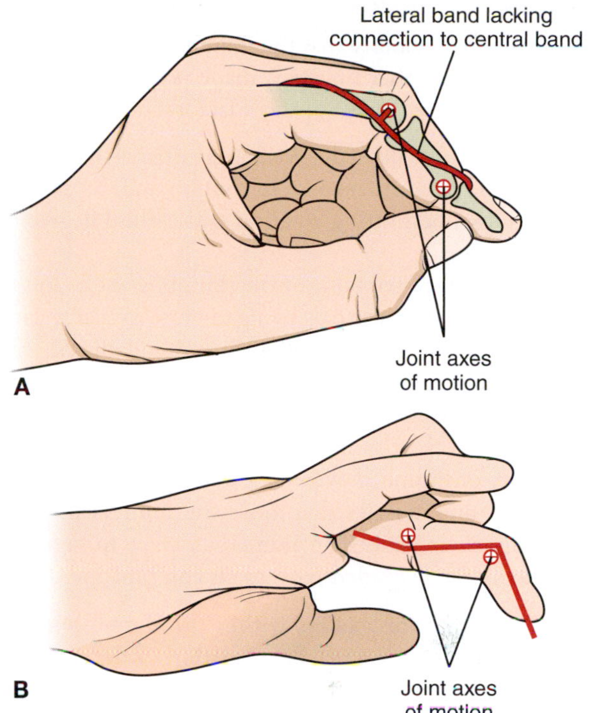

Figure 7.42 Finger deformities. When either a balance of forces of the three muscle groups of the hand does not exist or another force exceeds that of the muscle groups, deformity develops.

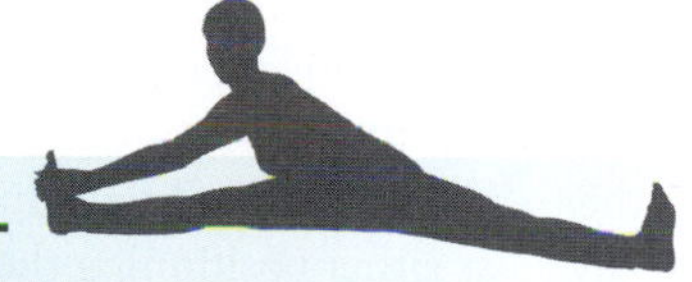

PRACTICE POINT

If balance is lost in the finger, deformity often becomes apparent. Two common deformities include a boutonnière deformity and a swan neck deformity. Either of these deformities may occur over time with progressive changes in soft tissue alignment or suddenly from acute trauma. A **boutonnière deformity** (Fig. 7.42A) occurs when the central slip of the extensor digitorum is injured at its insertion on the middle phalanx. The lateral bands lose their connection to the central band, so they drift more anterior toward the PIP joint, causing that joint to flex. The positions of the lateral bands on the distal phalanx remains intact, but because of the flexed position of the PIP, the lateral bands are now more posterior to the axis of motion of the DIP joint, so that joint becomes hyperextended. A **swan neck deformity** (Fig. 7.42B) occurs primarily with arthritis; with subsequent weakness of the intrinsic muscles, the PIP joints deform into hyperextension. The hyperextended position of the PIP moves the lateral slips of the extensor tendon dorsally relative to the joint. This causes increased tension on the flexor digitorum profundus so the DIP joint maintains a flexed position.

Mobility

The extensive mobility that the thumb possesses as compared with the other fingers is made possible through a number of factors. A list of these factors includes:

- The saddle-shaped CMC joint of the thumb has two degrees of freedom of motion and the capsule is loose, permitting rotation and a third degree of freedom;
- The metacarpal bone of the thumb is not bound to the other metacarpals by ligaments, so that a wide separation between index finger and thumb can take place;
- The movements that occur at the MCP and IP joints of the thumb add substantially to the versatility of thumb movements; and
- The nine muscles that move the thumb can combine their actions in numerous ways to generate many finely graded movement combinations.

The amount of motion within the thumb joints is presented following a brief explanation of the terminology used to describe thumb motions.

Nomenclature

Potential confusion in the description of thumb movements exists because of variations in terminology of these motions, especially for those movements of the CMC joint. Movements at this joint have been labeled variously as flexion, extension, abduction, adduction, palmar abduction, opposition, reposition, pronation, and supination, and have been described as taking place either in the plane of the palm or in a plane perpendicular to the palm. To add to the confusion, movements are sometimes defined as related to the entire thumb rather than to movements of its separate joints. Clinically, for example, opposition of the thumb means the ability to bring the palmar surface of the tip of the thumb in contact with the palmar surfaces of the other digits. Functionally, this is justifiable, but anatomically, each thumb joint has its own separate movement for opposition to occur.

The CMC joint of the thumb is a saddle joint (see Fig. 1.6C) with two degrees of freedom of motion. If this concept is followed, movements at this joint are defined as **opposition-reposition** and **abduction-adduction** (which occurs in a plane perpendicular to the palm of the hand). The term **flexion-extension** is then reserved for the two distal thumb joints; however, flexion-extension is frequently used when referring to carpometacarpal joint motion.

Motion and Function

It is important to recognize that a wide range of terminology exists for thumb motions. In this text, the terminology used in *Gray's Anatomy*[31] and by Kendall and associates[32] is followed (Fig. 7.8). Motions of the thumb are confusing because although many of the motions are the same as the other digits, the names of these motions are different. For example, the direction of thumb flexion and flexion of the second digit (index finger) are different. It may be easier to remember and identify thumb directions of movements if you first visualize the thumb rotated so you "see" it sitting in the same plane as the other digits. Once you have imagined the thumb in the frontal plane, visualize it flexing and once it flexes, visually "move" it back to its normal plane. Repeat this same mental image of moving the thumb and have it this time abduct and adduct in the frontal plane; once you perform this mental exercise, you see that the flexion-extension and abduction-adduction motions of the thumb are similar to those of the other digits.

The axes of the CMC joint are determined by the shape of the "saddle" of the trapezium; the "rider" in the "saddle" is the metacarpal bone. One axis passes longitudinally and the other transversely through the saddle, so that the "rider" may slide from side to side or tip forward and backward in the "saddle."

The MCP joint of the thumb is more stable than the MCP joints of the other digits. Approximately 50° to 60° of flexion can occur, whereas hyperextension and abduction-adduction at this joint are negligible.

The thumb contains only two phalanges and, therefore, has only one IP joint. Interphalangeal joint flexion is 90° or less. Passive hyperextension, as in pressing down on the thumb pad, may have a large range.

The thumb seldom acts alone except to press on a small object or play musical instruments. The thumb is mostly used against the fingers in gripping, pinching, or precision handling. Muscle function can be categorized as either positioning the thumb or stabilizing the thumb. In positioning, the extrinsic extensors and abductor pollicis longus reposition the thumb around objects and the intrinsic thenar muscles oppose the object (opponens and flexor and abductor pollicis brevis). Muscles used primarily for applying force for strength are the flexor pollicis longus, adductor pollicis, and the first dorsal interosseous. In most functional movements of the thumb, all of the thumb's muscles participate in varying degrees. All of the muscles of the thumb have an effect on first CMC joint movements and provide strong stabilization of the joint during forceful opposition and grasp. All of the muscles except the opponens and the abductor pollicis longus also cross the MCP joint.

Synergic Action of Wrist Muscles in Movements of the Thumb and Little Finger

Synergic actions of the wrist muscles should be noted in the following movements:

1. As the little finger is abducted (by abductor digiti minimi), the flexor carpi ulnaris contracts to furnish countertraction on the pisiform bone (Fig. 7.43A). During abduction of the little finger, the abductor pollicis longus contracts to prevent ulnar deviation of the wrist when the flexor carpi ulnaris contracts to stabilize the pisiform during the fifth digit motion. These tendons may be palpated as indicated in the illustration.
2. When the thumb extends to the position seen in Fig. 7.43B, the tensed tendon of the extensor carpi ulnaris is palpated on the ulnar side of the wrist. The extensor carpi ulnaris springs into action to prevent radial deviation of the wrist by the abductor pollicis longus. The points of palpation of the tendons of both muscles are indicated in Figure 7.43B. The tendon of the abductor pollicis longus lies close to, and is partially covered by, the tendon of the extensor pollicis brevis.
3. When the entire thumb is brought in a palmar direction (flexion) by the thenar muscles, the palmaris longus aids the movement by tensing the fascia of the palm. The extensor carpi radialis brevis contracts to prevent the palmaris longus from flexing the wrist.

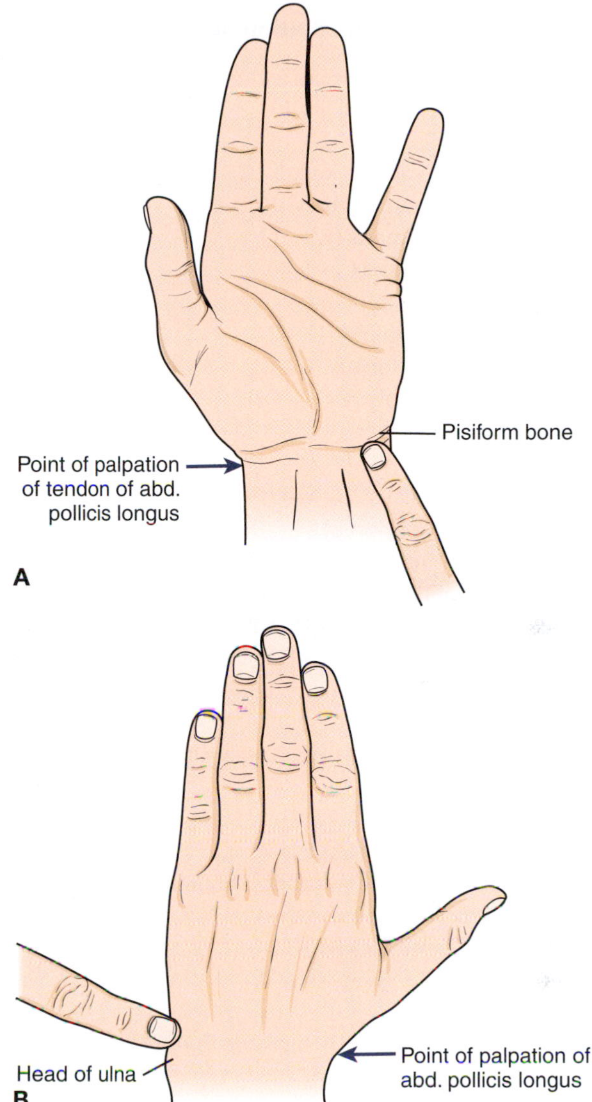

Figure 7.43 Synergistic wrist motions occur during thumb motions. **A)** With the forearm and hand relaxed on a table, palpation of flexor carpi ulnaris is made proximal to the pisiform bone during abduction of the little finger. The abductor pollicis longus contracts synergistically. **B)** Palpation of the extensor carpi ulnaris distal to the ulnar styloid process during extension of the thumb. Abductor pollicis longus may be palpated as indicated by the arrow.

Peripheral Nerves of the Wrist and Hand

In addition to nerve root levels, nerves innervating the wrist and hand are commonly identified by their peripheral nerve names. The three primary peripheral nerves sending motor and sensory innervation to the wrist and hand include the radial, median, and ulnar nerves.

Peripheral Nerve Innervations

The muscles may be thought of in groups, innervated as follows: The radial nerve supplies all the extensors of wrist and digits that have proximal attachments on the forearm and in the region of the lateral epicondyle; the median nerve supplies most of the flexors of the wrist and digits whose proximal attachments are on the forearm and in the region of the medial epicondyle; and the ulnar nerve supplies most of the small muscles in the hand. Exceptions include the "half-half" supply of flexor digitorum profundus and lumbricals (median and ulnar), the ulnar nerve supply to flexor carpi ulnaris, and the median nerve supply to thenar muscles.

BOX 7-1 | Motor Innervation of the Hand

The innervation of muscles acting on the wrist and digits is as follows:

Radial Nerve

Extensor carpi radialis longus (C_6–C_7)
Extensor carpi radialis brevis (C_6–C_7)
Extensor carpi ulnaris (C_7–C_8)
Extensor digitorum (C_6–C_8)
Extensor indicis (C_7–C_8)
Extensor digiti minimi (C_7–C_8)
Extensor pollicis longus (C_7–C_8)
Extensor pollicis brevis (C_7–C_8)
Abductor pollicis longus (C_7–C_8)

Median Nerve

Flexor carpi radialis (C_6–C_7)
Palmaris longus (C_7–C_8)
Flexor digitorum superficialis (C_7–T_1)
Radial half of flexor digitorum profundus (C_8–T_1) and the two radial lumbricals (C_8–T_1)
Flexor pollicis longus (C_8–T_1)
Superficial portion of flexor pollicis brevis (C_8–T_1)
Opponens pollicis (C_7–T_1)
Abductor pollicis brevis (may have ulnar innervation[33] (C_5–T_1)

Ulnar Nerve

Flexor carpi ulnaris (C_8)
Ulnar half of flexor digitorum profundus (C_8–T_1) and the two ulnar lumbricals (C_8–T_1)
All interossei muscles (C_8–T_1)
All hypothenar muscles (C_8–T_1)
Palmaris brevis (C_8–T_1)
Deep portion of flexor pollicis brevis (C_8–T_1)
Abductor pollicis (C_8–T_1)

Peripheral Nerve Injuries

In radial nerve paralysis, the extensors of the wrist and the long extensors of the digits are paralyzed. A wrist-drop develops causing a hand position much like the one seen in Figure 7.44A. The wrist cannot actively extend and since wrist extension is required to stabilize the wrist during grasping, an effective grasp is not possible. In the wrist-drop position, the digits are partially extended, but such extension is due to passive tendon tension, not to active contraction. The grasp becomes awkward and weak (Fig. 7.44A), but if the wrist is supported in extension by means of a splint (Fig. 7.44B), the strength of the grip is good when the wrist is passively positioned in extension because the flexor muscles are intact.

In ulnar nerve paralysis, the habitual position of the hand is known as the "claw hand" or "ulnar claw", based on its characteristic appearance that occurs when the intrinsic muscles are paralyzed (Fig. 7.45A). The fourth and the fifth digits are the ones mostly affected because the flexor digitorum profundus, the lumbricals, and the interossei belonging to these fingers are paralyzed and the hypothenar group is also not able to function. The extensor digitorum tends to keep the MCP joints of digits 4 and 5 hyperextended and the IP joints in partial flexion. If the examiner holds the MCP joints in a flexed position, however, the subject is capable of extending the IP joints by using the extensor digitorum. Figure 7.45B displays a brace used for this purpose. Although the abductor of the little finger is paralyzed, this finger is maintained somewhat abducted (by the extensor digiti minimi proprius), but it cannot be adducted because the action of the palmar interosseus cannot be taken over by any other muscle. Abduction and adduction movements of all digits served by the interosseous muscles are not possible with ulnar nerve paralysis. Occasionally, however, there is some median nerve supply to the more radially located interossei, in which case some movements may be preserved.

If the ulnar nerve is interrupted in the proximal forearm, the deformity is less than when the disruption

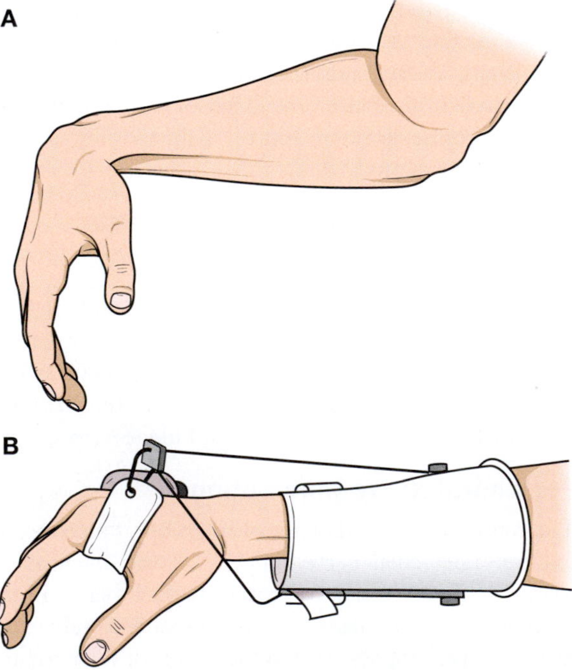

Figure 7.44 Radial nerve palsy creates an inability to extend the wrist and fingers. **A)** Wrist drop occurs with radial nerve palsy. **B)** With use of a wrist extension brace, grip is possible.

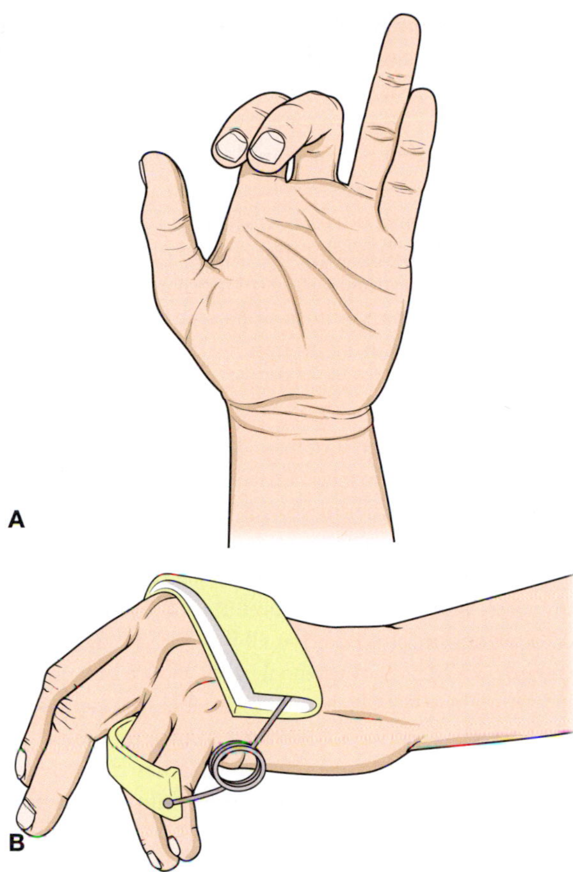

Figure 7.45 Ulnar nerve palsy. A) Claw hand occurs when the ulnar nerve function is lost. B) A splint to correct the claw hand deformity produces passive flexion of the fourth and fifth MCP to allow IP extension.

occurs in the hand. This fact may seem counterintuitive until we realize that the claw-hand deformation that occurs because of the unopposed pull of the flexor digitorum profundus on the distal fingers; when the ulnar nerve is damaged in the proximal forearm, the flexor digitorum profundus is affected, so there is no unopposed flexor force on the distal phalanges to create a claw hand. Such a condition is known as the "ulnar paradox" because of the lesser deformity.

A median nerve paralysis causes most of the flexors of the digits to lose action and, therefore, seriously affects the grasp. The digits on the radial side, having only median nerve supply, are affected to a greater extent than those on the ulnar side. Flexion and opposition of the thumb are lost, the thenar muscles atrophy, and the entire thumb is pulled in a dorsal direction by the extensor muscles so that it remains in the plane of the palm or is taken even farther back toward the dorsum of the hand. This hand is referred to as the "hand of Benediction" because of the position of the index and middle fingers; as the individual attempts to close the hand into a fist, the inability to flex the second and third digits causes them to remain extended, giving the appearance of an individual giving a Benediction. (Fig. 7.46). The adductor is the only useful thenar muscle and, with the first dorsal interosseous muscle, may enable the subject to hold a small object between the thumb and the index finger. Because the flexor digitorum superficialis and profundus, as well as the lumbricals of the index and middle fingers, have median nerve supply, these two fingers lose their ability to flex. The index finger tends to remain in an extended position whereas the middle finger may be drawn into some flexion when the two ulnar fingers flex. However, if the subject extends the wrist as far as possible, both index and middle fingers may flex by tendon action, but this is not an active grasp.

If the median nerve is injured proximal to the wrist, an "ape hand" becomes apparent. Since only the intrinsic muscles are affected with this more proximal nerve injury, the thumb is unable to oppose the other fingers, but the flexor digitorum superficialis and flexor digitorum profundus remain unaffected so flexion of the second and third digits occurs when the individual makes a fist.

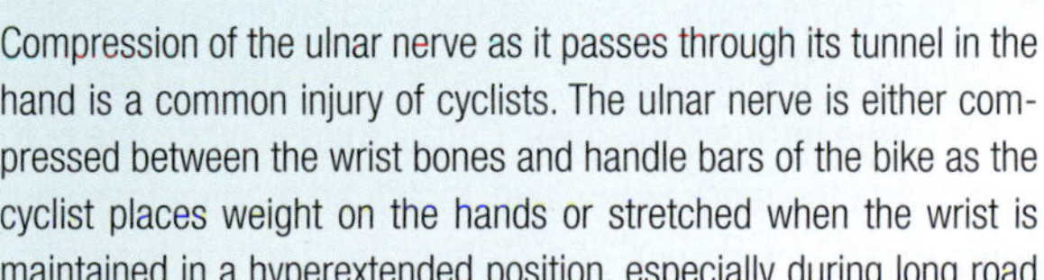

PRACTICE POINT

Compression of the ulnar nerve as it passes through its tunnel in the hand is a common injury of cyclists. The ulnar nerve is either compressed between the wrist bones and handle bars of the bike as the cyclist places weight on the hands or stretched when the wrist is maintained in a hyperextended position, especially during long road trips when a dropdown handlebar is grasped in the lower position. This condition is sometimes referred to as either "handlebar palsy" or "Guyon's canal syndrome." Initial signs and symptoms of the condition include numbness or tingling in the ring and little finger. Weakness may also occur.

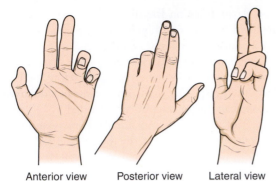

Anterior view Posterior view Lateral view

Figure 7.46 Median nerve palsy. Median nerve palsy is known as the "hand of Benediction". The index and middle finger positions in extension when a fist is made are the cause of the name.

Deficits in hand function are additionally influenced by sensory loss resulting from peripheral nerve injury. Hand rehabilitation programs have always included motor retraining; in recent years, these programs also emphasize the importance of sensory retraining. The effect of sensory loss resulting from peripheral nerve injuries is that of diminishing power and precision of hand function.[33, 34] Wynn-Parry divides re-education into stereognosis and localization of touch. He states that his experience has shown that patients can improve their sensory function remarkably, and their recovery occurs in too short a time to be explained by reinnervation.[34]

Summary

The wrist and hand is a complex organ of the upper extremity that has many responsibilities in daily activity. It is used as a sense organ to provide information about the environment. It grasps and carries objects from one destination to another, and it manipulates objects using many varied grasps. Because of its several joints and the complex relationship of its muscles, the hand is able to conform to any object within its grasp. The muscle groups that allow the hand its myriad functions and positions include the extrinsic flexors, extrinsic extensors, and intrinsic muscles. These muscle groups work in concert with each other to provide assistance, stabilization, and motion. Hand motion is dependent upon stabilization obtained from the wrist muscles, especially the wrist extensors. The position of function of the wrist is 20° to 35° of extension; this position allows optimal movement, strength, and dexterity of the fingers. When one of these three muscle groups is injured or unable to function, the entire hand's function is impaired. Injury to a joint, soft tissue, nerve, or bone within the hand has the potential to severely impede the individual's ability to perform even simple activities of daily living.

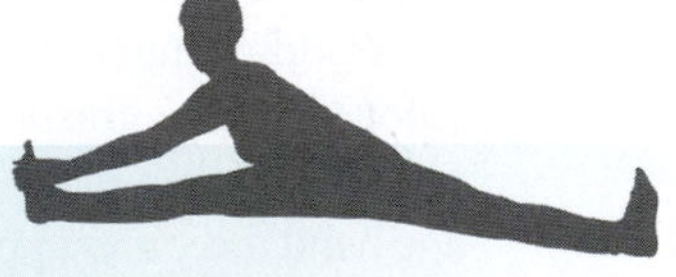

PRACTICE POINT

A lesser condition than median nerve palsy that commonly impacts the median nerve is carpal tunnel syndrome. Clinicians see this in individuals whose median nerve is compressed within the carpal tunnel at the wrist. Various etiologic factors may lead to this condition including performing tasks that involve repetitive or prolonged wrist flexion or extension such as typing or piano playing. Swelling within the carpal tunnel may also bring on carpal tunnel syndrome. This swelling may be caused by either injury or a systemic condition such as arthritis, hypothyroidism, pituitary pathology, diabetes, or pregnancy. The patient reports symptoms of numbness or tingling along the median nerve distribution in the hand, possible weakness of muscles innervated by the nerve, and sleep disturbances secondary to pain.

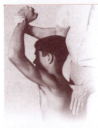

CLINICAL SCENARIO SOLUTION

Through strength testing and obtaining a thorough history from Lori, the clinician is able to identify symptoms of carpal tunnel syndrome, which is caused by compression of the median nerve. Symptoms include pain and paresthesia in the hand particularly in the area of the sensory distribution of the median nerve. Symptoms can also include weakness of the intrinsic muscles. Carpal tunnel syndrome is frequently observed in individuals whose jobs are characterized by repetitive, high load manual tasks such as the hand activities carried out by a busy hairdresser. Intervention would include use of a night splint keeping the wrist in neutral to slight extension to decrease the compression on the median nerve and some instruction in resting and moderate stretching activities between clients to decrease the pressure in the carpal tunnel.

Discussion Questions

1. Explain how the elbow and shoulder serve to position the hand for function. How does the forearm contribute to the hand's ability to perform its actions?
2. Since the ulna is not in direct contact with the proximal carpal bones, it is not a part of the wrist joint. Rather, the triangular fibrocartilaginous disc sits between the ulna and proximal carpal bones as well as the radius and ulna. If this disc was injured, how would it impact the wrist joint?
3. The interosseous membrane between the radius and ulna allows a transfer and distribution of forces from the wrist to more proximal extremity segments. Explain how this membrane distributes the forces when a person falls and lands on an outstretched arm. How does this membrane play a role in allowing a waiter to carry a heavy tray overhead? Why is it easier for this waiter to carry his tray in this overhead position rather than at his waist?
4. Now that you are familiar with the extensor hood mechanism, describe one hand activity in which the extensor hood mechanism plays a role in the hand's ability to perform that activity.
5. The long extrinsic tendons of the dorsal and palmar hand are different in design from one another. Identify these differences and how these characteristics add to their function.
6. Normal hand function is dependent upon normally functioning long finger flexors, long finger extensors, and intrinsic muscles. Discuss how deficiency in each element impairs normal hand function. In your discussion, explain a normal activity of the hand and how this function becomes impaired when an element (long finger flexors, long finger extensors, or intrinsic muscles) is injured.

Lab Activities

1. On disarticulated bones or the skeleton, identify the following bones and bony landmarks of the wrist and hand. Determine which of these are palpable and palpate them on yourself and on a partner.

   head of the ulna
   styloid process of the ulna
   styloid process of the radius
   dorsal radial tubercle
   eight individual carpal bones
   shafts of metacarpal bones
   heads of metacarpal bones
   phalanges

2. Examine and identify the following joint surfaces:

   radiocarpal
   midcarpal
   intercarpals
   carpometacarpal; 2–5
   metacarpophalangeal (MCP)
   interphalangeal (IP)
   carpometacarpal joint of the thumb (CMC)

3. Analyze wrist and finger movements (excluding thumb) on yourself and on a partner. Identify and palpate bony landmarks that locate axes of these movements.
4. Analyze all thumb movements (CMC, MCP, IP) on yourself and on a partner. Palpate in your own hand and in several subjects' hands the location of the "saddle" joint of the thumb.
5. Passively move the joints of your partner's wrist, fingers, and thumb through their ranges of motion in flexion, extension, and lateral motions (if present) and:
   a. State the approximate range of motion in degrees;
   b. Describe the end feel for each motion
6. Place your forearm and hand on a table, palm down. Extend and hyperextend your fingers actively (keeping the palm on the table), then passively perform the same motions. Notice that there is always slightly greater range of motion passively. If you observe a number of female and male subjects, you will find that the females usually have more flexibility in these joints.

7. Perform gentle passive accessory motions for the carpal bones and the joints of the fingers. Points to remember are that the subject's forearm and hand must be relaxed and the examiner must stabilize one bone and move the joint surface of the other bone in glides, rotation, and distraction.
8. On the skeleton, locate the points of proximal and distal attachments for these muscles:

extensor carpi radialis longus	extensor pollicis longus
extensor carpi radialis brevis	extensor pollicis brevis
extensor carpi ulnaris	flexor carpi ulnaris
extensor digitorum	flexor carpi radialis
flexor pollicis longus	flexor digitorum profundus
abductor pollicis longus	flexor digitorum superficialis

Identify the:
a. Joints these muscles cross;
b. Motions that these muscles can produce.

9. Palpate tendons and muscle bellies of wrist and finger flexors and extensors, tracing their action line to their proximal bony attachments in the region of the elbow. Palpate tendons about the wrist and analyze their relationships so that you can identify them accurately irrespective of forearm or hand position.
10. Using skin pencils, sketch on your own hand the extrinsic tendons, including those of the thumb. Next add the "short" (i.e., intrinsic) muscles and analyze their relationships to the extrinsic muscles. Determine hand, finger, and thumb movements performed by the intrinsic muscles. Analyze integrated action of intrinsic and extrinsic hand muscles.
11. Pick up or manipulate these objects: thumb tacks, straight pins, paper clips, cards, coins, keys, glass, weights, pencil or pen, briefcase, handbag, cup, doorknob, scissors, magazine, newspaper, screwdriver, book, ball. Analyze prehension patterns; note particularly the wrist positions, the specific finger movements, and the continuous transition from pattern to pattern (Figs. 7-35 and 7-36—power grips and precision grips).
12. With a hand dynamometer and a pinch meter, test the strength of your grip using these precision grips: three-prong chuck pinch, and lateral pinch. Test your dominant and your nondominant hand. Compile and compare results among all class members and determine average scores. Ensure standardization of the test procedure with respect to the number of repetitions and to the position and support (or nonsupport) of the forearm.
13. Predict dysfunction of the elbow, wrist, and hand that could occur when the:
    a. Radial nerve is severed in the region of the spinal groove of the humerus;
    b. Median nerve is cut at the wrist joint;
    c. Ulnar nerve is crushed at the elbow between the medial epicondyle of the humerus and the olecranon process;
    d. Lateral cord of the brachial plexus is damaged.
    In your analysis of each nerve injury, determine functions that will be lost, functions that will decrease, and functions that will remain.

References

1. Hoppenfeld S. *Physical examination of the spine and extremities*. East Norwalk, CT: Appleton-Century-Crofts, 1976.
2. Razemon JP, Fisk GR. *The Wrist*. Edinburgh: Churchill Livingstone, 1988.
3. Kapandji IA. *The Physiology of Joints. Upper Limb. Vol 1,* ed 5. Edinburgh: Churchill Livingstone,1982.
4. Moore KL, Dalley AF, II. *Clinically Oriented Anatomy*, ed 4. Philadelphia: Lippincott Williams & Wilkins, 1999.
5. Zancolli E. *Structural and Dynamic Bases of Hand Surgery*. Philadelphia: JB Lippincott, 1979.

6. Brand P, Hollister A. *Clinical Mechanics of the Hand*, ed 2. St. Louis: Mosby Year Book, 1992, p. 83.
7. Amadio PC, Lin GT, An K. Anatomy and pathomechanics of the flexor pulley system. *Journal of Hand Therapy* 2:138–141, 1989.
8. Lin GT, Amadio PC, An KN, Cooney WP. Functional anatomy of the human digital flexor pulley system. *Journal of Hand Surgery (Am)* 14(6):949–956, 1989.
9. Kuhlmann JN, Tubiana R. Mechanism of the Normal Wrist. In Razemon JP, Fisk GR (eds): *The Wrist*. Edinburgh: Churchill Livingstone, 1988.
10. Napier JR. The prehensile movements of the human hand. *Journal of Bone and Joint Surgery* 38B(4):902–913, 1956.
11. Schlesinger G. *Der mechanische Aufbau der kuntslichen Glieder*. Berlin: J Springer,1919.
12. Taylor CL, Schwarz RJ. The anatomy and mechanics of the human hand. *Artificial Limbs* 2(2):22–35, 1955.
13. Swanson AB, Matev IB, deGroot G. The strength of the hand. *Bulletin of Prosthetics Research* 10(14):145–153, 1970.
14. Toews JV. A grip-strength study among steelworkers. *Archives of Physical Medicine and Rehabilitation* 45:413–417, 1964.
15. Crosby CA, Marwan A, Wehbé MA, Mawr B. Hand strength: Normative values. *Journal of Hand Surgery (Am)* 19(4):665–670, 1994.
16. Petersen P, Petrick M, Connor H, Conklin D. Grip strength and hand dominance: Challenging the 10% rule. *American Journal of Occupational Therapy* 43(7):444–447, 1989.
17. Thorngren KG, Werner CO. Normal grip strength. *Acta Orthopaedica Scandinavica* 50(3):255–259, 1979.
18. Ertem K, Inan M, Yologlu S, et al. Effects of dominance, body mass index and age on grip and pinch strength. *Isokinetics & Exercise Science* 11:219–223, 2003.
19. Incel NA, Ceceli E, Durukan PB, Erdem HR, Yorgancioglu ZR. Grip strength: Effect of hand dominance. *Singapore Medical Journal* 43(5):234–237, 2002.
20. Klopsteg DE, Wilson PD. *Human limbs and their substitutes*. New York: McGraw-Hill, 1954.
21. Snijders CJ, Volkers AC, Mechelse K, Vleeming A. Provocation of epicondylalgia lateralis (tennis elbow) by power grip or pinching. *Medicine and Science in Sports and Exercise* 19(5):518–523, 1987.
22. Werremeyer MM, Cole KJ. Wrist action affects precision grip force. *Journal of Neurophysiology* 78:271–280, 1997.
23. Smith MA, Soechting JF. Modulation of grasping forces during object transport. *Journal of Neurophysiology* 93:137–145, 2005.
24. Backhouse KM, Catton WT. An experimental study of the function of the lumbrical muscles in the human hand. *Journal of Anatomy* 88:133–141, 1954.
25. Long C, Brown ME. Electromyographic kinesiology of the hand: Muscles moving the long finger. *Journal of Bone and Joint Surgery* 46A:1683–1706, 1964.
26. Landsmeer JM, Long C. The mechanism of finger control: Based on electromyograms and location analysis. *Acta Anatomica* 60(3):330–347, 1965.
27. Long C, 2nd. Intrinsic-extrinsic control of the fingers: Electromyographic studies. *Journal of Bone and Joint Surgery* 50A(5):973–984, 1968.
28. Long C, 2nd., Conrad PW, Hall EA, Furier SL. Intrinsic-extrinsic muscle control of the hand in power grip and precision handling: An electromyographic study. *Journal of Bone and Joint Surgery* 52A(5):853–867, 1970.
29. Fess EE. Convergence points of normal fingers in individual flexion and simultaneous flexion. *Journal of Hand Therapy* 2:12, 1989.
30. Inglis AE, Cooper W, Bruton W. Surgical correction of thumb deformities in spastic paralysis. *Journal of Bone and Joint Surgery* 52A(2):253–268, 1970.
31. Standring S, ed. *Grays Anatomy: The Anatomical Basis of Clinical Practice,* ed 40. New York: Elsevier Churchill Livingstone, 2008.
32. Kendall HO, Kendall FP, Wadsworth GE. *Muscles: Testing and Function*, ed 2. Baltimore: Williams & Wilkins, 1971.
33. Belson P, Smith LK, Puentes J. Motor innervation of the flexor pollicis brevis. *American Journal of Physical Medicine* 55(3):122–138, 1976.
34. Wynn-Parry CB. *Rehabilitation of the Hand*, ed 4. London: Butterworths, 1981.

Head, Neck, and Trunk

Christopher R. Carcia, PhD, PT, SCS, OCS

"An honorable man or woman will personally commit to live up to certain self-imposed expectations. They need no outside check or control. They are honorable in their inner core."
—James E. Faust (Ensign, May 1982)

CHAPTER OUTLINE

Learning Outcomes
Clinical Scenario
Introduction
Bones
Normal Curves of the Vertebral Column
Nonpalpable Structures
Palpable Structures
Vertebral Joints, Ligaments, and Motions
Vertebral Motions
Anterior Vertebral Joint Elements
Posterior Vertebral Joint Elements
Cervical Region
Thoracic Region
Lumbar Region
Sacrum
Sacroiliac Joint
Symphysis Pubis
Coccygeal Joints
Pelvic Balance
Muscles
Anterior Cervical Muscles
Posterior Cervical Muscles
Posterior Thoracic and Lumbar Muscles
Anterior and Lateral Trunk Muscles
Functions of the Head, Neck, and Trunk Muscles
Balancing of the Head and the Vertebral Column
Trunk Motions and Stabilization of the Vertebrae
Forward Bending and Lifting (Knees Extended)

LEARNING OUTCOMES

This chapter investigates the head, neck and trunk. By the end of this chapter, you should be able to:

- ❑ Identify the segments of the vertebral column;
- ❑ Express the differences in the various spinal regions;
- ❑ List the primary muscles of the cervical, thoracic, and lumbar regions and their functions;
- ❑ Explain the mechanisms of trunk motions and how the spine is stabilized during motion;
- ❑ Discuss the relationship between the pelvis, low back, and trunk and their contributions to functional movement;
- ❑ Demonstrate the motions of the pelvis: anterior and posterior pelvic tilt;
- ❑ Identify muscles and functions of the temporomandibular joints.

Squat Lifting
Functional Activities (Muscles of the Extremities and Trunk)
Breathing and Coughing
Temporomandibular Joints
Motions of the Temporomandibular Joint
Muscles
Temporomandibular Dysfunction
Summary
Clinical Scenario Solution
Lab Activities
References

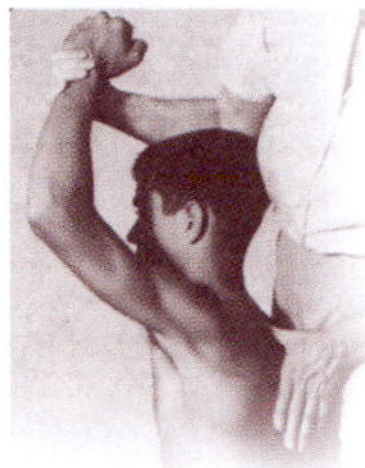

CLINICAL SCENARIO

Kamryn has been working with Matt, a patient who has been unable to work because of a back injury. Matt injured his back as he was moving a box onto a truck for delivery from the warehouse where he has been working for the past 10 years. This is his first injury on the job. Matt is anxious to get back to work, but before he can be released for full duty, Kamryn must instruct him in proper body mechanics. She is well aware of the stresses that poor mechanics place on the spine, and throughout his treatment course, she has tried to impress the importance of good body mechanics to her patient. Today, she will instruct him how to bend over to pick up a box the proper way so he does not risk another low back injury.

Introduction

Included in the axial skeleton are the head, vertebral column, sternum, and ribs. The head is closely related to the vertebral column, or spine, as its position influences the position of the spine, as we will learn in this chapter. The axial skeleton serves as an intermediary to transfer and absorb forces between the upper and lower extremities. As we move through this chapter, it should become readily apparent why the axial skeleton is so important to upper and lower limb function.

The vertebrae, ribs, and jaw have multiple purposes that frequently must be carried out simultaneously: protecting organs (spinal cord and viscera); providing the vital functions of breathing, chewing, and swallowing; supporting head, arms, and trunk (HAT) against the force of gravity; transmitting forces between upper and lower extremities; and providing stability and mobility for hand function, locomotion, and other activities. The anterior portion of the vertebral column (bodies and discs) provides for weight-bearing, shock absorption, and mobility in all directions. The posterior portion of the column provides for protection of the spinal cord, guidance and limitation of motion, and elongated processes to increase the leverage of muscles of the trunk and extremities.

Bones

The bones of the vertebral column, including the sacrum, are presented in this section. The pelvis is covered in Chapter 9. Although the sacrum functions with the pelvis, it is a component of the vertebral column, so it is presented in this chapter. The vertebral column is composed of several bones; this is a distinct advantage because such a design provides extensive spinal mobility. On the other hand, the disadvantage is that the spine must rely on muscles and ligaments for its stability. As we progress through this chapter, we will see how this advantage and disadvantage impact function, injury, and disease.

Normal Curves of the Vertebral Column

From a posterior view, the normal spine is vertical. Laterally, the normal spine exhibits anterior and posterior physiologic curves. These curves improve the vertebral column's resistance to axial compression.[1] At birth, the vertebral column is a single curve that is convex posteriorly (**kyphosis**; primary curve) (Fig. 8.1A). As the infant raises his or her head from the prone position and develops the ability to sit, the cervical spine becomes convex anteriorly (**lordosis**; secondary curve) (Fig. 8.1B). As the child achieves standing and walking, the lumbar spine likewise develops an anterior convexity; this lumbar curve develops largely because of the tension of the psoas muscles.[2] At about 10 years of age, the child's physiologic curves are similar to those found in the adult (Fig. 8.1C).[1] There are four curvatures in the adult spine: cervical (concave posteriorly); thoracic (convex posteriorly); lumbar (concave posteriorly); and sacral (convex posteriorly). Because the spine is originally convex posteriorly (kyphotic), this curve is referred to as the primary vertebral curve whereas the anterior convex curves (lordotic) that develop later in the cervical and lumbar regions are secondary curves. The center of gravity of the head and subsequent

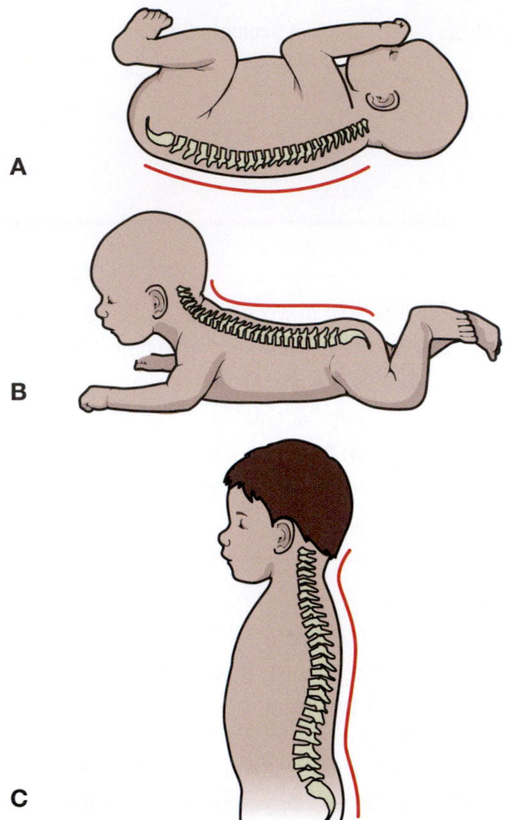

Figure 8.1 Changes in vertebral curves. **A)** An infant has a convex curve posteriorly. **B)** As the infant begins to pick up the head, a lordotic cervical curve develops. **C)** By the time the child is about 10 years old, all spinal curves are equal to adult spinal curves.

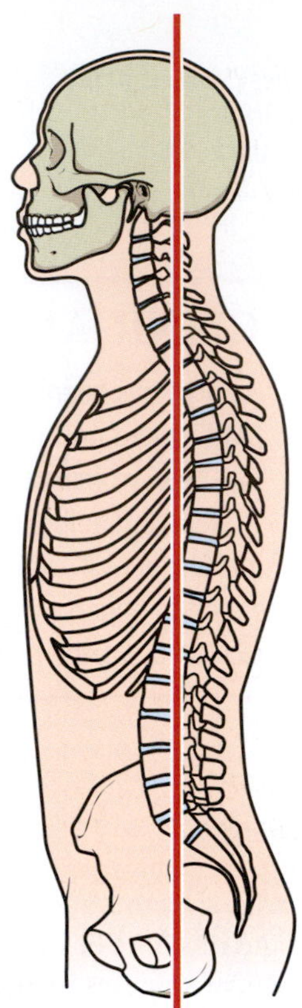

Figure 8.2 The line of gravity of the body falls on the concave side of the spinal curves.

superimposed segments fall on the concave side of the curves (Fig. 8.2). In the standing position, the lumbar spine is normally in a position of lordosis. In the erect sitting position, the pelvis and sacrum are rotated anteriorly and the lumbar curve is accentuated.

When a normal individual stands and slowly flexes the entire spine beginning at the neck and continuing caudally, a lateral view of the spinous processes reveals an unfolding of a posterior convexity without flattened areas or angulations (Fig. 8.3A). Lateral flexion to each side (viewed posteriorly) also produces symmetric curves of the spinous processes (Fig. 8.3B). Lack of symmetry, straightened regions, or angulations indicates skeletal deviations. Although these deviations are considered abnormal, they may or may not be accompanied by back pain and dysfunction.

Nonpalpable Structures

The vertebral column is imbedded in muscles posteriorly and laterally and is not available for palpation anteriorly; therefore, its general structure and the characteristics of its individual parts should be studied using a disarticulated bone set and an anatomic atlas. An appreciation of the anatomy and its orientation is fundamental to performing clinical palpation. Although your previous anatomic studies have covered these structures, it is recommended that you review the anatomy and include the following in your review study:

- The physiologic curves of the vertebral column:
  - cervical;
  - thoracic;
  - lumbar; and
  - sacrococcygeal.
- The general structure and specific characteristics of the seven cervical, 12 thoracic, and five lumbar vertebrae, comparing and contrasting the differences in shapes and positions of these vertebral parts:
  - body and arch, enclosing the vertebral foramen, and laminae;
  - transverse, articular, and spinous processes;
  - intervertebral discs.

- Ligaments that bind the vertebrae together:
  - anterior and posterior longitudinal ligaments, extending the entire length of the column;
  - ligamentum flavum (L., *flavus*, yellow) between the laminae of adjacent vertebrae;
  - ligamentum intertransversarium, interspinale, and supraspinale; and
  - ligamentum nuchae.

On the skull, the following structures should be identified (Fig. 8.4):

- the inferior nuchal line of the occipital bone, which is almost parallel with the superior nuchal line but is hidden from palpation by the overlying musculature;
- the occipital condyles, one on each side, which serve as a component of the atlanto-occipital joints;
- the jugular processes of the occipital bone, which are located lateral to the occipital condyles and serve as attachments to one of the short posterior neck muscles (rectus capitis lateralis); and
- the foramen magnum of the occipital bone, which transmits the medulla oblongata.

On the anterior side of the foramen magnum is the basilar part of the occipital bone. This portion of the bone lies on the anterior side of the axis of motion of the atlanto-occipital joints and serves as an attachment for the deep flexor muscles of the head (longus capitis, rectus capitis anterior).

On the mandible (lower jaw), the following parts should be identified (Fig. 8.5A):

- the body;
- the ramus;
- the convex condyles; and
- the coronoid process for attachment of the temporalis muscle.

At rest, the condyles of the mandible lie in the glenoid fossa of the temporal bone (Fig. 8.5B). When the mouth is opened, the condyles move down and forward to lie beneath the articular tubercle on the zygomatic process of the temporal bone (Fig. 8.5C).

Palpable Structures

If the fingers are placed behind the earlobes, the mastoid portion of the temporal bone can be palpated; its lowest part is the mastoid process (Gr., *mastor,* breast; *eidos,* resemblance) (Fig. 8.6). In the erect position, this process is best felt if the head is bent forward slightly so that the sternocleidomastoid (SCM) muscle, which attaches to it, is relaxed. When the head is tipped backward, the muscle tightens, and only part of the process may be palpated. If the fingers are moved in a posterior direction from the mastoid process, the occipital bone with its superior nuchal line is reached (Fig. 8.6A and B). The lateral portion of this ridge serves, in part, as a site for attachments of the SCM muscle and its medial portion, in part, as a site for attachment of the trapezius.

At the point where the two superior nuchal lines of the right and the left sides meet at the median line, there is a small eminence, the **external occipital protuberance** (Fig. 8.6); the external occipital crest extends from the protuberance to the foramen magnum, also in the median line. These bony eminences serve as sites for attachment of the **ligamentum nuchae,** a strong ligamentous band extending from the seventh cervical vertebra to the skull. This ligament is attached to the trapezius muscle and to a number of posterior neck muscles. It is best palpated when it is slack—when the head is tilted backward.

Just anterior to the external auditory canals, the **condyles of the mandible** can be palpated. When the

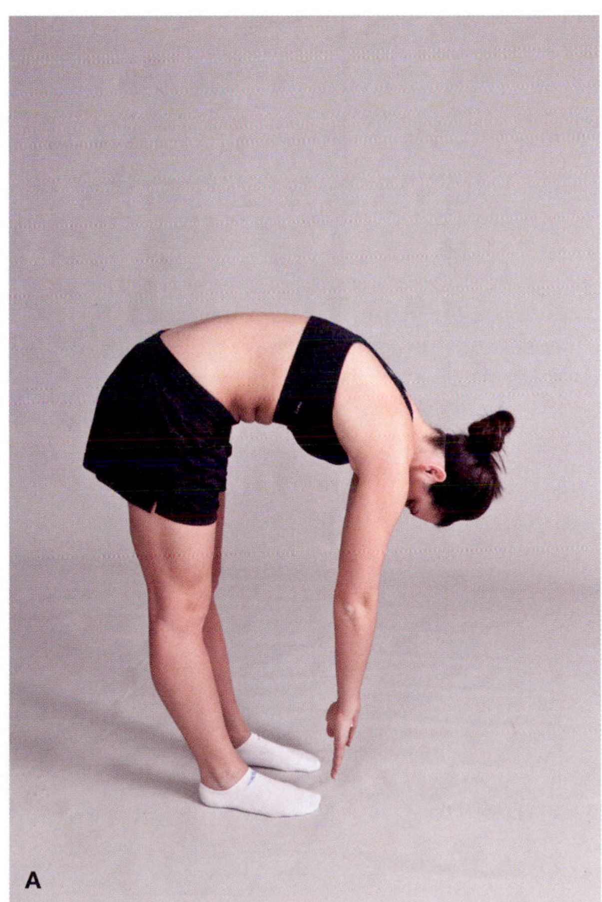

Figure 8.3 A) Spinal alignment in flexion.

continued

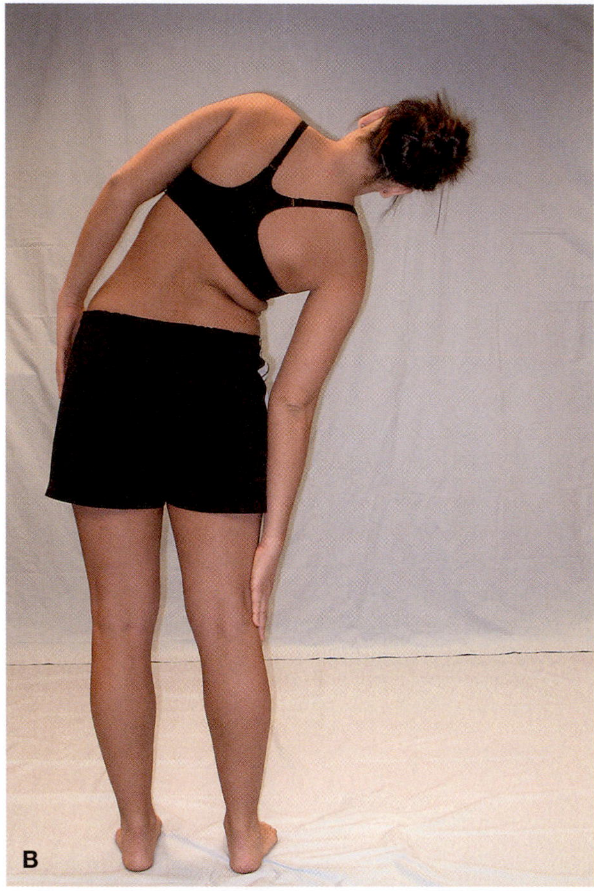

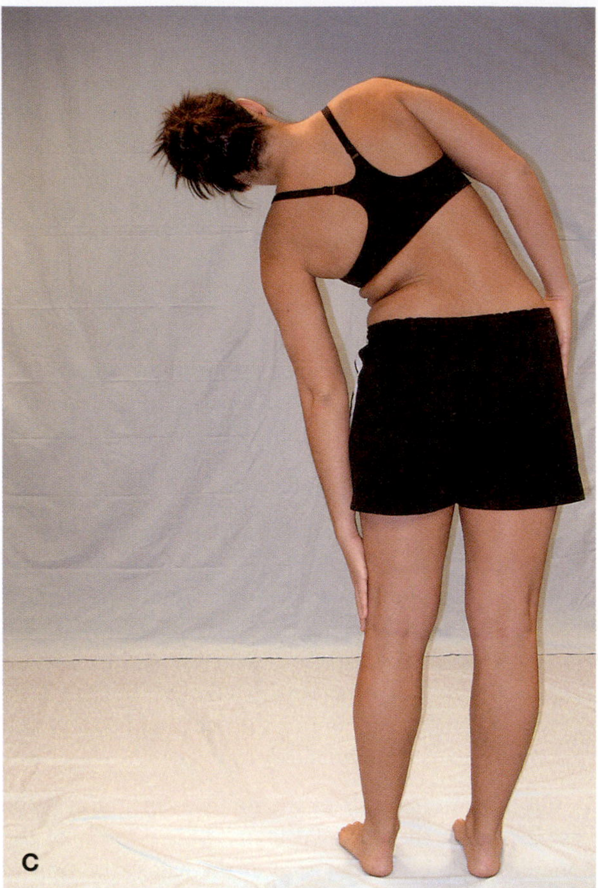

Figure 8.3—cont'd B) Lateral flexion to the right; C) Lateral flexion to the left.

subject opens the mouth or deviates the jaw, the condyles can be felt to move on the glenoid fossa and tubercle of the temporal bones. The mandibular condyles also can be felt by placing the finger in the ear canal and pressing anteriorly (Fig. 8.7).

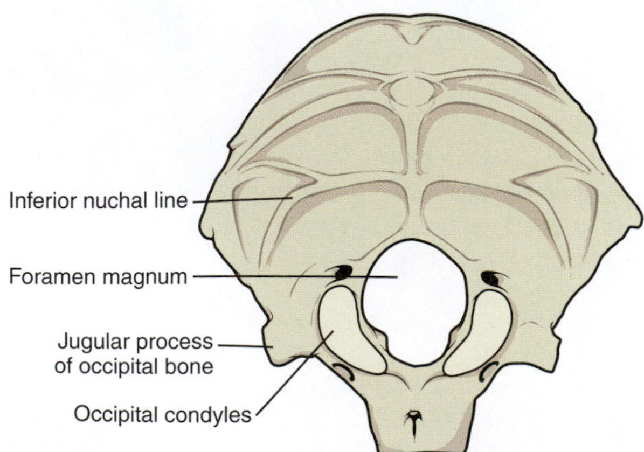

Figure 8.4 Nonpalpable inferior skull structures.

For clinical orientation and palpation, the following landmarks may be used to identify levels of specific vertebrae:

- C-3 is level with the hyoid bone, which can be palpated anteriorly just below the mandible;
- C-4 and C-5 are level with the thyroid cartilage;
- C-6 is level with the arch of the cricoid cartilage;
- body of T-4 is at the height of the junction of the manubrium and the body of the sternum;
- spinous process of T-7 is even with the inferior angle of the scapula;
- body of T-10 is even with the tip of the xiphoid process;
- spinous process of L-4 is level with the highest portion of the crest of the ilium;
- S-2 is at the height of the posterior superior iliac spines. (Table 8–1).

First and Second Cervical Vertebrae

The first cervical vertebra, the atlas, has a transverse process that protrudes more laterally than do those of

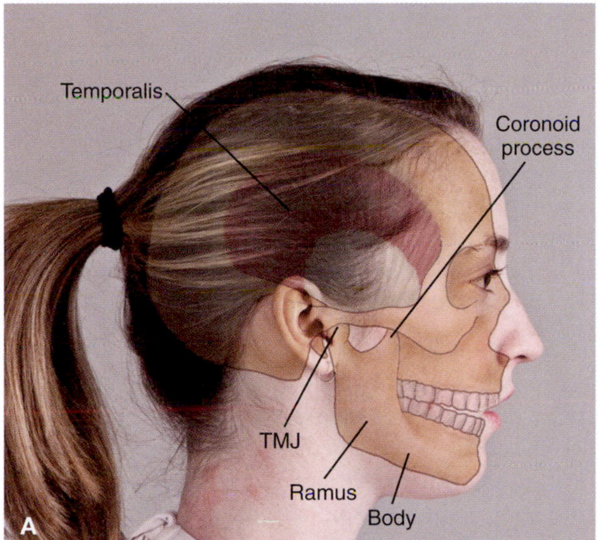

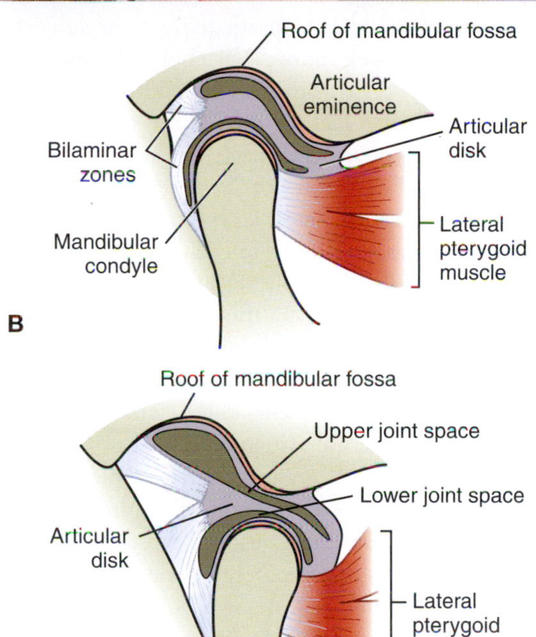

Figure 8.5 The lateral head and temporomandibular joint (TMJ). A) Bony landmarks and attachments of the temporalis and masseter muscles. Approximate lines of pull of these muscles that close the TMJ provide the leverage advantage of these powerful muscles. Note the close proximity of the TMJ to the ear. B) Schematic midsagittal section of the TMJ when the jaw is closed and the mandibular condyle is in the mandibular fossa of the temporal bone. C) The jaw is open and the mandibular condyle is beneath the articular eminence.

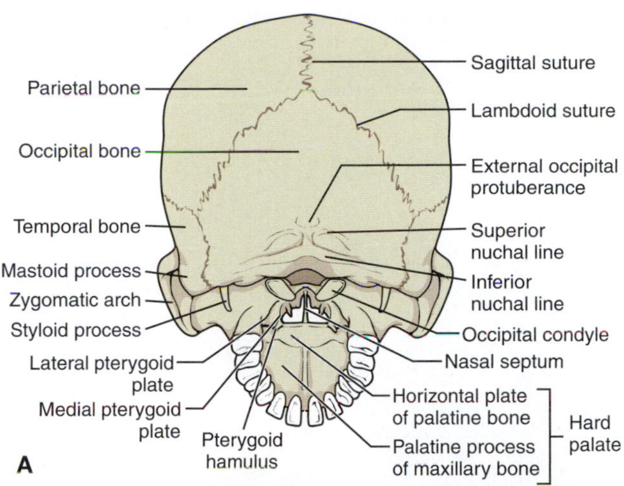

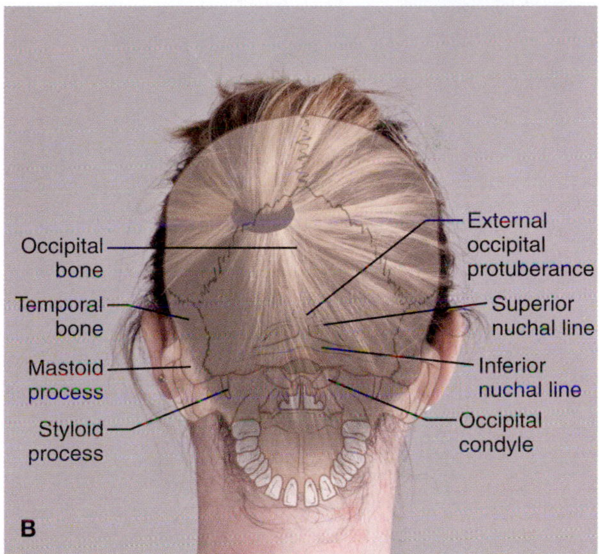

Figure 8.6 Posterior view of head landmarks.

the other vertebrae in this region. This process may be palpated and is found just below the tip of the mastoid process. This region is rather sensitive to pressure, so it is recommended that you palpate the process on yourself before palpating it on another person. The posterior tubercle of the atlas (with its rudimentary spinous process) lies deep but may be found relative to the second cervical vertebra. The spinous process of the axis, the second cervical vertebra, is strong and prominent and is therefore easy to identify.

Third to Sixth Cervical Vertebrae

The lateral portions of these vertebrae present a number of processes and tubercles that are best palpated with the subject supine to relax the muscles of the neck. These vertebrae have short and perforated transverse processes through which the vertebral arteries pass.

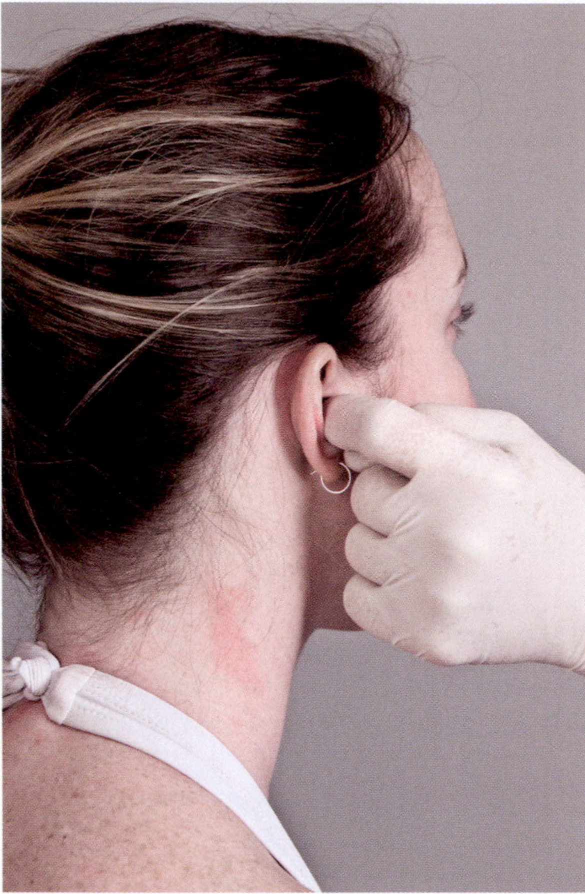

Figure 8.7 Palpation of the mandibular condyles occurs by placing the finger in the ear canal and pressing anteriorly.

TABLE 8-1 | VERTEBRAL LEVELS WITH CORRESPONDING ANATOMIC LANDMARKS

Vertebrae Level	Corresponding Anatomic Landmarks
C3	Hyoid Bone
C4–5	Thyroid Cartilage
C6	Cricoid Cartilage
T4	Manubrium / Body of Sternum Junction
T7	Inferior Angle of Scapula
T10	Tip of Xiphoid Process
L4	Iliac Crest – highest portion
S2	Posterior Superior Iliac Spines

Their articular processes protrude laterally; therefore, the palpable areas of these vertebrae feel very uneven. Their short, bifid spinous processes may be felt in the median line, although they are covered by ligamentum nuchae.

C-7 Vertebra Prominence

Because of the prominence of its spinous process, which is longer and sturdier than those of the other cervical vertebrae and not bifid, the vertebra prominence can be identified easily on most individuals. However, the spinous process of the first thoracic vertebra is often equally prominent. When the subject flexes the neck forward, these processes are identified more easily. When two processes in this region seem to be equal in size, they are identified as those of C-7 and T-1.

Thoracic and Lumbar Vertebrae

When the subject bends forward, flexing the entire spine, the spinous processes of the vertebral column become relatively separated from each other and may be more easily palpated throughout the thoracic and lumbar regions. The C-7 spinous process is used as a starting point for counting the vertebrae, which can be done accurately in most subjects, particularly if the subject is told to "make the back round." Vertebral columns, however, present a great deal of individual variation. Common anomalies include one or the other spinous process being less developed and more difficult to locate and minor lateral deviations of the processes.

In the thoracic region, the spinous processes are directed downward and overlap each other so that the spinous process of one vertebra is located approximately at the height of the body of the next lower one. In the lumbar region, the spinous processes are large and directed horizontally, so that the height of the spinous process more nearly represents the height of its body. The change in vertebral structure from one region of the spine to another is gradual. For example, the two lowest thoracic vertebrae resemble the lumbar vertebrae, having rather horizontally directed spinous processes that are approximately at the height of the intervertebral disc between its own body and the body of the next lower vertebra.

Sacrum and Coccyx

The surface of the sacrum is palpated as a direct continuation of the lumbar spine. The medial sacral crest represents the rudimentary spinous processes of the sacral vertebrae, with the processes fused with the rest of the bone. On both sides of the sacral crest are rough areas serving as attachment sites of ligaments, fascia, and muscles. The approximate boundaries of the sacrum may be palpated by following each iliac crest in a posterior direction, where the sacrum is inserted between the two ilia. The "dimples" medial to the posterior superior iliac spines indicate the location of the sacroiliac joints.

Caudally, the sacrum is continuous with the coccyx with the juncture of the two bone segments forming a marked posterior convexity so that the tip of the coccyx has a deep location between the two gluteal eminences. If an individual sits on the front portion of a hard chair and then leans against the back of the chair, the coccyx may be felt contacting the chair.

Thorax (Rib Cage)

The thorax consists of the 12 thoracic vertebrae posteriorly, the sternum anteriorly, and the 12 ribs. Most of the thorax bony structures may be palpated. Some difficulty arises in palpating the upper ribs, which are hidden by the clavicle and neck structures. In obese individuals, palpation of the last two, or "floating," ribs may also be difficult. Those portions of the ribs adjacent to the vertebral column are covered by muscles, but the ribs may be palpated beginning at their angles along their lateral, forward, and downward courses. It should be recalled from anatomy that the first to seventh ribs attach to the sternum, the eighth to tenth ribs join with each other by means of cartilage, and the eleventh and twelfth ribs have free ends.

When palpating the ribs on the left side, they are more easily palpated if the subject places the left hand on top of the head and stretches the left side laterally to separate the ribs somewhat from each other. In stretching the ipsilateral side of the thorax in this manner, the distance between the lower lateral rib cage and iliac crest increases, permitting the floating ribs to be more easily located. In the erect standing position, distance between these floating ribs is very narrow. In pathologic conditions such as severe lateral curvature of the spine, the ribs may actually come to rest on the ilium, causing nerves to become pinched and subsequently very painful.

Sternum

The sternum may be palpated from the xiphoid process at its most caudal point to its more cranially located manubrium and sternoclavicular joints. The sternum forms a closed system with the thoracic vertebrae and ribs that attach to it. Ribs 1–10 attach to the sternum with hyaline cartilage connections of ribs 1–7 forming a direct attachment on the lateral sternum through the sternocostal joints. The hyaline cartilage of ribs 8–10 attach indirectly to the sternum through a merging of their cartilage with the hyaline cartilage of the adjacent superior rib.

Vertebral Joints, Ligaments, and Motions

The joint between the intervertebral disc and vertebra is a cartilaginous joint while the facet joints are synovial (diarthrodial) joints. Biomechanically, the bony and ligamentous structures of the vertebrae are divided into anterior and posterior vertebral structures. The anterior structures function primarily to bear weight, and the posterior structures are responsible primarily for controlling motion.

Vertebral Motions

The spine is delineated into motion segments. A **motion segment** of the spine consists of two adjacent vertebrae, three intervertebral joints, the soft tissues of the intervertebral disc, longitudinal and intersegmental ligaments, and the capsules of the facet joints.[3] The disc and the left and right facet joints form a triangle whereby motion at one joint always produces motion at the other two joints. In most of the vertebral joints, three degrees of motion occur. These osteokinematic motions include flexion and extension in the sagittal plane, left and right side bending (lateral flexion) in the frontal plane, and left and right rotation in the transverse plane. Arthrokinematic motions also occur in the vertebral joints; these types of motions include anterior-posterior shear or slide, lateral shear or slide, and distraction-compression.

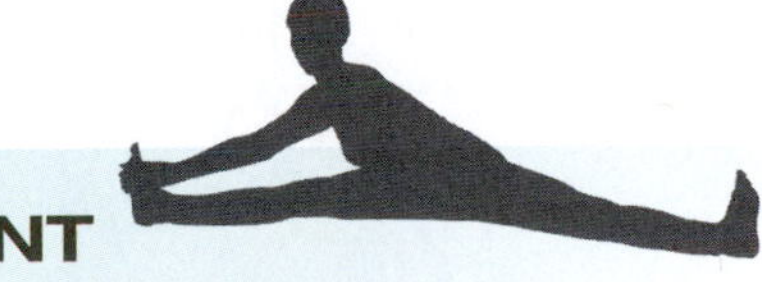

PRACTICE POINT

Identification of the spine levels is important in locating and palpating appropriate structures when examining patients. Palpation of the thoracic spine and ribs is made easier by the realization of the position of spinous structures relative to other easily located structures. For example, the inferior angle of the scapula is at the T7 level and the root of the spine of the scapula is directly across from T3. The costotransverse joints are located by first identifying the spinous process and then moving the palpating finger two finger-widths from the spinous process; the joint directly under the finger is the costotransverse joint. It must be remembered that when palpating a spinous process in the thoracic region, the vertebral body directly under that spinous process is one level below the level of the spinous process being palpated. For example, directly below the T7 spinous process is the vertebral body of T8.

Anterior Vertebral Joint Elements

The weight-bearing bodies of the vertebrae, the intervertebral discs, and the longitudinal ligaments form the anterior vertebral structures. Biomechanical functions of the vertebral bodies include resistance to the compressive forces of superincumbent weight; muscle contractions; and external loads that occur in lifting, pulling, or pushing. The intervening discs protect the facet joints from compression injury and permit—as well as limit—motions of the vertebrae. Each disc is composed of three parts: the **annulus fibrosus,** a series of fibroelastic cartilaginous rings that enclose the **nucleus pulposus,** a gel with an 80% or more water content (Fig. 8.8A); and two hyaline **cartilaginous plates** called **vertebral end plates** (Fig. 8.8B), which separate the nucleus and the annulus from the vertebral bodies and merge with the annulus fibrosus collagen fibers. The fibers in the annulus run obliquely from the inferior edge of the upper vertebrae to the superior margin of the lower vertebrae. Fiber direction is opposite in alternate layers, forming crossing patterns so that motions in opposite directions can be restrained. The circumference of the disc is basically the same as the bodies, but the height is greater in the lumbar area. In total, the intervertebral discs account for approximately 25% of the length of the vertebral column.

With weight-bearing or muscle contraction, forces are transmitted from the vertebral bodies to the disc. During these force transmissions, the pressure increases within the entire disc to exert forces on the elastic annulus fibrosus, which bulges (stretches) to absorb these forces and limit motion as the nucleus pulposus remains confined within the annulus fibrosus (Fig. 8.9A). In most loading situations, the force is not applied in the center but rather on the anterior, posterior, or lateral parts of the vertebral body. This produces compression of the annulus on its side near the force and tension on its opposite side, with each mechanism serving to limit vertebral compression (Fig. 8.9B).

Since the nucleus pulposus is composed largely of water, it is hydrophilic (loves water). Compression forces produced by standing and walking throughout the day cause the nucleus to lose small quantities of water. Fluid levels within the nucleus pulposus are restored during sleep and recumbency when pressure

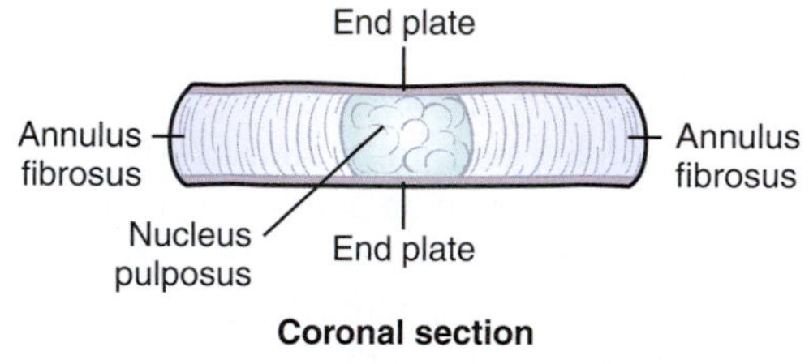

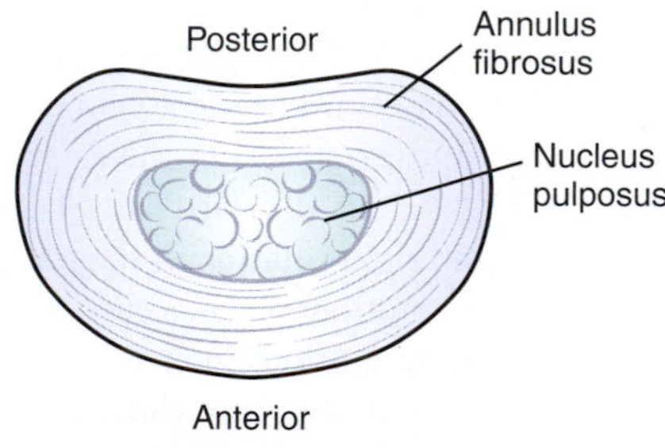

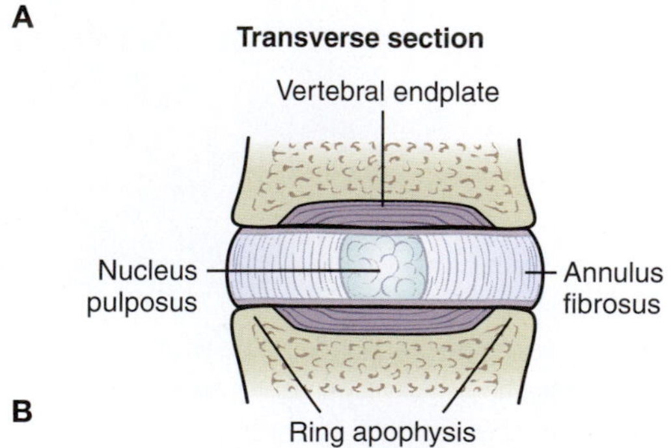

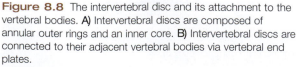

Figure 8.8 The intervertebral disc and its attachment to the vertebral bodies. **A)** Intervertebral discs are composed of annular outer rings and an inner core. **B)** Intervertebral discs are connected to their adjacent vertebral bodies via vertebral end plates.

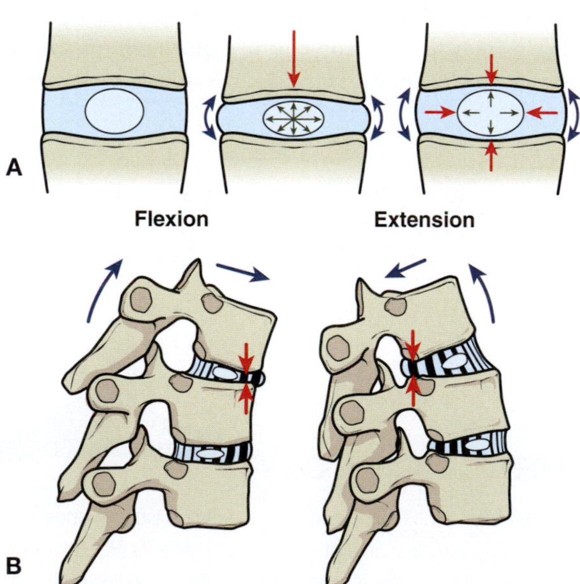

Figure 8.9 Pressure on the disc causes bulging of the disc. **A)** Axial pressure produces tension within the disc to stretch the annulus fibrosus to absorb and distribute forces and limit motion. **B)** Loads applied off center increase compression of the disc on the loaded side and tension on the opposite side.

inside the nucleus is reduced. It is for this reason that height of an individual may diminish as much as 2 cm from morning to evening. As the supply of blood vessels to the disc disappears in the second decade of life,[2] and the ability of the nucleus to restore lost water also begins to decrease. The normal aging process along with repeated microtrauma from lifting heavy objects and incorrect mechanics causes an increase in fibrous elements of the annulus and a decrease in the relative number of resilient elastic elements. In extreme cases, this degeneration may result in herniation of the nucleus onto the nerve roots in adults under 50 years old. Older adults (50 to 90 years old) with a propensity toward poor posture may be prone to developing thoracic kyphosis (Gr., *kyphos,* a hump), a prominent posterior convex curvature of the spine. As individuals age, we all lose height because of fluid loss in the vertebral discs.

Longitudinal Ligaments

Anterior and **posterior longitudinal ligaments** (ALL and PLL) cover the front and back of the vertebral bodies, respectively, from the axis to the sacrum (Fig. 8.10A). The broad and strong ALL attaches to the annulus and the edge of each vertebral body. Between the vertebral body and ligament are veins and arteries that pass into foramina to the vertebral body. The ALL limits backward bending, and in the lumbosacral area supports the anterior convexity (Fig. 8.10B). The narrower PLL attaches to the annulus fibrosis and the superior margin of the vertebral body, but covers a plexus of arteries, veins, and lymphatics as well as the nutrient foramina through which these vessels pass to the cancellous bone of the body. Forward flexion is somewhat restrained by the PLL but the leverage of the PLL is poor, and its tensile strength is relatively low.[4] With forward flexion the PLL becomes taut (Fig. 8.10C) to close the nutrient foramina and trap fluid in the cancellous vertebral body. This mechanism is thought to increase the vertebral body's ability to withstand compression forces.

The width of the PLL decreases as the ligament descends from the cervical to lumbar spines. Given this progressive narrowing, the PLL likely offers greater stabilization to the intervertebral disc in the cervical rather than lumbar spine. When these ligaments (as well as the ligamentum flavum) were removed from the spine, Tkaczuk[5] found them to retract. He suggested that normal discs are prestressed by the ligaments. In other words, the disc and the longitudinal ligaments together create a system of balanced forces and resistance to motion.

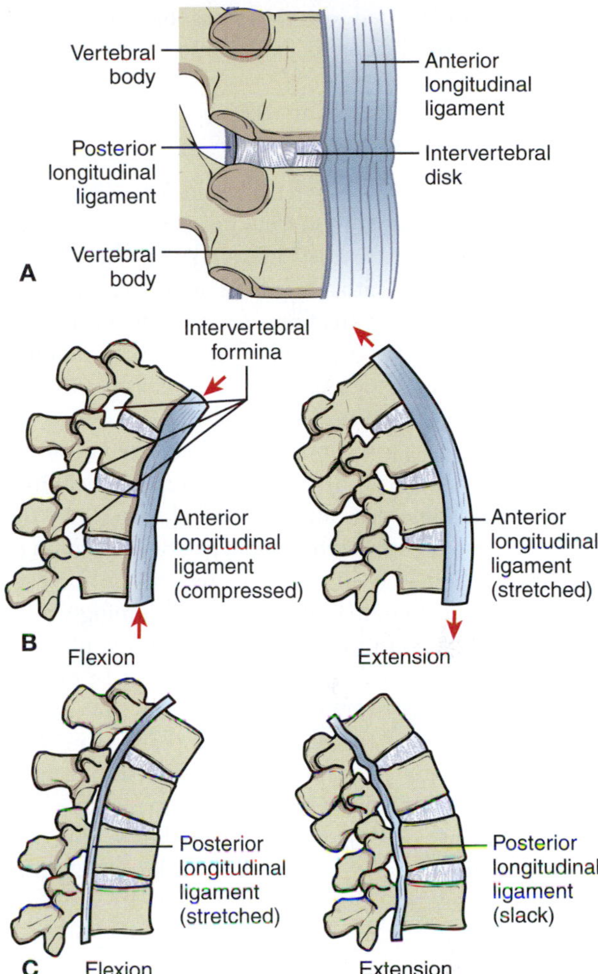

Figure 8.10 Anterior and posterior vertebral structures. **A)** Sagittal view of two vertebral bodies and associated soft tissues. **B)** Anterior longitudinal ligament is lax during spinal flexion and taut during extension. **C)** Posterior longitudinal ligament is taut during spinal flexion and lax during extension.

Disc Pressures

Pressures within the lumbar disc have been studied and recorded in both cadavers and live human subjects by Nachemson.[6–8] His work demonstrated that in normal discs:

- the center of the nucleus pulposus acts hydrostatically;
- disc pressure is linearly related to the compressive force up to 450 lb;
- the nucleus pulposus supports about one and a half times the compressive load and the annulus fibrosus supports half of the imposed load;

- pressures exerted on the sides of the annulus fibrosus reach four to five times the compressive load; and
- the bilateral facet joints can support one-fifth of the imposed load.

More recent studies by McNally and Adams[9] confirm that compressive forces are generally distributed across the nucleus pulposus in normal discs and that the annulus fibrosus may behave either as a fluid or as a tensile structure. Detailed exploration of pressures in different areas of the disc suggests that it actually functions with multiple fluid compartments possessing mechanical properties that vary with the load and the loading history.

Examples of approximate disc loads recorded by Nachemson at L-3 in different postures and activities are found in Table 8–2. The prestress of the disc by the ligaments can be seen in the supine position. Traction in the area of 500 N was needed to reduce the force to zero. As can be seen in Table 8–2, many seemingly mild activities, such as arm exercises in the supine position and unsupported sitting, create greater forces on the disc than occur when standing.

Further study of the disc suggests that the nucleus pulposus migrates in a reasonably predictable fashion during osteokinematic motion. Using magnetic resonance imaging (MRI), research has shown that the nuclear material of the disc in healthy subjects migrates anteriorly when the spine is extended and posteriorly when the spine is flexed in the sagittal plane.[10] Although not as consistent as in sagittal plane motion, the nucleus pulposus of a healthy lumbar disc deforms to the contralateral side in the majority of cases with axial rotation. This response was detected by MRI in nine of 12 asymptomatic female subjects by Fazey and colleagues.[11]

TABLE 8–2 | SOME EXAMPLES OF FORCES ON THE LUMBAR (L-3) INTERVERTEBRAL DISC

Position	Newtons	Ratio to Standing
Supine in traction (300 N)	100	–0.2
Supine	250	_0.5
Supine arm exercises (20 N)	600	+ 1.2
Standing at ease	500	1.0
Sitting unsupported	700	+ 1.4
Sitting in office chair	500	1.0
Cough in standing	700	+1.4
Standing forward bent 40°	1000	+2.0
Lifting 100 N (knees ext, back flex)	1700	+3.4
Lifting 100 N (knees flex, back ext)	1900	+3.8

Source: Data from Nachemson, A. Disc pressure measurements, Spine 6:93, 1981; and from Nachemson, A. Lumbar intradiscal pressure. In Jayson, M (ed): *The Lumbar Spine and Back Pain,* Edinburgh: Churchill Livingstone, 1987, pp 191–203.

Posterior Vertebral Joint Elements

Posterior vertebral structures comprise the arches, the transverse and spinous processes, the bilateral facet joints, joint capsules, and ligaments. The facet joints (apophyseal or zygapophyseal joints) are formed by the inferior articulating process of one vertebra with the superior articulating process of the vertebra below (Fig. 8.11). The major functions of the facet joints are to control vertebral motions and to protect the disc from excessive shear, flexion, side bending, and rotation. The direction and amount of motion permitted are determined by the planes of the joint surfaces, which change in their orientation from the cervical through the lumbar areas.

Ligaments

The **ligamenta flava** (L., *flavus,* yellow) are a series of 23 intersegmental ligaments that connect the lamina of two adjacent vertebrae from C-2 to the sacrum. Its yellow color reflects the high elastic content, which contributes to the prestress of the disc and resistance to forward flexion. Ligamentum flavum fibers cover the anterior surface of the capsule of the facet joint and provide tension on the capsule to prevent nipping and injury by the facet joints during movement. In addition, the fibers of the ligamentum flavum are continuous with the **interspinous ligaments,** which attach between adjacent

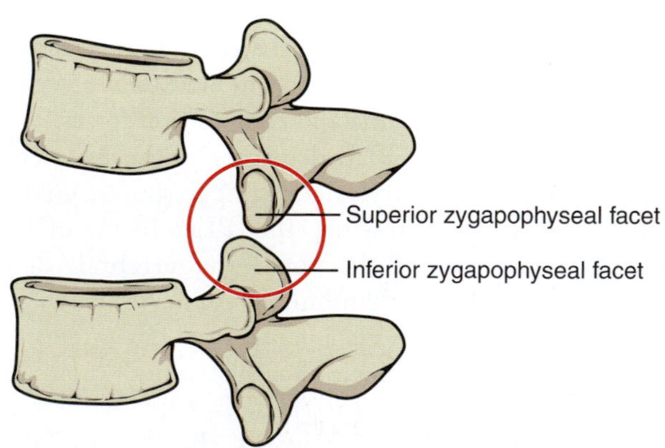

Figure 8.11 Facet joints of a vertebra are formed by the inferior articulating process of one vertebra with the superior articulating process of the vertebra below.

spinous processes. The interspinous ligaments are continuous with the **supraspinous ligament,** a strong, fibrous cord attaching to the tips of the spinous processes and continuous with the thoracodorsal fascia. Figures 8.12A and B illustrate these ligaments. In the cervical area, the supraspinous ligament becomes the **ligamentum nuchae** (L., *nucha,* nape or scruff of the neck). **Intertransverse ligaments** are segmental with attachments between adjacent transverse processes.

The interspinous and supraspinous ligaments resist motions of forward bending very effectively. This ligamentous system is attached farther from the vertebral bodies than some of the spinal muscles so it has a leverage advantage. In addition, the supraspinous ligament has great tensile strength, especially in the lumbar area.[4]

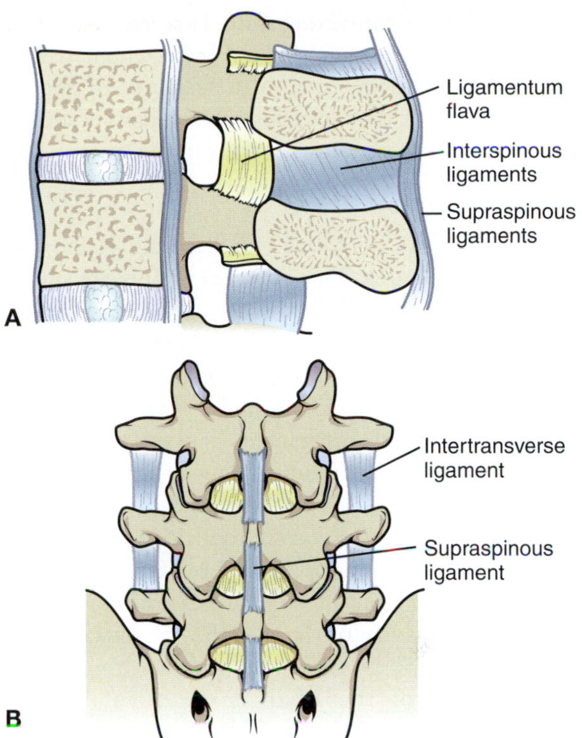

Figure 8.12 Posterior ligaments of the spine. **A)** The ligamentum flavum has a high amount of elastic fiber and is continuous with the interspinous ligament. The interspinous ligament is continuous with the supraspinous ligament. **B)** Posterior view of the intertransverse and supraspinous ligaments.

Coupling Motions

Motions in the vertebral joints seldom occur in pure planar motion but rather in combined motions called **coupling.** Coupling occurs because of the orientation of the planes of the left and right facet joints and limitation of motion provided by the disc, vertebral ligaments, fascia, and muscles. The greatest complexity of coupling in the spine is with side bending and rotation. After one or two degrees of motion, side bending is always accompanied by rotation, and rotation is always accompanied by side bending.[15] It has been traditionally viewed that coupling is influenced by the position the spine assumes in the sagittal plane.[16] When the spine is in neutral position and moves in the sagittal plane, rotation and side bending occur contralaterally. However, when the spine is either flexed or extended, rotation and side bending occur in an ipsilateral fashion.[16] More recently however, these views have been questioned. Research has identified that coupling motions of the spine vary not only by region (i.e., cervical versus lumbar) but within each region[17, 18] and is likely more complex (three motions occurring simultaneously) than previously thought.[19] Investigations of coupling motions of the spine have produced conflicting results. It is likely that variations in factors such as research methods, subjects' age ranges, flexibility, joint mobility, and the precision of start positions and motions performed are

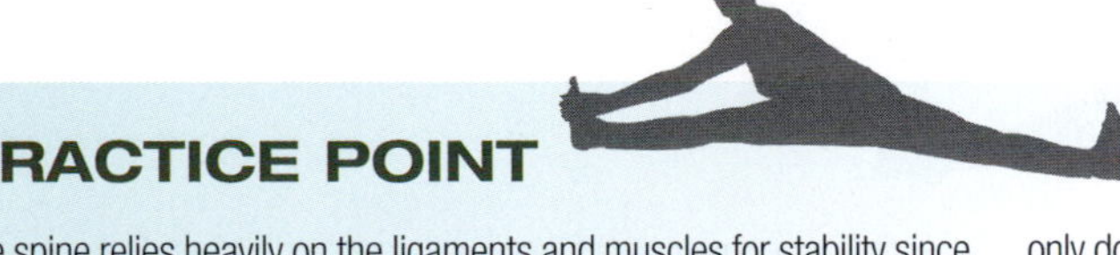

PRACTICE POINT

The spine relies heavily on the ligaments and muscles for stability since it is an inherently unstable structure without their support. If the ligaments and muscles are removed from a spine, the vertebrae are able to tolerate only 4 to 5 lb (1.8 to 2.3 kg) of vertical load before the spine collapses into flexion.[12] Because of the spine's flexibility and amount of weight it must support, Farfan[13] has likened the spine to balancing a 75-lb weight at the end of a rod that is 14 inches long and flexible. Not only do the ligaments have to be strong, but the muscles must also provide significant force to maintain both stability and function of the spine. It is no wonder that up to 84% of the population worldwide experience back pain at some point in their lives.[14] From a clinical standpoint, with such a large number of patients with low back pathologies, it is important to understand the spine and how it functions so proper treatment courses and prevention methods may be applied.

sources of these conflicting data. It seems that at this point, although there is dispute as to whether lateral flexion and rotation occur to the same or to opposite sides, it is agreed that coupling motion does occur with rotation and side bending motions in the spine.

Cervical Region

The occiput (0), atlas (C1), and axis (C2) form the **craniovertebral area.** Here the facet joints are specialized, two or three degrees of freedom exist, and the planes of motion are nearly horizontal. The **atlanto-occipital joints** have two degrees of freedom of motion (Fig. 8.13A). The two joints (0–C1 and C1–C2) work in unison to provide movements between the head and the vertebral column. The shallow, concave joint surfaces on the atlas (one on each side of the vertebral canal) support the two convex condyles of the occipital bone. This structure supports the head from below while providing head movement but without interfering with the passage of the medulla oblongata into the vertebral canal.

Movement of the head at the atlanto-occipital (0–C1) joint is mainly a nodding movement in the sagittal plane around a medial-lateral axis that passes through the two condyles. The approximate location of this axis is seen by placing the tips of the two index fingers pointing toward each other on the mastoid processes. Small lateral bending movements of the atlanto-occipital joint are also possible, but these motions are quite limited.

The **atlanto-axial joint** (C1–C2) is formed by one centrally located articulation and two facet joints (the inferior articular processes of the atlas and the superior articular processes of the axis) (Fig. 8.13B). Centrally, the dens of the axis (odontoid process) fits into a ring formed by the anterior arch of the atlas and its

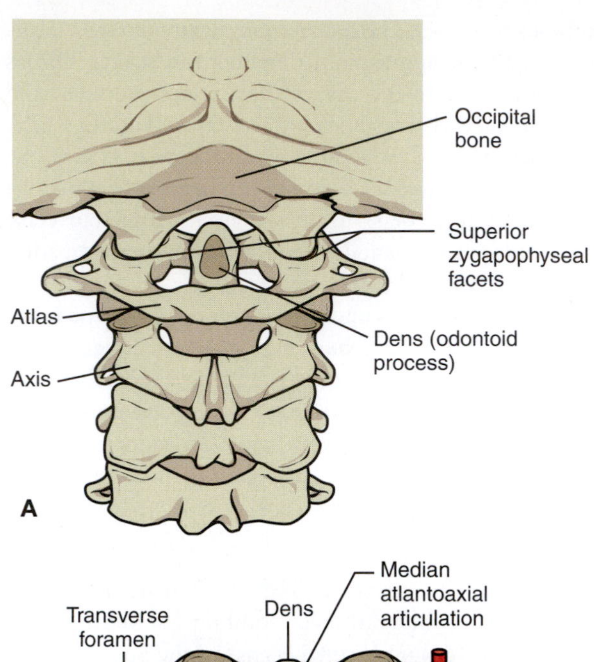

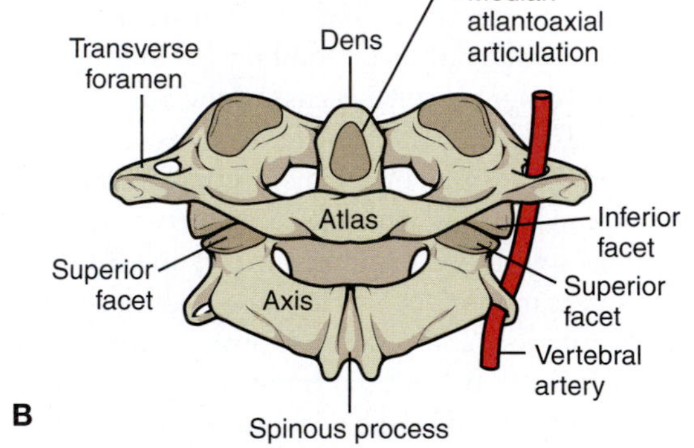

Figure 8.13 Craniovertebral joints. **A)** The shallow concave joint surfaces of the atlas support the convex condyles of the occipital bone to allow two degrees of freedom in the atlanto-occipital joints. **B)** One central articulation and two facet joints comprise the atlanto-axial joint between C1 and C2. Rotation occurs in this joint as the atlas rotates around the dens of the axis.

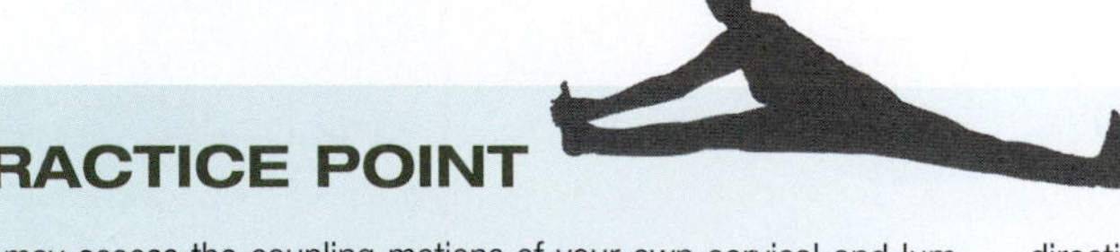

PRACTICE POINT

You may assess the coupling motions of your own cervical and lumbar spines. Sit in a properly aligned position and laterally flex your neck to one side, noting to which direction your neck rotates as you laterally flex. Now return to your starting sitting position. This time, before you laterally flex your neck, move into a slumped posture so your shoulders become rounded and your head moves forward. Once you are in a poor postural position, laterally flex your neck and observe which direction your head rotates. You may perform this test in the lumbar spine as well, laterally flexing in a properly aligned position and then repeating it in either an arched (lordotic) lumbar spine or a flat lumbar spine. Notice how the proper and improper alignment positions change the coupling motions and if the lumbar spine and cervical spine coupling motions are the same. You may also check other individuals to see how your coupling motions compare with theirs.

transverse ligament posteriorly, so that the atlas pivots around the dens. Since the axis of motion is vertical through the dens, the motion occurring on this axis is rotation. Approximately 50% of rotation in the cervical area occurs at this joint.

In the typical **cervical vertebral articulations** (C2–C3 through C6–C7), the articulating surfaces of the facet joints change from horizontal to a 45° angle between the horizontal and frontal planes. This facet orientation, along with loose and elastic capsules, permits motion in each plane. The superior articular facets slide superior and anterior in forward bending (flexion) and inferior and posterior in backward bending (extension). In side bending right, the left superior facet moves superiorly and anterior while the right superior facet moves inferior and posterior, producing a rotation of the vertebral body to the right and the spinous process to the left.[3] Although discussions on coupling motions presented earlier indicate that there are variable patterns in coupling of rotation and lateral bending, this combination of facet movements in the cervical spine has been frequently reported.[3]

Normally, the erect posture of the cervical spine is lordotic (concave posteriorly). Flexion occurs in a straight sagittal plane, and extension occurs until the spinous processes contact each other to limit further motion. Normal flexion range of motion enables the subject to touch the chin to the chest, and in a normal end range of extension, the anterior neck forms a vertical line from the chin to the chest.

Specific joint ranges of vertebral motion recorded between individual levels that have been cited in the literature vary considerably. When taken as a whole segment, however, there is greater consensus of cervical spine ranges of motion. Although it is accepted that range of motion declines with increasing age, normal active range of motion for the entire cervical spine collectively has been reported as listed in Table 8–3.

In addition to permitting and controlling motion, the facet joints in the cervical area also share some of the weight-bearing forces of the head because of their 45° orientation to the frontal plane. This function is significant because the head (~10 lb) requires support by the long lever arm of the cervical vertebrae to allow an individual to sit and stand for up to 16 or more hours per day without rest. Keep in mind that the cervical muscles are able to rest only when an individual is lying down. Since most people commonly stand, sit, and remain in an upright position for 16 or more hours a day, these cervical muscles must function for extended periods.

TABLE 8–3 | NORMAL RANGES OF CERVICAL MOTION[20]

Motion	Average Range
Flexion	50°
Extension	60°
Lateral Flexion—Right	45°
Lateral Flexion—Left	45°
Rotation—Right	80°
Rotation—Left	80°

Thoracic Region

Based on their position and design, the thoracic vertebrae have several varying responsibilities. They support and permit motion of the head and trunk; provide protection of the heart, lungs, and great vessels; supply articulations for respiration; and provide attachments for muscles of respiration, the trunk, and the extremities.

Facet Joints

The plane of the thoracic facet joints moves toward the vertical or frontal plane (Fig. 8.14). This facet orientation limits flexion and anterior shear motions but permits side bending. The ribs and the sternum, however, limit potential motions of the thoracic vertebrae. Extension of the thoracic spine also is limited by contact of the spinous processes to each other in backward bending. Total thoracic extension produces a straight-line alignment of the thoracic spine. Motion of lower thoracic vertebrae is less restricted by the ribs than higher thoracic vertebrae, and their facet joint planes are more sagittally oriented. Intervertebral motions of the thoracic spine as a whole more resemble lumbar motions, with increased flexion-extension and side bending and less rotation. Active range of motion for this region is reported in conjunction with lumbar spine range of motion as the two regions are difficult to dissociate (Table 8–4). As previously noted, range of motion also generally declines in the thoracic and lumbar as age increases.

Costal Joints

Two synovial joints are formed by the ribs on each side of the thoracic vertebrae posteriorly (Fig. 8.15A). The typical ribs 2 through 9 articulate with the adjacent body, the body above, and the disc between the two bodies to form the costovertebral joint. The exceptions to this arrangement are the atypical ribs 1, 10, 11, and 12 that articulate only with the corresponding body. In addition to these articulations, ribs 1 through 10 also articulate with their same-level transverse process to form the costotransverse joints (Fig. 8.15B). Both the

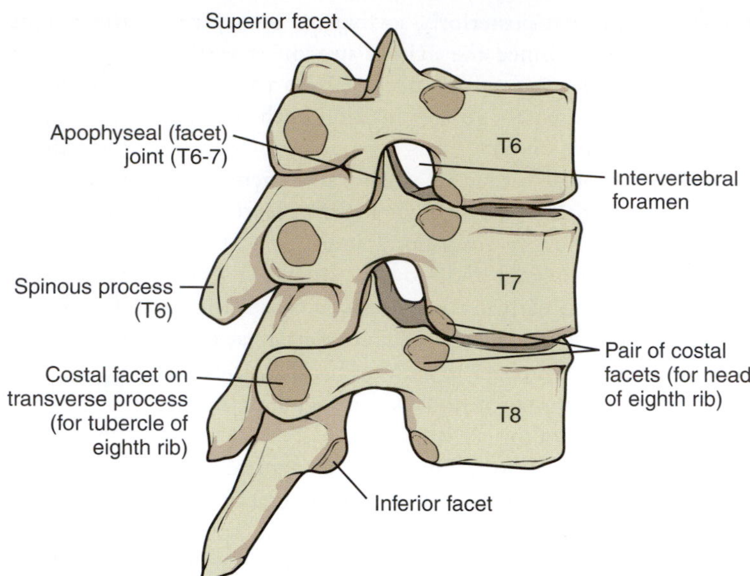

Figure 8.14 The thoracic facet joints are aligned near vertical in the frontal plane so they will limit flexion-extension shear motions.

costovertebral and costotransverse joints are reinforced by strong ligaments. Anteriorly, the cartilages of ribs 2 through 7 form synovial joints with the sternum. The costal cartilages of ribs 8 through 10 articulate with the cartilage above and the lateral ends of ribs 11 and 12 are free, or floating.

Elevation and depression of the ribs occur by a pivoting motion through an axis crossing the costovertebral and costotransverse joints. The orientation of the upper ribs is more horizontal, and the motion of elevation produces an increased anterior diameter of the rib cage. The lower ribs have a more oblique downward orientation, and elevation of the ribs increases the transverse diameter of the rib cage. Increase in the anterior diameter can be felt by placing one hand on the upper part of the sternum and the other hand on the back in the upper thoracic area and asking the subject to perform a vital capacity maneuver (maximum

TABLE 8-4 | THORACOLUMBAR RANGES OF MOTION[20]

Motion	Average Range
Flexion	60°
Extension	25°
Lateral Bending—Right	25°
Lateral Bending—Left	25°
Rotation—Right	30°
Rotation—Left	30°

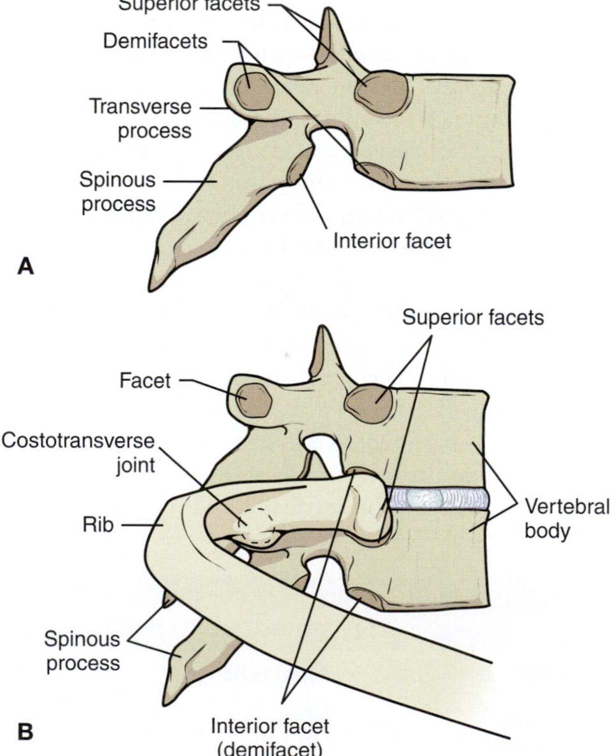

Figure 8.15 Costovertebral joints. A rib is joined with the vertebra above at the inferior demifacet (see glossary for definition) and with the rib's same-level vertebra at the superior demifacet and the facet on the transverse process.

inspiration followed by a maximum expiration). The larger changes that occur in the transverse diameter in the lower thoracic region can be felt by placing both hands over the lateral surfaces of the lower ribs and asking the subject to perform the same vital capacity maneuver.

In addition to participating in respiration, the articulations and structures of the rib cage protect vital organs and make significant contributions to the stability of the thoracic spine. Organs such as the kidneys, lungs, spleen, and liver are protected by the ribs, and the heart is protected by the ribs and sternum.[21] Stabilization of the thoracic spine is enhanced by the rib attachments to the vertebral bodies and transverse processes.[22] Additionally, mobility of the ribs allows for lung expansion and play a critical role in both inspiration and expiration.[23]

Lumbar Region

The large bodies and the intervertebral discs of the lumbar vertebrae along with the strong anterior longitudinal and iliolumbar ligaments normally bear most of the weight of the HAT in an erect posture. Lumbar facet joints are half-moon shaped, with articulating surfaces in both sagittal and frontal planes. The proportion of sagittal surface is greatest at T12 to L1. This facet alignment progressively changes to a more frontal-plane orientation at L5 to S1. This facet joint orientation prohibits motions of rotation and anterior shear. Although rotation is described as being 1° to 3°, Porterfield and DeRosa[24] consider this to be the result of cartilage deformation rather than true joint motion. Facet joint damage was demonstrated in a cadaver study when the lumbar spine was loaded and subjected to 1° to 3° of rotation.[25]

Lumbosacral Junction

Angulation of the vertebral column at the lumbosacral junction is evident in standing (Fig. 8.16A), and this joint is subjected to a great deal of anterior shear by the superimposed body weight on it (Fig. 8.16B). This joint is reinforced by strong iliolumbar ligaments from L-4 to L-5 and by sacrolumbar ligaments, which primarily restrict motions of lateral bending but also limit flexion, extension, and rotation.[26] The near frontal plane orientation of the L-5 to S-1 facet joints prevents excessive anterior shear of the fifth lumbar vertebra. Anatomic variations that weaken the joint may permit the lumbar vertebra to slide forward on the sacrum, a pathology known as **spondylolisthesis** (Gr., *spondylos,* vertebra; *olisthesis,* a slipping or falling).

Thoracolumbar Fascia

The **thoracolumbar fascia** (also called thoracodorsal fascia) is a strong, complex structure that acts like a

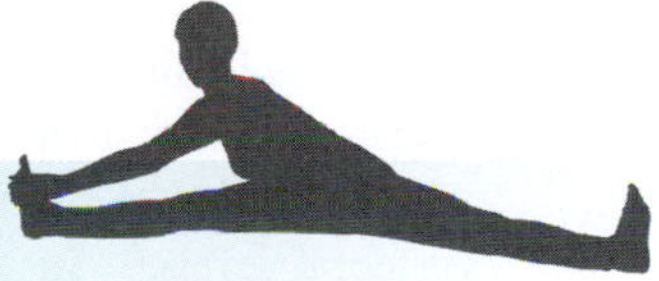

PRACTICE POINT

With narrowing of the intervertebral disc that occurs as people age, the tips of the facet joints come to rest on the lamina of the vertebrae above or below. This occurs with degenerative disc disease and results in up to 70% of the compression force being transmitted in the facets, which are not designed for weight-bearing.[25] Contact of the facet tips also may occur with prolonged standing in normal individuals because of the decrease in disc height that occurs combined with the lumbar lordotic position in standing. Adams and Hutton[25] postulate that the dull ache that can occur in the low back may be due to pressure and microtrauma on the facet joint capsules.

Spondylolisthesis occurs more frequently in females than in males between the ages of 10 and 20. The most common site for this pathology to occur is at L5–S1. It is seen in individuals who have excessive lumbar lordosis or participate in activities such as gymnastics, diving, weight lifting, rowing, and wrestling.[27] The L5–S1 joint has the greatest amount of shear under normal conditions, so increased lordosis and hyperextension-promoting activities occurring in these sports increase this shear stress. Thus, extension and rotation activities will exacerbate the condition. To minimize the likelihood of slippage (anterior shear), clinicians should teach a patient with spondylolisthesis trunk stabilization activities with emphasis on maintaining some degree of posterior pelvic tilt.

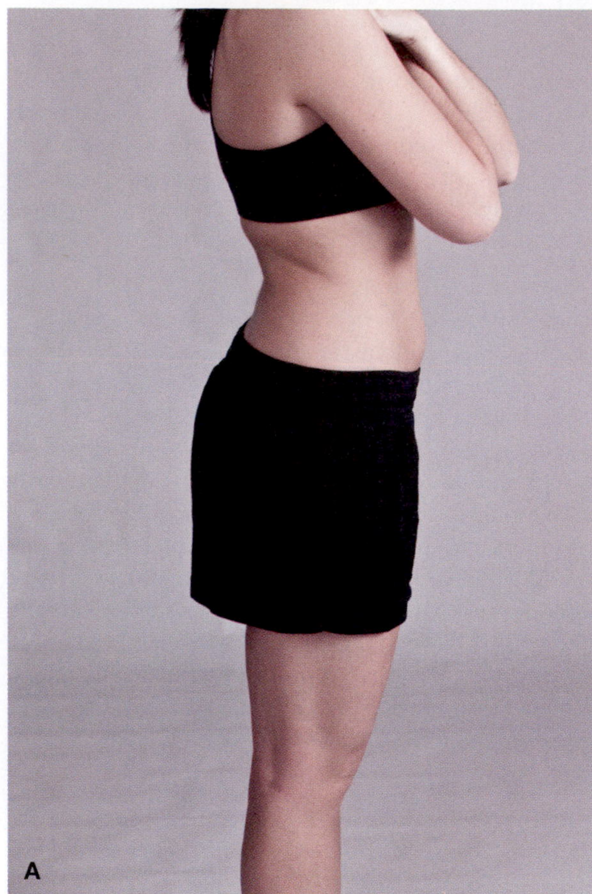

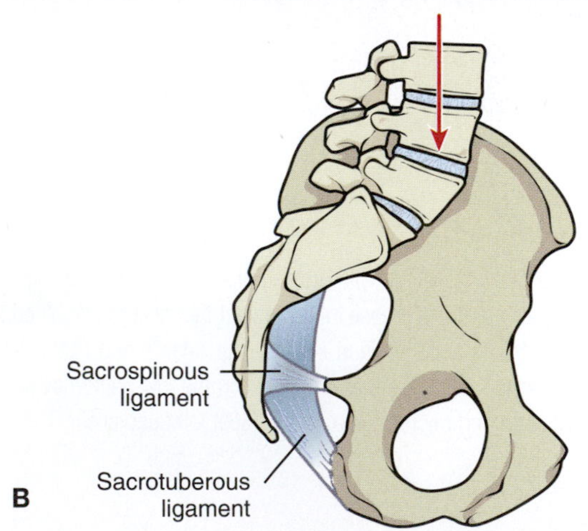

Figure 8.16 The change from lumbar spine to sacral spine is easily observed. **A)** Lateral view of the spine reveals the lordotic curve in the lumbar region. **B)** Sagittal view of the pelvic bones showing the direction of the force of the heads, arms and trunk through the lumbar vertebrae to the sacrum. Notice the normal increased angle between L5 and S1, which promotes shear at this joint.

huge ligament to connect the ribs, vertebrae, and sacrum; the posterior intervertebral ligamentous system; and three trunk muscles. This fascial system provides humans with the unique ability to lift heavy weights overhead as well as to stabilize the trunk for throwing objects with high velocities.[13] Detailed anatomic description of the fascia and biomechanical considerations are presented by Bogduk and Macintosh.[28]

The thoracolumbar fascia is composed of anterior, middle, and posterior layers (Fig. 8.17A). The **anterior layer** is deep and attaches to the transverse processes of the lumbar vertebrae to cover the quadratus lumborum muscle. The **middle layer** is composed of strong, transverse fibers, attaching to the lumbar transverse processes medially, the 12th rib, and the transverse abdominis muscle at the lateral raphe (Gr., seam). The **posterior layer** covers the back and attaches to the spinous processes and the supraspinous ligament medially. Superiorly, the fascia blends with that of the splenius muscles and distally attaches to the sacrum and fuses with the fascia of the gluteal muscles (Fig. 8.17B). Laterally, the posterior layer attaches to the ribs and the ilia, and it forms attachments at the lateral raphe with the internal abdominal oblique muscle.

The posterior layer of the thoracodorsal fascia is further divided into superficial and deep lamina. The **superficial lamina** is the broad aponeurosis of the latissimus dorsi muscle whose fibers angle inferiorly and medially from the lateral raphe to attach the latissimus muscle to the spinous processes. The deep lamina is fused to the superficial lamina and crosses it in the opposite direction. Together they form a series of strong triangular structures with apices on the lateral raphe and bases covering two vertebral levels.[28] In addition, the thoracodorsal fascia provides a retinaculum (L., a net) to envelop the erector spinae and multifidus muscles.

These connections permit a number of forces to be applied to the lumbodorsal fascia, the spinous processes, and the posterior ligamentous system to contribute to lumbar extension and resistance to lumbar flexion. These forces include contraction of the latissimus dorsi muscles when the hands are fixed; contraction of the transverse abdominis and internal abdominal oblique muscles; contraction of the erector spinae to make the fascial envelope rigid; and the motion of forward bending as in leaning over to pick something up from the floor. The ways in which the thoracodorsal fascial system is thought to function are discussed later in this chapter in the section on forward bending and lifting.

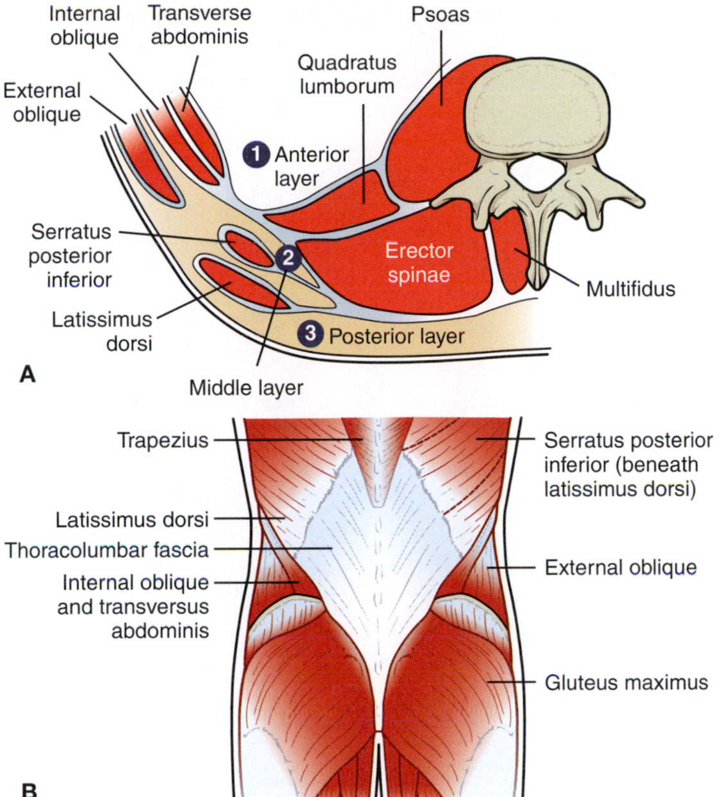

Figure 8.17 Thoracolumbar fascia. A) Cross-section showing the three layers of thoracolumbar fascia. B) Muscles attaching to the thoracolumbar fascia.

Sacrum

The sacrum is the link between the axial skeleton and the lower extremities. The sacrum connects to the lumbar spine at the lumbosacral junction, creating the L5–S1 joint. The sacrum has an intimate connection with the pelvic bones through the left and right sacroiliac joints. These joints along with the pelvic bones create a closed-ring system. The pelvic bones include the ischium, ilium, and pubis; these three bones form the socket portion of the most proximal lower extremity joint, the hip. The hip and pelvis are presented in Chapter 9. Only a cursory mention of the pelvis as it relates to sacral function is provided in this chapter.

Sacroiliac Joint

The sacroiliac joint (SIJ) was thought by ancient practitioners to be immobile except for slight motions occurring during pregnancy. In the 20th century, it was established that small motions in these joints occur in

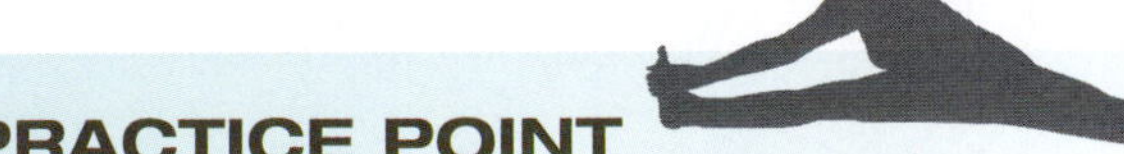

PRACTICE POINT

As we see, there are several important muscles that attach to the lumbosacral fascia. Some of the more important muscles include the gluteals, latissimus dorsi, transverse abdominis, internal obliques, multifidus, and erector spinae. Therefore, during clinical rehabilitation of individuals with back pain or injury, it is important to strengthen these muscles that attach to the lumbosacral fascia so both the muscles and lumbosacral fascia provide improved support of the lumbar spine. Likewise, part of the instructions to patients on proper lifting techniques should include tensing these muscles prior to lifting so additional lumbar support is provided and reduced lumbar spine stress occurs during the activity.

both men and women.[29–31] Because SIJ motions are small (1 to 3 mm) and difficult to measure, there is a tendency to consider the motions insignificant and unimportant. Many practitioners, however, consider injuries to the ligaments, hypermobility or hypomobility, and inflammatory conditions of the SIJ to be primary sources of low back pain,[29, 32, 33] with the most frequent problems occurring following childbirth.[31]

Type of Joint

Most authors classify the SIJ as a freely movable diarthrodial joint.[34–36] The sacral surface is covered in hyaline cartilage, and the iliac surface is covered in fibrocartilage. Synovial fluid is found in the joint cavity and the joint is covered with a capsule. With aging, the incidence of osteophytes and ankylosis of the SIJs is high, especially in men. Sashin[37] found gliding and anterior-posterior motion in the cadavers of men up to 30 years of age, slight motion in the cadavers of men up to 40 years, and ankylosis in most men older than 40. By contrast, slight motion was found in the cadavers of women up to 50 and 60 years of age, and none showed advanced ankylosis at any age.

Motions

Movements of the SIJ are small.[38] Although the joint's motions are small, the joint has three degrees of motion (Fig. 8.18). These motions include: 1) anterior-posterior rotation around a medial-lateral axis in a sagittal plane; 2) abduction-adduction around an anterior-posterior axis in a frontal plane; and 3) medial rotation-lateral rotation around a vertical axis in a transverse plane. In 32 fresh cadavers of persons who were under 29 years of age, Sashin[37] found superior-inferior gliding and slight anterior-posterior gliding of the sacrum on the fixed ilia or of the ilia on the fixed sacrum. The average combined motion of the SIJs was 4°, with a range from 2° to 8°. In a meta-analysis study, Goode and his associates[38] found in the seven manuscripts which were eligible for their study that maximal sacroiliac anterior-posterior rotation was just over 2°, motion around a vertical axis in a transverse plane was up to 8°, and rotation around an anterior-posterior axis in a frontal plane was up to 4°. Weisl[39] measured the movement of the sacral promontory radiographically in living people. He found that the greatest movement in the sacral promontory was 5.6 mm (±1.4mm) in the ventral direction when subjects moved from supine to a standing position. In another study, steel pins were imbedded in the posterior superior iliac spines of medical students by Colachis and his coworkers.[30] They found the greatest change between the right and left sides was 4 mm which occurred with movement from an erect standing position into full forward flexion.

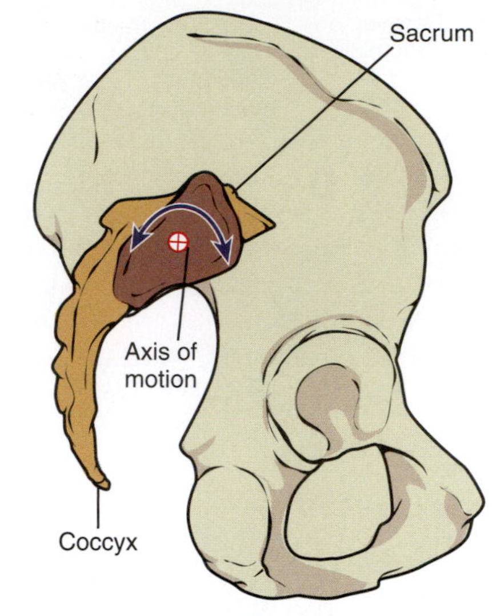

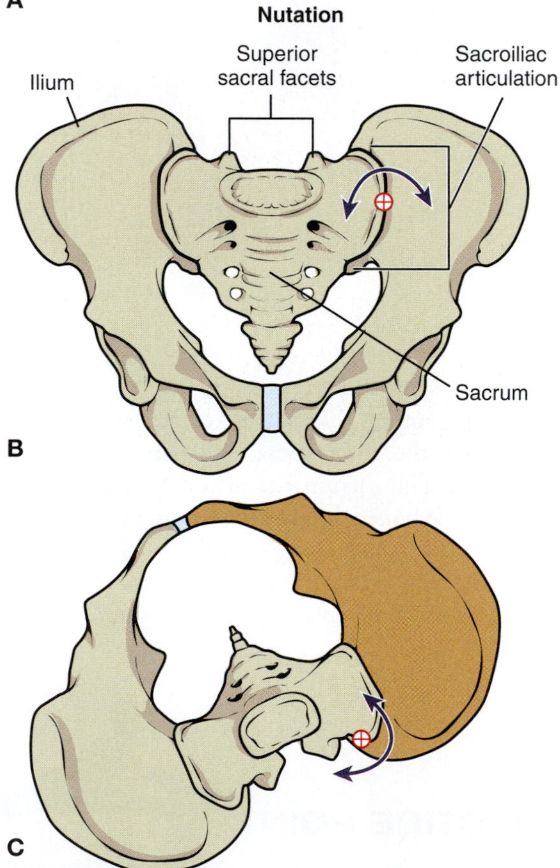

Figure 8.18 Motions of the SI joint. **A)** Anterior-posterior motion around a medial-lateral axis in the sagittal plane. **B)** Abduction-adduction around an anterior-posterior axis in the frontal plane. **C)** Medial rotation-lateral rotation around a vertical axis in the transverse plane.

Trigonometrically, the measurements indicate approximately 2° to 3.5° of movement per SI joint. Although the results of these studies vary, the important point of each of them is that the motions within the SI joint are small. That is not to say, however, that the SI joint should be ignored. Pathology in this joint is known to exist.[34, 40, 41]

As with several other segments of the body, unique motions occur at the sacrum that require use of distinctive terminology to define these motions. Kapandji[42] described the sacral motions of nutation (L., *nutare*, to nod) and counternutation. In **nutation**, the **promontory** on the base of the sacrum moves inferiorly and anteriorly while the distal aspect of the sacrum and the coccyx move posteriorly (Fig. 8.19A). In addition, the iliac crests are approximated and the ischial tuberosities move apart during nutation. Nutation causes the pelvic outlet to become larger. **Counternutation** is the opposite movement with the sacral promontory moving upward and posteriorly. Counternutation causes the coccyx to move anteriorly, the iliac crests to move apart, and the ischial tuberosities to approximate (Fig. 8.19B). Counternutation and its secondary motions enlarge the pelvic inlet. Secretion of the hormone relaxin during pregnancy causes ligamentous laxity and increases in the magnitude of the motions of the SIJs and the symphysis pubis.[35] Thus, the pelvic inlet becomes larger to accommodate the fetus, and the pelvic outlet becomes larger at birth. This excessive ligamentous laxity, however, can produce severe pain and sometimes spontaneous dislocation of the SIJs and the symphysis pubis. Following lactation, the secretion of relaxin ceases and the ligaments tighten up again. It is not uncommon to find that reapproximation of the joints occurs with an asymmetric alignment of the SIJs and the symphysis pubis, resulting in chronic low back and hip pain.

In standing and walking, the superincumbent weight of the HAT is distributed from the fifth lumbar vertebra to the sacrum, through the pelvis to the pubic symphysis and the heads of the femurs, and then down to the floor. In the sitting position, the weight is distributed to the

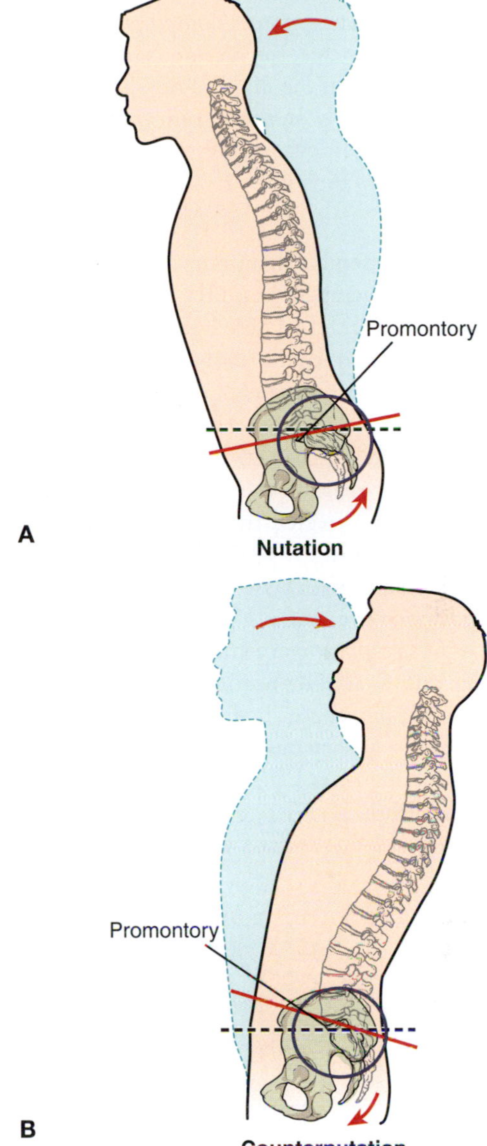

Figure 8.19 Nutation and counternutation of the sacrum. **A)** Nutation occurs when the promontory of the sacrum moves anteriorly and downward. **B)** Counternutation occurs with the posterior and upward motion of the sacral promontory.

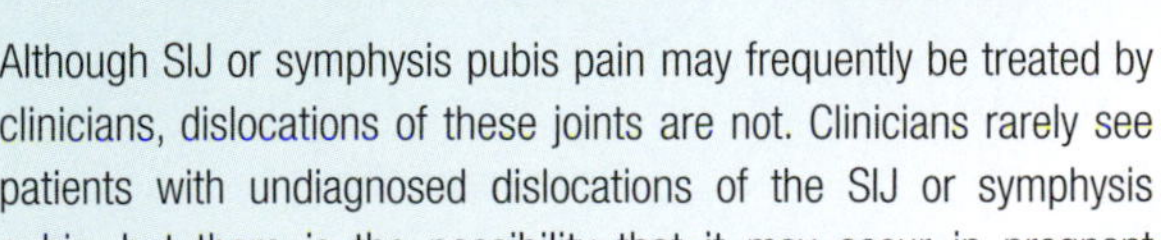

PRACTICE POINT

Although SIJ or symphysis pubis pain may frequently be treated by clinicians, dislocations of these joints are not. Clinicians rarely see patients with undiagnosed dislocations of the SIJ or symphysis pubis, but there is the possibility that it may occur in pregnant women. Dislocations of the SI joints or symphysis pubis are serious and very painful conditions. Pain is localized and intense with any movements. Weight-bearing is especially painful, particularly when standing on one leg. This condition requires referral to a physician.

pubic symphysis and the ischial tuberosities and then to the seat of the chair. These forces compress the sacrum and ilia together; in essence, the sacrum is driven distally and anteriorly between the ilia, and the ilia are driven proximally and posteriorly on the sacrum (Fig. 8.20). An extensive, strong ligamentous system limits these motions and stabilizes the joints.[36]

Ligaments

Posteriorly, interosseous ligaments fill the space between the lateral sacral crest and the inner side of the iliac tuberosity (Fig. 8.21B). These ligaments have multidirectional fibers and cover about one half of the length of the joint. Several layers of short and long posterior sacroiliac ligaments cover the interosseous ligaments and the posterior aspect of the sacrum. These attach on the tuberosity of the ilia (to the posterior gluteal line) and are directed medially and distally to attach on the sacrum. On the ventral side are the anterior sacroiliac ligaments, which are thin and not as extensive as the posterior ligaments (Fig. 8.21A). The anterior and posterior sacroiliac ligaments suspend the sacrum from the ilia, and as weight-bearing drives the sacrum distally on the ilia, these ligaments act as shock absorbers. This suspensory mechanism has caused some authors to describe the SIJs as nonweight-bearing joints.[43] In addition, the length of these ligaments places limits on the motion of counternutation. The strong anterior longitudinal ligament, which covers the lumbar vertebrae and attaches to the sacrum and the iliolumbar ligaments, has been discussed with the vertebrae.

The sacrotuberous and the sacrospinous ligaments are broad, long ligaments connecting the lower aspect of the sacrum to the tuberosity and spine of the ischium (Fig. 8.21). These ligaments have excellent leverage to hold the distal aspect of the sacrum in place against

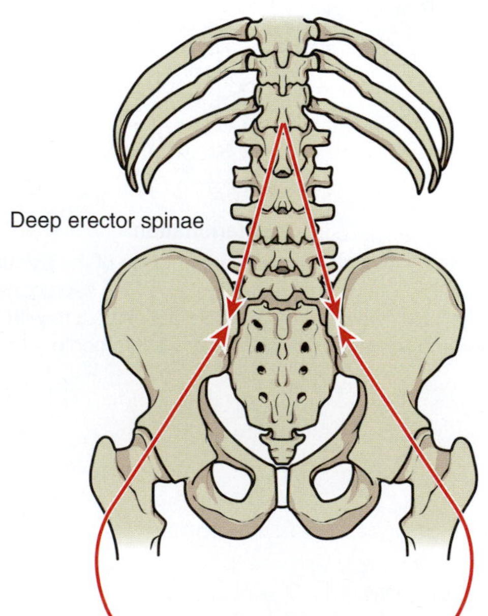

Figure 8.20 Compressive forces in the SI joint. Forces compress the sacrum and ilia together, driving the sacrum distally and anteriorly between the ilia and driving the ilia proximally and posteriorly on the sacrum.

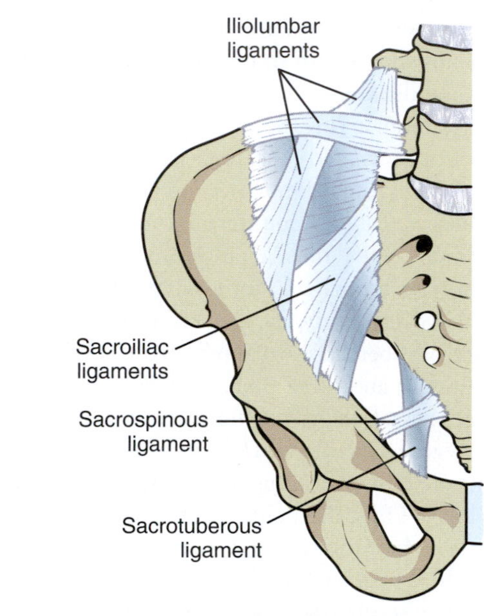

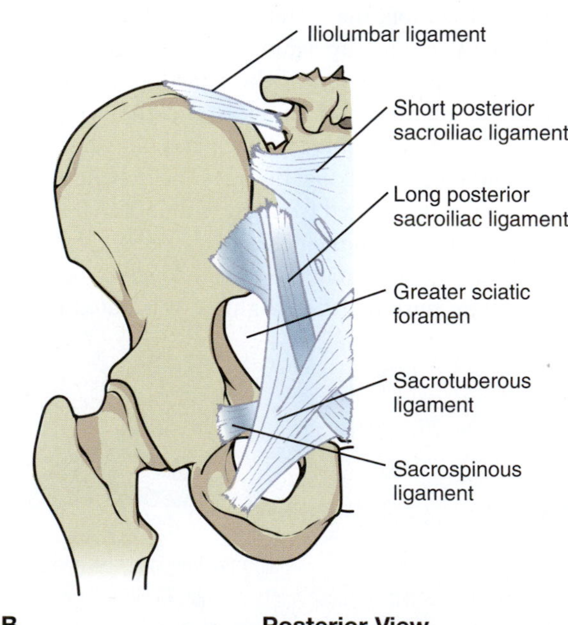

Figure 8.21 SI ligaments. A) Anterior view of sacroiliac ligaments. B) Posterior view of sacroiliac ligaments.

the anterior weight-bearing forces that tend to cause the sacral promontory to tilt anteriorly and inferiorly. The length of these ligaments controls the amount of nutation that is possible. The sacrotuberous ligament is palpated lateral to the coccyx and superior and medial to the ischial tuberosities. It is palpated as a thick cord angling from the ischial tuberosity medially and superiorly toward the base of the sacrum at about a 30° to 45° angle.

The combination of its bony architecture and its strong and extensive ligamentous system creates a self-locking mechanism for the SI joint. As forces increase to cause downward movement of the sacrum on the ilia, the posterior ligaments tighten and pull the ilia closer together like a clamp.

Symphysis Pubis

Articulating surfaces of the pubic bones are covered by hyaline cartilage and separated by fibrocartilaginous discs. The joint is protected by strong ligaments on all sides, and the fibrocartilage is reinforced by the attachments of the rectus abdominis, pyramidalis, and internal abdominal oblique muscles. The symphysis pubis completes the closure of the ring of the pelvic articulations of the sacrum and the innominate bones (Fig. 8.22). Thus, even small motions occurring at the SIJs must be accompanied by motion at the symphysis pubis. Generally, there is little motion at this joint. However, excessive forces may occur to produce injury or dislocation of the SIJ and the symphysis pubis. These forces can occur with landing on the feet from a jump, hitting the knees on the dashboard in an auto accident, walking with a leg-length discrepancy, or having a forceful motion of hip flexion suddenly obstructed as with a blocked football kick.

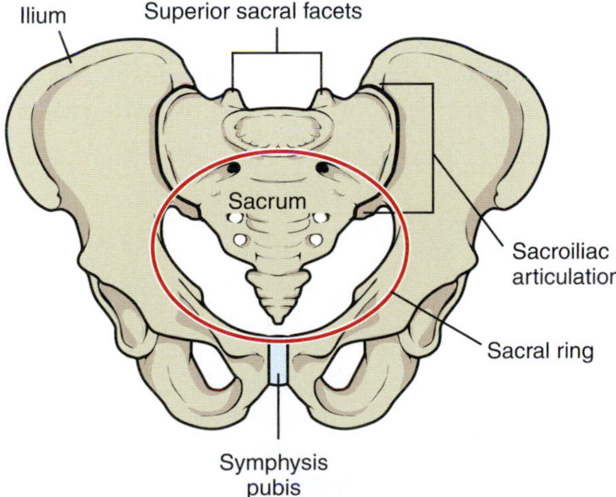

Figure 8.22 The sacral ring forms a closed unit of the pelvis. Since it is a closed unit, small movements at one joint within the ring affect other joints within the ring.

Coccygeal Joints

The sacrococcygeal and the intercoccygeal joints are classified as synarthroidal joints. Synarthroidal joints are defined as a line of fusion between bones that are separated in early development then later totally fuse.[44] The base of the coccyx joins the apex of the triangular sacrum at the sacrococcygeal joint. This joint is highly congruent, having a fibrocartilaginous disc and is completely surrounded by several small strong ligaments called the sacrococcygeal ligaments. There is a slight amount of passive anterior-posterior motion available that occurs only during defecation and labor at the time of childbirth. The joint actually fuses as part of the normal aging process. The intercoccygeal joints are the small articulations between the distal three vertebrae. These are typically fused by adulthood and no motion occurs there.[45]

Pelvic Balance

The rigid sacrum, firmly connected with the ilia, is part of the pelvis. The pelvis, interposed between the lower extremities and the flexible portions of the vertebral column, possesses movements of its own. Because of the firmness of the sacroiliac and lumbosacral junctions, however, whenever the pelvis moves, the spine also moves, especially in the lumbar region. Therefore, if the pelvis moves, it impacts the lumbar spine, and likewise, if the lumbar spine moves, then the pelvis is affected. Similarly, because the pelvis attaches to the hip, movement of either the hip or the pelvis affects the other.[46, 47] The relationship between the hip and pelvis is presented in Chapter 9.

Muscles

Head, neck, and trunk muscles are paired with a muscle on each side of the midline. When both of the paired muscles contract to produce movement, the motion is forward or backward bending in the sagittal plane. If only one of the muscles contracts, side bending or rotation occurs in the frontal or transverse planes. Most of the time, the neck and trunk muscles cocontract during activities to stabilize the vertebrae. Cocontraction of these paired muscles allows them to withstand applied weight, extremity muscle contractions, and ground reaction forces.

Kinesiologic knowledge of functions of the superficial muscles of the neck and trunk is almost equal to our knowledge of extremity musculature. Evidentiary knowledge of the actions and functions of the deep neck and trunk musculature, on the other hand, is limited because the three to five layers of muscles make it difficult to differentiate the individual muscles by manual palpation or surface electrode (EMG) recording. Most research performed on the axial skeleton muscles has utilized surface electrodes. Fine-wire electrodes are required to investigate activity of deeper muscles, but many research labs are either not equipped to perform fine-wire electrode investigations or do not have personnel qualified in fine-wire electrode application. Additionally, confirmation that the correct muscle has been inserted with the fine-wire electrode can be difficult. For these reasons, many unanswered questions regarding deeper axial skeleton muscles and their functions remain.

Anterior Cervical Muscles

There are several anterior cervical muscles that perform various functions, depending on whether the motion requires unilateral or bilateral muscle activity. When working bilaterally, the primary actions of these cervical muscles is head or neck flexion. Evidence now also points to the fact that these muscles, especially the smaller muscles which lie closer to the axes of motion, act as stabilizers or provide proprioception.[51] The cervical muscles along with their proximal and distal insertions, innervations, actions, and methods of palpation are identified in Table 8–5.

Primary Neck Flexors

With the exception of the sternocleidomastoid, muscles of the anterior neck can be paired with other muscles that are close in either function or location. These muscles include:

- Rectus capitis anterior and rectus capitis lateralis
- Longus capitis and longus colli
- Anterior, middle, and posterior scalenes

These muscles will be briefly presented here; Table 8–5 contains each muscle's specific information.

Of the two short **rectus capitis anterior** and **rectus capitis lateralis muscles,** the rectus capitis lateralis has excellent leverage for medial-lateral control of the head or lateral flexion with unilateral contraction. Fibers of the **longus capitis** cover the rectus capitis anterior. The **longus colli** is a complex three-part muscle covering the anterolateral surface of the vertebrae from the arch of the atlas to the third thoracic vertebra. Basmajian[50] states that EMG studies show the longus colli to be a strong flexor of the cervical spine. He hypothesized that the increase in longus colli activity found during talking, coughing, and swallowing represents stabilization of the neck for these functions. In addition to its anatomic action, more recent evidence has identified a substantial number of muscle spindles in the longus colli, suggesting that the muscle has a proprioceptive function as well.[51]

The **scalene muscles** (Gr., *skalenos,* uneven triangle) have **superior attachments** on the transverse processes of the lower six cervical vertebrae and **inferior attachments** on the anterior inner border of the first or second rib (scalene posterior). The superior attachments of the scalenes are adjacent to the inferior attachments of the longus capitis and the oblique portions of the longus colli so that there are direct lines of pull from the anterior aspects of the occiput through the cervical vertebrae to the first and second ribs.

The ventral roots of C_5–T_1 spinal nerves and the subclavian artery and vein pass between the scalenus anterior and the scalenus medius and above the first rib. Anatomic variation, hypertrophy, or spasm of these muscles can cause compression of the vessels or nerve roots, resulting in pain and dysfunction. This has been termed **thoracic outlet syndrome.**

The **sternocleidomastoid muscles (SCM)** are the most superficial of the anterior neck muscles

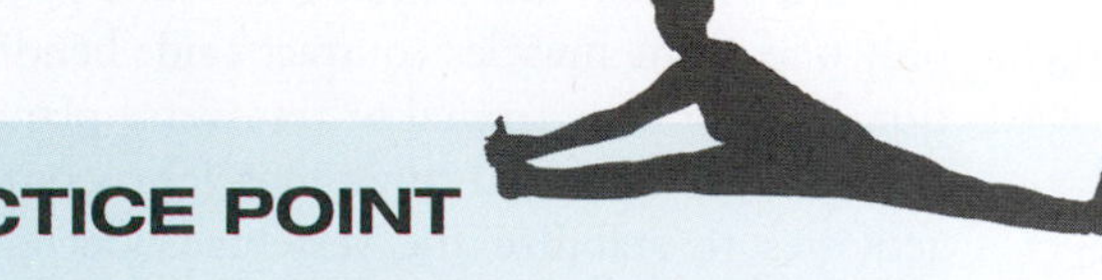

PRACTICE POINT

Results of current research investigations combined with theory have provided clinicians with a foundation of spine muscle function and methods to rehabilitate pathological dysfunctions in this area. Rehabilitation of acute and chronic lumbar sprains and strains now incorporate exercises that develop two types of muscle functions: trunk movement and trunk stabilization. The superficial trunk muscles such as the rectus abdominis and the erector spinae are the "movers" of the trunk whereas the deeper muscles, including the multifidus, transverse abdominis, and internal obliques, are the "stabilizers." As with extremity rehabilitation, the stabilizers are strengthened in advance of the mover muscles since stabilization is crucial before movement may occur safely and effectively.

(text continues on page 341)

TABLE 8–5 | MUSCLES OF THE CERVICAL SPINE

Group	Muscle	Proximal Insertion	Distal Insertion	Innervation	Action	Palpation/ Inspection
Anterior cervical muscles	Rectus capitis anterior	Base of the skull, immediately anterior to the occipital condyle	Anterior surface of C1	C1–C2	Flexes head but the muscle's line of pull may make it a poorly positioned flexor and a better head stabilizer or provider of proprioception.	Too deep to palpate.
Anterior cervical muscles	Rectus capitis lateralis	Occipital bone's jugular process	C1 transverse process	C1–C2	Stabilizes head and may provide proprioceptive feedback. It is able to provide medial-lateral control of the head.	Too deep to palpate.
Anterior cervical muscles	Longus capitis	Basilar portion of the occipital bone	Transverse processes of C3–C6	C1–C3	Bilaterally, the muscles produce head and neck flexion. Unilaterally, they produce lateral bending and rotation. Because they are close to the axis of motion, they provide significant joint compression.	They cover the rectus capitis. The longus capitis is palpated with the longus colli; see below for palpation description.

continued

TABLE 8-5 | MUSCLES OF THE CERVICAL SPINE—cont'd

Group	Muscle	Proximal Insertion	Distal Insertion	Innervation	Action	Palpation/ Inspection
Anterior cervical muscles	Longus colli	Anterior tubercle of C1, bodies of C1–C3, and transverse processes of C3–C6	Bodies of C5 through T3, transverse processes of C3–C5.	C2–C6	Cervical flexion. It works with the longus capitis to stabilize the head, especially when the upper trapezius moves the scapula.	Place your fingers medially and deep to the sternocleidomastoid (SCM) muscle near the anterolateral surface of the cervical vertebrae. Have the subject rotate the head to the same side to relax the SCM and then resist neck flexion with the other hand so that the muscle contraction can be felt by the palpating fingers.
Anterior cervical muscles	Anterior scalene	C4–C6 transverse processes	First rib	C4–C6	Bilaterally: forward flex the cervical spine. If the C/S is stabilized, elevates the first rib. Unilaterally: laterally flexes neck and rotates to same side.	Palpate just above the clavicle and behind the SCM.

Anterior cervical muscles	Middle scalene	Posterior aspects of C4–C6 transverse processes	Superior aspect of first rib	C3–C8	Bilaterally: forward flex cervical spine. Unilaterally: laterally flexes neck and rotates to same side. Elevates first rib during forced inspiration.	Palpated immediately lateral to anterior scalene, just above the clavicle.
Anterior cervical muscles	Posterior scalene	Posterior aspects of C4–C6 transverse processes	Anterior aspect of second rib	C7–C8	Bilaterally: flexes neck forward. Unilaterally: laterally flexes neck and rotates to same side. Elevates second rib during forced inspiration.	
Anterior cervical muscles	Sternocleidomastoid (SCM) 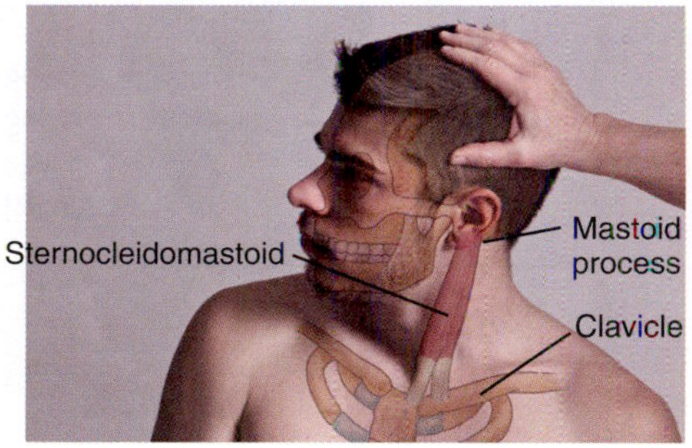 Sternocleidomastoid Mastoid process Clavicle	1) Upper border of manubrium of the sternum and 2) upper border of the clavicle	Mastoid process of temporal bone and superior nuchal line of occipital bone	Spinal accessory nerve (XI) C1–C3	Bilaterally: forward flexes the neck so chin thrusts forward when other muscles function to stabilize. Unilaterally: rotates neck to opposite side, lateral flexion to same side, extension of head and neck.	Easily observed when the subject rotates the head to the opposite side; it becomes the most prominent muscle of the anterior neck.

continued

TABLE 8-5 | MUSCLES OF THE CERVICAL SPINE—cont'd

Group	Muscle	Proximal Insertion	Distal Insertion	Innervation	Action	Palpation/ Inspection
Posterior cervical suboccipital muscles	Rectus capitis posterior major Rectus capitis posterior minor Inferior oblique Superior oblique	**RCP Major:** spinous process of axis. **RCP Minor:** Just above the atlas. IO & SO: axis spinous/transverse process.	**Rectus capitis major & minor:** inferior nuchal line of occiput. Inferior & superior oblique: occiput.	C1 (suboccipital nerve)	Bilaterally: head extension at atlanto-occipital joint. Unilaterally: lateral flexion and atlantoaxial joint rotation.	Palpated with finger tips when the subject is supine and the neck muscles are relaxed.
Posterior transversospinal muscles	Rotators Multifidus Semispinalis capitis Semispinalis cervicis	**Rotators:** Transverse process of 1 vertebra. **Multifidus:** Transverse processes of 2–5 vertebrae. **Semispinalis capitis & cervicis:** Transverse processes of T1–T6.	**Rotators:** the base of the spinous process above. **Multifidus:** Spinous processes above. **Semispinalis capitis:** above the inferior nuchal line. **Semispinalis cervicis:** C2–C5 Spinous processes.	Dorsal rami of spinal nerves	Bilaterally: extend head and neck. Unilaterally: laterally flex and rotate head to same side.	**Rotators:** deepest; **Multifidus:** covers the rotators; **semispinalis muscles:** most superficial of this group. Best palpated with the subject supine and the neck muscles relaxed. Difficult to palpate because of overlying muscles.

(Fig. 8.23). Most anatomic texts state that the bilateral action of the SCM is neck flexion. However, Kapandji[1] points out that the SCM, which spans the entire length of the cervical spinal segment, requires synergistic contractions of the vertebral muscles to stabilize the cervical spine so that the SCM can flex the cervical spine. In the absence of these synergistic contractions, isolated bilateral contraction of the sternocleidomastoid muscle causes extension of the head and an increase in the lordotic cervical curve. Normal unilateral contraction of the SCM causes ipsilateral side bending and contralateral rotation.

Because of the sternocleidomastoid's attachments on the sternoclavicular joint, the left and right SCM are considered accessory muscles of inspiration. Persons with attacks of asthma or other respiratory distress exhibit contractions of the SCM and other accessory muscles on inspiration.

Accessory Neck Flexors

A large number of small muscles essential for chewing, swallowing, and speaking also are classified as accessory neck flexors. These include the **platysma, suprahyoid muscles** (digastric, stylohyoid, mylohyoid, and geniohyoid), and **infrahyoid muscles** (sternohyoid, thyrohyoid, sternothyroid, and omohyoid). The primary function of these muscles is to position the hyoid bone, thyroid cartilage, and mandible. When the jaw is stabilized by the masseter muscles bilaterally, the suprahyoid and infrahyoid muscles will contract against resistance to neck flexion. With paralysis of the long neck flexors, however, the accessory muscles produce some stabilization of the neck, but they do not have sufficient leverage to lift the head when the body is in the supine position. Additionally, because these muscles contract ineffectively during inspiration, they are unable to offer assistance when a person is in respiratory distress.

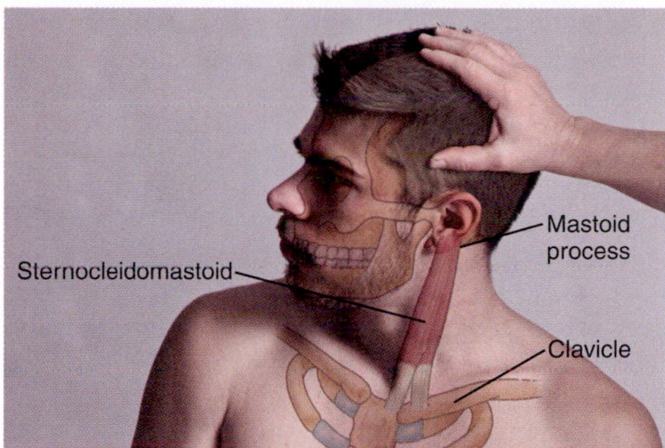

Figure 8.23 Testing the sternocleidomastoid muscle unilaterally. For strong activation of the left sternocleidomastoid muscle, the head is rotated to the right and resistance is given to lateral flexion of the head to the left.

Posterior Cervical Muscles

Numerous muscles are on the posterior aspect of the cervical spine. This group of posterior muscles has considerably more bulk than the anterior group, indicating that greater strength is needed to maintain neck extension. Cervical nerves exit between these posterior muscles and are sometimes compressed by the muscles, causing tension headaches or neck and shoulder pain.

Suboccipital Muscles

These four short, deep muscles connect the upper two cervical vertebrae and the occipital bone. They include the **rectus capitis posterior major, rectus capitis posterior minor, inferior oblique,** and **superior oblique** muscles. These and the short anterior muscles are thought to provide precise fine control of head posture.

Transversospinal Muscles

The transversospinal muscles are so named because they attach between the transverse and spinous processes. These four pairs of muscles include the **rotators,**

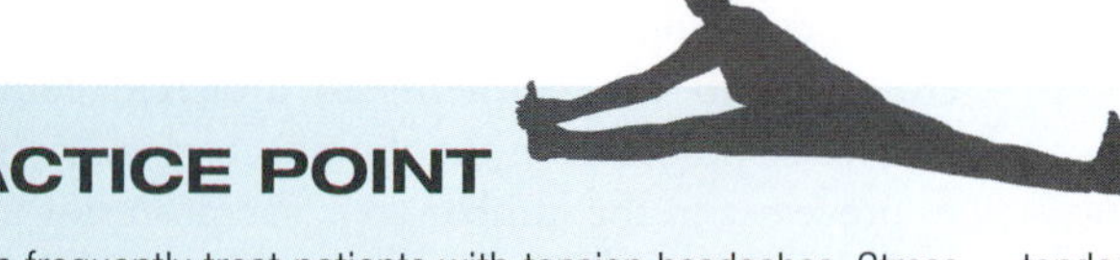

PRACTICE POINT

Clinicians frequently treat patients with tension headaches. Stress is the primary culprit, which causes sustained tension in the neck and upper back muscles. With persistent muscle tension, patients will report pain in these muscles and headaches. A tension headache typically produces pain in the frontal and/or temporal head regions. The clinician is able to palpate painful areas of tenderness, spasm, or trigger/tender points in cervical muscles. The muscles most often causing tension headaches include the suboccipital, transversospinal, erector spinae, and scalene muscles. Since one or more of these muscles may cause the patient's headaches, assessment of each of them is necessary before effective treatment begins.

multifidus (L., *multifid,* many parts), and the most superficial of these muscles, the **semispinalis capitis** and **cervicis.**

Erector Spinae Muscles

A large number of posterior spinal muscles are collectively called **erector spinae,** or **sacrospinalis muscles.** These muscles are continuous from the sacrum to the occiput, and their combined action is vertebral extension or prevention of flexion (Fig. 8.24). Medially-to-laterally from the spinous processes, their alignment is the **spinales, longissimus,** and **iliocostalis.** These three muscles are subtitled according to the area of the spine in which they are located with the muscle name first and the spinal segment second. The erector spinae muscle groups are identified from head to sacrum as **capitis, cervicis, thoracis** (dorsi), or **lumborum.** Not all erector spinae muscles occur in each of these segments. For example, there is a longissimus thoracis, longissimus cervicis, and a longissimus capitis but no longissimus lumborum.

The cervical erector spinae muscles include all three muscles. These are named the iliocostalis cervicis, longissimus capitis, longissimus cervicis, splenius capitis, and splenius cervicis. The **iliocostalis cervicis** is the most lateral of the cervical erector spinae muscles. The **longissimus capitis** and **cervicis** lie just medial to the iliocostalis cervicis. The most superficial and medial layer of the cervical erector spinae is the **splenius capitis** and **cervicis.** All of these muscles are covered by the upper trapezius and the levator scapulae, which can exert forces on the head and cervical spine as well as on the scapula. These muscles are described with the shoulder in Chapter 5.

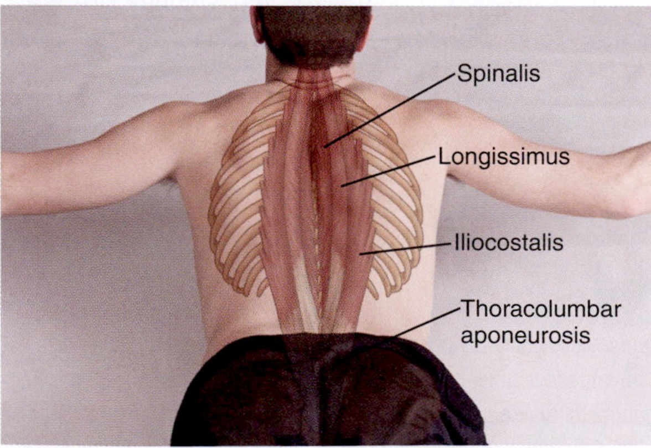

Figure 8.24 Although the erector spinae group runs throughout the length of the spine, it is best observed in the lumbar region. In the thoracic region, this group is covered by the rhomboids and the trapezius.

Posterior Thoracic and Lumbar Muscles

Many of the muscles in the posterior thoracic and lumbar regions of the spine are extensions of the posterior cervical muscles. The thoracic and lumbar areas also contain muscles that are unique to them and either affect the shoulder complex or work directly on the spine. Many of the deeper muscles have short moment arms so they are unable to provide significant motion but do work to stabilize the spine. The larger muscles that lie more distally from the spine's axes of motions are responsible for producing spinal movement.

Deep Muscles of the Back

The intrinsic muscles of the back are continuous with the posterior cervical muscles and include the deep transversospinal group and the more superficial erector spinae group. Their functions are to control the amount of extension and to prevent collapse of the vertebral column. These muscles are assisted in their functions by the quadratus lumborum, psoas major, latissimus dorsi, internal abdominal oblique, and transverse abdominis muscles as well as the thoracodorsal fascia.

Transversospinal Muscles

As in the cervical region, the transversospinal muscles are multiple, small intrinsic muscles of the thoracic and lumbar regions that lie between transverse or spinous processes, or both. Each muscle has fasciculi (L., small bundles) crossing from one to five vertebral segments. Actions of the **intertransversarii** and the **interspinalis** muscles are theorized from their mechanical lines of pull to include lateral flexion and extension of the trunk. However, these muscles have a very small cross-sectional area and poor leverage because their attachments are near the axis of motion, so it seems unlikely that these muscles produce sufficient forces or torques that are required for trunk movement or stabilization. Some investigators have proposed that these small muscles really function in proprioception to provide precise monitoring of intervertebral positions and length-tension relationships of muscles.[24, 52, 53]

The **multifidus muscles** are composed of fasciculi from a common tendon on the spinous processes, which cross two to five segments to attach distally on the transverse processes in the thoracic region, the mammary processes in the lumbar area, the posterior iliac crest, and the sacrum. The deep **rotators** are often included with the multifidus in the thoracic region. In the lumbar region, the multifidus has been categorized as having superficial and deep fibers.[54] The superficial fibers cross up to five segments whereas the deep fibers cross a maximum of two segments. Given their length and, hence, leverage, coupled with their nearly vertical line of pull which is at right angles to the spinous processes, the superficial fibers are capable of exerting high torques in lumbar extension. Conversely, because of the shorter span of the deep fibers, they act closer to the axis of rotation, so they function to provide local compression and, therefore, stability of the respective segments.[55] Research has identified preferential activation of the superficial and deep fibers of the multifidus.[56] In addition to providing local stability, the deep fasciculi of the multifidus also attach to the capsule of the facet joints; this capsular attachment allows the multifidus to protect the capsule from being nipped in movement.[57]

Thoracic and Lumbar Erector Spinae Muscles

Thoracolumbar erector spinae muscles have an extensive area of origin from their distal insertions. Strong tendons and fascia anchor the erector spinae or sacrospinalis distally to the spinous processes from T-11 through S-5, the sacrum, the sacrotuberous and sacroiliac ligaments, the posterior iliac crest, and muscle fibers of the gluteus maximus. From these attachments, deep and superficial muscles ascend through the lumbar, thoracic, and cervical areas. The deep part of the **longissimus lumborum** and the **iliocostalis lumborum** consist of muscle fascicles attaching near the posterior superior iliac spine and crest of the ilium. Their fascicles are lateral to the multifidus, with the longissimus attaching to the medial part of the lumbar transverse processes and the iliocostalis attaching to the tips from L-1 to L-4. Porterfield and DeRosa[24] suggest that in addition to spinal motion, these muscles function to provide strong stabilization and compression of the lumbar vertebrae on the ilium as well as posterior shear forces, particularly in the lower lumbar area.

Superficial to these muscles are the **longissimus thoracis** and the **iliocostalis thoracis.** These muscles have long tendons which arise from the sacrum, iliac crest, and lumbar spinous processes. Muscle fascicles arise on the tendons; the longissimus thoracis attaches to all the ribs and transverse processes of the thoracic vertebrae whereas the iliocostalis thoracis attaches to the lower six to eight ribs. The long tendons in the lumbar area form the aponeurosis that covers the deep layer of the erector spinae.[53]

Quadratus Lumborum

The **quadratus lumborum** is a large muscle on the posterior abdominal wall. The muscle lies between the posterior iliac crest and the 12th rib, lateral to the erector spinae attachments on the iliac crest. When an individual stands in an erect position and laterally flexes the trunk to the left or right side, the trunk lowering movement occurs from an eccentric contraction of the contralateral quadratus lumborum, and the return movement to the upright position is the result of a concentric contraction on the same muscle. The muscle is also in part responsible for hiking the ipsilateral hip; other muscles may assist in this activity, including the erector spinae and lateral abdominal muscles. If the humerus is stabilized, the latissimus dorsi may also assist in hip hiking. Additionally, the quadratus lumborum has excellent leverage and size to prevent collapse of the vertebral column in the frontal plane (i.e., **scoliosis**).

Anterior and Lateral Trunk Muscles

In addition to functioning as supporters of the abdominal viscera and breathing, the anterior and lateral trunk muscles (Table 8–7) move the trunk in flexion, lateral bending, and rotation. They consist of large sheaths of muscles in several layers. The fibers of the various layers run in different directions, a factor that contributes to the strength of the combined layers. A similar fiber arrangement is seen in the thoracic region: The external and internal intercostals represent two layers corresponding to the external and internal oblique abdominal muscles.

The linea alba is a fibrous band in the median line of the abdominal region, extending from the xiphoid process above to the pubis below. This line unites the aponeuroses of the muscles of the right and left sides.

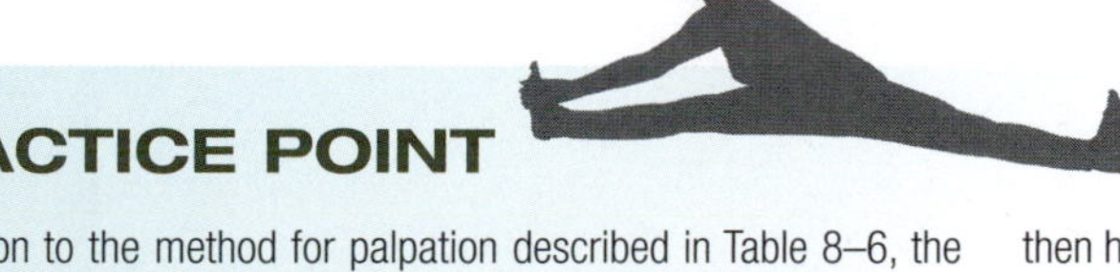

PRACTICE POINT

In addition to the method for palpation described in Table 8–6, the erector spinae may also be palpated with the subject in erect standing. In this position, the effect of swaying the trunk forward and backward is realized. While palpating the left and right erector spinae, have the subject sway forward and feel the muscles tense; then have the subject sway backward to feel the muscles relax. They may also be palpated in lateral bending and in trunk rotation. In walking and single-leg stance, the erector spinae contralateral to the weight-bearing leg are active.

(text continues on page 347)

TABLE 8-6 | MUSCLES OF THE ENTIRE SPINAL COLUMN

Group	Muscle	Inferior attachments	Superior attachments	Innervation	Action	Palpation/Inspection
Erector spinae, cervical section 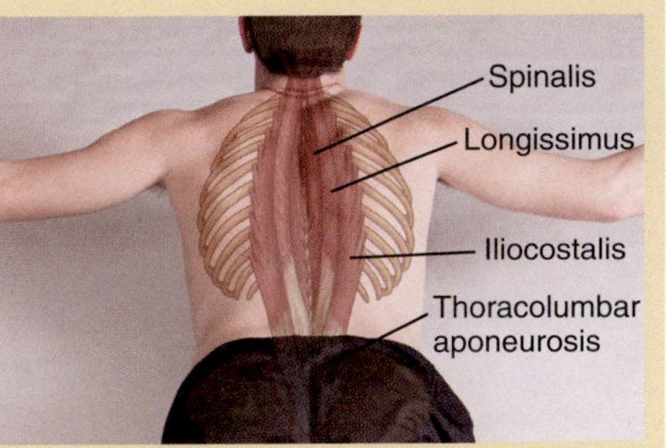	Iliocostalis cervicis	Angles of third to sixth ribs	C4–C6 transverse processes	C1–T4	Bilaterally: extend the cervical spine. Unilaterally: laterally flex the cervical spine. Some of these muscles may be aligned to also provide cervical rotation.	These muscles are difficult to palpate individually but are easy to palpate as a group. They are the most superficial of the posterior cervical muscles and form parallel ridges on either side of the spinous processes.
	Longissimus capitis & cervicis	Upper 5 thoracic transverse processes	Mastoid process and C2–C6 transverse processes			
	Splenius capitis & cervicis	Lower part of ligamentum nuchae and T1–T3 spinous processes	Splenius capitis: mastoid process and superior nuchal line. Splenius cervicis: upper cervical vertebrae's transverse processes			
Intrinsic back muscles: Transversospinals	Intertransversarii	One transverse process of a vertebra	One transverse process of an adjacent upper vertebra			

Intrinsic back muscles: Transversospinals	Interspinous	One spinous process of a vertebra	One spinous process of an adjacent upper vertebra on either side of the interspinous ligament	Dorsal rami of spinal nerves	Propriocept-ors of movement and position.	Palpated as the erector spinae group.
Intrinsic back muscles: Transversospinals	Multifidus	Cross 4-5 segments to attach distally on transverse processes in T/S, mammary processes in lumbar area, posterior iliac crest, sacrum.	A common tendon on the entire spinous processes	Dorsal rami of spinal nerves	Local spinal stability. Deep fasciculi of the muscle also protects the capsule from being pinched during movement.	Too deep to palpate.
Intrinsic back muscles: Transversospinals	Rotators	Transverse process of one vertebra	Root of spinous process of next 1-2 vertebrae superiorly	Dorsal rami of spinal nerves	Bilaterally: Local spinal stability. Unilaterally: Rotation to the same side.	This is the deepest of the transversospinal muscles. Too deep to palpate.

continued

TABLE 8-6 | MUSCLES OF THE ENTIRE SPINAL COLUMN—cont'd

Group	Muscle	Inferior attachments	Superior attachments	Innervation	Action	Palpation/Inspection
Erector spinae: Thoracic & Lumbar	Iliocostalis thoracis & iliocostalis lumborum		Upward to lower ribs and transverse processes			
	Longissimus thoracis & longissimus lumborum	Broad tendon and fascia from T11–S5, sacrum, sacrotuberous & sacroiliac ligaments, posterior iliac crest, gluteus maximus muscle fibers	Upward to ribs and transverse processes	Dorsal rami of spinal nerves	Bilaterally: extend spine. Unilaterally: laterally flex spine.	Action of the erector spinae as a group may be observed best in the lumbar and lower thoracic regions when the subject, in the prone position, raises the upper part of the body off the floor.
	Spinalis thoracis & spinalis lumborum		Upward to spinous processes			
	Quadratus lumborum	Iliac crest lateral to erector spinae attachments	12th rib and L1–L3 transverse processes	T12–L3	Depresses 12th rib. Laterally flexes the trunk.	With the subject supine, the palpating fingers are positioned above the iliac crest just lateral to the erector spinae attachments. The subject "hikes" the hip to activate the muscle.

Rectus Abdominis

The **rectus abdominis** is a superficial muscle and consists of two parts, one on each side of the linea alba. The longitudinally arranged muscle fibers are interrupted by three tendinous inscriptions (L., a mark or line), the lowest one at or slightly below the level of the umbilicus (Fig. 8.25). Because of this tendinous arrangement, this muscle is commonly referred to as the "six-pack" muscle. In the subject shown in Figure 8.25, the lowest inscription is well below the level of the umbilicus, and three "muscle hills" above this inscription can be seen. The widest portion of the linea alba is above the umbilicus. The lowest portion of the rectus is usually uninterrupted by inscriptions; however, in the illustration, the lowest portion of the rectus is hidden by the subject's shorts.

External Abdominal Oblique

The **external abdominal oblique muscle** constitutes the superficial layer of the abdominal wall (Fig. 8.26). It is located lateral to the rectus abdominis and covers the anterior and lateral regions of the abdomen. To activate the muscle on the left side, the trunk is rotated to the right; the muscle on the right side contracts in trunk rotation to the left. Bilateral action helps to produce flexion of the trunk without rotation. The external abdominal oblique muscles are also active bilaterally when one is "straining" or coughing.

Internal Abdominal Oblique

The **internal abdominal oblique muscle,** which is covered by the external abdominal oblique, belongs to the second layer of the lateral abdominal wall. The muscle extends essentially over the same area as the externus, but its fibers run at right angles to those of the external oblique. As the muscle fans out from its proximal to distal insertion, the direction of the fibers is continuous with those of the internal intercostals. Although the muscle is not easily palpated because it lies beneath the external abdominal oblique, its performance may be observed when the subject performs a rotational sit-up. In this activity as shown in Figure 8.26, the line of action of the external abdominal oblique on the left side and the internal abdominal oblique on the right side is a continuous one, both muscles contributing to the rotation.

Transverse Abdominis

The transverse abdominis is the innermost layer of the abdominal wall. This muscle has been named the "corset muscle" because it encloses the abdominal cavity like a corset. The direction of its fibers is transverse. From a clinical perspective, it has been identified that impairments of the transverse abdominis (and multifidus) are evident in patients with low back pain.[58]

The transverse abdominis is partly responsible for tension produced when the abdominal wall is tightened, an activity which involves all the layers of the abdominal wall.

External and Internal Intercostals

The **external and internal intercostal muscles,** as their names indicate, are located between the ribs. They may be looked upon as the thoracic continuation of the external and internal oblique abdominal muscles. Each intercostal muscle extends between two adjacent ribs, but all of them together compose a two-layered muscle sheath enclosing the thoracic cavity. The internal intercostals are deeper to and run at right angles to the external

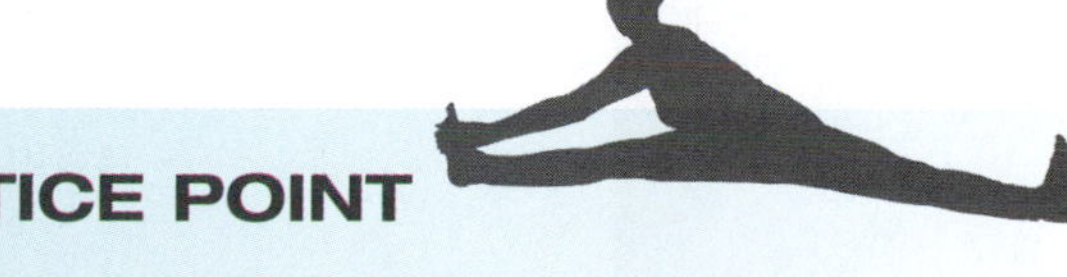

PRACTICE POINT

Through the results of investigative studies, clinicians have learned that the transverse abdominis is an important muscle in the prevention and treatment of low back pain. Although a patient may have a strong rectus abdominis, it does not mean he or she has sufficient transverse abdominis strength to provide lumbosacral stability. An easy way that a clinician may assess function of the transverse abdominis is to have the patient lie in a supine hooking-lying position. While palpating the transverse abdominis just cranially and medially to the ASIS, instruct the patient to "pull the navel to the spine." Palpate as the abdomen moves inward. While the patient maintains tension in the abdominals, have the patient curl so the neck and shoulders lift up and off the table. If the abdomen remains pulled inward, the transverse abdominis is working, but if the abdomen moves outward, the patient lacks sufficient transverse abdominis control.

(text continues on page 351)

TABLE 8-7 | ANTERIOR AND LATERAL TRUNK MUSCLES

Group	Muscle	Proximal attachments	Distal attachments	Innervation	Action	Palpation/ Inspection
Abdominals	Rectus abdominis 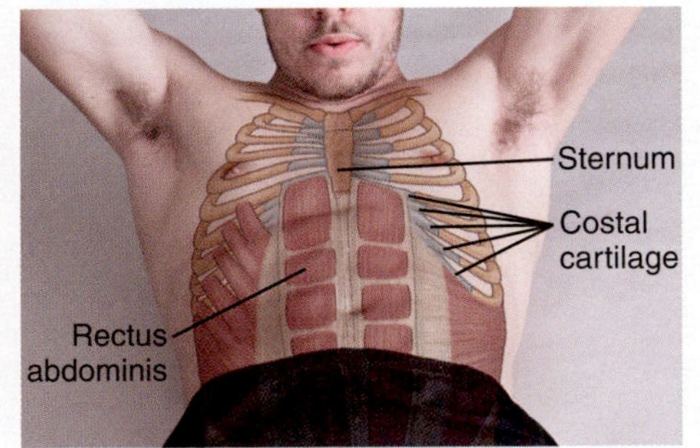	Xiphoid process of sternum & adjacent costal cartilages	Pubic bones, near the symphysis pubis	Ventral portions of fifth through 12th intercostals nerves	Trunk flexion	In well-developed subjects, the rectus abdominis may be observed and palpated throughout its length in flexion of the trunk. The tendinous inscriptions and the muscular portions between them are easily recognized. In obese individuals, the tendinous inscriptions and the boundaries of the muscle cannot be recognized very well but, when the subject raises the head while in the supine position, the tension in the muscle can always be palpated.

	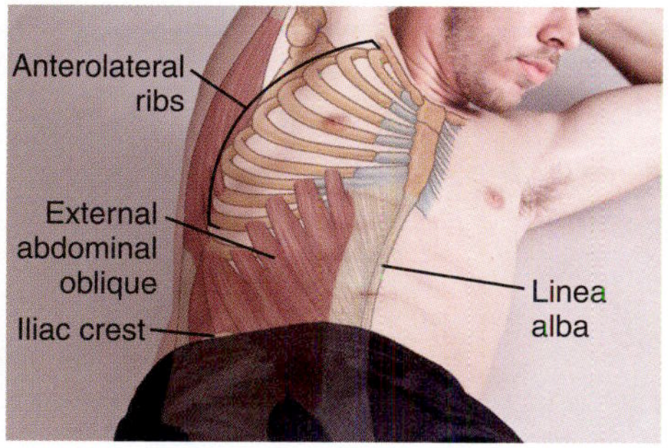 External oblique Anterolateral ribs External abdominal oblique Iliac crest Linea alba	Anterolateral ribs with fibers aligned in a downward-forward direction.	Aponeurosis that connects the muscle to the linea alba. The lower fibers are attached to the iliac crest.	Lower intercostals nerves T7–T12.	Bilaterally: trunk flexion without rotation. Unilaterally: trunk rotation to the opposite side and side bending to the same side.	Because of the oblique direction of the fibers of the muscle, flexion of the trunk combined with rotation brings out a strong contraction of external abdominal oblique, particularly if the movement is opposed by the weight of the upper part of the body.
	Internal oblique	Inguinal ligament, iliac crest, and thoracolumbar fascia. Fibers fan out to distal attachments.	Pubic bone, an aponeurosis connecting with the linea alba, and the last 3–4 ribs.	Lower intercostals nerves and branches from the iliohypogastric nerve (T9–L1).	Bilaterally: forward trunk flexion. Unilaterally: side bending and trunk rotation leading with the opposite shoulder.	The internal oblique cannot be well differentiated from the other layers of the abdominal wall. However, the tension of the abdominal wall (seen and felt on the left side of the abdomen when the trunk is rotated to the left) is due, at least in part, to the internal abdominal oblique.

continued

TABLE 8-7 | ANTERIOR AND LATERAL TRUNK MUSCLES—cont'd

Group	Muscle	Proximal attachments	Distal attachments	Innervation	Action	Palpation/ Inspection
	Transverse abdominis	Lower ribs, thoracolumbar fascia, iliac crest, and inguinal ligament.	Via an aponeurosis, it is partly fused with the other abdominal muscles into the linea alba.	Lower intercostal nerves, iliohypogastric, and ilioinguinal nerves	Abdominal compression	In forced expiration, a tightening of the abdominal wall is felt anterolaterally between the lower ribs and the crest of the ilium.
Respiratory muscle	Diaphragm	Inner surface of the xiphoid process of the sternum, the inner surface of the costal cartilages and adjacent parts of the lower six ribs, the tendinous lumbocostal arches covering the psoas and quadratus muscles, and two tendinous crus (L., legs) attaching to the anterior longitudinal ligament and the bodies of the first three lumbar vertebrae.	Central attachment: The muscular fibers of the right and left parts of the diaphragm ascend to form the dome with central tendinous attachments to each other.	Phrenic nerve (C3–C5)	Inspiration	It is palpated directly by placing the fingertips just under the anterior surface of the rib cage on either side.

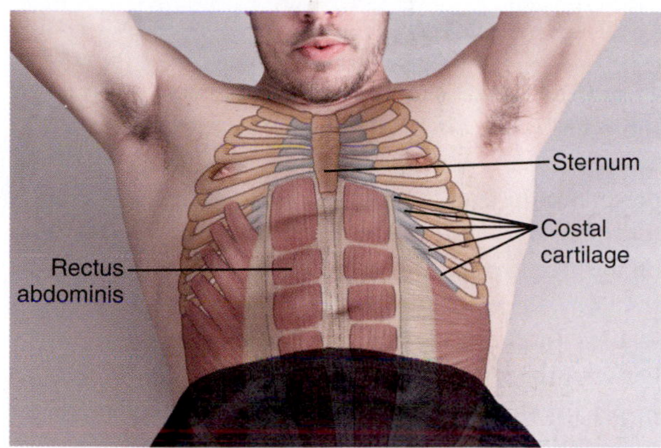

Figure 8.25 Activation of the rectus abdominis. In the supine position, the head and the shoulders are raised so that the spine flexes. The three tendinous inscriptions across the muscle are seen, the lowest slightly below the umbilicus.

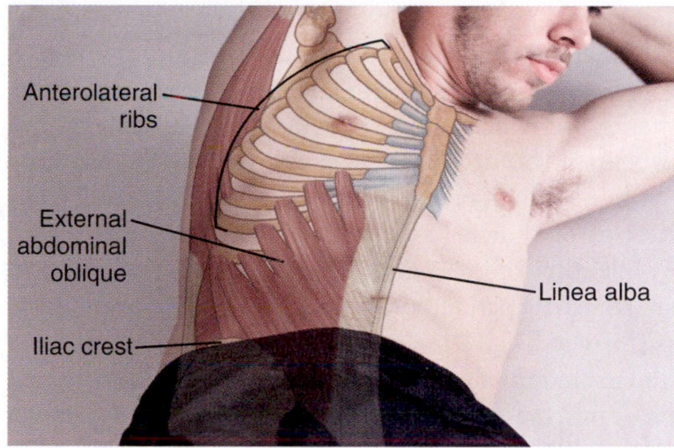

Figure 8.26 Activation of the right external abdominal oblique muscle. In the supine position, the head and the shoulders are raised and the trunk rotated to the left. The interdigitations of the left external oblique with the latissimus dorsi and serratus anterior are seen. The rectus abdominis is also contracting.

intercostals. Both muscles are innervated by the intercostal nerves. They function to elevate and depress the ribs during respiration. The intercostals may be palpated by inserting a fingertip between two ribs. When the ribs move, the muscles are activated and are palpated more easily. For example, in sitting or standing, have the subject reach overhead with the left arm, then flex the trunk laterally to the right; these motions will spread the ribs apart on the left side. Then have the subject return the trunk to the upright position. The intercostals on the left side may be identified during both parts of this movement.

Diaphragm

The **diaphragm** is a musculotendinous dome that separates the thoracic cavity from the abdominal cavity. The muscle is perforated by openings (hiatus, foramina, and arches), which permit passage of the aorta, vena cava, esophagus, nerves, psoas major, and the quadratus lumborum muscles. When a healthy person breathes in, the central portion of the diaphragm descends and puts pressure on the abdominal contents, causing the abdomen to rise outward. This is often mistakenly called "abdominal breathing." The subject should be supine and may need to be taught how to breathe with the diaphragm. When attention is called to breathing, it is common for subjects to voluntarily change their pattern to upper chest breathing.

Functions of the Head, Neck, and Trunk Muscles

As has been mentioned, the muscles of the head, neck, and trunk are vital not only for trunk motion, but for motions of the extremities as well. This section identifies

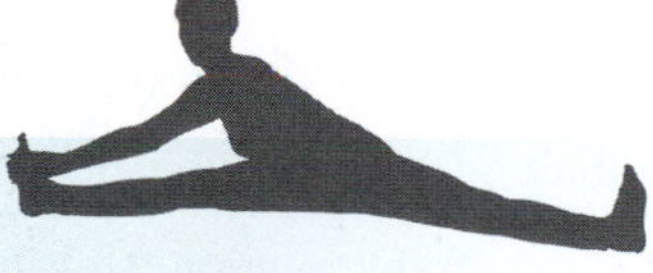

PRACTICE POINT

Clinicians working with patients with respiratory pathology such as emphysema or asthma may encounter individuals who use all of their available respiratory muscles for breathing. Normal breathing utilizes primarily the diaphragm for inhalation whereas expiration is a passive activity. However, during vigorous activity or respiratory pathology, accessory respiratory muscles are used. You are able to identify a patient's breathing pattern using a simple test. With the patient supine and relaxed, place one hand on the abdomen just below the diaphragm and the other on the upper chest over the ribs. As the person inhales, identify which of your hands is raised and which one is relatively unmoved. In resting breathing, normal individuals will raise and lower the abdomen as the diaphragm contracts and relaxes. However, patients who have difficulty breathing will also use the accessory muscles, so the chest elevates because of activity from the sternocleidomastoids, scalenes, intercostals, pectorals, and serratus anterior. In these cases, the clavicle elevates, the sternum rises, and the ribs expand.

some of the more common activities in which muscles of the axial skeleton play a role. In the last unit of this text, four chapters are devoted to additional functional movements in which more activities are identified and explained. Some of these activities include relatively "simple" actions such as walking, transferring, and activities of daily living whereas others are more complex. While some of the complex activities including running, sports participation, and recreational skills will not be performed by all patients, as clinicians, it is important to understand the demands of these endeavors so treatment programs are appropriately planned for those patients who do engage in them. As you read through the more basic activities in this section, appreciate the roles the muscles of the head, neck, and trunk must play, so when the more difficult motions presented later in this text are investigated you will appreciate the importance of these muscles in those motions as well.

Balancing of the Head and the Vertebral Column

The function of the muscles of neck and trunk in maintaining the upright position may be compared to guy wires supporting a vertical pole. As long as the pole remains vertical, the forces in the wires are balanced and minimal. However, if the pole is tilted from vertical, increased force is required from the guy wire on the side opposite to the tilt if the pole is to remain stable. Another way to maintain stability is to increase the forces of several of the wires to compress the pole into the ground. In the body, both of these mechanical stabilizing methods are used, often simultaneously. Axial muscles involved in providing and maintaining the body's upright position include:

- **Anterior muscles:** suboccipital, longus capitis and colli, scalenes, SCM, rectus abdominis, internal and external abdominal obliques, and psoas major;
- **Posterior muscles:** suboccipital, transversospinal, and erector spinae;
- **Lateral muscles:** scalenes, SCM, quadratus lumborum, psoas major, internal abdominal oblique, and intercostals.

In normal, relaxed, upright sitting or standing, these muscles show only minimal periodic activity related to postural sway (Fig. 8.27A). Any change in position of the body's center of gravity or an outside force such as a push or pull on the body immediately triggers a greater muscle contraction to either return the center of mass over its base of support or resist the destabilizing force.

If any of these groups of muscles listed above is paralyzed, the body assumes a posture in relation to gravity so that pathologic group is not required for the activity. In most cases, either other muscle groups work as substitutes for those muscles unable to contract or the body relies on passive structures for support. For example, if the abdominal muscles are paralyzed, the person sits or stands in slight trunk flexion so the erector spinae muscles are able to control the anterior motion of the trunk using either eccentric or concentric contractions, depending on where the center of gravity is relative to the body's base of support. The interplay between the trunk flexors and extensors can be realized by placing the fingers of one hand on the lumbar erector spinae and those of the other hand on the upper rectus abdominis when sitting on the edge of a chair. As the trunk moves forward of the hips, the erector spinae are palpated as they contract, but when the trunk sways backward from the hips, the rectus abdominis contracts and the erector spinae relax.

Trunk Motions and Stabilization of the Vertebrae

The transversospinal and erector spinae muscles have lines of pull that produce extension, rotation, and side bending of the vertebrae. It has been demonstrated by EMG that maximum activity of these muscles occurs during extension of the spine against gravity (Fig. 8.27C, D) or during eccentric contraction to control flexion (Fig. 8.27B). With paralysis of these muscles, the person is unable to extend the spine in the prone position or straighten it in the upright position (Fig 8.28).

Although the transversospinal and erector spinae muscles may have high activity during motions of side bending, rotation, maximum inspiration, and forced expiration, this does not mean that the muscles are prime movers for these activities. Most frequently, the back muscles act as synergists to stabilize the vertebrae in extension to prevent unwanted motion of the prime movers. For example, the external abdominal oblique muscles have excellent leverage for trunk rotation but also cause trunk flexion. Increased EMG activity of the lumbar multifidus on the contralateral side occurs with trunk rotation. However, this EMG activity is the same for both motions of rotation and the return to the midline position, indicating that the external abdominal oblique muscle's activity may be more for trunk stabilization than for rotation.[59] During side bending, EMG activity of the erector spinae and multifidus occur throughout the motion. If, however, care is taken to maintain the motion exactly in the frontal plane, electrical silence is found in these muscles.[60] In other words, this evidence indicates that the back extensors are not prime movers for side bending. Rather, the motion is accomplished by

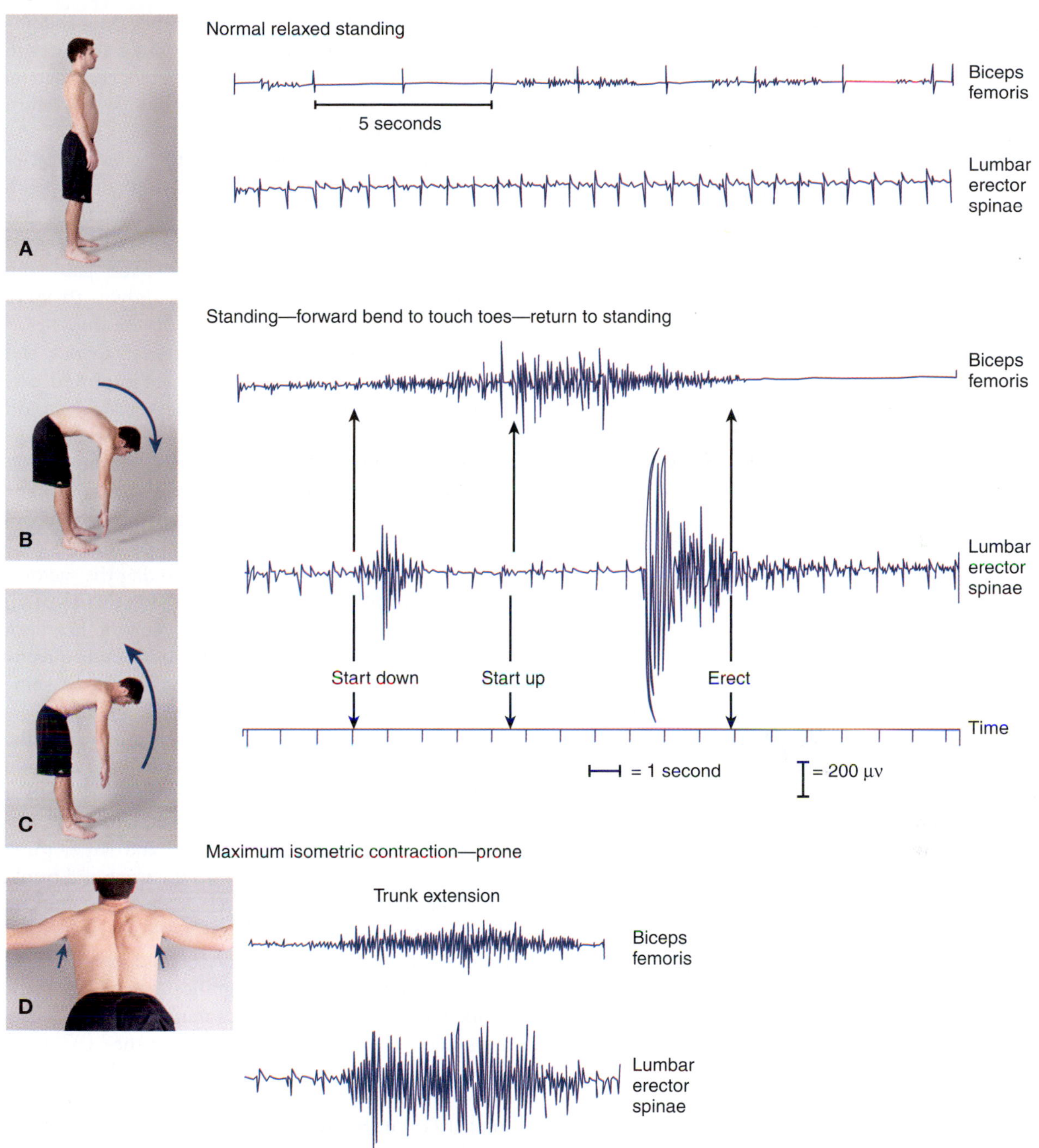

Figure 8.27 Surface electromyograms (EMG) of the right lumbar erector spinae (L. ER. SP) at L3 and of the right biceps femoris (BIC. FEM.) muscles paired with photographs depicting those movements. **A)** Normal, relaxed standing shows minimal intermittent activity in the biceps femoris. The erector spinae shows barely perceptible activity. The regular spikes in the baseline of this muscle are due to the electrocardiogram. **B)** Forward bending to touch the toes demonstrates the eccentric contraction in the biceps femoris to lower the body and the concentric contraction to raise the trunk by extending the hips. The erector spinae also shows **B)** eccentric and **C)** concentric contractions at the beginning and ending of the maneuver. The muscle becomes electrically silent about two-thirds of the way down and remains silent until about one-third of the ascent has been completed. **D)** Maximum isometric contractions produced by manual resistance provided when the subject is in an antigravity position demonstrate a standard for comparison of amplitude and frequency of the EMG activity. Notice the contraction of the biceps femoris during trunk extension to stabilize the pelvis on the thighs.

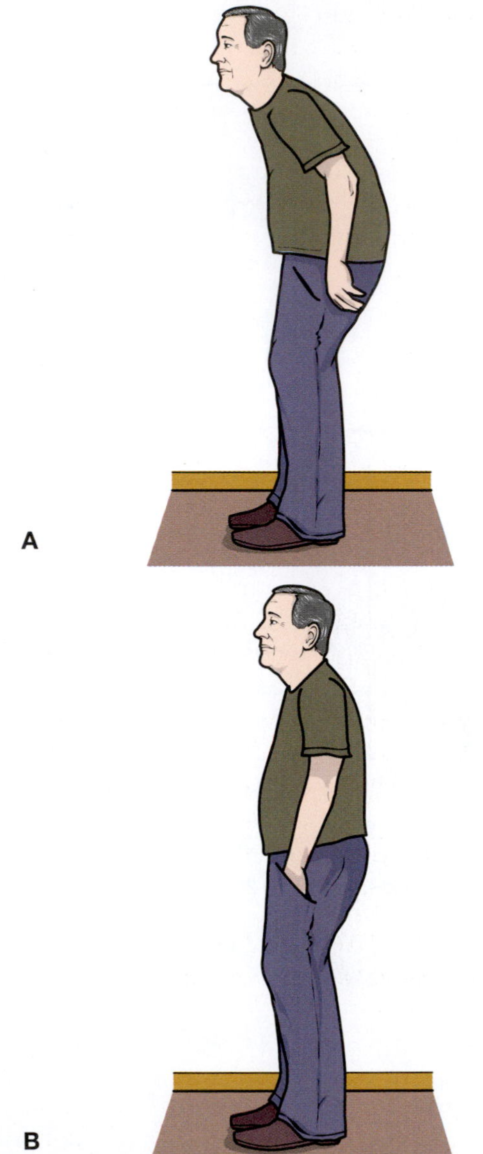

Figure 8.28 This man has paralysis of his abdominal and back extensor muscles that was caused by poliomyelitis when he was a young man. **A)** Demonstrates his inability to extend the spine. He is supporting his trunk with the posterior ligamentous system. Note that he has a posterior pelvic tilt to increase tension on the thoracolumbar fascia and the ligaments. **B)** He maintains a more erect posture when he can push down on his hands. Here he appears in a casual posture with his hands in his pockets. In reality, he is pushing down on his hips to extend his spine. He has precarious trunk balance unless he is grasping stable objects or supporting his trunk with his elbows or hands. He is unable to produce an effective push or pull on another object, such as a drawer or a door. He cannot lift or carry objects such as a plate of food because even this slight amount of weight changes the center of gravity of the head, arms, and trunk (HAT) beyond his control.

a contralateral eccentric contraction of the lateral abdominals, quadratus lumborum, and the psoas major with the trunk moving into lateral flexion and a contralateral concentric contraction of the same muscles to return the trunk to the erect position.

Investigations have identified the trunk muscles close to the spine as stabilizers of the trunk during both trunk and extremity activities.[61] Specifically, these stabilizing muscles include the multifidus and transverse abdominis.[62] Individuals with low back pain and sacroiliac dysfunction have been shown to have weakness or poor recruitment of these muscles.[62] Additionally, use of core stabilization activities and lower extremity strengthening exercises improved performance in healthy athletes during vertical take-off activities compared to just lower extremity strengthening exercises alone.[63] Part of trunk stabilization involves identifying and maintaining a neutral position of the spine.[64] A neutral spine is defined by Panjabi[65] as a position that places the least amount of stress on the spine; this position is found by positioning the sacroiliac approximately midway between the extremes of an anterior and a posterior pelvic tilt. Since it has been demonstrated that the lumbar spine position is directly related to the sacroiliac position,[46] the lumbar spine realigns as the pelvis realigns. As with shoulder performance and stability of the scapula, motions of the trunk and extremities are executed more accurately and safely when the trunk stabilizers perform their role of providing a stable base for functional activities.

In addition to the core stabilizers and larger trunk muscles, hip muscles also influence the spine and trunk. The psoas major is a large muscle with attachments on the vertebral bodies, discs, and transverse processes from T-12 to L-5. In closed-chain motions, the psoas major is a prime mover and significant stabilizer of the trunk. For example, the iliopsoas muscles raise the head, arms, and trunk in a sit-up and prevent the HAT from falling backward in unsupported sitting. In an analysis of the lines of pull of the psoas major with the trunk in lumbar flexion, Sullivan[66] found the muscle's line of pull to run either anterior to or through the vertebral axes of motion, whereas in lumbar extension, the lines run posterior to the axes of motion. Sullivan concludes that, regardless of the position of the lumbar spine, the psoas major is an active lumbar spine stabilizer.

An important function of the trunk musculature is to fixate the thorax, pelvis, and vertebrae so the proximal attachments of the muscles of the neck, shoulders, and hips are stabilized as the extremities move. When the body is supine, head and neck flexors are synergistically accompanied by a strong isometric contraction of the rectus abdominis to stabilize the rib cage during neck flexion. During a straight-leg lift exercise, all the abdominal muscles are activated to stabilize the pelvis and lumbar vertebrae. By varying the lever arm length of the lower extremity (flexing or extending the knee) and by using one or both extremities, a finely graduated exercise program for weak abdominal muscles can be developed using leg-raising and leg-lowering exercises. Manual resistance to shoulder motions such as moving from full flexion-abduction to extension-adduction causes abdominal muscle activity, most notably from the ipsilateral external abdominal oblique and the contralateral internal abdominal oblique.

In the prone position, similar activation of the erector spinae occurs. Hip extension produces a synergistic contraction of the back extensors to stabilize the pelvis. If the arms are placed in full elevation and then lifted, the back extensors automatically contract.

Forward Bending and Lifting (Knees Extended)

Forward bending and lifting with the knees straight from a standing position is a complex maneuver. It has been investigated by many researchers, and we have yet to fully understand all the elements involved. This section takes a brief look at some of the concepts and theories of the activity.

Just as the extensor muscles work when a standing person bends forward to touch the toes, so do the hip extensors (Fig. 8.29A). This motion occurs as a result of eccentric contractions of the hip extensor muscles (primarily the hamstrings) and the erector spinae muscles as they work to control hip flexion and forward bending of the vertebrae, respectively (Fig. 8.29B). Concentric contractions of these same muscles return the trunk to the upright position (Fig. 8.29C). An unusual phenomenon of sudden muscle inhibition of the erector spinae occurs on the EMG record when the trunk has completed about two-thirds of the range of trunk flexion motion on the way down. Silence of the EMG continues until the trunk extends about one-third of the range of movement on the return to standing. This point of inhibition has been named the "critical point" and has been found to have a mean value of 81° of trunk flexion.[69] The authors found this value to occur at 60% of maximum hip flexion and 90% of maximum vertebral flexion. When a weight was lowered or lifted from the floor, the angle of the critical point increased slightly. Fine-wire EMG studies of the deeper lumbar multifidus muscles revealed decreased activity at the critical point, but this did not always equate to electrical silence.[59] Inhibition of the erector spinae muscles during the highest torque requirements of forward flexion and extension of the vertebral column suggests that load bearing is produced by structures in addition to the extensor muscles of the spine, such as the facet joints and posterior ligaments. Although the physiological cause of reduced erector spinae EMG occurs at around 80° is not known, some theories presented have speculated that this decrease occurs because either the posterior spinal ligaments become stretched to cause a reflex inhibition of the muscles[70] or joints, ligaments, or muscle spindles are the source of reflex inhibition.[69] It has been noted that although EMG activity of the muscles decreases, substantial force is still generated through passive stretching of the muscles.[69]

It is known that the lower lumbar spine is able to withstand substantial flexion forces. Theories attribute this ability of the trunk to withstand large flexion moments to a combination of passive and dynamic forces produced by the posterior spinal ligaments, the thoracolumbar fascia, and the transverse abdominis and internal oblique muscles.[28, 53, 71, 72] This theory is based on the hip extensor muscles (hamstrings, gluteus

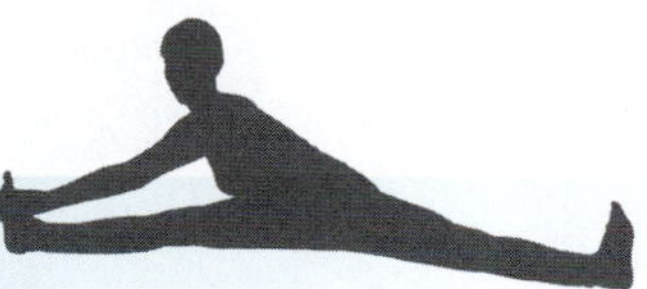

PRACTICE POINT

In recent years, clinicians have begun using "core stabilization" techniques as part of the rehabilitation process of low back injuries and pain. Part of core stabilization involves a cocontraction of trunk muscles that increases stiffness of those muscles, improving stability of the spine during activities.[67, 68] Terms such as "global" and "local" muscles, referring to the muscles farthest from the axes of motion and closest to the axes of motion, respectively, have been used to differentiate the "core" muscles, which are responsible for trunk stabilization, from the more distant muscles whose responsibility is trunk movement.[68] Persons with low back pain have demonstrated less core stability than normal subjects.[68] Since stabilization of the spine is important in both upper and lower extremity function, clinical programs that improve core muscles during treatment of extremity injuries may improve functional performance.[63]

maximus, hip adductors) providing the major forces to lower or elevate the trunk. Large forces can be generated by these muscles because of their size and leverage advantages. These forces must be transmitted to the upper body through the lumbar spine, which has relatively smaller muscles with shorter lever arms. When the lumbar spine is in flexion, the line of pull of the erector spinae muscles is almost parallel to the vertebrae with a minimal extension component. Erector spinae muscle contraction in this position would not be effective in producing lumbar extension but would increase disc compression to injurious levels.

Passively, the posterior ligaments and inert soft tissue, including the facet joint capsules, interspinous and supraspinous ligaments, and thoracolumbar fascia, can support large forces when the lumbar spine is in the forward flexed position. In this position, the trunk can be elevated by the hip extensor muscles, and, as the center of gravity of the head, arms, and trunk and any added weight moves closer to the axis of hip motion, the erector spinae are activated to complete vertebral extension. A dynamic lateral force on the thoracolumbar fascia is added by contraction of the transverse abdominis and internal abdominal oblique muscles through their attachments on the lateral raphe. This bilateral force and the increased intra-abdominal pressure prevent the passive elongation of the thoracolumbar fascia by the imposed load of HAT.

Finally, additional forces are provided by the geometry of the thoracolumbar fascia and its attachments in the lumbar region. The superficial and deep lamina of the fascia cross each other to form a series of strong triangles. The apex of each of these triangles lies on the lateral raphe, and each triangle base covers two vertebral levels. Forces from contraction of the transverse abdominis and the internal abdominal oblique are

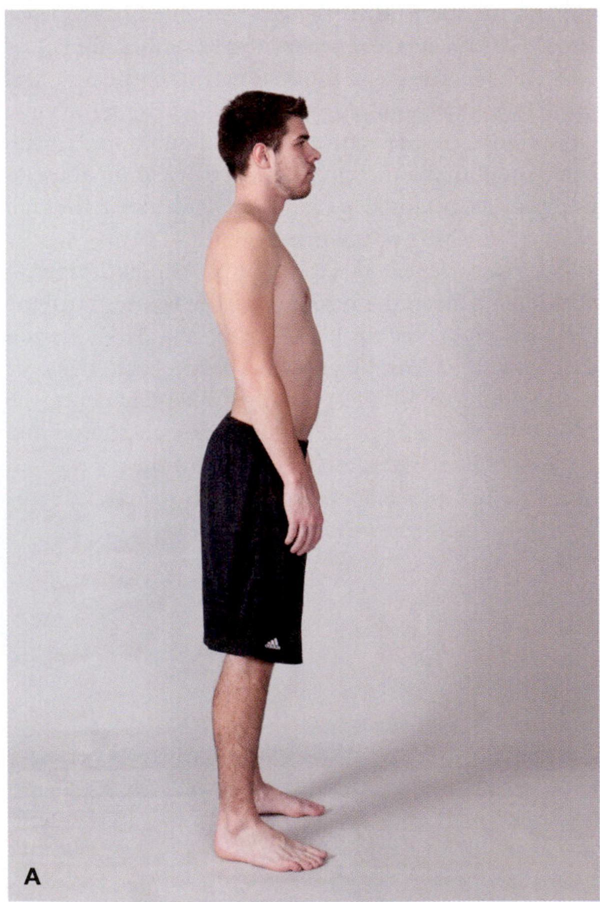

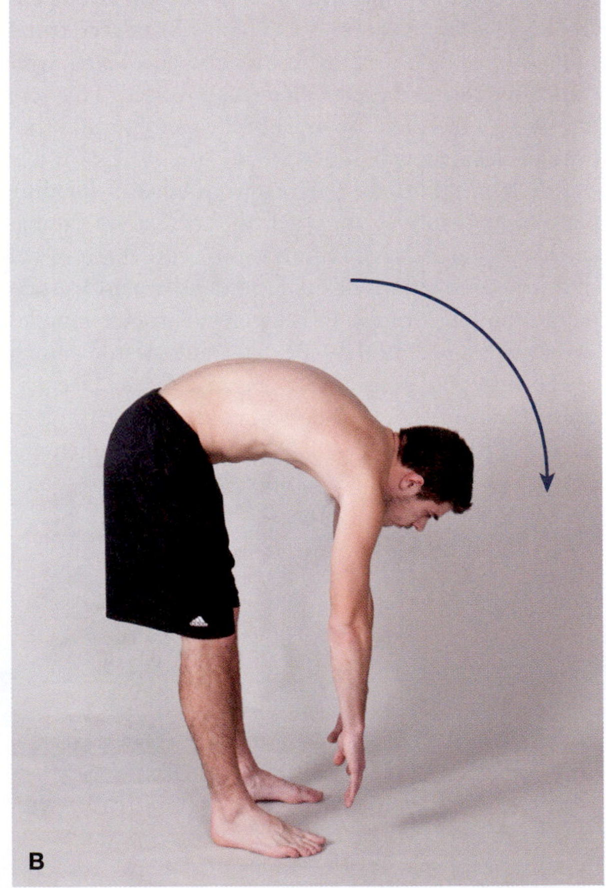

Figure 8.29 Hip extensors and trunk extensors work together. **A)** During quiet standing, these muscles provide low-level activity to maintain an erect standing position. **B)** As the individual flexes the trunk to touch the floor, the hip extensors and erector spinae muscles fire eccentrically to control the rate of descent of the trunk towards the floor.

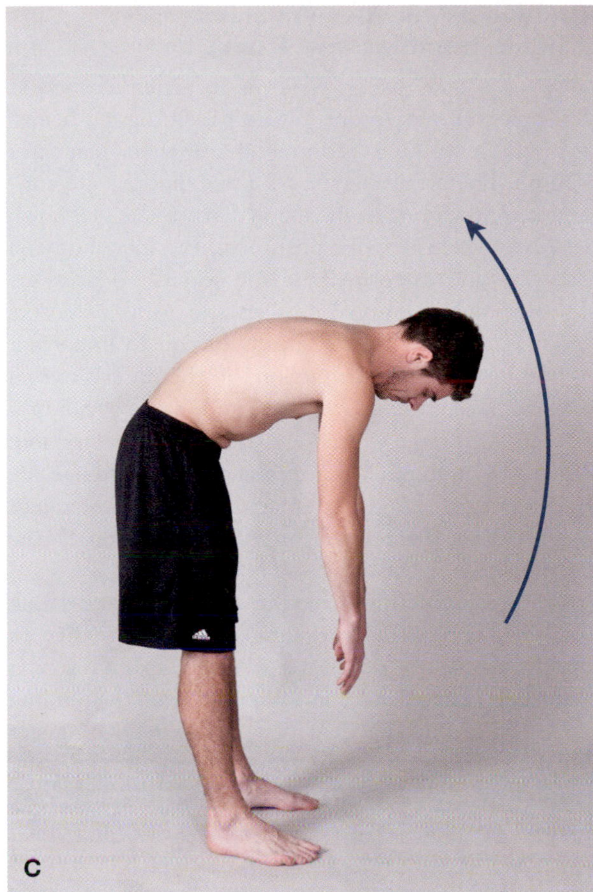

Figure 8.29—cont'd C) As the individual returns to a standing position, these same muscles contract concentrically.

transmitted posteriorly to cause the spinous processes to approximate each other, producing an extension torque on the lumbar vertebrae and a possible "bracing" force in the thoracic spine. Contraction of the latissimus dorsi when the arm is fixed, as in a pull-up maneuver, creates similar forces on the thoracolumbar fascia.[7, 71] This theory also includes the "hydraulic amplifier mechanism." This means that when the erector spinae muscles contract, they expand and put tension on the aponeurosis and fascial coverings of the muscles. This additional tension provides an anti-flexion force during forward bending and an extension force during trunk elevation similar to pressure forces in an elongated balloon.

As mentioned, although it is known that the back tolerates excessive forces applied to it, the reason for this tolerance is unknown. It is likely that a number of theories on various aspects affecting muscle, joint, and soft tissue structures along with complex biomechanical elements are correct and the actual cause is multifactorial.

Squat Lifting

Another way to lift objects from the floor is to flex at the knees and hips and dorsiflex the ankles. Squat lifting can be used with two positions of the pelvis and vertebrae: 1) anterior tilt of the pelvis with lordotic position of the lumbar spine (Fig. 8.30A); or 2) posterior tilt of the pelvis with kyphotic position of the vertebrae (Fig. 8.30B). EMG activity of the erector spinae muscles in lifting differs according to the position of the trunk. When the trunk is in the lordotic position, EMG activity is greater than that in the flexed position, and the maximum recruitment activity occurs at the initiation of the lift.[73] Lowering the body to pick up an object from the floor initially requires eccentric contractions of the gastrocnemius-soleus, quadriceps, and hip extensor muscles with isometric contraction of the erector spinae when the trunk is in the lordotic position. When the spine is more kyphotic, erector spinae EMG activity is decreased and inhibited as it is in bending with the knees straight, as was discussed above. When the squat-lift is performed in the kyphotic lumbar position, there is no contraction of the erector spinae at the initiation of the lift, and the peak activity of the erector spinae occurs in the middle of the lift.[74]

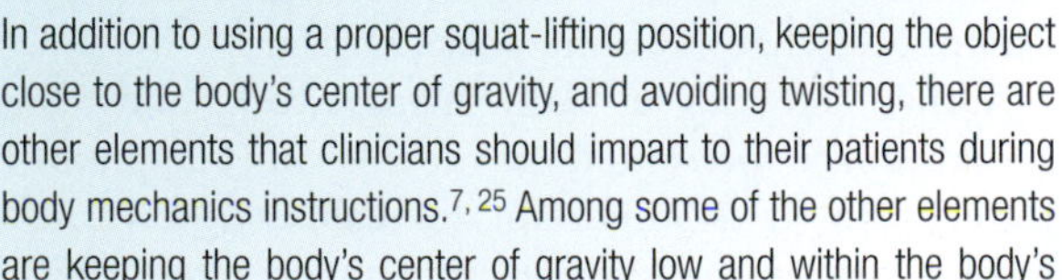

PRACTICE POINT

In addition to using a proper squat-lifting position, keeping the object close to the body's center of gravity, and avoiding twisting, there are other elements that clinicians should impart to their patients during body mechanics instructions.[7, 25] Among some of the other elements are keeping the body's center of gravity low and within the body's base of support, knowing the weight of the object to be lifted in advance, placing the feet in the direction of body movement, and preparing for the lift by "setting" the muscles prior to lifting the object. Lifting techniques and other functional activities are discussed in more detail in Chapters 13, 14, and 15.

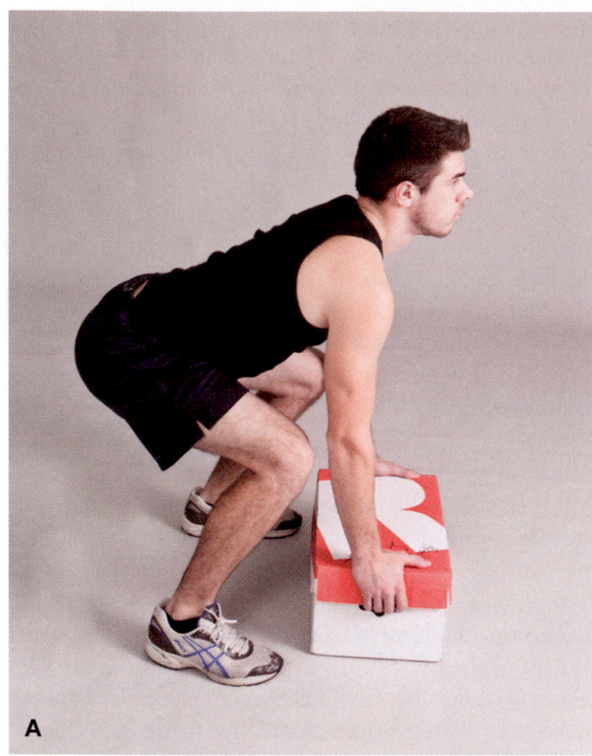

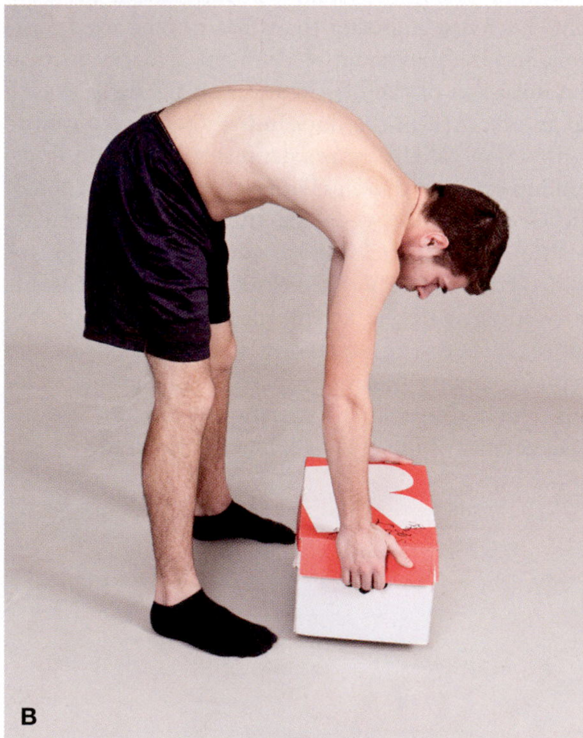

Figure 8.30 Squatting to pick up a box. **A)** Anterior tilt of the pelvis with lordotic position of the lumbar spine provides for greater recruitment of lumbar erector spinae muscles in a squat lift. **B)** A posterior pelvic tilt reduces the amount of erector spinae muscle recruitment, but in this position, greater stress is placed on the intervertebral discs.

Functional Activities (Muscles of the Extremities and Trunk)

Lifting the body using the arms in activities such as chin-ups, pull-ups, prone push-ups, sitting push-ups, and crutch-walking requires more than just arm strength. The prime movers for these motions are concentric contractions of the elbow flexors (for pull-ups), the elbow extensors (for push-ups), the glenohumeral adductors and extensors, and the scapular depressors. However, the abdominal muscles and trunk extensors working isometrically as synergists are equally important in both preventing distraction of the intervertebral joints with lengthening of the trunk and providing a stable platform from which the shoulder muscles function. When the abdominal muscles and erector spinae are paralyzed as in spinal cord injuries, the person may not be able to lift the body regardless of the strength the individual has in the arms.

As upper extremities require abdominal and trunk extensor muscle activity to complete their activities, so too, do the lower extremities. Rising up and sitting down, deep knee bends, and ascending and descending stairs have similar patterns of lower extremity muscle activity. Elevating the body from a sitting or squatting position or ascending a step (lead leg) requires knee extension with a concentric contraction of the quadriceps and hip extensors, especially the hamstring muscles. In addition, these activities require an isometric contraction of the erector spinae so the head and spine maintain an erect position. On the other hand, lowering the body to sit, squat, or descend a step (following leg) requires eccentric contractions of the quadriceps and the hamstring muscles, but these motions still require isometric contractions of the erector spinae to maintain the head and trunk in an upright position and provide stability of the trunk for lower extremity muscle performance

During forceful activities of either the upper or lower extremities, the abdominals and trunk extensors are used to stabilize the trunk and allow transmission of forces from lower to upper extremities. For example, pulling on an object such as a door or pushing something such as a football sled requires strong stabilization of the trunk to develop an effective force. Pushing activates the abdominal muscles and the hip flexors so that the trunk is not driven into extension. Pulling activates the back and hip extensors so that the trunk does not flex.

Other activities of daily living, work, and sports activities are presented in details in Chapters 13 through 15. It is important to realize, however, that most activities that involve the upper extremities or lower extremities require activation of the abdominals and/or trunk extensors. Stabilization of the trunk is important during extremity movements in that two purposes are achieved: the extremities are given a stable platform from which they move to provide their own efficiency of motion; and when forceful movements are required, transmission of forces through timed activities improves the total force available.

Breathing and Coughing

The primary muscles that are used in inspiration are the diaphragm, which produces about two-thirds of maximum inspiratory capacity; the external intercostals; and the scalene muscles. Muscles of forced expiration are the abdominals and the internal intercostals. In normal, quiet breathing, the only muscles that contract are the inspiratory muscles. Normal expiration is accomplished by the relaxation of these muscles and the passive recoil of the lung (elastic tissues and the surface tension produced by the fluid interface on the 3 million alveoli).

During exercise or forceful breathing activities such as a vital capacity maneuver or coughing, all the primary muscles of respiration are activated, along with accessory muscles and stabilizing muscles. Accessory muscles of inspiration are the SCM, the pectoralis minor, and the suprahyoid and infrahyoid muscles. The pectoralis major and the serratus anterior have also been found to be active in forced inspiration. During exercise or forced ventilation, expiration occurs by contraction of the abdominal muscles. The latissimus dorsi can assist with expiration when the arms are stabilized by placing the hands on the thighs or a table. During coughing, the latissimus dorsi can be seen to contract sharply.

The upper trapezius, erector spinae, and the quadratus lumborum are activated in forced breathing, probably more as stabilizers than as primary muscles of respiration. Trunk flexion motion, normally activated by abdominal muscle contraction, is prevented during strong coughing episodes by activation of the erector spinae muscles. Persons with back injuries often feel severe pain when they cough, sneeze, or strain because of the reflex stabilizing contraction of the back extensors.

Temporomandibular Joints

The temporomandibular joints (TMJ) or the craniomandibular articulations are among the most frequently used in the body. In their functions of chewing, talking, yawning, swallowing, and sneezing, the TMJs are estimated to move 1,500 to 2,000 times per day. These joints provide motions of opening, closing, protrusion, retraction, and lateral deviation of the mandible on the temporal bone. Normally, opening and closing of the mandible should be in a straight line without lateral deviations of the mandible on the temporal bone. Normal opening of the mouth allows a person to place the width of three fingers between the teeth. There should be no clicking or popping with joint motion or pain from palpation of the muscles of mastication.

The bilateral TMJs are synovial joints formed by the convex condyles of the mandible, the concave glenoid fossa (mandibular fossa), and the convex articular eminence of the temporal bone (Fig. 8.31A). In the adult, the mandibular condyles are about two times as wide in the frontal plane, as in the sagittal plane, providing a large articular area. The bony articulating surfaces are covered with fibrous cartilage and separated by a movable articular disc forming an upper and a lower joint space (Fig. 8.31B, C, Fig. 8.5B). Posteriorly, the disc is attached to thick connective tissue called the bilaminar zones, which are separated by spongy tissue with an extensive neural and vascular supply that normally is not subjected to large joint forces. The disc is attached medially and laterally to the sides of the condyles and anteriorly to the joint capsule and the lateral pterygoid muscle (Fig. 8.5). These attachments cause the disc to move forward with the condyle when the mouth opens. The joint is surrounded by a capsule that is reinforced laterally by the temporomandibular ligament running from the articular eminence and the zygomatic arch posteriorly to the neck of the mandible. The capsule and its ligaments limit motions of the mandible, particularly depression and retrusion. Protrusion of the mandible is limited by the stylomandibular ligament (the styloid process is seen below the TMJ in Fig. 8.31A).

Motions of the Temporomandibular Joint

As the mouth opens, rotation of the mandibular condyles occurs around the lower joint space, followed by translation of the articular disc on the upper joint space down to the articular eminence. Thus, the TMJ is like a hinge joint on a movable base. Closing of the mouth requires reversal of the translatory and rotational motions. These motions of the condyles can be felt by placing the index fingers flat against the side of the jaw with the fingertips touching the tragus of the ear and asking the subject to open the mouth slowly. The posterior part of the condyles can be felt by donning gloves and placing the fingertips inside the ears and pressing forward. When the mouth is opened, the condyles move away from the fingertips and then return when the jaw closes (Fig. 8.7). Other motions that can be made by the mandible are protrusion, or movement of the jaw forward; retrusion, or movement of the jaw posteriorly; and lateral shift to the left and to the right, which

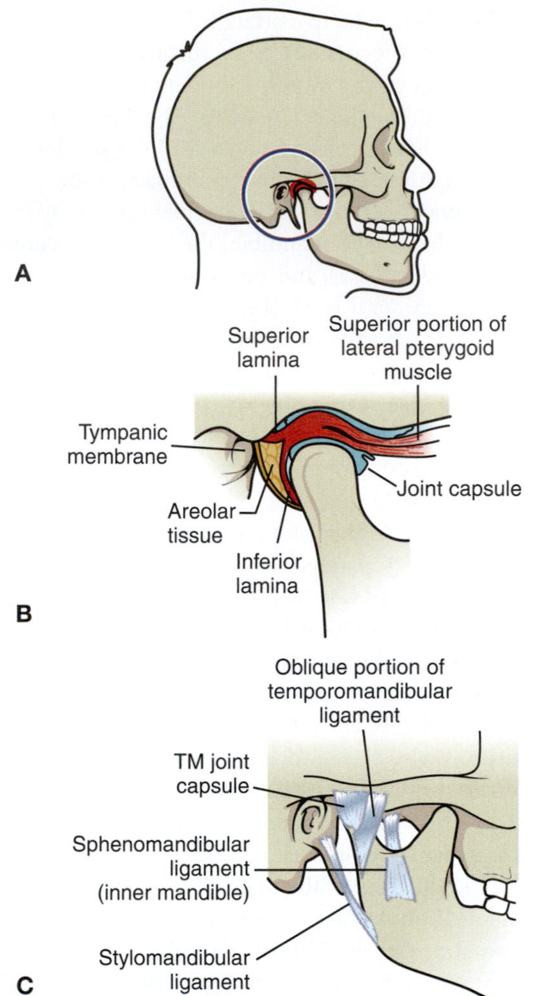

Figure 8.31 TMJ and its ligaments. A) View of the temporomandibular joint. B) Segments of the joint. C) Ligaments of the joint.

includes mediolateral translatory motion. Functional movements of the jaw are combinations of these motions. In chewing, these motions are called incision for cutting food and mastication for crushing and grinding.

Muscles

Jaw Closure

Three very powerful muscles that are all innervated by the trigeminal nerve (cranial nerve V) close the jaw. The **temporalis** muscle attaches to the temporal fossa and its fibers converge into a tendon running under the zygomatic arch to attach on the coronoid process of the mandible (Fig. 8.32). The muscle is palpated by placing the fingers over the temporal fossa and asking the subject to bite down. The muscle is also palpated with retrusion and lateral shift of the mandible. The **masseter** muscle attaches to the zygomatic arch and divides into superficial and deep parts that attach to the angle and ramus of the mandible (Fig. 8.32). To palpate the superficial part of the muscle, place the index finger just under the zygomatic arch and over the ramus of the mandible and then ask the subject to bite down. The deep part can be palpated by placing the gloved index finger inside the mouth between the teeth and the cheek as close to the ear as it will go. Have the subject bite down gently and the masseter's strong contraction is easily palpated. The masseter also provides a small lateral force component.

The **medial pterygoid** muscle (on the inside of the mandible) is almost a mirror image of the masseter muscle. The medial pterygoid attaches to the pterygoid (Gr., *pteron,* wing) fossa of the sphenoid bone and to the medial side of the ramus and angle of the mandible, often interdigitating with fibers of the masseter. Together, these muscles form a "sling" around the ramus of the mandible. In addition to the large vertical force component, the medial pterygoid has a medial force component to match the lateral component of the masseter. The medial pterygoid may be palpated extraorally by placing the index finger just superior to the ramus at the level of the mandibular angle and having the subject gently close the jaw.

Jaw Opening

The normal resting position of the mandible in an upright standing or seated position is with the lips closed and the teeth several millimeters apart. This is maintained by low levels of activity of the temporalis muscles.[75] Reduction of this muscle activity and the force of gravity are sufficient to cause the mouth to open. Rapid or resisted opening of the jaw is performed by a part of the lateral pterygoid, the digastric, and the suprahyoid and infrahyoid muscles.

The **lateral pterygoid** muscle has a horizontal direction of pull relative to the vertical direction of the masseter and the medial pterygoid (Fig. 8.30). The muscle attaches to the neck of the mandibular condyle and also frequently attaches to the articular disc. Two heads are formed with the superior head located medially and upward at about a 45° angle to attach on the greater wing of the sphenoid bone. The inferior head fans out in a more horizontal direction to attach on the distal lateral pterygoid plate of the sphenoid bone. The lateral pterygoid muscle is innervated by the trigeminal nerve (cranial nerve V).

Because the lateral pterygoid muscles are deep and difficult to palpate or record EMG activity, their actions

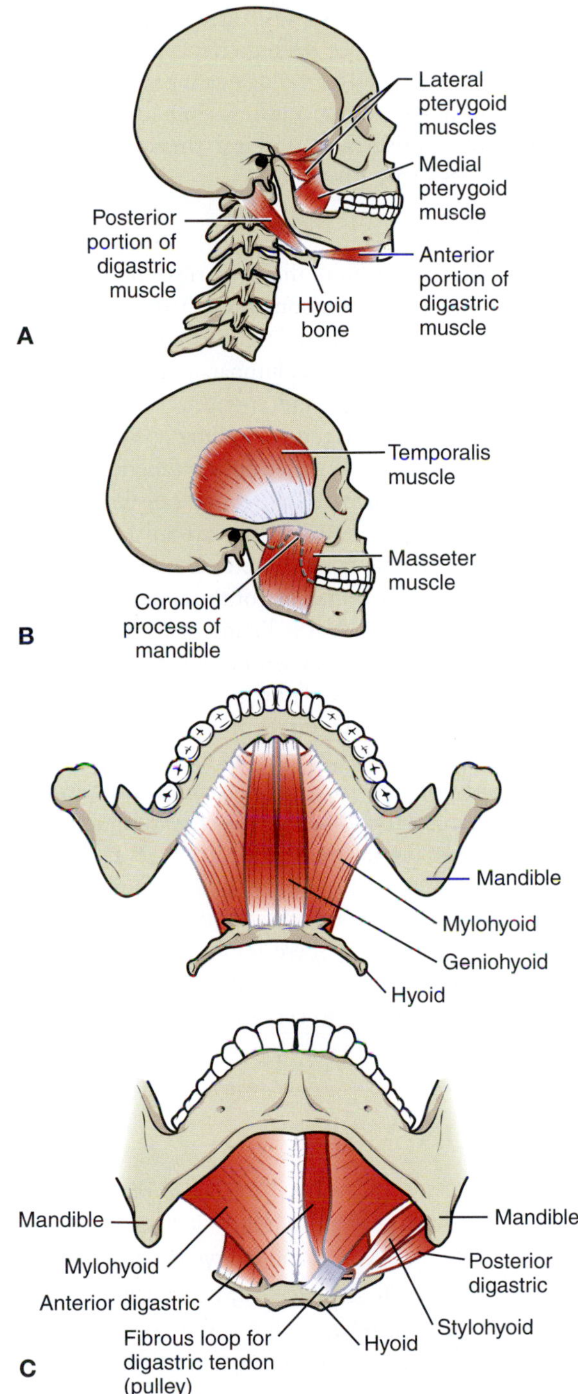

Figure 8.32 Muscles of the temporomandibular joint.

have been described based on their anatomic lines of pull rather than EMG evidence. Based on their anatomic orientation, their actions include protrusion, depression, and lateral shift of the mandible.[76] However, some EMG findings have revealed that activity in the superior head occurs with closing of the jaw, and activity in the inferior head occurs with opening of the jaw. This has led to investigators to conclude that the two heads have different actions.[77,78] These investigators propose that the probable function of the superior head of the lateral pterygoid is protrusion to stabilize the mandibular condyle against the posterior aspect of the articular eminence during mastication whereas the primary action of the inferior head is depression and protrusion of the mandible.

The **digastric** muscle has two muscle bellies lying on the underside of the chin. The anterior belly attaches to the inner border of the mandible near the midline, and the posterior belly attaches to the mastoid notch of the temporal bone. The two muscle bellies are joined in a tendinous loop that attaches to the hyoid bone. Marked EMG activity was recorded for jaw opening in both bellies of the muscle, and moderate activity was found with protrusion, retrusion, and lateral shift.[79] The authors found a complex pattern with high-amplitude, short-duration bursts of activity in this muscle during swallowing. In parts of the swallowing act, the two bellies of the digastric muscle contracted antagonistically. Each muscle belly has its own innervation: the posterior belly is innervated by the facial nerve (cranial nerve VII); the anterior belly is innervated by the trigeminal nerve (cranial nerve V).

Two other muscles of the jaw include the **mylohyoid** and the **geniohyoid**. These muscles may also participate in depression of the mandible when the hyoid bone is stabilized and may elevate the hyoid when the mandible is stabilized.

Temporomandibular Dysfunction

Abnormal signs or symptoms of TMJ involvement have been reported from 20% to 80% in a review of 25 studies of healthy subjects.[80] The incidence of problems is greater in females than in males and increases with age. The TMJs along with the muscles of mastication are a complex area to evaluate because of their close relation and attachments to head, neck, shoulder, and thoracic structures (upper quarter). Dysfunction in the TMJs is frequently unrecognized because pain may be referred to the ear, head, face, or other upper quarter areas.[81] Pathology in the other areas may also contribute to TMJ dysfunction. Although the causes of TMJ abnormalities are in most cases multifactorial, there is a high association of previous trauma[82] and postural abnormalities in the head and neck.[83]

Injuries produced by blows to the head such as whiplash in an auto accident, hitting the chin on bicycle handlebars, or falling and landing on the back of the head may lead to TMJ dysfunction. Often problems with the TMJ go unrecognized and untreated at the time because of more serious cervical, vascular, and cerebral concerns. Long-term repetitive microtrauma of the joint can occur from clenching and grinding the teeth **(bruxism)**, frequent gum chewing, cracking hard candy or nuts with the teeth, cervical traction, prolonged thumb-sucking or mouth breathing, malocclusion, or dental procedures that require wide and prolonged opening of the mouth. Repetitive, abnormal forces in occupational and athletic activities can also lead to TMJ pain and dysfunction. These types of activities include the extended head position of the professional scuba diver; the clenched jaw, forward-tilted head position of the symphony violinist; the clenched jaw of the weight lifter; and the asymmetric mouth breathing of the freestyle swimmer.[84]

Postural deviations such as a significantly shorter leg or scoliosis (lateral curvature of the spine) cause asymmetry in shoulder height and a head tilt that lead to altered craniovertebral forces. A forward-head posture in the sagittal plane produces major alterations in craniovertebral relationships. The forward-head position is a common postural abnormality that reveals a straight cervical spine on x-ray with loss of the normal cervical lordosis. The longus capitis and colli are shortened and often in some level of continuous tension. To be able to look forward, the head must hyperextend on the neck. This position then causes the suboccipital extensor muscles and the suprahyoids to shorten, and the infrahyoids to lengthen. These muscle length changes result in mandibular repositioning and hyperactivity of the muscles of mastication. Compression may occur posteriorly in the C-1 to C-2 area with craniofacial pain.[83] With all of these related effects and changes, it is easy to see why TMJ pathology cannot be considered in isolation and why a multidisciplinary treatment approach of dentists and physical therapists is often required to restoring function.

Summary

The axial skeleton includes the head, ribs, and spinal column from the cervical region through the sacrum and coccyx. The spinal column is divided into four basic units—the cervical, thoracic, lumbar, and sacral regions. It serves many functions and connects intimately with the upper and lower extremities. Among its functions, the spine serves to move the trunk during functional activities as well as stabilize it to permit transfer of forces between the upper and lower extremities. Motion between the vertebrae is permitted because of the intervertebral discs, whereas stability of the spine occurs from combined efforts of both ligaments and muscles. Although the spine moves within the three planes of movement, the positions of the vertebral facets are primary determinants of the direction and extent of movement provided in each of the spinal regions. Lateral bending and rotation motions are coupled movements seen in the spine. How these movements are coupled may depend on the alignment of the vertebrae at the time motion occurs. Motion of the temporomandibular joint occurs through activity of some of the body's strongest muscles. Dysfunction in these joints may occur from a variety of pathology such as irregularity within the joints themselves or secondary to cervical region pathology.

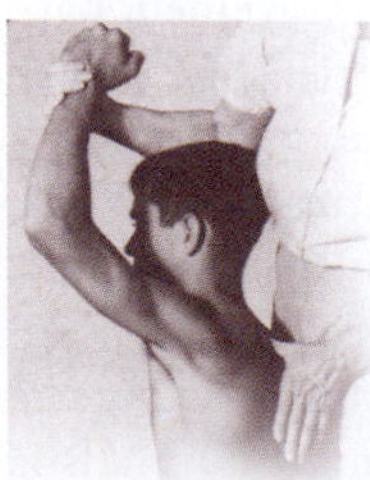

CLINICAL SCENARIO SOLUTION

Kamryn has decided that she will instruct Matt in the proper technique for lifting boxes. He is acquainted with placing himself in an appropriate anterior pelvic tilt position to reduce lumbar stresses, so increased knowledge about the muscular system will fit in well with what Kamryn has taught him so far in his rehabilitation program. She has worked with him on strengthening his abdominals, trunk extensors, hip, and thigh muscles, so she is confident that he is ready for this part of his rehabilitation program. She first instructs him to put his legs apart to provide a stable base of support. Reminding him to tighten his core muscles, she has him move into a squat position while maintaining a lumbar curve; in order to be able to get down to the floor while holding this position, it is necessary for him to flex his hips and knee and push his hips backwards so he can keep his center of gravity over his feet. When he is lowered sufficiently, Kamryn instructs him to move the box close to his body and grasp it securely before lifting it. Once Matt has the box, she instructs him to straighten his legs to stand erect. When he is able to perform this technique well, Kamryn will be to show Matt how to carry and move the box to another location without risk of reinjuring his back.

Lab Activities

1. On a skeleton and on a partner, observe and palpate the cervical, thoracic, and lumbar curves in the sagittal plane in standing. Have your partner bend forward and note that the thoracic curve increases in flexion, but that the cervical and lumbar areas move to a straight line. Have the subject bend backward (extend the trunk) and note that the lumbar curves increase and the thoracic curve moves to a straight line. Have your partner sit in a chair. Note the difference in the curves from the standing position.
2. Have your partner take off one shoe and stand with both feet on the floor while you view and palpate relative heights for symmetry:
   a. Shoulders
   b. Anterior superior iliac spines
   c. Crests of the ilia
   d. Posterior superior iliac spines
   e. Inferior angles of the scapula

   Trace by palpation the spines of the vertebrae from C-7 to the sacrum to see if there is any lateral deviation of the vertebrae. Have the subject put on the shoe and repeat the measurements. Explain how they vary.
3. With the subject standing in front of you, ask him or her to raise the right arm over the head and side bend the trunk to the left. Palpate the spines of the vertebrae from C-7 to the sacrum to determine if there is a smooth curve to the left without any straight segments. Repeat with side bending to the right.
4. Have a subject sit on a stool or table so that the pelvis is stabilized, and have the subject rotate the trunk to the right and then to the left. Where does the majority of the rotation occur?
5. On a disarticulated bone set, identify the following parts of the atlas, axis, and one each of the cervical, thoracic, and lumbar vertebrae: body, vertebral foramen, transverse processes, spinous process, lamina, pedicle, and all articulating surfaces. Identify how the same parts vary from one level of vertebra to another. How does a change in alignment of these bony parts alter the function of each of the three spinal segments?
6. Articulate pairs of the vertebrae (and the ribs) and simulate all the possible motions. Visualize the bony and ligamentous limiting structures.
7. On a partner, palpate the neck and trunk muscles as described in this chapter.
8. Palpate the abdominal and the lumbar erector spinae muscles in a subject who is lying down (supine). Have subject perform the following activities:
   a. Lift the head. Why do the abdominal muscles contract?
   b. Raise one lower extremity a few inches. Why do the abdominal muscles contract?
   c. Cough. Why do the abdominal muscles contract? The erector spinae muscles?
9. Palpate the erector spinae muscles in a subject who is prone with forehead resting on the table and arms flexed beside the head.
   a. Raise the arm a few inches. Why do the erector spinae contract?
   b. Lift one lower extremity a few inches and determine why the erector spinae contract.
10. Palpate the abdominal and erector spinae muscles on a subject sitting on a table or a stool and perform the following activities of the trunk (keep the hip position at 90° of flexion):
    a. Trunk flexion. Which muscle group is contracting and with what type of contraction while flexing and what type while returning to the upright posture?
    b. Perform side bending to the right and return to the upright position. Which side is contracting and with what type of contraction? Note that the contraction can be in either the abdominal or the erector spinae muscles with a small change in the position of the hips or trunk in the sagittal plane.

11. Analyze the following activities for the total body. State the prime mover(s) for each joint motion, the type of muscle contraction, and the essential stabilizing muscles:
    a. Supine: Perform a sit-up and return to the starting position.
    b. Prone: Raise head and shoulders and extend the trunk.
    c. Prone: Perform a push-up.
    d. Standing: Perform a chin-up.
    e. Standing: Bend forward and touch the floor and return.
    f. Standing: Sit down in a chair and return.
    g. Ascending stairs for lead leg and for following leg. Descending stairs.
12. Compare the position of the lumbar spine in supine with the hips and knees flexed so that the feet are flat to when the hips are knees are extended. Describe why the position of the lumbar spine changes with hip movement.
13. Describe how changes in arm position can make a partial sit-up progressively more challenging to the rectus abdominis.
14. While you palpate the rectus femoris tendon and the abdominals, have your partner perform a full sit-up with the legs straight. Then, have him or her perform a full sit-up with the hips and knees flexed so the feet are flat on the floor. Finally, have your partner perform an abdominal curl (partial sit-up). What differences did you feel when each muscle contracted and when it relaxed in the various exercises performed? Is there a benefit to performing a sit-up rather than an abdominal curl? Explain your answer.
15. On the skull, identify bony structures around the TMJs—temporal bone, acoustic meatus, glenoid fossa, articular eminence, and zygomatic arch. On the mandible, identify the coronoid process, ramus, body, and condyles. Note the shape and the angle of the condyles, and simulate articulation with the glenoid fossa and the articular eminence in opening and closing the jaw.
16. On a partner, palpate the condyles of the mandible as the jaw is slowly opened and then closed. Feel for rotation followed by descent on the eminence, presence of symmetry of motion and absence of jerks or pops. Observe whether the path of the lower teeth on opening is straight or deviates. Palpate the condyles and the tip of the chin while the subject slowly protracts and retracts the mandible and then deviates the mandible to each side.
17. Palpate the masseters and the temporalis muscles and ask the subject to clench the teeth to feel the muscles when they contract. Palpate the digastric muscle under the chin and give some resistance to jaw opening to feel the muscle contract.
18. Have your partner perform all active ranges of motion of the jaw. Palpate each group of muscles that perform the motions. Are your partner's motions equal and symmetrical?

References

1. Kapandji IA. *The Physiology of the Joints: The Trunk and Vertebral Column, Vol 3.* Edinbugh: Churchill Livingstone, 1974.
2. Cailliet R. *Low Back Pain Syndrome*, ed 3. Philadelphia: FA Davis, 1981.
3. White AA, III, Panjabi MM. The basic kinematics of the human spine: A review of past and current knowledge. *Spine* 3(1):12–20, 1978.
4. Myklebust JB, Pintar F, Yoganandan N, et al. Tensile strength of spinal ligaments. *Spine* 13(5):526–531, 1988.
5. Tkaczuk J. Tensile properties of human lumbar longitudinal ligaments. *Acta Orthopaedica Scandinavica* S115:1–69, 1968.
6. Nachemson A. Lumbar intradiscal pressure. *Acta Orthopaedica Scandinavica* 43:1–104, 1960.
7. Nachemson A. Disc pressure measurements. *Spine* 6(1):93–97, 1981.
8. Nachemson A. Lumbar intradiscal pressure. In Jayson M (ed): *The lumbar spine and back pain*. Edinburgh: Churchill Livingstone, 1987, pp 191–203.
9. McNally DS, Adams MA. Internal intervertebral disc mechanics as revealed by stress profilometry. *Spine* 17(1):66–73, 1992.

10. Fennell AJ, Jones AP, Hukins DWL. Migration of the nucleus pulposus within the intervertebral disc during flexion and extension of the spine. *Spine* 21:2753–2757, 1996.

11. Fazey PJ, Song S, Monsas A, et al. An MRI investigation of intervertebral disc deformation in response to torsion. *Clinical Biomechanics* 21:538–542, 2006.

12. Panjabi M, Yamamoto I, Oxland T, Crisco J. How does posture affect coupling in the lumbar spine? *Spine* 14(9):1002–1011, 1989.

13. Farfan HF. Biomechanics of the lumbar spine. In Kirkaldy-Willis WH, Burton CV (eds): *Managing Low Back Pain*. Edinburgh: Churchill Livingstone, 1988.

14. Walker BF. The prevalence of low back pain: A systematic review of the literature from 1966 to 1998. *Journal of Spinal Disorders* 13(3):205–217, 2000.

15. Grieve GF. *Common Vertebral Joint Problems*. Edinburgh: Churchill Livingstone, 1988.

16. Fryette HH. *Principles of osteopathic techniques.* Carmel, CA: Academy of Applied Osteopathy, 1954.

17. Edmondston SJ, Aggerholm M, Elfving S, et al. Influence of posture on the range of axial rotation and coupled lateral flexion of the thoracic spine. *Journal of Manipulative & Physiological Therapeutics* 30(3):193–199, 2007.

18. Mimura M, Moriya H, Watanabe T, Takahashi K, Yamagata M, Tamaki T. Three-dimensional motion analysis of the cervical spine with special reference to the axial rotation. *Spine* 14(11):1135–1139, 1989.

19. Harrison DE, Harrison DD, Troyanovich SJ. Three-dimensional spinal coupling mechanics: Part I. A review of the literature. *Journal of Manipulative & Physiological Therapeutics* 21(2):101–113, 1998.

20. American Medical Association. *Guides to the Evaluation of Permanent Impairment*, ed 3. Chicago: American Medical Association, 1988.

21. Thor CP, Gabler HC. The relationship between thoracic organ injuries and associated rib fractures. *Biomedical Sciences Instrumentation* 44:292–297, 2008.

22. Carrier G, Fréchette E, Ugalde P, Deslauriers J. Correlative anatomy for the sternum and ribs, costovertebral angle, chest wall muscles and intercostal spaces, thoracic outlet. *Thoracic Surgery Clinics* 17(4):521–528, 2007.

23. Cappello M, DeTrover A. On the respiratory function of the ribs. *Journal of Applied Physiology* 92(4):1642–1646, 2002.

24. Porterfield JA, DeRosa C. *Mechanical Low Back Pain Perspectives in Functional Anatomy*. Philadelphia: WB Saunders, 1991.

25. Adams MA, Hutton WC. The mechanical function of the lumbar apophyseal joints. *Spine* 8:327–330, 1983.

26. Yamamoto I, Panjabi MM, Osland TR, Crisco JJ. The role of the iliolumbar ligament in the lumbosacral junction. *Spine* 15(11):1138–1141, 1990.

27. McNeely ML, Magee TDJ. A systematic review of physiotherapy for spondylolysis and spondylolisthesis. *Manual Therapy* 8(2):80–91, 2003.

28. Bogduk N, Macintosh JE. The applied anatomy of thoracolumbar fascia. *Spine* 9(2):164–170, 1984.

29. Mennell JB. *Physical Treatment by Movement, Manipulation and Massage*. Philadelphia: The Blakiston Company, 1947.

30. Colachis SC, Jr., Worden RE, Bechtol CO, Strohm BR. Movement of the sacroiliac joint in the adult male: A preliminary report. *Archives of Physical Medicine and Rehabilitation* 44:490–498, 1963.

31. Ro CS. Sacroiliac Joint: Part I. Anatomy. In Cox JM (ed): *Low Back Pain*. Baltimore: Williams & Wilkins, 1990.

32. DonTigny RL. Anterior dysfunction of the sacroiliac joint as a major factor in the etiology of idiopathic low back pain syndrome. *Physical Therapy* 70(4):250–265, 1990.

33. Grieve GF. *Modern Manual Therapy of the Vertebral Column*. Edinburgh: Churchill Livingstone, 1986.

34. Cohen SP. Sacroiliac joint pain: A comprehensive review of anatomy, diagnosis, and treatment. *Anesthesia and Analgesia* 101(5):1440–1453, 2005.

35. Foley BS, Buschbacher RM. Sacroiliac joint pain: Anatomy, biomechanics, diagnosis, and treatment. *American Journal of Physical Medicine and Rehabilitation* 85(12):997–1006, 2006.

36. Forst SL, Wheeler MT, Fortin JD, Vilensky JA. The sacroiliac joint: Anatomy, physiology and clinical significance. *Pain Physician* 9(1):61–67, 2006.

37. Sashin D. A critical analysis of the anatomy and pathological changes of the sacroiliac joints. *Journal of Bone and Joint Surgery* 12A:891–910, 1930.

38. Goode A, Hegedus EJ, Sizer P, Jr., Brismee JM, Linberg A, Cook CE. Three-dimensional movements of the sacroiliac joint: A systematic review of the literature and assessment of clinical utility. *Journal of Manual & Manipulative Therapy* 16(1):25–38, 2008.

39. Weisl H. The movements of the sacroiliac joint. *Acta Anatomica* 23(1):80–91, 1955.

40. Gaskill M. A solid base of support. *Today in Physical Therapy* 4:42–45, 2007.

41. Lindsay DM, Meeuwisse WH, Vyse A, Mooney ME, Summersides J. Lumbosacral dysfunctions in elite cross-country skiers. *Journal of Orthopaedic and Sports Physical Therapy* 18(5):580–585, 1993.

42. Kapandji IA. *The Physiology of the Joints. Lower Limb, Vol 2* ed 5. Edinburgh: Churchill Livingstone, 1987.

43. DonTigny RL. Function and pathomechanics of the sacroiliac joint. *Physical Therapy.* 1985;65(1):35–44.

44. Starkey C. Taber's Cylopedic Medical Dictionary. In Starkey C (ed): *Taber's Cyclopedic Medical Dictionary*, ed 20. Philadelphia: FA Davis, 2005, p 2123.

45. Palastanga N, Field D, Soames R. *Anatomy and Human Movement. Structure and Function*. ed 4. Boston: Butterworth Heinemann, 2002.

46. Nakayama T, Yamamoto I, Fujiwara T, Yamada T. Sagittal kinematics and muscular activities of torso and hip during trunk flexion and extension. *Journal of Physical Therapy Sciences* 18(2):165–173, 2006.

47. Andersson E, Oddsson L, Grundström H, Thorstensson A. The role of the psoas and iliacus muscles for stability and movement of the lumbar spine, pelvis and hip. *Scandinavian Journal of Medicine in Science and Sports* 5(1):10–16, 1995.

48. Fick R. *Anatomie und Mechanik der Gelenke: Teil III, Spezielle Gelenk und Muskel Mechanik*. Jena, Germany: Fisher, 1911.

49. Prushansky T, Ezra N, Kurse N, Man L, Schneiderman Y. Reproducibility of sagittal plane pelvic tilt measurements in normal subjects using digital inclinometry. *Gait & Posture* 28:513–516, 2008.

50. Basmajian JV. Cyclobenzaprine hydrochloride effect on skeletal muscle spasm in the lumbar region and neck: Two double-blind controlled clinical and laboratory studies. *Archives of Physical Medicine and Rehabilitation* 59:58–63, 1978.

51. Boyd-Clark LC, Briggs CA, Galea MP. Muscle spindle distribution morphology, and density in longus colli and multifidus muscles of the cervical spine. *Spine* 27(7):694–701, 2002.

52. Abrahams VC. The physiology of neck muscles: Their role in head movement and maintenance of posture. *Canadian Journal of Physiology and Pharmacology* (55):332–338, 1977.

53. Macintosh JE, Bogduk N. The anatomy and function of the lumbar back muscles and their fascia. In Twomey LT, Taylor JR (eds): *Physical Therapy of the Low Back*. New York: Churchill Livingstone, 1987.

54. Moseley GL, Hodges PW, Gandevia SC. Deep and superficial fibers of the lumbar multifidus muscle are differentially active during voluntary arm movements. *Spine* 27(2):E29–E36, 2002.

55. MacDonald DA, Moseley GL, Hodges PW. The lumbar multifidus: Does the evidence support clinical beliefs? *Manual Therapy* 11(4):254–263, 2006.

56. Moseley GL, Hodges PW. Reduced variability of postural strategy prevents normalization of motor changes induced by back pain: a risk factor for chronic trouble? *Behavioral Neuroscience* 120(2):474–476, 2006.

57. Lewin T, Mofett B, Vidik A. The morphology of the lumbar synovial intervertebral joints. *Acta Morphologica Neerlando-Scandinavica* 4:299–319, 1962.

58. Kiesel KB, Underwood FB, Mattacola CG, Nitz AJ, Malone TR. A comparison of select trunk muscle thickness change between subjects with low back pain classified in the treatment-based classification system and asymptomatic controls. *Journal of Orthopaedic and Sports Physical Therapy* 37(10):596–607, 2007.

59. Valencia FP, Munro RR. An electromyographic study of the lumbar multifidus in man. *Electromyography and Clinical Neurophysiology* 25(4):205–221, 1985.

60. Pauly JE. An electromyographic analysis of certain movements and exercises: I. Some deep muscles of the back. *Anatomical Record* 155(2):223–234, 1966.

61. Hodges P, Richardson C. Inefficient muscular stabilization of the lumbar spine associated with low back pain: A motor control evaluation of transversus abdominis. *Spine* 21(22):2640–2650, 1996.

62. Richardson CA, Snijders CJ, Hides JA, Damen L, Pas MS, Storm J. The relation between the transversus abdominis muscles, sacroiliac joint mechanics, and low back pain. *Spine* 27(4):399–405, 2002.

63. Butcher SJ, Craven BR, Chilibeck PD, Spink KS, Grona SL, Sprigings EJ. The effect of trunk stability training on vertical takeoff velocity. *Journal of Orthopaedic and Sports Physical Therapy* 37(5):223–231, 2007.

64. Norris CM. Functional abdominal training: Part 2. *Journal of Bodywork and Movement Therapies* 3(4):208–214, 1999.

65. Panjabi MM. The stabilizing system of the spine. Part II: Neutral zone and instability hypothesis. *Journal of Spinal Disorders* 5(4):390–396, 1992.

66. Sullivan MS. Back support mechanisms during manual lifting. *Physical Therapy* 69(1):38–45, 1989.

67. Akuthota V, Nadler SF. Core strengthening. *Archives of Physical Medicine and Rehabilitation* 85(3):S86–S92, 2004.

68. Borghuis J, Hof AL, Lemmink KAP. The importance of sensory-motor control in providing core stability: Implications for measurement and training. *Sports Medicine* 38(11):893–916, 2008.

69. Kippers V, Parker AW. Posture related to myoelectric silence of erectores spinae during trunk flexion. *Spine* 9(7):740–745, 1984.

70. Floyd WF, Silver PH. Function of erectores spinae in flexion of the trunk. *Lancet* 257(6647):133–134, 1951.

71. Gracovetsky S, Farfan H, Helleur C. The abdominal mechanism. *Spine* 10(4):317–324, 1985.

72. Gracovetsky S, Kary M, Levy S, Ben Said R, Pitchen I, Hélie J. Analysis of spinal and muscular activity during flexion/extension and free lifts. *Spine* 15(12):1333–1339, 1990.

73. DeLitto SR, Rose SJ. An electromyographic analysis of two techniques for squat lifting and lowering. *Physical Therapy* 72(6):438–448, 1992.

74. Holmes JA, Damaser MS, Lehman SL. Erector spinae activation and movement dynamics about the lumbar spine in lordotic and kyphotic squat lifting. *Spine* 17(3):327–334, 1992.

75. Basmajian JV. *Muscles Alive: Their Function Revealed by Electromyography*, ed 4. Baltimore: Williams & Wilkins, 1978.

76. Gray H. *Anatomy of the Human Body*, ed 28. Philadelphia: Lea & Febiger, 1966.

77. McNamara JA, Jr. The independent functions of the two heads of the lateral pterygoid muscle. *American Journal of Anatomy* 138(2):197–205, 1973.

78. Sarnat BG, Laskin DM. *The Temporomandibular Joint: A Biological Basis for Clinical Practice*, ed 4. Philadelphia: WB Saunders, 1992.

79. Widmalm SE, Lillie JH, Ash MM, Jr. Anatomical and electromyographic studies of the digastric muscle. *Journal of Oral Rehabilitation* 15(1):3–21, 1988.

80. Burakoff R. Epidemiology. In Kaplan AS, Assael LA (eds): *Temporomandibular Disorders: Diagnosis and Treatment*. Philadelphia: WB Saunders, 1991.

81. Travell JG, Simons DG. *Myofascial pain and dysfunction: The trigger point manual,* Vol. 1. Baltimore: Williams and Wilkins, 1983.

82. Pullinger AG, Monteiro AA. History factors associated with symptoms of temporomandibular disorders. *Journal of Oral Rehabilitation* 15(2):117–124, 1988.

83. Mannheimer JS, Dunn J. Cervical spine-evaluation and relation to temporomandibular disorders. In Kaplan AS, Assael LA (eds): *Temporomandibular Disorders: Diagnosis and Treatment*. Philadelphia: WB Saunders, 1991.

84. Goldman JR. Soft Tissue Trauma. In Kaplan AS, Assael LA (eds): *Temporomandibular Disorders: Diagnosis and Treatment*. Philadelphia: WB Saunders, 1991.

INTRODUCTION TO

Unit 3: Lower Quarter

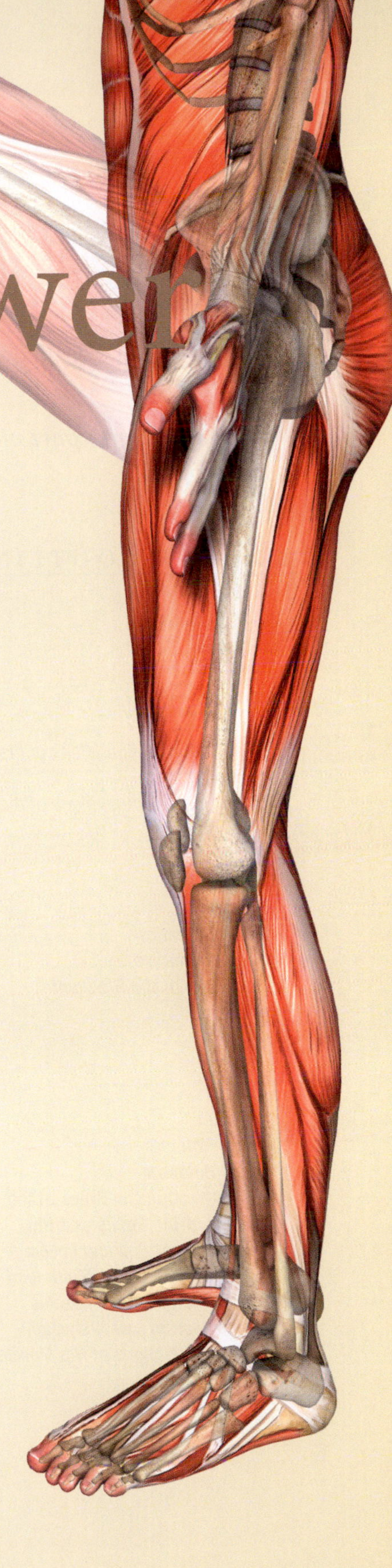

As the upper extremity and axial skeleton were presented in Unit 2, Unit 3 continues on to the lower extremity and provides information and investigations into the kinesiological functions of the pelvis, hip, knee, and ankle from a clinical perspective. Anatomy of these segments is summarized in tables to make reference to the information a matter of quick review. Emphasis in each of the chapters is placed on joint kinematics and osteokinematics along with important muscle functions of each of the segments.

Unit 3 begins with the hip in Chapter 9. Since the pelvis is an intimate part of the hip, it is presented here as it regards hip movement and function. The impact weight-bearing during stance and gait has on these structures is presented along with the influences of single-limb weight-bearing.

Chapter 10 addresses the knee complex. The knee includes the tibiofemoral joint and the patellofemoral joint, both of which are investigated in this chapter. How forces affect these joints and the impact of neural influences are also discussed. Hip and knee muscle interaction is also presented in this chapter.

In Chapter 11, the foot and ankle are discussed. The multiple joints of these structures and their separate and combined actions are presented along with changes in their function and motion during open and closed kinetic chain activities. Unique motions of the foot are discussed along with how these impact other body segments.

Pelvis and Hip

Dolores B. Bertoti, MS, PT, and Christopher R. Carcia, PhD, PT, SCS, OCS

"Knowing in part may make a fine tale, but wisdom comes from seeing the whole."
—Asian Proverb

CHAPTER OUTLINE

Learning Outcomes
Clinical Scenario
Introduction
Bones
Pelvis
Femur
Biomechanical Angulations of the Femur
Biomechanical Angulations of the Acetabulum
Joints
Pelvis
Hip Joint
Osteokinematics
Arthrokinematics
Soft Tissue at the Hip Joint
Muscles
Flexors
Adductors
Extensors
Abductors
Lateral Rotators
Medial Rotators
Factors Affecting the Roles of the Muscles of the Pelvis and Hip
Muscle Line of Pull and Leverage
Muscular Sufficiency: Multi-Joint versus Single-Joint Muscles
Weight-bearing and Nonweight-bearing Functions of Hip Muscles

LEARNING OUTCOMES

This chapter investigates the pelvic and hip region. By completion of this chapter, the reader should be able to:

- ❑ Identify the bones, joints, soft tissue, and muscles of the pelvic and hip region;
- ❑ Discuss the relationship between the pelvis, hip, low back, and trunk and their contributions to functional movement;
- ❑ Demonstrate the motions of the pelvis on the femur—anterior and posterior pelvic tilt, lateral tilt, and forward and backward rotation;
- ❑ Demonstrate the motions at the hip joint and list the muscles that are responsible for motion of the femur on the pelvis at the hip joint—flexion, extension, abduction and adduction, lateral and medial rotation;
- ❑ Name the prime muscles that move the pelvis and hip to accomplish specific functional activities;
- ❑ List the muscles at the hip that contribute to motions in varying planes and describe the uniqueness of these contributions to functional movement;
- ❑ Describe the function of the hip and its musculature in closed kinematic chain as compared to open kinematic chain movements;
- ❑ Explain frontal plane control of the pelvis including the role of the gluteus medius and adductor muscles in unilateral stance and describe the implications for function;
- ❑ Describe commonly encountered pathological conditions of the pelvic and hip region and their functional consequences.

Analysis of Muscle Activity at Pelvis and Hip
Analysis of Sagittal Plane Motion at the Hip and Pelvis
Analysis of Frontal Plane Motion and Control at the Hip and Pelvis
Analysis of Transverse Plane Motion at the Hip and Pelvis
Summary
Clinical Scenario Solution
Discussion Questions
Lab Activities
References

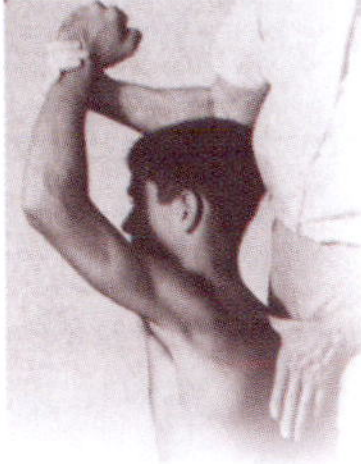

CLINICAL SCENARIO

Noelle notices that the retired man she is working with is walking with an unsteady gait. Every time he takes a step onto his left lower extremity, he laterally leans his trunk over to that side. Noelle is concerned with the long-term effects that this gait deviation will have on Mr. Reyes' lumbar spine. What assessment steps should Noelle take to evaluate the underlying cause of this gait pattern? What should she recommend to Mr. Reyes, and why?

Introduction

Similar to the shoulder region, the pelvic and hip region integrally intertwine their structure and function. However, in contrast to the shoulder area, this region's primary responsibility is not mobility during open chain activities; rather, it is power production during closed chain functions. Just as there is a direct relationship between the trunk and scapula and the scapula and glenohumeral joint, there is also an association between the trunk and pelvis and the pelvis and hip.

In anatomical terms, "girdle" signifies an anatomical structure that acts as a functional brace or girder from which a segment moves.The shoulder complex is an incomplete girdle whereas the pelvic girdle forms a complete girdle. The pelvic girdle includes the right and left pelvic bones that are joined to the axial skeleton via the sacrum and fifth lumbar vertebra posteriorly, with the left and right hemipelvis meeting at the pubic symphysis anteriorly. Similar to how the humeral head articulates with the glenoid fossa, the femoral head articulates with the pelvic girdle fossa—the acetabulum. Beyond these basic similarities, the pelvic girdle is unique from the shoulder girdle in both structure and function.

The term *pelvis* comes from Latin, meaning "bowl" or "basin;" quite literally the pelvis forms a bony bowl that holds crucial visceral contents. Additonally, its musculoskeletal anatomy forms a bridge between the lower extremities and the entire head, arm, and trunk complex (HAT). The pelvis has multiple functions including: 1) providing a stable base for HAT; 2) containing and supporting the visceral contents; and 3) transmitting and absorbing forces to and from both HAT superiorly and the lower extremities inferiorly. In addition to providing these important stability functions, however, the pelvic girdle also offers a highly prescribed degree of mobility so that it works in concert with the lumbar spine, sacrum, and hip to move the body efficiently and effectively. Since the pelvic articulation with the sacrum at the sacroiliac joint and with the fifth lumbar vertebra at the iliolumbar area were covered in depth in the previous chapter, please refer to that chapter for details. These joints are mentioned here only as they relate to pelvic control and motion.

As we shall see, the hip, or acetabulofemoral joint is very stable structurally; it is also very mobile. In addition to transmitting large forces between the trunk and the ground, the hip region is a major player in the body's locomotor system. For example, the hip abductor muscles on the weight-bearing leg must create a force to counterbalance about 85% of body's weight during each step taken. The hip also serves a major role in elevating and lowering the body, as in climbing, rising from a chair, or lifting the limb, as when the foot is elevated to tie a shoelace.

Remember that a muscle can act at a joint by either moving the proximal end or moving the distal end. The hip is no exception; hip muscles may function by moving the femur on the pelvis (e.g., flexing the hip to step up onto a step) or by moving the pelvis over the femur (e.g., leaning over to pick up an object from the floor). These variations in mucle activity, depending upon which segment of the joint is stabilized and which one is moving, enable the hip to provide unique and important contributions to daily functional movement.

Bones

The primary bones presented in this chapter are the bones comprising the hip joint: the pelvis and femur.

Although the sacrum, coccyx, and lumbar spine are also involved in pelvic motion, they have already been described in the Chapter 8. Bony prominences that are essential to understanding hip and pelvic muscle function are presented here for review.

Pelvis

The pelvis has several important functions, some for organ purposes and others for kinesiological purposes. Providing support and protection of viscera and providing a bony support for the birth canal are its two organ functions. Kinesiological functions of the pelvis include:

- Supporting and transfering the weight of the HAT to the femurs in standing or to the ischial tuberosities in sitting;
- Rotating during walking to create a rhythmic pelvic swing so a smooth translation of both the trunk and the lower extremities occurs; and
- Providing a broad area for muscular attachment.

The **pelvis** is made up of a right and left innominate bone, or os coxa (L., hip bone), which are joined to the sacrum posteriorly. The word "innominate" is actually quite descriptive because it means "nameless" (L., *innominatum)*, illustrating that the pelvic bone is not really a single named bone but is made up of three bones that are fused together. These fused segments include the anterior and superior ilium, the posterior ischium, and the anterior-inferior pubis (Fig. 9.1). Although these three bones are individual bones, they all join together as a unit to form the bony pelvis and to contribute to the formation of the **acetabulum** (L., a shallow vinegar vessel or cup). The acetabulum is the cup into which the head of the femur fits to form the hip joint. This is an interesting stability feature in this region, ensuring that the hip joint is actually structurally comprised of portions of *all three* pelvic bones. Other bony formations of note of the pelvis include the **greater sciatic notch** and the **obturator foramen**. The sciatic nerve travels through the greater sciatic notch, and the piriformis muscle spans across it. Several vessels and nerves on their way to the lower extremity travel through the obturator foramen, which is formed by the ischium and pubis (Fig. 9.1).

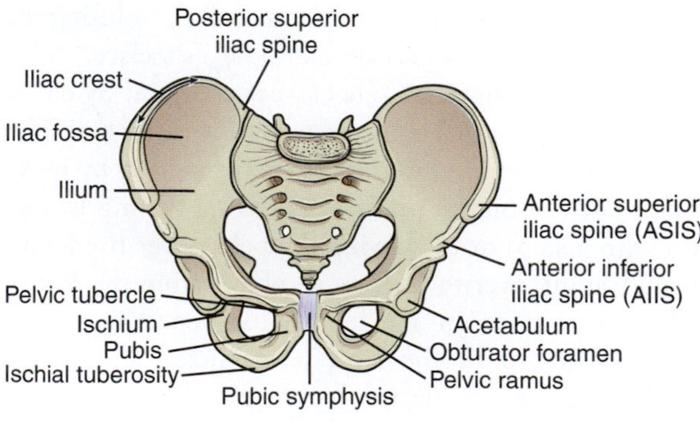

Figure 9.1 Drawing of pelvis with landmarks marked, including acetabulum; ilium—iliac crest, iliac fossa, ASIS, AIIS; ischium—ischial tuberosity; and pubis—rami, pubic symphysis, pubic tubercle.

Ilium

The **ilium** is the more anterior and superior of the three pelvic bones, the bone that you feel when you "put your hands on your hips"—an interesting colloquialism because, obviously, now you realize that the ilium is not your hip but rather is your pelvis (Fig. 9.2A). The body of the ilium contributes approximately 40% to the formation of the acetabulum.

You can palpate your ilium by placing the thumbs on the **iliac crests**, the very prominent superior bony border of the ilium, one on the right and one on the left side. The ilium's large surface area provides attachment sites for many muscles that cross the abdominal region and the hip joint. Under normal conditions, crests of the ilia are level to one another in the standing position. The most anterior and superior aspect of the crest is the **anterior superior iliac spine (ASIS)**. The ASIS is the attachment site for the sartorius and tensor fascia latae muscles and is an important landmark for assessing pelvic position, leg length, and Q-angle. If the iliac crest is followed in a posterior direction, the **posterior superior iliac spine (PSIS)** can be identified. The left and right PSIS prominences are broader and sturdier than the ASIS and feel rough under the palpating fingers. Immediately inferior to each PSIS is a depression; this is the posterior landmark for the sacroiliac joint (Fig. 9.2B).

Inferior to the ASIS and the PSIS are the **anterior inferior iliac spine (AIIS)** and **posterior inferior iliac spine (PIIS),** respectively. These landmarks are not easily palpated. The AIIS serves as the proximal attachment for the rectus femoris muscle. The **iliac fossa** is the large concave inner surface of the ilium, which provides a deepened large surface area to which a portion of the large, powerful iliacus muscle attaches. The posterior, anterior, and inferior gluteal lines on the outer ilium are not palpable, but it is important to realize that they separate the areas of attachment of the three gluteal muscles (Fig. 9.3).

Ischium

The ischium is the posterior inferior bone of the pelvis. The body of the ischium makes up approximately 40% of the acetabulum. Its most notable palpable feature is the large **ischial tuberosity** located at the bone's most

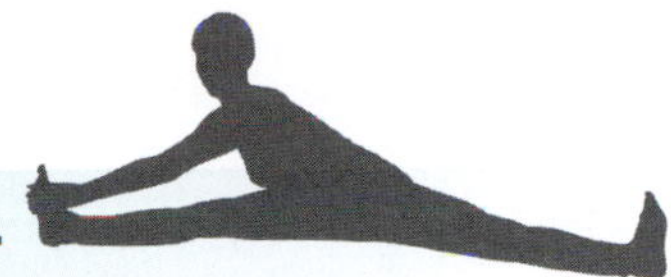

PRACTICE POINT

Clinically, a frontal plane lateral tilt of the pelvis can be assessed by checking the height of the crests of the ilia. The symmetry of the pelvis also may be checked anteriorly by placing the thumbs on each ASIS. In most individuals, the ASIS are easily located, often visible under the skin.

inferior aspect (Fig. 9.3). This is an important landmark because it is the weight-bearing prominence when sitting, and it is the proximal attachment site for the hamstring muscles and a portion of the adductor magnus.

Not easily palpable, the **ischial ramus** (L., *branch,* or as used when describing a ram's horns) extends medially from the body of the ischium to connect to the ramus of the pubis. This is an additional attachment site for the adductor magnus and also some of the small lateral rotators of the hip (Fig. 9.1). There is also a spine on the posterior ischium which provides a firm attachment for the sacrospinous ligament, a major reinforcer of the sacroiliac joints.

Pubis

The pubic bone is the anteroinferior portion of the pelvis. The body of the pubis contributes the remaining 20% to the formation of the acetabulum. When viewing

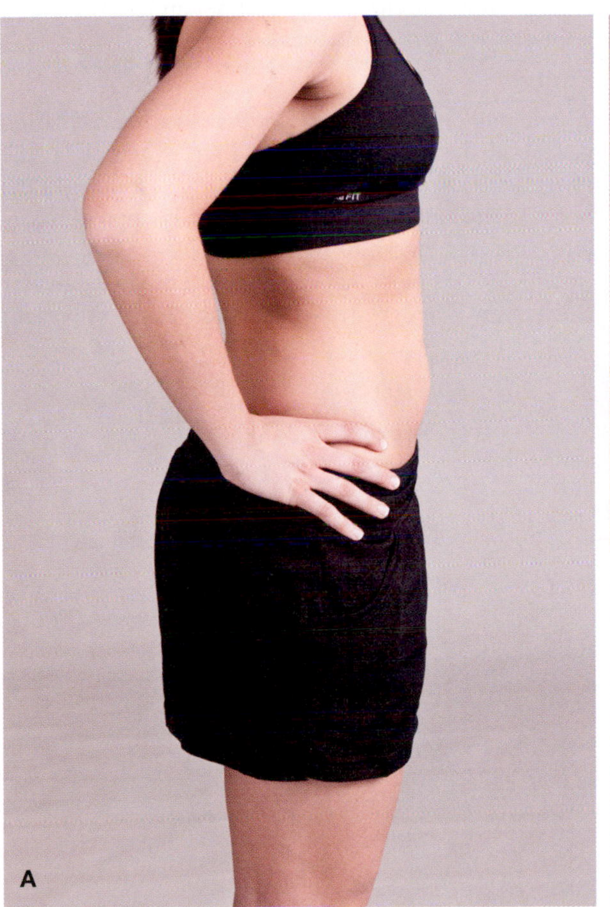

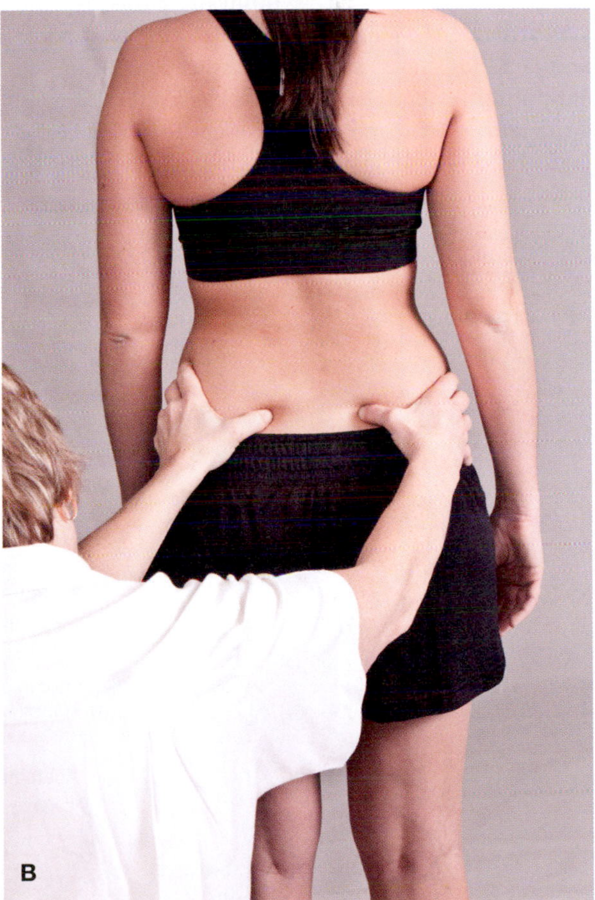

Figure 9.2 **A)** Subject with "hands on hips" so that whole hand depicts the location of the iliac crest with the index finger on the ASIS and thumb on the PSIS. **B)** The PSIS is palpated by following the iliac crest posteriorly. Immediately inferior to each PSIS is a depression indicating the location of the SI joint.

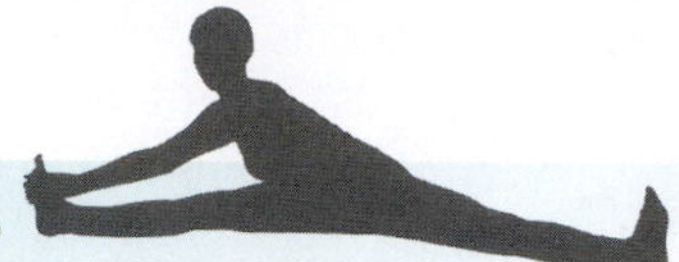

PRACTICE POINT

The ischial tuberosities are easy to locate when sitting on a hard chair or lying on the side with hips and knees flexed. Once located in these positions, the tuberosities can also be palpated in the standing position by approaching them from below the gluteal folds. The tuberosities may be palpated when a subject stands in front of a table or in parallel bars. He or she flexes the trunk forward while supporting the weight of the trunk on the hands. The ischial tuberosities are palpated when the individual is in this position and then returns to the erect posture, using the arms to push up the trunk into extension rather than the hip extensor muscles. The ischial tuberosity is an important consideration for two groups of individuals: those who use a wheelchair for locomotion and those with an above-knee (AK) amputation. The individual who sits in a wheelchair for prolonged periods must be cautious in preventing skin breakdown from prolonged pressure on the ischial tuberosities. Reducing pressure may occur with proper seat-pad selection and instruction in periodic pressure relief techniques. Individuals with an AK amputation use a prosthesis that contains a shelf that is incorporated into the design on which the isichial tuberosity "sits" to provide some of the limb's weight-bearing surface during standing and walking.

the pubic bone from the front, it is easy to see that it is comprised mainly of a **superior** and **inferior ramus.** These serve as attachment sites for most of the hip adductor muscles. The **symphysis pubis** is the amphiarthrodial connection between the two pubic bones anteriorly and will be discussed later with the joints of this region. The pubis also has a **pubic tubercle** on the most medial and superior aspect of the superior ramus. The inguinal ligament attaches here (Fig. 9.1).

Acetabulum

The acetabulum is the name given to that part of the pelvis that articulates with the head of the femur to form the hip joint. This concave partner of the acetabulofemoral joint will be described further in the section under joint function but it is mentioned here because it is a combination bony feature, actually formed from the three bony components of the pelvic bones (Box 9-1).

Femur

The femur, or thigh bone (Fig. 9.4), is the articulating partner at the hip proximally and with the tibia at the knee distally. It is the longest and strongest bone in the body. Interestingly, a person's height is approximately four times the length of the femur.[1]

The femur's most palpable prominence is its **greater trochanter**. The greater trochanter is an important

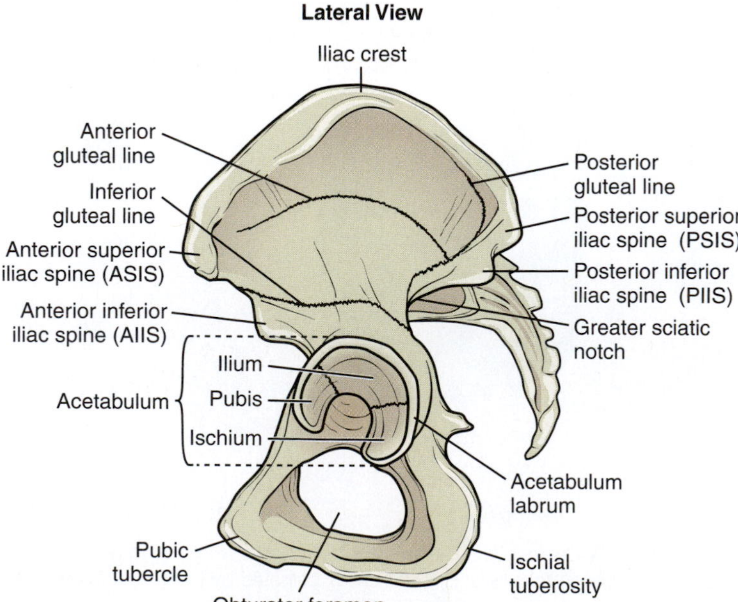

Figure 9.3 Lateral view of pelvis with landmarks marked, including the anterior, the posterior and inferior gluteal lines, and the ischial tuberosity.

BOX 9-1 | Distinctive Bony Features of the Pelvis

Ilium
- Iliac crest
- Iliac fossa
- ASIS
- AIIS
- PSIS
- PIIS

Ischium
- Ischial ramus
- Ischial tuberosity
- Spine

Pubis
- Superior and inferior ramus
- Symphysis pubis
- Pubic tubercle

From combinations of ilium, ischium and pubis
- Acetabulum
- Greater sciatic notch
- Obturator foramen

clinical landmark because it provides the attachment for the gluteus medius and lateral rotator muscles; it is also a marker used in measuring leg length. In normal adults, the greater trochanter is level with the center of the femoral head.[2] Because it is a lateral projection of the femur, the greater trochanter increases the leverage of many hip muscles that attach here by increasing their moment arm. These muscles include the gluteus medius, gluteus minimus, gluteus maximus; and the lateral rotators. The greater trochanter increases the moment arm of these muscles by deflecting their line of pull away from the axis of hip motion, thereby increasing the torque able to be produced by these muscles.

Because the femur is surrounded by large muscles, palpation of most of its proximal features is difficult. Proximal bony features that are not palpable include the following: the **lesser trochanter**, located medially and inferiorly to the greater trochanter. The lesser trochanter is an attachment site for the iliopsoas muscle. The **linea aspera** is a prominent ridge running almost the entire length of the posterior femur, serving as an attachment for some of the adductor muscles. Between the greater trochanter and the linea aspera is a smaller **pectineal line**, so named because the pectineus muscle attaches here. The distal femur is more easily palpated. These distal femoral prominences are discussed in Chapter 10.

Although the femoral **head** and **neck** are nonpalpable proximal features, they are important hip structures. The large rounded head of the femur is almost entirely covered in hyaline cartilage. A small central foveal pit is a section of the femoral head that is devoid of hyaline cartilage. The ligamentum teres and its accompanying blood vessels travel through the fovea from the acetabulum to the femur. The head of the femur is connected to the femoral shaft by the femoral neck. The femoral neck angulates the head of the femur so it faces medially, superiorly, and posteriorly. The acetabulum faces a correspondingly lateral, inferior, and anterior direction. Although the discrepancy is not as great as we saw in the glenohumeral joint, the ball portion of this joint also has more articular surface than its corresponding socket; for this reason, several anatomical and biomechanical features are present to increase the fit and stability of the hip joint (Box 9-2).

Biomechanical Angulations of the Femur

The femur demonstrates two unique angulation features: one in the frontal plane and one in the transverse plane. Both of these angulating designs improve the femur's mechanical efficiency.

Angle of Inclination

In the frontal plane, the **shaft of the femur** angles medially to align the knee and femoral head within the same

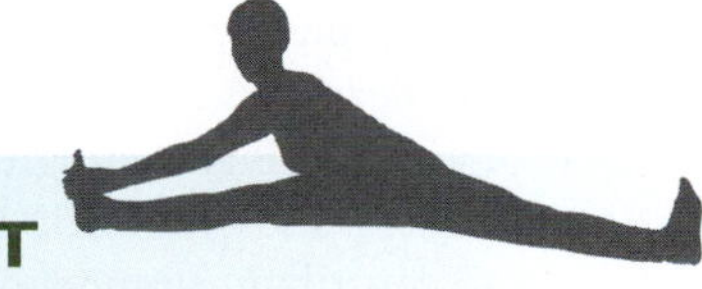

PRACTICE POINT

To locate the prominent femoral greater trochanter, position the subject supine with the lower extremities extended. Place your thumb on the lateral iliac crest over its most proximal point and extend your fingers down the lateral thigh as far as possible. As you passively rotate the subject's thigh medially and laterally with the other hand, the greater trochanter may be felt moving under your middle finger. Once located, the greater trochanter may be more accurately palpated as a large bony prominence over which the fingers may slide from side to side and upward and downward. In the standing position, the height of the greater trochanter should be the same for both legs.

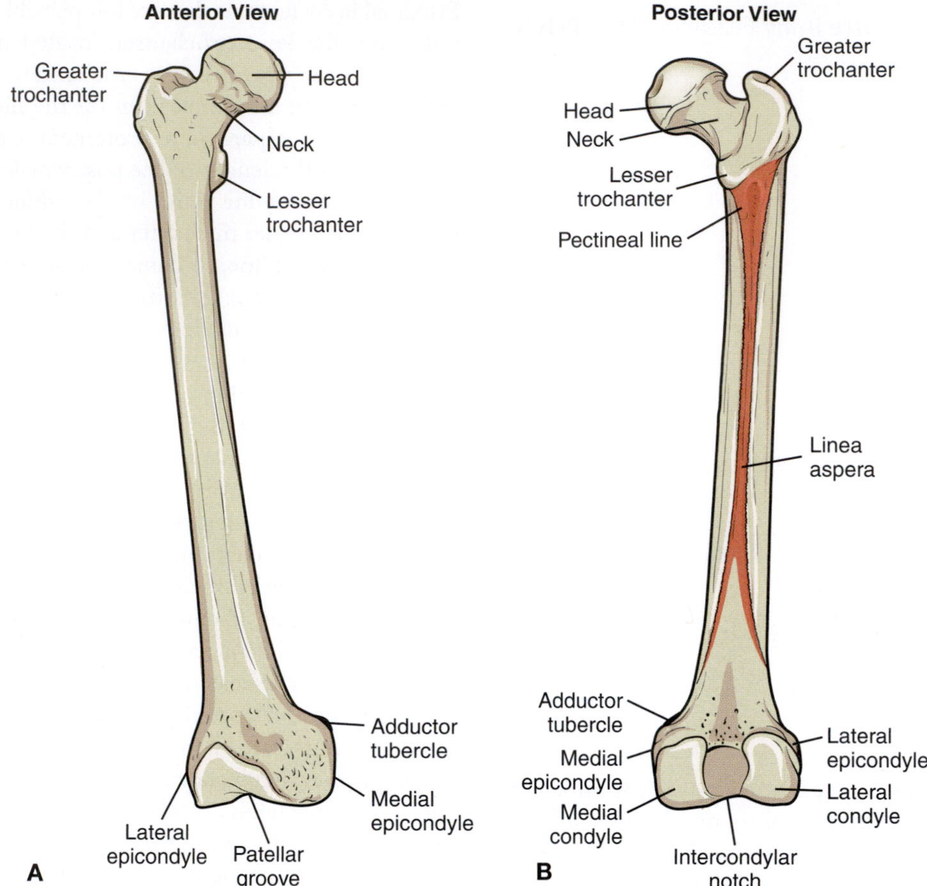

Figure 9.4 A) Anterior and B) posterior view of femur with landmarks marked, including the greater trochanter, the lesser trochanter, the pectineal line, the head, the neck and shaft of femur, the linea aspera, the adductor tubercle, and the medial and lateral condyles and epicondyles.

weight-bearing line (Fig. 9.5). This frontal plane angulation or neck-shaft angle is the **angle of inclination.** The angle of inclination undergoes developmental changes throughout the life span, but by age 2 and throughout adulthood, it averages 125°.[3] These life span changes are a good illustration of the harmony that exists in the body between structure and function. At birth, the typical angle of inclination is usually 150° and the acetabulum is rather shallow, placing the hip in a position of incongruency and relative instability. The compressive and tensile forces into and across the joint occurring during infancy and early childhood exerted by normal muscle tone, muscular contraction secondary to movement, and the compressive forces of weight-bearing create two important changes: 1) the acetabulum deepens; and 2) the angle of inclination decreases. The developmental sequence of movements from that of a supine infant, progressing to quadruped rocking on all fours, and eventually moving from standing to walking contribute to modeling the immature cartilaginous bone so the acetabulum deepens and the angle of inclination decreases with the progressive stresses placed upon the bones and joint. Both of these changes improve the congruency between the acetabulum and femoral head and align muscles that cross the joint for optimal leverage.

BOX 9-2 | Distinctive Bony Feature of the Femur Relative to Hip Function

Head of femur
Neck of femur
Greater trochanter
Lesser trochanter
Linea aspera
Pectineal line
Shaft (body) of femur
Adductor tubercle

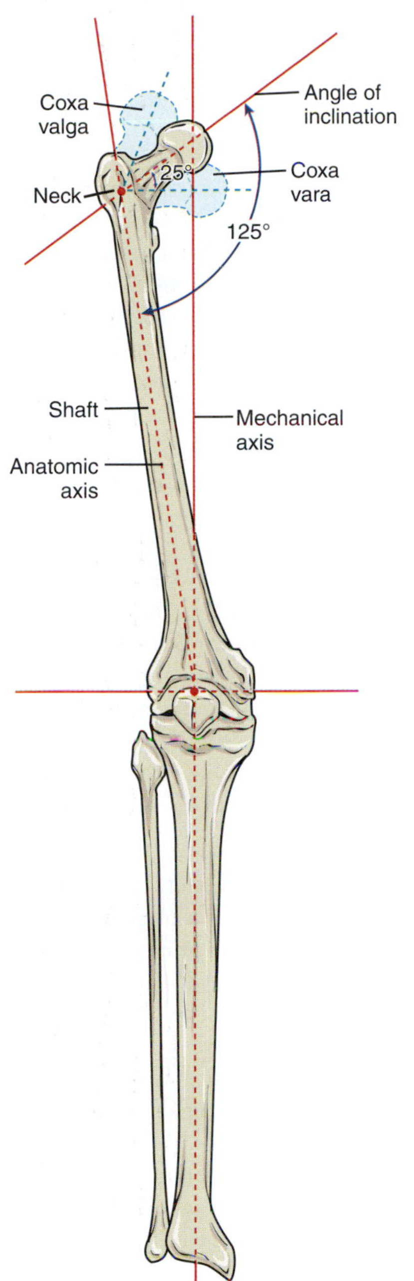

Figure 9.5 Anatomic and mechanical axes of the femur; angle of inclination. Typical adult angle of inclination is 125°; coxa valga is an angle greater than normal whereas coxa vara is an angle less than normal.

An excessive angle of inclination between the femoral neck and shaft, beyond 130° is **coxa valga** (Fig 9-5). Coxa valga results in functional consequences such as hip instability with a predisposition to dislocation or subluxation. The limb may also appear longer. An increased angle of inclination places the limb in an adducted position during weight-bearing to create a functional increase of limb length.[4–6] Coxa valga also reduces the distance of the greater trochanter from the joint's axis of motion, thereby contributing to decreased leverage of the muscles that attach to the greater trochanter. Such a reduction in moment arm length of the hip abductor muscles contributes to hip abductor weakness and reduces pelvic stability.

At the other end of the life span, the angle of inclination may decrease slightly secondary to normal aging changes. At this time the femoral head becomes more congruent with the acetabulum to increase joint stability. Such a change may result in a decrease in apparent leg length with the limb in a more abducted position and widened base of support.

If the angle of inclination is less than 125°, it is abnormal and is called **coxa vara** (Fig. 9.5). Coxa vara causes an increase in tensile forces across an acutely angled femoral neck, predisposing the femoral neck to fracture. Coxa vara is more likely to occur later in the life span as arthritic changes decrease the angle of inclination.[6] Both of these structural changes, coxa valga or coxa vara, contribute to decreased muscle strength because of changes in torque. These torque reductions are due to alterations in moment arm length and length-tension relationships.

Angle of Torsion

In the transverse plane, another angulation of the femur is seen, called the **angle of torsion** (Fig. 9.6). The angle of torsion is an innate medial twist of the femur. Viewing the femur from a superior-to-inferior "birds' eye view," imagine one line bisecting the femoral head and neck on the proximal femur and another line connecting the medial and lateral femoral condyles at the femur's distal end. The line between the condyles is medially rotated relative to the line between the femoral head and neck. This medial rotation of the femur is reflective of the natural changes that occur during embryonic development. When the limb buds first form, they are abducted from the developing trunk. As the fetus develops *in utero*, the arms stay somewhat laterally rotated (recall Chapters 5 and 6 and the carrying angle), but the lower extremities medially rotate as the baby folds into a fetal position and the lower extremities continue to develop. During infancy, the angle of torsion may be as high as 40°. The angle of torsion decreases during early development so the angle by adulthood is a 10° to 20° anterior rotation of the head and neck relative to the femoral shaft.[3, 7–11] An angle greater than normal is **anteversion** and results in joint incongruency to produce relative instability of the hip joint. Someone with excessive femoral anteversion

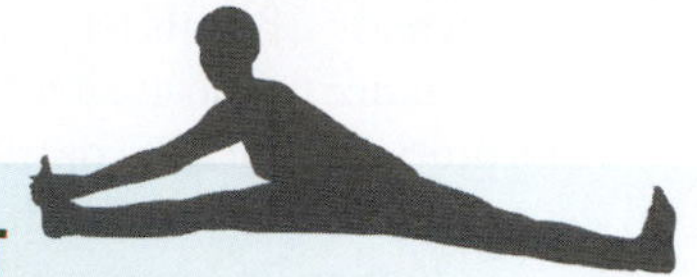

PRACTICE POINT

A discussion of coxa valga and coxa vara offer an opportunity to appreciate how structure and function of the human body are intertwined and how varying risks for altered function can occur at different stages in the life span. Children with developmental disorders, specifically cerebral palsy or spina bifida, will often present with coxa valga. In the face of delayed motor development, limited movement and abnormal muscular forces pulling on their malleable bones, the 150° angle of inclination seen at birth is retained and does not diminish to the typical adult angle of 125°. This greater angle of inclination creates obvious consequences, including hip instability, decreased muscle leverage, and reduced force production capability.

In older persons, normal aging and development of an acute angle of inclination can present an increased risk of hip fracture. Interestingly, if you were to ask patients who have sustained a hip fracture about their injury, many will say that it wasn't really a fall that seemed to actually cause the fracture, but rather, they experienced a feeling of their hip giving way and then they fell. In other words, perhaps the coxa vara predisposed the hip to fracture first, resulting in a fall.

clinically presents as "in-toeing" and demonstrates an apparent increase in hip medial rotation with a concomitant limitation of hip lateral rotation motion.[7] Less commonly seen is **retroversion,** a decrease in this angle that presents with a "out-toeing," or lateral hip rotation, during standing and walking.[8]

Biomechanical Angulations of the Acetabulum

Similar to the femur, the acetabulum demonstrates two unique angulation features: one in the frontal plane and one in the transverse plane. Both angles serve to provide containment and, hence, stability of the femoral head within the acetabulum. Stability of the hip joint is of particular importance given the magnitude of the forces that cross this joint during simple tasks such as walking and running.

Center Edge Angle

In the frontal plane, the center edge angle, also commonly referred to as the Angle of Wiberg, is defined by the angle formed by two lines that originate at the center of the femoral head (Fig. 9.7). One line extends vertically forming the reference whereas the other line extends to the lateral aspect of the acetabulum.[9] Larger angles reflect greater containment of the femoral head by the acetabulum whereas smaller angles imply lesser coverage of the femoral head. Angles vary during development although after age 5, angles less than 20° suggest hip dysplasia.[10] Angles greater than 25° are considered normal.[9]

Acetabular Anteversion Angle

In the transverse plane, the acetabular anteversion angle is formed by two lines which originate at the posterior rim of the acetabulum. The reference line extends in an anterior direction parallel with the sagittal plane while the second line extends obliquely to the anterior margin of the acetabulum (Fig. 9.8). The angle formed by the intersection of these two lines is defined as the acetabular anteversion angle. Normal acetabular anteversion angles are between 15° to 20°.[11] Angles greater than 20° are associated with less containment of the femoral head by the acetabulum whereas angles less than 15° signify excessive coverage of the femoral head by the

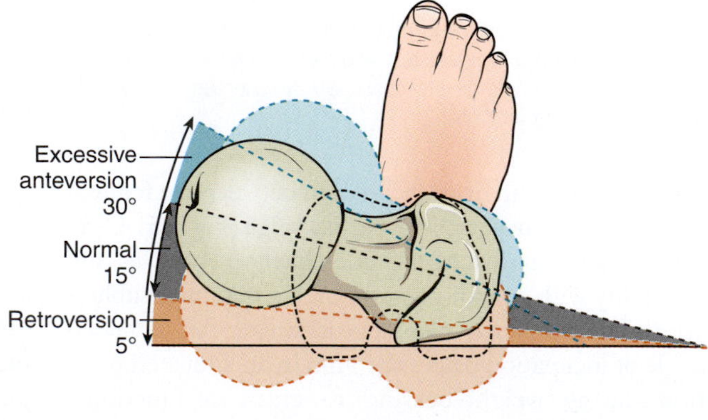

Figure 9.6 Angle of femoral torsion can be visualized by taking a superior view of the femur and superimposing a line drawn along the frontal axis between the head and the neck of the femur proximally onto a line drawn between the femoral condyles distally. Natural angle of 15° is contrasted with anteversion and retroversion.

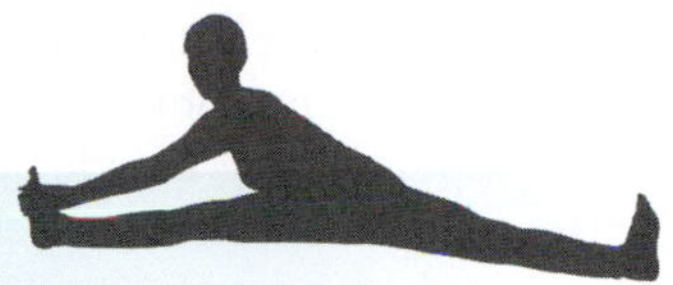

PRACTICE POINT

Femoral torsion and the angle of inclination are good illustrations of our effective biomechanical design. The innate torsion or twist of the femur allows for some resiliency and the ability to absorb and transmit forces. You can imagine that a lever, or in this case a femoral shaft, that possesses some degree of resiliency and ability to bend with force will be able to sustain greater applied forces than would an absolutely straight shaft. The angle of inclination increases leverage of the muscles that connect the pelvis to the greater trochanter. This angle also allows forces to dissipate through the acetabulum and distribute over the entire bony pelvis.

acetabulum. There is also evidence to indicate that individuals with acetabular anteversion angles greater than 20° put significantly more stress on the hip joint, especially when going down stairs, making them more susceptible to osteoarthritic joint changes.[12]

Joints

Pelvic and hip function is dependent on the smooth interaction of other articulations immediate to this region. For example, the lumbosacral and sacroiliac joints impact the pelvis and hip joints. Their relevance to pelvic function is presented later in this chapter. This section, however, focuses on the osteokinematic motions occurring primarily at the hip joint. Presentation of hip joint motions must be identified as either *pelvic motions* whereby the pelvis moves on the femur or *hip motions* whereby the femur moves on the pelvis. Pelvic motions (pelvis on femur) include: anterior pelvic tilt and posterior pelvic tilt; lateral tilt on the left or right, up or down; and forward rotation, or protraction, and backward rotation, or retraction. On the other hand, hip motions (femur on pelvis) include: flexion and extension; abduction and adduction; and medial and lateral rotation. Regardless of whether the pelvis is moving over a stationary femur or the femur is moving under a stable pelvis, three degrees of motion are available at this triaxial articulation between the pelvis and proximal femur. The motions simply change names, depending on which bony segment moves and which is stationary.

Pelvis

Since the pelvis is the bony link between the lower extremities and the trunk, pelvic motion and control is intimately related to motions at both the low back and the hip. Because of these interrelationships, multiple joints participate when the pelvis moves. In total, seven joints participate: lumbosacral (1), left and right sacroiliac (2), sacrococcygeal (1), symphysis pubis (1), and both hips (2). As has been previously mentioned in Chapter 8, although motions are small at the sacroiliac,

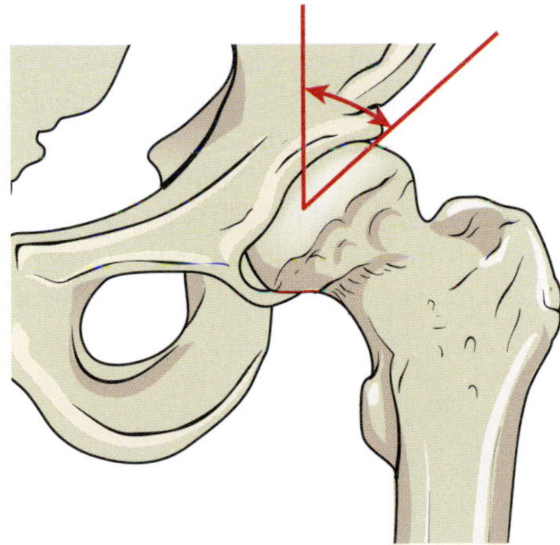

Figure 9.7 Center-edge angle. This angle is formed by two lines which originate at the center of the femoral head. One line extends vertically forming the reference whereas the other line extends to the lateral aspect of the acetabulum. This angle indicates how much of the femoral head is covered by the acetabulum. Normal acetabular coverage of the femoral head provides at least a 25° angle.

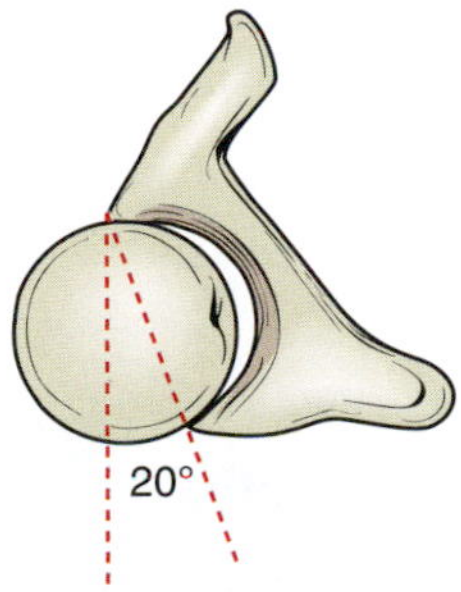

Figure 9.8 Acetabular anteversion angle. This is the angle formed by a reference line that is parallel to the sagittal plane and drawn from the posterior acetabulum and the other line that is drawn from the posterior to the anterior acetabulum. Normal acetabular anteversion angle is 15° to 20°.

symphysis pubis, and sacrococcygeal joints, movement at these joints is very important. These joints are subject to injury and may become hypomobile or hypermobile with resulting pain and dysfunction. For a complete discussion of the lumbosacral, sacroiliac, and sacrococcygeal joints, refer to the previous chapter. The pubic symphysis articulation is discussed here but the primary focus of this chapter is the pelvis and hip motions.

As mentioned in Chapter 8, the pelvic ring is formed by connections of the ilia, sacrum, and pubic symphysis. Detail of the sacroiliac joints is provided in Chapter 8. The symphysis pubis is the anterior connection between the left and right pubic bones (Fig. 9.1). The articulating surfaces of these pubic bones are covered with hyaline cartilage and separated by a fibrocartilagenous disc. As you recall from Chapter 1, the pubic symphysis is an amphiarthrodial joint whose primary function is stability. The joint is protected by strong ligaments on all sides and, additionally, is reinforced by attachments of the rectus abdominus, pyramidalis, and internal abdominal oblique muscles (Chapter 8). The pubic symphysis closes the pelvic ring anteriorly. Because the pelvic ring is a closed system with all its bones forming a complete ring, motions occurring at the SI joints will affect pubic symphysis motion, and vice versa.

Hip Joint

The hip joint, or acetabulofemoral articulation, is a diarthrodial triaxial joint with three degrees of freedom. The hip joint is a ball-and-socket joint. The joint surfaces of the femoral head and acetabulum correspond better to each other and have firmer connections than the joint surfaces of the body's other ball-and-socket joint, the glenohumeral joint. This high congruency and the presence of firm connective tissue between the articulating partners promotes joint stability. The hip joint moves in three planes to produce the following motions: flexion-extension, abduction-adduction, and medial rotation-lateral rotation. In most activities, hip motion occurs as a combination of these three planes of movement. Additionally, these hip motions are accompanied by movements of the pelvis and the lumbar spine during functional activities.

The acetabulum portion of the hip joint (Fig. 9.9) is a deep sphere-shaped cavity rimmed by a strong, fibrocartilagenous acetabular labrum, which adds to the joint's depth and stability. The acetabulum faces anteriorly and inferiorly, forming a roof over the head of the femur. At birth, the acetabulum is actually quite shallow. The concavity deepens secondary to the forces of weight-bearing that occur during the normal developmental advancement in locomotion.

The articulating surface of the acetabulum includes only its anterior, superior, and posterior sides. The superior periphery of the acetabulum, easily visualized as a horseshoe, is thicker and lined with hyaline cartilage; this is where the weight-bearing occurs.[15, 16] Inferior to this horseshoe-shaped articular cartilage is the center of the **acetabular fossa.** This central area of the socket is not lined with hyaline cartilage. The acetabular fossa does not bear weight and is deep enough that it does not come in contact with the femoral head, but it makes other important contributions. The acetabular fossa contains a fibroelastic fat pad that contains proprioceptors providing valuable joint sensory input. The acetabular fossa also serves as a reservoir for synovial fluid when the hip is heavily loaded.[17] As the joint compresses during lower extremity weight-bearing, synovial fluid is secreted to lubricate the joint.[18, 19] When the forces on the joint decrease, synovial fluid returns to the reservoir. The acetabular fossa contains the ligamentum teres, further described with the joint's other soft tissue. Along with its labrum, the acetabular fossa establishes a partial vacuum so that negative atmospheric pressure helps to maintain the contact between the two articulating partners.[20, 21]

The femoral head is two-thirds of a sphere, and the acetabulum is a hemisphere. Similar to the glenohumeral joint, the femoral head has a larger articulating surface than the acetabulum. At the center of the head of the femur is a small pitted foveal area devoid

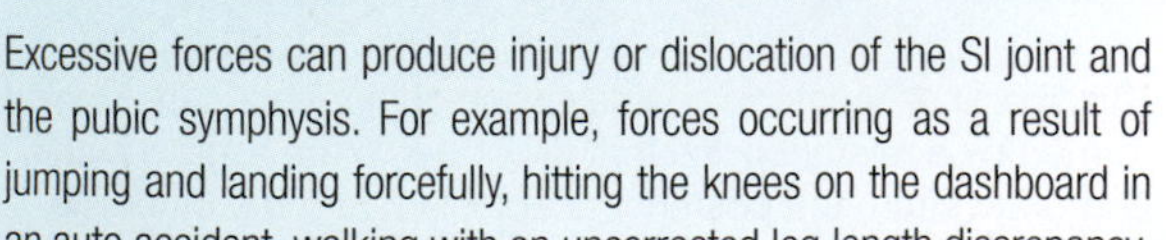

PRACTICE POINT

Excessive forces can produce injury or dislocation of the SI joint and the pubic symphysis. For example, forces occurring as a result of jumping and landing forcefully, hitting the knees on the dashboard in an auto accident, walking with an uncorrected leg length discrepancy, or producing forceful hip flexion motion during a soccer kick that is suddenly blocked by an opponent can all result in secondary injury to the pubic symphysis.

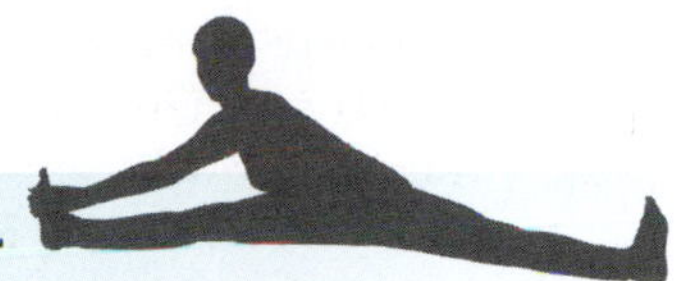

PRACTICE POINT

The acetabular labrum is a vital structure of the hip joint that provides important joint stability. It is susceptible to injury in sports that require sudden and powerful flexion-extension movements of the hip such as dance, ice hockey, baseball, soccer, martial arts, and golf.[13] A high correlation has been found between labral tears and femoroacetabular impingement primarily because of the types of repetitive stresses placed on the hip during these sports activities.[13, 14] The average age range of subjects experiencing these injuries is from the midteens to 40, an age range consisting of active individuals. Symptoms include pain with scouring tests (checking for pain while axial load is placed on the femur) and passive end range motions in hip extension, abduction, and lateral rotation. Most repairs are performed arthroscopically with patients returning to pre-injury activities.[14]

of hyaline cartilage. This femoral fovea reciprocates with the acetabular fossa as the connection point of the ligamentum teres and blood supply (Fig. 9.10). When weight-bearing in the quadruped position with the hips flexed, slightly abducted, and laterally rotated, the femoral heads are completely covered by the acetabulum (Fig. 9.9). In nonweight-bearing, however, the hip joints are incongruent because the femoral heads are larger than the acetabula. The soft tissue surrounding the hip provides significant stability and support for the joint, as we will see in a subsequent section of this chapter.

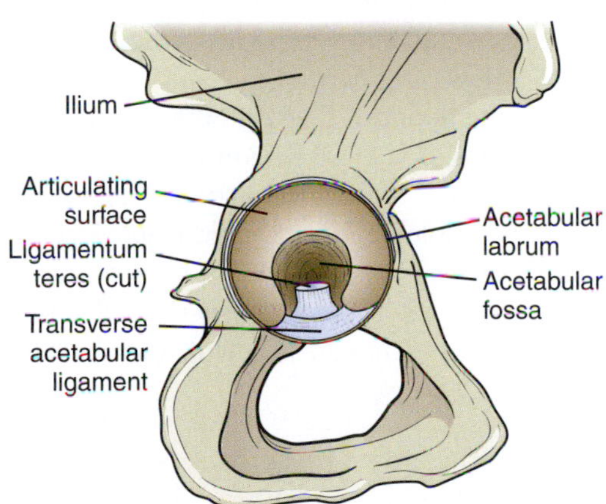

Figure 9.9 Articulating surface of acetabulum with key features noted, including: acetabular articulating surface, acetabular labrum, acetabular fossa, ligamentum teres, and transverse acetabular ligament.

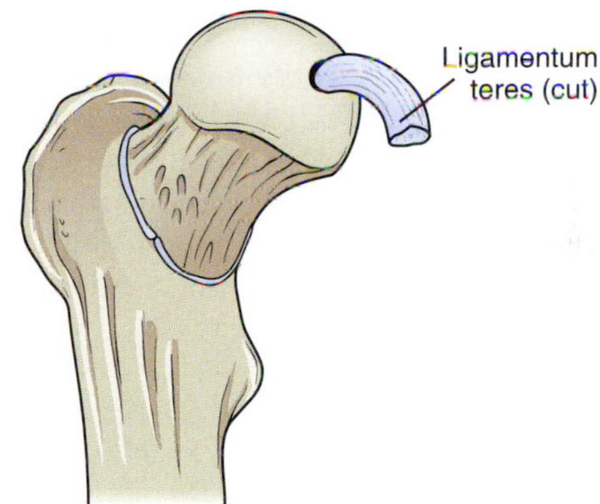

Figure 9.10 Articulating surface of femur illustrating the relationship of the ligamentum teres that attaches to the head of the femur at the fovea and then to the acetabular fossa.

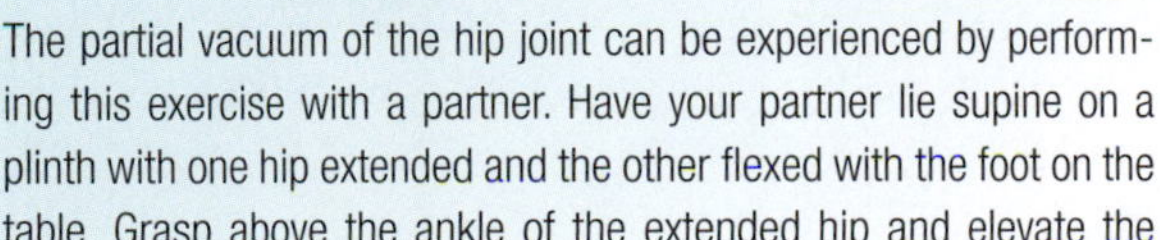

PRACTICE POINT

The partial vacuum of the hip joint can be experienced by performing this exercise with a partner. Have your partner lie supine on a plinth with one hip extended and the other flexed with the foot on the table. Grasp above the ankle of the extended hip and elevate the extremity about 30° off the table. Lean back to apply a distraction force on the hip. Now, relax the distraction force and feel the suction force pulling the femur back into the joint.

Osteokinematics

The osteokinematics of this region change according to which bony segment is the moving segment. In open kinematic activity, the hip joint's motions in all three of its cardinal planes occur as movement of the convex femoral head within the concave acetabulum. However, when hip motion occurs in closed chain positions, osteokinematic motion involves the concave acetabulum moving on the convex femoral head. Since the proximal acetabular segment of this joint is the pelvis, which is functionally and structurally linked with the trunk and low back, motion of the hip also produces motions at its neighboring segments in closed chain positions. Remember that, at all joints, motion between the articular surfaces is the same whether the distal or the proximal bony segment moves. If the proximal segment is stabilized, then motion results at the distal segment, but if the distal segment is anchored, then the proximal segment is the moving segment. We will look at osteokinematic motion of this joint from both perspectives: *pelvic motion,* or motion at the pelvis on the femur, and *hip motion,* or motion of the femur on the pelvis.

Pelvic Motion on the Femur

Unique to this body segment, there are additional specific terms used to identify the joint motion when the pelvis rather than the femur is the moving segment. These terms describe pelvic motion: anterior and posterior pelvic tilt in the sagittal plane; lateral tilt in the frontal plane; and protraction (anterior rotation) and retraction (posterior rotation) in the transverse plane (Fig. 9.11). At rest, the pelvis is in a neutral position (Fig. 9.11A1). A neutral position is when the ASIS are horizontally aligned with the PSIS and in vertical alignment with, or slightly posterior to, the pubic symphysis.[22, 23]

Sagittal plane motion of the pelvis is either an *anterior* or *posterior pelvic tilt* (Fig. 9.11A2 and 9.11A3). In an anterior pelvic tilt, the pelvis tilts or inclines forward so that the ASIS move in an inferior direction anterior to the pubis. Associated with this movement is lumbar spine extension so that the low back becomes lordotic. As we shall see when we discuss the muscles of this region, the primary muscle responsible for an active anterior pelvic tilt is the iliopsoas. A posterior pelvic tilt occurs when the pelvis moves or inclines posteriorly; the ASIS moves in a superior and posterior direction, and the lumbar spine flexes to reduce lumbar lordosis. This action is the result of a force couple whereby the abdominal muscles rotate the pelvis upward and anteriorly in concert with the gluteus maximus muscle which rotates the pelvis posteriorly and into extension. Anterior and posterior pelvic tilts are motions of the entire pelvic ring in the sagittal plane around a medial-lateral axis. To illustrate the concept described earlier related to articulating partner motions, these pelvic tilt motions on the femur in the sagittal plane are really the same as motions of femoral flexion and extension on the pelvis. An anterior pelvic tilt occurs when the pelvis moves on the stable femur, and hip flexion occurs when the femur moves on the stable pelvis; likewise, a posterior pelvic tilt occurs when the femur is the stable segment and the pelvis is the moving segment, and hip extension

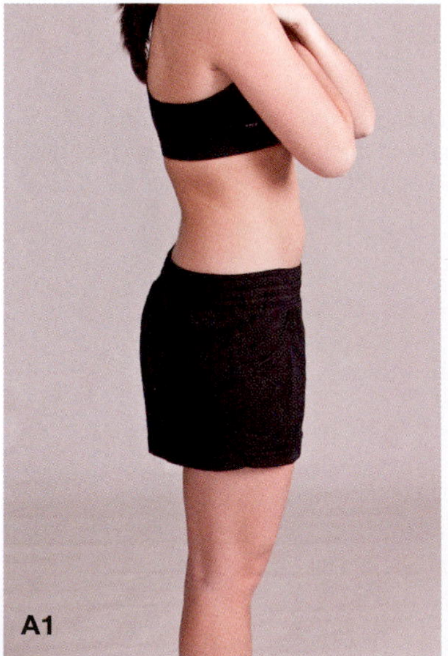

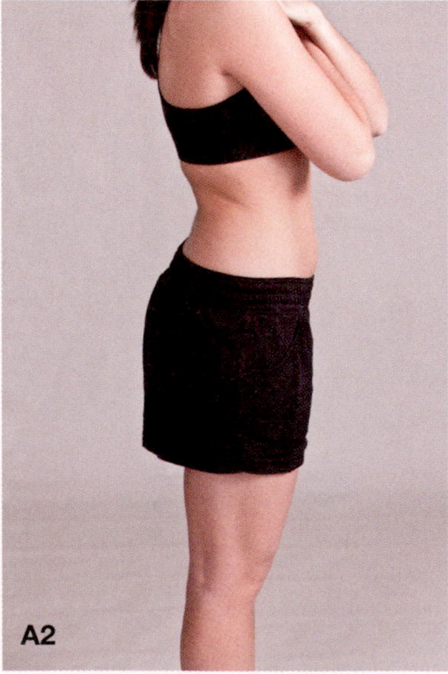

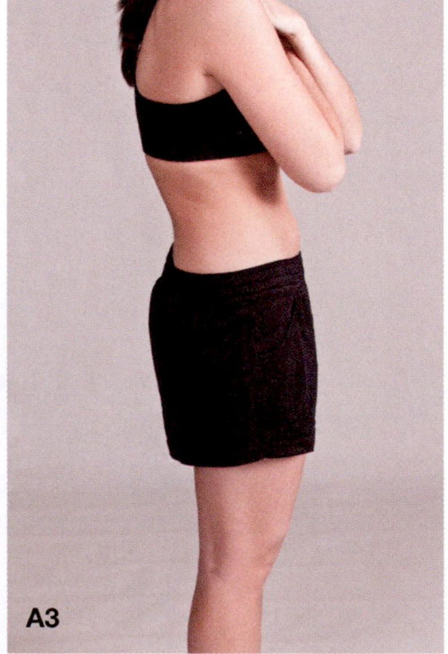

Figure 9.11 Pelvic motions. **A1)** Neutral position. **A2)** Anterior pelvic tilt. **A3)** Posterior pelvic tilt.

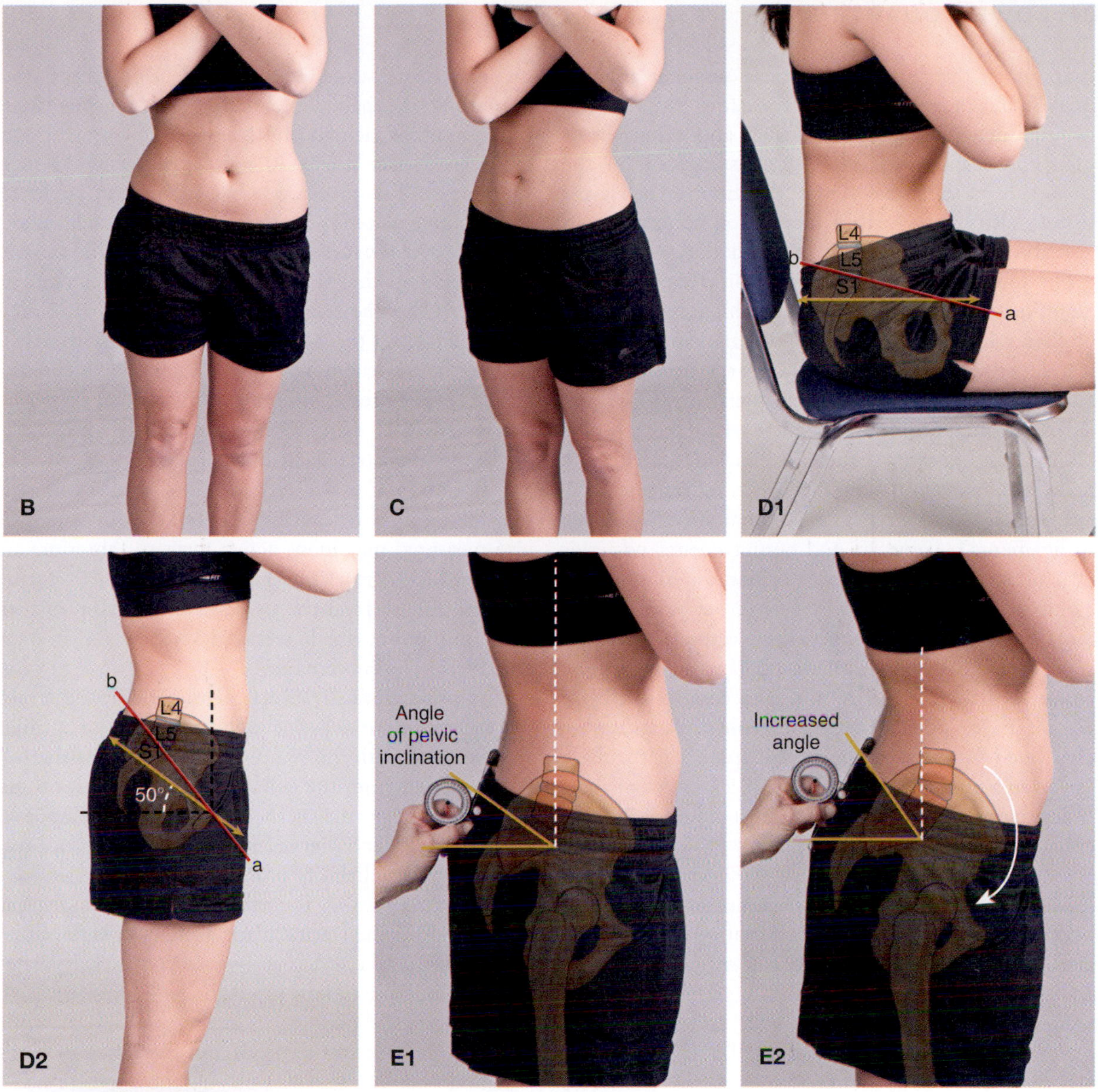

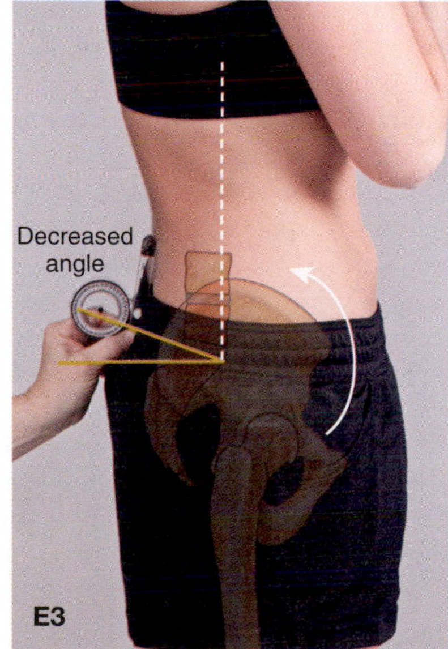

Figure 9.11—cont'd B) Lateral tilt. C) Anterior rotation or protraction (left) and posterior rotation or retraction (right). D) Pelvic inclination in sitting contrasted with position in standing. Arrows on the drawing in D1 and D2 contrasts original method used by Fick[24] to determine pelvic inclination by drawing a line between the PSIS and pubic symphysis to the later use of the "plane of the inlet" represented by line a-b, between L-S junction and pubic symphysis. E) Current clinical method to evaluate pelvic inclination using an inclinometer.

occurs when the pelvis is the stable segment and the femur is the moving segment. Therefore, anterior and posterior pelvic tilt produce flexion and extension of both hips, respectively, in bilateral stance or on the stance side in unilateral stance. An anterior pelvic tilt position also occurs with a hip flexion contracture or weak abdominal control during hip motion.

The amount of posterior pelvic tilt in erect standing is determined by the tension of the two hip joint's capsules and their reinforcing ligaments. The ligament having the greatest influence is the iliofemoral, or Y ligament; this ligament is discussed later this chapter (Fig. 9.12A and 9.13). If greater posterior pelvic tilt is attempted, it occurs only by compensatory motion that includes flexing the knees simultaneously with the pelvic movement. This knee flexion causes hip flexion so the tightened anterior hip ligaments become lax and permit greater posterior pelvic tilt motion. In the sitting position, anterior hip ligaments become lax and no longer restrict pelvic movement, and the pelvis tilts backward causing the plane through the PSIS and symphysis pubis to be more horizontal. A posterior pelvic tilt is accompanied by a decrease in, or obliteration of, the physiologic lumbar curve. Such flattening of the lumbar spine is particularly marked in sitting. On the other hand, a forward inclination of the pelvis, as is often seen in standing, is accompanied by an increased lumbar curve.[14–16]

Clinical Evaluation of Pelvic Inclination

A determination of the amount of range of motion of anterior and posterior pelvic tilt (inclination in degrees) can be made by visualizing or drawing a line representing an oblique plane through the PSIS and the foremost portion of the symphysis pubis (Fig. 9.11D). The angle created by this plane intersecting with the transverse plane is called the **angle of pelvic inclination**. This method of measuring pelvic inclination was first advocated by Fick,[24] who considered the amount of sagittal plane tilt range for adult men to be between 50° and 60° and somewhat larger for women. Fick's method of measuring the angle of pelvic inclination has been used by many investigators but has not been universally adopted. Sometimes, the "plane of the inlet" (inlet to the lesser pelvis) is used as a reference plane. This plane, indicated by the line a-b in Figure 9.11D, passes through the lumbosacral junction and through the foremost portion of the symphysis pubis. If this plane is used, the angle of pelvic inclination is greater than when it is determined by Fick's method.

It is difficult to measure the angle of pelvic inclination in the living subject. Therefore, a more clinically applicable method to determine normal or abnormal inclination of the pelvis is needed. One recent study examining the pelvic inclination angle using digital inclinometry yielded both good intratester and intertester reliability in 30 healthy subjects (15 male, 15 female).[49] To measure pelvic inclination angle, the investigators placed the inferior peg of the inclinometer centrally over the sacrococcygeal joint with the superior peg touching the skin superiorly, as illustrated in Figure 9.11E. The researchers defined the pelvic inclination angle as the angle between that of the inclinometer and a true horizontal. Mean pelvic inclination angles between testers in females ranged between 73.8° ± 6.1° and 76.1° ± 6.1° whereas mean pelvic inclination angles between testers in males ranged between 70.1° ± 5.7° and 75.4° ± 4.2°. In addition to measuring the neutral pelvic inclination angle, the investigators also measured maximum active forward (anterior) and backward (posterior) tilt (Fig. 9.11E2, 3). This further allowed the researchers to calculate total pelvic tilt range of motion, which averaged 13.85° ± 4.1° in males and 19.1° ± 7.3° in females.

A simple clinically practical method to determine normal or abnormal pelvic inclination is done by aligning the ASIS with the symphysis pubis. When the subject is viewed from the side, the pelvic inclination may be considered normal if these two points are approximately in vertical alignment. Walker and associates[25] confirmed the reliability of this method.

Lateral tilt is either the left or right pelvis moving up or down along the frontal plane around an anteroposterior axis (Fig. 9.11B). When one side of the pelvis laterally tilts, the contralateral hip is the pivot point or axis of motion. Lateral tilt will occur in a reciprocal relationship between one side of the pelvis and the other, such that when one side of the pelvis tilts up, the opposite side of the pelvis will tilt slightly down, or drop. In unilateral stance, if you place a hand on each ASIS, you will feel a slight tilt of your pelvis up on the unsupported side in order to resist the natural downward pull of gravity when your leg is in the nonweight-bearing position. This lateral pelvic tilt in unilateral stance is described later in this chapter and again in Chapter 12 when we discuss aspects of stance and gait.

Pelvic rotation is an anterior (or forward) and posterior (or backward) motion of the pelvis in the transverse plane around a superior-inferior axis. During pelvic rotation, as with lateral tilt, the contralateral hip is the pivot point around which the motion occurs. This reciprocal relationship between the left and right pelvis exists in all pelvic motions occurs because of its closed system—one side moves and the opposite must move in the contralateral direction if full motion is to occur. In pelvic rotation, as one side of the pelvis rotates anteriorly, or protracts, the opposite side rotates posteriorly, or retracts (Fig. 9.11C). These transverse plane rotational motions are vital pelvic motions during gait and will be discussed later.

Hip Motion on the Pelvis

Primary motions of the femur at the hip include flexion and extension in the sagittal plane, abduction and adduction in the frontal plane, and medial and lateral rotation in the transverse plane. Typical ranges of motion for adults are displayed in Table 1–2. The anatomic axis of the femur is represented by a line drawn through the femoral shaft (Fig. 9.5). The mechanical axis is represented by a line connecting the centers of the hip and knee joints. For typical adults in standing, the mechanical axis is vertical because of the angle of inclination. A line connecting the centers of the two femoral heads in the standing position is called the common hip axis. At the hip joint, movement may take place about any of its three axes, each of which pass through the center of the femoral head and neck area.[26]

Flexion and *extension* at the hip occur in the sagittal plane; the axis for flexion and extension is in a medial-lateral direction. Typical range of motion in adults is 120° of flexion and 10° to 20°of extension[2, 16–21] (Table 1–2). Normal unilateral hip flexion with the knee flexed occurs until the anterior thigh contacts the anterior surface of the trunk. When the knee is extended, the muscle length of the hamstrings limits full hip flexion. Hip extension is limited by the iliofemoral ligament to 10° to 20°; this ligament is discussed later. When an individual extends the hip beyond its limits, excessive pull of the psoas major on its proximal attachment on the lumbar vertebrae moves the lumbar spine into increased lumbar lordosis.

Abduction and *adduction* at the hip occur in the frontal plane around an anteroposterior axis. Hip abduction is approximately 45° and is usually accompanied by some degree of lateral tilt (elevation) of the pelvis; this pelvic movement is also called hip hiking. Hip adduction is clinically described as contact of the two thighs at the body's midline (0°). However, the lower extremities may cross over the midline into additional adducted positions of 30° to 40°[2, 16–21] (Table 1–2). Since the hip must be in slight flexion to allow clearance for full adduction, adduction is not a pure planar motion; however, it is an important motion during many functional activities such as in running, kicking, pivoting, and crossing the thighs during relaxed sitting.

Medial and *lateral rotation* at the hip in standing occur in the transverse plane around a vertical axis, which is identical to the mechanical axis of the femur. This axis runs through the centers of the femoral head and the knee joint (Fig. 9.5). In medial rotation, the greater trochanter moves forward in relation to the anterior part of the pelvis. Lateral rotation is a movement in the opposite direction. To illustrate the close relationship between pelvic and hip motion, in standing, forward rotation of the pelvis produces medial rotation of the weight-bearing hip whereas backward rotation produces lateral rotation of the supporting hip. When the knee and hip are both flexed to 90° (as in sitting), hip rotation is defined by the amount of tibial motion from 0°, the neutral position with the leg hanging over the plinth. Typical ranges of motion in adults is 0° to 45° in hip lateral rotation and 0° to 35° in medial rotation[2, 16–21] (Table 1–2).

Passive ranges of hip joint motion vary considerably with age and may deviate markedly from the average values found in Table 1–2. For example, because of the fetal position prior to birth, the normal hip posture of a full-term newborn baby is flexion with marked limitation of hip extension. Several studies have documented the restriction in extension typically measured at a 28° average (SD = 8.2) of flexion in a newborn.[27] During infancy and early childhood, this newborn "flexion contracture" disappears as the baby moves about, progresses from the supine to the prone position, and develops extension antigravity control. As development proceeds, the amount of hip extension increases so a residual flexion contracture of 19° is present by six weeks and only 7° persists by six months of age.[28, 29] On the other hand, flexibility of other hip motions gradually decreases throughout childhood, adolescence, and into adulthood. At the other end of the developmental time line, hip ranges of motion in active, healthy people 60 years and older show decreases from younger averages (Table 1–2).[30] Decreases in all hip motions is seen between ages 70 and 92, with the largest loss (33%) occurring in hip abduction motion (Table 9–1).[31] Studies have found that normal subjects have no significant difference in motion between the right and left hips.[27, 29, 32] This finding validates the clinical practice of using the contralateral unimpaired joint's measurement as a guide in determining the individual's normal ranges of motion.

End feels of hip ranges of motion usually are firm because of ligamentous limitations. The exception is hip flexion in knee flexion, which may be limited by abdominal adipose tissue, yielding a soft end feel. In severe obesity, this limitation can limit functions such as tying shoes or driving a car, as well as the ability to reach for objects. Hip flexion performed with the knee extended is limited by the length of the hamstring muscles.

(text continues on page 388)

TABLE 9–1 | HIP JOINT LIGAMENTS

Image	Joint	Ligament	Proximal Attachment	Distal Attachment	Motions it Limits
Anterior View Iliofemoral ligament Pubofemoral ligament Intertrochanteric line	Hip	Iliofemoral ("Y" ligament or ligament of Bigelow)	AIIS and iliac portion of acetabulum	As a thickening of the anterior and superior joint capsule, attaches to the intertrochanteric line of femur	Hip extension, especially hyperextension; superior portion limits adduction and lateral portion limits some lateral rotation;[63] also limits pelvic posterior tilt.
Anterior View Iliofemoral ligament Pubofemoral ligament Intertrochanteric line	Hip	Pubofemoral	Pubis (anterior aspect of superior ramus) and anterior-medial or pubic portion of acetabular rim	As a thickening of anterior and inferior capsule, attaches to anterior intertrochanteric fossa and to neck of femur, posteriorly	Hip extension, abduction and lateral rotation; also limits ipsilateral pelvic lateral tilt.

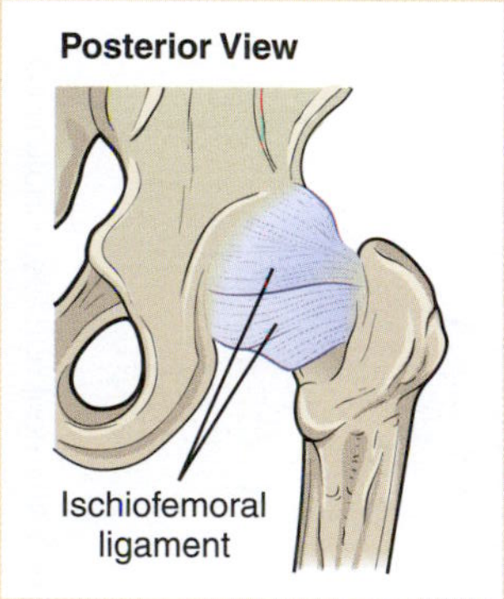 Posterior View Ischiofemoral ligament	Hip	Ischiofemoral	Ischial portion of acetabulum rim and labrum, posteriorly and inferiorly	As a thickening of posterior and lateral capsule, attaches to posterior aspect of femoral neck near apex of greater trochanter medially	Hip extension, abduction and medial rotation; limits hyperflexion; superior fibers limit extreme adduction (especially when hip is flexed); also limits ipsilateral pelvic rotation.
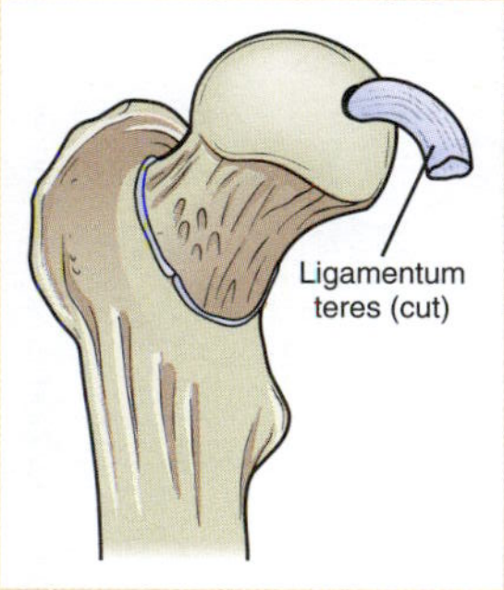 Ligamentum teres (cut)	Hip	Ligamentum teres (means ligament to the head; *teres* meaning round as in femoral head)	Center of acetabular fossa	Fovea of femoral head	Prevents extreme limits of adduction, flexion and lateral rotation or adduction, extension and medial rotation.[3] Primary function: serves as a conduit for a branch of obturator artery (foveal artery) to deliver blood supply to femoral head.

Arthrokinematics

A convex, spherical femoral head moves within a concave acetabular cup. Therefore, the joint abides by the convex-on-concave principle: The convex head glides in the concave acetabulum in a direction opposite to the distal femur's motion. During sagittal plane hip motions, the femoral head spins posteriorly during flexion and anteriorly during extension. When sagittal plane motion is combined with motion in another plane both spinning and gliding of the articular surfaces occur. For example, when flexion combines with abduction-adduction or medial-lateral rotation, the femoral head spins and glides within the acetabulum.

The accessory motions of the hip include distal traction and lateral, dorsal, and ventral glides. The negative atmospheric pressure within the joint usually limits the amount of joint distraction. In one study, a force of 45 lb was required in adult cadavers to laterally distract the joint 3 mm, but when the joint capsule was incised to release the vacuum, the femur could be distracted about 8 mm without significant traction force.[33] In adults, Arvidsson found that traction forces above 90 lb are required to produce a significant joint separation in the open-packed position.[34] However, when the hip is in the close-packed position of full extension, medial rotation, and abduction, the capsule and ligaments are taut and produce additional resistance to accessory motions and joint distractions. Because of the weight of the limb and the large forces needed to apply joint mobilization, the techniques usually require additional mechanical stabilization and external straps to support body parts during their application.[35]

Soft Tissue at the Hip Joint

The soft tissue of the hip joint includes an acetabular labrum, several bursae, a joint capsule, and four main ligaments. As previously mentioned, the strong, fibrocartilagenous labrum encircles the rim of the acetabulum like a horseshoe to deepen the joint cavity and grip the head of the femur; this configuration increases bony congruency and enhances stability. The labrum's horseshoe ends are connected in the inferior socket by the transverse acetabular ligament (Fig. 9.9). The joint capsule is a strong structure attaching to the outer rim of the acetabulum, enclosing the neck of the femur like a tube. The capsule attaches its distal border along the trochanteric line anteriorly and just above the trochanteric crest posteriorly. This thick joint capsule is strongest and thickest superiorly and anteriorly, lending maximum stability to the hip during weight-bearing.

Strong ligaments reinforce the capsule on all sides and are named according to their attachment sites: iliofemoral, ischiofemoral, and pubofemoral ligaments (Table 9–1). All three ligaments are embedded within the capsule, arising from pelvic attachments and spiraling around the femoral head and neck to provide tremendous reinforcement and stability (Fig. 9.12). Interestingly, in addition to offering individual unique contributions to hip stability, all three ligaments stabilize the extended hip, limiting extension and contributing to the ability to stand upright with minimal muscle activity. The iliofemoral ligament covers the hip joint anteriorly and superiorly. This ligament is also called the Y ligament because it resembles an inverted letter "Y." The pubofemoral ligament lies over the anterior

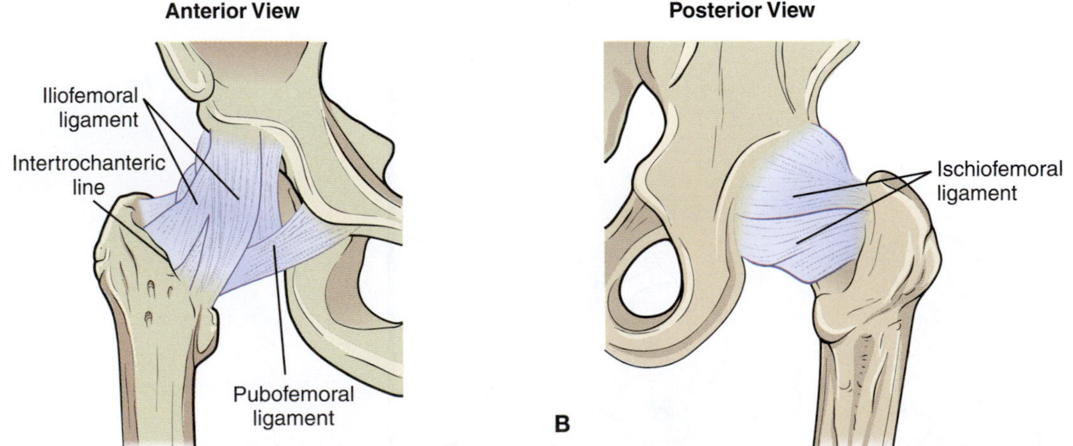

Figure 9.12 Ligaments of the right hip joint. **A)** Anterior view demonstrates the iliofemoral or Y ligament and the pubofemoral ligament. **B)** Posterior view illustrates the ischiofemoral ligament.

and inferior hip joint and the ischiofemoral ligament covers the posterior and inferior joint. All of these ligaments are lax when the hip is flexed and are taut when the hip is extended. In the standing position, the iliofemoral ligament, particularly its inferior band, prevents both posterior motion of the pelvis on the femur and extreme extension of the hip (Fig. 9.12). The anterior ligaments, especially the pubofemoral ligament, limit lateral hip rotation, and the ischiofemoral ligament limits medial rotation. Abduction of the hip is limited by tension on the pubofemoral and ischiofemoral ligaments. Adduction is limited by tension of the superior, or iliotrochanteric, portion of the Y ligament. Spanning the pelvis and the hip, these ligaments likewise offer stability to the pelvis.

The ligamentum teres is not strong enough to add significantly to the stability at this joint. The word *teres* means "head" in Latin; the other name for this ligament is *ligament of the head of the femur*. It is an interesting structure, encased in a flattened sleeve of synovial membrane, functioning primarily as a conduit for the small artery that helps to supply the femoral head and additionally as a small elastic guy wire for the head of the femur in the acetabular fossa. Its mechanical role is minimal because it is a weak structure and tension on it does not occur until the hip reaches extreme positions of hip abduction and flexion with lateral rotation or hip adduction and extension with medial rotation.[3] See Table 9–1 for a complete list of the ligaments, their attachments and functions.

There have been as many as 20 bursae described at the hip. As you would expect, they are all associated with musculotendinous regions that are subjected to high friction or compressive forces. Three main bursae are the most important in this region: over the greater trochanter, over the iliopsoas tendon, and in the iliopectineal region.[22,36,37]

Muscles

It is important to remember when studying the muscular function of the pelvic and hip region, that these muscles work to either move the pelvis on the femur or move the femur on the pelvis. For example, the hip flexors will either flex the hip on the stable pelvis or tilt the pelvis anteriorly on the stable femur. These functions of the muscles at the pelvis and hip are determined by whether the limb is moving in weight-bearing or non-weight-bearing. In weight-bearing, the femur is stationary and movement occurs as the pelvis moves on the femur. On the other hand, in the open chain or non-weight-bearing position, the femur moves on the stable pelvis. The pelvic and hip muscles are adaptable and utilize their structural features, such as their size, length, or line of pull, to meet the joint's functional task demands.

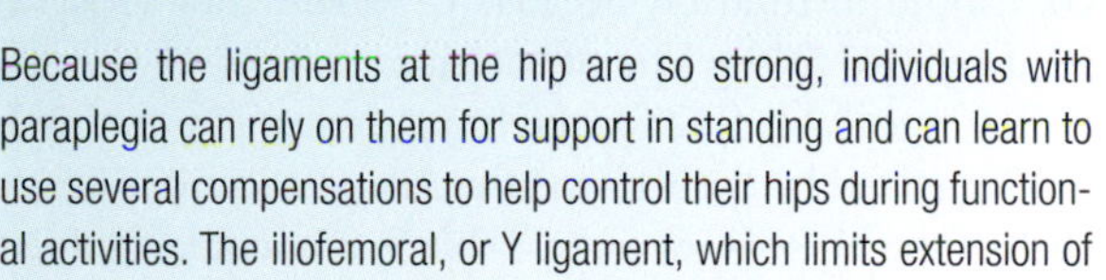

PRACTICE POINT

Because the ligaments at the hip are so strong, individuals with paraplegia can rely on them for support in standing and can learn to use several compensations to help control their hips during functional activities. The iliofemoral, or Y ligament, which limits extension of the hip, is so strong that it permits persons with paraplegia to maintain standing balance when the knees and ankles are stabilized with orthoses (Fig. 9.13). The upper body's center of gravity is moved posterior to the axis of the hip joint so the individual can then lean the upper body weight against the hip's Y ligaments. In this position, the pelvis remains in extension on the femur.

Greater trochanteric bursitis is a commonly encountered clinical condition. Comprised actually of several smaller bursa and a larger bursal sac spanning between the greater trochanter and iliotibial band over the posterior aspect of the greater trochanter, their role is to reduce friction between the greater trochanter and gluteus maximus and between the iliotibial band and greater trochanter. Greater trochanteric bursitis is sometimes associated with malalignment such as a leg length discrepancy and femoral anteversion. It also can result from either a trauma such as falling and landing on the lateral hip or from repetitive microtrauma to the lateral hip, seen frequently in runners. In the aging hip, it can occur secondary to degenerative changes.

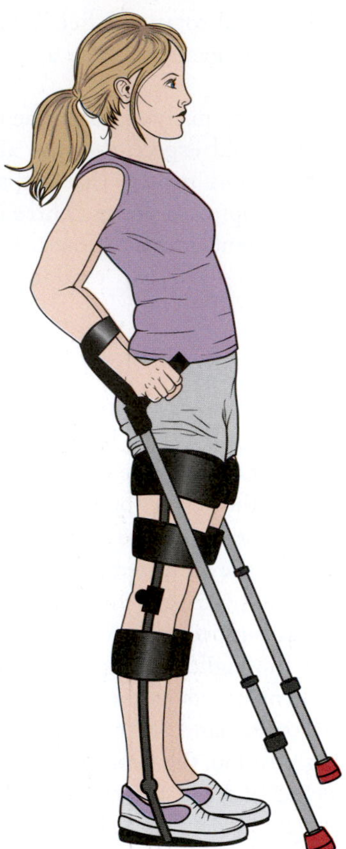

Figure 9.13 In the presence of paralysis of active hip extension, functional standing balance is achieved by placing the center of gravity of the head, arms, and trunk (HAT) posterior to the hip joint axis and leaning against the iliofemoral ligaments. Such a posture is accompanied by an increased lumbar curve.

Before we can learn about the hip muscles in relation to their specific functions, such as single-limb support, we must first understand their anatomical plane actions. Therefore, the primary hip muscles and their primary roles as flexors, extensors, adductors, abductors, and lateral or medial rotators are presented first. It will be helpful to recall from your anatomy studies where the muscles cross the joint so you may more easily visualize muscle function. The following generalizations of hip muscles can be made:

- Most of the muscles in the anterior area which cross the front of the hip joint flex the hip and are innervated by the femoral nerve. This "anterior" group includes:
  - Iliopsoas
  - Rectus femoris
  - Sartorius
  - Pectineus (listed here as a flexor but is also a primary adductor)
  - Tensor Fascia Latae (listed here as a flexor but is also a primary abductor).
- Most of the muscles in the medial region adduct the hip and are innervated by the obturator nerve. This "medial" group includes:
  - Adductor longus
  - Adductor brevis
  - Adductor magnus
  - Gracilis
  - Pectineus (listed here as a adductor but is also a primary flexor).
- Most of the muscles that cross the hip posteriorly extend the hip and are innervated by the sciatic nerve. This "posterior" group includes:
  - Gluteus maximus
  - Biceps femoris
  - Semitendinosus
  - Semimembranosus
  - Adductor magnus (posterior fibers).
- Most of the muscles in the lateral hip region abduct the hip. This "lateral" group includes:
  - Gluteus medius
  - Gluteus minimus
  - Tensor fascia latae (listed here as a primary abductor but also flexes and to a lesser degree, medially rotates the hip).

The actions of hip lateral and medial rotation are performed by some "prime" movers responsible solely for those actions, such as the deep lateral rotators. Several other muscles also act as lateral rotators in addition to their primary motion. Medial rotation is not performed by any solo prime mover but by muscles which have other "primary" anatomical actions; they contribute to rotation because of where they cross the joint relative to the axis of rotation.

Refer to Table 9–2 for the hip muscles. These muscles are organized by their prime functional contributions for each of the hip's six motions. Table 9–3 is a quick guide to the primary motions at the hip. Box 9-3 summarizes the key weight-bearing functions of the hip muscles.

Flexors

The hip flexors act primarily as a mover of the limb in the open kinematic chain by advancing the lower extremity during the swing phase in gait, lifting the limb up steps, and propelling objects in various activities such as in kicking. There are actually nine muscles that cross the anterior hip joint. Of those nine, five muscles are primary hip flexors. Listed in order of their significant

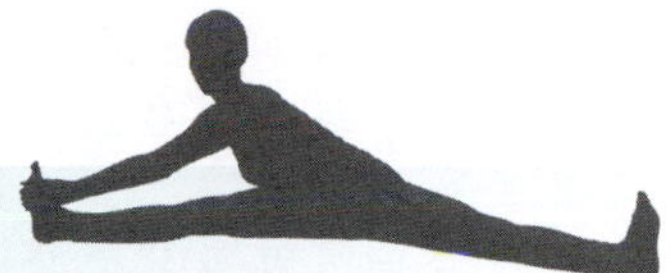

PRACTICE POINT

The nerves that innervate the muscles of the hip arise from spinal nerves L_1 through S_3 that form the lumbosacral plexus. These nerves and the muscles they innervate are easy to remember because their names are very descriptive of their anatomic locations and functions. The femoral nerve innervates most of the flexors of the anterior thigh; the obturator nerve passes through the medial and inferiorly located obturator foramen and innervates the adductor group; the superior and inferior gluteal nerves innervate the gluteal muscles and the sciatic nerve supplies the posterior hamstring muscles.

contribution, these muscles include the iliopsoas, rectus femoris, sartorius, pectineus, and tensor fascia latae (TFL). Of these five, the iliopsoas is the strongest and most consistent hip flexor. It crosses over the anterior middle aspect of the joint, so its line of pull is always well aligned to act as a hip flexor. The sartorius, TFL, and pectineus cross either laterally or medially to the midline of the joint; therefore these muscles also act in either the frontal or transverse plane or both, depending on their position to these axes. The pectineus and sartorius have anteromedial locations whereas the tensor fasciae is located anterolaterally. Although the TFL flexes and medially rotates the hip, because its position makes it is a very strong abductor, it is discussed along with the other abductors. The rectus femoris, sartorius, and tensor fascia latae cross two joints, the hip, and the knee, and are therefore subject to active and passive insufficiency.

Iliopsoas

The iliopsoas (Fig. 9.14A), aptly named because of its location (*ilio,* ilium, and Gr., *psoa,* the loins), consists of two parts—the iliacus and the psoas major. These two muscles have separate proximal attachments but a common distal attachment (Fig. 9.14B). The portion of the iliopsoas that lies distal to the hip joint is located medial to the sartorius and is partially covered by the upper portion of the sartorius. The psoas major muscle fibers form a round, rather long belly that lies medial to the iliacus.

As a single joint hip flexor, the contribution of iliopsoas is quite powerful; it is the most important flexor of the hip. Functionally, the iliopsoas contributes to limb shortening and limb advancement during the swing phase of gait. Because of its proximal attachment on the lumbar vertebrae, the iliopsoas tilts the pelvis anteriorly and works with the abdominal muscles to maintain pelvic stability during functional activity. When the legs are fixed in the supine position, the combined bilateral action of the iliopsoas muscles elevates the trunk and flexes the pelvis on the femur, motions occurring when performing a full sit-up. Some sources indicate that the iliopsoas contributes weakly to rotation, especially lateral rotation of the abducted hip, but its leverage to act in hip rotation is so small that it is functionally negligible.[38, 39] For our purposes, we will consider its primary role as a strong hip flexor when the femur moves on the pelvis and as a muscle producing anterior pelvic tilt when the pelvis moves on the femur.

Rectus Femoris

The rectus femoris, a bipennate shaped muscle, is so named because it runs "straight" down the anterior aspect of the femur. It is the only muscle of the quadriceps group that crosses both the hip and the knee (Fig. 9.15). Acting as both a hip flexor and knee extensor, the rectus femoris can develop considerable force as a hip flexor but runs the risk of active insufficiency when hip flexion is performed with knee extension. The rectus femoris is a strong contributor to hip flexion and applies most of its force at the hip when the knee is flexed, such as in climbing stairs.

Sartorius

Considered the longest muscle in the body, the sartorius (L., *sartor,* a tailor) is a superficial, strap-like muscle extending obliquely from the lateral pelvis and thigh (ASIS), across the anterior and medial thigh down to the proximal anteromedial tibia (Fig. 9.16). The sartorius is a two-joint muscle, passing on the flexor side of the knee, where it forms the pes anserine along with the gracilis and semitendinosus tendons (see Chapter 10). Its nickname, "tailor muscle," is descriptive of the hip's seated position when the muscle performs its three hip actions of flexion, abduction, and lateral rotation in the "tailor" or cross-legged sit. This muscle's additional functions at the knee are described in the Chapter 10.

The perpendicular distance from the axis of hip flexion-extension to the line of action of the sartorius is considerable. Therefore, even though this muscle's cross section is relatively small, it can exert a comparatively large torque. As the muscle contracts, it rises from the

(text continues on page 400)

TABLE 9–2 | MUSCLES OF THE PELVIC AND HIP REGION

Group	Muscle	Proximal attachment	Distal attachment	Nerve	Action	Palpation
Flexors (5 primary)	Iliopsoas 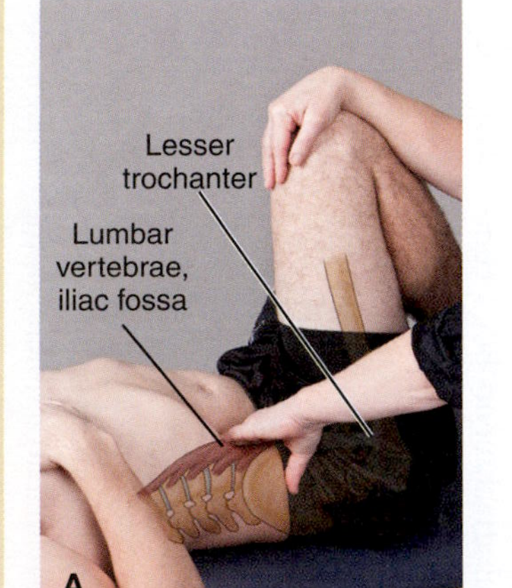 	**Iliacus:** iliac fossa, inner sides anterior spines of ilium, covers anterior and medial hip joint and femoral neck; winds around neck in a posteromedial direction; **Psoas major:** vertebral bodies, intervertebral discs, transverse processes T_{12}–L_5	Lesser trochanter	**Iliacus:** branches of femoral nerve (L_1–L_4); **Psoas major:** branches of lumbar plexus (L_1–L_4).	Hip flexion; Anterior pelvic tilt	**Iliacus:** Deep and difficult to palpate; rather flat lying behind abdominal viscera, following and partly filling out the iliac fossa; **Psoas major:** With subject in supine or sitting, subject relaxes abdominal muscles. The palpating fingers are placed at waist, between lower ribs and iliac crest, probing deeply but gently toward posterior wall of abdominal cavity, near vertebral column. The round, firm belly of the psoas major may be felt as the muscle contracts.

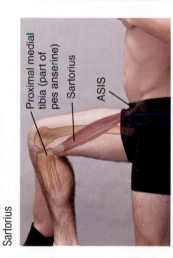

Flexor	Rectus femoris 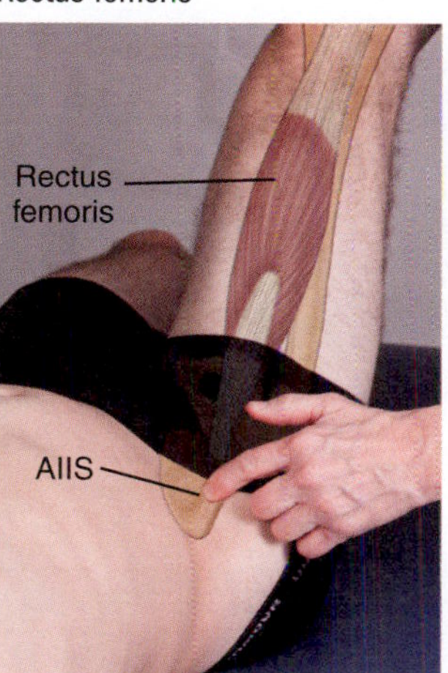	**AIIS and above the acetabulum**	Deep aponeurosis narrowing to broad tendon attaching to superior aspect of patella and to tibial tuberosity via patellar tendon	Femoral nerve (L_2–L_4)	Hip flexion; knee extension	With subject supine, resist hip flexion and knee extension: rectus femoris tendon is palpated proximally in the "V" formed between laterally running TFL and medially running sartorius; muscular portion can be palpated and followed down the anterior thigh to attachment onto superior patella.
Flexor	Sartorius	**ASIS**	Medial surface of tibia close to crest; anterior to distal attachments of gracilis and semitendinosus tendons	Femoral nerve (L_2–L_3).	Hip flexion, abduction and lateral rotation; knee flexion and medial rotation	The lower portion of the muscle cannot be observed well but may be followed by palpation if the subject alternately isometrically contracts and relaxes the muscle once the examiner passively positions the hip in lateral rotation with both the knee and hip in flexion to 90°. Sartorius can also be palpated at its distal attachment as part of the Pes Anserine (see Chapter 10).

Continued

TABLE 9–2 | MUSCLES OF THE PELVIC AND HIP REGION—cont'd

Group	Muscle	Proximal attachment	Distal attachment	Nerve	Action	Palpation
Flexor	Tensor fascia lata	Crest of ilium, ASIS lateral to proximal attachment of sartorius	Iliotibial tract, about one-third of the way down the thigh to the iliotibial tract, which then attaches to lateral condyle of tibia	Branch of the superior gluteal nerve (L_4–L_5, S_1)	Hip flexion, abduction, and medial rotation	Identified near hip joint, lateral to the upper portion of sartorius, while flexing, abducting, and medially rotating hip.
Flexor	Pectineus	Superior ramus of pubis	Along a line (pectineal line) between lesser trochanter and linea aspera on upper posteromedial femur	Femoral nerve (L_2–L_4).	Hip flexion and adduction	Flat muscle bordering laterally to iliopsoas and medially to adductor longus; palpation of the pectineus as a separate muscle is difficult, but it may be felt contracting with other muscles. Pectineus has a muscular attachment palpable on superior ramus of pubis.
Adductors (5 primary)	Adductor longus	Pubis	Linea aspera (middle third)	Obturator (L_3–L_4)	Hip adduction	Suggestion: palpate on yourself, as follows: In sitting, palpating fingers are placed in proximal groin distal to the pubic ramus, where some of the adductor tendons can be grasped from front to back; flex your hip

						with adduction and lateral rotation, continuing motion until your legs are crossed. The tendon of the adductor longus is prominent and easily distinguished from the others.
Adductor	Adductor brevis	Pubis	Proximal linea aspera and pectineal line	Obturator (L_3–L_4)	Hip adduction	Muscular attachment of adductor brevis palpated by adducting thigh and locating belly lateral to prominent adductor longus tendon.
Adductor	Adductor magnus	Pubic and ischial rami, ischial tuberosity	Linea aspera (entire length) and adductor tubercle	Obturator (L_2–L_4) and sciatic (L_4)	Hip adduction	While resisting hip adduction, palpate adductor magnus along entire medial thigh and follow to distal attachment on adductor tubercle of femur.

Continued

TABLE 9–2 | MUSCLES OF THE PELVIC AND HIP REGION—cont'd

Group	Muscle	Proximal attachment	Distal attachment	Nerve	Action	Palpation
Adductor	Gracilis 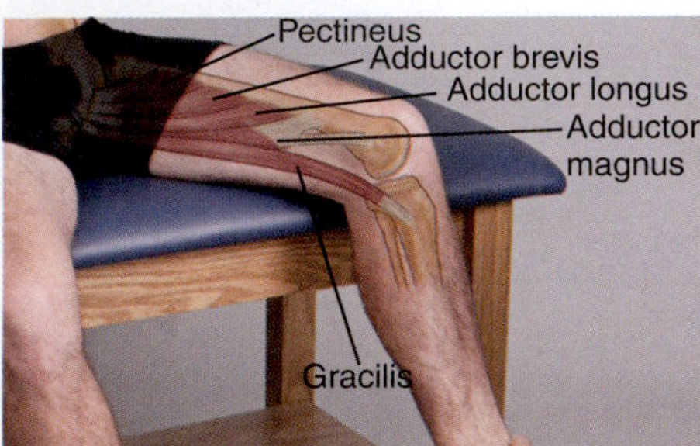	Pubis	Anterior medial surface proximal tibia	Obturator (L_2–L_3)	Hip adduction	Gracilis crosses knee attaching on anteromedial side of tibia beside sartorius and semitendinosus; resistance to knee flexion activates hamstrings and gracilis; hamstrings run laterally to ischial tuberosity while gracilis belly is medial, attaching on inferior pubic ramus.
Extensors (4 primary)	Pectineus* Gluteus maximus 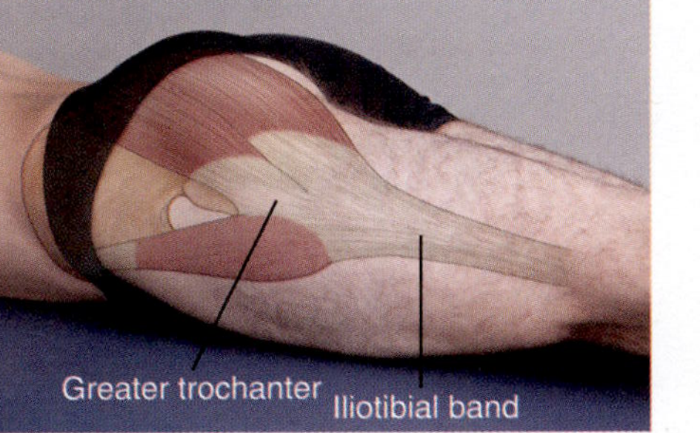	Posterior iliac crest, lumbodorsal fascia, sacrum, coccyx, sacrotuberous ligament	Posterior aspect femur onto gluteal tuberosity (distal to greater trochanter); into iliotibial tract	Inferior gluteal nerve (L_5, S_1–S_2).	Hip extension, and lateral rotation; posterior pelvic tilt	In prone or standing, gluteus maximus is easily observed by simply "setting" it without any joint motion being carried out; stronger activation of the muscle seen with hip extension and lateral rotation. Strong contraction of the gluteus maximus also observed in climbing stairs, in running and jumping.

*see flexors

Extensors	Biceps femoris (lateral hamstring) 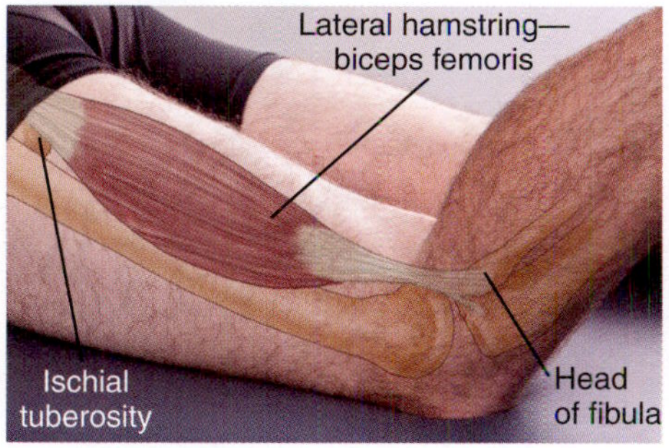	Two heads: 1) Ischial tuberosity; 2) lateral lip linea aspera	Head of fibula and lateral condyle of tibia	Sciatic nerve (L_4–L_5, S_1–S_2)	Hip extension; knee flexion and lateral rotation	Easily palpated when knee flexion or knee flexion with tibial lateral rotation is resisted, on posterior lateral thigh running from ischial tuberosity to fibular head.
Extensors	Semimembranosus and Semitendinosus (medial hamstring) 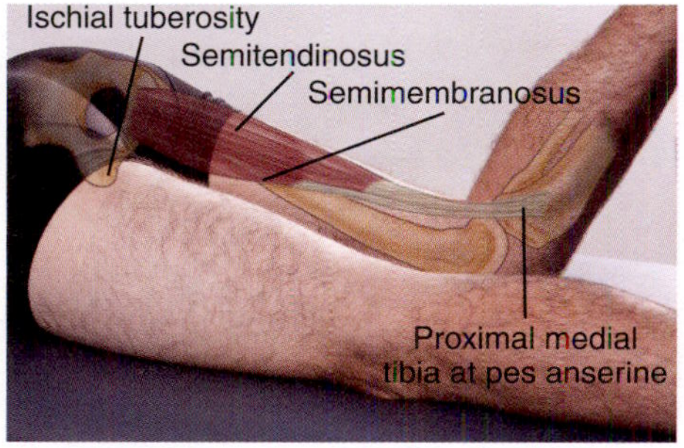	Ischial tuberosity	Posterior surface medial condyle of tibia distal to the gracilis	Sciatic nerve (L_4–L_5, S_1-S_2)	Hip extension; knee flexion and medial rotation	Semitendinosus tendon is palpated just proximal to the posterior medial knee with the knee flexed. Most of the semimembranosus is covered by semitendinosus and adductor magnus. With subject prone, the distal portion of both muscles can be palpated while resisting knee flexion or knee flexion with medial tibial rotation.

Continued

TABLE 9-2 | MUSCLES OF THE PELVIC AND HIP REGION—cont'd

Group	Muscle	Proximal attachment	Distal attachment	Nerve	Action	Palpation
Abductors (3 primary)	Gluteus medius	Fan-shaped from iliac crest and outer surface of the ilium and anterior gluteal line, a line that separates its origin from that of the gluteus minimus.	Greater trochanter, near tip	Superior gluteal nerve (L_4–L_5, S_1).	Hip abduction; anterior portion flexes and medially rotates, posterior portion extends and laterally rotates. In stance, maintains pelvic stability by preventing opposite side of pelvis from dropping.	Palpated laterally below crest of ilium superior to greater trochanter during active abduction. Can also be easily palpated on stance side in unilateral stance, contracting to support HAT.
Abductors	Gluteus minimus	Fan-shaped, outer surface of ilium, between anterior and inferior gluteal lines	Anterior border of greater trochanter	Superior gluteal nerve (L_4–L_5, S_1).	Hip abduction and medial rotation	Cannot be well differentiated from medius since both muscles contract simultaneously in abduction and medial rotation; anterior portion of muscle is thickest part and is felt, together with the medius, when the hip is medially rotated.
	Tensor fascia latae*					
Lateral rotators	Piriformis	Ventral surface of sacrum, sciatic notch, sacrotuberous ligament.	Fibers take a downward lateral course, following posterior border of gluteus medius, attaching onto inner portion of greater trochanter.	Branch derived from first and second sacral nerves (L_5, S_1–S_2).	Hip lateral rotation	Palpated in lateral rotation, especially if the gluteus maximus is relaxed, as when the limb is raised into slight flexion. The palpating fingers are placed posterior to greater trochanter and moved about somewhat until the best spot for palpation is located.

*see flexors

	Deep lateral rotators: piriformis (also listed separately above because of its strong action), inferior and superior gemellus, obturator internus and externus, quadratus femoris	Posterior gluteal region with horizontal fibers attaching to posterior sacrum, ischium and pubis; covered by gluteus maximus. Uppermost is piriformis and lowermost is quadratus femoris with other four located between those two.	Greater trochanter	Varying but generally branches from S_1–S_2	Hip lateral rotation	Palpated as a group but not well individually; can palpate piriformis (uppermost of the group) and quadratus femoris (lowermost) with fair accuracy. Quadratus femoris: palpated between ischial tuberosity and greater trochanter, contracting when performing or resisting hip lateral rotation.
Lateral Rotators	Gluteus maximus	See above				Gluteus maximus and sartorius are large muscles whose secondary responsibility is hip lateral rotation.
	Sartorius	See above				
Medial rotators	Multiple contributors Gluteus medius* Gluteus minimus* Tensor fascia latae Pectineus Adductor group					

*act most consistently as medial rotators

TABLE 9-3 | PRIME MOVERS AT THE HIP BY ANATOMIC ACTION

Hip Action	Prime Movers
Flexion	Iliopsoas Rectus Femoris • Especially with knee extension Sartorius • Especially with hip abduction and lateral rotation Pectineus • Especially with hip adduction Tensor fascia latae • Especially with hip abduction and medial rotation
Extension	Gluteus Maximus Biceps femoris Semimembranosus Semitendinosis Adductor magnus (posterior fibers)
Adduction	Adductor longus Adductor brevis Adductor magnus Gracilis Pectineus (also a flexor)
Abduction	Gluteus medius Gluteus minimus Tensor fascia latae (also flexes and medially rotates)
Lateral Rotation	Gluteus maximus Deep lateral rotators Sartorius • Especially with hip flexion and abduction
Medial Rotation No muscle acts as a primary mover; all are secondary movers in medial rotation	Gluteus minimus, anterior fibers Gluteus medius, anterior fibers Tensor fascia latae • Especially with hip flexion and abduction

underlying structures; this movement away from the joint mechanically increases its moment arm length to increase its torque. Because of its great length, the sartorius can shorten a long distance. Due to the way the sartorius crosses both the hip and knee, it is most effective in simultaneous hip and knee flexion, especially

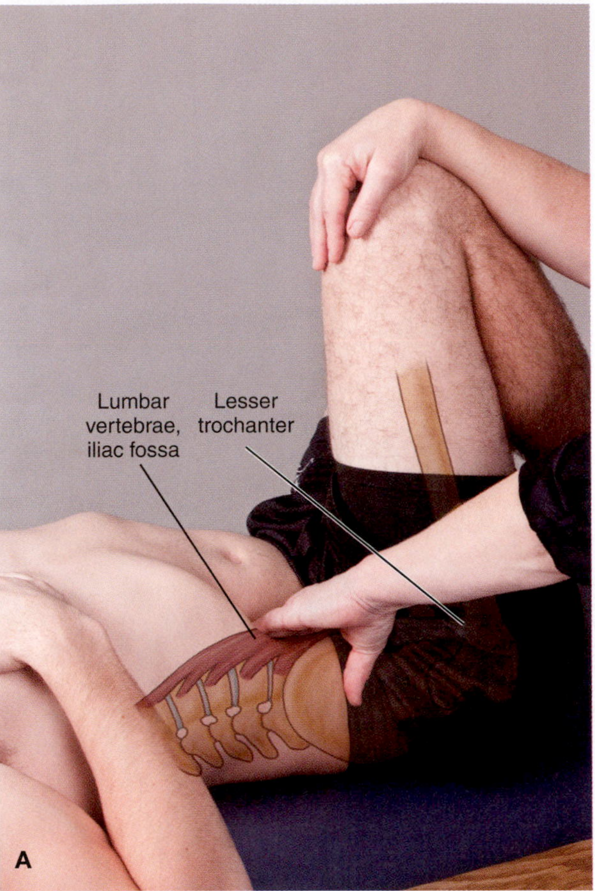

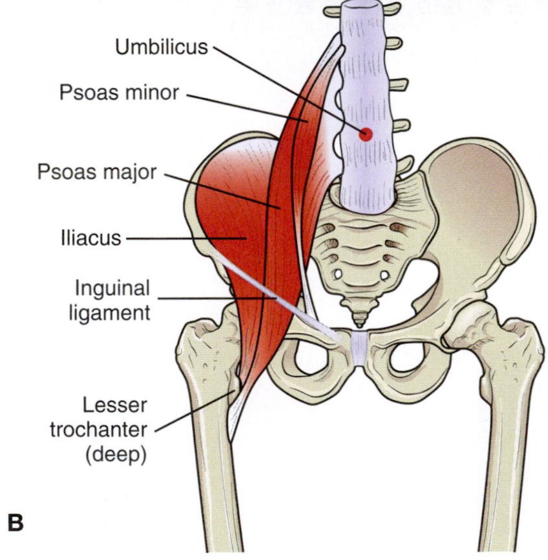

Figure 9.14 A) Identification of the iliopsoas and palpation of the psoas major. If the subject's abdominal muscles are relaxed, the examiner may place the palpating fingers deep enough to feel the contraction of the psoas major when the subject flexes the hip against mild resistance. B) Line drawing of iliopsoas depicting attachments and line of muscle pull.

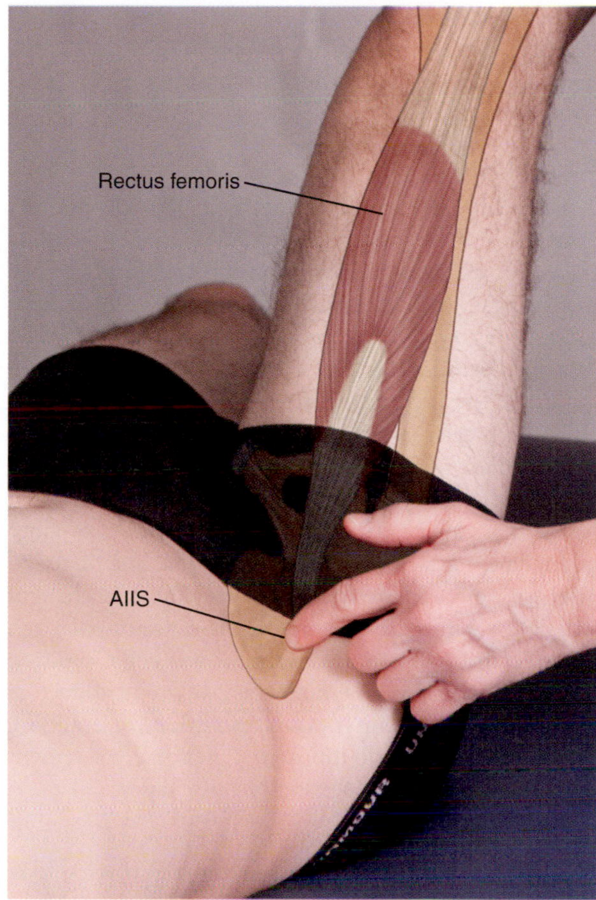

Figure 9.15 Rectus femoris. Model demonstrates a contraction of the rectus femoris muscle and the artwork overlay draws attention to the attachments and line of muscle pull.

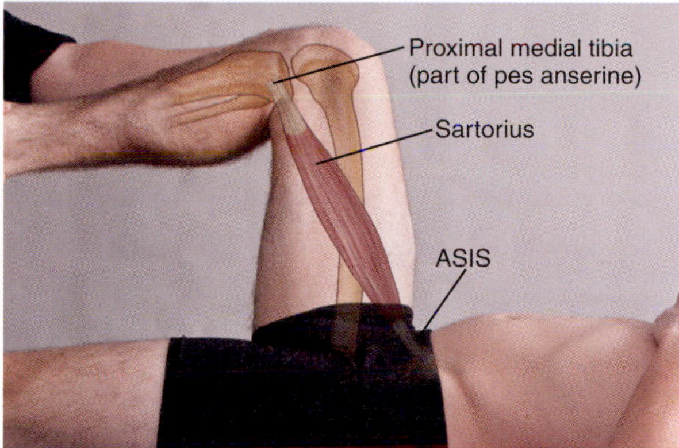

Figure 9.16 Sartorius. Model demonstrates a contraction of the sartorius muscle and the artwork overlay draws attention to the attachments and line of muscle pull.

when hip lateral rotation is added to provide foot clearance, such as when stepping over to mount a horse, motorcycle, or bicycle.[22, 40]

Tensor Fasciae Latae

Lateral to the sartorius on the anterolateral thigh is the tensor fasciae lata (TFL). This muscle is named because one of its primary actions is to "tense" the "fascia lata" or iliotibial band, which stabilizes the lateral thigh and knee. The tensor fascia lata's small muscle belly is only a few inches long, but its tendinous attachment is long, forming the iliotibial band or tract (ITB or ITT) (Fig. 9.17). The tensor fascia lata has been nicknamed as the "pocket muscle" because if you put your hand in your side pants pocket, your hand will rest on the muscle's belly. This muscle, like the sartorius, affects both the hip and knee. At the hip, the tensor fascia lata flexes, abducts, and to a small degree, medially rotates the thigh.

Pectineus

The pectineus muscle is located at the anteromedial hip. The pectineus (L., *pecten, comb)* is a rather flat muscle located deep in the groin. The area of its distal attachment is approximately as wide as its proximal attachment, giving the muscle a quadrangular or comb-like shape, hence its name (Fig. 9.18). The pectineus belongs essentially to the adductor group of muscles, its fibers running approximately parallel to those of the adductor longus, but it also flexes and medially rotates the hip.

Secondary Flexors

In addition to the five primary hip flexors listed above, including the tensor fascia lata, which will be further discussed as a hip abductor, there are several muscles that can act to flex the hip because they cross the joint anteriorly but more medially. The adductor longus,

PRACTICE POINT

If the iliotibial band becomes tight, it "snaps" as it moves over the greater trochanter, when the hip moves between flexion and extension. This "snapping hip syndrome" of a tight iliotibial band is often associated with greater trochanteric bursitis, a condition commonly seen in distance runners.

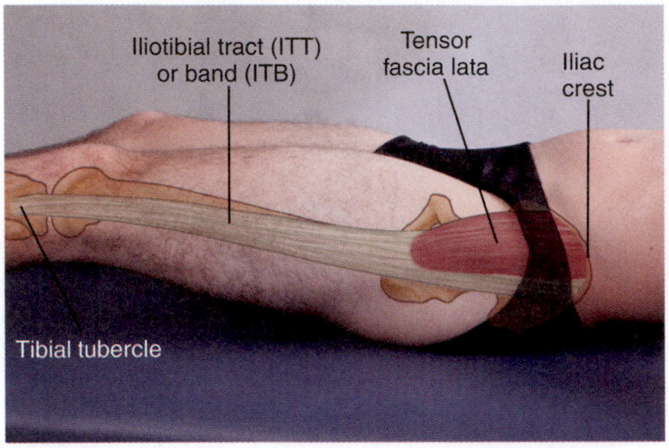

Figure 9.17 Tensor fascia lata contracting as the subject abducts, slightly flexes and medially rotates the hip. The artwork overlay draws attention to the attachments and line of muscle pull as well as highlights the long, wide iliotibial tract. The location of the TFL to the anterior portion of the gluteus medius should also be noted; the two muscles lie side by side in the anterolateral hip region.

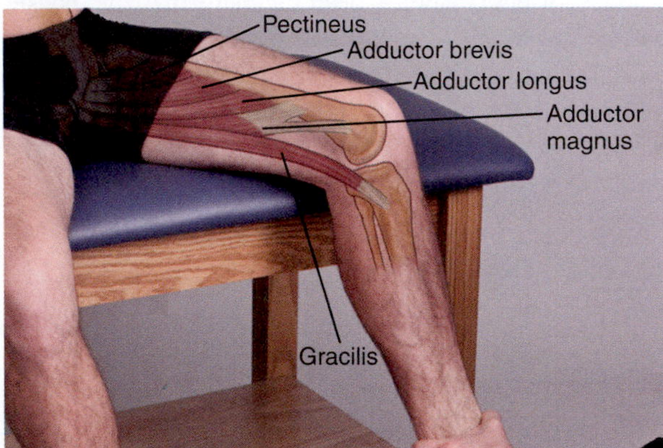

Figure 9.18 The hip adductor group: pectineus, adductor longus, adductor brevis, adductor magnus, and gracilis. The artwork overlay illustrates the relationships between these muscles and their attachments and lines of pull.

adductor magnus, and gracilis muscle are capable of flexing the hip, but with the exception of the adductor magnus, it depends on the hip's position at the time they contract.[41]

Adductors

The hip adductor group is identified as the large muscular mass of the medial thigh, bordered anteriorly by the vastus medialis and sartorius and posteriorly by the hamstrings. The pectineus, located on the anteromedial thigh is also an adductor but has been previously described because it is also a flexor. The adductor group includes the adductor magnus, adductor longus, adductor brevis, and gracilis. With the exception of the gracilis, these adductor muscles are collectively triangle-shaped, originating at fairly narrow attachments on the pelvis and giving rise to a broad triangular fiber arrangement attaching on the femur. The line of action of these muscles in relation to the joint axis changes when the hip flexes; therefore, the action of each muscle can be determined only for a specific position of the joint. In certain positions, different adductors may also produce hip flexion, extension, or rotation. These varying contributions to functional movement are discussed in a later section of this chapter.

Adductor longus and brevis

As its name indicates, the adductor longus is a long strap-like muscle. This muscle is easily located by its very thick prominent tendon in the anterior groin. It is a strong, single-joint hip adductor; its smaller synergist is the adductor brevis (Fig. 9.18).

Adductor magnus

So named for its massive size, the deeply located adductor magnus is actually made of two portions. Its more

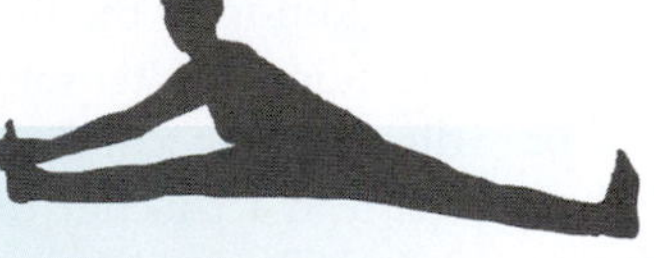

PRACTICE POINT

The adductor group can be palpated on the thigh's medial side from the pubis to the distal thigh when hip adduction is resisted. Press your knees together to palpate your own adductors. Palpating the individual muscles is difficult and proper identification requires palpating the muscles toward their attachments. Refer to Table 9–2 for additional palpation information.

The adductor group's nerve supply is primarily the obturator nerve, although the posterior fibers of the adductor magnus are also innervated by a branch from the sciatic nerve.

The adductor longus tendon is the very prominent tendon that is palpable at the groin in the anteromedial aspect of the thigh. It is so prominent that in prosthetic limb design, a well needs to be bevelled out in the prosthesis' proximal medial aspect, allowing for pressure relief for this tendon.

medial portion is a strong adductor whereas its posterior fibers assist in hip extension (Fig. 9.18).

Gracilis

The slender gracilis muscle (L., *gracilis*, slender or grace-like) is a synergist to the other hip adductors for adduction (Fig. 9.18). As part of the pes anserine, its strong distal tendinous attachment onto the proximal medial tibia provides knee stability.

Extensors

The primary hip extensor muscles are located in the posterior hip and thigh and include the gluteus maximus, biceps femoris, semitendinosus, semimembranosus, and posterior portion of the adductor magnus.

Gluteus Maximus

The gluteus maximus (Gr., *gloutos*, buttock) is the large, superficial muscle that is responsible for the roundness of the buttock region. As described in Table 9–2, its fibers run laterally from the posterior pelvis to attach to the proximal femur (Fig. 9.19). By visualizing its line of action, it is easy to imagine its primary role in weight-bearing as a stabilizer. This powerful muscle exerts a strong contraction in activities such as stair climbing, running, and jumping.[42] During walking and running, it acts both concentrically to extend the hip and eccentrically to decelerate leg swing, especially during running.[42] At the pelvis, the gluteus maximus works in concert with the abdominal muscles as a force couple to tilt the pelvis posteriorly. A strong contraction of the gluteus maximus can be palpated if an individual stands in weight-bearing hip flexion and suddenly extends the hip to bring the body upright.[43]

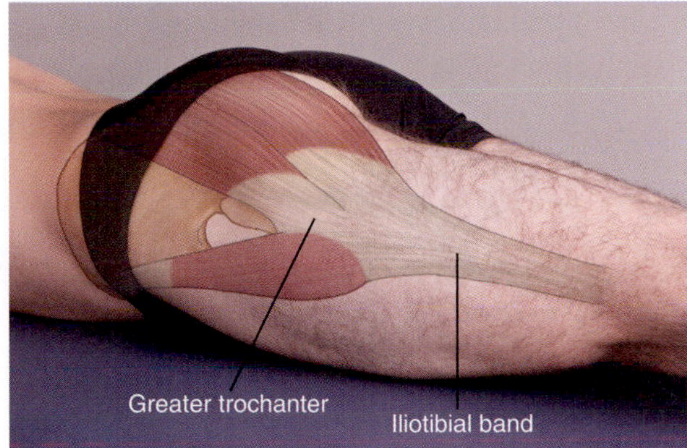

Figure 9.19 The gluteus maximus is strongly activated when the hip is extended and laterally rotated. The artwork overlay draws attention to the attachments and line of muscle pull.

Biceps Femoris, Semitendinosus and Semimembranosus

The biceps femoris, semitendinosis, and semimembranosus muscles are all part of the posterior group known as the hamstrings. This group extends the hip and flexes the knee. With their proximal attachments on the ischial tuberosity and their distal attachments on the proximal tibia, these large and powerful two-joint muscles are able to exert tremendous hip extension force; however, they are at risk for insufficiency because they cross two joints. These muscles are discussed at length in the next chapter because of their powerful actions at the knee. They are also powerful, strong hip extensors, synergistically working with the gluteus maximus.

Known as the "lateral hamstring" because of its lateral location on the posterior thigh, the biceps femoris muscle, as its name implies, has two heads. The medial hamstrings includes two muscles: the fusiform-shaped semitendinosus and the semimembranosus (Fig. 9.20 A, B). The contribution of all three hamstrings muscles to hip extension varies and is discussed in a later section of this chapter. The hamstrings rather than the gluteus maximus provide small-range anteroposterior balance of the pelvis.[43]

Abductors

Muscles of this group are located on the lateral hip and include the gluteus medius, gluteus minimus, and tensor fascia latae. Described previously, the tensor fascia lata muscle is located anterolaterally and is also a flexor and medial rotator.

PRACTICE POINT

Proper body mechanics and posture are important considerations during all functional activity. Maintaining pelvic neutrality by contracting the gluteus maximus along with the transverse abdominus and multifidus will stabilize the lumbar spine and core control during functional activities such as lifting a heavy barbell or simply standing at the kitchen sink to wash dishes.

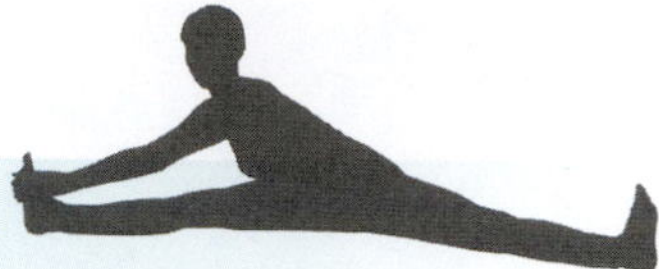

PRACTICE POINT

Similar to how a hip flexion contracture with a tight iliopsoas muscle can pull the pelvis in the sagittal plane into an anterior pelvic tilt, a comparative situation can occur with tight hamstrings. Because they attach at the ischial tuberosities, shortened hamstrings will pull the pelvis into a posterior pelvic tilt.

Both hip abductor and adductor torques demonstrate rather marked age-related changes.[44] Because of the primary role that these muscles play in standing balance, functional approaches to rehabilitation and prevention programs should emphasize balance training as well as strengthening of these muscle groups to improve pelvic stability and to prevent falls, especially in older adults.

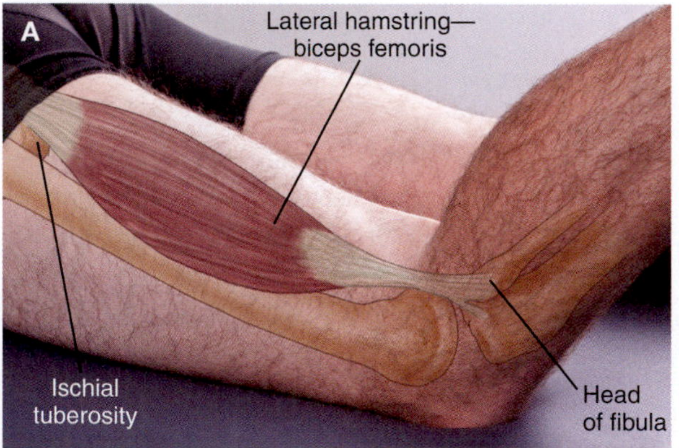

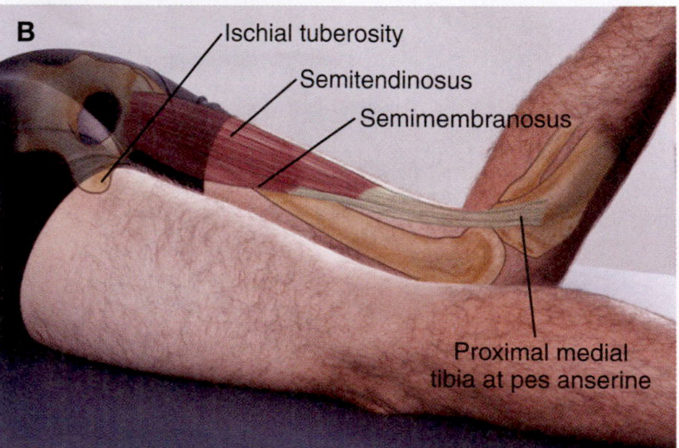

Figure 9.20 A) Biceps femoris (lateral hamstring) and B) medial hamstrings: semitendinosus and semimembranosus. The artwork overlay draws attention to the attachments and line of muscle pull.

Gluteus Medius

The gluteus medius is the largest of the lateral hip muscles. It is partly covered by the gluteus maximus posteriorly and tensor fascia lata anteriorly, but its upper middle portion is superficial, covered only by thick fascia (Fig. 9.21). Like the deltoid at the glenohumeral joint, this fan-shaped muscle has anterior, middle, and posterior portions, but these portions are not as clearly separated from each other as is the deltoid muscle. Also similar to the deltoid, all portions of the gluteus medius act as strong abductors. All portions of the gluteus medius also act as strong pelvic stabilizers. The anterior portion assists in hip flexion and medial rotation whereas the posterior portion assists in hip extension and lateral rotation. The posterior portion is comparatively small and is supplemented in hip lateral rotation by the small but powerful piriformis muscle. The piriformis is discussed later in this chapter.

In the open chain, the gluteus medius muscle is an abductor of the hip. In single-leg stance, the gluteus medius provides lateral stabilization of the pelvis to prevent dropping of the pelvis on the opposite, non-weight-bearing side (Fig. 9.22). This is by far the most important functional contribution of the gluteus medius and is elaborated on later in this chapter.

Gluteus Minimus

The fan-shaped gluteus minimus is in the deepest layer of the gluteal muscles. This muscle lies close to the capsule

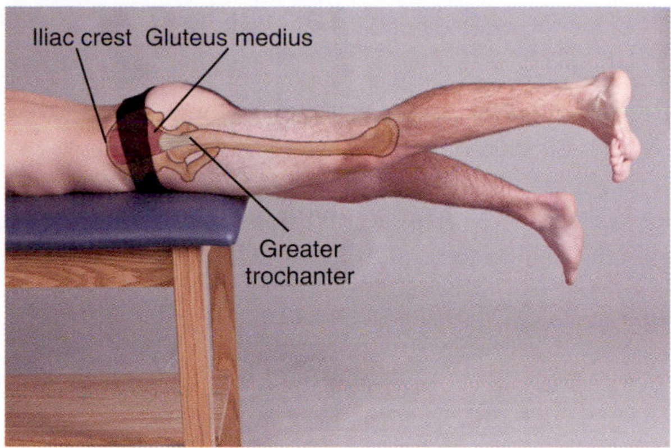

Figure 9.21 The gluteus medius is seen contracting as the subject abducts the left hip. The artwork overlay draws attention to the attachments and line of muscle pull.

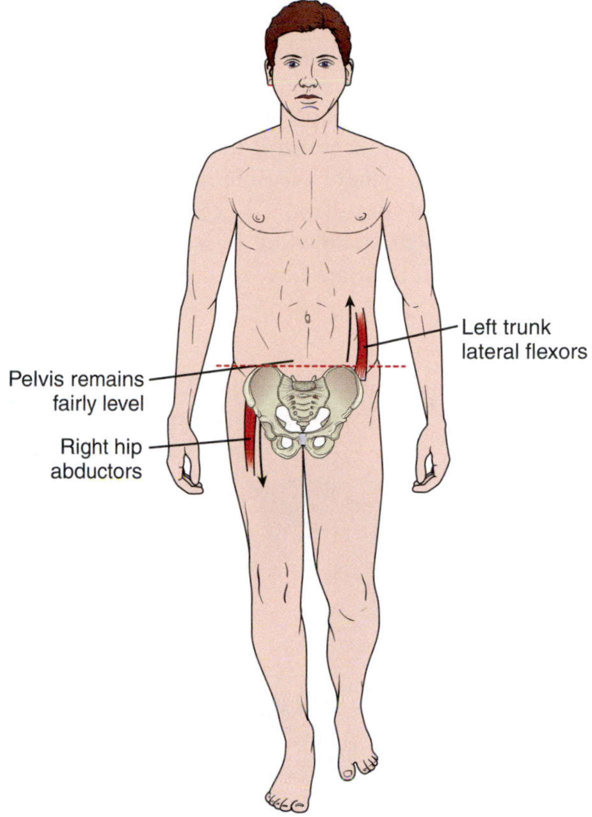

Figure 9.22 Hip abductors in single limb stance. In single leg stance, the gluteus medius provides lateral stabilization of the pelvis to prevent dropping of the pelvis on the unweighted side. With the supporting limb in adduction during single leg stance, the hip abductors are stretched, thereby placing them at their optimal length to offer a strong contraction.

of the hip joint and is covered by the gluteus medius. It is a synergist with the gluteus medius in hip abduction and can also medially rotate the hip. The gluteus minimus has also been credited with two interesting additional functional tasks: 1) contracting to keep the folds of the joint capsule from pinching; and 2) applying pressure on the femoral head to stabilize the femoral head firmly against the acetabulum.[45]

Tensor Fasciae Latae

Discussed previously because of its action as a hip flexor, the tensor fascia lata (TFL) also acts as a strong abductor and lateral thigh stabilizer. In fact, its main contribution may be to maintain tension on the large iliotibial band (ITB). By so doing, the TFL offers lateral stabilization to the thigh and knee joint during weight-bearing activities. The TFL's specific action and ability depends on the position at the hip and the forces required. Additionally, the TFL assists in medial hip rotation. As an abductor, it abducts best when the hip is also flexing. The attachment of the gluteus maximus and TFL to the iliotibial band enable these muscles to assist as knee stabilizers during weight-bearing in closed chain activities. These muscles add ITB tension without lateral knee motion to aid the knee's lateral passive support structures.

Lateral Rotators

The six small lateral rotators of the hip are located in the posterior gluteal region and are covered by the gluteus maximus, which is also a primary lateral rotator. They have proximal attachments on the pelvis and sacrum, with fibers running in a nearly horizontal direction, and distal attachments in the greater trochanter area to place them in good alignment to provide compression and, therefore, stability to the joint. Their line of pull is almost perpendicular to the vertical hip axis in standing, so they are positioned well as lateral rotators. The uppermost of the six lateral rotators is the piriformis; the lowermost is the quadratus femoris. The piriformis (Fig. 9.23), a pear-shaped muscle (L., *pirum,* pear) belongs to the second layer of muscles in this region, as does the gluteus medius, both of which are covered here by the gluteus maximus. The gemellus superior, gemellus inferior, and obturator internus share a common tendon and lie between the piriformis and the quadratus femoris. The obturator externus lies anterior to these muscles. Because of their insertion in the posterior greater trochanter region, their line of pull is collectively posterior to the axis of motion, so they serve as a lateral rotator. These rotators are considered by many to be the "rotator cuff" of the hip, providing a "fine tuning" role during hip motion.[46]

Medial Rotators

There are no specific muscles whose line of pull provides pure hip medial rotation in the transverse plane; rather, medial rotation is performed by several muscles that also provide other primary motions. These multipurpose muscles include the anterior gluteus medius, gluteus minimus, pectineus, TFL, and adductors. In addition, the medial hamstring muscles can also contribute to medial rotation.

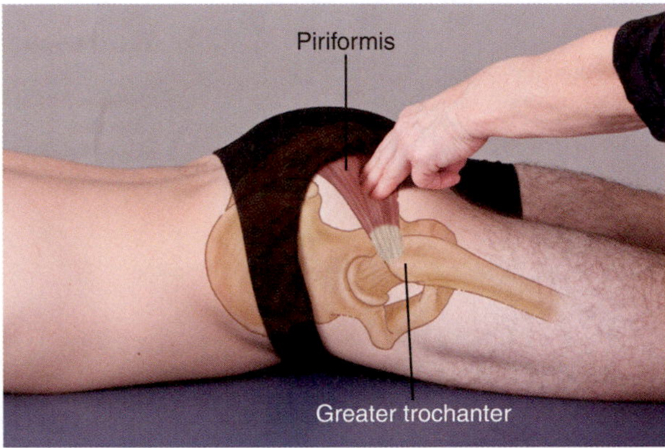

Figure 9.23 Location and palpation of piriformis.

Factors Affecting the Roles of the Muscles of the Pelvis and Hip

Remember from discussions in previous chapters that muscles may provide functional activity in various ways, acting as an agonist, antagonist, synergist, stabilizer, or neutralizer so that the desired functional action occurs effectively and efficiently. A muscle's role is determined by several factors, including the:

- number of joints it crosses;
- position of the other joints which the muscle crosses;
- size and cross section of the muscle, including fiber type/arrangement;
- leverage, determined by length and distance of attachment and line of pull from joint axis;
- type of muscle contraction—eccentric, concentric, or isometric;
- segment's position relative to gravity;
- movement task requirement;
- load being moved or stabilized; and
- speed of motion.

In addition to these factors, the pelvis and hip provide an important functional contrast in the lower extremity between the weight-bearing and nonweight-bearing demands and how those demands are met. When

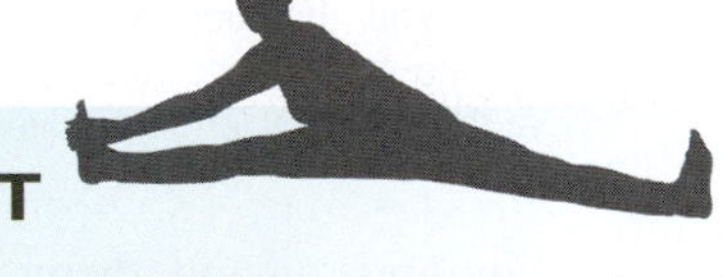

PRACTICE POINT

Clinically, the piriformis is a frequent site of pathology secondary to irritation or overuse. The sciatic nerve passes beneath the piriformis as it exits the greater sciatic foramen on its way to supply the posterior thigh musculature. Muscle spasm or tightness of the deep lateral rotators, especially the piriformis, results in tenderness in the deep gluteal region with accompanying decreased range of motion in hip medial rotation and irritation of the sciatic nerve. Either muscle trigger points or sciatic nerve irritation may cause radiating pain down the posterior leg. Subsequent pain results in functional limitations.

In a study by Delp and colleagues,[39] 15 of the 18 hip muscles studied demonstrated a tendency to provide medial rotation during excessive hip flexion. The moment arm for medial rotation increased with hip flexion whereas the moment arm for lateral rotation is decreased. This change occurs because some muscles switch roles from lateral rotators to medial rotators when the hip is more flexed.[39] With the hip in flexion, the small lateral rotators align anterior to the vertical axis of rotation and become hip medial rotators, essentially "switching" their action (Fig. 9.24). For this reason, a typical stretch of these muscles is performed with the hip and knee flexed and the hip stretched into lateral rotation.

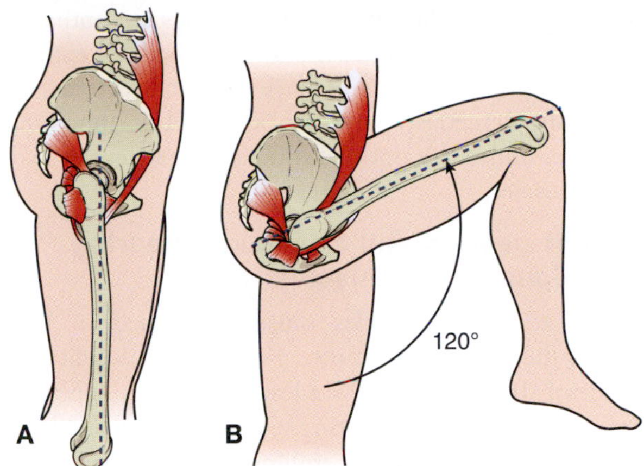

Figure 9.24 The small posterior rotators move from a posterior to an anterior position relative to the axis of rotation when the hip moves from extension to flexion. This change in position results in a change of activity. **A)** In hip extension, these muscles are lateral rotators. **B)** In hip flexion, they are medial rotators.

analyzing the functional contributions of various muscles of the pelvis and hip, it is important to consider all of the factors listed above with a special emphasis on three important kinesiological concepts: 1) the line of pull and leverage affecting the muscle's action; 2) one-joint versus two-joint muscles; and 3) whether the motion is an open kinematic chain or a closed kinematic chain activity. The following section elaborates on these concepts and offers examples of how these factors impact the pelvis and hip.

Muscle Line of Pull and Leverage

A muscle's action is determined by its line of pull relative to an axis of motion. Since the hip joint's ranges of motion are large, changes in the hip's position may change a muscle's line of pull to allow that muscle additional functions or changes in its function. For example, the gluteus medius and the tensor fascia lata are hip abductors. They both also medially rotate the hip; the anterior fibers of the gluteus medius and the tensor fascia lata medially rotate the hip when it is in flexion. Also, they do provide some medial rotation force on an extended hip, but their leverage for medial rotation is much greater when the hip is flexed to 90°.

In addition to providing muscles with opportunities for additional functions when the hip changes position, a muscle's line of pull may change so profoundly when the hip position changes as to allow it to perform actions of its antagonistic muscle.[47] The piriformis is a good example of this phenomenon. The piriformis is a lateral rotator when the hip is extended, but it becomes a medial rotator when the hip is flexed (Fig 9.24).[3, 47] Another example of this inversion of functional action occurs with the hip adductors. The line of pull of the adductor muscles is anterior to the hip joint axis in hip extension and posterior to the joint axis in hip flexion. A hip adductor may act as a hip flexor with the joint in neutral but will assist in hip extension when the hip is already flexed. For example, when the hip is in flexion, as in rock climbing, the hip adductors are forceful hip extensors; however, when the hip is extended, the adductors have more leverage as flexors (Fig 9.25). The exact position of this change from flexor to extensor varies with the specific adductor muscle, but this shift in action generally occurs between 50° and 70° of hip flexion.[47] Inversion of functional muscle action occurs in other body segments, but it is more frequently seen during functional activities at the hip.

As with other body segments which possess large muscles, there are several pelvic and hip muscles whose segments function both in cooperation and in opposition to one another. This contrast in functions within the same muscle occurs because the line of pull of the muscle at one segment is opposite to the line of pull of the muscle's other segment. Such an arrangement allows one muscle to essentially serve as its own force couple. For example, the main action of the gluteus maximus is hip extension. Upon closer assessment, however, we see that the upper portion of the gluteus maximus abducts the hip while the muscle's lower portion is an adductor. Similarly, the gluteus medius as a whole abducts the hip, but the anterior gluteus medius is a medial rotator while posterior gluteus medius is a lateral rotator. This method of performance, utilizing one muscle to provide multiple functions, provides efficiency during movement, recruiting fewer muscles than would otherwise be required.

Muscular Sufficiency: Multi-Joint versus Single-Joint Muscles

At the pelvis and hip, there are several muscles which cross two joints. These muscles include the rectus femoris, sartorius, tensor fascia lata, gracilis, and hamstring group. Recall from previous chapters that based on the principle of length-tension, a two-joint muscle's abiltiy to function is substantially influenced by the positions of the two joints it crosses. Remember that all muscles are able to shorten only so far, to about 70% of their resting length (Chapter 4). Since two-joint muscles also abide by this law, they create their greatest force at one joint if they are lengthened at the other joint. When a two-joint muscle shortens over both of its joints

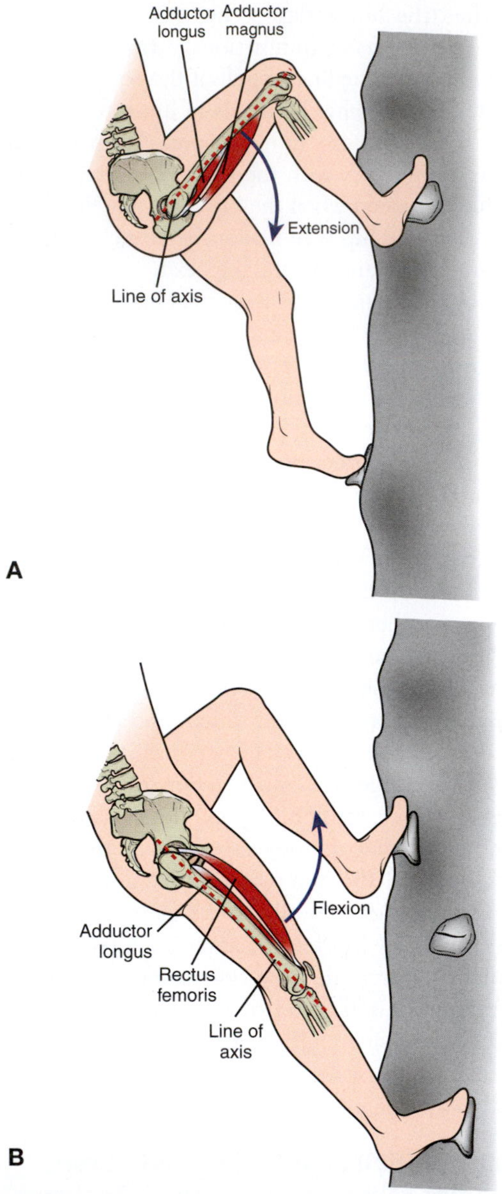

Figure 9.25 The hip adductors also serve as either hip flexors or hip extensors, depending upon the position of the muscle's line of pull relative to the joint's axis of motion. A) When the hip is in flexion, the adductors work as extensors. B) When the hip is in extension, the adductors are in a position to flex the hip.

simultaneously, it encounters active insufficiency. For example, the rectus femoris is actively insufficient when hip flexion occurs with knee extension. The rectus femoris becomes optimally sufficient as a hip flexor if the knee is flexed during hip flexion. Likewise, the rectus femoris is optimally sufficient as a knee extensor when the hip is extended during knee extension. Similarly, the hamstrings become actively insufficient if hip extension occurs with knee flexion. The hamstrings are optimally sufficient either as hip extensors when the knee extends during hip extension or as knee flexors when the hip flexes simultaneously with the knee. Most functional activities utilize this optimal sufficiency concept of two-joint muscles.

Weight-bearing and Nonweight-bearing Functions of Hip Muscles

Lower extremity muscles must be studied in both weight-bearing and nonweight-bearing situations. Some of the most important lower extremity contributions to function occur during weight-bearing and body movement. The task of controlling and supporting body weight of the head, arms, and trunk (HAT) involves controlling and supporting approximately two-thirds of one's body weight (e.g., 100 lb in a 150-lb individual). On the other hand, the mass moved when moving a single lower extremity is equal to only approximately one-sixth of one's body weight (e.g., 25 lb in a 150-lb individual). Obviously, the amount of force and control required to support the trunk and upper body are much greater than that of a single extremity. Nonweight-bearing (NWB) lower extremity movements provide speed of movement, such as swinging the leg during kicking, running, or walking. However, during weight-bearing (WB) activities, the muscles of the lower extremity are required to perform forceful contractions upon the extremity's fixed distal segment. Such movement relies on hip and pelvic muscles to provide pelvic stability on the moving extremity. In functional terms, even slight to moderate muscle weakness results in noteably diminished ability to perform proper closed chain functions although open chain motions without resistance may appear unimpaired.

Analysis of Muscle Activity at Pelvis and Hip

This section examines and describes ways in which hip and pelvic muscles work together to accomplish a multitude of functional tasks. Motions in each cardinal plane followed by discussions of primary motions as either the pelvis moving on the femur or the femur moving on the pelvis are included here.

Analysis of Sagittal Plane Motion at the Hip and Pelvis

Sagittal plane motion is hip joint flexion and extension when the femur moves on the pelvis and anterior and posterior pelvic tilt, respectively, when the pelvis moves on the femur. Either may occur in open or closed chain activities.

Overview of Hip Flexion Function

The hip flexors connect the pelvis and the low back to the femur. In pelvis-on-femur motion, the hip flexors tilt the pelvis anteriorly. They work as a force couple with low back muscles to rotate the pelvis anteriorly and secondarily increase lumbar lordosis. When moving the femur on the pelvis, the hip flexors contract synergistically with the abdominal muscles, as when performing a forceful sit-up.

Hip Flexion in Standing

In unilateral stance with NWB hip flexed and the ipsilateral knee raised toward the chest, the iliopsoas, the rectus femoris, the sartorius, and the tensor fascia lata all contribute to the hip flexion action. In the pure sagittal plane, medial rotation produced by the tensor fascia lata is neutralized by the lateral rotation action of the sartorius; likewise, knee extensor action of the rectus femoris is resisted by gravity and neutralized by the knee flexors to prevent passive insufficiency of the rectus femoris. The combined action of the iliopsoas, rectus femoris, sartorius, and TFL muscles results in pure hip flexion. Maximum isometric torque of the hip flexors is greatest when the muscles are on slight stretch (optimal length), as in a kicking motion when the hip begins flexing from an initial position of extension. As hip motion continues from extension into flexion, torque decreases with progressive hip flexion. The adductor muscles may also act as flexors during early hip flexion motion, especially if resistance is applied.[49]

Hip Flexion in the Sitting Position

Regardless of hip position, the iliopsoas contributes most of the hip flexion force. Although the sartorius is considered a primary hip flexor; because of its length and strap-like anatomy, its most important function is likely to occur when simultaneous hip flexion and knee flexion occur, as when climbing stairs. In an acute hip angle, as when sitting, the sartorius and tensor fascia lata contract, but they lose much of their ability to develop tension, making them incapable of contributing to hip flexion in this position.

Sit-ups and Straight Leg Raises

When performing sit-ups or straight leg raises, the abdominal muscles act synergistically with the hip flexors: One muscle group performs the activity while the other muscle group provides stabilization. For example,

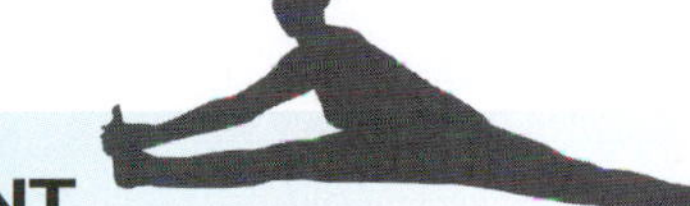

PRACTICE POINT

Hip flexors work most of the time in an open kinetic chain to provide lower extremity progression and powerful hip flexion forces during activities such as walking, running, and kicking. However, if the individual is standing so that the lower extremities are both in a closed kinetic chain position, the iliopsoas is anchored at its distal insertion on the femur. If the iliopsoas is tight, it will pull on its proximal insertions. What results is an anterior pelvic tilt from the iliacus' pull on the pelvis and an anterior positioning of the lumbar vertebrae from the psoas major's pull on the lumbar vertebrae. Therefore, when examining patients presenting with an anterior pelvic tilt and lumbar lordosis posture, assessment of hip flexor range of motion is indicated.

The iliopsoas is the only hip flexor that can produce enough tension to flex the hip beyond 90° in the sitting position. Patients with a severely weak iliopsoas can sometimes flex the hip sufficiently to walk since the amount of hip flexion required is only about 30° during gait (see Chapter 12). When sitting, however, these patients must use their hands to lift and move the thigh. In the sitting position, the iliopsoas also functions to stabilize the lumbar vertebrae and pelvis on the femur as the person leans back and then returns to the upright position. If the iliopsoas muscles are paralyzed bilaterally, the person may fall backward as soon as the line of gravity of HAT falls behind the hip joint axis. Therefore, persons with paraplegia typically need to use trunk and upper extremity support to prevent falling over backward when sitting.

during a typical sit-up, the neck flexors and abdominal muscles perform concentric contractions until the trunk is flexed sufficiently so the scapula clears the surface; while these muscles perform the motion, the hip flexors act concentrically to stabilize and maintain position of the hips. If the individual continues the sit-up maneuver to a full sitting position, the abdominal muscles maintain isometric contractions while the iliopsoas performs concentrically to raise the trunk and pelvis on the fixed femur. Substantial torque is produced by the weight of HAT, so the iliopsoas must produce large forces to complete the sit-up to a full sitting position. If the abdominal muscles are not strong enough to maintain lumbar spine stabilization, the psoas major portion of the iliopsoas pulls the lumbar spine into hyperextension. The resulting increased lumbar lordosis places additional stress on the lumbar spine and positions the back for potential injury during this activity.

As we have just seen, an abdominal crunch requires stabilization by the hip flexors as the abdominals move the trunk. The muscle groups are reversed in their responsibilities during a straight leg raise. In this motion, the femur flexes on the pelvis, so the abdominals provide the lumbopelvic stabilization that allows the hip flexion motion. This activity requires sufficient force from the iliopsoas to counteract the torque provided by the lower extremity's weight. As with any activated muscle, this force is transmitted throughout the muscle (e.g., iliopsoas), pulling both proximal and distal insertion sites towards each other as the muscle contracts.[50] A straight leg raise is normally performed unilaterally while the contralateral lower extremity is flexed at the hip and knee with the foot and pelvis stabilized. In this position, the abdominals provide stabilization of the proximal insertion site of the iliopsoas (pelvis and lumar spine) so the extremity can be raised by the muscle.

Overview of Hip Extension Function

Like the hip flexors, the hip extensors either move the pelvis on the femur or the femur on the pelvis. However, unlike the hip flexors, the hip extensors either tilt the pelvis posteriorly or extend the hip. The powerful gluteus maximus works as a force couple in concert with the abdominal muscles to posteriorly tilt the pelvis on the femur and flatten the lumbar spine, decreasing lumbar lordosis. As a mover of the femur on the pelvis, the gluteus maximus works with the three hamstring muscles to extend the hip. The gluteus maximus is the most powerful hip extensor, regardless of knee position.[42] Similar to that of the rectus femoris, the ability of the hamstrings to act at the hip is influenced by the knee's position since hamstrings also act as a knee flexor. The hamstrings function primarily to extend the hip when the knee is extended. When the hamstrings extend the hip during knee flexion, they become actively insufficient. The best knee position that provides optimal hamstrings function at the hip is knee extension. As

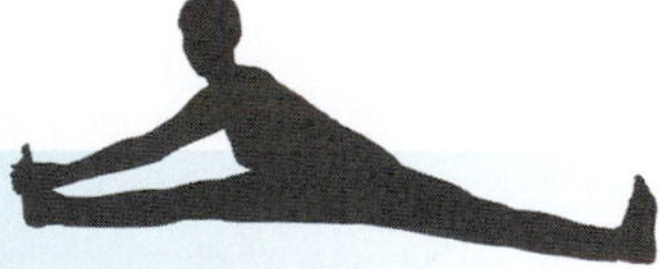

PRACTICE POINT

A powerful iliopsoas can exert tremendous force on a vulnerable low back unless the abdominal muscles have sufficient strength to provide adequate support. Since the abdominals contract isometrically once the scapulae are off the floor, it is usually not necessary to perform a full sit-up to strengthen the abdominals. Maintaining hip flexion at 90° during the abdominal curl limits the amount of force the hip flexors produce during the exercise.

For an average-height, 150-lb adult, the weight of a single lower extremity is approximately 25 lb; the torque produced by the weight and length of the lower extremity is almost 75 ft-lb. If this individual raises both legs simultaneously, the lower extremity torque that the hip flexors must overcome is approximately 150 ft-lb. If the abdominal muscles are too weak to stabilize the pelvis and lumbar spine, the pelvis tilts anteriorly, and the lumbar vertebrae are pulled into hyperextension, causing significant lumbar stress and risk of injury.

has already been mentioned, other muscles that pass behind the medial-lateral hip axis that can also extend the hip include the adductor group. Although the adductor magnus is a hip extensor in most hip positions, the other smaller adductors may also provide extension force when their lines of pull are posterior to the axis of motion.

Hip Extension in Prone

The prone position is an easy position within which to isolate hip extension muscle activity. Both hip and pelvis motions may occur in this position.

Unilateral hip extension is characterized by a contraction of the gluteus maximus. With the knee in flexion, strong action is required of the gluteus maximus to move the hip into extension. Such a position makes the hamstrings actively insufficient so hip extension occurs as a result of gluteus maximus activity. In spite of its actively insufficient position, the hamstrings are still able to provide a minimal contribution to hip extension, so an isolated action of the gluteus maximus is by no means guaranteed. Patients often complain of a cramp-like feeling in the posterior thigh region when full range hip extension is performed with the knee flexed, due to active insufficiency of the hamstrings.

The hamstrings and gluteus maximus each contribute to hip rotation. The gluteus maximus is a strong lateral rotator during patient examination in prone. Hip rotation in the transverse plane facilitates increased gluteus maximus activity during lateral rotation and decreased activity in medial rotation. In contrast, the medial hamstring group is more active in medial rotation during hip extension.

Although we generally address either hip motion or pelvic motion as separate activities, there are occasions when they occur together. Hip extension to approximately 20° occurs without pelvic motion. However, once the hip moves beyond this 20°, the pelvis rocks forward into an anterior pelvic tilt. When performing unilateral hip extension in prone, the pelvis remains comparatively stable with mild synergistic contraction of the paraspinal vertebral extensors. However, when both limbs are raised simultaneously, the pull on the pelvis from the contracting hip extensors and the weight of the limbs causes marked changes in pelvis and spine positions. This bilateral hip extension increases the demand on the vertebral column extensors and creates a stretch of the hip flexors without providing stabilization, causing an increase in both lumbosacral angle and lumbar lordosis.

Hip Extensors in Stance and in the Sitting Position

Forward and backward inclination of the trunk and pelvis in the sitting or standing position is controlled at the hip joint by eccentric and concentric activity of the hip extensors. For example, the forward trunk motion required to retrieve an object from the floor occurs in part because of an eccentric contraction of the hip extensors (see Fig. 2.33A), whereas a concentric contraction of the same muscles produces a return to the erect position. Such hip extensor muscle activity occurs in a more subtle form in other activities, such as ascending and descending stairs, rising from a sitting position, and walking. These activities are associated with simultaneous contraction of the quadriceps as they extend the knee and the hamstrings as they extend the hip. Functional motions such as leaning forward while sitting, bending over to touch the toes while standing, climbing stairs, or rising from a chair all use the hamstrings as the primary muscles controlling the hip. When these motions are rapid or are accompanied by moderate or maximum resistance, the gluteus maximus also participates.[51]

Analysis of Frontal Plane Motion and Control at the Hip and Pelvis

Frontal plane motion is hip abduction and adduction when the femur is moving on the pelvis and lateral pelvic tilt when the pelvis is moving on the femur.

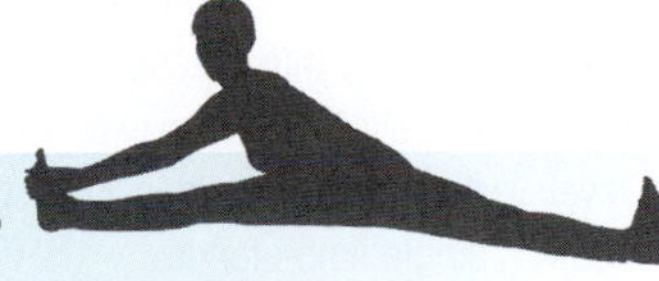

PRACTICE POINT

Weakness of the gluteus maximus or hamstrings accompanies several clinical conditions and is often seen in patients with orthopedic and sports injuries who have undergone prolonged periods of non-weight-bearing. Walking with gluteus maximus weakness is often characterized by a slight forward trunk lean, occurring when the limb accepts weight. Another common compensation is a gluteus maximus "lurch." Clinicians performing gait assessment of patients who have significant gluteus maximus or hamstring weakness should be observant for this gait deviation or its compensation and confirm gluteus maximus and/or hamstring weakness during the muscle testing portion of the examination.

Overview of Abduction Function

Once again, either the pelvis moves on the femur or the femur moves on the pelvis. During pelvic-on-femoral motion, such as in a lateral pelvic tilt, the pivot point is the side of the pelvis that is contralateral to the motion. A unilateral hip hike is an example of a lateral pelvic tilt motion. A lateral pelvic tilt also occurs during single limb stance and walking. When the femur moves on the pelvis, the hip abducts away from the midline or adducts towards the midline.

The gluteus medius, gluteus minimus, and tensor fascia lata provide the primary force to accomplish femur-on-pelvic motion in the frontal plane whereas the sartorius, piriformis, and upper fibers of the gluteus maximus assist in hip abduction when the hip is in specific positions. For example, the sartorius and piriformis are strong abductors when the hip is in flexion.

Of the primary hip abductors, the gluteus medius is by far the most powerful. Investigations demonstrating the importance of the gluteus medius have shown that the gluteus medius comprises 60% of the hip abductor cross-sectional area compared to a 20% contribution from the gluteus minimus, supplemented by small contributions from both the tensor fascia lata and piriformis, at 10% each.[52] Interestingly, however, the mean total cross-sectional area of all of these abductors is still relatively small compared to other thigh muscle groups. For example, a study by Fick demonstrated the abductor cross-sectional area in typical adults to be 43 cm^2, compared to 175 cm^2 for the quadriceps and 58 cm^2 for the hamstrings muscles.[24] In light of this information, a question arises: How do these abductor muscles provide the tremendous forces needed to accomplish their vital function during stance?

The answer to this question lies in understanding the mechanics of this area specifically related to the leverage these muscles possess. Although their cross-sectional size is relatively small, the hip abductors have a large mechanical advantage. By virtue of their distal attachments on the greater trochanter, their line of pull is deflected laterally by the greater trochanter such that the muscle action line is approximately two to three inches from the center of rotation of the hip. As a result, the gluteus medius has a moment arm angle of 72°, the relatively small tensor fascia lata moment arm angle is 83°, and gluteus minimus has a leverage angle of 61°. This is *significant* leverage. Compare those values to the patellar tendon moment arm angle which is only 15° to 20°.[52] Because of these leverage advantages, a large torque can be produced by these relatively small hip abductor muscles. The hip abductors exert their greatest torque when contracting in the lengthened position and the torque decreases linearly as the muscle shortens. In fact, in unilateral stance, the supporting limb adducts to 15°, putting the abductors at optimal length so they are able to provide tremendous force-producing potential and serve as functional pelvic stabilizers (Fig 9.22, 9.26). As the center of gravity of the body shifts laterally over the supporting foot in unilateral stance, the hip becomes adducted. Fortunately, this factor coincides with the high functional demands placed on the muscle in unilateral stance, so optimal muscle function coincides with the muscle's highest demands.

During pelvic motion on the femur, the abductors laterally tilt the pelvis. As we know from our study of muscular function in Chapter 4, the greatest maximum isometric force of a muscle occurs when there is strong stabilization of the muscle's fixed attachment site.

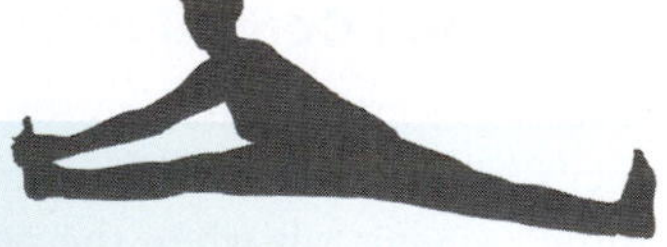

PRACTICE POINT

Basmajian discovered that when a muscle contracts, both the proximal and distal insertion ends move towards the center of the muscle.[50] Since this is evident, we can exercise a muscle by stabilizing either the proximal end and moving the distal end or vice versa. Therefore, if a patient is unable to maintain a level pelvis during ambulation because of weak hip abductors, we can strengthen the muscle by having the patient perform either a hip abduction motion or a lateral pelvic tilt motion while stabilizing the opposite muscle end. Once the muscle gains sufficient strength in these open chain exercise positions, it is then vital to develop functional activities that promote gluteus medius strength in single limb stance.

Mean values of maximum isometric torques for the gluteus medius have been reported to be from 92 to 114 ft-lb for men and 58 to 76 ft-lb for women, with variations due to differences in positions, types of stabilization, and ages.[39–42] In male subjects, Neumann and associates measured a maximum isometric mean torque of 100 ft-lb when these muscles were on stretch in 10° of adduction.[53] This position in relaxed unilateral stance amounts to relatively slight hip adduction, but the position puts the hip abductors on a stretch sufficient to provide optimal length-tension positioning, giving them a large advantage over body weight forces.

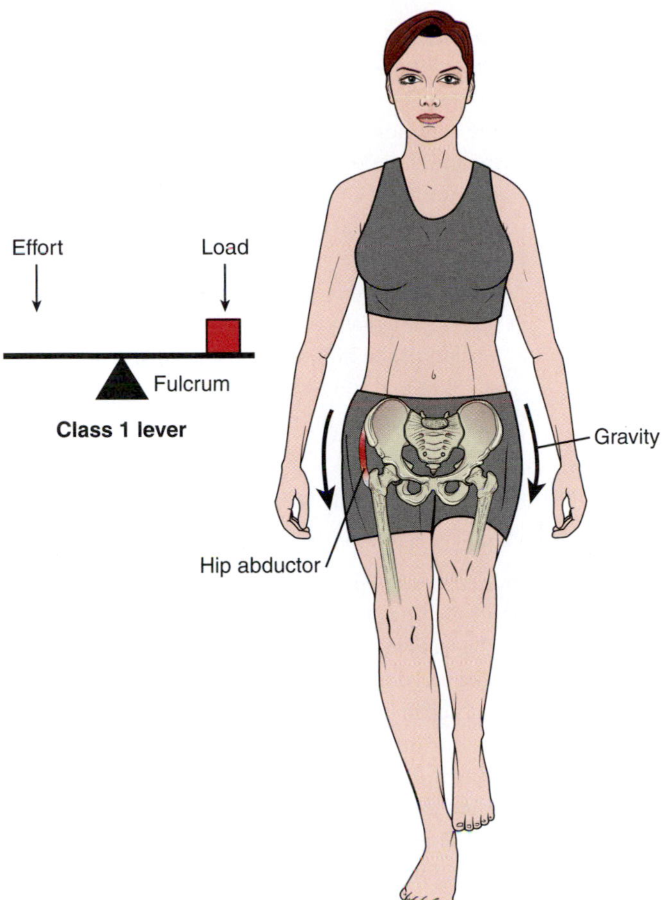

Figure 9.26 The hip abductors are a first-class lever during single-limb stance since the hip joint is the fulcrum and the abductors and body weight are on either side of the fulcrum.

Because the pelvis is a closed system, unilateral pelvic motion is difficult to stabilize. The contralateral hip abductors provide the best pelvic lateral stabilization. Such stabilization requires an equal maximum isometric contraction of the bilateral hip abductors.

A major function of the hip abductors occurs in the closed kinematic chain: They maintain a level pelvis during unilateral stance. Functionally, the abductors, mainly the gluteus medius, contracts on the weight-bearing side when standing on one leg. When standing on one foot as during walking, 85% of the weight of the body, including HAT and the contralateral lower limb, must be balanced by the hip abductors around the femoral head. In this way, the femoral head is a fulcrum in a first-class lever system (Fig. 9.26). Therefore, the hip abductors provide a primary functional source of control and balance at the pelvis.

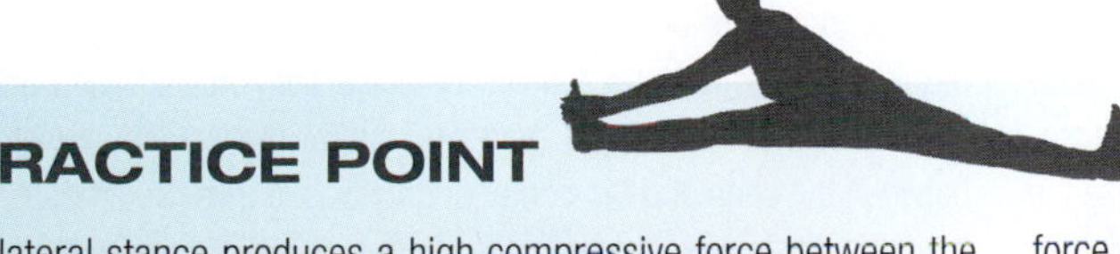

PRACTICE POINT

Unilateral stance produces a high compressive force between the femoral head and acetabulum; this has been calculated to be from 2.5 times body weight to as high as more than four times body weight.[54–56] Forces of four times body weight occur during gait at the end of loading response.[57] Imagine the amount of compressive force on a painful hip. If obesity is also a factor, imagine the large compressive forces! As clinicians, we must offer solutions to reduce such high compressive forces on a painful hip. One suggestion you can give a patient is to carry a heavy object in the ipsilateral hand (Fig. 9.27).

BOX 9-3 | Hip Muscle Function at a Glance

Hip Extensors: Two joint hamstring muscles compared with single joint gluteus maximus

- Hamstrings primarily extend hip when knee is extended, because with the knee flexed they become actively insufficient;
- Single joint muscles, such as the gluteus maximus, will function regardless of knee position; therefore they are most active during movements when the knee is flexed and the hamstrings are actively insufficient.

Hip Abductors

- Major function of hip abductors, such as gluteus medius, minimus, and TFL is to maintain a level pelvis during unilateral stance;
- In unilateral stance, which occurs with every step, 85% of the body weight must be balanced by the hip abductors around the femoral head, forming a first class lever; producing a high compression force at the hip joint, calculated to be as high as 2.5 times the body weight;
- As the COG is shifted laterally over the supporting foot, the hip assumes an adducted position;
- Hip abductors produce the greatest torque at 15° of hip adduction where the length tension relationship is the most favorable, a position coinciding with the functional demands placed on the muscle in unilateral stance.
- Hip Abductor Weakness
  - Unilateral stance with the pelvis level is not possible (Trendelenberg sign)
  - Three common methods of compensation:
    1. Inclining the trunk laterally toward the stance side until the COG lies vertically over or slightly lateral to the hip joint;
    2. Allowing the pelvis to sag laterally toward the unsupported side until the hip on the stance side is maximally adducted, at which point tension in the hip joint capsule, ligaments and iliotibial tract prevents further motion;
    3. Placing a cane in the opposite hand to provide an upward force at a long distance from the joint axis.

Gait Deviations: typically seen in midstance, when the body weight is centered over the stance leg

1. Trendelenburg or Gluteus medius gait—the pelvis opposite the side of the weak gluteus medius drops while the weak leg is in stance and/or the weak medius forces the individual to laterally lean the trunk over the involved side in order to place the COG over the hip.
2. Gluteus maximus lurch—weak gluteus maximus forces the individual to "lurch" the trunk backward by leaning the trunk posteriorly during stance on the weak side to keep the COG posterior to hip and to maintain hip extension.

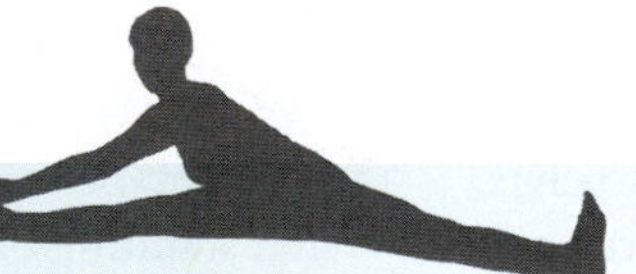

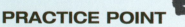

PRACTICE POINT

Hip abductor weakness makes it difficult to ambulate with a level pelvis (Fig. 9.28). The positive clinical sign for gluteus medius weakness is dropping of the pelvis on the nonweight-bearing side during unilateral stance. This is a **Trendelenberg sign** (Fig. 9.28C). For example, in the case of a severely weakened gluteus medius on the right, when the patient or client attempts to stand on the right limb unilaterally, the left pelvis drops. The weight-bearing hip is adducted, and its motion is limited by the joint's capsule and ligaments. Patients with hip abductor weakness can compensate in a variety of ways. One of the most common compensations is lateral flexing the trunk during the stance phase of gait. This maneuver shifts the center of gravity and the weight of HAT over the weight-bearing hip joint to minimize the torque demand on the weakened abductors. This gait compensation is known as a **Trendelenberg** or **gluteus medius gait.** Because the compensatory lateral trunk lean decreases joint compression forces throughout the entire stance limb, this type of gait may be seen also in people with pain in the hip, knee, or foot. Regardless of the underlying pathology or impairment, gait compensations require an increase in energy expenditure and creates the demand for compensatory or substituted abnormal forces in the trunk and lower extremities. As clinicians, an appropriate recommendation may be the use of an assistive device. A cane or one crutch is commonly used to reduce joint compression forces. Using the device in the contralateral hand provides a force platform through which the pelvis remains level (Fig. 9.28D). During ambulation, the contralateral device and weakened lower extremity bear weight at the same time. The upward force transmitted from the floor, through the assistive device, onto the upper extremity, and then through the trunk will assist in maintaining a level pelvis on the swinging, nonweight-bearing side. Even a small upward force provides considerable assistance in reducing the force required by the gluteus medius because the force of the cane is applied at a long distance from the axis of motion. The lever arm between the cane and the center of gravity is four to five times longer than the lever arm between the center of gravity and hip joint;[58] the large mechanical arm from the cane to the axis of motion requires minimal force (2% to 10% of body weight) exerted through the cane to provide sufficient support during ambulation to avoid a pathological gait. [58] (Fig. 9.28E).

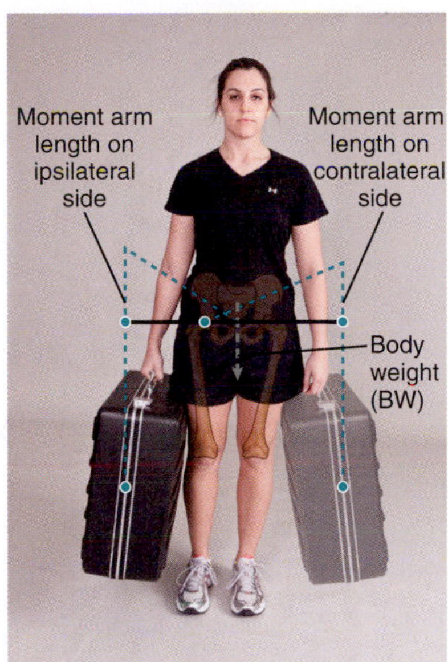

Figure 9.27 An individual with unilateral hip pain or degeneration should carry an object with the ipsilateral arm since it will place less compression force on the hip joint. Its moment arm is shorter than an object carried with the contralateral arm, so its joint reaction force will also be less. On the other hand, the moment arm and subsequent torque of an object carried with the contralateral arm is significantly greater, so the joint reaction force applied by the torque of the object is concomitantly greater.

Overview of Adduction Function

As with the other hip muscles we have studied, the adductors will move either the pelvis on the femur or the femur on the pelvis. During pelvic motion, the hip adductors are primarily pelvic stabilizers, cocontracting with the hip abductors. When they move the femur on the pelvis, these muscles, as their collective name implies, adduct the femur in the frontal plane. Because these muscles essentially originate from the same location and insert along the femur at various levels, their lines of force also varies. This variation in alignment allows most of the adductors to have secondary actions. For example, the posterior fibers of the adductor magnus can act as a hip extensor, the pectineus flexes the hip, and most of the adductors contribute to medial rotation. Against resistance or in pure frontal-plane adduction, all five adductors adduct the hip. During functional activities, the five primary adductor muscles all contribute to hip adduction and contribute as secondary muscles to the other hip motions of flexion, extension, and rotation.

Analysis of Transverse Plane Motion at the Hip and Pelvis

Transverse plane motion occurs either as rotational motion of the pelvis on the femur or as femoral rotation on the pelvis. Transverse plane motion of the pelvis on the femur is anterior rotation (or protraction) and posterior rotation (or retraction). When the femur rotates on the pelvis, it is medial and lateral hip rotation.

Pelvic Rotation

Since the pelvis is a closed system, the transverse plane motions of pelvic anterior rotation (protraction) and posterior rotation (retraction) occur as paired motions. In other words, as one side of the pelvis protracts or rotates anteriorly, the contralateral side of the pelvis retracts or rotates posteriorly. The muscles responsible for this pelvic rotation include not only the muscles that we have listed and described as hip rotators, but also include some of the trunk musculature such as the abdominal oblique muscles and some deep back muscles. These muscles and their functional actions have been described previously in Chapter 8. Pelvic rotation is further described in Chapter 12, in which its importance is most apparent during the gait cycle.

Overview of Hip Medial and Lateral Rotation Function

Many muscles surrounding the hip joint make a contribution to hip rotation. Which of these muscles laterally or medially rotate depends on the hip's position in the sagittal and frontal planes. For example, the gluteus

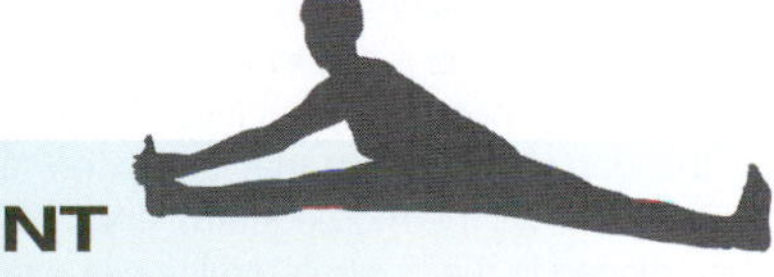

PRACTICE POINT

Interestingly, the total cross-sectional area of the adductor group far surpasses that of the abductors. At first glance, this might appear illogical because the abductors play a greater role during stance and gait compared to the adductors, and during these activities the hip abductors must work against gravity, but gravity assists the adductors in their effort. Adduction activities such as squeezing an object between the knees and climbing a rope are relatively rare activities and hardly warrant such a large muscle cross section. The explanation for the adductors' large bulk is found in their additional responsibilities as hip flexors, extensors, and rotators and in the role they provide as hip stabilizers.

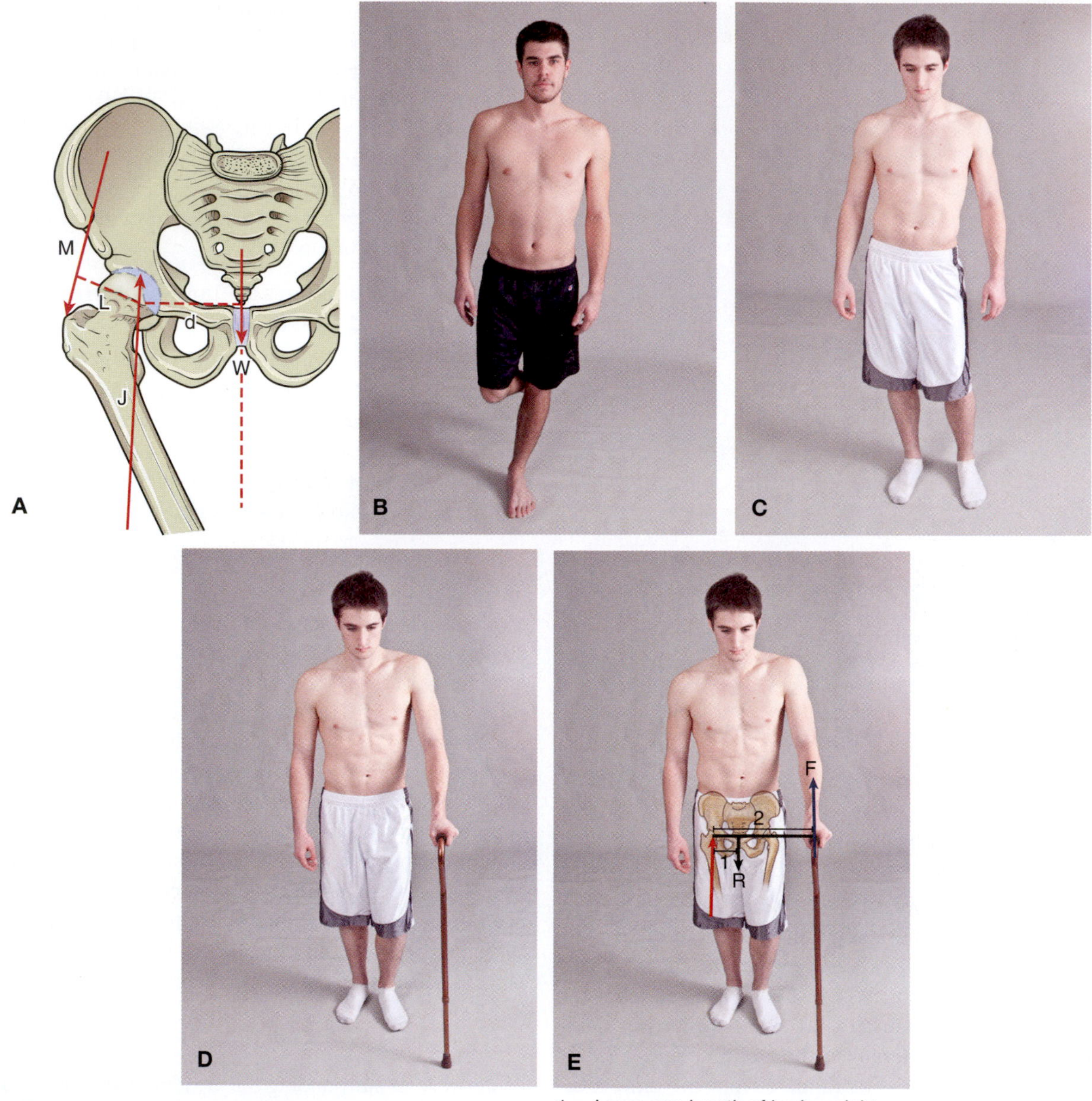

Figure 9.28 Gluteus medius function in unilateral stance. **A)** Forces on the pelvis when standing on one leg. W = 85% of body weight (head, arms, trunk, and opposite leg); M = force of the hip abductors required to maintain a level pelvis; J = joint reaction force between the head of the femur and the acetabulum; d = 4.25 inches (lever arm distance for W); L = 2.75 inches (lever arm for M). Lever arm distances were measured from x-rays and are provided so that the student can solve for the actual forces of M and W. **B)** Pelvic alignment in unimpaired unilateral stance. **C)** With hip abductor weakness on the right, an attempt to raise the left leg off the floor results in pelvic drop on that side (Trendelenberg sign). **D)** Placing a cane in the individual's left hand (contralateral to the weak gluteus medius on the right) provides a force platform through which the pelvis remains level. **E)** Artwork depiction: With the cane used in the hand contralateral to the affected lower extremity, the long moment arm that is created requires little force exerted through the cane to provide sufficient support during ambulation. 1 shows the moment arm length of the body weight and 2 represents the moment arm length of the assistive device when placed in the contratateral upper extremity; notice the significantly larger moment arm with the device on the opposite side to the affected lower extremity.

maximus is a strong lateral rotator with the hip extended, but when the hip is flexed, the line of pull of the muscle's upper fiber is conducive for medial rotation.[47] The six small lateral rotators (piriformis, gemellus superior, gemellus inferior, obturator internus, obturator externus, and quadratus femoris) have an effective angle of pull for lateral rotation, but their ability to act as strong lateral rotators decreases as the hip moves into flexion; at 90° of flexion their line of pull actually favors abduction rather than rotation, and the piriformis becomes a medial rotator.[3, 47]

Of all the hip muscle groups, EMG studies have demonstrated that the adductors contribute significantly more consistently to hip medial rotation than either the glutei or tensor fascia lata.[51, 59] This is because the axis of rotation goes through the mechanical axis from the femoral head to the medial femoral condyle (Fig. 9.5), and the natural femoral angulation puts the linea aspera (where the muscles insert) anterior to the longitudinal axis of hip rotation. When the femur rotates medially, the linea aspera approaches the pubis. With lateral rotation, the distance between these attachment sites becomes longer, putting the adductors on a slight stretch and placing them in an their optimal length-tension position, thereby allowing them to act as effective medial rotators. Additional medial rotators include the anterior portion of the gluteus medius, anterior portion of the gluteus minimus, and tensor fasciae latae. The medial rotation moment arms of these muscles increase when the hip is flexed.

As with other single-joint muscles, the maximum isometric torque for both the medial and lateral rotators occurs at their lengthened positions and decreases as the muscles shorten.[60] Their forces are equal when the hip is near neutral relative to the sagittal and frontal planes. An interesting change in maximum medial rotation torque occurs when the hip is in either flexion or extension. In hip flexion, the medial rotators produce almost three times the torque they can when the hip is extended.[61, 62] Conversely, the lateral rotators show little difference in hip flexion or extension. This large difference in medial rotation torque is thought to occur with a change in line of action of the gluteus medius, gluteus minimus, and piriformis; these muscles assist in medial rotation when the hip is flexed.

Summary

This chapter described the basic anatomy and kinesiology of the pelvic and hip region. This region is described with an emphasis on its dual role in the provision of both stability and mobility for the entire lower extremity. Surface anatomy and guides to palpation are described and displayed in table format. The focus of the chapter was on the functional relationships between the pelvis and hip with a thorough discussion of pelvic and hip motion and the relationship between the two. The primary muscles that produce pelvic and hip movement in its three axes of motion were described and summarized. Key concepts related to the specific kinesiological demands of this region, such as muscle leverage and line of pull, muscular sufficiency, and the unique demands of weight-bearing and nonweight-bearing, were summarized, compared, and contrasted. Common functional movements were described and kinematically analyzed. Pathological conditions were included as an illustration of the functional consequences encountered when the mechanics of this area are compromised.

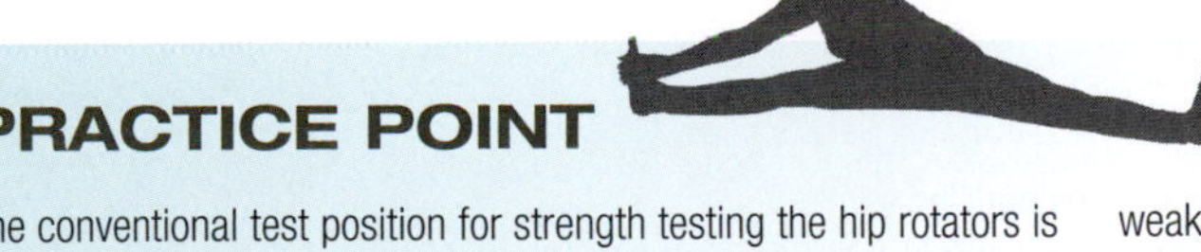

PRACTICE POINT

The conventional test position for strength testing the hip rotators is the sitting position. This position may provide misleading information about functional strength of the medial rotators that are used in activities such as walking, running, cutting, or pivoting. A person with weak medial rotators may appear to have normal strength in sitting when actual strength is inadequate for the activities performed in an upright position with the hip extended.

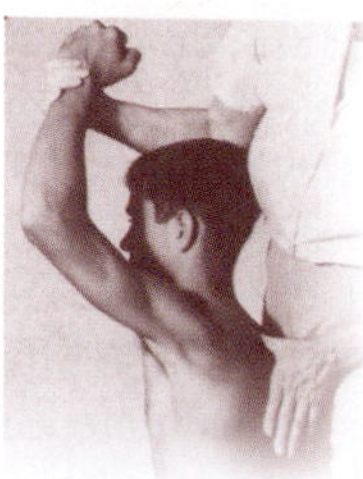

CLINICAL SCENARIO SOLUTION

Noelle knows that the hip abductors, specifically the gluteus medius, exert their primary role to stabilize the pelvis during the unilateral stance phase of gait by preventing the pelvis on the side of the swinging leg from dropping. She evaluates Mr. Reyes by asking him to stand on his left leg and notes that he immediately attempts to laterally lean his trunk over that leg. When Noelle gives him manual support at the trunk and prevents this compensatory trunk lean, she sees that the right side of his pelvis drops during left unilateral stance. Noelle recognizes this as a Trendelenberg sign, indicative of left hip abductor (gluteus medius) weakness. To confirm this observation, she performs a manual muscle test on Mr. Reyes' hip abductors. She gives Mr. Reyes a cane to use in his right hand and demonstrates how he should use it. She explains to Mr. Reyes that over time, his compensatory lateral trunk lean may eventually contribute to soft tissue and bony degenerative changes in his lumbar spine if the cane is not used and the weakness is not corrected. She explains that until the muscles are strengthened, the cane will allow him to maintain a level pelvis while he walks, thereby decreasing the stress on his lumbar spine.

Discussion Questions

1. What is the relationship of pelvic and hip motions, and how do they contribute to function in this region?
2. As you stand, contract your gluteus maximus bilaterally. What motions occur at the hip and the pelvis, and how do these motions contribute to functional stability in stance?
3. What muscle at the glenohumeral joint is similar in structure and function to the gluteus medius? How are they similar and how are they unique?
4. Why is the ischial tuberosity such an important landmark to consider in rehabilitation?
5. Compare and contrast hip function during weight-bearing and nonweight-bearing activities.

Lab Activities

1. Using a skeleton or a disarticulated skeleton, identify these landmarks. Which are palpable? Locate them on yourself and on another individual.

Pelvis

ilium
iliac crest
anterior superior iliac spine (ASIS)
anterior inferior iliac spine (AIIS)
posterior superior iliac spine (PSIS)
posterior inferior iliac spine (PIIS)
posterior gluteal line
anterior gluteal line
inferior gluteal line
greater sciatic notch
obturator foramen
iliac fossa
acetabulum
ischium
ramus of ischium
ischial tuberosity
pubis
ramus of pubis
symphysis pubis
pubic tubercle

Femur

head, including fovea
greater trochanter
lesser trochanter
neck
shaft of femur
pectineal line
gluteal tuberosity
linea aspera
adductor tubercle
medial condyle and epicondyle
lateral condyle and epicondyle
patellar groove

2. In standing, rest your hands on your hips as depicted in Fig. 9.2 and perform the following motions of the pelvis on the femur: anterior pelvic tilt, posterior pelvic tilt, lateral tilt, anterior rotation or protraction, and posterior rotation or retraction. Notice how each hand moves in relation to the other as you perform each pelvic motion.
3. With your partner supine, locate the ASIS and greater trochanter. Measure the distance between those two landmarks on each side and compare. Although we haven't studied the knee and ankle yet (Chapters 10 and 11), use both as the proximal landmark and measure leg length to the medial tibial plateau (Fig. 10.4C) and the medial malleolus (Fig. 11.5). Discuss how these measurements will discern differences or similarities in length at the pelvis, femur and tibia, as well as giving an overall functional leg length.
4. With your partner supine, passively perform all of the range of the motions of hip flexion, lateral and medial rotation, abduction, and adduction. Note the available ranges of motion, using Table 1–2 as a guide. Describe the end feels.
5. On your partner, palpate the hip muscles, using Table 9–2 as your guide.
6. Differentiate hip extension from pelvic and lumbar motion. With your partner lying prone on a plinth, extend his or her hip passively and then ask him or her to do the motion actively while you observe where the motions are taking place. Next, ask your partner to move to the side edge of the table so that the hip can be flexed to 90°, allowing the foot to be supported by the floor. Extend the opposite hip passively and note the range of motion and the end feel and then ask your partner to actively extend his or her hip. What are the differences in hip extension in this position and the first position? What is the reason for the differences?
7. Differentiate the range of motion of hip flexion with the knee flexed and then with it extended. Passively flex the hip through its full range permitting the knee to flex. Then passively flex the hip with the knee straight. Note the differences in range and end feels. Why is there a difference in range of motion and what is this mechanical limitation called? What are the structures that limit hip flexion when the knee is in extension?
8. On your partner, place the following muscles in their shortest position and in their longest position (stretched). Study and analyze the effects at the pelvis, low back, and hip.

iliopsoas	biceps femoris
pectineus	semimembranosus
rectus femoris	semitendinosus
tensor fascia lata	sartorius

9. Analyze the following hip muscle actions:
   a. Sit sideways on a chair so that you can lean forward and backward. Palpate your hamstring muscles at their distal tendons behind the knee. As you lean back, performing hip extension, the tendons should be relaxed, and when you lean forward they contract when you cross the vertical position. The hamstring muscles continue to contract with the forward lean as you move into hip flexion as well as on the return to the upright position, as you perform hip extension. What type of muscle contraction is occurring in the hamstrings as you lean forward and what type occurs to bring you back to the erect position? What muscle of the hip controls leaning back and then returning to the erect position?
   b. Stand upright and palpate the hamstrings at their proximal attachments on the ischial tuberosity. Lean the trunk back and feel the relaxation of the muscles and then lean forward. Note the relative inactivity of the gluteus maximus.
   c. Stand upright and palpate your gluteus medius muscles just above the greater trochanters. When standing comfortably on both feet, the muscles should be relaxed. Gently shift your body weight to the right foot. Note the strong contraction of the gluteus medius. What is the purpose of this contraction? Note also the adducted position of your stance leg. What mechanical purpose does this adduction position fulfill and for what muscle?

d. Palpate the gluteus medius bilaterally when you walk. When does each muscle contract? Analyze the hip muscle actions of the gluteus medus in nonweight-bearing and weight-bearing. Use Figure 9.28 as a guide. Analyze the function of the hip abductors—primarily the gluteus medius—in unilateral stance: Stand in unilateral stance and explain the effect on balance and pelvic stability in this position as a result of the weight of HAT and the unsupported limb. What muscle activity counteracts this effect? Identify the lever system working during this functional task by naming and visualizing the fulcrum, or axis, the weight lever arm, and the force lever arm. Model a Trendelenberg sign. Demonstrate, visualize, and discuss the functional significance of this by allowing your pelvis to drop on your unsupported side. Demonstrate, visualize, and discuss the common compensations of lateral trunk flexion over the stance limb and use of a cane on the side of the unsupported limb.

10. Analyze multiple actions of the hip adductors. Palpate the adductors on yourself during the following positions and motions:

a. Sit on a table with your feet unsupported and flex your hip; laterally rotate your hip, then medially rotate it.

b. Stand erect with the left foot on a block or a book and the right foot hanging free and unsupported. Palpate the right adductors while you abduct the right hip and then adduct it against the left leg. Note that the muscles do not contract until resistance occurs. What muscle is controlling the motion of adduction in this position and what type of contraction is it using? Now, flex your hip, keeping the trunk erect. Then laterally and medially rotate the hip. What is the difference in the activity of the adductors when hip rotation is performed with the hip in flexion versus extension? Is there a contraction of the adductors when the hip flexes?

c. Stand with one foot on a high step or a chair in order to place the hip in flexion. Press down with your foot as if to lift your body up, such as in climbing, and note the strong contraction in the adductors.

d. Using the skeleton model of the pelvis and femur, attach a piece of string to the proximal attachment of the adductors and hold the free end near the middle or at a specific distal attachment. Keep the string taut but let it slide to represent the line of pull as you perform the motions in a, b, and c above. Note the changing relationships between the axis of motion and the line of pull as you place the hip in flexion and extension. Notice that the axis for rotation of the hip is the mechanical axis rather than the anatomic axis.

11. Analyze hip rotator function in different positions.

a. Palpate your lab partner's piriformis with your partner in standing. Have your partner medially and laterally rotate the hip and identify when the piriformis contracts.

b. Now have your partner supine with hips and knees flexed so the feet are flat on the plinth. Have your partner lift one leg towards his or her chest as you palpate the piriformis. With the hip and knee each at 90°, have your partner move the hip into medial and lateral rotation. Identify when the piriformis is contracting in this position.

c. Explain in your own words why the differences between these positions changes the muscle's activity.

References

1. Moore K. *Clinically Oriented Anatomy*. Baltimore: Williams & Wilkins, 2004.
2. Iglič A, Antolic V, Srakar F. Biomechanical study of various greater trochanter positions. *Archives of Orthopaedic and Trauma Surgery* 114:76–78, 1995.
3. Kapandji IA. *The Physiology of the Joints, Vol 2, Lower Limb*, ed 5. Edinburgh: Churchill Livingstone, 1987.
4. Brenneman SB, Stanger M, Bertoti D, eds. Musculoskeletal system: Age related issues: Pediatric. In Myers RS (ed): *Saunders Manual of Physical Therapy Practice*, Philadelphia: WB Saunders, 1994, pp 1229–1283.
5. Bertoti D. Cerebral Palsy: Lifespan management. In *Orthopaedic Interventions for the Pediatric Patient, Orthopaedic Section Home Study Course*, Alexandria: American Physical Therapy Association, 2000, pp 1–10.
6. Bertoti DB. *Functional Neurorehabilitation through the Life Span*. Philadelphia: F. A. Davis Company, 2004.

7. Neely FG. Biomechanical Risk Factors for Exercise-Related Lower Limb Injuries. *Sports Medicine* 26(6):395–413, 1998.
8. Crane L. Femoral torsion and its relation to toeing-in and toeing-out. *Journal of Bone and Joint Surgery* 41A:421–428, 1959.
9. Manaster BJ, Radiological Society of North America. Adult chronic hip pain: Radiographic evaluation. *Radiographics* 20:S3–S25, 2000.
10. Crockarell JR, Jr., Trousdale RT, Guyton JL. The anterior centre-edge angle: A cadaver study. *Journal of Bone and Joint Surgery Br* 82(4):532–534, 2000.
11. Tönnis D, Heinecke A. Acetabular and femoral anteversion: Relationship with osteoarthritis of the hip. *Journal of Bone and Joint Surgery Br* 81(12):1747–1770, 1999.
12. Daniel M, Iglič A, Kralj-Iglič V. Hip contact stress during normal and staircase walking: The influence of acetabular anteversion angle and lateral coverage of the acetabulum. *Journal of Applied Biomedicine* 24(1):88–93, 2008.
13. Kang C, Hwang DS, Cha SM. Acetabular labral tears in patients with sports injury. *Clinincal Orthopaedic Surgury* 1(4):230–235, 2009.
14. Streich NA, Gotterbarm T, Barié A, Schmitt H. Prognostic value of chondral defects on the outcome after arthroscopic treatment of acetabular labral tears. *Knee Surgery Sports Traumatology, Arthroscopy* 17(10):1257–1263, 2009.
15. Ipavec M, Brand R, A, Perdersen D, R, Mavcic B, Kralj-Iglic V, Iglic A. Mathemechanical modeling of stress in the hip during gait. *Journal of Biomechanics* 32:1229–1235, 1999.
16. Carter DR, Wong M, Orr T, E. Musculoskeletal ontogeny, phylogeny, and functional adaptation. *Journal of Biomechanics* 24:3–16, 1991.
17. Palastanga N, Field D, Soames R. *Anatomy and Human Movement*. London: Heinemann Medical Books, 1989.
18. vonEisenhart-Rothe R, Eckstein F, Mueller-Gerbl M. Direct comparison of contact areas, contact stress and subchondral mineralization in human hip joint specimens. *Anatomy and Embyology* 195:279–288, 1997.
19. Oatis CA. *Kinesiology The Mechanics & Pathomechanics of Human Movement*, ed 2. Philadelphia: Lippincott Williams & Wilkins, 2008.
20. Kronrath G, Hamel A, Olson S. The role of the acetabular labrum and the transverse acetabular ligament in load transmission of the hip. *Journal of Bone and Joint Surgery Am* 80:1781–1788, 1998.
21. Wingstrand H, Wingstrand A, Krantz P. Intracapsular and atmospheric pressure in the dynamics and stability of the hip. *Acta Orthopaedica Scandinavia* 61:231–235, 1990.
22. Levangie PK, Norton CC. *Joint Structure & Function: A Comprehensive Analysis*, ed 4. Philadelphia: FA Davis, 2005.
23. Kendall FP, McCreary EK, Provance PG. *Muscles: Testing and Function*, ed 4. Baltimore: Williams & Wilkins, 1993.
24. Fick R. *Anatomie und Mechanik der Gelenke: Teil III, Spezielle Gelenk und Muskel Mechanik*. Jena, Germany: Fisher, 1911.
25. Walker ML, Rothstein JM, Finucane SD, Lamb RL. Relationships between lumbar lordosis, pelvic tilt and abdominal muscle performance. *Physical Therapy* 67(4):512–516, 1987.
26. Begon M, Monnet T, Lacouture P. Effects of movement for estimating the hip joint centre. *Gait Posture* 25(3):353–359, 2007.
27. Hass SS, Epps CH, Jr., Adams JP. Normal ranges of hip motion in the newborn. *Clinical Orthopaedics and Related Research* 91:114–118, 1973.
28. Coon V, Donato G, Houser C, Bleck EE. Normal ranges of hip motion in infants six weeks, three months and six months of age. *Clinical Orthopaedics and Related Research* 110:256–260, 1975.
29. Boone DC, Azen SP. Normal range of motion of joints in male subjects. *Journal of Bone and Joint Surgery Am* 61(5):756–759, 1979.
30. Walker JM, Sue D, Miles-Elkousy N, Ford G, Trevelyan H. Active mobility of the extremities in older subjects. *Physical Therapy* 64(6):919–923, 1984.
31. James B, Parker AW. Active and passive mobility of lower limb joints in elderly men and women. *American Journal of Physical Medicine and Rehabilitation* 68(4):162–167, 1989.
32. Svenningsen S, Terjesen T, Auflem M, Berg V. Hip motion related to age and sex. *Acta Orthopaedica Scandinavica* 60(1):97–100, 1989.
33. Wingstrand H, Wingstrand A, Krantz P. Intracapsular and atmospheric pressure in the dynamics and stability of the hip. *Acta Orthopaedica Scandinavica* 61(3):231–235, 1990.
34. Arvidsson I. The hip joint: Forces needed for distraction and appearance of the vacuum phenomenon. *Scand J Rehabil Med* 22:157–161, 1990.
35. Kaltenborn FM. *Manual Mobilization of the Joints. The Kaltenborn Method of Joint Examination and Treatment*, ed 6. Oslo, Norway: Olaf Norlis Bokhandel, 2002.

36. Paluska SA. An overview of hip injuries in running. *Sports Medicine* 35(11):991–114, 2005.

37. Pfirrmann C, Chung CP, Theumann B. Greater trochanter of the hip: Attachment of the abductor mechanism and a complex of three bursae—MR imaging and MR bursography in cadavers and MR imaging in asymptomatic volunteers. *Radiology* 221:469–477, 2001.

38. Basmajian JV, DeLuca CJ. *Muscles Alive: Their Functions Revealed by Electromyography,* ed 5. Baltimore: Williams & Wilkins, 1985.

39. Delp S, Hess W, E, Hungerford D, S, Jones L, C. Variation of rotation moment arms with hip flexion. *J Biomech* 32:493–501, 1999.

40. Williams P. *Gray's Anatomy*, ed 38. New York: Churchill Livingstone, 1999.

41. Dostal WF, Andrews JG. A three-dimensional biomechanical model of hip musculature. *Journal of Biomechanics* 14(11):803–812, 1981.

42. Lieberman D, Raichlen D, Pontzer H, Bramble D, Cutright-Smith E. The human gluteus maximus and its role in running. *Journal of Experimental Biology* 209(11):2143–2155, 2006.

43. Joseph J. *Man's Posture: Electromyographic Studies*. Springfield, IL: Charles C Thomas, 1960.

44. Johnson ME, Mille ML, Martinez KM, Crombie G, Rogers MW. Age-related changes in hip abductor and adductor joint torques. *Archives of Physical Medicine and Rehabilitation* 85(4):593–597, 2004.

45. Beck M, Sledge JB, Gautier E, Dora CF, Ganz R. The anatomy and function of the gluteus minimus muscle. *Journal of Bone and Joint Surgery Br* 82(3):358–363, 2000.

46. Torry MR, Schenker ML, Martin HD, Hogoboom D, Philippon MJ. Neuromuscular hip biomechanics and pathology in the athlete. *Clinics in Sports Medicine* 25:179–197, 2006.

47. Steindler A. *Kinesiology of the Human Body Under Normal and Pathological Conditions*. Springfield, IL: Charles C Thomas, 1955.

48. Basmajian JV, Greenlaw RK. Electromyography of iliacus and psoas with inserted fine-wire electrodes. *Anatomical Record* 160:130, 1968.

49. Janda VSV. The role of the thigh adductors in movement of the hip and knee joint. *Courrier* 15:1–3, 1965.

50. Basmajian JV. Electromyography of two-joint muscles. *Anatomical Record* 129:371–380, 1957.

51. Basmajian JV. *Muscles Alive: Their Function Revealed by Electromyography*, ed 4. Baltimore: Williams & Wilkins, 1978.

52. Clark JM, Haynor DR. Anatomy of the abductor muscles of the hip as studied by computed tomography. *Journal of Bone and Joint Surgery Am* 69(7):1021–1031, 1987.

53. Neumann DA, Soderberg GL, Cook TM. Comparison of maximal isometric hip abductor muscle torques between hip sides. *Physical Therapy* 68(4):496–502, 1988.

54. Inman VT. Functional aspects of the abductor muscles of the hip. *Journal of Bone and Joint Surgery* 29:2, 1947.

55. LeVeau B. *Williams and Lissner: Biomechanics of Human Motion*, ed 3. Philadelphia: WB Saunders, 1992.

56. Frankel VH, Nordin M. *Basic Biomechanics of the Skeletal System*, ed 2. Philadelphia: Lea & Febiger, 1989.

57. Maquet PGJ. *Biomechanics of the Hip as Applied to Osteoarthritis and Related Conditions*. Berlin: Springer-Verlag, 1985.

58. Inman VT, Ralston HJ, Todd F. *Human Walking*. Baltimore: Williams & Wilkins, 1981.

59. Williams M, Wesley W. Hip rotator action of the adductor longus muscle. *Physical Therapy Review* 31(3):90–92, 1951.

60. May WW. Maximum isometric force of the hip rotator muscles. *Physical Therapy* 46(3):233–238, 1966.

61. Jarvis DK. Relative strength of the hip rotator muscle groups. *Physical Therapy Review* 32(10):500–503, 1952.

62. Woodruff G. *Maximum Isometric Torque of the Hip Rotator Muscles in Four Positions of Hip Flexion-Extension.* Denton, TX: Texas Woman's University, 1976.

63. Neumann DA. *Kinesiology of the Musculoskeletal System: Foundations for Physical Rehabilitation*. St. Louis: Mosby Inc., 2002.

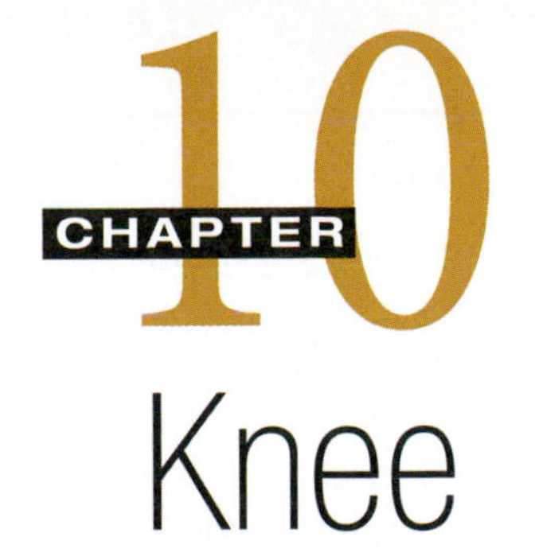

Knee

"Don't be afraid to take a big step if one is indicated; you can't cross a chasm in two small jumps."

—David Lloyd George, 1863–1945,
British politician and prime minister of United Kingdom

CHAPTER OUTLINE

Learning Outcomes
Clinical Scenario
Introduction
Bones
- *Femur*
- *Tibia*
- *Patella*

Joints
- *Tibiofemoral Joint*
- *Patellofemoral Joint*
- *Q Angle*

Muscles
- *Knee Extensors*
- *Knee Flexors*
- *Tibial Rotators*

Functions of Muscles of the Knee
- *Knee Extensors*
- *Knee Flexors*
- *One-Joint and Two-Joint Muscles Acting at the Knee*

Joint Forces
- *Tibiofemoral Joint Forces*
- *Patellofemoral Joint Forces*
- *Torque of Muscles Acting at the Knee*

Interaction of Muscles and Ligaments in Function
- *Sensory Innervation and Reflexes*
- *Static and Dynamic Connections*
- *Muscle Protection of Ligaments*

Summary
Clinical Scenario Solution
Discussion Questions
Lab Activities
References

LEARNING OUTCOMES

By the end of this chapter, you should be able to:

- ❑ Identify the bones, joints, soft tissue, and muscles of the knee;
- ❑ Discuss the relationship between the tibiofemoral and patellofemoral joints and their contribution to functional movement;
- ❑ List muscles that are prime movers of the knee;
- ❑ Discuss the influence of gravity and body position in determining muscles acting on the knee during functional motions;
- ❑ Name muscle groups that function to position and move the knee in specific functional activities;
- ❑ Describe commonly encountered movement disorders of the knee joints and their functional consequences;
- ❑ Explain how the knee impacts motions at the hip and ankle during closed chain activities.

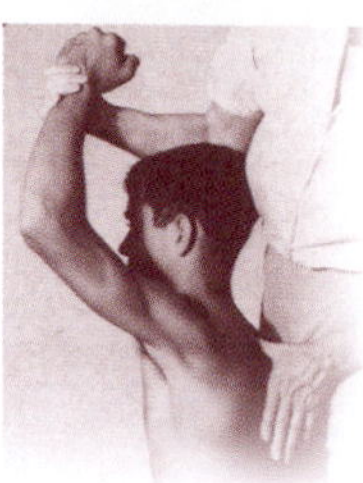

CLINICAL SCENARIO

Logan experiences pain when he goes up and down stairs, squats, and kneels. He enjoys going on long mountainous climbs but notices his left knee was painful for several days following the weekend that he hiked up and down the mountains in Yosemite National Park. Today is his first day with a clinician with whom he made an appointment to see if he can get rid of his knee pain. Cole, his clinician, has just taken Logan's history and is about to begin his examination. Cole tells Logan that he has a good indication of what Logan has but wants to perform a few tests before talking over treatment options.

Introduction

The knee is a complex joint (Figs. 10.1 and 10.2) with three bones (femur, tibia, and patella), two degrees of freedom of motion, and three articulating surfaces: the medial tibiofemoral, lateral tibiofemoral, and patellofemoral articulations, which are enclosed by a common joint capsule. However, not all of its ligaments lie within the capsule.

Functionally, the knee can support the body weight in the erect position without muscle activity; an individual is able to rely on the joint's ligaments to maintain quiet standing. The knee plays a primary role in lowering and elevating body weight during sitting, squatting, and climbing, and it permits rotation of the body when turning on the planted foot as a football receiver does when avoiding a pursuing tackler. In walking and running, the normal knee reduces vertical and lateral oscillations of the center of gravity of the body[1] while sustaining vertical forces equal to four to six times body weight.[2, 3] Some of the muscles that control the knee joint also cross either the hip or the ankle, so there is an intimate relationship between the knee and both of these other joints.

Although it is the largest joint in the body, the knee is among the more frequently injured joints within athletic and industrial environments.[4, 5] One factor that

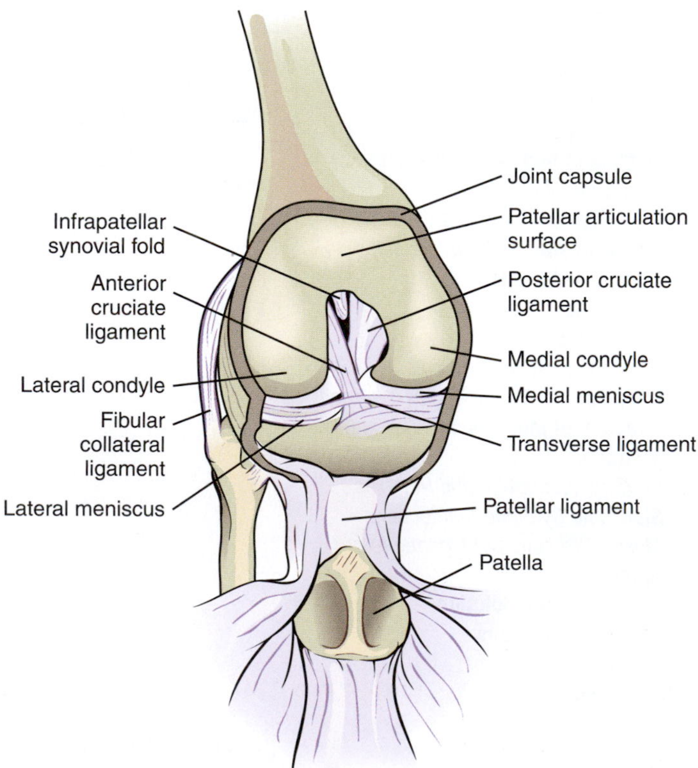

Figure 10.1 The anterior view of a right knee of a young adult flexed to about 90°. The anterior capsule is excised and the patella turned down to view the joint.

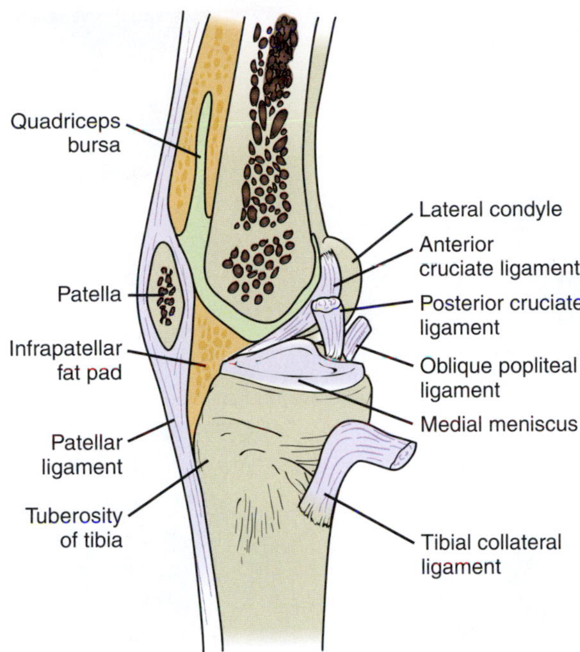

Figure 10.2 Medial perspective of a right knee with the femur and patella split in half sagittally.

places the knee at risk is the large torques it receives because of its position between two long lever arms, the femur and tibia. The multiple functions of normal knees—to withstand large forces, to provide great stability, and to afford large ranges of motion—are achieved in a unique way. The relatively shallow joint provides for extensive motion, but the joint configuration means that the knee must rely on soft tissue structures for it primary support and stability.

Bones

The three bones comprising the knee include the femur, tibia, and patella. Although the proximal fibula is near the knee joint, it is not considered part of the knee; however, it does play a role in ankle function, so it is presented in Chapter 11. Because of the soft tissue surrounding the knee, it is easier to palpate the bony structures anteriorly than it is to palpate the posterior structures, which are covered by the hamstrings and gastrocnemius muscles. It is easiest to palpate these anterior structures with the subject sitting on a table and with the knee relaxed in 90° of flexion.

Femur

The distal femur forms the proximal end of the knee joint. The distal femur changes to expand its design in a medial-lateral direction. This medial-lateral distal femoral expansion is referred to as the medial and lateral **condyles** (Gr., *kondylos,* knuckle; a rounded projection on a bone). These condyles are covered with articular cartilage and are connected to each other anteriorly but are separate posteriorly. Because the femur is obliquely positioned relative to vertical, the medial condyle is larger and extends more distally than the lateral condyle so their distal alignment in the frontal plane is level to each other (Fig. 10.3). On average, the medial condyle is 1.7 cm larger than the lateral condyle in adults.[6] The anterosuperior aspect of the condyles forms a groove between them known as the **intercondylar groove** or **trochlear groove**. This is where the posterior patella articulates with the femur. The articular cartilage of the femoral condyles for the patellofemoral joint is continuous with that of the femoral condyles for the tibiofemoral joint, but there is a slight medial-lateral ridge that distinguishes one from the other.[7] The anterior aspect of the lateral condyle which articulates with the patella juts more anteriorly than the medial condyle; it has been demonstrated that lateral femoral condyles that have an inadequate anterior projection may precipitate lateral patellar dislocations.[8–10] An **intercondylar fossa** separates the two condyles at their most inferior aspects and posteriorly. It is through this fossa that the cruciate ligaments traverse.

Immediately superior to the femoral condyles are the **epicondyles** (Gr., *epi,* upon). As shown in Figure 10.4B, they are distal enlargements of the femur immediately proximal to the condyles. The condyles can be palpated anteriorly on either side (Fig. 10.4A) of the patella and followed proximally to the epicondyles (Box 10-1). When the palpating fingers then reverse direction and move

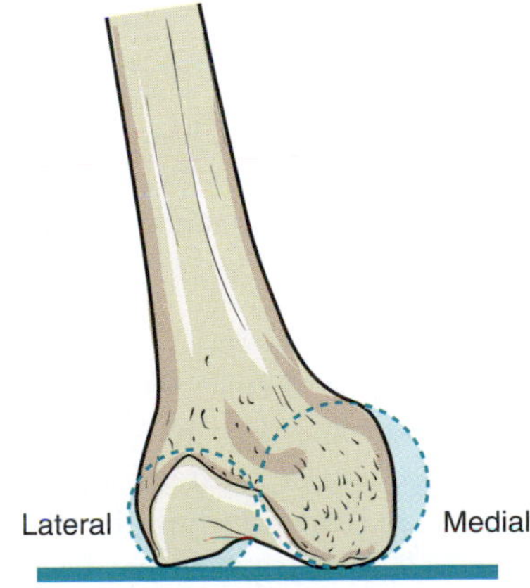

Figure 10.3 The medial condyle is larger than the lateral condyle to compensate for the femoral alignment to the vertical, thereby allowing the distal femur to lie horizontal in the frontal plane.

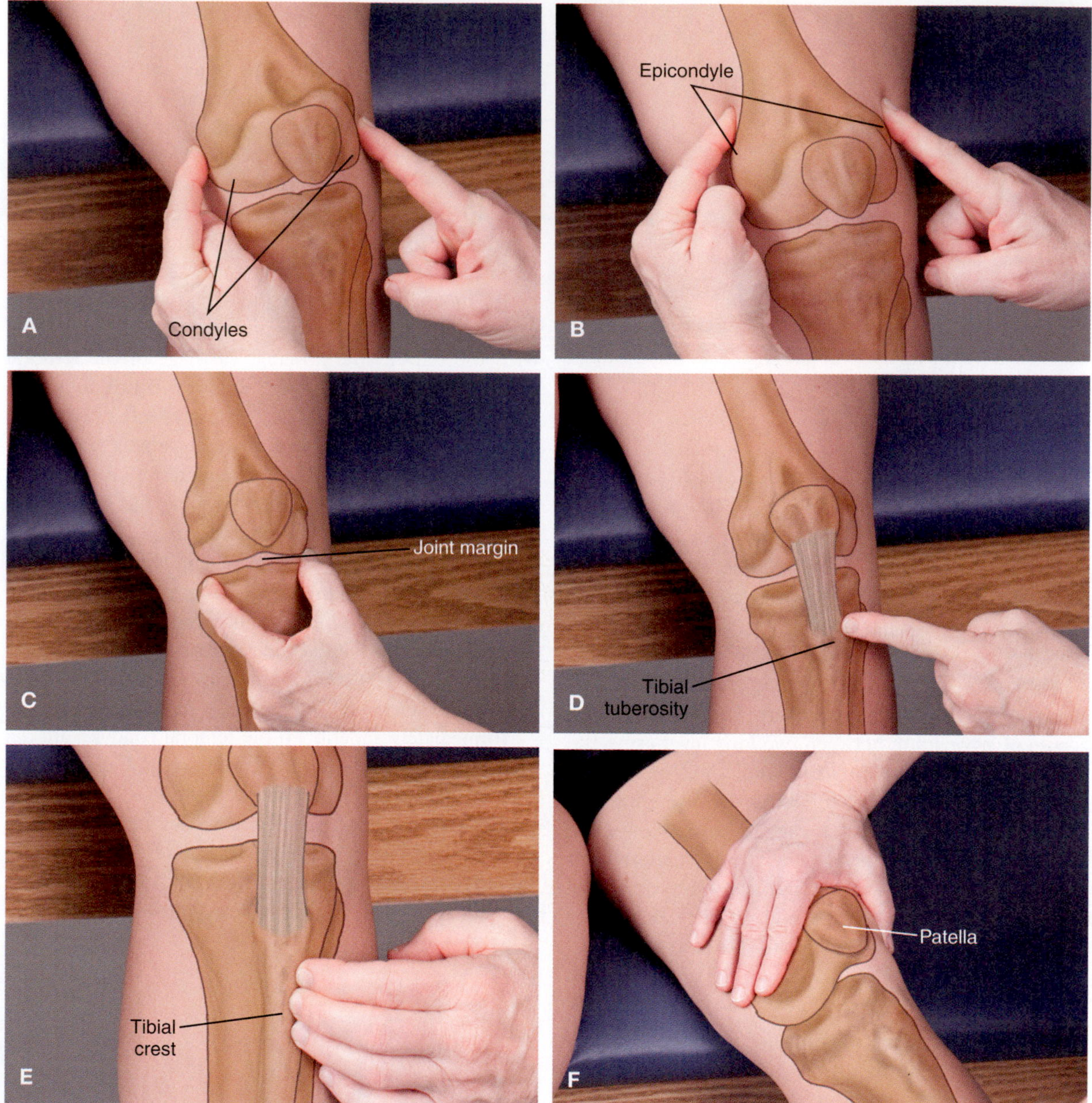

Figure 10.4 Surface anatomy. A) Condyle. B) Epicondyle. C) Joint margin. D) Tibial tuberosity. E) Tibial crest. F) Clinician grasping the patella.

inferiorly from the femoral condyles, the depression for the **tibiofemoral joint line** (Fig. 10.4C) is encountered. With a normal knee relaxed in extension, the joint line is palpated laterally and medially just inferior from the patella's inferior pole. This joint line can be confirmed by passively rotating or extending the knee while feeling the motion of the tibial condyles on the femur.

The surface of the anterior femoral condyles articulating with the patella is concave. On the other hand, the distal and posterior condyle surfaces which articulate with the tibia are slightly convex, somewhat similar to the runners on a rocking chair.

Tibia

The tibia flares at its proximal end as it meets the femur to form the distal portion of the tibiofemoral joint. The articular surfaces of the tibia are significantly smaller than those of their counterparts of the femur. The tibia has two slightly concave plateaus, or condyles, corresponding to the medial and lateral femoral condyles. As

BOX 10-1 | Palpable Bony Features of the Distal Femur

- Medial epicondyle
- Lateral epicondyle
- Medial condyle
- Lateral condyle
- Tibiofemoral joint line

BOX 10-2 | Palpable Bony Features of the Proximal Tibia and Fibula

- Medial condyle or plateau
- Lateral condyle or plateau
- Tibial tuberosity
- Crest of the tibia
- Fibular head

with the femur, the tibia's medial condyle is larger than its lateral condyle. This is an important anatomical design since the medial knee bears more pressure in standing, so having a greater surface area reduces the amount of stress applied to it.[11] Between the two tibial condyles is an intercondylar eminence that contains two small spines, the medial and lateral tubercles. This intercondylar eminence sits within the femoral intercondylar fossa when the knee is in extension.

Anteriorly on the tibia and inferior to the tibial condyles is a large roughened area, the **tibial tuberosity** (Fig. 10.4D), which serves as the distal attachment for the quadriceps muscle's tendon. Just distal and slightly posterior to the middle of the lateral tibial plateau, about two finger widths from the lateral joint margin, is the tibial fossa where the proximal fibula attaches. On the medial aspect of the proximal tibia slightly distal from the level of the fibular head is the site of the **pes anserine,** an important support structure to be described later.

The shaft of the tibia is triangular in its cross-sectional shape. The sharp **crest of the tibia** (Fig. 10.4E) divides the medial and lateral aspects of the bone and may be palpated distally to the ankle. The medial aspect of the tibia is not covered by muscle and is also easily palpated (Box 10-2). On the other hand, the lateral and posterior aspects are covered by muscle so they cannot be palpated.

Patella

The patella (L., *patina*, small plate) begins its ossification process by the third to fifth year to ultimately become the largest **sesamoid bone** in the body. Sesamoid bones are small bones that lie within a tendon to protect the tendon and change the tendon's angle of pull. Since the continuation of this tendon connects two bones, the patella and tibia, this distal structure between the patella and tibia is the patellar ligament. The patella loosely resembles an inverted triangle with the apex at the inferior pole with a rounded proximal base. Anteriorly, the patella's surface is convex. The posterior surface is oval, articulating with the femur and divided into two facets by a vertical ridge that runs from its superior border to its apex. This vertical ridge corresponds to the trochlear groove of the femur. The lateral facet is the larger of the two and is concave, conforming to the corresponding surface of the femur. Medial to the medial facet is a small region called the odd facet. The patella's articular surface is covered by some of the thickest articular cartilage in the body;[12,13] reports of as much as 4.7 to 6.6 mm[14] and up to 7.75 mm[15] thick have been noted in previous studies.

The patella has several important functions at the knee. According to Heegaard and associates,[16] the patella serves to:

1. Improve the efficiency and increase torque of the knee extensors throughout the knee's range of motion;
2. Centralize the forces of the four quadriceps muscles into one concerted direction of pull;
3. Provide a smooth gliding mechanism for the quadriceps muscle and tendon to reduce compression and friction forces during activities such as deep knee bends;
4. Contribute to the overall stability of the knee; and
5. Provide bony protection from direct trauma to the femoral condyles when the knee is flexed.

Therefore, the patella contributes to overall knee function. If the patella is injured or absent, direct consequences are experienced at the tibiofemoral joint.

The patella is best palpated when the subject is supine with the knee extended and relaxed (Box 10-3).

BOX 10-3 | Palpable Bony Features of the Patella

- Apex (inferior pole)
- Base
- Anterior surface
- Posterior surface of lateral facet
- Posterior surface of medial facet
- Posterior surface of odd facet

The thick patellar ligament may be felt from the tuberosity of the tibia to the apex of the triangular patella. When the quadriceps is relaxed and the knee is in full extension, the patella can be easily mobilized laterally and distally and can be compressed on the femur without discomfort (Fig. 10.4F).

The following are nonpalpable structures of the knee and are illustrated in Figures 10.1, 10.2, and 10.5: articular surfaces and patellar articulation surfaces on the condyles of the femur; intercondylar fossa; lateral and medial supracondylar lines, extending proximally from the condyles and enclosing an area that forms the floor of the **popliteal fossa** (L., *poples,* posterior knee); articular surfaces of the condyles of the tibia ("tibial plateau"), separated by the intercondylar eminence; lateral **meniscus,** nearly circular in form (Gr., *meniskos,* crescent); medial meniscus; anterior and posterior cruciate ligaments; and transverse ligament, connecting the menisci anteriorly.

Joints

The knee complex contains two joints—the tibiofemoral joint and the patellofemoral joint—surrounded by one capsule. As mentioned, the proximal tibiofibular joint is not technically part of the knee complex since it does not lie within the joint capsule, so it will be presented in Chapter 11.

Tibiofemoral Joint

As the largest joint in the body, the tibiofemoral joint is made from the two longest bones of the body. Because of the knee joint's complexity and of how the medial and lateral femoral condyles function with their corresponding tibial counterparts, it is considered by some to actually be two joints, a medial and a lateral joint.[17]

The tibiofemoral joints achieve their greatest stability and two degrees of freedom of motion in a remarkable way. The medial and lateral femoral condyles are convex both longitudinally and transversely. They are connected anteriorly by the femur's patellar articulation surface and separated distally and posteriorly by the intercondylar notch. These femoral condyles articulate with the two smaller tibial condyles, which have only a slight concavity; hence, they are commonly referred to as plateaus. The lateral tibial condyle is also convex anteriorly and posteriorly. The congruity of the articulations is increased slightly by the intercondylar eminence of the tibia and the wedge-shaped medial and lateral menisci (semilunar cartilages), which form an incomplete ring, or crescent, on each tibial condyle. The longitudinal articulating surface of the femoral condyles is approximately twice the length of the surface of the tibial condyles. Therefore, the motions of knee flexion and extension cannot be pure rolling or hinge motions. Instead, the condyles execute both rolling and sliding movements, with the ratio of each changing throughout the range of motion (Fig. 10.6). Rolling is predominant at the initiation of flexion, and sliding occurs more at the end of flexion.[6] Because the length of the articular surface of the lateral femoral condyle is longer than that of the medial condyle, the movements of the two condylar surfaces differ. The impact of this size difference on condylar motion is presented later in this chapter.

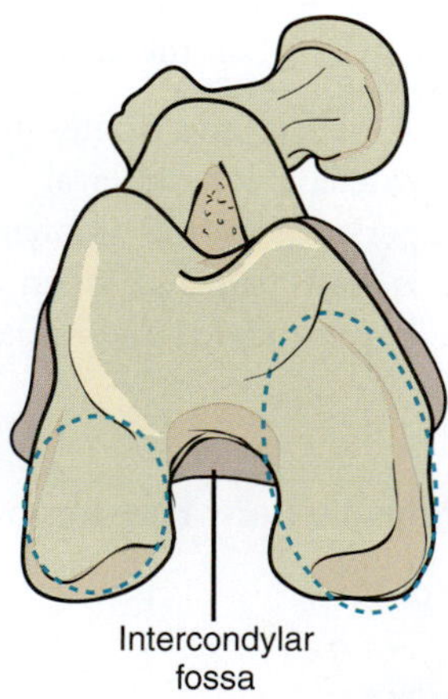

Figure 10.5 The intercondylar fossa separates the two condyles at their most inferior aspect and posteriorly. This is the site through which the cruciate ligaments traverse. Note the difference in size/articulating surface area (dotted circles) between the medial and lateral femoral condyles.

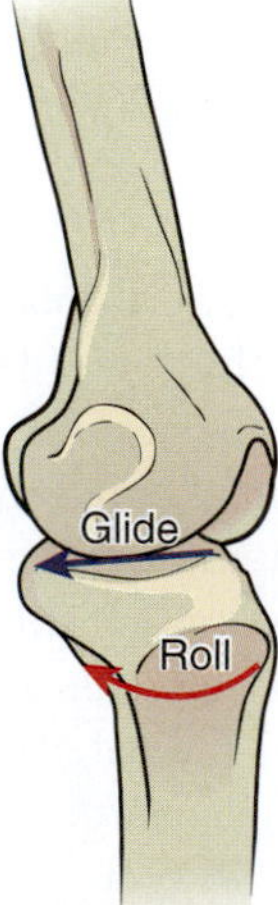

Figure 10.6 The roll and glide of the knee during open chain motion. As the knee joint moves into flexion, the tibia rolls posteriorly and glides in the same direction on the femur.

Menisci

The menisci provide the knee joint with important properties. The fibrocartilaginous menisci are attached to the tibia to deepen the joint's socket, improving the joint's congruency. Although increased congruency usually leads to less mobility, the menisci provide for both more congruency and a larger range of knee flexion.[18] Each meniscus is attached to the tibia at its anterior and posterior ends, or poles (Fig. 10.7). The lateral meniscus's configuration is nearly a circle whereas the medial meniscus is more of a C-shape. Each meniscus is anchored along its lateral rim to the tibia and joint capsule by a loose **coronary ligament**. These ligaments are also known as **meniscotibial ligaments**. The horns of the menisci at the anterior and posterior intercondylar fossae and through the coronary ligaments are the only bony attachments of the menisci; these ligaments also attach the peripheral margins of the menisci to the joint capsule. Since the menisci are not attached to the tibia except at these points, they have mobility during knee motion; the lateral meniscus has more mobility during knee motion than the medial meniscus. There are several additional attachments of both ligaments and muscles to these menisci. In summary, these attachments include:

1. The transverse ligament connects the anterior horns of the two menisci together.
2. Fibrous bands connect the anterior horns of both menisci to the retinaculum of the patellar tendon (meniscopatellar fibers).
3. Deep fibers of the medial collateral ligament attach to the medial meniscus.
4. The tendon of the semimembranosus muscle sends fibers to the posterior edge of the medial meniscus.
5. The popliteus muscle sends fibers to the posterior edge of the lateral meniscus.
6. The meniscofemoral ligament extends from the lateral meniscus (posteriorly) to the inside of the medial condyle near the posterior cruciate ligament.

Each meniscus is wedge-shaped with the thickest portion on the outer rim of the meniscus. As the meniscus continues towards the center of the condyle, it becomes thinner. This design with the thickness on the rim and the thinness on the inner border allows the menisci to improve the joint's congruity and stability. According to Clark and Ogden,[19] the lateral meniscus takes up more space on its tibial condyle than does the medial meniscus, and the lateral meniscus extends closer to the center of its condyle (Fig. 10.7).

Since the menisci are attached to the tibia, their movement is controlled by knee movement, both passively and actively. Passively, they are pushed anteriorly by the femur as the knee extends and the contact of the femoral condyles is more anterior on the tibial condyles. Conversely, the menisci move posteriorly with knee flexion. According to Kapandji,[6] a total movement of 6 mm occurs in the medial meniscus and 12 mm in the lateral meniscus. In addition, the menisci move or deform according to the direction of movement of the femoral condyles during axial rotation. Edges of the menisci are moved by their ligamentous and muscular attachments. For example, anterior movement is caused by the meniscopatellar fibers to the extensor mechanism, and posterior movement is caused by their attachments to the knee flexors (the semimembranosus and the popliteus muscles). If a meniscus fails to move with the femoral condyles, as may occur with sudden twisting or forceful motion, the meniscus may be crushed or torn by the condyles.

The menisci serve several purposes for the knee joint:

1. The menisci deepen the knee joint and thereby add stability to it.[18]
2. The menisci absorb and distribute forces of impact.[20]
3. The menisci are able to distribute forces of impact by increasing the surface contact area and congruency of the joint.[21] By increasing the surface contact area, the load is distributed over a larger area. Therefore, when the menisci are removed, the load-bearing surface must endure the same load as it did

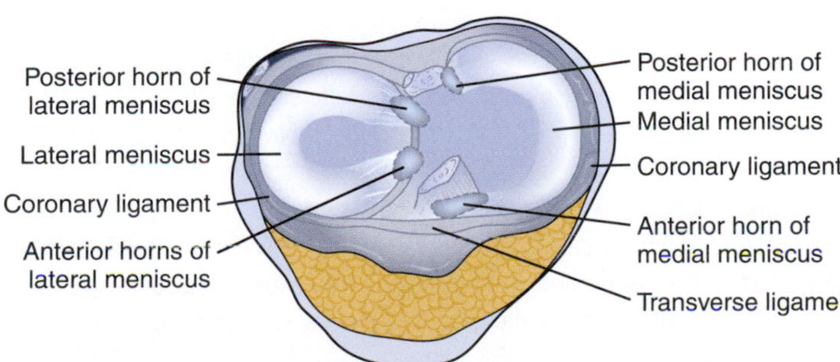

Figure 10.7 Medial and lateral meniscus and their attachments to the right tibial plateau. Each meniscus is attached to the tibia at its anterior and posterior poles. Other attachments along the rim of each meniscus secure it to the tibia, but the medial meniscus is more securely anchored than the lateral meniscus.

with the meniscus; this stress is about three times the magnitude it was when the menisci were present.[18]

4. The menisci promote joint lubrication by spreading a film of synovial fluid over the articular surfaces.[18,22]
5. The menisci prevent the joint capsule from intruding into the joint space.[18]
6. Although the ligaments provide most of the protection against knee hyperextension, the menisci provide partial protection to this excessive movement.[18]

Weight-bearing areas of the knee are almost equal on the medial and lateral tibiofemoral surfaces with the largest area occurring when the knee is in hyperextension.[2] With knee flexion, the weight-bearing area moves posteriorly on the tibial condyles and becomes smaller. Surgical removal of the menisci decreases the surface area and causes pressure to increase on the femoral and tibial condyles, which may lead to later osteoarthritis.[23]

Ligaments and Capsule

Several ligaments surround the tibiofemoral joint to provide protection for this relatively shallow joint. In addition to the capsule, there are two pairs of ligaments, collateral and cruciate ligaments, which are responsible for providing integrity to joint stability. These ligaments are summarized for your review in Table 10–1. The collateral ligaments provide stability in a medial-lateral direction whereas the cruciate ligaments provide anterior-posterior stability. Both groups of ligaments are extracapsular and taut in full knee extension.

Collateral Ligaments

The attachments of the collateral ligaments on the femoral condyles are offset posteriorly and superiorly to the knee's axis for flexion. This offsetting causes the ligaments to become taut when the knee moves into extension and slack as the knee flexes (Fig. 10.8). The collateral ligaments thus provide stability to terminal rotation of the extended knee and yet permit axial rotation in the flexed knee. Axial rotation also is facilitated by a decrease in the congruency of the joint surfaces when the knee is flexed. The posterior aspects of the femoral condyles have a greater convexity, and the intercondylar notch is wider at this point. Thus, when the knee is flexed, the mating surfaces with the tibial intercondylar tubercles and the menisci are reduced, and the condyles have more freedom to rotate.

The medial collateral ligament (MCL) is a broad, flat ligament that is a thickening of the medial joint capsule and attaches to the tibia at two points; this attachment allows the ligament to provide joint stability in both flexion and extension. The anterior portion of the ligament is about 10 cm in length and is taut in flexion whereas the posterior portion is shorter and taut in extension.[27] A bursa is located between the superficial and deep layers of this ligament. When a **valgus** force is applied to the knee, the medial collateral ligament provides less than 60% of the restraining force, but when the force is applied to the knee when it is in 25° of flexion, the ligament applies almost 80% of the protective restraining force.[28] Other structures such as the capsule and cruciate ligaments provide resistance to valgus forces when the knee is in extension, but the medial collateral ligament is the primary structure protecting the knee in flexion.

In contrast to the medial collateral ligament, the lateral collateral ligament (LCL) is a shorter, cord-like structure. It sits outside the joint capsule and is easily palpated when the foot rests on the opposite knee and a **varus** force is applied to the joint; fingers placed along the lateral joint margin easily palpate the ligament as the varus force is applied. It also provides protection to

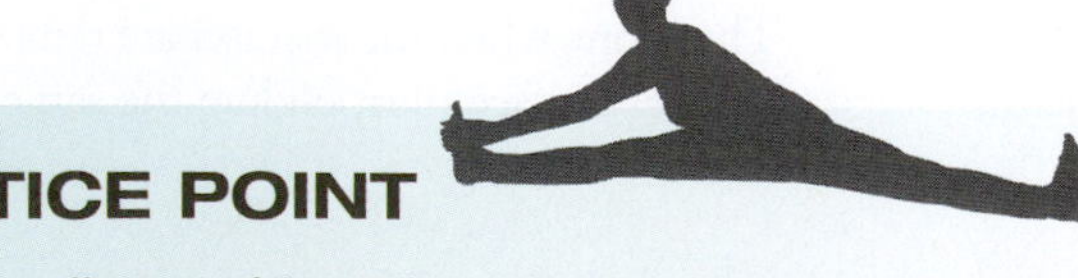

PRACTICE POINT

Individuals who suffer tears of the meniscus often find the tear is not an acute one but one that has occurred over time. With repeated stresses of knee flexion during athletic activities such as weight-resisted squats and sport activities that require weight-bearing in knee flexion, the posterior aspect of the menisci begins to wear and tear. Over time, the posterior aspects of the menisci show evidence of macroscopic tears. Patients who report signs and symptoms of meniscus lesions without a frank injury often demonstrate on MRI lesions of the posterior meniscus, medial more frequently than lateral.[24] However, which meniscus suffers lesions more frequently is disputable since some investigators have found no difference between the medial and lateral meniscus in the frequency of lesions[25] whereas others have found more lateral lesions in athletes who participate in sports such as basketball,[26] in which lateral joint stresses occur more frequently. It may depend upon the population studied as to the prevalence of one meniscal lesion over the other.

(text continues on page 434)

TABLE 10–1 | LIGAMENTS OF THE KNEE

Image	Joint	Ligament	Proximal Attachment	Distal Attachment	Motions it limits
	Tibiofemoral	Medial (Tibial) Collateral ligament	Medial epicondyle of femur	Posterior section attaches on the medial epicondyle; anterior section attaches along the middle superior aspect of medial tibia distal to the pes anserine.	Protects against a valgus force in the frontal plane.
	Tibiofemoral	Lateral (Fibular) Collateral ligament	Lateral epicondyle of the femur	Head of the fibula on its lateral aspect. It also merges with the biceps femoris tendon.	Protects against a varus force in the frontal plane.
	Tibiofemoral	Anterior cruciate ligament	Anterior intercondylar tibial fossa behind anterior attachment of medial meniscus	Posteromedial aspect of lateral femoral condyle.	Prevents anterior displacement of tibia on femur and protects against hyperextension.
	Tibiofemoral	Posterior cruciate ligament	Posterior tibial spine	Travels medial to the ACL to the anterolateral surface of medial femoral condyle.	Prevents posterior displacement of the tibia on the femur and protects against hyperflexion.

Continued

TABLE 10-1 | LIGAMENTS OF THE KNEE—cont'd

Image	Joint	Ligament	Proximal Attachment	Distal Attachment	Motions it limits
Gastroc heads; Medial collateral ligament; Lateral collateral ligament; Arcuate popliteal ligament; Oblique popliteal ligament; Popliteus	Tibiofemoral	Arcuate ligament	Posterior capsule and popliteal tendon on lateral femoral condyle	Forms a Y-insertion with one head on the posterior fibular head and the other on the oblique popliteal ligament.	Protects the posterolateral capsule against hyperextension and rotational forces.
	Tibiofemoral	Oblique popliteal ligament	Posteromedial tibia near semimembranosus insertion	Posterolateral femur near lateral gastrocnemius head	Protects posterior knee from hyperextension.
	Fibulofemoral	Popliteofibular ligament (Not pictured)	Musculotendinous junction of popliteus near lateral femoral epicondyle[168]	Tip of the fibular styloid process	Resists posterolateral tibial rotation and posterior tibial translation.[169]

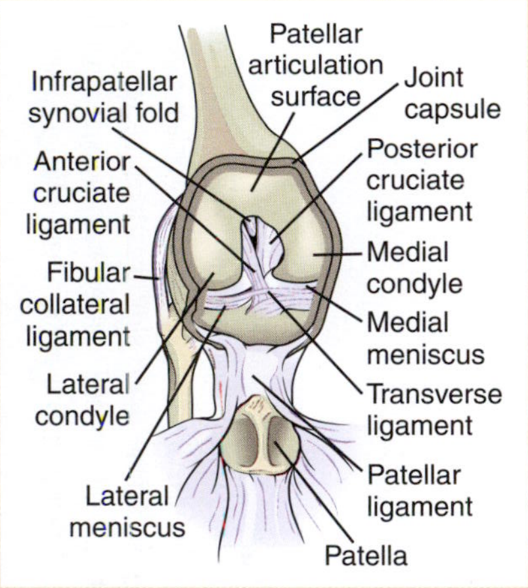	Patellofemoral	Patellar ligament	Apex of the patella	Tibial tuberosity	Serves as a continuation of the quadriceps tendon and protects the anterior knee.
	Meniscofemoral	Ligament of Humphrey (anterior meniscofemoral ligament) (Not pictured)	Posterior horn of lateral meniscus	Distal portion of PCL attachment to the femur	Anchors lateral meniscus. Note: It is common to have either the Ligament of Humphrey or Wrisberg, but not both.
	Meniscofemoral	Ligament of Wrisberg (posterior femoral ligament) (Not pictured)	Posterior horn of lateral meniscus	Medial femoral condyle	Stabilizes lateral meniscus.

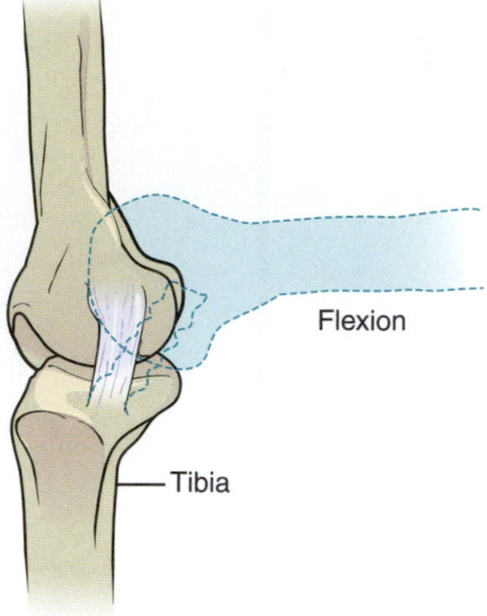

Figure 10.8 Because of their offset attachment on the femur relative to the axis of motion, the collateral ligaments are taut in knee extension and lax in flexion. This arrangement allows them to provide stability to rotation during extension but allow rotation when the knee is flexed.

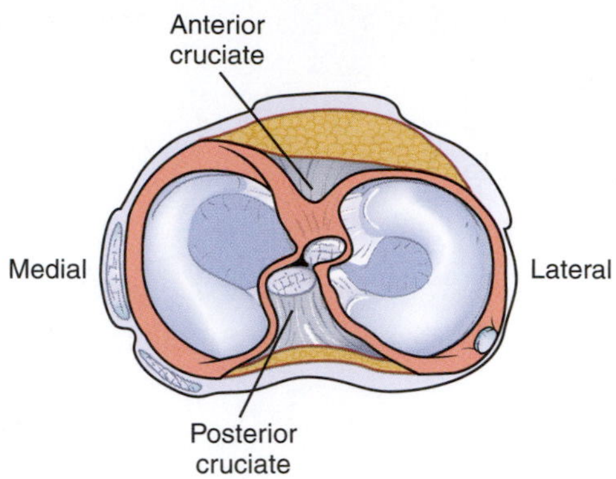

Figure 10.9 A view of the cruciate ligaments from overhead makes them appear as if they are parallel rather than that they cross one another within the knee joint.

the knee, but in the opposite direction of the medial collateral ligament. The lateral collateral ligament assists in providing varus stress protection when the knee is in full extension by offering just over half of the total protection, but when the knee is in partial flexion at 25°, it provides almost 70% of the protection against varus stresses.[28]

Cruciate Ligaments

The anterior and posterior cruciate ligament (L., *crux*, cross) provide control and stability to the knee throughout the motions of flexion and extension. These ligaments lie in the center of the joint within the femoral intercondylar fossa (Figs. 10.1 and 10.2). They receive their name because they form a cross when viewed from the side or from the front. However, they appear parallel when viewed from above (Fig. 10.9). These ligaments lie within the fibrous capsule but are outside of the synovial joint capsule, so they are intracapsular but extrasynovial. The cruciate ligaments maintain a relatively constant length throughout the motions of flexion and extension even though not all of their parts are taut at the same time. In this way, these ligaments help to force the sliding motions of the condylar surfaces to occur.

Both of the cruciate ligaments arise from the tibia and attach to the distal femur within the knee joint. The anterior cruciate ligament (ACL) is more oblique whereas the posterior cruciate ligament (PCL) follows a more vertical course. The anterior cruciate ligament is longer, but the posterior cruciate ligament is thicker and stronger. Each has bundles of fibers that are twisted to form spirals along their course; this arrangement allows some part of each ligament to remain taut throughout knee motion.[29] Each ligament also has two bands, or bundles, of fibers that are labeled according to their sites of attachment or their relative position; the anterior cruciate ligament bundles are labeled according to their

PRACTICE POINT

The medial collateral ligament is unique to most ligaments in that it is well endowed with a blood supply. For this reason, injuries to medial collateral ligaments are rarely repaired surgically. Clinicians who treat these injuries follow a rehabilitation protocol that includes a cautious plan to allow healing and provides gradual stresses to the ligament only after it has progressed through the healing phases and is able to tolerate those stresses. If other structures are also injured along with the medial collateral ligament, the surgeon may or may not opt to repair the medial collateral ligament. Clinicians dealing with surgical repair of other knee structures must be aware of whether or not the medial collateral ligament has also been repaired and make appropriate adjustments in the rehabilitation program.

sites of attachment and include an anteromedial band (AMB) and a posterolateral band (PLB)[30] whereas the posterior cruciate ligament bundles are identified according to their relative position and are identified as the anterolateral (AL) bundle and the posteromedial (PL) bundle.[29]

Anterior and posterior translation of the knee is restricted by anterior and posterior cruciate ligaments, respectively. Severance of the anterior cruciate ligament allows anterior displacement of the tibia on the femur or posterior displacement of the femur on the tibia.[31,32] Severance of the anterior cruciate ligament in cadavers demonstrated an anterior displacement of the tibia on the femur of 7 mm.[33,34] Such movement in subjects with non-injured ACLs is far less; mean values of this motion in healthy young adults were measured from 1.2 to 2.7 mm at 90° of flexion.[35]

On the other hand, the posterior cruciate ligament provides stability in the opposite direction to the anterior cruciate ligament. In closed chain motion as when the foot is planted in running, the posterior cruciate ligament helps prevent anterior displacement (dislocation) of the femoral condyles on the tibial condyles or posterior displacement of the tibia on the femur. Normally the posterior cruciate ligament permits only minimal passive movement between the tibia and femur. The average displacements in normal young adults ranged from 0.6 to 1.0 mm in men and from 1.2 to 1.9 mm in women when the knee was at 90° of flexion.[35] The posterior cruciate ligament produces its most restriction to tibial posterior displacement between 90° and 120° of flexion.[29]

Capsule and Other Inert Soft Tissue Structures

The largest capsule of the body is the knee's joint capsule. The joint capsule forms a sleeve around the joints, attaching just above the femoral condyles and below the tibial condyles. Anteriorly, there is a cutout for the patella and posteriorly, and there is a central fold that almost divides the joint space (Fig. 10.10). Retinacula and ligaments reinforce and become integral parts of the capsule. The proximal tendon of the popliteus muscle pierces the capsule to attach on the lateral femoral condyle. The semimembranosus muscle forms part of the oblique popliteal ligament and gives off fibers to the medial collateral ligament as well as to its large bony attachment. These are a few examples of the complex passive and active connections among the menisci, ligaments, retinacula, bones, muscles, and the capsule (Fig. 10.11).

As with other joint capsules, the knee joint capsule has an inner synovial layer and an outer fibrous layer.

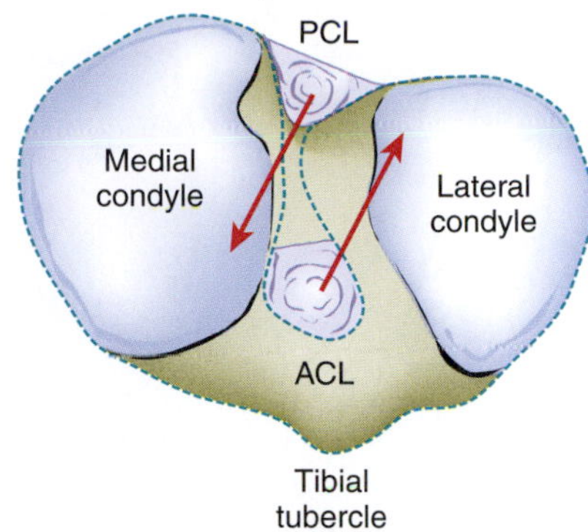

Figure 10.10 The tibia viewed from above. The dotted line is the attachment of the synovial lining as it folds in and around the attachments of the anterior and posterior cruciate ligaments. From this perspective, it is seen that the cruciate ligaments are within the joint but remain outside the synovial portion of the capsule.

However, these two capsular layers do not adhere to each other like those capsular layers of other joints. The posterior aspects of the synovial layer extend more proximally and may also extend distally from the fibrous layer above and below the knee joint. The synovial layer follows the fibrous layer around the medial and lateral aspects of the knee, but it separates from the fibrous layer at the superior patella and expands to form a large pouch proximal to the patella under the quadriceps muscle. This area is the **suprapatellar pouch** and is frequently identifiable when the knee joint is injured and experiences extensive swelling. The synovial aspect of the capsule has been found to hold over 260 ml (9 ounces) of fluid.[36] In knees that become very swollen, this pouch is enlarged to become noticeable, extending about 5 cm proximal to the patella.[37]

In addition to the collateral and cruciate ligaments, other ligaments, particularly in the posterior knee, lend support to the joint capsule. These primary and most consistently present ligaments include the arcuate ligament complex and popliteofibular ligament. These are expansions of the posterior capsule that add support during torsional stresses applied to the posterior capsule (Fig. 10.12). The arcuate ligament complex often includes a head that originates on the posterior fibular styloid process and traverses upward between the biceps femoris tendon and lateral gastrocnemius head to merge and insert with the oblique popliteal ligament on the posterior femur near the condyles. These structures along with the lateral collateral ligament provide the greatest stability to the posterolateral corner of the joint capsule.[38,39]

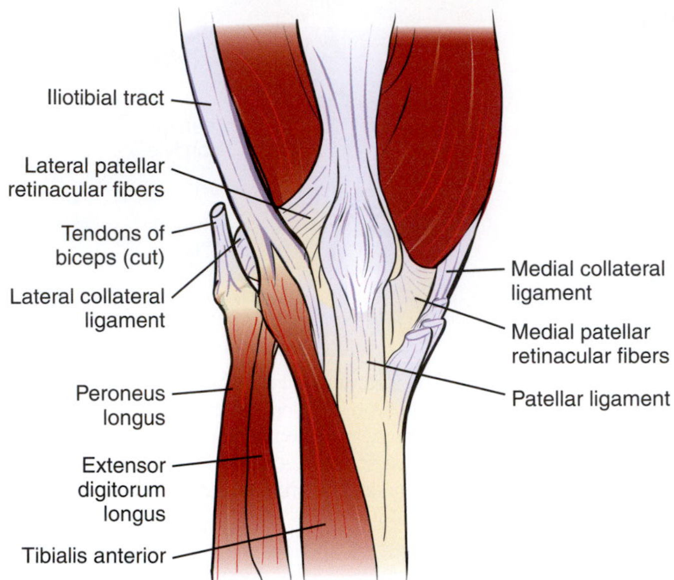

Figure 10.11 There is an intimate relationship among the capsule, ligaments, and tendons within the anterior knee. Retinacula and ligaments reinforce and fuse with the capsule.

There are also 12 bursae around the knee joint.[37] However, some of these bursae are extensions of the synovial lining of the knee. They, along with the fat pad around the knee, serve to reduce friction between adjacent structures and protect the knee.

Kinematics of the Tibiofemoral Joint

The knee joint (*articulatio genu,* L., *genua,* knee or any structure bent like the knee) possesses two degrees of freedom: flexion-extension and axial rotation. The amount of flexion is from 120°to 150° depending on the size of the muscle mass of the calf in contact with the posterior thigh. However, the average expected range of motion is 135°.[43] When the hip extends, the range of motion of knee flexion decreases because of limitation by the two-joint rectus femoris muscle, which has its proximal attachment on the anterior inferior spine of the ilium. Knee hyperextension is minimal and does not normally exceed 15°.

Normal passive motion end feel for knee flexion is soft from contact of the tissues of the posterior calf with the thigh or from a shortened rectus femoris muscle if calf-thigh contact is not made. The end feel for extension or hyperextension is firm from tension on ligamentous and posterior capsular structures. If the hip is flexed to 90°, knee extension may be limited if the hamstring muscles lack normal extensibility.

Axes for Flexion and Extension

From a clinical perspective, the axis of motion is located a few centimeters above the joint line passing medially-laterally through the femoral condyles. Because the condyles of the femur are so much larger than those of the tibia, the femoral condyles not only roll over the tibial condyles when the knee moves from extension into flexion in weight-bearing, but they must also glide so they don't roll off the tibia. Since the femur glides as it moves in flexion-extension, the center of axis of

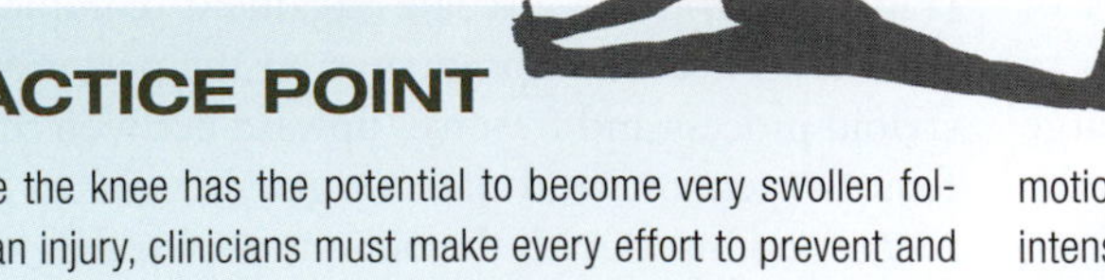

PRACTICE POINT

Because the knee has the potential to become very swollen following an injury, clinicians must make every effort to prevent and reduce the amount of fluid within the knee joint as soon as possible following an injury. Extensive swelling in the joint causes a number of deleterious results including reducing the amount of motion through which the joint is able to move,[40] diminishing the intensity of muscle activity of the quadriceps muscle,[41] and increasing pain from the fluid's pressure placed on nerve receptors.[42] Full recovery following an injury cannot occur until these issues are resolved.

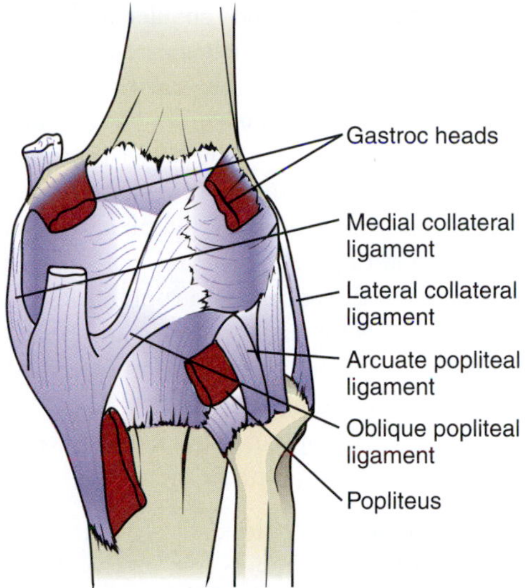

Figure 10.12 Posterior ancillary ligaments of the knee include the arcuate ligament complex and popliteofibular ligament. These ligaments are expansions of the posterior capsule and provide necessary additional support to the posterior capsule during torsional stress applications. Posterior muscles also interact with ligaments to aid in posterior support. The proximal tendon of the popliteus muscle goes through the capsule to attach on the lateral femoral condyle. The semimembranosus muscle becomes a portion of the oblique popliteal ligament and gives off fibers to the medial collateral ligament and patellar retinacular fibers.

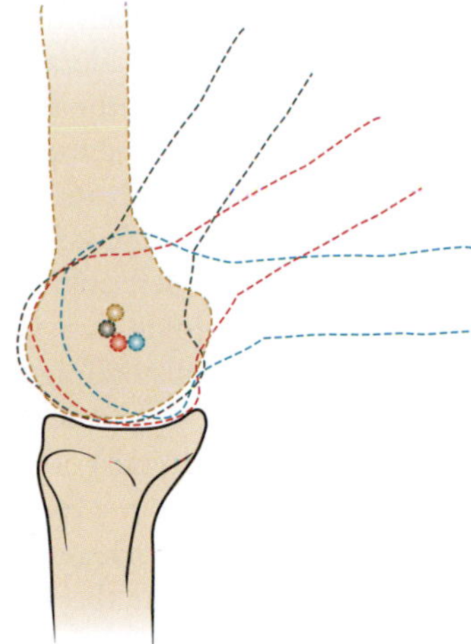

Figure 10.13 Instantaneous center of rotation of a joint. This is a theoretical axis of rotation that changes when a joint glides and rolls through its range of motion.

motion changes as the range of motion changes. For example, when you flex your knees to sit down, your femur rolls backward; however, the surface of the tibia is used up during this rolling maneuver before the knee is done flexing, so the femur must glide forward to a new location on the tibia so it can continue rolling backward to allow your knee to flex sufficiently to allow you to sit in the chair. When you stand to get out of the chair, your knees perform a reverse maneuver during closed chain activities, starting a forward roll of the femur on the tibia and then gliding posteriorly as the femoral condyles run out of space on the tibia but need to continue to roll forward until you are fully standing. This continual change in the center of axis of rotation (Fig. 10.13) is called the **instantaneous center of rotation (ICR).** This may be of concern for engineers or biomechanists, but the instantaneous center of rotation has no clinical application regarding either range of motion measurements or treatments.

The glides we have been discussing occur during closed chain or weight-bearing activities when the tibia is stabilized and the femur moves. The relationship between the glide and direction of roll during flexion and extension changes when the tibia moves and the femur is stabilized because the surface that is moving is different. This is discussed in the arthrokinematic section.

The change that occurs in the knee joint's center of rotation is one reason it has been difficult to design either an artificial knee that is able to closely resemble a normal knee or external devices that are applied to the joint. Because of the shifting axis of motion of the human knee, problems occur when devices with mechanical hinge joints such as an isokinetic dynamometer, knee-ankle-foot (long-leg) orthosis, or above-knee prosthesis are applied to the knee. When a human knee joint is moved from extension to flexion, the anatomic axis of the knee moves about 2 cm while the mechanical axis of the attached device remains fixed. Thus, the arms of the mechanical device cannot remain parallel to the thigh and leg, and motions or pressures between the mechanical and anatomic parts will occur. Compromise and careful alignment are required to prevent discomfort and abrasions. Misalignment of an orthotic knee joint can cause pressure from the device cuffs on the extremity during knee flexion and gapping during knee extension (or vice versa). This change in the anatomic axis of the knee is also the reason why a prosthetic knee is positioned more forward of the contralateral normal knee of the individual when he or she sits, even though the hips and ankles are aligned.

Axial Rotation

Axial rotation occurs in the transverse plane when the knee is flexed. When the knee is fully extended, the medial and lateral collateral ligaments are relatively tense, contributing to the stability of the joint, preventing rotation. These ligaments slacken when the joint flexes; this is one of the reasons why a considerable amount of transverse rotation may take place in the flexed position. In Figure 10.14, the position when the medial and lateral knee is extended is compared with its position when the knee is flexed. Note that the distance from the points of insertion of the ligaments is less in flexion than in extension. During knee flexion, more slack is produced in the lateral than in the medial collateral ligament; therefore, the movement between the femoral and tibial condyles is more extensive laterally than medially. Transverse rotation takes place about a longitudinal axis located medial to the intercondylar ridge of the tibia so that, roughly, it may be stated that the lateral condyle rotates around the medial one.

Although many conflicting values are reported for this motion, the results of published studies indicate the average total rotation to be approximately 40°.[44, 45] A later study found similar result at 90°of knee flexion.[46] Additionally, lateral rotation was approximately twice as large as medial rotation. Axial rotation decreases as the angle of knee flexion becomes smaller and cannot be performed as the knee approaches extension. Rotation of the tibia on the femur can be performed voluntarily in the sitting position and is useful in placing and positioning the foot. The major functional importance of the motion, however, is in closed chain motion, in which the femur rotates on the fixed tibia, as in turning from kneeling, sitting, or squatting positions and in sudden changes in direction when running.

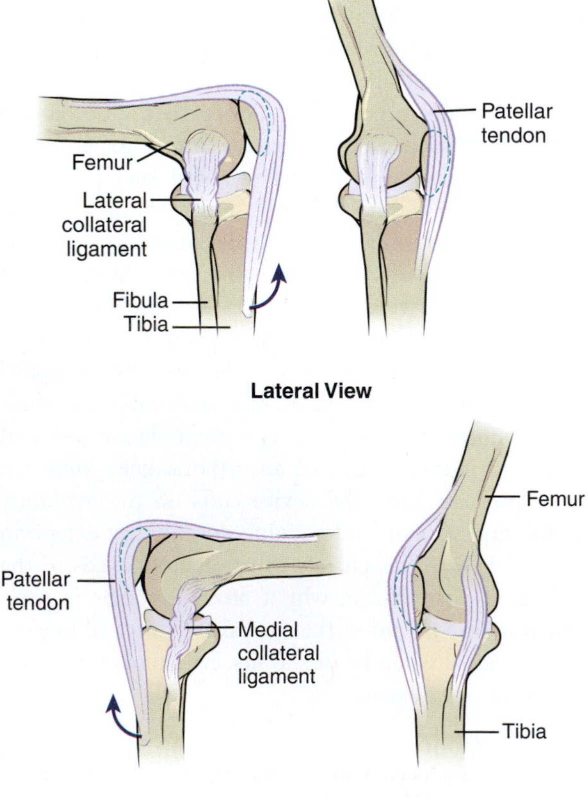

Figure 10.14 Collateral ligaments are taut in extension and slack in flexion to allow axial rotation of the knee in flexion.

Normal end feels for passive medial and lateral rotation of the knee are firm. Motion is limited by capsular and ligamentous structures, including the collateral, cruciate, and oblique popliteal ligaments as well as the retinacula and the iliotibial tract.

Terminal Rotation of the Knee

Normally, when the knee moves into extension, the tibia laterally rotates about 20°on the fixed femur. This motion occurs in the last 20°of knee extension and is called **terminal rotation of the knee,** or the **screw home mechanism.** It is purely a mechanical event that occurs with both passive and active knee extension and cannot be produced (or prevented) voluntarily. Since terminal rotation must occur with knee extension, this lateral rotation of the tibia with knee extension is a coupled movement, similar to adjacent spinal vertebral levels discussed in Chapter 8. Medial tibial rotation occurs with knee flexion and lateral tibial rotation occurs with knee extension in the open chain. Some observation of femoral abduction/adduction was also noted, but the occurrence of this additional coupling motion of this movement with flexion/extension was inconsistent.[47] In closed chain motion such as rising from a chair, terminal rotation occurs as medial rotation of the femur on the fixed tibia, whereas lateral femoral rotation occurs when returning to the chair as the knee moves from extension to flexion.

Although many species such as chimpanzees, orangutans, and birds walk on flexed knees, terminal rotation provides humans with an exquisite and energy-efficient mechanism for the extended knee. This screw home mechanism provides mechanical stability since it locks the knee; therefore, in this position the knee is able to withstand forces occurring in the sagittal plane. The locked knee also permits humans to stand erect without the need for quadriceps muscle contraction, and it allows the extended knee to withstand anterior-posterior forces with reduced muscle force. Many believe that this is one of the primary reasons for the screw home mechanism.[48] Although the amount of both axial rotation and terminal rotation of the knee is modest, it must occur for normal knee function.[49] Therefore, both terminal rotation and axial rotation motions must be clinically evaluated and regained for successful rehabilitation of the knee.

The screw home mechanism occurs as a result of various mechanical and structural factors of the knee. These altering factors include the anterior cruciate ligament, posterior cruciate ligament, and surface architecture of the femoral condyles.[48–51] It seems that each plays a role in terminal rotation to varying degrees.[48] Of these, the surface architecture plays the greatest role.[49] As the tibial condyles move on the femoral condyles during open chain knee extension, the motion on the shorter lateral femoral condyle is completed before the motion on the medial femoral condyle is completed. Since the available surface area of the lateral femoral condyle is used before movement on the medial femoral condyle is finished, pivoting of the tibia on the femur occurs between the lateral condyles to allow the medial aspect of the knee to complete its motion. This pivoting produces passive lateral rotation of the tibia on the femur in the last 15° of extension. When the knee extends during closed chain activities, motion of the femur rather than the tibia occurs; as with open chain activities, movement of the shorter lateral femoral condyle is completed before that of the medial femoral condyle but now the femur rotates medially on its lateral condyle to allow full terminal extension to occur at the knee. Unlocking the knee in either an open or closed chain produces reverse rotation motions to those of their respective terminal knee extension functions.

Arthrokinematics of the Tibiofemoral Joint

The close-packed position of the knee is full extension. In full extension, terminal rotation produces tightening of the ligamentous and capsular structures to provide strong stabilization of the joint. The tibiofemoral joint is at its most congruent position in full extension. However, if the femur is stabilized with the knee placed in 25° or more of flexion, the tibia can be distracted several millimeters on the femur, moved 1 to 3 mm in anterior or posterior glides and medial or lateral glides, and in abduction or adduction. This flexed position is the knee's resting position, or the position in which the joint is least congruent.

The concave tibial surface slides or glides in the same direction as the roll, or joint motion, when the tibia moves on the femur during open kinetic chain activity. Therefore, when the tibia rolls forward on the femur into extension, it also glides forward; likewise, when the tibia rolls backward as the knee moves into flexion, the tibia glides posteriorly. When joint motion occurs in the closed kinetic chain as during a sit-to-stand activity, the convex femoral condyles move on concave tibial condyles. During closed chain motions, then, as the knee moves into extension, the roll of the femur on the tibia, or joint motion, is anterior (forward) while the glide is posterior. Reverse directions of movement of the roll and glide occurs when the weight-bearing knee moves into flexion: the roll of the femur is posterior and the glide is anterior.

Patellofemoral Joint

The patella lies within the common tendon of the quadriceps, which extends above and on the sides of the patella as well as attaching to it. From the apex of the patella, the patellar ligament is the continuation of the quadriceps tendon and extends to the tibial tuberosity. On the sides of the patella, tendinous fibers spread out to form the medial and lateral retinacula, which attach to the condyles of the tibia.

As previously mentioned, the patella is a sesamoid bone set within the knee's joint capsule. It articulates with the anterior and distal saddle-shaped surfaces of the femoral condyles (trochlear surfaces). You may also recall that the articulating surface of the patella has a prominent vertical ridge dividing the medial and lateral articular facets; however, there is considerable variation of the patella's osseous shape that does not always reflect the cartilaginous surface.[52]

Although it does not have a stable joint to keep it in place, the patella is protected by both active and passive constraints. When the knee is in full extension, patellar stability relies primarily on soft tissues which surround it.[53] The extensor, or quadriceps, mechanism actively stabilizes the patella on all sides and guides the motion between the patella and the femur. From 20° to 0°, the primary responsibility of the vastus medialis oblique (VMO) muscle is to serve as a dynamic stabilizer of the patella.[54] The patella receives additional stability from its other surrounding structures. Distally, the patella is anchored to the tuberosity of the tibia by the strong patellar ligament, connecting the patella to the tibial tuberosity. Dense fibrous medial and lateral retinacula as well as muscles anchor the patella on each side and also aid in its stability.[55] Laterally, the patella is passively stabilized by superficial and deep retinacula, the iliotibial band, and the vastus lateralis muscle. These lateral forces are balanced on the patella's medial aspect actively by the VMO and passively by the forces of the patellofemoral ligament and the medial meniscopatellar ligament. Additionally, superior stability occurs actively from attachments of the rectus femoris and the vastus intermedius to the base of the patella whereas inferior stability is provided to the patella by the patellar ligament. When the knee flexes, the lateral structures move posteriorly and create lateral and tilting forces on the patella. Therefore, the patella is affected by both static (fascia) and dynamic (muscle) forces. In essence, the minimal congruency between the posterior patella and anterior femoral condyles forces the patella to rely on the soft tissues for its stability.[53]

Kinematics of the Patellofemoral Joint

The patellofemoral joint is intimately connected to the tibiofemoral joint, not only in anatomy but also in function. When the tibiofemoral joint moves, the patellofemoral joint must also move, but if restriction of either joint occurs, the other joint's mobility is also affected. Likewise, weakness of muscles controlling the tibiofemoral joint also has an affect on the patellofemoral joint. Essentially, both injury and health of one joint directly impacts the other joint.

Patellofemoral Contact

As the knee moves from extension into flexion, the patella and femur move relative to one another—which moves depends on whether it is an open or closed chain motion. During open chain activities when the tibia is moving and the femur is stationary, the patella moves over the femoral condyles. On the other hand, when the femur moves during closed chain activities, the femoral condyles glide along the patellar surface. In either case, as the knee moves from extension into flexion, the contact surface on the patella moves from its inferior aspect to its superior aspect, and the contact surface on the femur moves from the superior aspect of its intercondylar groove, distally towards the inferior and posterior condylar surfaces.

When the knee is fully extended, the patella sits at the proximal end of the intercondylar groove. When the quadriceps muscle is relaxed, the only contact the posterior patella has is with its inferior pole on the suprapatellar fat pad. As the knee moves into flexion, it contacts the femur at about 25° of knee flexion. The lower margin of the patella makes initial contact with the intercondylar groove's superior aspect at this time.[56] As shown in Figure 10.15, as the knee continues to flex and the patella moves inferiorly and progressively increases the patellofemoral contact area until at about 90° of knee flexion, a maximum contact area between the patella and femur occurs.[57] When the knee flexes to 115°, the patella makes contact with the medial and lateral femoral condyles at a point at which the intercondylar sulcus is present, so the contact surface area between the two bones decreases.[56] By the time the knee flexes to 135°, the odd facet and lateral facet of the posterior patella are the only areas in contact with the femoral condyles.[55]

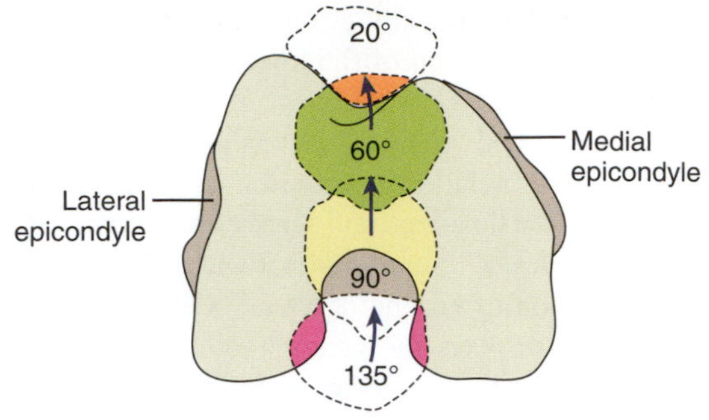

Figure 10.15 Contact areas between the patella and femoral condyles from full extension to full knee flexion. As the knee moves from full extension into flexion, the point of contact between the posterior surface of the patella and the anterior surfaces of the femoral condyles changes. The contact area on the patella moves from the inferior surface to the superior surface, whereas the contact area on the femur moves from the superior femoral condyles to their inferior aspects.

Patellofemoral Static and Dynamic Alignment

As mentioned, when the tibiofemoral joint is in full extension, the patella rests at the proximal aspect of the intercondylar groove. Because its position is maintained by the surrounding soft tissues, the health and condition of these soft tissues is important to the patella's alignment. Both inert (connective tissue) and active tissue (muscle) impact patellar alignment. Therefore, if inert structures are tight or muscles are weak or tight, these dysfunctions will alter the patella's position either at rest or during activity; such imbalances may lead to injury of the patellofemoral joint.

With the knee relaxed in full extension, the patella lies in the proximal intercondylar groove. When the knee flexes and extends, the patella moves in several directions: flexion-extension, medial-lateral tilt, medial-lateral shift, and medial-lateral rotation (Fig. 10.16).[58] Of these motions, the greatest excursion occurs in flexion and extension as it moves proximally and distally in the intercondylar groove; the patella travels from full knee extension to full flexion a distance of 5 to 7 cm.[59] Unfortunately, results of the timing and quantity of these motions lack consistency in the literature.[60] These differences are likely because of the variations in methodology of the studies, differences between *in vivo* and *in vitro* results, ranges of motion analyzed, whether the muscle activity was eccentric or concentric, and whether the knee was moving into extension or into flexion.[58, 61–67] The majority of studies report that when the knee is at about 90° of knee flexion, the patella is in a flexed, lateral shift, and lateral tilt position.[58, 64]

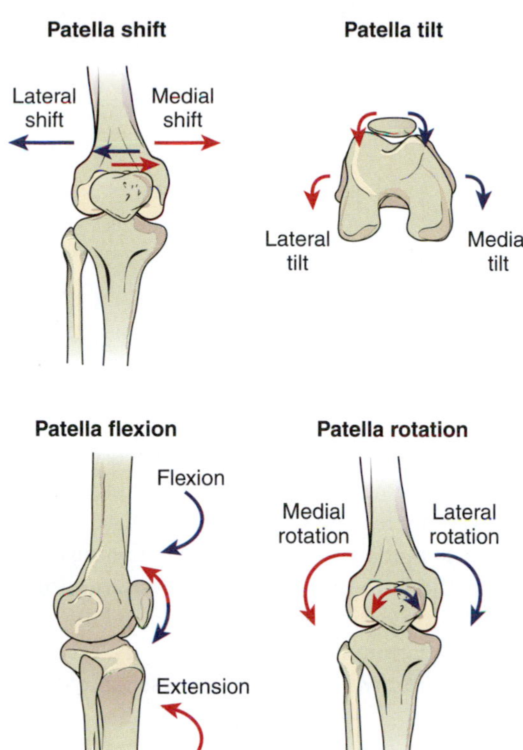

Figure 10.16 Patellar motions of right knee. The patella is able to move within the intercondylar groove in a medial-lateral shift, medial-lateral tilt, medial-lateral rotation, and flexion-extension. Note that medial and lateral refer to patella motion, not knee position. Tilt and rotation refer to the relative motion of the patella apex.

As mentioned in the anatomy segment of this chapter, the apex of the patella lies near the tibiofemoral joint margin when the knee is fully extended. If the patella lies more distally on the femur, it is a **patella baja**; if it lies more proximally, it is a **patella alta.** Either pathological alignment will cause anterior knee pain and abnormal patellar tracking during knee flexion and extension.

Excessive lateral displacement of the patella as it tracks on the trochlear surfaces is normally prevented by the congruence of the joint surfaces, the elevated lateral trochlear facet, and by the medial soft tissue stabilizers. Imbalances such as tightness of the iliotibial band or weakness of the VMO cause the patella to track more laterally with muscle contraction of the quadriceps during knee movement and may lead to changes in joint contact areas and pressures with resulting pain and dysfunction.

Arthrokinematics of the Patellofemoral Joint

The posterior patellar surface is concave and moves on a convex femoral surface. Therefore, the patellofemoral joint abides by the concave-on-convex principle. The resting position of the patellofemoral joint is full extension and the close-packed position is flexion. As the knee flexes and extends, the patella glides within the intercondylar groove. As the knee moves into flexion, the patella glides inferiorly, and as the knee extends, the patella glides superiorly.

Patellar rotation, medial-lateral shifting, and medial-lateral tilting occur during knee flexion and extension. The specific timing and occurrence of each of these motions is yet to achieve consensus among investigators. There is some evidence to indicate that the amount of passive medial-lateral motion of the patella with the knee resting in extension is about half the width of the patella in each direction.[59] With the quadriceps resting in full knee extension, the patella is unrestricted as it sits in the proximal intercondylar groove. It may be passively mobilized medially, laterally, superiorly, inferiorly, and rotated medially and laterally a few centimeters.[59]

Q Angle

An anterior view of the extended knee reveals an angle, open laterally, between the shafts of the femur and the tibia. This is the quadriceps angle, or **Q angle** (Fig. 10.17). The size of the angle is variable for both sexes; studies place the range of values for men from about 10° to 14° whereas measures for women are larger and range from about 15° to less than 23°.[68–70] Women have been shown to have consistently larger Q angles than men.[71] It was speculated that one reason for this discrepancy between the sexes is because of the women's wider pelvis which causes a greater angle between the femur and tibia, but this reason has been disproven.[72] There are more recent indications that the smaller Q angles in men may be the result of either differences in strength[72] or differences in height.[73] Although there may be some differences between the sexes, this Q angle occurs in both groups as the femoral shaft adducts so the tibia is able to transmit the body's weight perpendicularly to the foot and ground. Therefore, when we stand on one leg, forces are directed toward the medial side of the knee. An excessive Q angle is referred to as **genu valgum,** or knock knee. Conversely, if the Q angle is closer to 0° or the knee joint is convex laterally, the alignment is referred to as **genu varum,** or bowleg. Q angles have been found to be greater in those individuals reporting patellofemoral pain than in nonpainful groups.[74,75]

Muscles

Many of the muscles that cross the knee joint also cross either the hip or the ankle. Therefore, how well they perform at the knee is dependent upon their other joint's position. Recall these three factors: 1) Active insufficiency occurs when a multijoint muscle shortens

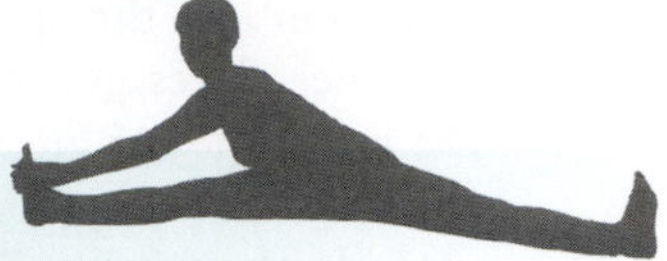

PRACTICE POINT

It is likely that although Q angles may be larger in those individuals who experience patellofemoral pain syndrome, this condition may have more of a multifactorial basis. Investigators have found that those with large Q angles do not necessarily have patellofemoral pain syndrome.[71] Other conditions that contribute to patellofemoral pain syndrome include rearfoot pronation, quadriceps weakness, hamstring tightness, iliotibial band restriction, and femoral anteversion.[70, 74–81] The important relevance of this fact is that the clinician who encounters a patient with patellofemoral pain syndrome should be mindful of the plethora of potential causes for this condition and evaluate the individual accordingly.

but is unable to shorten sufficiently to allow full joint motion at all the joints it crosses; 2) Passive insufficiency occurs when a multijoint muscle is unable to stretch sufficiently to allow both joints it crosses to fully shorten; and 3) Optimal sufficiency occurs when opposing muscles at one end where a multijoint muscle attaches, positions that joint to allow optimal function of the multijoint muscle. These principles are used frequently during knee motions. We will identify the muscles surrounding the knee and then see how these principles apply to knee function. Specific anatomical information of muscles surrounding the knee is in Table 10–2. Additional information regarding these muscles is provided below.

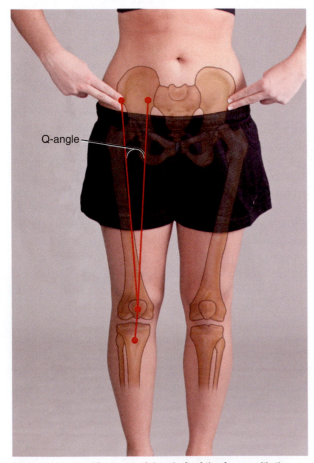

Figure 10.17 Alignment of the shaft of the femur with the tibia form the Q angle (quadriceps angle). It is the angle created by drawing a line from the anterior superior iliac spine to the center of the patella and extending another intersecting line from the tibial tuberosity to the center of the patella upward.

Knee Extensors

The quadriceps femoris muscle group extends the knee and includes four muscles: rectus femoris, vastus lateralis, vastus medialis, and vastus intermedius. These four muscles form a single, strong distal attachment to the patella, capsule of the knee, and anterior proximal surface of the tibia. In well-developed subjects in whom little adipose tissue is present, the rectus femoris, the vastus medialis, and the vastus lateralis may be observed as separate units (Fig. 10.18), whereas in other subjects, the boundaries of these muscles are less distinct. The vastus intermedius is deeply located and cannot be observed from the surface.

The rectus femoris occupies the middle of the thigh, is superficial, and takes a straight course down the thigh. It is the only quadriceps muscle which also moves the hip joint. The vastus lateralis is the largest of the four quadriceps muscles and is located on the lateral side of the rectus femoris. The vastus lateralis fibers converge toward the patella at a 12° to 15° angle, which is even greater in its distal portions.[82] The vastus medialis lies in a position medial to the rectus femoris. The vastus medialis has two different fiber directions, and therefore, two different functions.[82] The more proximal fibers are longitudinal and work with the other quadriceps muscles in knee extension, whereas the more distal oblique fibers provide patellar stabilization, especially during terminal extension.[82, 83] There are some investigators, however, whose evidence indicates that the

(text continues on page 449)

TABLE 10–2 | MUSCLES OF THE KNEE

Group	Muscle	Proximal Insertion	Distal insertion	Innervation	Action	Palpation
Quadriceps 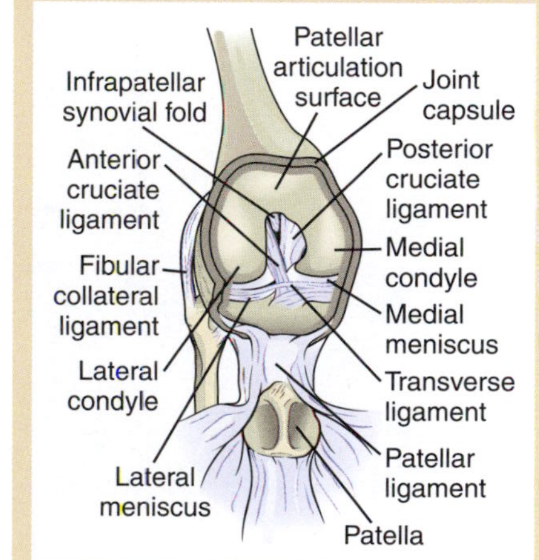	Rectus femoris	**1)** The anterior or "straight" tendon, from the anterior inferior spine of the ilium; and **2)** the posterior or "reflected" tendon from just above the brim of the acetabulum; as this tendon swings forward, it courses close to the hip joint and is blended with the capsule. The two tendons unite, covering part of the capsule anteriorly.	The muscle fibers attach to a deep aponeurosis narrowing to a broad tendon that attaches to the superior border of the patella, and by means of the patellar ligament, into the tuberosity of the tibia.	Two branches of the femoral nerve (L_2–L_4).	Hip flexion and knee extension	When the hip is flexed, the tendon of origin may be observed and palpated in the V-shaped area between the sartorius and the tensor fascia lata. The muscular portion is superficial and may be followed down the thigh to its attachment on the patella.
Quadriceps 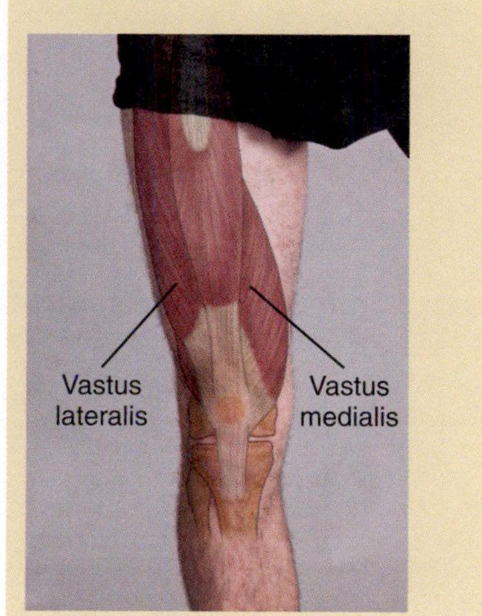	Vastus lateralis	By a broad aponeurosis on the lateral and posterior aspects of the femur, as high up as the greater trochanter and as far posterior as the linea aspera.	The lateral border of the patella, the lateral patellar retinaculum, and by means of the patellar ligament, the tuberosity of the tibia.	Branches of the femoral nerve (L_2–L_4).	Knee extension	The muscle may be seen and palpated from just below the greater trochanter down to the patella.

Continued

TABLE 10-2 | MUSCLES OF THE KNEE—cont'd

Group	Muscle	Proximal Insertion	Distal insertion	Innervation	Action	Palpation
Quadriceps	Vastus medialis	Medial and posterior aspects of the femur, as high up as the intertrochanteric line and as far posterior as the linea aspera	Medial portion of superior border of patella, medial patellar retinaculum, and by means of the patellar ligament, the tuberosity of the tibia.	Branches of the femoral nerve (L_2–L_4).	Knee extension and patellar stability	The distal portion of the muscle is quite bulky and is palpated medially in the lower third of the thigh (see Fig. 10.18).
Quadriceps	Vastus intermedius	Anterior and lateral surfaces of the femur, as high up as the lesser trochanter and as far posterior as the linea aspera. The muscle fibers are aligned parallel to the long axis of the femur	Superior border of the patella, fused with the tendons of the two other vasti muscles, and directly into the capsule of the knee joint.	Branches of the femoral nerve (L_2–L_4).	Knee extension	If the rectus is grasped and lifted somewhat, the vastus intermedius may be palpated underneath the rectus if approached from the medial or lateral side of the rectus.

Active during knee extension	Genu articularis	Sometimes part of the vastus intermedius but often separate, attaching to the distal anterior femur	Synovial membrane and wall of suprapatellar bursa.	Branches of the femoral nerve (L_2–L_4).	Pulls the synovial capsule and bursa superiorly during knee extension to move them out of the way of the joint to prevent the capsule from being compressed between the femur and patella	Too deep to palpate.
Hamstrings 	Biceps femoris	**1)** The long head to the tuberosity of the ischium, having a common tendon of attachment with the semitendinosus; **2)** the short head, to the lower portion of the shaft of the femur and to the lateral linea aspera.	The two heads unite to be attached to the head of the fibula, to the lateral condyle of the tibia, and to the fascia of the leg.	Branches of the sciatic nerve (L_4–L_5, S_1).	Hip extension, lateral hip rotation, knee flexion, lateral knee rotation	When knee flexion is resisted (subject prone), the long head of the biceps femoris may be observed and palpated from its attachment on the head of the fibula to the ischial tuberosity. The short head is covered largely by the long head and is, therefore, difficult to identify. The biceps tendon is easily palpated with the subject in the sitting position if the leg is laterally rotated with respect to the femur.

Continued

TABLE 10-2 | MUSCLES OF THE KNEE—cont'd

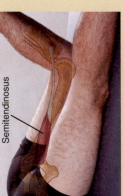

Group	Muscle	Proximal Insertion	Distal insertion	Innervation	Action	Palpation
Hamstrings	Semitendinosus	Tuberosity of the ischium, having a common tendon with the long head of the biceps.	Medial aspect of the tibia near the knee joint, distal to the attachment of the gracilis.	Branches of the sciatic nerve (L_5, $S_{1,2}$).	Hip extension, hip medial rotation. Knee flexion, knee medial rotation	With the subject prone, the tendon may be observed and palpated posteriorly on the medial side of the knee when knee flexion is resisted. Palpation of the tendon also may occur with the subject in the sitting position. The palpating fingers are placed in the "fold" of the knee, medially, where several relaxed tendons may be distinguished. If the muscles of this region are then tightened without joint movement, the tendon of the semitendinosus rises markedly from the underlying tissue, as it is the most prominent tendon in the back of the knee. The tendon may be followed proximally toward the muscle belly as it proceeds obliquely toward the ischial tuberosity.
Hamstrings	Semimembranosus	Ischial tuberosity	Medial condyle of the tibia	Branches of the sciatic nerve (L_5, $S_{1,2}$).	Hip extension, hip medial rotation. Knee flexion, knee medial rotation	The muscular portion of the semimembranosus extends farther distally than that of the semitendinosus; therefore, its lower portion may be palpated on both sides of the semitendinosus tendon. As the semimembranosus approaches its distal attachment, its tendon lies deep and can be palpated only with difficulty.

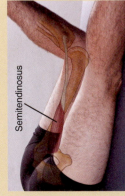

Knee flexor Gastrocnemius Soleus	Gastrocnemius	Above the medial and lateral femoral condyles and span the knee joint posteriorly on the flexor side.	Posterior surface of calcaneus	Tibial nerve (S_1 and S_2).	Knee flexion and ankle plantarflexion	The muscular portion of the gastrocnemius may be seen contracting in resisted flexion of the knee.
Knee flexor	Plantaris (No image)	Above the lateral condyle of the femur, where it lies between the lateral head of the gastrocnemius and the popliteus, close to, and partially blended with, the capsule.	Into the calcaneus and calcaneal tendon	Tibial nerve (L_5, S_1).	May serve as a weak flexor of the knee	This muscle is not always present. It follows along the medial border of the soleus.

Continued

TABLE 10-2 | MUSCLES OF THE KNEE—cont'd

Group	Muscle	Proximal Insertion	Distal insertion	Innervation	Action	Palpation
Knee flexor	Popliteus	Lateral aspect of the lateral femoral condyle and lateral meniscus.	Widespread in a proximal-to-distal direction into the medial, proximal posterior tibia and into the distal medial collateral ligament.	Tibial nerve (L_4–S_1).	Unlocking and medially rotating the knee during initiation of knee flexion, assist in balance and posture control in single leg stance.	This muscle lies deep in the posterior knee and is too deep to palpate.
Knee medial rotator	Sartorius	See Chapter 9				
Knee medial rotator	Gracilis	See Chapter 9				
Knee medial rotator	Semitendinosus	See above				
Knee lateral rotator	Biceps femoris	See above				
Knee lateral rotator	Tensor fascia lata	See Chapter 9				

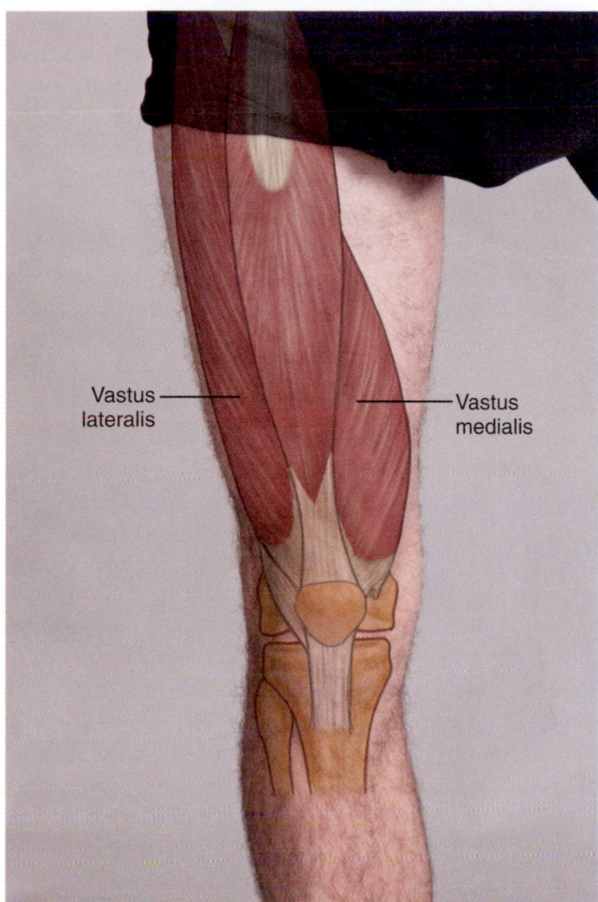

Figure 10.18 Rectus femoris, vastus lateralis, and vastus medialis are visualized in an anterior view of the thigh and may be easily identified with strong contraction of the quadriceps with the knee in extension.

oblique portion of the vastus medialis (VMO) does not function in knee extension but serves only as a patellar stabilizer.[54, 82] The fourth and deepest quadriceps, the vastus intermedius, is located under the rectus and is partially fused with the two other vasti muscles.

The **articularis genu** is a small, flat muscle with attachments on the anterior lower portion of the shaft of the femur and the capsule of the knee joint or on the superior edge of the patella. The muscle lies beneath the vastus intermedius and sometimes merges with it. This muscle is innervated by a branch of the nerve to the vastus intermedius. It is believed that the function of the articularis genu is to pull the joint capsule (and synovial membrane) superiorly as the knee extends to prevent an impingement or crushing of these structures in the patellofemoral joint.[37] The anterior-superior capsule must move and pleat during knee extension to avoid injuries to the capsule and **plica,** so this muscle serves an important function.

Knee Flexors

A number of muscles pass posterior to the flexion-extension axis of the knee, contributing to a variable extent of knee flexion. The primary muscles are the hamstrings (biceps femoris, semitendinosus, and semimembranosus), but other muscles also contribute to knee flexion. These muscles include the gastrocnemius, plantaris, popliteus, gracilis, and sartorius. These muscles are presented in Table 10–2.

The biceps femoris (Fig. 10.19) lies on the posterior thigh and is also known as the "lateral hamstring." The semitendinosus is one of the medial hamstrings with its muscular portion positioned medial to that of the long head of the biceps in the posterior thigh. Although the semimembranosus has the largest cross section of the hamstrings, it is not easily palpated as an individual muscle because most of it is covered by the semitendinosus and, proximally, by the adductor magnus. Together with these muscles, the semimembranosus makes up the large muscular mass of the medial and posterior thigh.

Once the distal tendon of the semitendinosus is identified (Fig. 10.20), another small, firm, round tendon may be palpated medially to the semitendinosus. This is the tendon of the gracilis (Fig. 10.21). Once the tendon is identified, the gracilis muscle may be distinguished from the semitendinosus by palpating the muscle belly toward its proximal attachment. The gracilis remains medial in its course toward the pubis. In the sitting position, medial rotation of the leg with respect to the thigh also brings out the tendons of both the semitendinosus and gracilis. The gracilis and sartorius provide assistance to knee flexion.[37] These hip muscles are presented in more detail in Chapter 9.

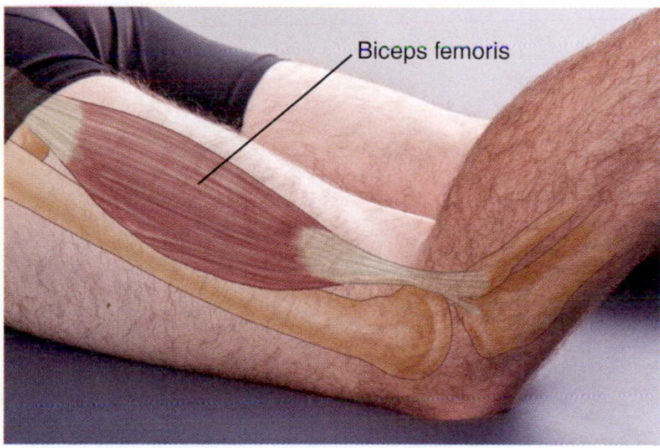

Figure 10.19 Biceps femoris. The prominent tendon of this lateral hamstring is seen on the lateral side of the posterior thigh region when knee flexion is resisted.

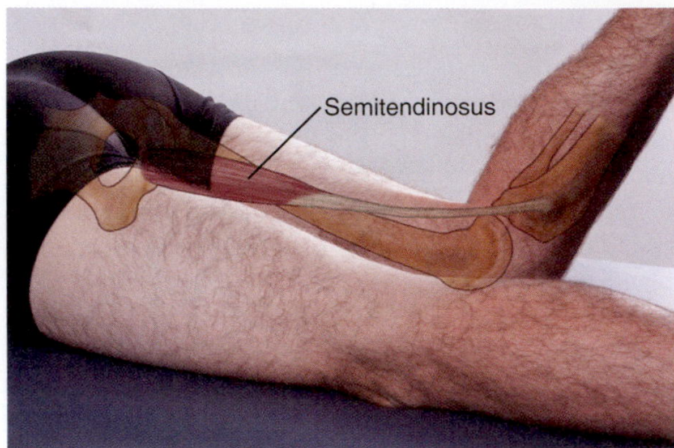

Figure 10.20 Semitendinosus. Prominence of this tendon is seen on the medial side of the posterior thigh area when knee flexion is resisted. Although the semimembranosus may be palpated beneath the semitendinosus tendon, it is more difficult to distinguish given its flat configuration.

Although the major role of the gastrocnemius is that of a plantarflexor of the ankle, it also plays a role in knee flexion. Its activity at the knee occurs more in the near-extension positions of flexion than in positions of greater flexion.[84, 85] The gastrocnemius assists in stabilizing the knee by cocontracting with the quadriceps from about 30° of flexion until the knee moves into extension.[86] Because the gastrocnemius is more important as a plantarflexor of the ankle than as a knee flexor, it is discussed in more detail in Chapter 11.

The **plantaris** is a small muscle in the posterior knee region and plays little if any role at the knee. The muscle belly is at times large and at times atrophied, and its specific function is unknown.

The **popliteus** is a small but important muscle to the posterior knee. It is the most deeply located muscle in the region, attaching to the femoral condyle and lateral meniscus. It lies close to the capsule, covered by the plantaris and the lateral head of the gastrocnemius. From its proximal attachment, the muscle fibers take a downward and medial course to the medial posterior tibia (Fig. 10.22). The popliteus aids in providing both static and dynamic posterolateral knee joint stabilization.[87] During muscle activation, the popliteus produces rotation of the tibia medially on the femur in an open kinetic chain or lateral rotation of the femur on the weight-bearing tibia.[88] It also stabilizes the knee by preventing forward dislocation of the femur on the tibia and protects the lateral meniscus from an impinging injury by pulling it posteriorly during knee flexion.[89]

Tibial Rotators

The muscles that act as tibial medial rotators include the semitendinosus, semimembranosus, popliteus, gracilis, and sartorius. The tibial lateral rotator is the biceps femoris which is possibly aided by the tensor fasciae latae. The biceps femoris is a strong lateral rotator. Contraction of the biceps femoris may be isolated from the medial hamstrings by placing the subject prone with the knee flexed slightly beyond 90°. The muscle will contract when performing tibial lateral rotation.

As was introduced in Chapter 9, the distal attachments of the tendons of the sartorius, gracilis, and semitendinosus are on the anterior medial surface of the tibia below the medial condyle (Fig. 10.23), forming the

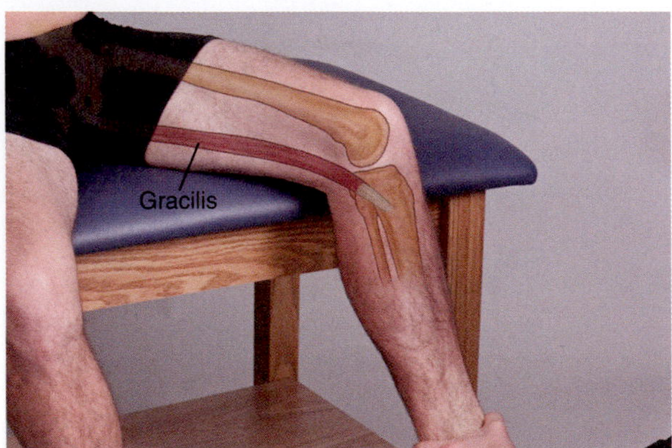

Figure 10.21 Gracilis. This muscle lies medial to the semitendinosus and is more easily observed with the subject sitting and resistance provided to knee flexion and simultaneous tibial medial rotation.

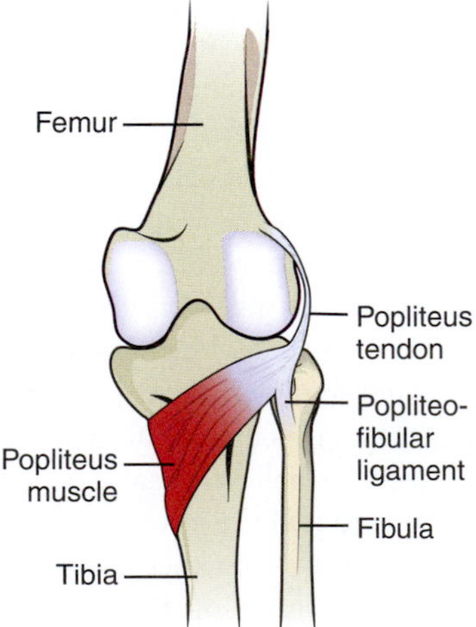

Figure 10.22 Popliteus. It lies deep and is close to the capsule. The plantaris and lateral gastrocnemius head cover the popliteus fibers as they course in a downward and medial direction from their proximal insertion.

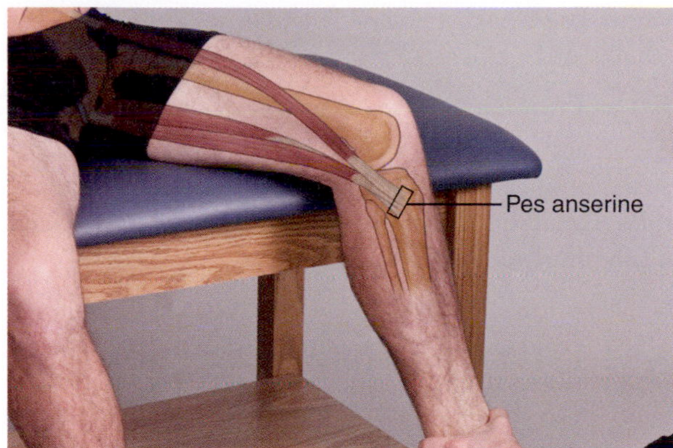

Figure 10.23 Pes anserine: insertion point for the sartorius, gracilis, and semitendinosus on the anteromedial tibia.

pes anserinus (L., *pes,* foot; *anserinus,* goose). Some of the fibers of these three tendons blend with each other and with the deep fasciae of the leg. The three muscles are thought to be important for medial stabilization of the knee.

Functions of Muscles of the Knee

The two main muscle groups of the knee include the knee extensors and knee flexors. Although the tibia also rotates on the femur, this rotation occurs from contraction of the knee flexors. Since many of the muscles crossing the knee also cross another joint, how they work at the knee during functional activities is dependent upon the position of the other joints these muscles cross. Since there are so many two-joint muscles operating at the knee, they also impact the responsibilities of the single-joint knee muscles during functional activities. This section investigates this interaction of muscle function.

Knee Extensors

The quadriceps femoris is a large muscle group (Fig. 10.24) that is responsible for stabilizing, accelerating, and decelerating the knee during functional activities. For example, it will provide an isometric muscle contraction to stabilize the knee during a downhill ski run, or will produce a sudden concentric activity during a jump up, or it will decelerate knee flexion when the body lands from a jump. Stabilization activity usually requires isometric contraction whereas acceleration demands concentric contraction, and eccentric work occurs during a deceleration activity. In many activities these types of contractions continually alternate as the demand changes. For example, a sprinter uses an isometric quadriceps contraction at the start of a race while in the blocks, but once the race begins, the quadriceps

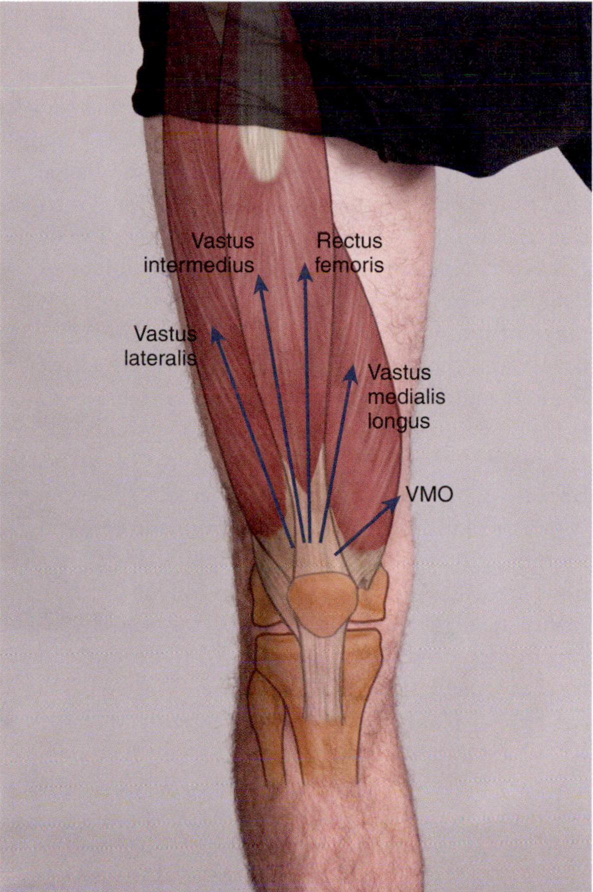

Figure 10.24 The pull of the quadriceps muscles extends the knee. The VMO pull provides lateral stability for the patella in terminal extension.

explode into a concentric contraction as the leg pushes off from the blocks and suddenly works eccentrically to control knee flexion when the foot hits the ground.

By necessity, the quadriceps is not only large but it is also a powerful muscle group that is capable of generating in excess of 1000 lb (4450 N or 2200 kg) of internal force. Such great force is needed in closed chain motion to elevate and lower the body, as in rising from a chair, climbing, and jumping, and to prevent the knee from collapsing in walking, running, or landing from a jump. Additionally, the quadriceps provides an active restraint to complement the knee's passive restraints such as the cruciate ligaments, which maintain the femoral condyles in position on the tibial plateau.

We know that one of the quadriceps muscles, the rectus femoris, crosses the hip and is a hip flexor as well as a knee extensor. Relying on our recall of two-joint muscles, we would expect this muscle to become more active as a knee extensor if the hip is placed in an extended position, allowing the rectus femoris to apply maximum torque in knee extension. This effect can be observed when a seated subject experiences difficulty extending the knee against resistance; if the subject leans back to place a stretch on the rectus femoris, increased force in knee extension becomes available.

At one time it was thought that the vastus medialis was responsible for the last 20° to 30° of knee extension. EMG studies have shown, however, that all four of the quadriceps muscles are active early and throughout the range of motion.[82, 90, 91] Basmajian[92] and others[83, 93–99] have found that although the onset of EMG activity in the four muscles is variable when knee extension is performed against little or no resistance, working against resistance caused all four muscles to be activated. Because there are two distinct fiber directions of the vastus medialis, there is a distinction made between the more longitudinal fibers and oblique fibers; these sections are called the vastus medialis longus (VML) and vastus medialis oblique (VMO), respectively.[82] The superior longitudinal fibers of the VML are directed 15° to 18° medially from their attachment on the patella in the frontal plane; the prominent inferior fibers of the VMO are more obliquely directed to form an angle of 50° to 55°.[82] Because of the oblique angle of muscle fibers of the VMO, it is unable to act as an effective knee extensor; it is believed to provide medial stability to the patella in terminal extension.[82, 83] In a mechanical study on cadavers, Lieb and Perry[82] found that each of the quadriceps muscles except the VMO could extend the knee and that the vastus intermedius was the most efficient (required the least force). They also found that it was impossible to extend the knee by contracting the VMO. The vastus medialis oblique is believed to play an important role in keeping the patella on track in gliding between the femoral condyles (tracking mechanism).[82, 83] The medially directed forces of the VMO may also counteract the laterally directed forces of the vastus lateralis to prevent lateral displacement of the patella in the trochlear groove.

Knee Flexors

There are several muscles that serve as flexors in the posterior knee. These muscles, however, have additional roles, including that of providing rotation to the knee during functional activities.

Hamstrings

Open chain motions of knee flexion and rotation require little muscle force to execute. On the other hand, great forces are required of these muscles as they act on the knee in closed chain motions or on the other joints they cross. The hamstring muscles are primary hip extensors and contract strongly to stabilize the pelvis during prone trunk extension. As was discussed in Chapter 8 and confirmed by electromyographic activity, the hamstrings also work to control the pelvis on the femur as the seated or standing subject leans forward to touch the feet and then returns to the upright position (Fig. 8.29). The hamstrings also serve to stabilize the knee by restricting an anterior glide of the tibia on the femur.[100]

Additionally, the hamstrings, sartorius, and the gracilis muscles have rotary actions at the hip and knee, and the popliteus is a rotator at the knee. After the foot is planted on the ground during the stance phase of walking, the knee and hip must rotate to allow forward motion of the body onto the supporting foot. The rotation is initiated and controlled by these rotator muscles. In activities such as running, turning, cutting, or maintaining balance on an unstable base of support (such as uneven ground or a rocking boat), the force required of these rotator muscles increases markedly. Activities carried out in the kneeling or squatting position (such as gardening, welding, mining, or playing football) require strong forces from these muscles to initiate and control hip and knee motions including rotation on the fixed

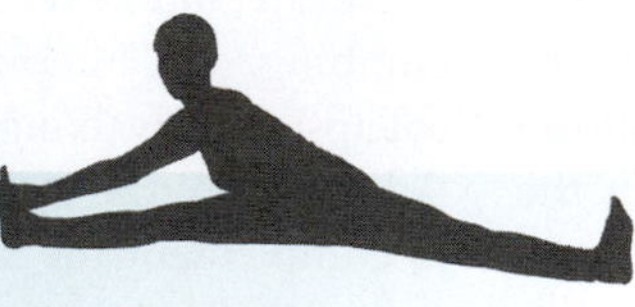

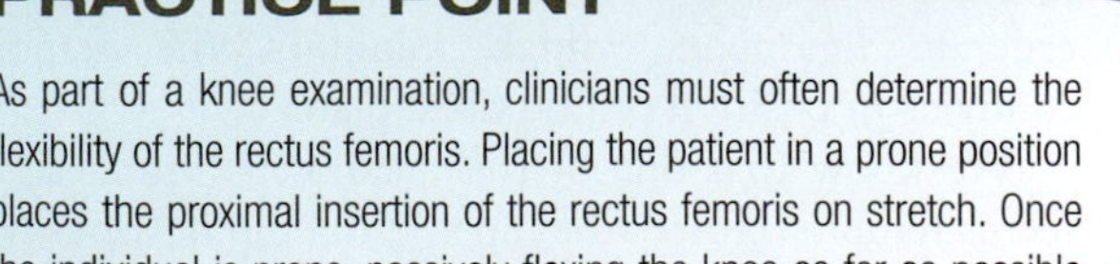

As part of a knee examination, clinicians must often determine the flexibility of the rectus femoris. Placing the patient in a prone position places the proximal insertion of the rectus femoris on stretch. Once the individual is prone, passively flexing the knee as far as possible while placing the hip in additional extension stretches the rectus femoris optimally. The clinician must, however, be sure to maintain a neutral frontal alignment of the hip during this stretch since moving the hip into abduction reduces the stretch on the muscle's proximal insertion at the anterior inferior iliac spine and allows the knee to be moved into more flexion, giving the clinician a false assessment.

tibia in response to necessary twists of the trunk and upper extremities. Thus, injuries to the knee flexors such as a hamstring strain are more commonly due to their actions as rotators or as decelerators of limb motion than as flexors of the knee.

Popliteus

You may recall that the popliteus muscle is deeply set in the calf and difficult to palpate or study, and although it is a small muscle, it has important functions. The arrangement of its distal insertion on the tibia gives the muscle a somewhat triangular shape, and its insertion into the medial collateral ligament also leads some anatomists to refer to this muscle as the popliteus muscle-tendon unit (PMTU)[87] or popliteal muscle-tendon complex (PMTC).[89] The popliteus is classified as a knee flexor, but its leverage is poor for this motion. Basmajian and Lovejoy[101] reported finding only 10% to 15% of maximum EMG activity of the popliteus associated with knee flexion-extension movement. On the other hand, when these motions were performed with voluntary medial rotation of the knee, the activity of the popliteus increased to 40% to 70% of maximum activity. Since Basmajian and Lovejoy's investigation, others have concurred with his conclusion that the popliteus does not contribute substantially to knee flexion.[48, 89, 102–104]

Rather than contributing substantially to knee flexion, the popliteus seems to have a more important dual function of initiating the unlocking of the extended knee and contributing to posterolateral stability of the knee.[87, 88, 105] The oblique angle of the popliteus muscle provides optimal alignment to initiate tibial rotation to unlock the extended knee. Because terminal knee extension requires lateral rotation of the tibia on the femur, initiation of knee flexion requires the reverse action of medial rotation of the tibia on the femur; this action is thought to be performed by the popliteus muscle. Additionally, the popliteus has been investigated electromyographically by Barnett and Richardson.[102] These investigators recorded large amounts of EMG activity from the popliteus when "knee bends" were performed from the standing position. When the knee approached a right angle, the popliteus became active and maintained this activity as long as a crouching posture was maintained; the investigators concluded that since the weight of the body tends to cause the femoral condyles to slide forward on the tibial plateau when the body is in a full squat position, the popliteus functioned to assist the posterior cruciate ligament in stabilizing the knee. Since their investigation, others have confirmed this initial finding and demonstrated through their own studies that the popliteus is an important active stabilizer of the posterolateral knee.[39, 87, 105, 106] Recall that the PCL attaches to the medial condyle of the femur, whereas the popliteus attaches to the lateral condyle. The action of the popliteus, therefore, is an important complement to that of the posterior cruciate ligament in preventing a forward sliding of the condyles in weight-bearing on flexed knees. One final responsibility that has been attributed to the popliteus muscle is providing kinesthetic information during functional activity.[89] Since the popliteus muscle has attachments that approximate the collateral ligaments, it is hypothesized that the muscle is able to respond quickly when a collateral ligament is stressed to protect knee structures such as the lateral meniscus.[89] This hypothesis is based, in part, on the fact that the popliteus has a larger than average number of muscle spindles; this fact is important since it is thought that small muscles that have a high density of muscle spindles provide proprioceptive information to the central nervous system when they are in a parallel arrangement to larger muscles that have a low concentration of muscle spindles.[107]

One-Joint and Two-Joint Muscles Acting at the Knee

Only five of the muscles that act on the knee are one-joint muscles: the three vasti, the popliteus, and the short head of the biceps femoris. The remaining muscles cross both the hip and knee (rectus femoris, sartorius, gracilis, semitendinosus, semimembranosus, long head of the biceps femoris, and the iliotibial tract of the tensor fasciae latae), or the knee and ankle (gastrocnemius). Thus, motions or positions of the hip and ankle influence the range of motion that can occur at the knee as well as the forces that these two-joint muscles can generate (passive and active insufficiency).

There may be important reasons why the knee has primarily two-joint muscles. One-joint muscles usually function synergistically with its two-joint agonist.[108] For example, the vasti portions of the quadriceps are active when the rectus femoris also works to extend the knee. However, when the single-joint muscle group's moment arm shortens as knee extension continues, its force output is reduced, but as the rectus femoris continues to work at the knee, additional force may be added at the knee by placing the hip in more extension, thereby lengthening the muscle at its proximal insertion.

Using single-joint muscles is also less efficient, requiring more muscle activity and, therefore, more energy for stability during functional motions.[108, 109] For example, if a two-joint muscle such as the rectus femoris works during an activity such as rising from a chair, it shortens at its distal end as it lengthens at its proximal end so length change is not as great as it would be for two single-joint muscles performing each activity. By using a two-joint muscle, positive work is produced at one end while negative work is produced at the opposite end, thereby reducing energy needs.[110] If only single-joint muscles were used, then more work would be required to perform the same motions.

One-joint muscles usually produce motion in only one plane. For example, the vastus intermedius produces knee extension. On the other hand, biarticular muscles also produce a transverse component.[111] One-joint, or monoarticular, muscles are usually used to produce force whereas the biarticular (two-joint) muscles determine direction of movement.[112] As we have discussed in earlier chapters, our muscular system is one of redundancy; there are many more muscles available to perform an action than is required for movement. This redundancy, however, is important since it allows the body to perform functional activities efficiently. Studies have shown that a two-joint muscle has its greatest activation when it shortens simultaneously from both of its attachment sites; its least activation level occurs when both attachment ends are lengthened; and it has a moderate activation level when one attachment site is lengthened while the other shortens.[108] When a multiple-joint limb like the lower extremity moves, the most efficient motions occur with a lengthening of a biarticular muscle at one of its insertions while its opposite insertion site is shortened; such activities are common occurrences during functional motions. If we relied only on one-joint muscles to provide force and motion, activities would require much more energy and would prove to be very inefficient.[111, 113] For a one-joint muscle to perform functional activities, not only would several other muscles also work to allow that one-joint muscle to perform its desired task, but it would require a lot more energy and control to determine exact muscle performance needs for each task. Fortunately, our two-joint muscles control our motions for us; as they provide torque production at one joint, they simultaneously reduce torque production at their other joint.[114]

Under ordinary functional activities, two-joint muscles are seldom used to move both joints simultaneously, especially during motions requiring force. More often, the action of two-joint muscles is prevented at one joint by resistance from gravity or the contraction of other muscles, thereby providing stability at one joint so the agonist muscle is able to produce optimal function at the desired joint. If a two-joint muscle was to shorten over both joints simultaneously and to complete the range at both joints, it would have to shorten a long distance and would rapidly lose tension as it shortened; as you recall this is based on the length-tension principle. Indeed, if a two-joint muscle does shorten at both ends, neither joint it crosses is able to achieve full motion because active insufficiency of the muscle prevents such a position from occurring. The two joints a muscle crosses usually move in directions that gradually elongate the muscle over one joint while shortening at the other joint. This occurrence is important since it allows favorable length-tension relations of the muscle to be maintained. Since there are so many two-joint muscles crossing the knee, it is important to identify how each muscle performs relative to the other joint it crosses as it performs its function as the knee. The action of the two-joint muscles is considered in the following movement combinations.

Knee Flexion Combined with Hip Extension

If the subject is lying prone or standing erect and flexes the knee while extending the hip, the hamstring muscles must shorten over both joints simultaneously, and difficulty is experienced in completing knee flexion. Some subjects complain of a cramp in the muscles of the posterior thigh when performing this motion. All subjects lose strength rapidly as knee flexion proceeds with the hip extended. The range of useful excursion becomes almost exhausted because of the length-tension factor; in multijoint muscles such as the hamstrings, the inability to fully flex the knee and simultaneously extend the hip is because of active insufficiency of the hamstrings.

Another element that often limits full excursion of the hamstrings is the inability of the rectus femoris, which is being stretched over the hip and knee simultaneously, to elongate sufficiently. This inability to fully stretch the hip in extension and the knee in flexion occurs because of passive insufficiency of the rectus femoris. If the rectus femoris is tight and the subject is placed in the prone position and the knee is then passively flexed, the hip will move into flexion to accommodate for the stretch on the rectus femoris unless the hip is passively stabilized prior to the stretch application.

Knee Extension Combined with Hip Flexion

An active straight leg raise may be performed in a supine or standing position. A straight leg raise (SLR) includes moving the hip into flexion while maintaining an extended knee. As the hip moves through its motion, the individual reaches a point at which either hip motion cannot continue or if it does, the knee flexes. Most of the time, the difficulty in continuing the motion occurs from passive insufficiency of the hamstrings; the hamstrings do not have the ability to further elongate to allow the motion to continue. Less frequently, the rectus femoris muscle is unable to continue shortening simultaneously at the hip and the knee, so either the hip motion stops or the knee flexes to allow further contraction of the rectus femoris at the hip. In this case, active insufficiency of the rectus femoris prevents full hip flexion and knee extension motion. The clinician is able to identify the reason a full straight leg raise is unattainable by performing a passive movement of hip flexion, first with the knee extended and then with the knee flexed; not only will the motion be substantially greater with the knee flexed, but the resistance to the passive straight leg raise will be palpable when the hamstring interference in hip flexion is the cause of a reduced SLR. If a straight leg raise is limited by muscle inflexibility, joint contracture (e.g., 30°), or spasticity, normal step length is diminished in walking. The individual is limited to short steps and usually walks with the knees flexed. Gait is more thoroughly discussed in Chapter 12.

Knee Flexion Combined with Hip Flexion

Fortunately, hip flexion with knee extension or hip extension with knee flexion is not a normal functional position for the lower limb. A more functional combination is knee flexion with hip flexion. This combination provides for elongation of the hamstrings over the hip while knee flexion is carried out, resulting in favorable length-tension relations and efficiency of torque production. During hip-knee flexion motion, the hip flexors and the hamstrings act synergistically to provide a functionally useful movement whereas in other movement combinations, these two muscle groups may act as antagonists. In these situations, the hip flexors provide hip flexion positioning to allow optimal sufficiency in hamstrings function.

We use this combination to our advantage during walking, running, and hopping activities. This synergistic movement occurs during these activities during the swing or nonweight-bearing phases of these activities to swing and advance the limb forward.

Knee Extension Combined with Hip Extension

Another common combination of hip and knee motions and torque production during functional activities is knee extension with hip extension. This is a most useful combination that occurs in activities such as rising from the sitting position, climbing stairs, running, and jumping to propel the body forward or upward. This positioning of knee extension, usually by contraction of the quadriceps, allows the hamstrings to elongate over the knee and act as hip extensors. In this movement, as in knee flexion with hip flexion, an effective portion of the length-tension curve is used to optimize muscle function.

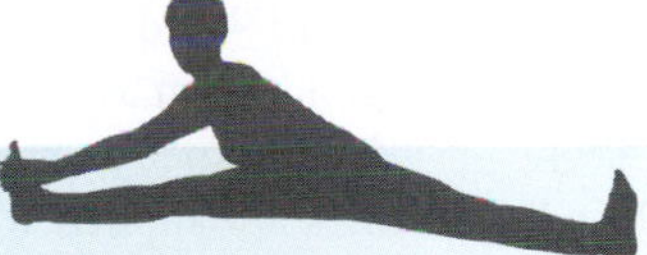

PRACTICE POINT

Quadriceps muscle paralysis occurs with severance of the femoral nerve from a gunshot or other trauma. In these cases, the person is unable to extend the knee in the sitting position or perform a straight leg raise when supine. When the person is prone, the knee can be flexed and extended by concentric and eccentric contractions of the hamstring muscles.

However, various compensations can be used by these individuals so they can walk and function in a safe manner without a noticeable limp. Momentum from the hip can be used to straighten the knee in walking. The big problem an individual without quadriceps activity faces is keeping the knee from buckling when weight is placed on the extremity in the stance phase of gait. A very effective compensation is to use the gluteus maximus to extend the knee in closed chain motion. This occurs in the stance phase of walking at the time of and following heel strike (initial contact). Some people develop such strength and control of the knee with the gluteus maximus that they can prevent the knee from buckling when they are standing, even if a strong push is applied to the back of the knee. When more force is needed, such as in stair climbing, the hand on the side of the weak quadriceps is used to push on the anterior thigh. This can be done in a casual manner and is seldom noticed as an abnormality by others. Some individuals develop a form of hop-and-skip run by using the gluteus maximus together with the hand to keep the weak knee straight. Rising up from low chairs usually can be accomplished by the uninvolved leg and assisted by the hands in pushing on the chair arms, if needed. A very discrete compensation often seen in walking is a slight forward lean from the hips; this move places the center of gravity of HAT in front of the knee's axis of motion in the sagittal plane so quadriceps muscle force is not needed to keep the knee extended. The hyperextension force that results from this motion is limited by the posterior capsule, PCL, and hamstring muscles. Unfortunately, hyperextension of the knee occurs as a result of this repetitive posterior force application and increase joint stresses.

An orthosis (brace) is usually a better alternative to reduce risk of eventual development of ligamentous laxities and bony deformities through the repetitive hyperextension force. Although the forward-leaning posture required for the gait described is slight, it can cause low back pain over time.

In closed chain motion, cocontraction of the hamstrings and quadriceps occurs to elevate the body (using knee extension and hip extension) or lower the body (using knee flexion and hip flexion). When a person stands up from a chair, the quadriceps performs a concentric contraction to extend the knee, and the hamstrings perform a concentric contraction to extend the hip. When the person sits down, eccentric contractions of both muscle groups control the rate of knee flexion (quadriceps) and hip flexion (hamstrings).

Knee Flexion Combined with Ankle Plantarflexion

The gastrocnemius is capable of performing motions of knee flexion and ankle plantarflexion simultaneously, but if full range at both joints is attempted, the muscle has to shorten a long distance, and tension falls rapidly. As with other two-joint muscles, it quickly faces active insufficiency and is unable to fully flex both joints simultaneously. Therefore, as in simultaneous knee extension with hip flexion or knee flexion with hip extension, it is not a very useful movement.

Knee Extension Combined with Ankle Plantarflexion

The quadriceps extends the knee whereas the gastrocnemius and the soleus plantarflex the ankle. As the quadriceps extends the knee, the gastrocnemius becomes elongated over the knee, and optimal conditions result for plantarflexion of the ankle. This functional combination is commonly seen, for example, in rising on tiptoes, running, and jumping. Once again, the synergistic relationship between muscles provides for optimal sufficiency to permit functional motion to occur most efficiently.

Joint Forces

Even in normal activity, the articulating surfaces of the knee sustain forces that far exceed body weight and are thus subject to microtrauma and its subsequent degenerative results.[115] During open chain exercises, maximum isometric knee extension was calculated by Smidt[116] to produce a tibiofemoral compression force of 1.6 times the body weight when the knee was extended and 3 times the body weight when the knee was in a position of 60°. Symptomatic inflammatory responses may occur when these forces are accompanied by overuse of the knee (e.g., gardening, jogging, or roofing) and by hypermobility or hypomobility of joint structures from the foot to the spine, which call for compensatory motion or stabilization at the knee during weight-bearing activities.[115] For example, excessive pronation at the ankle produces increased medial rotation of the tibia and repetitive abnormal stresses on tibiofemoral and patellofemoral joint structures.

Tibiofemoral Joint Forces

The body weight vector passes between the knees when standing on both feet, and each tibial plateau has a compressive force of 45% of body weight (68 lb in a 150-lb person) (Fig. 10.25A). In unilateral stance, however, the compressive force increases to about twice the body weight. In standing, this compressive force is equally distributed over the weight-bearing surfaces of the tibia.[2] The knee supports the weight of the thigh, HAT, and the opposite lower extremity during single limb stance. This weight acts through a center of gravity that is slightly higher than S_2 and projects to the base of support; when the body is in a single limb stance position, this line of gravity passes on the medial side of the knee causing a varus thrust (Fig. 10.25B). These tibiofemoral compressive forces increase with stair climbing, running, jumping, and squatting. During normal walking, tibiofemoral compression forces reach almost four times body weight with the majority of that force (60%) borne by the medial compartment.[117] It may be for this reason that the medial tibial condyle has about three times as much articular cartilage as its lateral counterpart.[118] The force of the weight is counterbalanced by dynamic and static forces of the iliotibial band. Dynamic forces occur at both the hip and knee in unilateral stance through the attachments of the gluteus maximus and the tensor fasciae latae muscles. Tension of the IT band can be palpated on the lateral thigh to the tibia when a person stands on one leg.

As the knee moves from extension to flexion, shear stresses are applied to the tibiofemoral joint, especially in moving from full extension to about 90° of flexion.[119] The menisci assist in both absorbing some of the forces applied to the knee and dissipating the forces over a larger area. However, the primary restraints against shearing forces encountered by the knee are the muscles and cruciate ligaments. The anterior cruciate ligament provides protection against forward movement of the tibia on the femur. When the knee is at 90° of flexion, the hamstrings are able to assist in this task. On the other hand, the posterior cruciate ligament restricts posterior shearing at end ranges of posterior tibial motion on the femur, and the quadriceps assist the PCL. At what point in the motion these shear forces occur depends upon whether the knee is weight-bearing or nonweight-bearing. In a weight-bearing condition, ACL stress progressively decreases from 0° to 90°.[120] Recent studies have demonstrated that peak strain on the ACL occurs similarly in OKC and CKC activities (Fig. 10.26), but increases in resistance during OKC exercises added to the ACL strain whereas additional weight during CKC activities did not.[121]

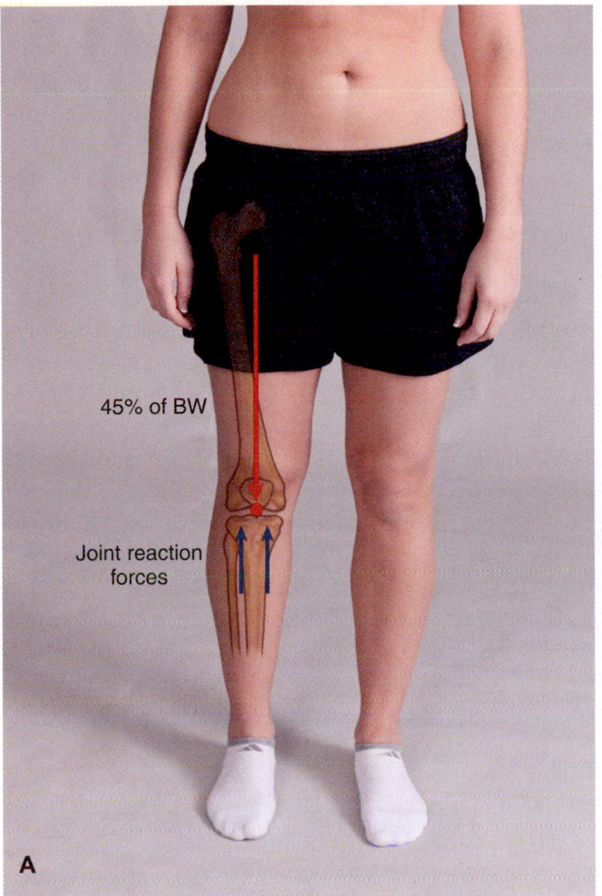

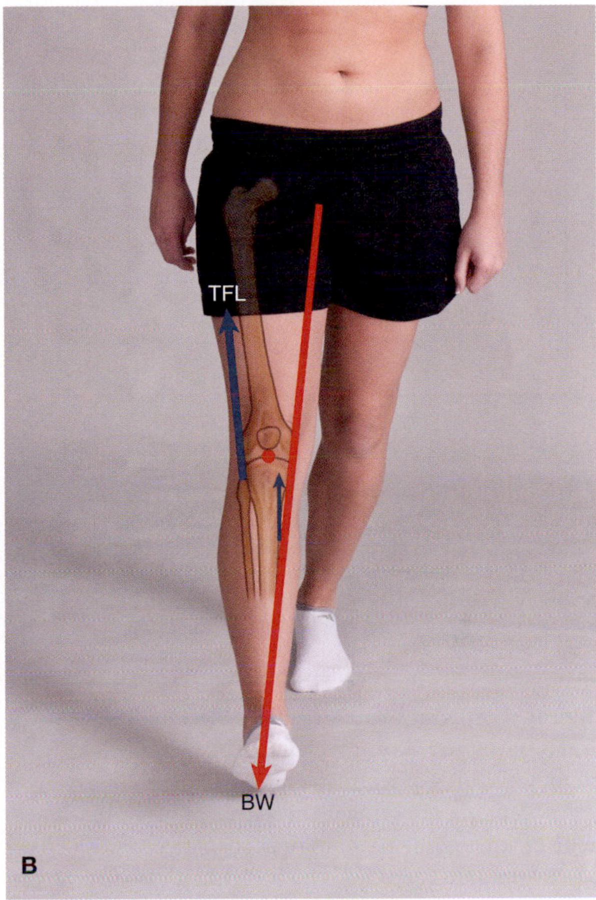

Figure 10.25 Reaction forces at the knee are located in the central joint in standing and move medially in walking and running. A) Joint reaction forces in bilateral standing go through the center of the knee joint. B) During unilateral weight-bearing as in walking or running, the joint reaction force moves medially within the knee joint to create a varus stress on the knee, increasing medial joint pressures.

Abnormalities that alter the torque of the body weight or the iliotibial band result in movement of the central joint force medially or laterally to produce an unequal distribution of compression forces.[2] Areas receiving excessive physiologic pressure over many years may develop pain, destruction of articular cartilage, and osteoarthritis. Conditions that can change the forces or the moment arms to produce these problems include paralysis of the tensor fascia lata muscle; iliotibial band tightness; obesity; genu varus or valgus; traumatic or

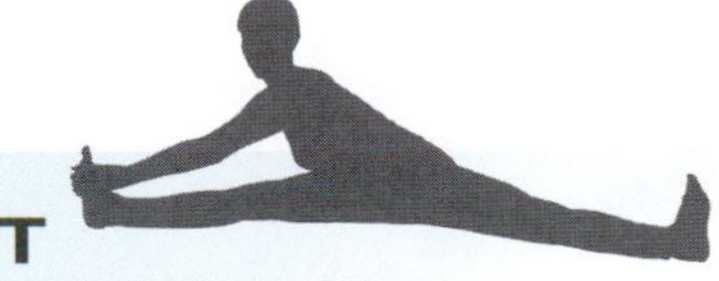

PRACTICE POINT

Menisci are vital structures to knee stability and force absorption. It has been determined that the menisci provide about 45% of a knee's ability to absorb forces.[122] If menisci are removed, the knee's stress increases by two to three times normal levels.[123] Various investigations have provided consistent evidence indicating eventual osteoarthritic changes in the knee following full or partial meniscectomies.[23, 124] It makes sense, then, for surgeons to salvage as much of an injured meniscus as possible. Arthroscopic repairs are now commonplace occurrences following meniscal injuries. Clinicians treating these patients postoperatively must respect the tissue's healing process and know where in the range of motion caution must be taken to protect the healing meniscus, especially during the early weeks of recovery.

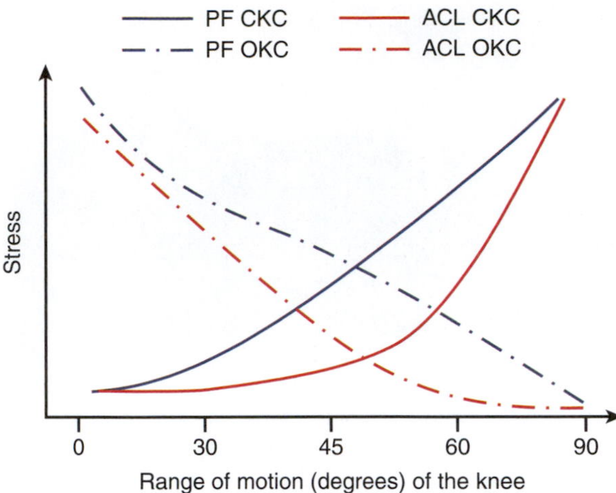

Figure 10.26 Shear stresses on the ACL and patellofemoral joint stresses in OKC and CKC motions. Weight-bearing activities provide less stress to the ACL and patellofemoral joint in the first half of knee motion from extension whereas nonweight-bearing activities offer the least amount of stress to these structures during the last half of knee flexion motion.

surgical shortening of the neck of the femur; excessive pronation of the foot; or changes in alignment of the femur, tibia, or foot from fractures.

An example of biomechanical causes in the development of knee joint pathology is seen in obesity.[125] As the weight gain increases, the individual can be seen to shift the trunk more and more laterally with each step in walking. If you recall information from Chapter 9, you will also recall that this maneuver decreases the force that the hip abductor muscles must generate to balance the increased weight. The tensor fascia lata is one of these hip abductor muscles, so its contributions to counteracting the compressive forces on the knee are decreased (Fig. 10.25). In addition, the excessive lateral trunk shift causes the force of the body's weight to move from the medial side of the knee joint toward the lateral side, with the joint reaction force moving laterally as well. This produces asymmetric distribution of condylar pressures with excess pressure on the lateral condyles and a valgus thrust. In time, these abnormal forces can lead to a knock-knee deformity, cartilaginous and meniscal thinning and destruction, and osteoarthritis.[2]

Patellofemoral Joint Forces

One of the purposes of a pulley is to change the direction or angle of a force. The patella may be thought of as a pulley for the quadriceps since it does change the angle of force of the quadriceps. Looking at Figure 10.27, the change in the angle of pull created by the patella does not seem significant, but the actual calculations tell a different story. Throughout the range of motion, the knee loses 15% to 30% strength following a **patellectomy**.[126] In other words, without a patella, the quadriceps must work 15% to 30% more to exert the same amount of force it does when the patella is intact. Because the patella attaches to both the quadriceps tendon and the patellar ligament, it becomes tethered when the quadriceps contracts. These two forces pulling on the patella from opposite directions creates a compression of the patella against the femur (Fig. 10.28). With the knee extended, the resultant force is small because the forces of the tendon and the ligament are almost on a straight line (Fig. 10.28A). When the knee flexes, the resultant force becomes large and can easily exceed the force of the muscle. As the knee flexion angle increases, the joint reaction force within the patellofemoral joint increases because the vector length becomes larger (Fig. 10.28B and C). Smidt[116] calculated patellofemoral joint reaction force in maximum isometric quadriceps contractions as 0.8 times body weight when the knee was in the 15° position. The force increased to 2.6 times body weight when the knee was at a 90° angle. During level walking, the joint reaction forces are 0.5 to 1.5 times

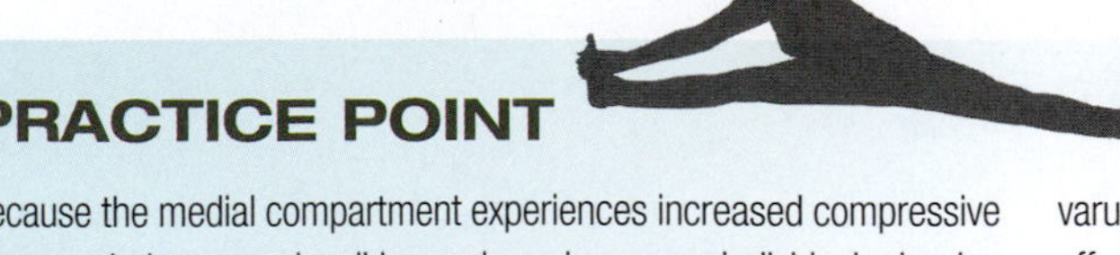

PRACTICE POINT

Because the medial compartment experiences increased compressive stresses during normal walking and running, some individuals develop osteoarthritis of the medial compartment. As the articular cartilage wears down over time and medial compressive forces continue, additional exaggeration of varus knee stress results, creating a cycle of increased wear and tear of the medial compartment with increased varus stress application. Short of surgical correction, clinicians may offer these individuals some relief with the application of orthotic devices to reduce medial compartment stress. These orthoses are applied either in the shoe as a foot orthosis or to the knee as an unloading brace. Additionally, therapeutic exercises to increase muscle strength of surrounding muscle groups may also be beneficial.

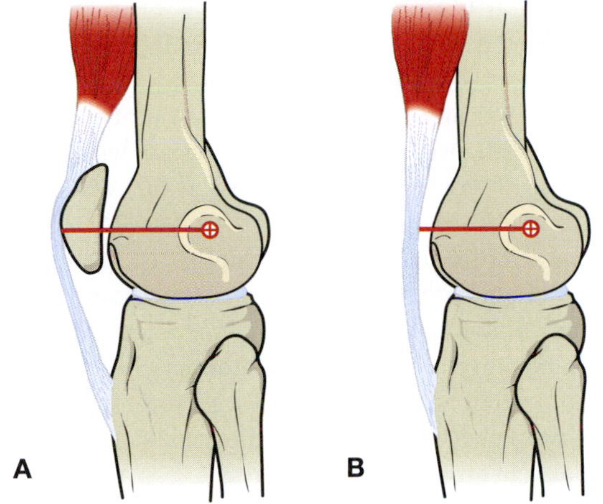

Figure 10.27 Pulley system of the patella and quadriceps. A) With a patella the lever arm of the quadriceps is larger. B) When the patella is absent, the moment arm of the quadriceps reduces significantly, causing a reduction in potential force provided by the quadriceps.

body weight.[119] When doing a squat, the joint reaction force increases to 7 to 8 times body weight.[119] It is no wonder that patients with patellofemoral pain syndrome report that their pain increases when going up or down stairs and in kneeling or squatting activities.

As with the tibiofemoral stress, there is stress at the patellofemoral joint as the knee moves throughout its range of motion. The stress the patellofemoral joint encounters occurs from the force that compresses the patella into the femur; this is also known as the patellofemoral joint reaction force. As with the tibiofemoral joint, this joint reaction force also changes depending on whether the knee is moving in open or closed chain functions. Patellofemoral compressive force in open kinetic chain activities is greatest at 0° and decreases as the knee moves to 90° (Fig. 10.26); in a closed kinetic chain motion, patellofemoral stress is greatest at 90° and decreases as the knee moves into full extension.[127]

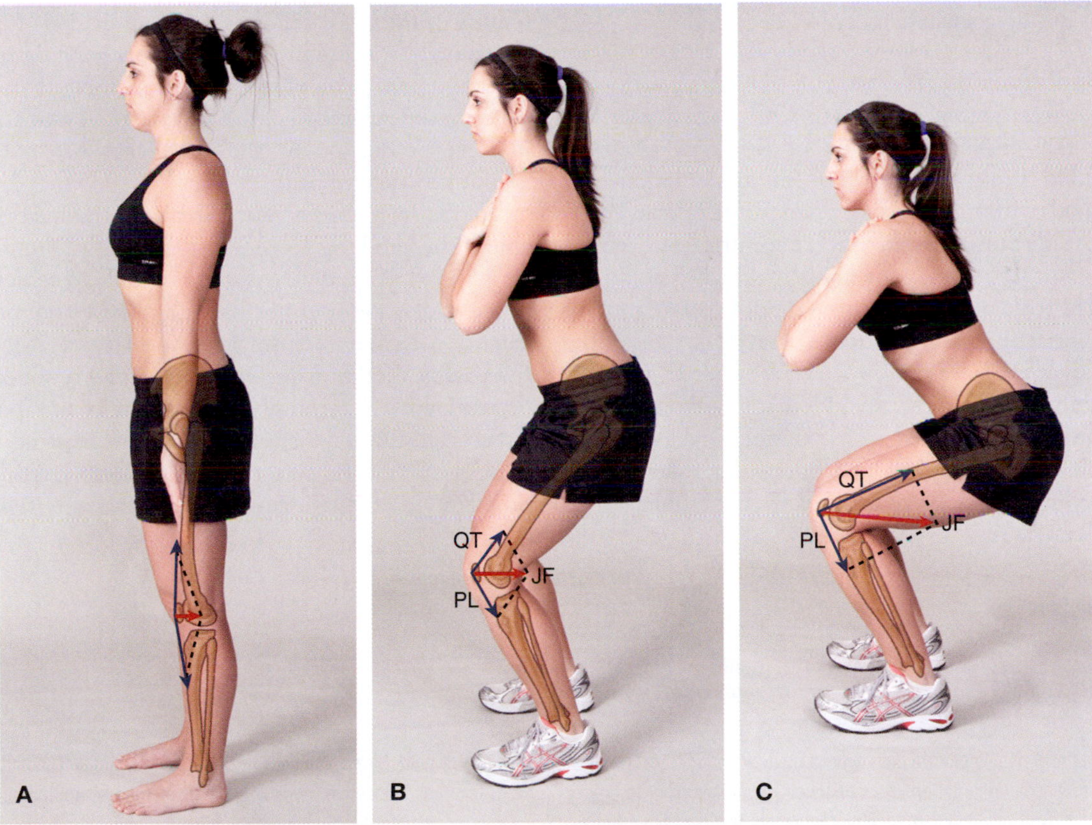

Figure 10.28 Patellofemoral compression force is a resultant vector between the patella and femur, which occurs during quadriceps activity as the quadriceps pulls on the patella superiorly and the quadriceps tendon pulls on the patella from the opposite direction. A) In full standing, little resultant vector force occurs. B) In a partial squat, the resultant vector force produced by the quadriceps muscle and quadriceps tendon increases, increasing compression of the patella against the femur. C) There is a significant resultant vector force pushing the patella against the femoral condyles when the individual squats to 90°.

Recall from our earlier discussion and Figure 10.15 that as the knee moves throughout its range of motion, the amount of contact the patella and femur have with each other also varies. This is important because as the pressure pushing the patella into the femur increases, the area of contact also tends to increase. With a larger area accepting this joint reaction force, the patella and femur are able to tolerate this increased stress. The ratio of joint reaction force and the area of contact is **contact pressure.** So, although the joint reaction force increases with increasing knee flexion to 90°, the contact pressure remains manageable by the patellofemoral joint since the contact area between the patella and femur increase as well.

Torque of Muscles Acting at the Knee

Since muscle forces applied to the knee create arcs of motion, the force created is torque. Torque forces applied to the knee are substantial. The quadriceps muscle group produces torque equivalent to one to three times body weight during walking, four times body weight during stair climbing, and five times body weight during a squat activity.[128]

Quadriceps Femoris Torque

Early investigators using isometric measurements found that maximum torque of the knee extensors reached a peak at about 60° of knee flexion and decreased with further extension of the knee.[129–131] Later studies using isokinetic concentric contractions also demonstrated that the angle at which peak torque occurred remains constant around 50° to 60° of motion when corrections for the effect of gravity (weight of the limb) were made.[132]

Recall from Chapters 2 and 3 that muscle strength is in large part determined by its physiological length and its moment arm length. The quadriceps is able to maintain about 90% of its maximum strength from 80° to 30° of flexion[116] (Fig. 10.29); this is a large range of motion for this muscle group to maintain such a high level of strength. How does it do it? Quadriceps strength is optimized through a utilization of the combined strength principles of physiological length and moment arm length. With the knee at 80° where the quadriceps provides high strength levels, there is a favorable length-tension relationship of the vasti muscles; combined with this factor, the change occurring in the patella's moment arm length as the knee continues through its range of motion allows for better quadriceps strength output as the knee moves into extension. When the knee is fully flexed, the patella lies in the intercondylar groove and close to the axis of motion, and the rectus femoris, as a two-joint muscle, provides for maintained strength levels. As the knee extends, the patella moves out of the groove to reach a maximum lever arm distance at 45° of flexion. Smidt[116] measured mean patellar lever arm distances of 3.8 cm at 90° of flexion and 4.9 cm at 45°. The lever arm distance then decreased to 4.4 cm at full extension. We have already discussed the advantage that occurs to the rectus femoris if the hip extends as the knee extends to allow the muscle to maintain a relatively unchanging length. The argument as to which of these factors (physiological or moment arm length) plays a predominant role in force production by the quadriceps has not been definitively determined.

As the knee moves near extension, the quadriceps's ability to produce force is significantly diminished (Fig. 10.29). An individual who is unable to achieve full active knee extension but has full passive motion into extension has an **extensor lag**. An extensor lag, when full passive motion is present, may be the result of pain or weakness. If incomplete extension is not possible either actively or passively, then there may be either joint restriction or soft tissue restriction causing the problem. Joint restriction may occur from tightness

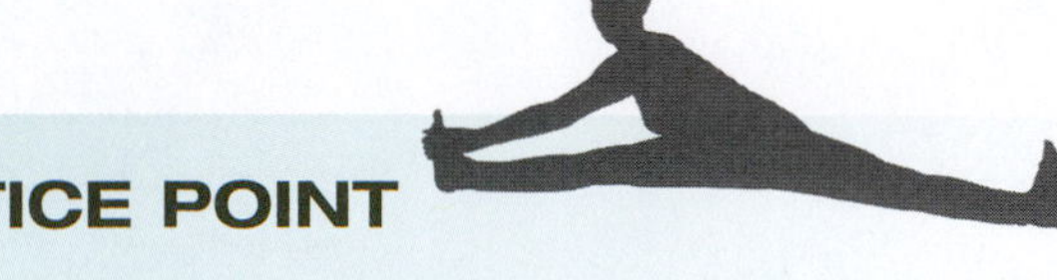

PRACTICE POINT

Patients with patellofemoral pain syndrome (PFPS) have classic symptoms that include anterior knee pain with stair climbing, kneeling, squatting, and other activities which increase pressure between the patella and femur. Quadriceps resistive exercises through a full arc of knee extension may be impossible for these individuals to complete because of pain. Strengthening the quadriceps of these patients with PFPS is often a challenge for clinicians. Oftentimes, strength gains are initially made by providing resistance with the knee in extension and through a short arc of terminal extension, the first 20° of flexion, before the patella engages in the femoral intercondylar groove.

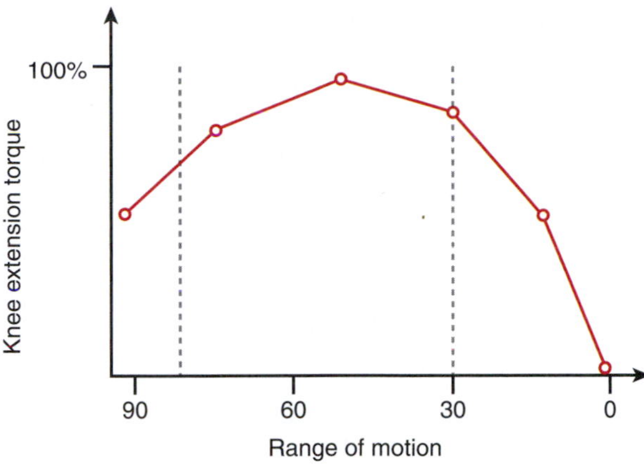

Figure 10.29 Based on data from Smidt.[116] knee extension torque is maintained at least at 90% throughout the knee's ROM from 80° to 30°. As the knee approaches full extension, the ability of the quadriceps to produce force diminishes.

within the joint capsule or a bony block preventing movement. Soft tissue restrictions are usually caused by scarring around or near a joint, by an inflexible muscle, or by edema.

Full knee extension is important to regain following injury or the presence of restricting structures. In the case of an extensor lag, if pain is the cause, treatment must be instituted to relieve the pain. If the cause is weakness of the quadriceps, various techniques are used to restore full active knee extension. Full knee extension must be achieved following most injuries before the patient is allowed to ambulate without assistance of either bracing or assistive devices such as crutches. Full weight-bearing ambulation that is permitted without full knee extension is likely to accelerate knee joint degeneration and add to instability.[133–135]

Functionally, the greater torque output of the quadriceps muscle at the 50° to 60° position coincides with a need for large torques in elevation of the body, as in rising from a chair and climbing. In these activities, a perpendicular line from the center of gravity of the body falls well posterior to the knee axis and, therefore, exerts a large resistance torque for the quadriceps to match (Fig. 10.30). Very little torque is required of the quadriceps in erect standing.

Knee Flexor Muscle Torque

The maximum isometric torque measurement of the hamstring muscles shows that the greatest torque occurs when the muscles are elongated at both the hip and knee (hip flexion and knee extension) and that the lowest torque occurs when the muscles contract in its shortened position of hip extension and knee flexion. This should be no surprise since the quadriceps and other two-joint muscles function the same way, utilizing the length-tension principle. The length-tension factor seems to be the predominant strength factor in hamstring torque production even though there are changes in the muscle's moment arm distances that occur as the muscle shortens. Smidt[116] found mean moment arm distances for the knee flexors of 2.5 cm at 90° of flexion, 4.1 cm at 45°, and 2.5 cm at full extension. A reduction in strength in spite of changes occurring in the hamstrings' moment arm may lend additional argument to the idea that the patella plays an important role in maintaining high strength output of the quadriceps throughout a significant range of motion. Functionally, the need for great torque in the knee-extended-during-hip-flexing position occurs in closed chain motion when the hamstring muscles are the primary muscle group used to lower and raise the weight of the HAT when a person

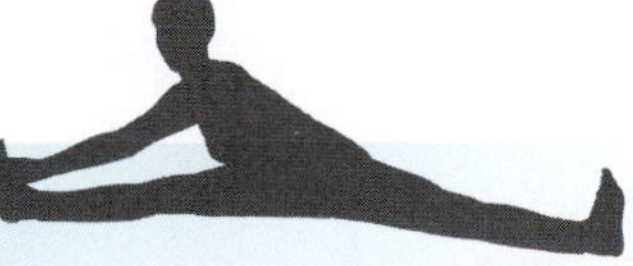

PRACTICE POINT

Although both the hamstrings and quadriceps are used in moving from a seated to a standing position, the quadriceps plays a major role in knee extension motion of this activity.[136] An individual who is unable to bear weight on one leg because of an injury restricting weight-bearing or an individual who is older and has lost muscle strength as a function of aging may find it difficult to get out of a chair. The lower the seat of the chair is positioned, the more difficult it is to rise to a standing position. Clinicians must be aware of the strength needs of the quadriceps muscle in transferring from sitting to standing and provide for adaptations which may be necessary for those individuals who find it difficult to perform such a task. Instructing them to sit in higher chairs may be one way to avoid difficulty getting out of a chair in social situations.

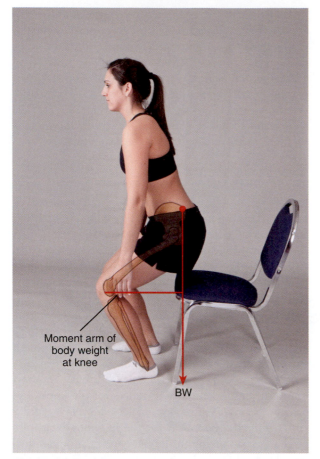

Figure 10.30 Large torque output is required of the quadriceps to rise from sitting because of the moment arm of the body's weight.

is reaching over to touch the floor or bending forward in the sitting position (see Figs. 2.27 and 2.33).

Hamstrings to Quadriceps Torque Ratio

The peak torques for the quadriceps muscles are greater than those of the knee flexors.[137] This is not unexpected because the knee extensors have over twice the cross-sectional area of the knee flexors,[138] and the knee extensors have a longer moment arm distance than the flexors.[116] Strength imbalance between these muscle groups has been suggested as a basis for injuries such as hamstring strains. Normative values for hamstring/quadriceps ratios (peak torque of hamstrings divided by peak torque of quadriceps) are 0.60 to 0.69 at 60° per second, increasing to 0.85 to 0.95 at 300° per second, not corrected for gravity.[139] However, when force output is corrected for gravity, the ratio is lower (i.e., 0.45 to 0.55) and does not change with speed.[132, 140] A 2006 study compared female and male soccer players and divided them into four groups of prepubescent and adolescent ages and males and females.[141] In this study, the more mature males demonstrated a greater percentage of strength increase in their hamstrings whereas the more mature females increased quadriceps strength. The mature females had a greater quadriceps strength ratio to put them at risk for an ACL injury.[141]

Interaction of Muscles and Ligaments in Function

Although the static ligamentous and capsular structures of the knee can limit manual passive joint movements, these structures are unable to withstand extreme high forces. Chronically applied end range forces also have an eventually detrimental effect on static structures. For example, knee hyperextension is the common result of relying on solely passive joint structures for support and stability. Normally, both the dynamic contraction of muscles and the static forces of the ligaments and capsule are used to stabilize the knee. The ligaments and other soft tissues additionally provide a sensory system for proprioception and kinesthesia (see Chapter 3), as well as input for producing reflex muscle contraction to unload and protect ligaments.[142–144]

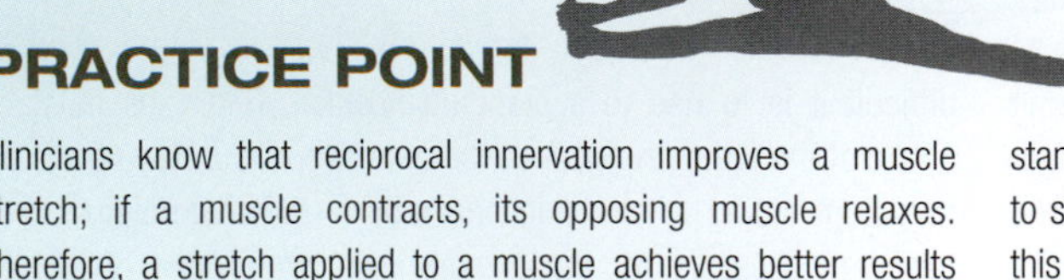

PRACTICE POINT

Clinicians know that reciprocal innervation improves a muscle stretch; if a muscle contracts, its opposing muscle relaxes. Therefore, a stretch applied to a muscle achieves better results when it is relaxed and its antagonist contracts. For example, to stretch the hamstrings, more flexibility is achieved when the hamstrings is relaxed and the quadriceps contracts. Since the hamstrings are primary muscles involved in bending over from a standing position to touch the floor, this may not be a very good way to stretch the hamstrings. Many individuals, however, seem to use this as a flexibility exercise. The hamstrings are felt by the individual stretching, but the individual feels the muscle contracting, not stretching. Clinicians should educate individuals who use this method to "stretch" the hamstrings and provide alternative—and more effective—means of doing so.

In recent years, attention has been drawn to the anterior cruciate ligament and the role it plays in proprioception. The frequency of progressive instability and disability after ACL injury and reconstruction has directed attention to investigation of sensory functions of ligaments and joint tissues in human subjects.[142, 145–151]

Sensory Innervation and Reflexes

Ligaments, capsule, and other soft tissues of the knee are richly innervated with sensory nerve fibers and receptors (see Fig. 3.9). Mechanoreceptors have been found in human cruciate and collateral ligaments, the capsule, and synovial lining and on the outer edges of the menisci.[152, 153] Reflexes from joint mechanoreceptors to muscles have been demonstrated in human subjects, including facilitation of the hamstrings and inhibition of the quadriceps with loading of the ACL.[154]

Swelling in the joint capsule has long been known to produce inhibition of the quadriceps muscle and a sudden collapse of the knee.[41, 155–158] This inhibition has been considered to be caused by deformation of the mechanoreceptors in the ligaments and capsule. Infusion of only 60 ml of normal saline solution into the joint capsule produced a 30% to 50% decrease of the EMG amplitude of the quadriceps muscle.[152] Inhibition secondary to joint effusion is detrimental to recovery following injury.

When ACL injuries occur, there is a decrease in the individual's proprioceptive abilities.[148, 159] Clinically, Barrack, Skinner, and Buckley[160] demonstrated over a 25% increase in the threshold for proprioception (of slow passive motion) in knees with complete ACL tears compared to the normal knee. When a joint's ligament is injured, there is a delay in the time to respond to perturbations.[161] These studies indicate that an ACL deficient knee is unable to react to stresses within a safe time response; since it takes an individual longer to respond to stresses applied to the joint, the knee is at increased risk of injury.

Static and Dynamic Connections

In addition to neural elements, there are important local connections between the dynamic and static structures that were described earlier in this chapter. These interconnections include the numerous attachments to the menisci, the reinforcement of the capsule by ligaments and retinacula, the extensive soft tissue attachments of the semimembranosus and the iliotibial band, and the penetration of the capsule by the popliteus muscle.

Muscle Protection of Ligaments

Sometimes muscles are used naturally to protect ligaments and sometimes the situation is pathological. An example of a naturally occurring use of muscles to reduce ligamentous stress is seen in walking. At the end of the swing phase, the hamstrings contract to decelerate the swinging limb and reduce stress on the cruciate ligaments.

Muscles also work to assist ligaments in providing knee support and stability. We have already discussed the fact that medial and lateral knee muscles assist the medial and lateral ligaments in providing stability to varus and valgus stresses, especially during single limb stance and movements. As mentioned previously, the hamstrings provide the ACL additional support against forward stress of the tibia on the femur and the quadriceps assist the PCL in restricting posterior movement of the tibia on the femur. The popliteus not only serves to initiate unlocking the knee from full extension, but it is an important active stabilizer of the knee as well.[164] In stance, the soleus, a one-joint muscle that crosses the ankle, also lends secondary assistance at the knee. When the soleus contracts during weight-bearing, the anchored foot remains in place, but the tibia moves posteriorly, causing the knee to move into extension. The gastrocnemius then plays an important role in controlling the amount of knee extension and preventing hyperextension.[84]

Pathological situations usually arise when a muscle must substitute for an injured ligament. In these situations, the muscle's increased activity requires increased

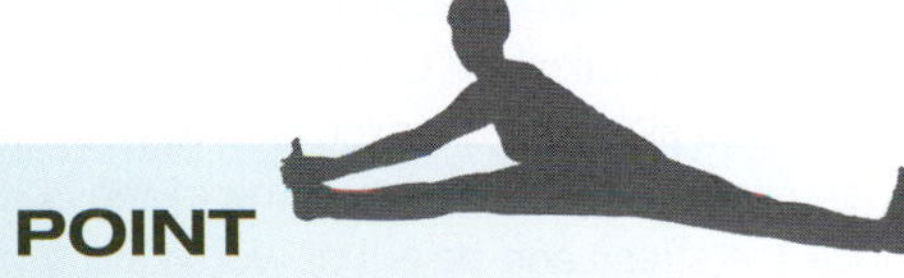

PRACTICE POINT

One concern early in the rehabilitation process following knee injuries is to reduce any effusion that may be present following either injury or surgery. Substantial quadriceps strength gains are not possible until the effusion is resolved. Clinicians must make efforts to resolve the effusion before expecting strength gains in rehabilitation. Additionally, clinicians dealing with patients who have had ACL injuries must be concerned about restoring lost proprioception. Joint proprioceptor function must be included as part of the rehabilitation program.[162, 163]

energy expenditure. Individuals with complete ACL ruptures have been found to have higher EMG amplitudes of the medial gastrocnemius and earlier onset of activation of hamstrings and quadriceps muscles.[165] Although voluntary reaction time for muscular protection of the knee is too slow in many sports situations, rehabilitation programs should include coordination and muscle timing training. Decreased hamstring reaction time in individuals with knee injuries has been demonstrated with a 12-week dynamic closed chain coordination program.[166] Although muscles may not provide sufficient protection during rapid sport activities, they may offer sufficient substitutions to protect the knee during daily activities.

Summary

In appearance, the knee does not seem complex, composed of the tibia, femur and patella, but the patellofemoral and tibiofemoral joints which make up the knee complex are anything but simple. These two joints work together to create knee function which is vital for body mobility. Many of the muscles that act at the knee are biarticular, so they are influenced by other joints and their positions. Since the lower extremity is most often used in closed chain activities, these two-joint muscles have significant influences on not only the knee and the other joints they cross but on the function of the entire lower extremity. Terminal knee extension must be accompanied by tibial rotation for full extension to occur. In the open chain position, the tibia rotates laterally on the femur, and in weight-bearing, the femur rotates medially on the tibial to achieve full knee extension. Tremendous muscle forces act at the knee to provide it with motion and power. The quadriceps and hamstrings provide for significant force delivery during running and jumping because of their arrangement and the motions produced synchronously at the knee and hip. Patellofemoral joint reaction force is generated by the quadriceps muscle pulling on the patella at one end and the patellar ligament pulling on it from the other end. This compressive force increases as the knee flexes, but the joint is able to tolerate these forces because of the extraordinarily thick articular cartilage covering the surfaces and the expanded area of patella and femur contact which changes as the knee moves through its range of motion.

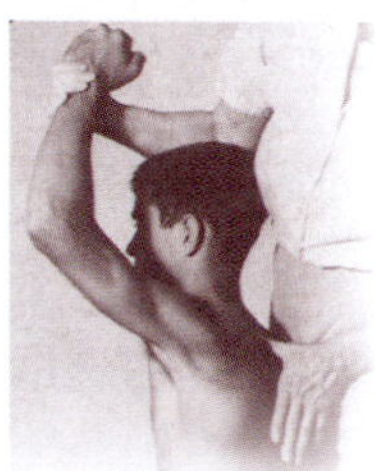

CLINICAL SCENARIO SOLUTION

As it turns out, the tests Cole performed on Logan reproduced Logan's pain. The test results also indicated that Logan has weakness in his quadriceps, hip abductors, and hip extensors. He also has some flexibility restrictions in his hamstrings and calf muscle groups. Logan reported pain to resistance in the range of 60° to 30° of flexion. Cole tells Logan that he has patellofemoral pain syndrome which is treated with several various rehabilitation options. He explains to Logan that the goal they are working toward is for Logan to strengthen the quadriceps without causing his pain. Cole develops an exercise program in Logan's pain-free ranges of motion using a combination of open and closed kinetic chain exercises. Cole also instructs him in flexibility exercises.

Discussion Questions

1. Using the Clinical Scenario and its solution, what degrees of motion will Cole have Logan perform during both his open kinetic chain exercises and his closed kinetic chain exercises to put the least amount of stress on the patellofemoral joint? If Logan experiences pain with some of the open and closed chain exercises, what could Cole do to reduce the stress and pain that would still allow Logan to perform the exercises?
2. If you are to instruct Logan in a hamstring stretch, what type of stretch would you instruct him to perform? Why have you selected this exercise? Be specific with your answer. What are the key points that need to be considered when stretching the hamstrings?

3. You have a patient who is unable to fully extend the knee into its last 15°, but you are able to move it passively into full extension. What are the possible reasons that your patient is unable to fully straighten the knee? What types of activities could you provide this patient to help achieve these last few degrees?
4. If the inferior pole of an individual's patella sits about an inch proximal to the joint margin, how may this affect the person's knee?
5. You are going to passively stretch the knee extensor muscles of an individual. How will you position him or her and what stretch application will you use? What alignments must you be aware of to be sure you are providing an optimal stretch?
6. You are working with a patient who has had a PCL reconstruction. What motions in open and closed kinetic chain should you avoid in the early portion of the rehabilitation program? Explain your answer.
7. When you are home over the holidays, your grandfather complains to you about the struggle he has been recently experiencing getting out of his favorite armchair. You know that his favorite armchair has a deep seat, big and soft cushioning, and sits low to the floor. What advice could you give him that would allow him to get out of his favorite armchair with less difficulty?
8. Explain in your own words why the tibia laterally rotates in its last few degrees of motion when an individual is performing an open chain knee extension motion, but when the individual stands and extends the knee while weight-bearing, the femur rotates medially on the tibia. What is the impact on function if the knee is unable to move through this rotation?
9. A patient you are treating has patellofemoral pain syndrome. During your observation, you notice that he has genu recurvatum. Based on this observation, what aspect of the posterior patella do suspect will be most tender to palpation for him, and why?[167]

Lab Activities

1. On the bones, identify the following bony landmarks and determine those that are palpable.

Femur

medial and lateral condyles
epicondyles
adductor tubercle
linea aspera
medial and lateral
  supracondylar lines
intercondylar notch
popliteal surface
patellar surface
distal articular surfaces

Tibia

medial and lateral condyles
tibial plateau
  intercondylar eminence
tibial tuberosity
  anterior border
  interosseous border
  proximal articular surfaces

Fibula

head, neck, shaft

Patella

anterior and posterior surfaces

2. When seated with the knee flexed, palpate on a classmate the patella, anterior border of the tibia, head of the fibula, tibial tuberosity, medial and lateral epicondyles of femur, and lateral condyle of tibia. Locate medially and laterally the joint space between the tibia and femur. With the knee extended and the quadriceps relaxed, grasp the patella and move it passively from side to side and in an up-and-down movement from proximal to distal end. Keep the quadriceps muscle completely relaxed to accomplish this maneuver. Describe the relative amount of motion in each direction.

3. With a partner in the prone position, passively flex the knee. Note the range of motion and the end feel. Have the partner turn on one side and flex the hip, and then repeat passive knee flexion. Why is there more motion when the hip is flexed? What is the limiting structure to knee flexion when the hip is extended?
4. Have your partner sit in a chair. Observe terminal rotation of the tibia on the femur when the knee is slowly extended. Then observe the femur medially rotating on the fixed tibia as the partner slowly stands up. Explain the difference between the two motions.
5. Have your partner perform axial rotation of the knee while sitting in a chair with the heel touching the floor. Observe as you palpate the movement of the medial and lateral malleoli and then the tibial condyles. Repeat your observation and palpation at four other positions of knee flexion and then in full knee extension. Note that as the knee is placed more toward extension, rotation is less, and when the knee is in full extension, axial rotation of the knee is impossible. Attempts cause rotation in the hip. Explain why this change in available axial rotation occurs.
6. Select a partner. Following the descriptions in this chapter, palpate the following knee muscles and tendons and identify their actions as you do:
   quadriceps femoris
   biceps femoris
   semimembranosus
   semitendinosus
   adductor gracilis
   proximal attachments of gastrocnemius
   distal attachments of sartorius and tensor fascia lata
7. Have your partner stand in a normal (relaxed) manner with eyes straight ahead (if the subject looks down, the muscle activity changes). Palpate the quadriceps and hamstring muscles during the following activities. Note whether the muscles are relaxed or have a slight or strong contraction:
   a. Normal relaxed standing.
   b. Sway forward from the ankles, return, and then sway back slightly.
   c. Stand on one leg.
   d. Hyperextend the knees.
   e. Bend forward at the hips to touch floor. Return to erect position.
   f. Perform a deep knee bend (squat) and return.
8. Palpate the hamstrings and the quadriceps with the subject sitting in a chair, slowly rising to the standing position, standing, and then slowly returning to the sitting position. Why do both the quadriceps and the hamstrings contract when rising up and sitting down? What type of contraction is occurring in the quadriceps on rising and on sitting down?
9. Analyze quadriceps and hamstring muscle activity in ascending and descending stairs for both the lead leg and the following leg.
10. Draw the Q angle on your partner's knee. Measure the angle with your partner in supine. Now have your partner stand only on one leg and measure it again. Does it change? Explain.

References

1. Inman VT, Ralston HJ, Todd F. *Human Walking*. Baltimore: Williams & Wilkins, 1981.
2. Maquet PG. *Biomechanics of the Knee*. Berlin: Springer-Verlag, 1983.
3. Morrison JB. The mechanics of the knee joint in relation to normal walking. *Journal of Biomechanics* 3(1):51–61, 1970.
4. Louw QA, Manilall J, Grimmer KA. Epidemiology of knee injuries in adolescents: A review. *British Journal of Sports Medicine* 42(1):2–10, 2008.

5. Clayton RAE, Court-Brown CM. The epidemiology of musculocutaneous tendinous and ligamentous injuries. *Injury* 39(12):1338–1343, 2008.

6. Kapandji IA. *The Physiology of the Joints, Vol 2, Lower Limb*, ed 5. Edinburgh: Churchill Livingstone, 1987.

7. Kwak SD, Colman WW, Ateshian GA, Grelsamer RP, Henry JH, Mow VC. Anatomy of the human patellofemoral joint articular cartilage: Surface curvature analysis. *Journal of Orthopaedic Research* 15(3):468–472, 1997.

8. Carrillon Y, Abidi H, Dejour D, Fantino O, Moyen B, Tran-Minh VA. Patellar instability: Assessment on MR images by measuring the lateral trochlear inclination-initial experience. *Radiology* 216(2):582–585, 2000.

9. Fucentese SF, Schöttle PB, Pfirrmann CW, Romero J. CT changes after trochleoplasty for symptomatic trochlear dysplasia. *Knee Surgery, Sports Traumatology, Arthroscopy* 15(2):168–174, 2007.

10. Post WR, Teitge R, Amis A. Patellofemoral malalignment: Looking beyond the viewbox. *Clinics in Sports Medicine* 21(3):521–546, 2002.

11. Levine HB, Bosco JA, 3rd. Sagittal and coronal biomechanics of the knee: A rationale for corrective measures. *Bulletin of the NYU Hospital for Joint Diseases* 65(1):87–95, 2007.

12. Adam C, Eckstein F, Milz S, Putz R. The distribution of cartilage thickness within the joints of the lower limb of elderly individuals. *Journal of Anatomy* 193:203–214, 1998.

13. Shepherd DE, Seedhom BB. Thickness of human articular cartilage in joints of the lower limb. *Annals of the Rheumatic Diseases* 58(1):27–34, 1999.

14. Weckbach S, Mendlik T, Horger W, Wagner S, Reiser MF, Glaser C. Quantitative assessment of patellar cartilage volume and thickness at 3.0 tesla comparing a 3D-fast low angle shot versus a 3D-true fast imaging with steady-state precession sequence for reproducibility. *Investigative Radiology* 41(2):189–197, 2006.

15. Eckstein F, Winzheimer M, Hohe J, Englmeier KH, Reiser M. Interindividual variability and correlation among morphological parameters of knee joint cartilage plates: Analysis with three-dimensional MR imaging. *Osteoarthritis and Cartilage* 9(2):101–111, 2001.

16. Heegaard J, Leyvraz PF, Curnier A, Rakotomanana L, Huiskes R. The biomechanics of the human patella during passive knee flexion. *Journal of Biomechanics* 28(11):1265–1279, 1995.

17. Blaha JD, Mancinelli CA, Simons WH. Using the transepicondylar axis to define the sagittal morphology of the distal part of the femur. *Journal of Bone and Joint Surgery Am* 84(suppl 2):48–55, 2002.

18. Seedhom BB. Loadbearing function of the menisci. *Physiotherapy* 62(7):223, 1976.

19. Clark CR, Ogden JA. Development of the menisci of the human knee joint: Morphological changes and their potential role in childhood meniscal injury. *Journal of Bone and Joint Surgery Am* 65(4):538–547, 1983.

20. Fukuda Y, Takai S, Yoshino N, et al. Impact load transmission of the knee joint-influence of leg alignment and the role of meniscus and articular cartilage. *Clinical Biomechanics* 15(7):516–521, 2000.

21. Messner K, Gao J. The menisci of the knee joint: Anatomical and functional characteristics, and a rationale for clinical treatment. *Journal of Anatomy* 193:161–178, 1998.

22. MacConaill MA. The function of intra-articular fibrocartilages, with special reference to the knee and inferior radio-ulnar joints. *Journal of Anatomy* 66:210–227, 1932.

23. Aagaard H, Verdonk R. Function of the normal meniscus and consequences of meniscal resection. *Scandinavian Journal of Medicine in Science and Sports* 9(3):134–140, 1999.

24. Metcalf MH, Barrett GR. Prospective evaluation of 1485 meniscal tear patterns in patients with stable knees. *American Journal of Sports Medicine* 32(3):675–680, 2004.

25. Smith JP, III, Barrett GR. Medial and lateral meniscal tear patterns in anterior cruciate ligament-deficient knees: A prospective analysis of 575 tears. *American Journal of Sports Medicine* 29(4):415–419, 2001.

26. Krinksy MB, Abdenour TE, Starkey C, Albo RA, Chu DA. Incidence of lateral meniscus injury in professional basketball players. *American Journal of Sports Medicine* 20(1):17–19, 1992.

27. Chen L, Kim PD, Ahmad CS, Levine WN. Medial collateral ligament injuries of the knee: Current treatment concepts. *Current Reviews in Musculoskeletal Medicine* 1(2):108–113, 2008.

28. Grood ES, Noyes FR, Butler DL, Suntay WJ. Ligamentous and capsular restraints preventing straight medial and lateral laxity in intact human cadaver knees. *Journal of Bone and Joint Surgery Am* 63(8):1257–1269, 1981.

29. Papannagari R, DeFrate LE, Nha KW, et al. Function of posterior cruciate ligament bundles during in vivo knee flexion. *American Journal of Sports Medicine* 35(9):1507–1512, 2007.

30. Girgis FG, Marshall JL, Monajem A. The cruciate ligaments of the knee joint: Anatomical, functional and experimental analysis. *Clinical Orthopaedics and Related Research* 106:216–231, 1975.

31. Hoppenfeld S. *Physical examination of the spine and extremities*. East Norwalk, CT: Appleton-Century-Crofts, 1976.

32. McCluskey G, Blackburn TA. Classification of knee ligament instabilities. *Physical Therapy* 60(2):1575–1577, 1980.

33. McQuade KJ, Crutcher JP, Sidles JA, Larson RV. Tibial rotation in anterior cruciate deficient knees: An in vitro study. *Journal of Orthopaedic and Sports Physical Therapy* 11(4):146–149, 1989.

34. Shoemaker S, Daniel D. The limits of knee motion. In Daniel DM, Akeson WH, O'Connor JJ (eds): *Knee Ligaments: Structure, Function, Injury and Repair*, New York, 1990, Raven Press.

35. Chandler TJ, Wilson GD, Stone MH. The effect of squat exercise on knee stability. *Medicine & Science in Sports and Exercise* 21(3):299–303, 1989.

36. Clunie G, Hall-Craggs MA, Paley MN, et al. Measurement of synovial lining volume by magnetic resonance imaging of the knee in chronic synovitis. *Annals of the Rheumatic Diseases* 56(9):526–534, 1997.

37. Moore K. *Clinically Oriented Anatomy*. Baltimore: Williams & Wilkins, 2004.

38. Veltri DM, Warren RF. Anatomy, biomechanics, and physical findings in posterolateral knee instability. *Clinical Sports Medicine* 13(3):599–614, 1994.

39. LaPrade RF, Ly TV, Wentorf FA, Engebretsen L. The posterolateral attachments of the knee: A qualitative and quantitative morphologic analysis of the fibular collateral ligament, popliteus tendon, popliteofibular ligament, and lateral gastrocnemius tendon. *American Journal of Sports Medicine* 31(6):854–860, 2003.

40. van der Wees PJ, Lenssen AF, Hendriks EJ, Stomp DJ, Dekker J, de Bie RA. Effectiveness of exercise therapy and manual mobilisation in ankle sprain and functional instability: A systematic review. *Australian Journal of Physiotherapy* 52(1):27–37, 2006.

41. Stokes M, Young A. Investigations of quadriceps inhibition: Implications for clinical practice. *Physiotherapy* 70:425–428, 1984.

42. Herrington L, Al-Shammari RA. The effect of three degrees of elevation on swelling in acute inversion ankle sprains. *Physical Therapy in Sport* 7:175, 2006.

43. Hislop HJ, Montgomery P. *Daniels and Worthingham's Muscle Testing: Techniques of Manual Examination*, ed 7. Philadelphia: WB Saunders, 2002.

44. Ouellet R, Lévesque HP, Laurin CA. The ligamentous stability of the knee: An experimental investigation. *Canadian Medical Association Journal* 100(2):45–50, 1969.

45. Ross RF. A quantitative study of rotation of the knee joint in man. *Anatomical Record* 52:209, 1932.

46. Mossberg K, Smith LK. Axial rotation of the knee in women. *Journal of Orthopaedic and Sports Physical Therapy* 4(4):236–240, 1983.

47. Wilson DR, Feikes JD, Zavatsky AB, O'Connor JJ. The components of passive knee movement are coupled to flexion angle. *Journal of Biomechanics* 33(4):465–473, 2000.

48. Fuss FK. Principles and mechanisms of automatic rotation during terminal extension in the human knee joint. *Journal of Anatomy* 180:297–304, 1992.

49. Johal P, Williams A, Wragg P, Hunt P, Gedrovc W. Tibiofemoral movement in the living knee: A study of weight-bearing and nonweight-bearing knee kinematics using "interventional" MRI. *Journal of Biomechanics* 38(2):269–276, 2005.

50. Rajendran K. Mechanism of locking at the knee joint. *Journal of Anatomy* 143:189–194, 1985.

51. Rehder U. Morphometrical studies on the symmetry of the human knee joint: Femoral condyles. *Journal of Biomechanics* 16(5):351–356, 1983.

52. Fulkerson JP, Hungerford DS. *Disorders of the Patellofemoral Joint*. Baltimore: Williams & Wilkins, 1990.

53. Waryasz GR, McDermott AY. Patellofemoral pain syndrome (PFPS): A systematic review of anatomy and potential risk factors. *Dynamic Medicine* 7:9, 2008.

54. Goh JC, Lee PY, Bose K. A cadaver study of the function of the oblique part of the vastus medialis. *Journal of Bone and Joint Surgery Br* 77(2):225–231, 1995.

55. Amis AA. Current concepts on anatomy and biomechanics of patellar stability. *Sports Medicine and Arthroscopy Review* 15(2):48–56, 2007.

56. Fujikawa K, Seedhom BB, Wright V. Biomechanics of the patellofemoral joint. Part I: A study of the contact and the congruity of the patellofemoral compartment and movement of the patella. *Engineering in Medicine* 12(1):3–11, 1983.

57. Von Eisenhart-Rothe R, Siebert M, Bringmann C, Vogl T, Englmeier KH, Graichen H. A new in vivo technique for determination of 3D kinematics and contact areas of the patellofemoral and tibiofemoral joint. *Journal of Biomechanics* 37(6):927–934, 2004.

58. Brunet ME, Brinker MR, Cook SD, et al. Patellar tracking during simulated quadriceps contraction. *Clinical Orthopaedics and Related Research* 414:266–275, 2003.

59. Carson WG, Jr., James SL, Larson RL, Singer KM, Winternitz WW. Patellofemoral disorders: Physical and radiographic evaluation. Part I: Physical examination. *Clinical Orthopaedics and Related Research* 185:165–177, 1984.

60. Wilson T. The measurement of patellar alignment in patellofemoral pain syndrome: Are we confusing assumptions with evidence? *Journal of Orthopaedic & Sports Physical Therapy* 37(6):330–341, 2007.

61. Doucette SA, Child DD. The effect of open and closed chain exercise and knee joint position on patellar tracking in lateral patellar compression syndrome. *Journal of Orthopaedic & Sports Physical Therapy* 23:104–110, 1996.

62. Brossmann J, Muhle C, Schröder C, et al. Patellar tracking patterns during active and passive knee extension: Evaluation with motion-triggered cine MR imaging. *Radiology* 187(1):205–212, 1993.

63. Sheehan FT, Zajac FE, Drace JE. In vivo tracking of the human patella using cine phase contrast magnetic resonance imaging. *Journal of Biomechanical Engineering* 121(6):650–656, 1999.

64. Koh TJ, Grabiner MD, DeSwart RJ. In vivo tracking of the human patella. *Journal of Biomechanics* 25(6):637–643, 1992.

65. Cheng C-K, Yao N-K, Liu H-C, Lee K-S. Influences of configuration changes of the patella on the knee extensor mechanism. *Clinical Biomechanics* 11(2):116–120, 1996.

66. Lin F, Makhsous M, Chang AH, Hendrix RW, Zhang L-Q. In vivo and noninvasive six degrees of freedom patellar tracking during voluntary knee movement. *Clinical Biomechanics* 18(5):401–409, 2003.

67. Katchburian MV, Bull AM, Shih Y-F, Heatley FW, Amis AA. Measurement of patellar tracking: Assessment and analysis of the literature. *Clinical Orthopaedics and Related Research* 412:241–259. 2003.

68. Woodland LH, Francis RS. Parameters and comparisons of the quadriceps angle of college-aged men and women in the supine and standing positions. *American Journal of Sports Medicine* 20:208–211, 1992.

69. Omololu BB, Ogunlade OS, Gopaldasani VK. Normal Q angle in an adult Nigerian population. *Clinical Orthopaedics and Related Research* 467(n8):2073–2076, 2009.

70. Horton MG, Hall TL. Quadriceps femoris muscle angle: Normal values and relationships with gender and selected skeletal measures. *Physical Therapy* 69(11):897–901, 1989.

71. Livingston LA. The quadriceps angle: A review of the literature. *Journal of Orthopaedic and Sports Physical Therapy* 28:105–109, 1998.

72. Byl T, Cole JA, Livingston LA. What determines the magnitude of the Q angle? A preliminary study of selected skeletal and muscular measures. *Journal of Sport Rehabilitation* 9(1):26–34, 2000.

73. Grelsamer RP, Dubey A, Weinstein CH. Men and women have similar Q angles: A clinical and trigonometric evaluation. *Journal of Bone and Joint Surgery Br* 87(11):1498–1501, 2005.

74. Näslund J, U.B. N, Odenbring S, Lundeberg T. Comparison of symptoms and clinical findings in subgroups of individuals with patellofemoral pain. *Physiotherapy Theory and Practice* 22(3):105–118, 2006.

75. Doucette SA, Goble EM. The effect of exercise on patellar tracking in lateral patellar compression syndrome. *American Journal of Sports Medicine* 20:434–440, 1992.

76. Lathinghouse LH, Trimble MH. Effects of isometric quadriceps activation on the Q angle in women before and after quadriceps exercise. *Journal of Orthopaedic and Sports Physical Therapy* 30:211–216, 2000.

77. Boucher JP, King MA, LeFebvre R, Pépin A. Quadriceps femoris muscle activity in patellofemoral pain syndrome. *American Journal of Sports Medicine* 20:527–532, 1992.

78. Host JV, Craig R, Lehman RC. Patellofemoral dysfunction in tennis players: A dynamic problem. *Clinics in Sports Medicine* 14:177–203, 1995.

79. Tyson AD. The hip and its relationship to patellofemoral pain. *Strength and Conditioning* 20:67–68, 1998.

80. Kerrigan DC, Riley PO, Nieto TJ, Della Croce U. Knee joint torques: A comparison between women and men during barefoot walking. *Archives of Physical Medicine and Rehabilitation* 81:1162–1165, 2000.

81. Livingstone LA, Mandigo JL. Bilateral rearfoot asymmetry and anterior knee pain syndrome. *Journal of Orthopaedic and Sports Physical Therapy* 33(1):48–55, 2003.

82. Lieb FJ, Perry J. Quadriceps function: An electromyographic study under isometric conditions. *Journal of Bone and Joint Surgery Am* 53A:749–758, 1971.

83. Toumi H, Poumarat G, Benjamin M, Best TM, F'Guyer S, Fairclough J. New insights into the function of the vastus medialis with clinical implications. *Medicine & Science in Sport & Exercise* 39(7):1153–1159, 2007.

84. Li L, Landin D, Grodesky J, Myers J. The function of gastrocnemius as a knee flexor at selected knee and ankle angles. *Journal of Electromyography and Kinesiology* 12(5):385–390, 2002.

85. Arampatzis A, Karamanidis K, Stafilidis S, Morey-Klapsing G, DeMonte G, Brüggemann GP. Effect of different ankle and knee joint positions on gastrocnemius medialis fascicle length and EMG activity during isometric plantar flexion. *Journal of Biomechanics* 39(10):1891–1902, 2006.

86. Azegami M, Yanagihash R, Miyoshi K, Akahane K, Ohira M, Sadoyama T. Effects of multijoint angle changes on EMG activity and force of lower extremity muscles during maximum isometric leg press exercises. *Journal of Physical Therapy Sciences* 19(1):65–72, 2007.

87. Ullrich K, Krudwig WK, Witzel U. Posterolateral aspect and stability of the knee joint. I. Anatomy and function of the popliteus muscle-tendon unit: An anatomical and biomechanical study. *Knee Surgery, Sports Traumatology, Arthroscopy* 10(2):86–90, 2002.

88. Pasque C, Noyes FR, Gibbons M, Levy M, Grood E. The role of the popliteofibular ligament and the tendon of the popliteus in providing stability in the human knee. *Journal of Bone and Joint Surgery Br* 85(2):292–298, 2003.

89. Nyland J, Lachman N, Kocabey Y, Brosky J, Altun R, Caborn D. Anatomy, function, and rehabilitation of the popliteus musculotendinous complex. *Journal of Orthopaedic and Sports Physical Therapy* 35:165–179, 2005.

90. Isear JA, Erickson JR, Worrell TW. EMG analysis of lower extremity muscle recruitment patterns during an unloaded squat. *Medicine & Science in Sport & Exercise* 29(4):532–539, 1997.

91. Pocock GS. Electromyographic study of the quadriceps during resistive exercise. *Journal of the American Physical Therapy Association* 43:427–434, 1963.

92. Basmajian JV. *Muscles Alive: Their Function Revealed by Electromyography*, ed 4. Baltimore: Williams & Wilkins, 1978.

93. Dionisio VC, Almeida GL, Duarte M, Hirata RP. Kinematic, kinetic and EMG patterns during downward squatting. *Journal of Electromyography and Kinesiology* 18:134–143, 2008.

94. Qi Z. Influence of knee joint position on cocontractions of agonist and antagonist muscles during maximal voluntary isometric contractions: Electromyography and Cybex measurement. *Journal of Physical Therapy Sciences* 19:125–130, 2007.

95. McClinton S, Donatelli G, Weir J, Heiderscheit B. Influence of step height on quadriceps onset timing and activation during stair ascent in individuals with patellofemoral pain syndrome. *Journal of Orthopaedic and Sports Physical Therapy* 37(5):239–244, 2007.

96. Ebersole KT, O'Connor KM, Wier AP. Mechanomyographic and electromyographic responses to repeated concentric muscle actions of the quadriceps femoris. *Journal of Electromyography and Kinesiology* 16(2):149–157, 2006.

97. Babault N, Pousson M, Ballay Y, Van Hoecke J. Activation of human quadriceps femoris during isometric, concentric, and eccentric contractions. *Journal of Applied Physiology* 91(6):2628–2634, 2001.

98. Pincivero DM, Gear WS. Quadriceps activation and perceived exertion during a high intensity, steady state contraction to failure. *Muscle & Nerve* 23(4):514–520, 2000.

99. Blanpied PR. Changes in muscle activation during wall slides and squat machine exercise. *Journal of Sport Rehabilitation* 8(2):123–134, 1999.

100. Withrow TJ, Huston LJ, Wojtys EM, Ashton-Miller JA. Effect of varying hamstring tension on anterior cruciate ligament strain during in vitro impulsive knee flexion and compression loading. *Journal of Bone and Joint Surgery Am* 90(4):815–823, 2008.

101. Basmajian JV, Lovejoy JF, Jr. Functions of the popliteus muscle in man: A multifactorial electromyographic study. *Journal of Bone and Joint Surgery Am* 53(3):557–562, 1971.

102. Barnett CH, Richardson AT. The postural function of the popliteus muscle. *Annals of Physical Medicine* 1:177–179, 1953.

103. Mann RA, Hagy JL. The popliteus muscle. *Journal of Bone and Joint Surgery Am* 59(7):924–927, 1977.

104. Prado Reis F, Ferraz de Carvalho CADE. Electromyographic study of the popliteus muscle. *Electromyography and Clinical Neurophysiology* 13(4):445–455, 1973.

105. Harner CD, Höher J, Vogrin TM, Carlin GJ, Woo SL. The effects of a popliteus muscle load on in situ forces in the posterior cruciate ligament and on knee kinematics: A human cadaveric study. *American Journal of Sports Medicine* 26(5):669–673, 1998.

106. Shahane SA, Ibbotson C, Strachan R, Bickerstaff DR. The popliteofibular ligament: An anatomical study of the posterolateral corner of the knee. *Journal of Bone and Joint Surgery Br* 81:636–642, 1999.

107. Peck D, Buxton DF, Nitz A. A comparison of spindle concentrations in large and small muscles acting in parallel combinations. *Journal of Morphology* 180(3):243–252, 1984.

108. Prilutsky BI. Coordination of two- and one-joint muscles: Functional consequences and implications for motor control. *Motor Control* 4(1):1–44, 2000.

109. Bobbert MF, van Soest AJ. Two-joint muscles offer the solution, but what was the problem? *Motor Control* 4(1):48–52, 2000.

110. Elftman H. Biomechanics of muscle with particular application to studies of gait. *Journal of Bone and Joint Surgery Am* 48(2):363–377, 1966.

111. Hof AL. The force resulting from the action of mono- and biarticular muscles in a limb. *Journal of Biomechanics* 34(8):1085–1089, 2001.

112. van Ingen Schenau GJ, Bobbert MF, Rozendal RH. The unique action of biarticular muscles in complex movements. *Journal of Anatomy* 155(1):1–5, 1987.

113. McNitt-Gray JL. Subject specific coordination of two- and one-joint muscles during landings suggests multiple control criteria. *Motor Control* 4(1):84–88, 2000.

114. Nozaki D. Torque interaction among adjacent joints due to the action of biarticular muscles. *Medicine & Science in Sport & Exercise* 41(1):205–209, 2009.

115. Davies GJ, Wallace LA, Malone T. Mechanisms of selected knee injuries. *Physical Therapy* 60(12):1590–1595, 1980.

116. Smidt GL. Biomechanical analysis of knee flexion and extension. *Journal of Biomechanics* 6(1):79–92, 1973.

117. Wimby CR, Lloyd DG, Besier TF, Kirk TB. Muscle and external load contribution to knee joint contact loads during normal gait. *Journal of Biomechanics* 42(14):2294–2300, 2009.

118. Kettlekamp DB, Jacobs AW. Tibiofemoral contact area—Determination and implications. *Journal of Bone and Joint Surgery Am* 54(2):349–356, 1972.

119. Nisell R. Mechanics of the knee: A study of joint and muscle load with clinical applications. *Acta Orthopaedica Scandinavica: Supplementum* 216:1–42, 1985.

120. Beynnon B, Johnson R, Fleming B, Stankewich C, Renstrom P, Nichols C. The strain behavior of the anterior cruciate ligament during squatting and active flexion-extension: A comparison of an open and a closed kinetic chain exercise. *American Journal of Sports Medicine* 25(6):823–829, 1997.

121. Fleming BC, Oksendahl H, Beynnon BD. Open or closed kinetic chain exercises after anterior cruciate ligament reconstruction? *Exercise and Sport Sciences Reviews* 33(3):134–140, 2005.

122. Shrive NG, O'Connor JJ, Goodfellow JW. Load-bearing in the knee joint. *Clinical Orthopaedics and Related Research* 131:279–287, 1978.

123. Kurosawa H, Fukubayashi T, Nakajima H. Load-bearing mode of the knee joint: Physical behavior of the knee joint with and without menisci. *Clinical Orthopaedics and Related Research* 149:283–290, 1980.

124. Rangger C, Kathrein A, Klestil T, Gloetzer W. Partial meniscectomy and osteoarthritis: Implications for athletes. *Sports Medicine* 23(1):61–68, 1997.

125. Bourne R, Mukhi S, Zhu N, Keresteci M, Marin M. Role of obesity on the risk for total hip or knee arthroplasty. *Clinical Orthopaedics and Related Research* 465:185–188, 2007.

126. Kaufer H. Mechanical function of the patella. *Journal of Bone and Joint Surgery Am* 53(8):1551–1560, 1971.

127. Steinkamp LA, Dillingham MF, Markel MD, Hill JA, Kaufman KR. Biomechanical considerations in patellofemoral joint rehabilitation. *American Journal of Sports Medicine* 21:438–444, 1993.

128. Buchbinder MR, Napora NJ, Biggs EW. The relationship of abnormal pronation to chondromalacia of the patella in distance runners. *Journal of the American Podiatry Association* 69(2):159–162, 1979.

129. Mendler HM. Postoperative function of the knee joint. *Journal of the American Physical Therapy Association* 43:435–441, 1963.

130. Mendler HM. Knee extensor and flexor force following injury. *Physical Therapy* 47(1):35–45, 1967.

131. Williams M, Stutzman L. Strength variation through the range of joint motion. *Physical Therapy Review* 39(3):145–152, 1959.

132. Westring SH, Seger JY. Eccentric and concentric torque-velocity characteristics, torque output comparisons, and gravity effect torque corrections for the quadriceps and hamstring muscles in females. *International Journal of Sports Medicine* 10(3):175–180, 1989.

133. Schmitz RJ, Kim H, Shultz SJ. Effect of axial load on anterior tibial translation when transitioning from non-weight bearing to weight bearing. *Clinical Biomechanics* 25(1):77–82, 2010.

134. Hurley MV. The role of muscle weakness in the pathogenesis of osteoarthritis. *Rheumatic Diseases Clinics of North America* 25(2):283–298, 1999.

135. Slemenda C, Brandt KD, Heilman DK, et al. Quadriceps weakness and osteoarthritis of the knee. *Annals of Internal Medicine* 127(2):97–104, 1997.

136. Van der heijden MM, Meijer K, Willems PJ, Savelberg HH. Muscles limiting the sit-to-stand movement: An experimental simulation of muscle weakness. *Gait & Posture* 30(1):110–114, 2009.

137. Hiemstra LA, Webber S, MacDonald PB, Kriellaars DJ. Hamstring and quadriceps strength balance in normal and hamstring anterior cruciate ligament-reconstructed subjects. *Clinical Journal of Sports Medicine* 14(5): 274–280, 2004.

138. Lehmkuhl LD, Smith LK. *Brunnstrom's Clinical Kinesiology*, ed 4. Philadelphia: FA Davis, 1983.

139. Davies GJ. Isokinetic approach to the knee. In Mangine RE (ed): *Physical Therapy of the Knee*, New York: Churchill Livingstone, pp. 221–243, 1988.

140. Fillyaw M, Bevins T, Fernandez L. Importance of correcting isokinetic peak torque for the effect of gravity when calculating knee flexor to extensor muscle ratios. *Physical Therapy* 66(1):23–31, 1986.

141. Ahmad CS, Clark AM, Heilmann N, Schoeb JS, Gardner TR, Levine WN. Effect of gender and maturity on quadriceps-to-hamstring strength ratio and anterior cruciate ligament laxity. *American Journal of Sports Medicine* 34(3):370–374, 2006.

142. Barrack RL, Lund PJ, Skinner HB. Knee joint proprioception revisited. *Journal of Sport Rehabilitation* 3:18–42, 1994.

143. Jerosch J, Prymka M. Knee joint proprioception in normal volunteers and patients with anterior cruciate ligament tears, taking special account of the effect of a knee bandage. *Archives of Orthopaedic and Traumatic Surgery* 115:162–166, 1996.

144. Hewett T, Paterno M, Myer G. Strategies for enhancing proprioception and neuromuscular control of the knee. *Clinical Orthopaedics* 402:76–94, 2002.

145. Lephart SM, Kocher MS, Fu FH, Borsa PA, Harner CD. Proprioception following ACL reconstruction. *Journal of Sports Rehabilitation* 1:188–196, 1992.

146. Beard DJ, Dodd CA, Trundle HR, Simpson AH. Proprioception enhancement for anterior cruciate ligament deficiency: A prospective randomised trial of two physiotherapy regimes. *Journal of Bone and Joint Surgery Br* 76(4):654–659, 1994.

147. Risberg MA, Beynnon BD, Peura GD, Uh BS. Proprioception after anterior cruciate ligament reconstruction with and without bracing. *Knee Surgery, Sports Traumatology, Arthroscopy* 7(5):303–309, 1999.

148. Roberts D, Zätterström R, Lindstrand A, Fridén T, Moritz U. Proprioception in people with anterior cruciate ligament-deficient knees: Comparison of symptomatic and asymptomatic patients. *Journal of Orthopaedic and Sports Physical Therapy* 29(10):587–594, 1999.

149. Risberg M, Mork M, Jenssen H, Holm I. Design and implementation of a neuromuscular training program following anterior cruciate ligament reconstruction. *Journal of Orthopaedic and Sports Physical Therapy* 31(11):620–631, 2001.

150. Beynnon BD, Good L, Risberg MA. The effect of bracing on proprioception of knees with anterior cruciate ligament injury. *Journal of Orthopaedic and Sports Physical Therapy* 32(1):11–15, 2002.

151. Cascio BM, Culp L, Cosgarea AJ. Return to play after anterior cruciate ligament reconstruction. *Clinics in Sports Medicine* 23(3):395–408, 2004.

152. Kennedy JC, Alexander IJ, Hayes KC. Nerve supply of the human knee and its functional importance. *American Journal of Sports Medicine* 10(6):329–335, 1982.

153. Schutte MJ, Dabezies EJ, Zimny ML, Happel LT. Neural anatomy of the human anterior cruciate ligament. *Journal of Bone and Joint Surgery Am* 69(2):243–247, 1987.

154. Solomonow M, Baratta R, Zhou BH, et al. The synergistic action of the anterior cruciate ligament and thigh muscles in maintaining joint stability. *American Journal of Sports Medicine* 15(3):207–213, 1987.

155. Spencer JD, Hayes KC, Alexander IJ. Knee joint effusion and quadriceps reflex inhibition in man. *Archives of Physical Medicine and Rehabilitation* 64:171–177, 1984.

156. Fahrer H, Rentsch HU, Gerber NJ, Beyeler C, Hess CW, Grunig B. Knee effusion and reflex inhibition of the quadriceps: A bar to effective retraining. *Journal of Bone & Joint Surgery* 70:635–638, 1988.

157. Bolgla LA, Keskula DR. A review of the relationship among knee effusion, quadriceps inhibition, and knee function. *Journal of Sport Rehabilitation* 9(2):160–168, 2000.

158. Torry MR, Decker MJ, Viola RW, O'Connor DD, Steadman JR. Intra-articular knee joint effusion induces quadriceps avoidance gait patterns. *Clinical Biomechanics* 15:147–159, 2000.

159. Meunier A, Odensten M, Good L. Long term results after primary repair or nonsurgical treatment of anterior cruciate ligament rupture: A randomized study with a 15-year follow-up. *Scandinavian Journal of Medicine and Science in Sports* 17(3):230–237, 2007.

160. Barrack RL, Skinner HB, Buckley SL. Proprioception in the anterior cruciate deficient knee. *American Journal of Sports Medicine* 17:1–6, 1989.

161. Lofvenberg R, Karrholm J, Sundelin G, Ahlgren O. Prolonged reaction time in patients with chronic lateral instability of the ankle. *American Journal of Sports Medicine* 23:414–417, 1995.

162. Myer G, Paterno M, Ford K, Quatman C, Hewett T. Rehabilitation after anterior cruciate ligament reconstruction: Criteria-based progression through the return-to-sport phase. *Journal of Orthopaedic and Sports Physical Therapy* 36(6):385–402, 2006.

163. Laskowski ER, Newcomer-Aney K, Smith J. Proprioception. *Physical Medicine and Rehabilitation Clinics of North America* 11(2):323–340, 2000.

164. Recondo JA, Salvador E, Villanúa JA, Barrera MC, Gervás C, Alústiza JM. Lateral stabilizing structures of the knee: Functional anatomy and injuries assessed with MR imaging. *Radiographics* 20:S91–S102, 2000.

165. Lass P, Kaalund S, LeFevre S, Arendt-Nielsen L, Sinkjaer T, Simonsen O. Muscle coordination following rupture of the anterior cruciate ligament. *Acta Orthopaedica Scandinavica* 62(1):9–14, 1991.

166. Ihara H, Nakayama A. Dynamic joint control training for knee ligament injuries. *American Journal of Sports Medicine* 14(4):309–315, 1986.

167. Bard G. Energy expenditure of hemiplegic subjects during walking. *Archives of Physical Medicine and Rehabilitation* 44:368–370, 1963.

168. Brinkman J-M, Schwering PJA, Blankevoort L, Koolos JG, Luites J, Wymenga AB. The insertion geometry of the posterolateral corner of the knee. *Journal of Bone and Joint Surgery Br* 87(10):1364–1368, 2005.

169. Veltri DM, Deng XH, Torzilla PA, Maynard MJ, Warren RF. The role of the popliteofibular ligament in stability of the human knee: A biomechanical study. *American Journal of Sports Medicine* 24(1):19–27, 1996.

CHAPTER 11

Ankle and Foot

"Progress always involves risks. You can't steal second base and keep your foot on first."
—Frederick B. Wilcox, American Author

CHAPTER OUTLINE

Learning Outcomes
Clinical Scenario
Introduction
Bones
Leg Bones
Tarsal Bones
Metatarsal Bones
Phalanges
Joints
Motion Terminology
Tibiofibular Joints
Talocrural Joint
Subtalar Joint
Transverse Tarsal Joint
Tarsometatarsal Joints
Intermetatarsal Joints
Metatarsophalangeal and Interphalangeal Joints
Muscles of the Ankle and Foot
Posterior Group of Muscles
Lateral Group of Muscles
Anterior Group of Muscles
Intrinsic Muscles of the Foot
Function of Leg and Foot Muscles and Joints
Pronation and Supination
Arches of the Foot
Loading of the Foot
Deformities of the Foot
Summary
Clinical Scenario Solution
Discussion Questions
Lab Activities
References

LEARNING OUTCOMES

This chapter investigates the ankle and foot complex. By the end of this chapter, you should be able to:

- ❑ Identify the bones, joints, soft tissue, and muscles of the foot and ankle complex;
- ❑ Discuss the relationship between the rearfoot and midfoot and their contribution to functional movement;
- ❑ List muscles of the anterior, lateral, superficial posterior calf, and deep posterior calf;
- ❑ Discuss the influence of the foot position during gait;
- ❑ Describe the windlass function of the foot and provide examples of its use;
- ❑ Describe commonly encountered movement disorders of the foot and how they impact the rest of the joints during closed chain function.

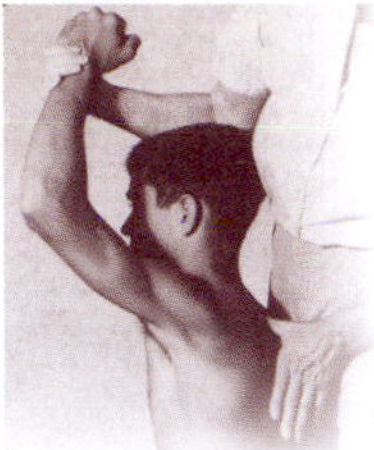

CLINICAL SCENARIO

Chaz Michaels graduated last spring and has been working at his first professional job for about six months. Today he is scheduled to work with a patient who has pain from plantar fasciitis. Although he saw a couple of patients with this diagnosis as a student, this will be the first one he will treat on his own. He feels he knows what the examination process will include, but he is nervous about it just the same. He wants to be prepared for what he might find, so he starts to make a mental review of the items he will include in his assessment.

Introduction

The ankle and foot is a complex system. It consists of 26 bones, 34 joints, and over 100 muscles, tendons, and ligaments. The ankle and foot joints can change within a single step from a flexible structure conforming to the irregularities of any terrain to a rigid weight-bearing structure in fractions of a second. The flexible-rigid characteristics of the ankle and foot complex provide many important, daily functions, including:

- Support of the body's weight;
- Control and stabilization of the leg on the planted foot;
- Adjustments to irregular surfaces;
- Compensation for more proximal segment malalignment or pathomechanics;
- Elevation of the body, as in standing on the toes, climbing, or jumping;
- Shock absorption in walking, running, or landing from a jump;
- Operation of machine tools; and
- Substitution for hand functions in persons with upper extremity amputations or muscle paralysis.

Ankle injuries, foot pain, and ankle and foot dysfunctions are common and result from the large forces that occur in the foot and ankle, even in quiet standing. Ankle joint forces up to 4.5 times body weight occur when walking on a level surface.[1] As the foot sustains these large forces, it is also making final adjustments to the terrain and must compensate for motions or deviations at the knee or hip to keep the center of gravity within the small base of support. When the foot is not protected by a shoe, it is subjected to trauma and temperature extremes. If the foot is enclosed in a shoe, it may be subjected to abnormal pressures and friction, as well as to a warm, humid environment conducive to bacterial and fungal growth, other infections, and skin breakdown.

Bones

There are 26 bones of the foot and ankle. These bones are divided into the leg, tarsals, metatarsals, and phalanges (Fig. 11.1). The leg bones include the tibia and fibula. There are seven tarsal bones, five metatarsal bones, and 14 phalanges.

Leg Bones

The tibia bears about 90% of the body weight whereas the fibula is essentially considered a nonweight-bearing bone, carrying only 10% of the body weight. Such a minimal amount of weight borne by the fibula allows an individual to ambulate on a fractured fibula with minimal or no pain.

Tibia

The tibia is easily palpated from the tibial tuberosity then distally along the anterior ridge, or "shin." Since its medial aspect is not covered by muscle, it is also palpated along its length to the proximal ankle. The most distal aspect of the tibia is the **medial malleolus** (L., diminutive of *malleus,* hammer). It is a prominent process of the enlarged distal portion of the tibia that forms a prominent landmark on the medial side of the ankle. Although the lateral aspect of the medial malleolus articulates with the talus, it is not a weight-bearing portion of the tibia.

The tibial shaft is rotated laterally in the transverse plane as it traverses distally. By the time the body matures in adulthood, the lateral rotation has increased to anywhere from 15° to 40°.[2–4] This lateral rotation places the medial malleolus more anteriorly, and, in turn, this positions the foot in slight lateral rotation relative to the frontal plane during standing and walking.

The lateral aspect of the distal end of the tibia has a triangular-shaped concavity into which the fibula sits. The inferior aspect of the tibia is a saddle-shaped structure called the **plafond**. The plafond is the "ceiling" or distal end of the tibia which forms the

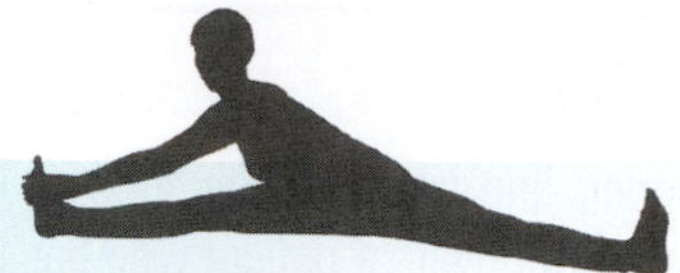

PRACTICE POINT

As infants, our shin bones are smooth. As we get older and begin creeping, crawling, walking, and running, we often hit the shin on any number of objects. Once we achieve our teen years, the shin is usually no longer smooth. Running your finger along your own shin, you are likely to realize the roughness of it. This roughness occurs as the shin is hit and receives contusions. Those contusions develop areas of swelling between the bone and periosteum covering it. Once the contusion heals, there is no pain, but there is the remnant of scar tissue; this is the roughness you feel under the shin.

proximal surface of the talocrural joint. The plafond is convex medially-to-laterally and concave anteriorly-to-posteriorly. It is this surface that bears 90% of the body's weight.

Fibula

The fibula is a small bone that serves primarily as a site for muscle and ligament attachments. The most distal end of the bone is the **lateral malleolus,** an easily observed landmark on the lateral aspect of the ankle. Palpation of the malleoli reveals that the lateral malleolus projects farther distally than the medial one. This more distal positioning causes lateral motion of the ankle to be more limited than medial motion. If the individual stands with the patella pointing straight forward with the knee in the

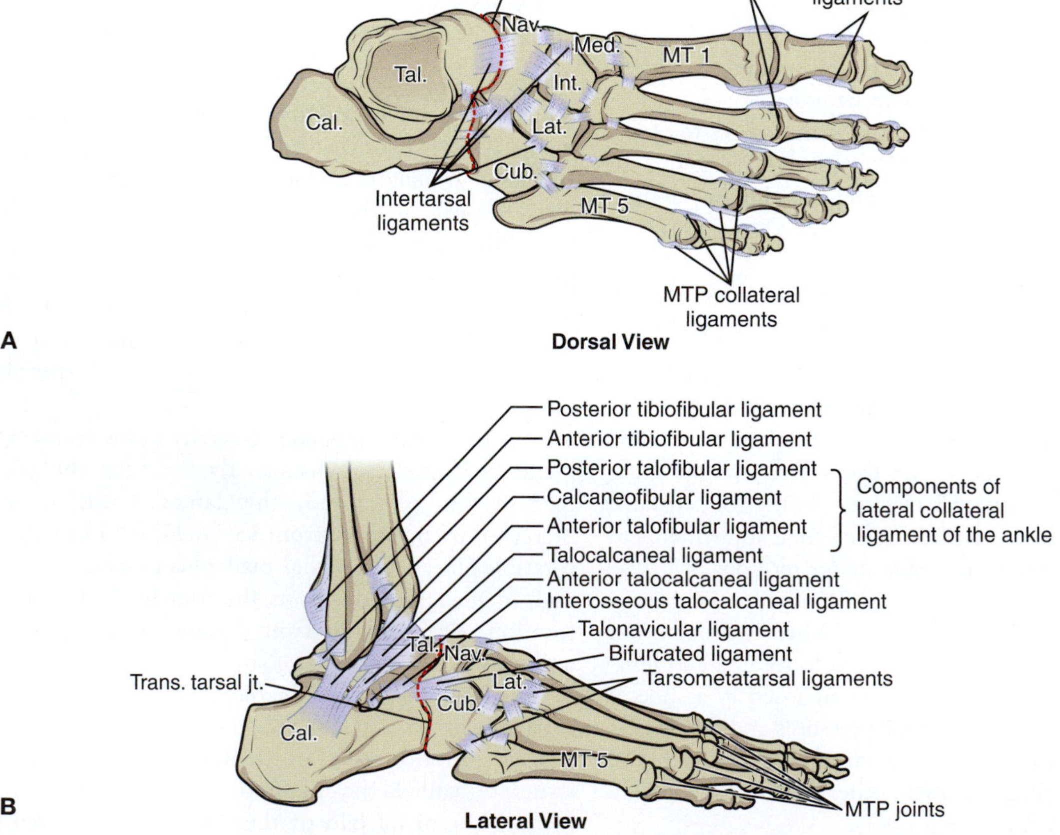

Figure 11.1 Bones of the foot and ankle. **A)** Dorsal view of the foot and ankle. **B)** Lateral view of the foot and ankle.

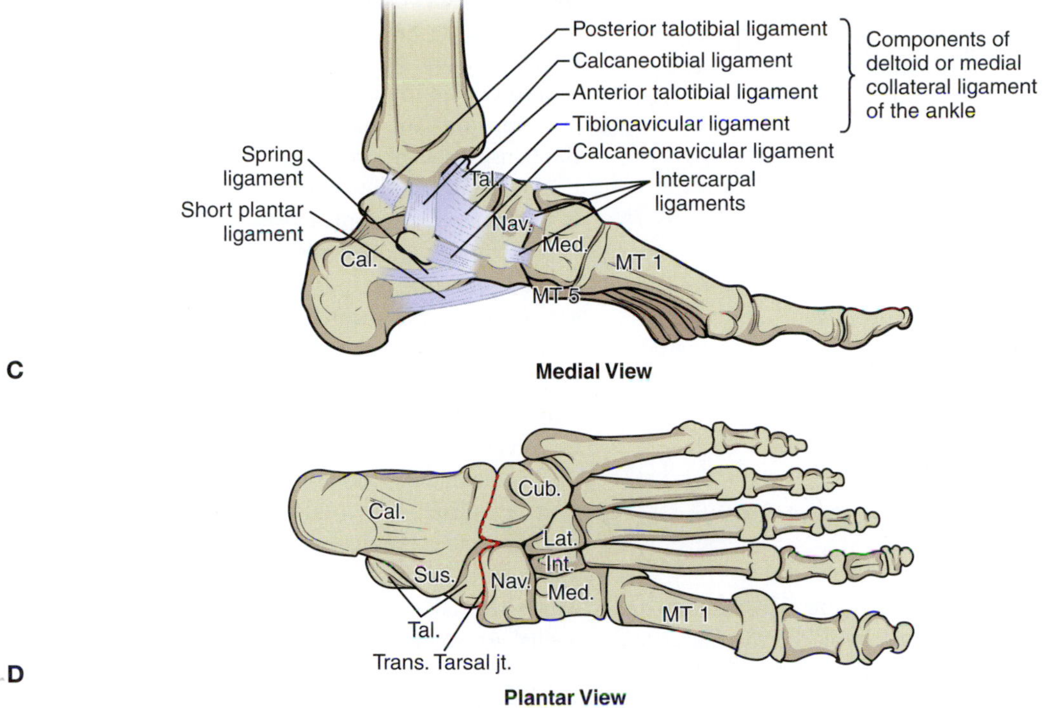

Figure 11.1—cont'd C) Medial ankle and foot ligaments. D) Plantar foot.

sagittal plane, it is easy to realize as it is palpated that the lateral malleolus lies in a more posterior position than the medial malleolus.

The more proximal aspect of the convex lateral malleolus is wedged within the fibular notch of the lateral distal tibia. The more distal aspect of the medial side of the lateral malleolus articulates with the talus.

Tarsal Bones

The foot is divided into three sections, the rearfoot, midfoot, and forefoot. The tarsal bones are divided into two sections of the foot, the **rearfoot** and the **midfoot**. The rearfoot comprises the talus and calcaneus whereas the midfoot includes the other five tarsal bones: the navicular, cuboid, and three cuneiforms. As we will learn later, the rearfoot plays an important role in motions and positions of the midfoot. The bones of the foot and the associated ligaments form three arches: the **medial longitudinal arch,** the smaller **lateral longitudinal arch,** and the **transverse arch.**

Talus

All of the body's weight is transferred through the talus during single limb weight-bearing. The talus is an unusual bone in several aspects. For one, it is one of the few bones of the body that has no muscle attachment to it. It is also oddly shaped because it connects the leg to the foot. Because it articulates with other bones on its superior, inferior, medial, lateral, and anterior aspects, more than half of its surface is covered with articular cartilage. The anterior portion of its body is the head with a short neck behind it that connects the head to the bone's body. The head is angled slightly medially to the sagittal plane (about 30°) to face the navicular. The superior aspect of the body is the dome of the talus. The dome is shaped to coincide with the saddle-shape of the inferior tibia; the dome is convex anteriorly-to-posteriorly and concave medially-to-laterally. The dome is a little wider anteriorly than it is posteriorly (Fig. 11.2).

Inferiorly, the talus articulates at three facets with the calcaneus, the anterior, medial, and posterior facets. The lateral and medial aspects of the talus articulate with the lateral and medial malleoli, respectively. The anterior aspect of the head of the talus articulates with the navicular. The medial posterior talus possesses a groove that is formed by the medial and lateral talar tubercles; running through this groove is the flexor hallucis longus tendon.

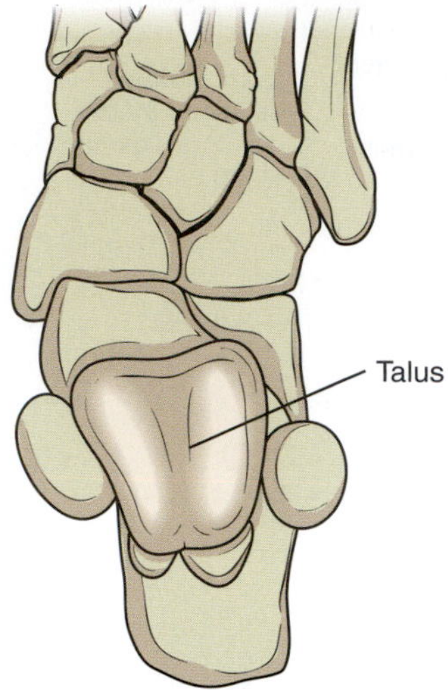

Figure 11.2 Talus is wider anteriorly than it is posteriorly.

The anterior aspect of the dome may be palpated with the subject's ankle passively placed in plantarflexion; the dome is palpated immediately distal to the articulation between the tibia and talus. Slightly distal and lateral to this point is a depression that lies over the **sinus tarsi,** which is a channel that runs between the articulations of the talus and the calcaneus. If the foot is inverted, the neck of the talus may become more prominent. The talus can also be palpated by placing the palpating finger between the navicular tuberosity and the distal end of the medial malleolus. The medial talus becomes more prominent when the foot is passively everted but then disappears as the foot is passively inverted. Immediately posterior to the distal end of the medial malleolus, the small prominence of the medial tubercle of the talus can sometimes be palpated.

Calcaneus

The other bone of the rearfoot is the calcaneus, the largest and strongest of the tarsal bones. The calcaneus sits inferior to, or under, the talus and articulates with it at three facets corresponding to those of the talus. The calcaneus is the first bone through which ground reaction forces are imparted during walking. The calcaneus also transmits the majority of the body's weight from the talus to the ground. The calcaneus is protected by a thick fat pad the lies between the bone and the skin. Unfortunately, as people age, the fat pad loses its thickness, so older individuals may have a difficult time standing for long periods. The rear aspect of the plantar surface of the calcaneus is the section that contacts the ground in weight-bearing. It is this section of the calcaneus that also provides the Achilles with a long moment arm so the calf muscle group is able to provide powerful forces for running and jumping.

It is the middle section of the calcaneus with which the talus articulates. This middle section also has a medial extension called the **sustentaculum tali** (L., *sustenataculum,* a support). The sustentaculum tali is a horizontal shelf on which the talus is supported. It supports the inferior medial aspect of the talus and where the two bones form one of their three articulations, the middle facet. Just distal to the tip of the medial malleolus, the edge of the sustentaculum tali may be felt as a slight protuberance (about the distance of a finger width).

Anteriorly, the calcaneus articulates with the cuboid (Fig. 11.1). There are two tubercles on the plantar surface of the posterior calcaneus: the medial and lateral tubercles. These serve as sites of insertion for the plantar fascia and several intrinsic foot muscles. The medial tubercle is the tubercle that is in contact with the ground during weight-bearing.[5]

Navicular

As its name implies, the navicular (L., *navicula,* diminutive of navis, ship) is a boat-shaped bone (Fig. 11.1). It lies between the head of the talus and the three cuneiforms. The navicular articulates with the talus posteriorly and the three cuneiforms anteriorly. Medially, it

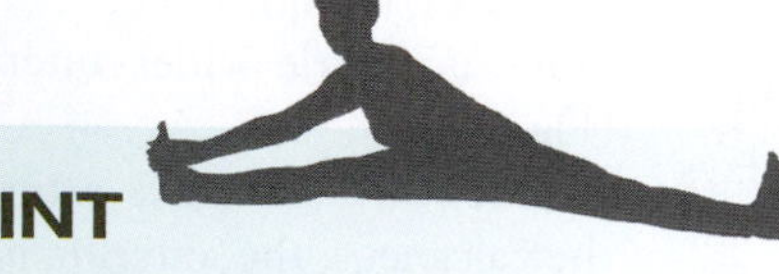

PRACTICE POINT

Elderly individuals often report heel pain with prolonged standing or walking. As mentioned, the fat pad thins as people age. It also flattens out with the repetitive stresses it receives from standing, walking, and running over the years. Clinicians may offer suggestions for these older individuals that may provide some relief to them. Wearing shoes with a little higher heel may relieve the direct stress upon the calcaneus with its diminished fat pad. Also, shoes that contain a deep seat for the heel may cup the heel, allowing the fat pad edges to conform more directly under the calcaneus and provide a little more padding where it is needed. Individuals who place most of their weight on their heels should be instructed to balance their weight more equally between the forefoot and rearfoot.

contains the navicular tuberosity. This tuberosity is prominent and palpated about a finger's width anterior to the sustentaculum tali. It may also be located about an inch in each direction inferiorly and anteriorly from the inferior aspect of the medial malleolus.

Three Cuneiforms

The three cuneiform (L., *cuneus,* wedge) bones are just anterior to the navicular (Fig. 11.1). They are so named because of their wedge shape. From medial to lateral, they are the medial, intermediate, and lateral cuneiforms. The cuneiforms lie across the instep of the foot to form the arched part of the dorsum of the foot, known as the transverse arch of the foot. The height of this arch varies considerably from one individual to another. The medial cuneiform bone is the largest of the three and identified by its medial position between the tuberosity of the navicular bone and the base of the first metatarsal bone. The intermediate and lateral cuneiform bones lie in line with the second and third metatarsal bones, respectively, articulating proximally with the navicular bone. The intermediate cuneiform is the smallest of the cuneiforms. The lateral cuneiform articulates with the medial cuboid.

Cuboid

As its name implies, this bone is six-sided. Three of its sides serve as articulations with other bones. Its posterior side articulates with the calcaneus; the medial side articulates with the lateral cuneiform; and the anterior side articulates with the fourth and fifth metatarsals (Fig. 11.1). Its lateral and plantar surfaces contain a groove through which the peroneus longus tendon travels to the plantar foot.

Metatarsal Bones

Whereas the tarsal bones make up the rearfoot and midfoot, the metatarsal and phalangeal bones comprise the **forefoot**. Similar to the metacarpal bones of the hand, there are five metatarsal bones of the foot. Although each metatarsal bone is similar to the others, there are some distinguishing characteristics among them. The metatarsals are numbered sequentially from medial to lateral, one through five. The first metatarsal is the shortest but thickest of the five; the second is the thinnest and longest. The second metatarsal is firmly wedged at its proximal end by the cuneiforms and the metatarsal bones on either side of it, making it the most securely anchored of the metatarsals. The fourth metatarsal is positioned more posteriorly relative to the third metatarsal, and the fifth metatarsal is the most posteriorly positioned of the metatarsals (Fig. 11.1). The fifth metatarsal has a tuberosity on its lateral aspect and is the site of the insertion for the peroneus brevis tendon. This tuberosity at the base of the fifth metatarsal bone may be felt as a large, easily identified prominence on the lateral side of the foot near the sole just distal to the indentation of the cuboid.

Each metatarsal has a base, shaft, and convex head with the base larger than the head. The structure of each of these metatarsals is similar, albeit different in size. Each metatarsal articulates with the distal row of tarsal bones proximally at its base, with the metatarsal on its proximal medial and lateral sides, and with the proximal phalanx at its head. The metatarsal shafts are concavely arched on the plantar aspect; this is important since it allows for increased load absorption by the metatarsals during weight-bearing. Immediately posterior to the first metatarsal head's plantar surface are two small grooves within which two sesamoid bones are contained. The fibrous sheath of the flexor hallucis longus tendon attaches to them.[6] Although the flexor hallucis longus tendon runs between them, the abductor and adductor hallucis tendons do insert into these sesamoids.[6] The sesamoids serve to protect and guide the flexor hallucis longus tendon and protect the first metatarsal head by absorbing shock. They also serve to increase the moment arm of the flexor hallucis brevis, absorb weight-bearing forces, and reduce friction.[7]

The heads of the metatarsal bones are felt both on the dorsal and the plantar aspects of the foot. By passively moving the toes in flexion and extension, the heads of the metatarsal bones are particularly easily palpated on the plantar foot. Their plantar surfaces constitute the ball of the foot on which weight is carried when standing on tiptoes. In the region immediately proximal to the head of the first metatarsal bone, the sesamoid bones, especially the medial one, can sometimes be palpated and moved slightly from side to side. The shafts of the metatarsal bones are best palpated on the dorsum of the foot.

Phalanges

As in the hand, there are 14 phalangeal bones, two in the great, or first toe, and three in each of the remaining lateral toes. They, along with the metatarsals comprise the forefoot. Each phalange has a concave base proximally, a small shaft and a convex head distally. The great toe has a proximal and a distal phalange whereas the lateral toes have proximal, middle, and distal phalanges. The heads of the proximal phalanges are trochlear, which fit into the bases of their adjacent phalanges. The middle phalanges are broader than the proximal phalanges but shorter whereas the distal phalanges are flatter and smaller. These bones are easily palpated in the toes.

Joints

The 26 bones of the foot and ankle comprise 34 joints. Many of these bones and joints may be compared to those of the wrist and hand. However, the joints of the foot serve primarily weight-bearing functions and are able to create or compensate for pathologies more proximal in the kinematic chain. As we go through the joints of the foot, we will focus on the joints that produce overall foot motion. Keep in mind, however, that there are also joints between adjacent bones that will not be discussed. For example, we will later discuss the tarsometatarsal joints, the articulations between the distal row of tarsal bones and the metatarsals, but there are also joints between the cuneiform bones and between the lateral cuneiform and cuboid. There is also an articulation between the navicular and cuboid. These joints have little if any motion during functional foot movement, so we do not take the time to discuss them but realize that they are present. From a kinesiological perspective, they do not impact functional motion unless they have suffered pathology. In rare instances when the ligaments connecting these joints together are injured, the clinician must appreciate this anatomy.

Since many of the joints of the foot and ankle are not in a pure plane but rather are oblique to the pure plane, the motions of these joints are actually multiplanar. These motions have names that are unique to the foot and ankle complex. Before we can discuss the various joints, it is important that these motions are identified and defined.

Motion Terminology

As we will realize shortly, the axes of motions of the foot and ankle are skewed from the pure planes of movement that we have come to know. In other words, the axes of motions are oblique to these traditional planes of motion. As a result, the movements that occur around these axes are not pure flexion-extension, abduction-adduction, or medial rotation-lateral rotation. Since these axes of motions are different from the traditional motions, the names of these motions are also different. These motions were presented in Chapter 1 and are briefly repeated here as points of review. Movements of the foot and ankle that occur close to the sagittal plane around a medial-lateral axis are dorsiflexion and plantarflexion. **Dorsiflexion** occurs as the two segments of the joint move closer together. In the pure sagittal plane this motion is known as flexion. **Plantarflexion** occurs when the two segments move farther apart. Extension is the term familiar and equivalent to plantarflexion. Ankle and foot joints also move in a frontal plane around an anterior-posterior axis. These motions include inversion and eversion. **Inversion** motion is a rotation movement so the bottom of the foot rolls to face the opposite limb. **Eversion** is the opposite motion; the plantar foot rolls laterally to face away from the opposite limb. The final motions occur in a transverse plane around a vertical (superior-inferior) axis. These motions are abduction and adduction, similarly named to the more traditional movements but occurring in a different plane around a different axis than abduction and adduction as we normally think of them. Throughout other body segments, abduction and adduction occur in the frontal plane, but in the foot, they occur in the transverse plane around a vertical axis. In the foot, **abduction** is the motion of the foot away from the midline whereas **adduction** occurs when the foot moves towards the midline. These motions are depicted in Figure 11.3.

Although these individual motions are often measured clinically, they are not functional movements. Functional motion usually incorporates all three movements simultaneously. A single joint axis that is not perpendicular to the cardinal planes but intersects all three planes is called a **triplanar axis.**[8] Motion around this axis occurs in all three planes. In the foot and ankle, these triaxial motions are called pronation and supination. **Pronation** and **supination** are the triaxial motions that include plantarflexion or dorsiflexion, inversion or eversion, and abduction or adduction occurring at one time (Fig. 11.4). The reason the talocrural joint and, more markedly, the subtalar joint function in triplanar motions is that their axes are oblique to true planes of motion. The combined motions that occur during pronation or supination vary depending on whether the foot is in an open or closed kinetic chain. For now, we will describe the combined motions making up pronation and supination in the open kinetic chain. Under an open kinetic chain condition, the combined movements of eversion, abduction, and dorsiflexion produce pronation whereas supination occurs with the combined movements of inversion, adduction, and plantarflexion. Pronation and supination are discussed in more detail later in this chapter.

Tibiofibular Joints

There are two joints that firmly hold tibia and fibula to each other: the proximal tibiofibular joint and the distal tibiofibular joint. The interosseous membrane, a sheet of dense connective tissue, also runs between the two bones and assists in maintaining alignment of the two bones. It also serves as a site of attachment of several leg muscles. Although the proximal or superior tibiofibular joint is a synovial joint, the distal or inferior

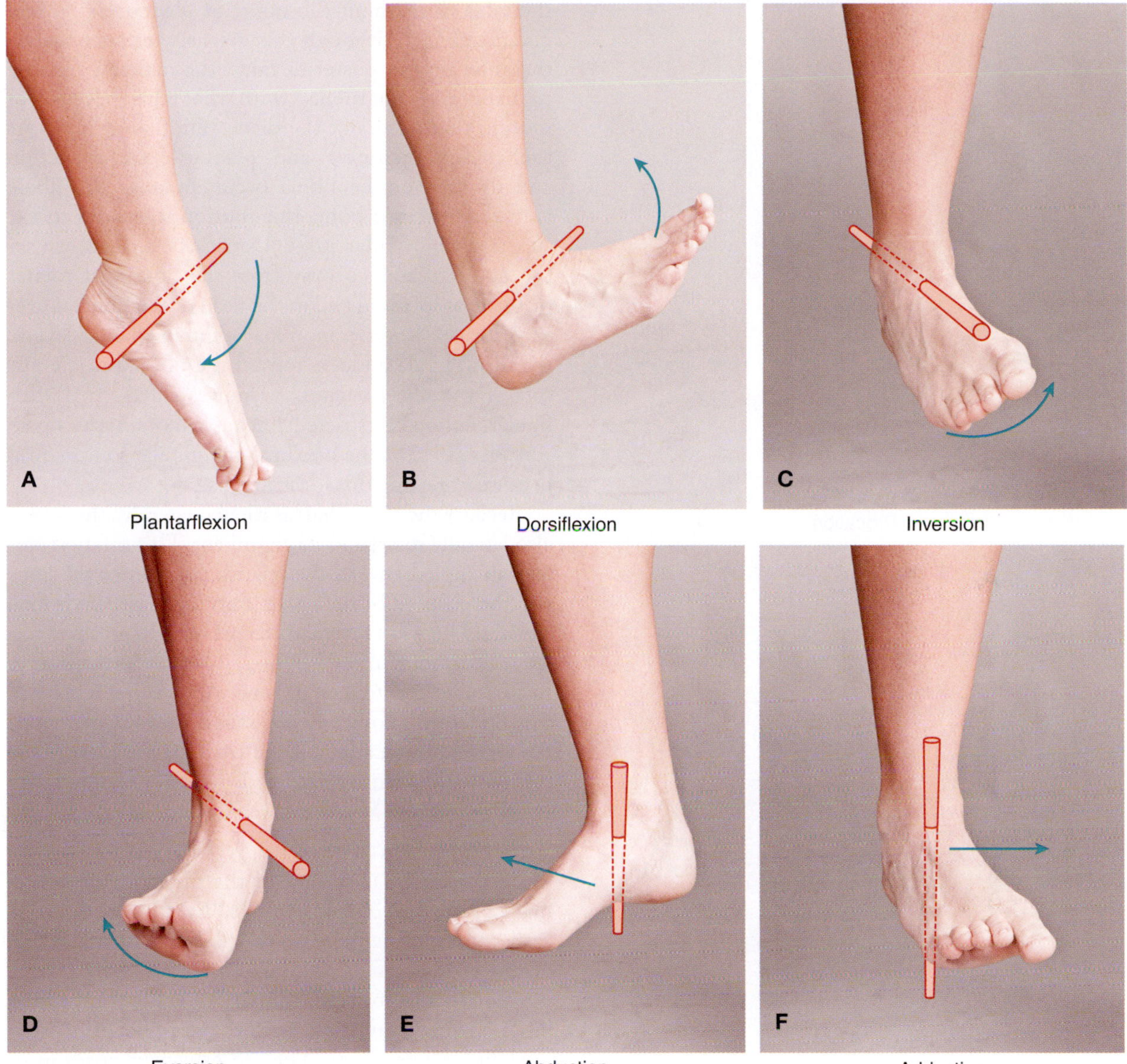

Figure 11.3 Motions of the talocrural and subtalar joints: A & B) plantarflexion-dorsiflexion; C & D) inversion-eversion; E & F) and abduction-adduction.

tibiofibular joint is a syndesmosis (Gr., *syndemos,* band or ligament) joint. Because the distal tibiofibular joint is a fibrous joint, the primary structure holding this joint together is the interosseous ligament, which is an extension of the distal interosseous membrane. The anterior and posterior tibiofibular ligaments also provide support to the distal tibiofibular joint.

Kinematics

Although the proximal tibiofibular joint is just distal to the knee joint, it is not impacted by the knee but rather by the ankle. Movement at this joint occurs with dorsiflexion and plantarflexion ankle motions as the fibula moves relative to the tibia. Although the motions of these two joints are only a few degrees, their movement is vital to the motions of ankle dorsiflexion and plantarflexion.

At the superior tibiofibular joint, motion is restrained by the distal attachments of the biceps femoris tendon, the lateral collateral ligament, and the tendon of the popliteus muscle as well as the tibiofibular ligaments and the fascia. Slight gliding movement in the joint can be felt when the ankle dorsiflexes. Knee injuries or surgery treated with immobilization can lead

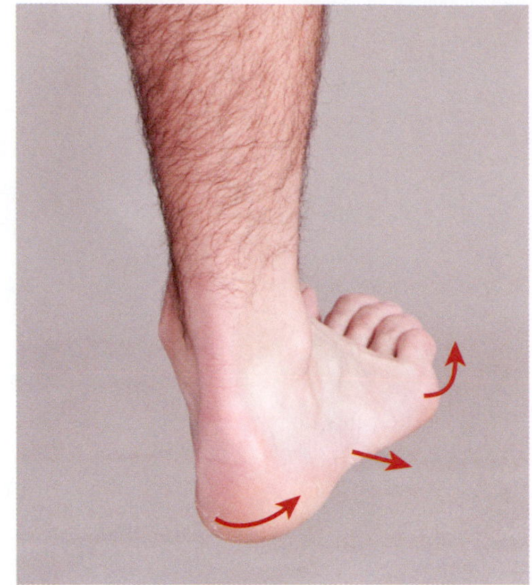

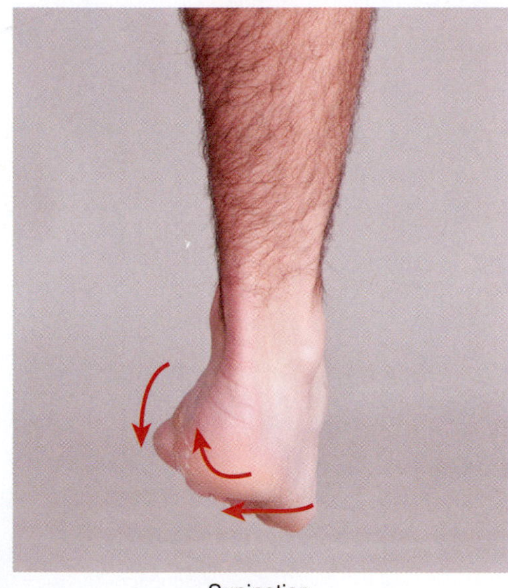

Figure 11.4 Supination and pronation are triaxial motion of the foot and ankle. These shown are in the open kinetic chain. **A)** Pronation includes the motions of eversion, abduction, and dorsiflexion. **B)** Supination includes the motions of inversion, adduction, and plantarflexion.

to restricted motion in the superior tibiofibular joint, which results in limitation of ankle dorsiflexion. The importance of the superior tibiofibular joint is described by Helfet[9] and its clinical relevance is presented by Radakovich and Malone[10] as the "forgotten joint."

Although the talar dome is wider anteriorly than posteriorly, the malleoli maintain congruence with the talus throughout the range of plantarflexion and dorsiflexion.[11] Although this disparity exists between the anterior and posterior talus, the malleoli are able to maintain congruency with the talus because of motion that occurs at the distal tibiofibular joint. As the ankle dorsiflexes and plantarflexes, abduction and rotation of the fibula occur; because the fibula is one continuous bone, this motion translates to the superior tibiofibular joint. Dorsiflexion, then, causes the fibula to abduct away from the tibia as it rotates medially at its distal end as the head of the fibula moves superiorly.[12] Reverse motions occur in plantarflexion: the distal fibula adducts toward the tibia as it laterally rotates and the fibular head moves inferiorly. If this fibular motion is restricted, full ankle motion is not possible. End feel of the proximal tibiofibular joint is firm because of ligamentous restrictions.

Because the tibial shaft is rotated laterally, the foot is also laterally rotated in its alignment. This rotation creates an angle between the relative position of the knee and the position of the ankle. This angle is called **tibial torsion**. There are several different ways to measure this angle of alignment.[13–17] Because of the numerous ways to measure tibial torsion, it is no wonder that reports in the literature show a wide range of measurements. Average values in adults range from 20° to 23° of tibial torsion with extensive variations in the literature ranging from –4° to +56°.[2,11,14,16,17]

Arthrokinematics

Since the articular surface of the fibula at the proximal tibiofibular joint is concave, it abides by the concave-convex principle. The roll and glide of the fibula on the tibia occur in the same direction. The resting position for the joint is about 10° of ankle plantarflexion. The knee joint position does not impact the proximal tibiofibular joint. The close-packed position of the proximal tibiofemoral joint is full dorsiflexion. Gliding motion of the tibia within this joint is minimal. With the medial and lateral malleoli stabilized in one hand, the talus can be moved passively in a posterior or anterior direction and distracted a few millimeters. Two to three millimeters of motion are considered normal.[18]

Talocrural Joint

The talocrural joint is commonly referred to as the ankle joint. The talocrural joint, between the talus and the **crus** (L., leg), is a hinge joint with one degree of freedom of motion. As previously mentioned, the trochlea of the talar dome is the superior weight-bearing surface that articulates with the distal end of the tibia whereas the medial and lateral surfaces articulate with the medial malleolus of the tibia and the lateral malleolus of the fibula, respectively. Because the tibiofibular ligaments hold the tibia and fibula firmly in place, their malleoli form a strong mortise for the trochlea of the wedge-shaped talus (Fig. 11.5).

The joint has a thin capsule surrounding it. There are anterior and posterior folds within the capsule to allow for the joint's sagittal plane motions. The capsule is reinforced medially and laterally by ligaments. The medial collateral ligament is also known as the deltoid ligament. It is a large structure that has superficial and deep components. Its purpose is to restrict end range eversion, or valgus tilting of the ankle.[18] Although they are difficult to delineate, the deltoid ligament has three large primary segments to it. Table 11–1 lists the ligaments of the talocrural joint.

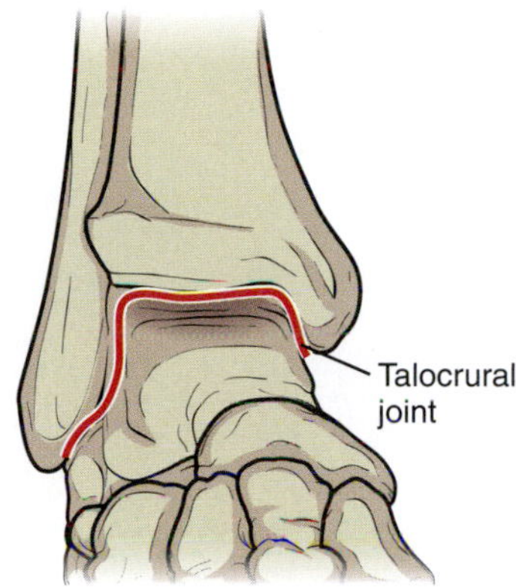

Figure 11.5 Talocrural joint. This joint is composed of the talus, tibia, and fibula. This joint is commonly referred to as a mortise joint because of its design.

Lateral collateral ligaments of the talocrural joint are not as strong or as melded together as those on the joint's medial aspect. These ligaments include the anterior and posterior talofibular ligaments and the calcaneofibular ligament. Although the anterior talofibular ligament is a flat band and rather weak, the calcaneofibular and posterior talofibular ligaments are stronger and thicker. The anterior talofibular ligament passes over the sinus tarsi on the anterolateral ankle and is the most often injured of these ligaments; injury to this ligament occurs when the ankle is plantarflexed and a varus or adduction stress is applied to it, as when an individual jumps up and lands on another person's foot.

Kinematics

A line connecting points just distal to the tips of the malleoli is the approximate ankle joint axis. When the medial-lateral axis of the knee is perpendicular to the midline of the body in the sagittal plane, the tip of the medial malleolus is usually anterior and superior

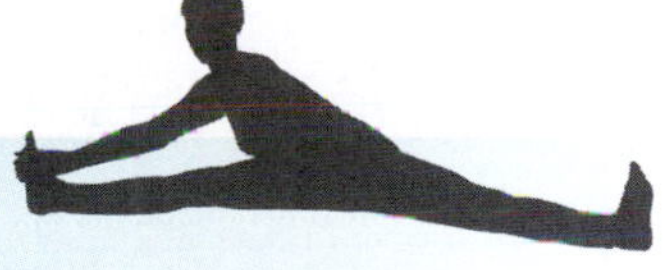

PRACTICE POINT

Injury to the anterior tibiofibular ligament is a common injury, and unfortunately, it can be a very significant injury. Unlike the other ligaments in the ankle region, the anterior tibiofibular ligament is stressed with each step an individual takes. When weight is borne on the foot, the ligament is stressed as the weight-bearing force on the talus tends to wedge the tibia and fibula apart. When this ligament is injured, it is stressed with each step. If the injury is not recognized and steps taken to protect it, especially during the first several days following injury, the individual may suffer prolonged pain and discomfort since the ligament is not allowed to heal properly, receiving repetitive stress with each step taken.

When an individual suffers a lateral collateral ligament injury of the ankle, occasionally a "goose egg" swelling about the size of a table tennis ball or golf ball occurs over the anterolateral ankle. Blood vessels coming off the lateral malleolar and lateral tarsal vessels lie within the sinus tarsi. If this goose egg appears rapidly following a sprain, it is likely that some of these vessels have ruptured. Within several hours, the goose egg disappears and is replaced by generalized edema and ecchymosis around the ankle.

(text continues on page 489)

TABLE 11-1 | LIGAMENTS OF THE ANKLE AND FOOT COMPLEX

Figure	Joint	Ligament	Proximal Attachment	Distal Attachment	Functions
	Talocrural and subtalar	Deltoid (medial collateral) ligament	Medial malleolus of the tibia	Fan-like attachment forms four ligaments: 1) to anterior medial talus (anterior tibiotalar ligament); 2) to sustentaculum tali of calcaneus (tibiocalcaneal ligament); 3) to navicular (tibionavicular); and 4) to posterior medial talus (posterior tibiotalar ligament)	Stabilizes during eversion to protect against valgus stresses to the talocrural, subtalar, and talonavicular joints.
	Talocrural and subtalar	Anterior talofibular ligament	Lateral malleolus	Neck of the talus	Part of the lateral collateral ligament group. Restricts combined motion of plantarflexion with inversion or adduction.

	Talocrural and subtalar	Calcaneofibular ligament	Tip of the lateral malleolus	Lateral aspect of calcaneus	Part of the lateral collateral ligament group. Restricts inversion or varus stress of the talocrural and subtalar joints.
	Talocrural and subtalar	Posterior talofibular ligament	Lateral malleolar fossa on posteromedial lateral malleolus	Lateral tubercle of talus	Part of the lateral collateral ligament group. Provides stability to the talus within the joint and restrict abduction during dorsiflexion.
	Subtalar	Lateral, posterior, and medial talocalcaneal ligament	Inferior aspect of the talus on its lateral, posterior, and medial aspects	Lateral, posterior, and medial aspects of the proximal calcaneus. Each ligament merges with their respective collateral ligaments	Although not key stabilizers, they do assist in providing some support to the subtalar joint.
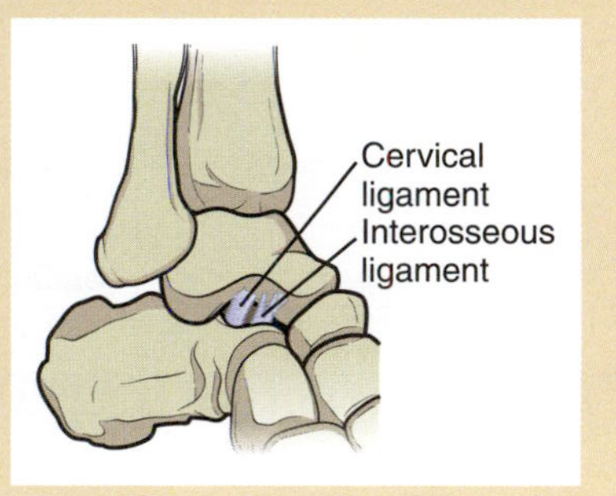	Subtalar	Interosseous (talocalcaneal) ligament	Two bands (anterior and posterior) that attach to the talar sulcus within the sinus tarsi	Calcaneal sulcus within the sinus tarsi	Restricts end-range eversion motion

Continued

TABLE 11-1 | LIGAMENTS OF THE ANKLE AND FOOT COMPLEX—cont'd

Figure	Joint	Ligament	Proximal Attachment	Distal Attachment	Functions
	Subtalar	Cervical ligament	Neck of the talus on its inferior-lateral aspect	Lateral to the interosseous ligament on the neck of the calcaneus	Restricts end-range inversion motion.
Trans. tarsal jt. MTP joints IP collateral ligaments Nav. Med. MT 1 Tal. Int. Cal. Lat. Cub. MT 5 Intertarsal ligaments MTP collateral ligaments **Dorsal View**	Transverse tarsal: Talonavicular	Talonavicular ligament	Dorsal neck of talus	Navicular, dorsal aspect	Restricts movement of talus on navicular. Allows rotation.
		Plantar calcaneonavicular ligament (spring ligament) and lateral calcaneonavicular ligament	Sustentaculum tali	Navicular	Maintains the medial longitudinal arch, especially during weight-bearing.
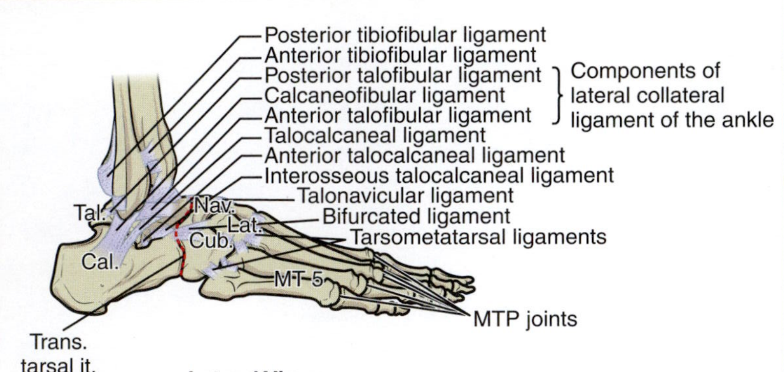 Posterior tibiofibular ligament Anterior tibiofibular ligament Posterior talofibular ligament Calcaneofibular ligament Anterior talofibular ligament Components of lateral collateral ligament of the ankle Talocalcaneal ligament Anterior talocalcaneal ligament Interosseous talocalcaneal ligament Talonavicular ligament Bifurcated ligament Tarsometatarsal ligaments Tal. Nav. Lat. Cub. Cal. MT-5 MTP joints Trans. tarsal jt. **Lateral View**	Transverse Tarsal: Calcaneocuboid	Bifurcated ligament	Anterior portion of superior calcaneus	Distal insertions for a Y-shaped ligament with two insertions. Calcaneocuboid portion (medial): dorsomedial aspect of cuboid. Calcaneonavicular (lateral): dorsolateral aspect of navicular.	Supports transverse tarsal joint. Permits rotation (inversion/eversion of foot).

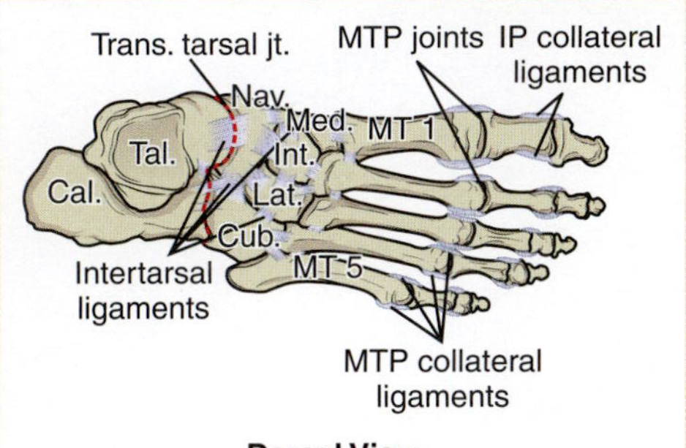

		Long plantar ligament	Plantar calcaneus anterior to the greater tubercle	Plantar cuboid	Limits depression of the lateral longitudinal arch.
		Short plantar ligament (Plantar calcaneocuboid ligament)	Deep to long plantar ligament, from plantar calcaneus	Plantar cuboid	Maintains the lateral longitudinal arch.
		Dorsal ligaments	1st MT: Dorsal aspect of medial cuneiform 2nd MT: Dorsal aspect of each cuneiform 3rd & 4th MT: Dorsal aspect of lateral cuneiform 5th MT: Dorsal cuboid	Dorsal bases of each metatarsal	Protect and support the tarsometatarsal joints. Permit gliding between tarsals and metatarsals.
Not shown	Tarsometatarsal joints	Plantar ligaments	1st MT: Longitudinal band from medial cuneiform 2nd & 3rd MT: Oblique bands from medial cuneiform 4th & 5th MT: some fibers from cuboid	Plantar bases of each metatarsal	Protect and support the tarsometatarsal joints. Permit gliding between tarsals and metatarsals.
	Tarsometatarsal joints	Interosseous cuneometatarsal ligaments	1: medial cuneiform 2: lateral cuneiform 3: lateral cuneiform	1 and 2: 2nd MT 3: 4th MT base	Protect and support the tarsometatarsal joints. Permit gliding between tarsals and metatarsals.

Continued

TABLE 11–1 | LIGAMENTS OF THE ANKLE AND FOOT COMPLEX—cont'd

Figure	Joint	Ligament	Proximal Attachment	Distal Attachment	Functions
Cal. Cub. Lat. Int. Sus. Nav. Med. MT 1 Tal. Talonav. jt. **Plantar View**	Intermetatarsal joints	Dorsal, plantar, and interosseous ligaments	Each metatarsal (except #1) is connected to its adjacent MT	Each metatarsal (except #1) is connected to its adjacent MT	Protect and support the intermetatarsal joints. Permit slight gliding between the metatarsals.
	Metatarsophalangeal joints	Collateral ligaments	Medial and lateral tubercles of metatarsal heads	Corresponding medial and lateral bases of proximal phalanges	Support capsule and restrict lateral motion of the respective joint. Allow flexion and extension.
		Plantar ligaments	Plantar metatarsal heads	Plantar bases of phalanges	Assist collateral ligaments with which they blend.
		Deep transverse metatarsal ligament	Plantar ligament of adjacent metatarsophalangeal joint	Plantar ligament of adjacent metatarsophalangeal joint	Supports the joint capsule and MTP joint.
	Interphalangeal joints	Collateral ligaments	Proximal medial and lateral interphalangeal heads	Corresponding medial and lateral bases of adjacent distal phalanges	Protect and support joint capsule.
		Plantar ligament	Plantar aspects of the heads of the proximal phalange	Plantar base of adjacent distal phalange	Assist collateral ligaments with which they blend.

to the lateral malleolus. Therefore, the ankle axis is oblique to both the sagittal and frontal planes (Fig. 11.6). Its vertical axis is also oblique to the horizontal plane.[11]

In the ankle joint, Lundberg and coworkers[19] produced 30° of plantarflexion from the neutral position. They measured motions of up to 28° in the sagittal plane (plantarflexion), 1° in the horizontal plane (in the direction of medial rotation), and 4° in the frontal plane (pronation). With 30° of dorsiflexion, these authors measured 23° in the sagittal plane, 9° in the horizontal plane (in the direction of lateral rotation), and 2° in the frontal plane (supination). In essence, this study and others[20, 21] have demonstrated that dorsiflexion and plantarflexion are actually coupled movements that require these motions in the other planes for complete dorsiflexion and plantarflexion to occur. From a clinical standpoint, it is sufficient to realize that because of the oblique orientation of the talocrural joint, dorsiflexion and plantarflexion are not pure plane motions but require movement in other planes in addition to the sagittal plane.

Normal range of dorsiflexion motion ranges from 0° to 30° in the anatomic position.[12, 22, 23] In one study, active range of dorsiflexion of 13° (SD = 4) was measured in healthy male subjects age 18 months to 54 years;[24] however, this measurement was made with the subjects in a supine position; with the knee in extension. In such a position, the gastrocnemius muscle, which crosses the knee and the ankle joints, is in a lengthened position at the knee to limit dorsiflexion at the ankle (passive insufficiency). Although this is an important functional measurement related to walking, in which the knee extends and the ankle dorsiflexes in the stance phase, it is equally important to determine the range of motion permitted by joint structures alone. When measuring ankle motion alone, it is best measured with the knee flexed. With the gastrocnemius on a slack at the knee, the range of motion in dorsiflexion is larger and not affected by limitations in gastrocnemius flexibility.

Plantarflexion ranges from 30° to 58°.[19, 22, 24, 25] Plantarflexion range of motion is not altered by the position of the knee because there are no dorsiflexor muscles that cross the knee. Although these measurements for both dorsiflexion and plantarflexion may vary by a few degrees from one investigator to another, depending on the techniques used and the population investigated, it is accepted that passive motion is greater than active motion, and individuals lose ankle mobility with age.[26]

The normal end feel for dorsiflexion of the joint is firm. When the knee is flexed, limitation is due to ligamentous structures; however, when the knee is extended, limitation is due to the length or resistance of the gastrocnemius muscle. The end feel of plantarflexion is firm because of resistance of the capsule, ligaments, and dorsiflexor muscles.

Arthrokinematics

For now, we will discuss the talocrural joint's arthrokinematics relative to the open kinetic chain, such as would be used during most joint mobilization techniques. The talus rolls and glides within the mortise joint formed by the tibia and fibula during dorsiflexion and plantarflexion. When the joint moves in dorsiflexion, the talus abides by the convex-concave principle, so as it rolls anteriorly, it glides posteriorly (Fig. 11.7). The opposite motions occur during plantarflexion: The talus rolls posteriorly as it glides or slides anteriorly. The resting position for the joint is about 10° of plantarflexion whereas the close-packed position is full dorsiflexion. A capsular pattern of motion observed when the capsule loses mobility appears as a loss of more planter flexion than dorsiflexion.

Subtalar Joint

Small but critical motions occur in all of the tarsal and metatarsal joints during open and closed chain motions of the ankle and foot. These joints must undergo instantaneous changes to allow the arches to remain flexible to absorb forces during weight acceptance in walking or running and also provide rigidity of the foot during propulsion (Fig. 11.8). If these joints lose their mobility because of injury, surgical fusion, or replacement with prosthetic segments, the loss of function of these small motions become readily apparent. The forces that are normally absorbed by these joints must be transferred along the kinetic chain and eventually produce compensatory hypermobility at the knee and other joints of the foot.[27]

As mentioned previously, the superior surface of the calcaneus has three facets (posterior, middle, and anterior) that articulate with corresponding facets on the inferior surface of the talus. The posterior calcaneal facet is convex (Fig. 11.9), whereas the middle and anterior facets of the calcaneus are concave. This anatomical configuration prevents anterior or posterior displacement of the talus on the calcaneus. The subtalar joint has two capsules. One encloses the posterior articular facets of the talus and the calcaneus. The second encloses the middle and anterior facets of the subtalar joint as well as the talonavicular joint. However, the talonavicular joint is not considered a part of the subtalar joint but is part of the transverse tarsal joint. Table 11–1 identifies the ligaments supporting the subtalar joint.

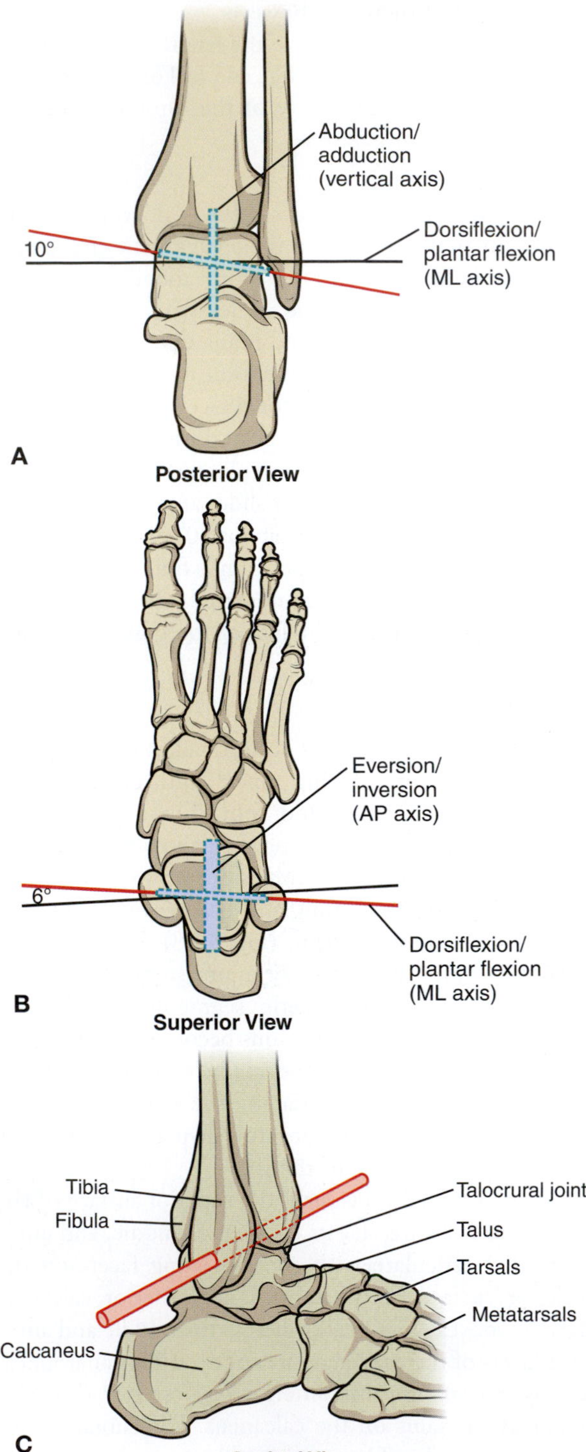

Figure 11.6 Axis of plantarflexion-dorsiflexion the talocrural joint from a A) frontal, B) superior, and C) sagittal view. Red lines in A and B indicate the joint's actual axis of motion while the black lines indicate the cardinal axis of motion.

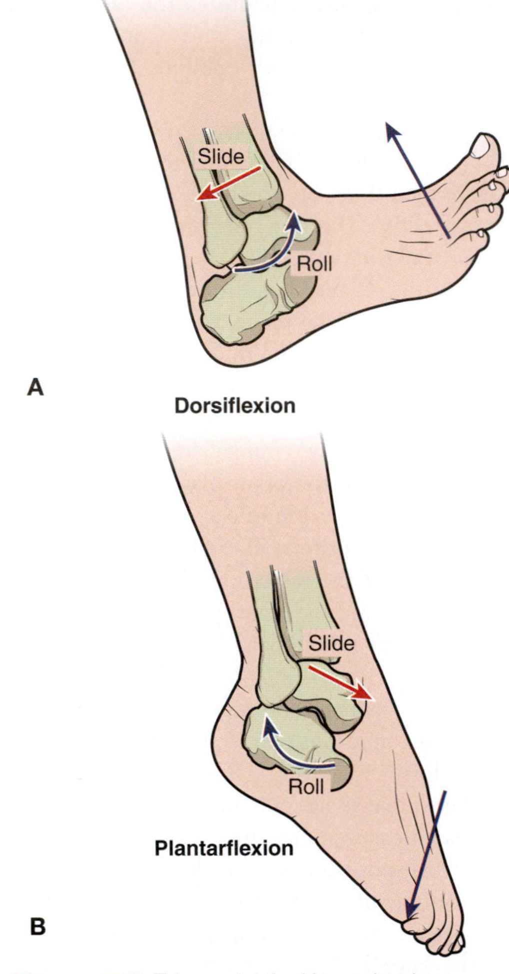

Figure 11.7 Talocrural arthrokinematics. In an open kinetic chain, the talus rolls and slides in opposite directions during A) dorsiflexion and B) plantarflexion.

A cone-shaped sulcus (groove or trench) runs between the posterior and middle articular surfaces of the talus to form the sinus tarsi. This sulcus, or tarsal canal, runs from the sinus tarsi on the lateral ankle to the ankle's medial side between the medial malleolus and sustentaculum tali and separates the posterior and anterior capsules of the subtalar joint. The sinus tarsi is the widest end of the sulcus and located just anterior to the lateral malleolus (Fig. 11.10). Short, thick, and strong interosseous talocalcaneal ligaments and the cervical ligament course the length of the sinus tarsi and provide the greatest forces to bind the talus and the calcaneus firmly together (Fig. 11.11). These ligaments and the adipose tissue in the sinus tarsi have been found to be richly endowed with neural receptors and nerve fibers traced to the cerebellum.[28] Valenti[28] hypothesized from this and additional

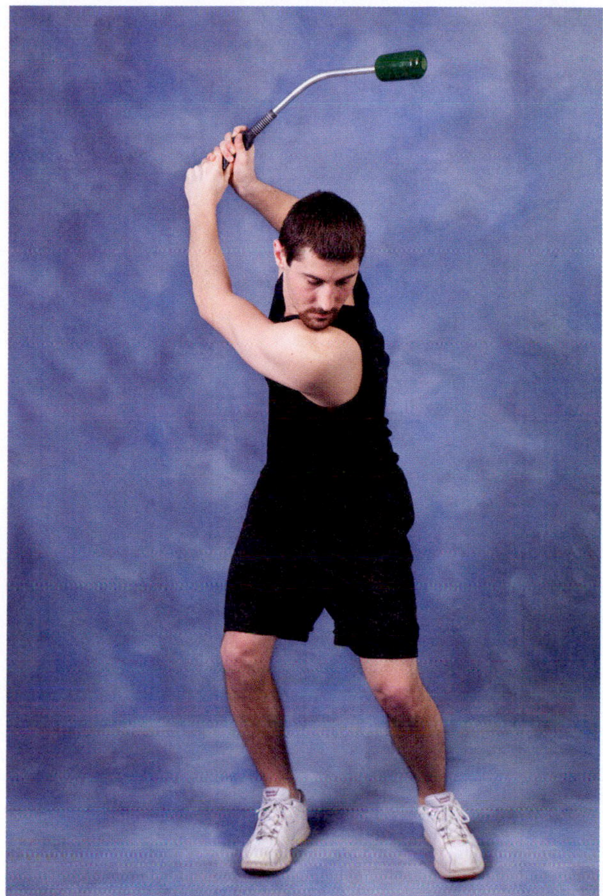

Figure 11.8 The foot and ankle undergo many various stresses and must instantaneously adapt to them during different closed chain activities.

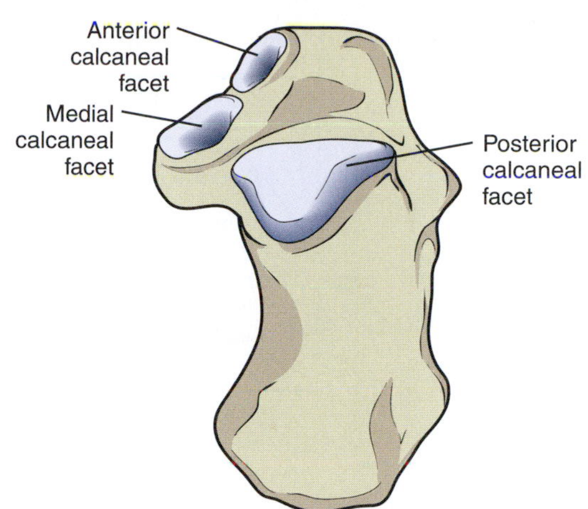

Figure 11.9 Dorsal surface of the calcaneus showing the facets that articulate with the inferior talus surface. The posterior calcaneal facet is convex, whereas the middle and anterior facets of the calcaneus are concave.

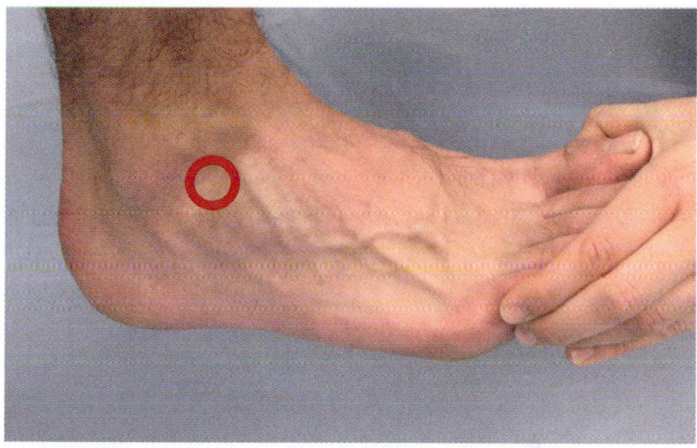

Figure 11.10 Sinus tarsi of the lateral ankle is the widest opening of the cone-shaped tarsal tunnel which runs obliquely to the medial aspect of the ankle, ending at its narrow opening between the medial malleolus and sustentaculum tali.

clinical and EMG evidence that the interosseous ligaments are the "proprioceptive subtalar center" responsible for rapid reflex response to closed chain motion.

Kinematics

As is the case of the talocrural joint, the subtalar joint does not move in a straight plane but produces movement on an axis that creates multiplanar motion. Although the subtalar joint has multiplanar movement, it is an uniaxial joint because of the oblique alignment of its axis.[33] The triplanar axis of the subtalar joint is represented by a line beginning on the lateroposterior aspect of the calcaneus and going in a forward-upward-medial direction through the subtalar joint and

PRACTICE POINT

Lateral ankle sprains commonly affect the ankle joint proprioceptors. Clinicians find balance deficiencies common in individuals who have a history of ankle sprains. Part of a complete rehabilitation program following ankle sprains is the incorporation of proprioception exercises to facilitate restoration of balance and agility control.[29–32]

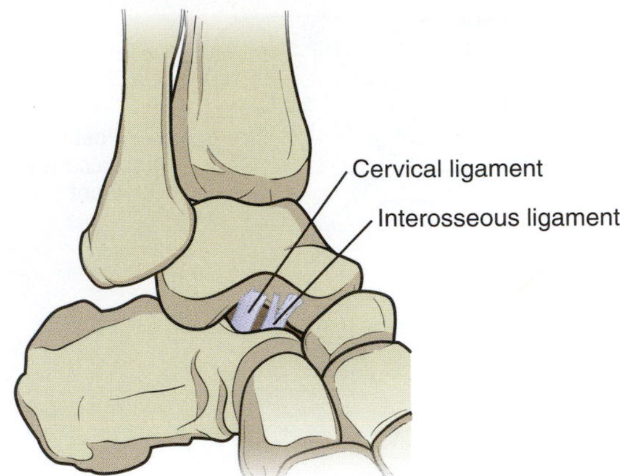

Figure 11.11 The interosseous and cervical ligaments are the ligaments most responsible for holding the talus and calcaneus together.

the superomedial aspect of the neck of the talus as seen in Figure 11.12.[11, 34–37] Various investigators have sought to identify the precise angle of the subtalar joint axis. Using different methods, they have arrived at near-similar results: The subtalar axis lies at about 45° (±5°) in the sagittal plane and about 25° (±9°) in the transverse plane.[11, 36, 38, 39]

Subtalar joint range of motion is described by those who have studied the subtalar joint in cadavers and normal human subjects as a rotation or a screw-like motion around the joint's triplanar axis. There is a wide range of motions attributed to the subtalar joint, with investigations ranging in their results from 5° to 65° of motion.[38] This large disparity is likely the result of a number of factors including differences in methods used, conditions of the investigations, populations identified, and rigor of analysis. A rigorous study has identified inversion and eversion to be 30° and 18°, respectively.[40] As demonstrated from this and other studies, several clinicians and investigators have identified total inversion-eversion motion to be about a 2:1 or 3:2 ratio of inversion-to-eversion movement.[11, 35, 41–45] One additional but important reason for the wide variation in recording range of motion of the subtalar joint may be that the subtalar joint rarely moves independently of the talocrural joint. Isolating motion of the subtalar joint from the talocrural joint, especially when looking at functional motion is very difficult. This intimate relationship between the two joints is discussed later in this chapter.

Arthrokinematics

The largest talocalcaneal facet interface has a convex calcaneal surface moving over a concave talar surface when in an open kinematic position. Therefore, the arthrokinematic motion of this joint abides by the convex-concave principle. In other words, as the calcaneus rolls into inversion, it also slides or glides laterally, and when it rolls into eversion, it slides or glides medially (Fig. 11.13). With the talus stabilized, the calcaneus can also be passively glided anteriorly, posteriorly, and distally (distraction).

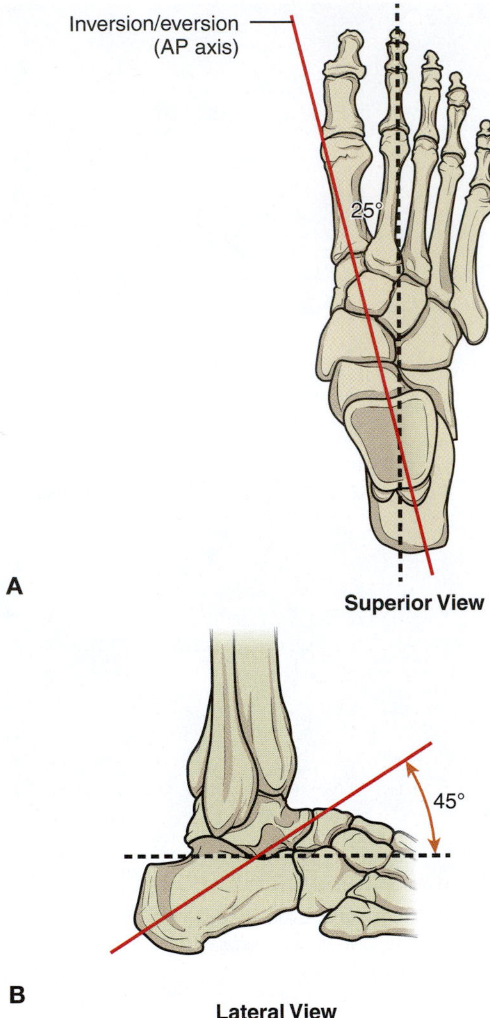

Figure 11.12 Axis of motion of the subtalar joint. It is an oblique axis which runs from the lateroposterior calcaneus in a forward-upward and medial direction through the sinus tarsi. The black dotted line indicates the pure axis of motion and the red line is the cardinal plane of motion for inversion-eversion.

Transverse Tarsal Joint

The transverse tarsal joint is also called the midtarsal joint, or **Chopart's joint**. When viewed from above, the joint line is S-shaped and is formed by two articulating surfaces, the talonavicular and calcaneocuboid joints (Fig. 11.14A). Independent motion of these joints, however, does not normally occur; therefore, although

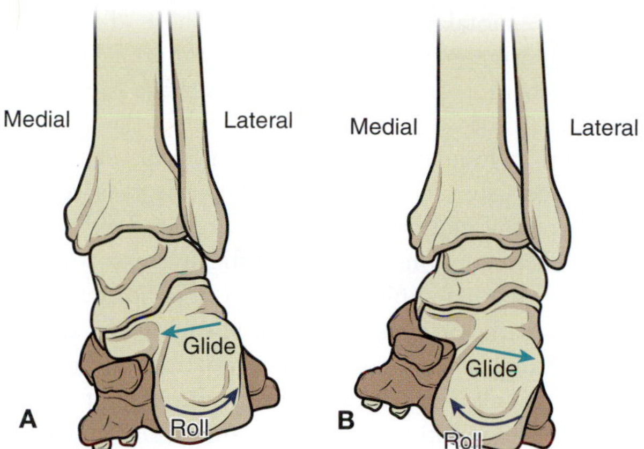

Figure 11.13 Arthrokinematics of the subtalar joint. Roll and glide (slide) are in opposite directions to one another. **A)** Subtalar eversion and **B)** Subtalar inversion in an open kinetic chain.

they are two joints, they are referred together as one—the transverse tarsal joint. Before we discuss the transverse tarsal joint, let us look briefly at each of the joints that make up this joint.

Talonavicular Joint

The talonavicular joint has a rounded anterior talar head that fits into a concave navicular, nearly like a ball-and-socket joint (Fig. 11.14B). The capsule of the talonavicular joint is the same capsule that encompasses the two anterior talocalcaneal articulations. See Table 11–1 for detailed information of the ligaments of this joint. The inferior aspect of this capsule is supported and reinforced by the spring ligament. The spring ligament, also known as the plantar calcaneonavicular ligament, is a rather thick and inelastic triangular-shaped ligament with a fibrocartilaginous lining of its surface adjacent to the talus;[46] its structure allows it to serve as a platform or hammock-like support for the head of the talus. In standing, the body's weight on the foot pushes the talar head towards the floor; the spring ligament provides the support the talar head needs to maintain its position and the alignment of the longitudinal arch.[5]

The spring ligament may be palpated by locating the sustentaculum tali and moving anteriorly but keeping the palpating finger posterior to the navicular tubercle. Applying some pressure under the arch between the sustentaculum tali and navicular bone will locate the ligament. An appreciation of the amount of mobility of this joint is also possible by stabilizing the talus by cupping the rearfoot and rotating the navicular or midfoot around the rearfoot; the navicular is easily rotated around the talus because of the configuration of the joint.

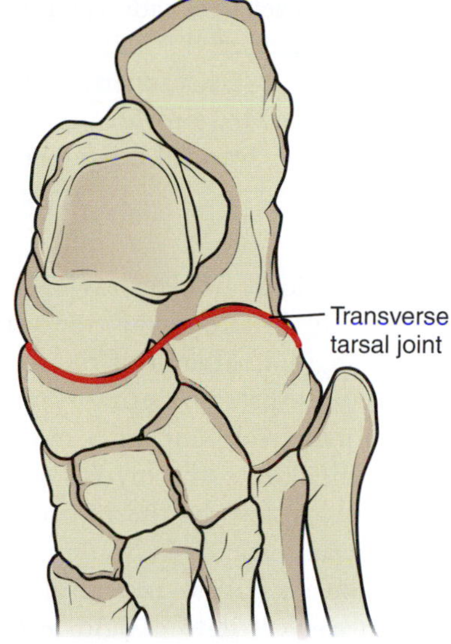

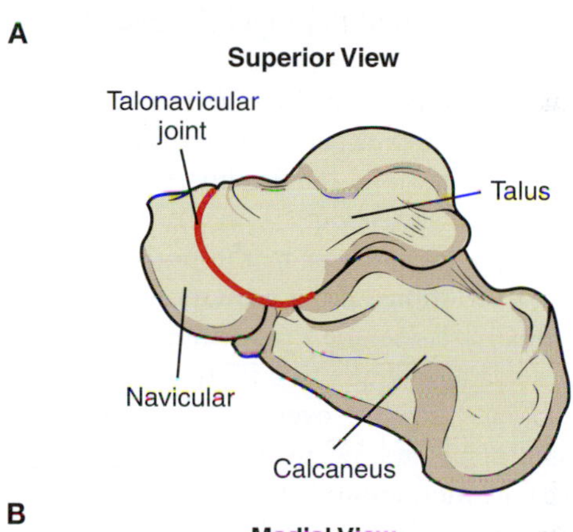

Figure 11.14 Transverse tarsal joints. The two joints of the transverse tarsal joint include the talonavicular joint medially and the calcaneocuboid joint laterally. **A)** Transverse tarsal joint is S-shaped. The calcaneocuboid joint has little movement because of the design of its joint surfaces; **B)** the talonavicular joint has more motion because of its ball-and-socket-like joint.

Calcaneocuboid Joint

Unlike the talonavicular joint, the calcaneocuboid joint has its own capsule. Also unlike the talonavicular joint, the calcaneocuboid joint formed is almost wedge-like in its structure so little motion occurs between the joint segments. The segmental ends of the anterior calcaneus and posterior cuboid that form this lateral joint of the transverse tarsal joint interlock with each other. They each have a concave and convex aspect of their surface that forms well with its corresponding opposing surface to create a joint that is convex vertically and concave transversely, thereby limiting the amount of movement within this joint.[47]

This joint is a modified sellar, or saddle, joint. The primary supporting ligament of this joint is the plantar ligament which has two layers, a superficial long and a deep short layer.[47] Table 11–1 provides detailed information on this and the other the ligaments of the calcaneocuboid joint.

Kinematics

The transverse tarsal joint participates in movement of the forefoot on the hindfoot; the transverse tarsal joint lowers the longitudinal arch of the foot during pronation and elevates the arch during supination. In other words, this midtarsal joint unlocks the foot to allow it to accommodate to the myriad surfaces the foot contacts and also absorbs the impact forces of weight-bearing during standing, walking, running, and jumping. Conversely, the midtarsal joint also locks the foot to convert it to a rigid lever for the transfer of forces required to propel the body forward or upward.

Because there are two joints of the transverse tarsal joint, its motion is complex and rotates around two axes of motion. One axis is a longitudinal axis that lies close to the subtalar axis, about 10° medial to the longitudinal plane and 15° superior to the horizontal plane (Fig. 11.15A).[36] Motions of the midtarsal joint around this longitudinal axis include inversion and eversion.[11] The other axis is an oblique axis that is similar to the talocrural axis and lies just over 50° (52°) superior to the horizontal plane and 57° to the longitudinal plane (Fig. 11.15B). Motion around the oblique axis include dorsiflexion with abduction and plantarflexion with adduction of the forefoot.[11] The two axes of the transverse tarsal joint move to become either parallel to each other when the joint pronates or cross each other when the joint supinates; the relative position of these joints to each other provide the unlocking (when they become parallel) and locking (when they cross) of the midtarsal joint (Fig. 11.16).

Since half of the bones of the transverse tarsal joint comprise the subtalar joint, the position of the subtalar joint bones determines the position of the transverse tarsal joints. For example, when the talus and calcaneus of the subtalar joint roll into supination, the other half of the bones making up the transverse tarsal joint—the navicular and cuboid—are also pulled along into supination, and when pronation of the subtalar joint occurs, the navicular and cuboid are likewise rolled by their corresponding bones into pronation. So, rather than just the subtalar joint moving into supination and pronation, other joints move into the same directions; this results in creating a sum of all of these joints' motions to produce a larger range of foot supination and pronation than would occur if only the subtalar joint moved in these directions. Such an arrangement allows the foot more adaptability in accommodating to whatever surface the foot is on at the time.

Keep in mind that motion of the transverse tarsal joint occurs simultaneously to different degrees in three true planes of motion because of the oblique angle of its axes. These motions are very difficult to isolate and measure. From a clinical standpoint, it is not necessary to identify the degrees of motion in each plane at each joint during foot supination and pronation. Suffice it to realize that all joints distal to the talocrural joint participate in these motions with the talonavicular joint providing the greatest rotation.[48] As in the subtalar joint, the amount of supination to pronation is approximately a 2:1 or 3:2 ratio.

Arthrokinematics

As you might suspect, the arthrokinematics of the midtarsal joint are complex due to the mere fact that the midtarsal joint is two joints. It may be easiest if we approach each of the two joints separately. Since the talonavicular joint has a concave distal surface moving on a convex proximal joint surface, the joint's roll and glide will move in the same direction. Therefore, as the navicular rolls or moves on the talus, it also glides or slides in the same direction. Since the calcaneocuboid joint is a saddle joint, it will depend on which way the cuboid moves on the calcaneus as to which way the roll and glide occur relative to one another. Fortunately, during flexion-extension motion, the cuboid is concave, similar to the navicular, and the calcaneus is convex, similar to the talus. Therefore, the roll and glide for the calcaneocuboid joint is the same as for the talonavicular joint for dorsiflexion-plantarflexion motions (Fig. 11.17). This point is important for clinicians who must mobilize a restricted midtarsal joint; they may have the option of mobilizing both joints as one transverse tarsal joint rather than individually and still achieve the desired results. For abduction-adduction movement of the calcaneocuboid joint, the cuboid is convex and the calcaneus is concave; therefore, roll or motion of the joint is in one direction whereas the glide or slide of the joint is in the opposite.

A capsular pattern of the transverse tarsal joint demonstrates a loss of dorsiflexion, plantarflexion, adduction, and medial rotation. The resting position for this joint is midway between the extremes of motions. The close-packed position places the transverse tarsal joint in full supination.[49] In a pronated position, the tarsal bones are more flexible. Small gliding motions can be achieved by fixating one bone and moving the

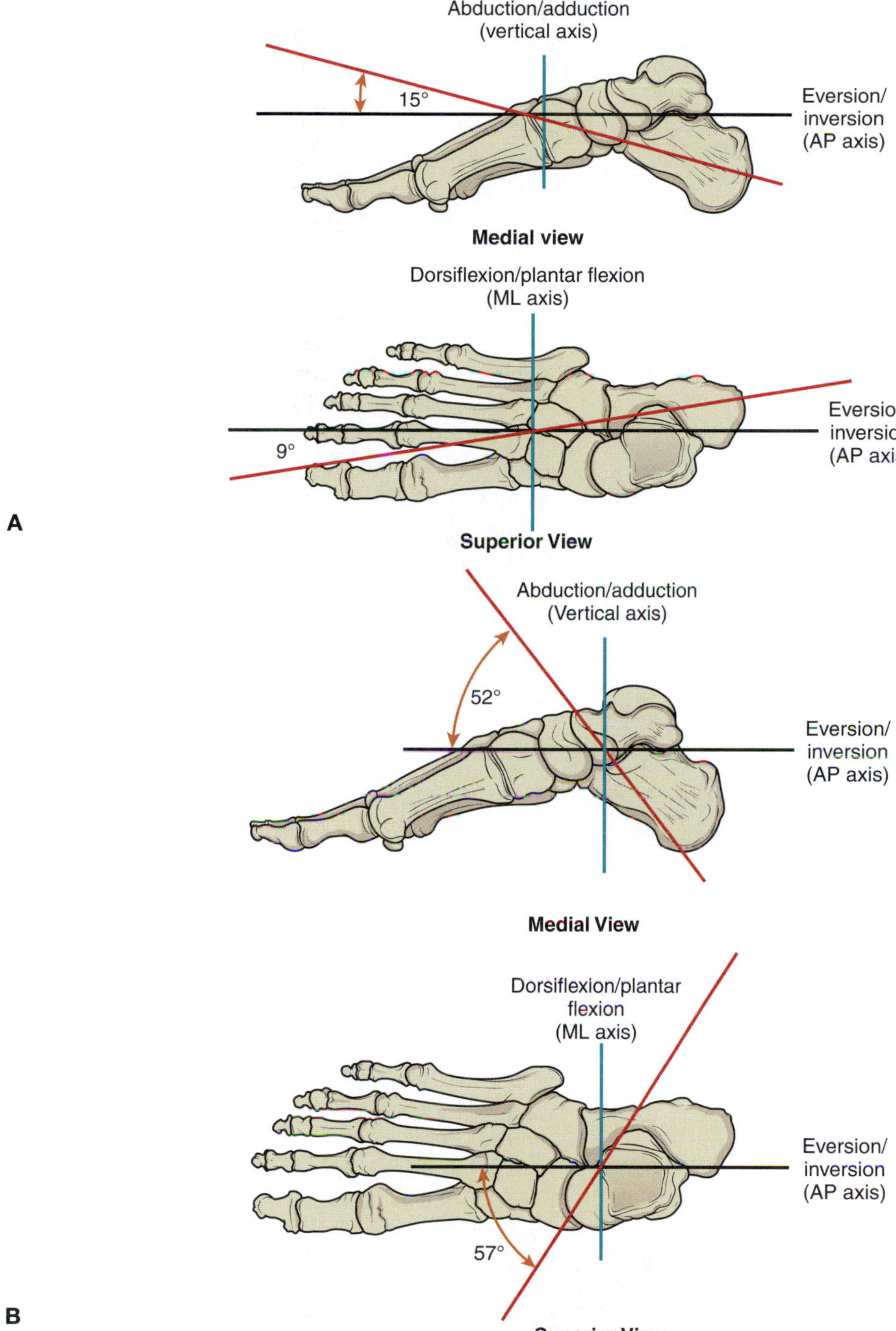

Figure 11.15 Axes of motion of the transverse tarsal joint. Two axes of motion are present in this joint. **A)** One is a horizontal axis; **B)** the other is an oblique axis. In each figure, the red line indicates the joint's actual axis of motion and the blue and black lines indicate the cardinal axes of motion.

adjacent bone. The talonavicular, calcaneocuboid, and naviculocuneiform joints can be moved in dorsal and plantar gliding movements when one bone is stabilized and the adjacent bone moved on it. There is little intercuneiform motion.

Tarsometatarsal Joints

The tarsometatarsal joints are the link between the rearfoot and forefoot. They form the transverse metatarsal arch and provide some contribution to the longitudinal arch.[50] The cuboid and the three cuneiform bones

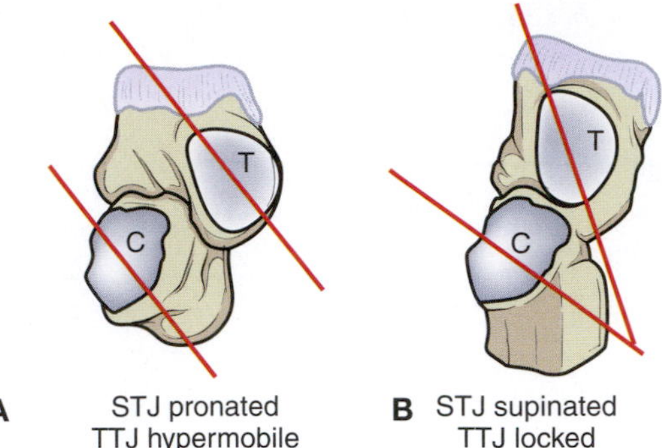

Figure 11.16 Relative position of the axes of motion of the two joints of the transverse tarsal joint impact the joint's mobility. **A)** When the transverse tarsal joint is in pronation, the talonavicular and calcaneocuboid axes of motion are parallel, allowing the transverse tarsal joint to move freely. **B)** When the transverse tarsal joint is supinated, the two axes converge, locking the joint and restricting movement. T = talus; C = calcaneus; STJ = subtalar joint; TTJ = transverse tarsal joint.

articulate with the bases of the five metatarsals to form the **tarsometatarsal joints** (Fig. 11.1). The tarsometatarsal joints are also called **Lisfranc's joint,** an **eponym** of this French surgeon who noted the occurrence of an injury to this joint when members of Napoleon's army fell off their horses with their foot trapped in the stirrup. Each of these joints is a plane synovial joint. The first, second, and third metatarsal each form their own tarsometatarsal joint with the medial, middle, and lateral cuneiforms, respectively. The fourth and fifth metatarsals articulate with the distal aspect of the cuboid to form their respective tarsometatarsal joints. The first metatarsal joint is the largest of these joints and has its own capsule. A strong mortise formed between the medial and lateral cuneiforms by the second metatarsal with the intermediate cuneiform creates a secure and strong articulation for the base of the second metatarsal; this configuration permits little motion of the second metatarsal. This joint lies more posteriorly towards the ankle than the other metatarsal joints. The second and third metatarsal joints share one joint capsule. The most mobile of the metatarsal joints include the fourth and fifth metatarsals. These two joints share the same capsule and have about 10° of total motion in dorsiflexion-plantarflexion and supination-pronation.[51] The ligaments supporting these joints are listed in Table 11–1.

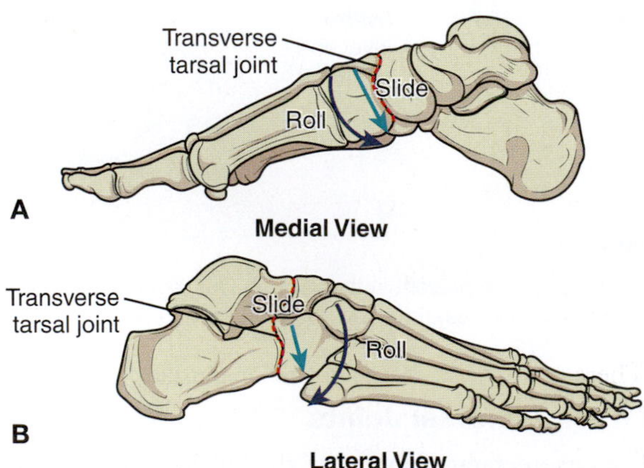

Figure 11.17 Arthrokinematics of the transverse tarsal joint. Plantarflexion-dorsiflexion roll or motion occurs in the same direction as the glide or slide in both joints of the midtarsal joint.

Rays are the functional unit of the forefoot. The three medial rays include the metatarsal and its corresponding cuneiform. Therefore, the first ray is the medial cuneiform and the first metatarsal, the second ray is the middle cuneiform and the second metatarsal, and the third ray is the third metatarsal and lateral cuneiform. The fourth ray is the fourth metatarsal by itself, and, like the fourth, the fifth ray includes only the fifth metatarsal.

Since the second metatarsal has the least amount of movement of the metatarsals, it is used as a reference point of motion for the forefoot. The second ray is also a stable platform from which the foot pushes off during locomotion. The medial forefoot has limited mobility compared to the lateral forefoot. The first ray has little movement, and it occurs primarily in flexion and extension motions; this mobility allows the medial foot to rotate around the second ray, allowing the foot to adapt to varying surfaces. First ray dorsiflexion occurs with foot inversion whereas first ray plantarflexion occurs with foot eversion. The lateral forefoot has the most mobility since the metatarsal bases are not as tightly wedged together as they are in the medial forefoot.

The tarsometatarsal joints are almost plane joints. Their mobility, however, is limited because of the close approximation of the adjacent metatarsals. Although motion at the tarsometatarsal joints is limited, motion of the first tarsometatarsal joint is most obvious and most useful to foot function. Motions of the first tarsometatarsal joint include plantarflexion (flexion) and dorsiflexion (extension) in the sagittal plane with minimal inversion and eversion in the frontal plane and even less abduction and adduction in the transverse plane. As the first metatarsal moves into plantarflexion, it usually also everts; conversely, as it moves into dorsiflexion, it also inverts.[52]

Intermetatarsal Joints

Implied in the discussion of the tarsometatarsal joints is the fact that each metatarsal base forms a joint with its adjacent metatarsal base(s). There are in fact, synovial joints between the second and third and between the third and fourth metatarsal bases. Although there is no synovial joint between the first and second metatarsal bases, there are ligaments connecting the two structures.

See Table 11–1 for information on these ligaments. This relationship between adjacent metatarsal bases provides for related motion between the adjacent bones, and the ligaments connecting the structures provide support to them.

The first, third, fourth, and fifth metatarsals rotate around the most stable metatarsal: the second metatarsal. Inversion and eversion of these bones are identified relative to the second metatarsal rather than the body's midline, similar to the third metacarpal of the hand as the reference for movement of the metacarpals and digits of the hand. Similar to the intertarsal joints, these intermetatarsal joints can be moved in dorsal and plantar gliding movements when one bone is stabilized and the adjacent bone is moved on it. The heads of the metatarsals normally can be moved in short arcs around each other if one segment is stabilized, or they can be moved together in arcs around the rigid second metatarsal segment. This motion occurs at the tarsometatarsal joints and is restricted in mobility by their joint structure as well as the transverse metatarsal ligaments. As indicated in Table 11–1, these ligaments attach between the heads. These ligaments are important since they limit the amount of abduction or "splaying" of the metatarsal heads.

Metatarsophalangeal and Interphalangeal Joints

These joints correspond in structure to those in the fingers, but they possess some functional differences. Each convex metatarsal head matches the corresponding concave base of the proximal phalanx to form the metatarsophalangeal (MTP) joints of the foot. These joints are biaxial, moving in the sagittal and transverse planes. In the fingers, the metacarpophalangeal (MCP) joints permit 90° of flexion and from 0° to 30° of hyperextension. At the metatarsophalangeal (MTP) joints of the toes, however, these relationships are reversed; hyperextension is 90°, and flexion is only 30° to 45°. The large range of hyperextension is required when standing on the toes and during walking in the late phase of stance after the heel comes off the ground. Although muscles are present to perform the actions, abduction and adduction movements of the toes have less range of motion and muscular control than in the hand.

The interphalangeal (IP) joints of the toes are similar to those of the fingers. They are essentially hinge joints with one degree of motion. The first, or great, toe possesses one such joint between a proximal and a distal phalange, and the four lesser, or lateral, toes have three phalanges with proximal and distal IP joints. Similar to the fingers, these joints have collateral ligaments that reinforce the joint's capsule. Table 11–1 contains a list of the ligaments for these joints.

The toes and fingers also have other similarities and differences when it comes to their arthrokinematic motions. In the great toe, the close-packed position is hyperextension of the metatarsophalangeal joint (its position at the end of stance during push-off in gait) and the four lateral metatarsophalangeal joints are in maximum flexion in their close-packed position. The metacarpophalangeal joints of the hand have the same close-packed positions: The thumb's position is maximum extension whereas the close-packed position of the other four digits is maximum flexion, the position required to produce a firm grasp of an object.[49] In one important sense, the first toe's MTP and the hand's MCP joints are similar (even though they are in opposite positions) since their most stable positions occur when force production is most required. Although the resting position of all of the metatarsophalangeal joints is slight (10°) extension, the resting position of the metacarpophalangeal joints is slight flexion. These joints in the feet and hands, however, have the same capsular pattern: a loss of flexion. The exception to this rule is the great toe, which has a loss of motion more in extension than flexion.

The interphalangeal joints in both the fingers and toes also have similarities and differences. These joints in both the hands and feet are in a close-packed position when they are in full extension. Their resting positions are also the same: slight flexion. Although the capsular pattern for toes and fingers is restriction of motion in all directions, the toes have more limitation of mobility in extension whereas the fingers have more limitation in flexion.

Muscles of the Ankle and Foot

The muscles that pass over the ankle joints have proximal attachments on the tibia and the fibula, with the exception of the gastrocnemius and the plantaris, which are attached to the femur. Because no muscles attach to the talus, the muscles passing from leg to foot act simultaneously on both the ankle and subtalar joints. Like the hand, the digits are moved and controlled by extrinsic muscles, which originate above the ankle joints, and by intrinsic muscles originating within the foot.

The muscles that act on the ankle or on the ankle and the toes, and that have proximal attachments primarily on the leg are divided into three groups: posterior, lateral, and anterior.

Posterior Group of Muscles

There are two groups of posterior muscles, the superficial and deep groups. The superficial group includes the gastrocnemius, soleus, and plantaris; the deep group of posterior muscles includes the long toe flexors and tibialis posterior. Table 11–2 presents information on these muscles regarding the proximal and distal insertions,

(text continues on page 501)

TABLE 11-2 | POSTERIOR MUSCLES

Figure	Group	Muscle	Proximal insertion	Distal insertion	Innervation	Action	Palpation
Gastrocnemius Soleus	Superficial	Gastrocnemius	Lateral head: Lateral femoral condyle Medial head: Posterior (popliteal) femoral surface proximal to medial femoral condyle	Posterior calcaneus via the Achilles (calcaneal) tendon	Branches of the tibial portion of the sciatic nerve (S_1–S_2).	Plantarflexion of the ankle and knee flexion	The gastrocnemius is largely responsible for the characteristic contour of the calf. It is easily seen contracting when the subject rises on tiptoes.
Gastrocnemius Soleus	Superficial	Soleus	Popliteal line of the tibia and the upper one-third of the posterior surface of the fibula	By means of a tendinous aponeurosis covering the posterior surface of the muscle, which narrows distally and unites with the tendon of the gastrocnemius to form the Achilles tendon	Tibial portion of sciatic nerve (S_1–S_2)	Plantarflexion of the ankle	The soleus is covered largely by the gastrocnemius, but in the lower portion of the calf it protrudes on both sides of the gastrocnemius so that it may palpated. When the subject rises on tiptoes, both gastrocnemius and soleus contract strongly. A comparatively isolated contraction of the soleus is seen if the subject lies prone with knee flexed and plantarflexes the ankle against slight resistance. The clinician places palpating fingers just distal to the gastrocnemius heads. The foot should be slightly resisted on the plantar side.
Not shown	Superficial	Plantaris	Lateral supracondylar line of the femur	Merges with the gastrocnemius and soleus to form the Achilles tendon	Tibial portion of sciatic nerve (S_1–S_2)	Presumed to be a weak assister of plantarflexion	Unable to palpate this muscle since it lies under the gastrocnemius.

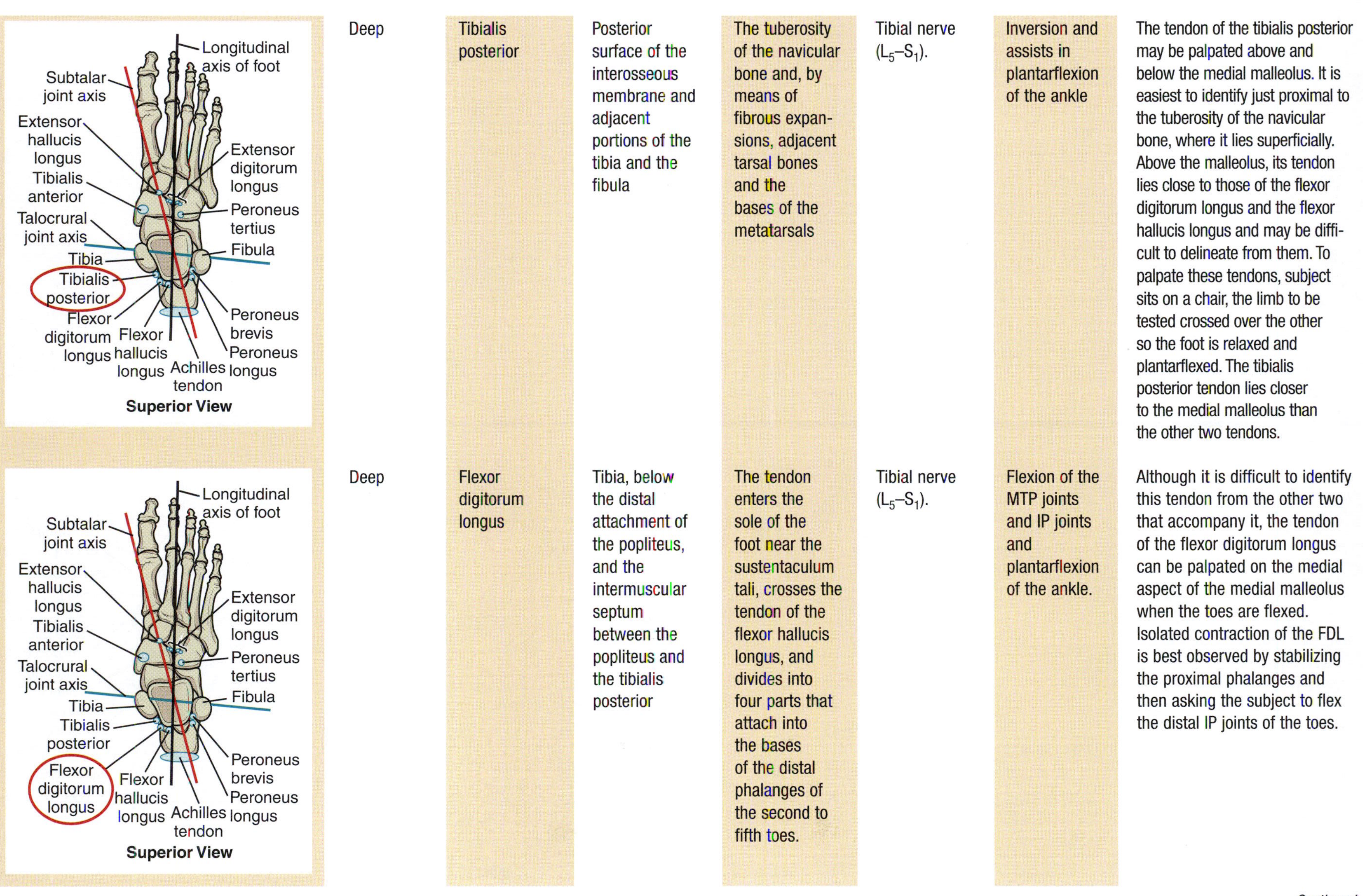

Deep	Tibialis posterior	Posterior surface of the interosseous membrane and adjacent portions of the tibia and the fibula	The tuberosity of the navicular bone and, by means of fibrous expansions, adjacent tarsal bones and the bases of the metatarsals	Tibial nerve (L_5–S_1).	Inversion and assists in plantarflexion of the ankle	The tendon of the tibialis posterior may be palpated above and below the medial malleolus. It is easiest to identify just proximal to the tuberosity of the navicular bone, where it lies superficially. Above the malleolus, its tendon lies close to those of the flexor digitorum longus and the flexor hallucis longus and may be difficult to delineate from them. To palpate these tendons, subject sits on a chair, the limb to be tested crossed over the other so the foot is relaxed and plantarflexed. The tibialis posterior tendon lies closer to the medial malleolus than the other two tendons.
Deep	Flexor digitorum longus	Tibia, below the distal attachment of the popliteus, and the intermuscular septum between the popliteus and the tibialis posterior	The tendon enters the sole of the foot near the sustentaculum tali, crosses the tendon of the flexor hallucis longus, and divides into four parts that attach into the bases of the distal phalanges of the second to fifth toes.	Tibial nerve (L_5–S_1).	Flexion of the MTP joints and IP joints and plantarflexion of the ankle.	Although it is difficult to identify this tendon from the other two that accompany it, the tendon of the flexor digitorum longus can be palpated on the medial aspect of the medial malleolus when the toes are flexed. Isolated contraction of the FDL is best observed by stabilizing the proximal phalanges and then asking the subject to flex the distal IP joints of the toes.

Continued

TABLE 11-2 | POSTERIOR MUSCLES—cont'd

Figure	Group	Muscle	Proximal insertion	Distal insertion	Innervation	Action	Palpation
Longitudinal axis of foot; Subtalar joint axis; Extensor hallucis longus; Extensor digitorum longus; Tibialis anterior; Peroneus tertius; Talocrural joint axis; Fibula; Tibia; Tibialis posterior; Peroneus brevis; Flexor digitorum longus; Flexor hallucis longus; Peroneus longus; Achilles tendon; **Superior View**	Deep	Flexor hallucis longus	Posterior surface on the fibular and intermuscular septa. Its tendon passes behind the medial malleolus, through a groove in the talus, and then under the sustentaculum tali.	Base of the distal phalanx of the great toe.	Tibial nerve (L_5–S_2).	Flexion of the first MTP joint, IP joint, and ankle plantarflexion.	Although it is difficult to identify this tendon from the other two that accompany it, the tendon of the flexor hallucis longus can be palpated on the medial aspect of the medial malleolus when the toes are flexed. Isolated contraction of the FHL is best observed by stabilizing the proximal phalange and then asking the subject to flex the distal IP joint of the great toe.

innervation, and function. Information within the table also indicates how to palpate each muscle. Since this information is anatomical rather than kinesiological, it is presented in table format for your review. Information on these muscles that is pertinent to function or their relationships with other muscles or joints is presented below.

Gastrocnemius

The gastrocnemius (G., *gaster,* belly, and *kneme,* knee) makes up the major bulk of the calf muscles. The proximal attachments of the muscle partly adhere to the capsule of the knee joint. The medial gastrocnemius head is larger than the lateral head, and its muscular portion descends farther distally (Fig. 11.18).

Soleus

The soleus (L., *soles,* sole, sandal), like the gastrocnemius, belongs to the superficial posterior group of the leg. These two muscles together are also called the **triceps surae,** or three-headed muscle of the calf. It lies deep to the gastrocnemius and plantaris muscles and is easily observed just distal to the muscle bellies of the medial and lateral gastrocnemius (Figs. 11.18 and 11.19).

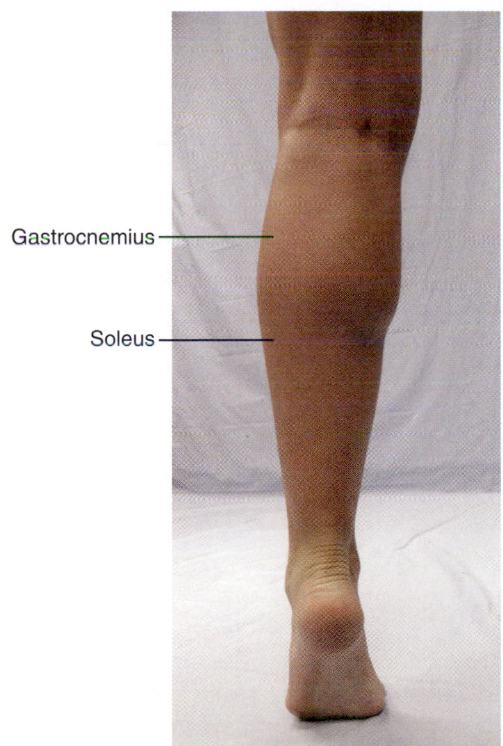

Figure 11.18 Gastrocnemius. Both gastrocnemius and soleus muscles contract when the subject rises up on the toes. Notice that the medial gastrocnemius head extends farther distally than the lateral head. Also notice the inversion of the heel.

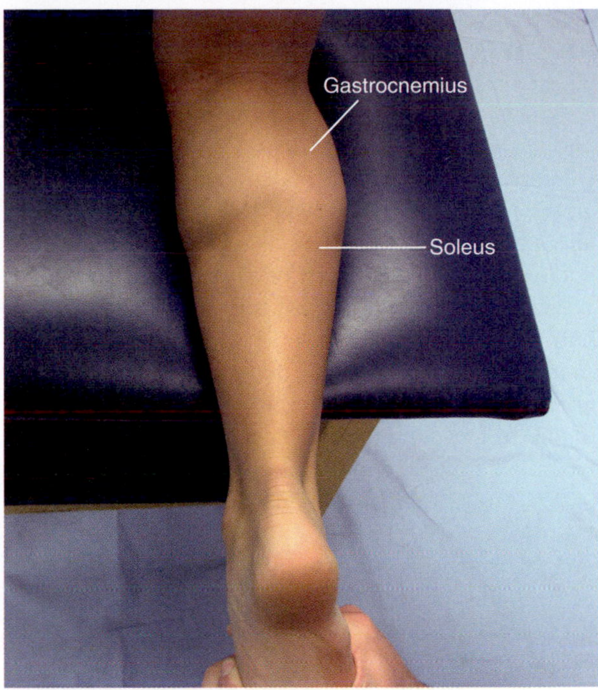

Figure 11.19 Soleus. The soleus is easily identified when the subject kneels with the knee flexed. When the subject points the toes, the soleus becomes apparent just distal to the gastrocnemius muscle.

As the tendons of the soleus and gastrocnemius merge to become the tendo calcaneus, or Achilles tendon, its fibers spiral about 90° so its medial fibers become positioned posteriorly by the time it reaches the calcaneus;[53] it is thought that this design both lengthens the tendon and provides it with additional elastic recoil, which is used during propulsive activities of the lower extremity.[53] The Achilles tendon is about 15 cm long from its origin at midleg level to its distal insertion on the calcaneus.[53]

Plantaris

The plantaris is the only other ankle/foot muscle besides the gastrocnemius whose proximal insertion is proximal to the knee joint. It is a very small muscle of the superficial calf group. It lies between the gastrocnemius and soleus but is not consistently present. Although the frequency of its presence has not been well documented, it has been found to be absent in anywhere from 6% to 60% of individuals.[54, 55] It is a very small muscle, about 7 to 10 cm long, with a fusiform fiber arrangement and very thin but long tendon.[53] Its true purpose is not known, but it presumed to provide some assist to the gastrocnemius and soleus in ankle plantarflexion.[53]

Function of the Triceps Surae

Plantarflexion of the ankle is performed mainly, and almost exclusively, by the triceps surae; this group provides 80% of the total plantarflexion torque.[56] These muscles have both a large cross-sectional area (43 cm^2 as compared with 33 cm^2 for all the other muscles of the ankle combined) and excellent leverage for plantarflexion. The perpendicular distance from the Achilles tendon to the ankle joint axis is approximately 5 cm (2 inches). Although it is difficult to isolate the maximum forces and torques that are produced by the triceps surae, forces which produce maximum isometric plantarflexion have been determined. Forces measured or calculated at the metatarsophalangeal joint area during maximum isometric plantarflexion range from 225 to 440 lb (1000 to 1780 N) in men.[57–60] A very large investigation was conducted to measure plantarflexion force in the sitting position in over 3,000 normal subjects ranging in ages from 5 to 70 years.[58] Their data revealed that the mean value of the force exerted by the triceps surae is equivalent to 2.4 times body weight. After the age of 30 years old, the triceps surae strength decreases gradually, becoming about 1.7 times body weight by the time an individual is 70 years old. When translated into amounts of force, the average strength for young adult men in this study was approximately 390 lb and 280 lb for young adult women. Keep in mind that even greater forces can be expected if the knee is in extension, placing the gastrocnemius muscle in a more favorable length-tension position. Two studies making this very comparison of torque production with the knee is flexed and extended were performed using young adult women subjects. With subjects in the sitting position and knees flexed to 90°, torque produced was an average of 98 ft-lb.[61] When the subjects were in the long sitting position with the knee extended, there was an average production of 122 ft-lb of torque.[62]

The soleus has been found to contain a higher proportion of slow-twitch muscle fibers than the gastrocnemius, which possesses predominantly fast-twitch muscle fibers.[63, 64] These results indicate that the soleus is concerned more with stabilization at the ankle and control of postural sway than is the gastrocnemius. Because it is composed of slow-twitch, fatigue-resistant motor units, the soleus operates economically. In other words, the soleus is able to maintain a sustained level of activity with less fatigue than the gastrocnemius, which contains predominantly fast-twitch and fast-fatiguing motor units.

Therefore, it makes sense to think of the soleus as a postural muscle; in fact, this has been confirmed in an EMG study. Subjects were asked to maintain a "standing-at-ease" position while EMG recordings were made of the muscles.[65] During this activity, continuous electrical activity in the soleus in all of the subjects occurred whereas activity in the gastrocnemius was detected in only a little more than half of the subjects.

The gastrocnemius and the soleus are both involved in activities requiring forceful plantarflexion of the ankle. In rising on tiptoes, both muscles contract simultaneously. In running, hopping, and jumping, the action of the gastrocnemius is essential since it has predominantly fast-twitch fibers that are required to produce a rapid rise in tension. The function of the triceps surae in walking is discussed in Chapter 12.

Other extrinsic muscles have tendons that pass posterior to the axis of motion of the talocrural joint, but they do not have long moment arms, making them fairly ineffective as plantarflexors. These muscles do not act on the calcaneus but attach to more distal parts of the foot so their specific actions occur at other joints. For example, the tendons of the tibialis posterior and the peroneal muscles lie so close to the malleoli that

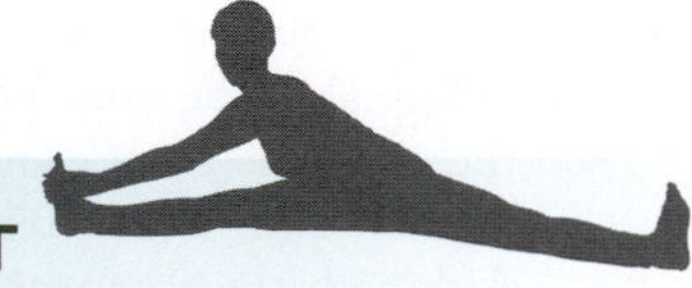

PRACTICE POINT

When clinicians begin treatment of patients, a common question they are asked is, "How long will this rehabilitation program take me to complete?" Before that question may be answered, the clinician must consider the individual's current status, including strength. Given the results from these studies mentioned above, it would be safe for a clinician to make a rough estimate that normal strength of the gastrocnemius-soleus will be present when the patient is able to lift about 2.5 times his or her own body weight if the patient is young and less than twice the body weight if the patient is older. Such information will provide the clinician with one tool that will assist in answering the patient's question.

they barely pass posterior to the axis. The tendon of the flexor digitorum longus lies only slightly farther back. The flexor hallucis longus has somewhat better leverage, but its action as a plantarflexor of the ankle still is insignificant compared with that of the triceps surae (Fig. 11.20).

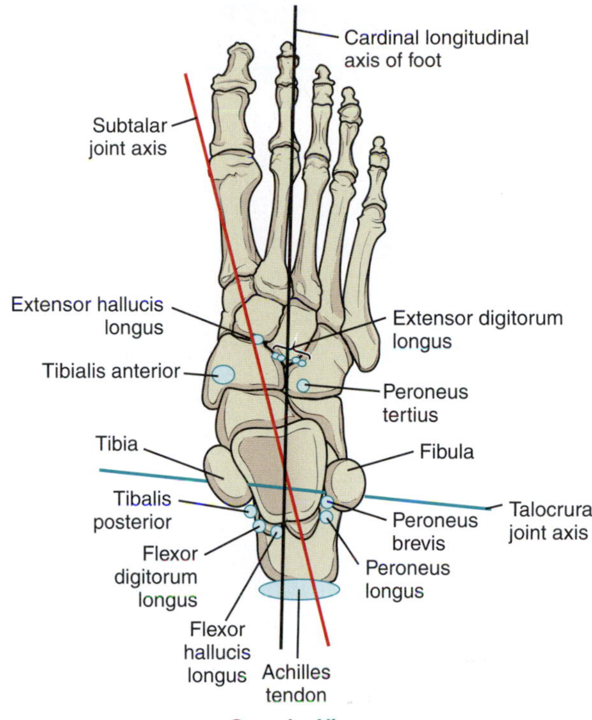

Figure 11.20 The ankle and subtalar joint axes and the muscles that run across them. Those muscles farthest from the axis of motion will have the greatest impact on the movement around that axis. Those muscles closest to the axis will have little or no impact on the motions around the axis since their moment arms are too short to be effective.

Tibialis Posterior

The tibialis posterior (TP) is the deepest muscle of the calf. It lies close to the interosseous membrane between the tibia and the fibula and is covered by the soleus and the gastrocnemius. In the upper calf, it occupies a central position between the flexor digitorum longus medially and the flexor hallucis longus laterally. In the lower calf, it takes a more medial course. Its tendon lies in a groove on the medial malleolus and is held down by the flexor retinaculum (Fig. 11.21). It then continues to the sole of the foot. The spreading out of its distal attachments provides a tendomuscular support on the plantar side of the foot, which assists in maintaining the mechanical integrity of the medial longitudinal arch.[66]

Flexor Digitorum Longus and Flexor Hallucis Longus

The flexor digitorum longus (FDL) is a deep muscle lying medially in the calf, covered by the soleus and the medial head of the gastrocnemius. In the leg, the FDL crosses over the tibialis posterior so that at the malleolus it comes to lie behind the tendon of the tibialis posterior. On the way to its distal attachments, each tendon perforates the corresponding tendon of the short toe flexor; you may recall that this arrangement is similar to that of the hand.

The flexor hallucis longus (FHL) is located under the soleus on the lateral side of the calf. The FHL is a strong muscle with a cross section that is almost two times that of the flexor digitorum longus. After entering the sole of the foot, the FHL tendon crosses to the medial side of the tendon of the FDL. At the first MTP joint, the tendon passes between the two sesamoid bones.

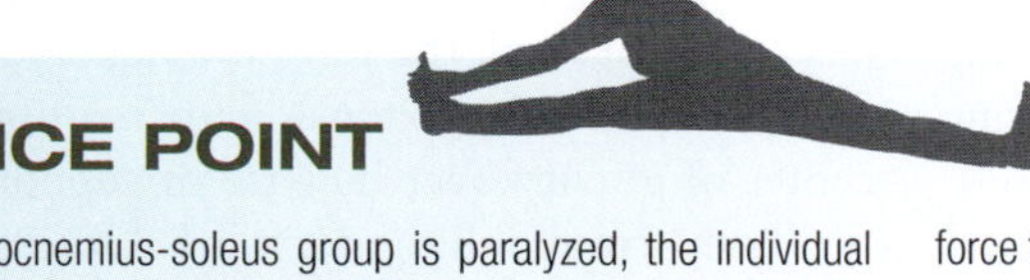

PRACTICE POINT

When the gastrocnemius-soleus group is paralyzed, the individual cannot rise on tiptoes, and gait is severely affected (see Chapter 12). The act of climbing stairs is difficult, and activities such as running and jumping are all but impossible. The deep calf muscles and the peroneals are used in these situations as substitutes for the nonfunctioning triceps surae.

In instances of bilateral paralysis of the triceps surae, there is a deficiency of standing balance because there is insufficient muscle force to prevent the tibia from dorsiflexing and collapsing on the foot. People with such weakness are often thought to be nervous because they do not stand still and are constantly moving their feet to get their base of support under their center of gravity. They can stand still only if they are holding onto a stable object or leaning against a wall. People with bilateral amputations have the same problem when standing in prostheses because they have no muscles to control closed chain positions of the feet and ankles.

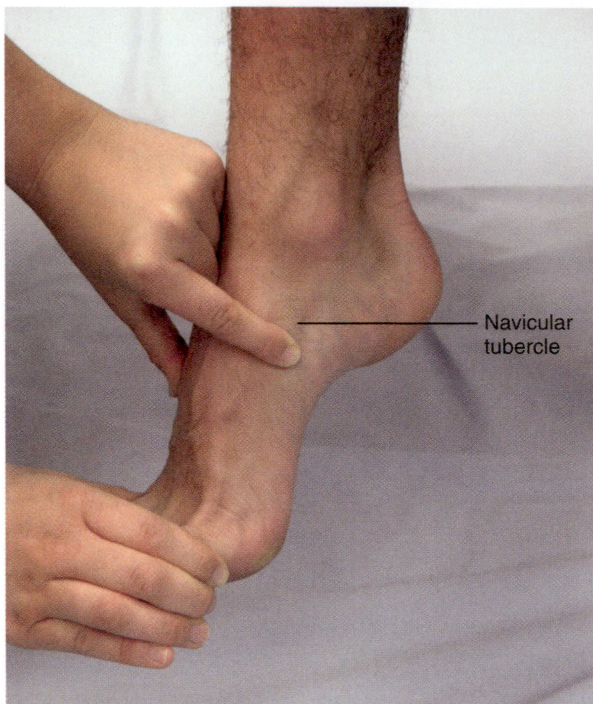

Figure 11.21 Tibialis posterior. Although the muscle is too deep to palpate, its tendon is identified as it passes around and distal to the medial malleolus. It is most easily palpated just behind the navicular tuberosity.

Functions of the Deep Muscles of the Calf

The flexor retinaculum is like the transverse carpal ligament of the wrist; it maintains the position of the tendons crossing the joint during movement and forms a tunnel through which the tendons travel. Through this tarsal tunnel, the tibialis posterior, flexor digitorum longus, and flexor hallucis longus all pass, along with the tibial nerve and artery. From anterosuperior to posteroinferior, the placement of these tendons is the TP, FDL, and FHL; the memory-jogging phrase used to recall this arrangement is "Tom, Dick, and Harry"—the TP, FDL, and FHL.

As the active inverter of the subtalar joint, the tibialis posterior produces this motion in either dorsiflexion or plantarflexion. Other muscles may assist in producing inversion motion but only in a limited range or during open chain motion. Because it passes medial to the subtalar joint axis, contraction of the triceps surae produces inversion of the calcaneus; notice the inverted position of the calcaneus in Figure 11.18. The tibialis anterior, FDL, and FHL may invert weakly from an everted position to neutral.

The tibialis posterior is an important muscle to the dynamic function and control of the foot. The extensive distal attachments of the tibialis posterior on the sustentaculum tali, navicular tuberosity, cuneiforms, cuboid, and bases of the metatarsals allow it to provide an important function in dynamic support of the foot arches.[66] This recruitment of the tibialis posterior occurs when increased loads are placed on the foot, and muscle contraction is needed to stabilize the arches during walking, standing on one foot, running, or jumping. In addition to providing stabilization of the hindfoot, midfoot, and forefoot joints, contraction of the tibialis posterior also causes the navicular to move slightly inferior and medially; this navicular movement stabilizes the navicular against the talus. This motion prevents the large torques produced by the triceps surae from moving the talonavicular and tarsal joints at a time when they need to be locked in place to allow foot propulsion. The tibialis posterior is the most active inverter throughout the stance phase of gait. When the foot lands on the ground, the tibialis posterior eccentrically contracts to control the rate at which the medial longitudinal arch is lowered towards the ground to absorb the impact forces of contacting the ground. In the later phase of stance, it concentrically contracts to lift the medial longitudinal arch upward, thereby assisting in moving the bones into position to lock the foot so it may be used as a lever of propulsion at push-off. In subjects who have either an isolated paralysis or chronic weakness of the tibialis posterior, the downward forces repetitively applied to the foot stretch the medial and plantar foot ligaments and eventually cause the navicular to roll to the floor, flattening the arch and making the navicular a weight-bearing bone.

The function of the FDL and FHL muscles becomes important primarily in closed chain activities such as walking, running, and standing on the toes. In these activities, they perform two important functions: 1) They contract to support the longitudinal arch; and 2) they apply a force to provide stability and control during standing and ambulation. When a subject leans forward, the long toe flexors resist metatarsophalangeal joint extension to maintain the body's center of gravity over its base of support and prevent the body from falling forward. During ambulation, the long toe flexors are active in the final phase of stance, again acting eccentrically on the metatarsophalangeal joints to control the rate at which the MTP joints hyperextend and maintain the body's center of gravity within its base of support. This force exerted by these muscles can be felt by placing the fingertips under the toes of a person who is standing. When the person then sways forward slightly from the ankles, the powerful gripping force will be felt.

Lateral Group of Muscles

This muscle group is located on the lateral side of the leg, anterior to the calf group, occupying a comparatively small area and separated from the anterior and posterior muscle groups by an intermuscular septum. There are two muscles in this group: the peroneus longus and peroneus brevis (Fig. 11.22). These muscles are also known as the fibularis longus and fibularis brevis, respectively. Detailed information on the insertions, innervations, actions, and palpation of these muscles is found in Table 11–3.

Peroneus (fibularis) Longus and Brevis

In its location, the peroneus longus (Gr., *perone,* brooch, fibula) appears as a direct continuation of the biceps femoris. It is about twice as large in its cross-sectional size and has a greater moment arm than the peroneus brevis, so it is able to produce significantly more torque.[67–70] Its muscle fibers converge to form a tendon that passes in a groove behind the lateral malleolus and then to the cuboid bone, where it enters the sole of the foot. In the plantar foot, the tendon follows a groove of the cuboid bone; the groove has an oblique direction coursing forward and medially.

The peroneus brevis, as its name indicates, is shorter than the peroneus longus. Its tendon passes behind the lateral malleolus, then across the calcaneus and the cuboid. From halfway down the leg to the ankle, the two peroneal muscles lie close together. Nearly all the brevis is covered by the longus, but in the lower part of the leg, the brevis can be felt separately from the longus.

Both peroneal muscles contract when eversion is resisted (Fig. 11.22). The tendon of the peroneus brevis stands out more than the tendon of the peroneus longus and can be followed to its attachment on the fifth metatarsal bone. At the malleolus, the tendons of the peroneal muscles appear as if they may slip over the malleolus, but they are anchored firmly in position by the peroneal retinaculum. Proximal to the malleolus, the peroneus longus tendon lies slightly posterior

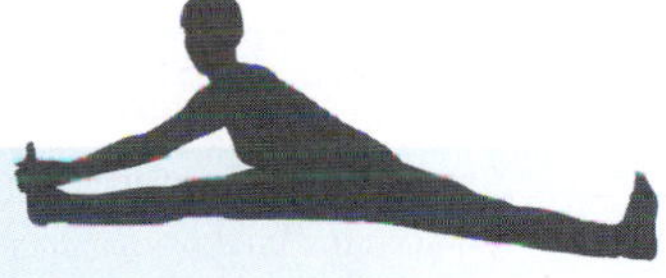

PRACTICE POINT

Since the tibialis posterior works throughout most of the time of weight-bearing in ambulation, it has little time to rest. This becomes an important consideration for clinicians who are treating individuals with excessive pronation of the foot. In these cases, the medial longitudinal arch is lowered for an extended amount of time during the gait cycle. This means that it is very likely that the tibialis posterior is working even longer than it does in a normal foot. It is no wonder that these individuals are often seen clinically for complaints of tendinopathy of the tibialis posterior. Clinicians working with these individuals must not only treat the diagnosis but must also attend to the reason the tibialis posterior is overworked.

As indicated in Table 11–3, both peroneal muscles are innervated by the superficial branch that comes off the common peroneal nerve. The common peroneal nerve becomes superficial as it winds around the neck of the fibula. At this point, the nerve is vulnerable to compression, which can cause loss of sensation and muscle paralysis. This frequently occurs if a person sits for a time with one leg crossed over the opposite knee. When the person stands up to walk, he or she finds that the leg has "gone to sleep," the foot cannot be controlled, and the ankle may collapse with weight-bearing. Usually, after the person moves to relieve the pressure on the nerve, sensation and function recover rapidly. In cases in which continued compression occurs, however, such as with a cast that is too tight under the fibular head, more permanent disability may result. If the pressure is not relieved promptly, permanent loss of sensation and paralysis of the peroneal and dorsiflexor muscles may occur.

TABLE 11–3 | LATERAL MUSCLES

Figure	Muscle	Proximal insertion	Distal insertion	Innervation	Action	Palpation
Peroneus brevis tendon	Peroneus longus	Its principal attachment is to the head of the fibula near the distal attachment of the biceps femoris. It also has additional proximal attachments, including the neighboring area of the tibia, the shaft of the fibula, and intermuscular septa.	Plantar surface of first cuneiform bone and base of first metatarsal	Superficial branch (L_5, S_1 and S_2) of the common peroneal (fibular) nerve	Eversion and plantarflexion of the ankle and depression of the head of the first metatarsal	The muscular portion of the peroneus longus is identified just below the head of the fibula and may be followed down the lateral side of the leg. Its tendon may be palpated over the lateral-plantar aspect of the cuboid when the foot is plantarflexed and everted.
Peroneus brevis tendon	Peroneus brevis	Fibula, lower than the longus, and intermuscular septa	The dorsal surface of the styloid process of the fifth metatarsal bone	Superficial branch (L_5, S_1 and S_2) of the common peroneal (fibular) nerve	Eversion and plantarflexion of the ankle	Its tendon may be palpated over the styloid process of the fifth metatarsal when the foot is plantarflexed and everted.

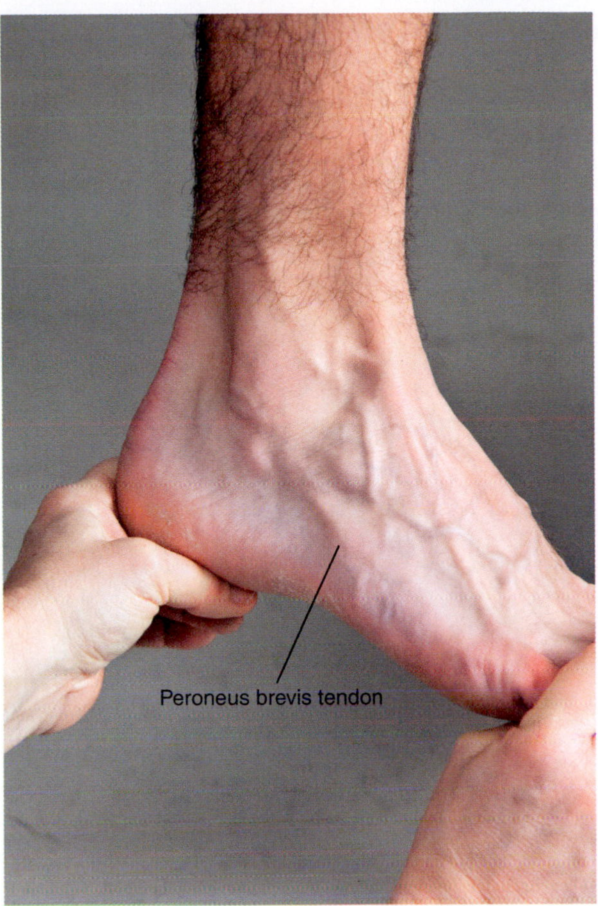

Figure 11.22 Peroneal muscles. The tendons of the peroneus longus and brevis both pass posteriorly to the lateral malleolus. The brevis tendon may be followed to its attachment on the fifth metatarsal base.

to that of the brevis and may be palpated at this location in some individuals. Distal to the malleolus, the peroneus longus tendon is held down close to the bone. It lies on the plantar side of the peroneus brevis tendon but the two are difficult to differentiate until they split at the cuboid at which point the longus tendon traverses the plantar foot to its insertion and the brevis ends at the styloid process of the fifth metatarsal.

Functions of the Peroneal Muscles

In open chain motion, the peroneus longus, brevis, and tertius (if present) are the main everters of the subtalar joint and do so whether the ankle is in dorsiflexion or plantarflexion. Their major functions, however, occur in closed chain motions such as standing on one foot, walking, jumping, and running. In these activities, the peroneal muscles provide major support of the arches of the foot, adjustment of the foot to the ground, and control of the leg on the planted foot. The peroneus longus is a significant supporter of the lateral longitudinal arch and the transverse metatarsal arch because of its insertion onto the plantar aspect of the first ray. It plays an important role in stabilizing the first tarsometatarsal joint, counteracting the lateral pull of the tibialis anterior on the joint.[71]

The peroneus longus is in good alignment to provide a pronation force to the foot. As the muscle contracts to evert the subtalar joint, it also pulls on the first ray to pronate the forefoot. You may experience this on your own foot in nonweight-bearing: Evert the subtalar joint to activate the peroneals and notice that your first metatarsal moves towards pronation.

The peroneals are active to provide important functions during the stance phase of gait. They are most active during the last half of the stance phase.[72] The peroneus longus isometrically pushes the first ray into the ground to stabilize it as the body's center of mass travels from the rearfoot to the forefoot.[67, 73, 74] The peroneus longus also coordinates with the tibialis anterior at the first ray to provide stability to the longitudinal arch at push-off (Fig. 11.23).[66, 75]

Although the peroneals are classified as plantarflexors, their leverage is poor to offer any significant contribution to that motion. The ineffectiveness of the peroneals as plantarflexors can be seen in Figure 11.20. Nevertheless, normal torque of plantarflexion requires strong contraction of both the peroneals and the deep calf muscles to stabilize the tarsal and metatarsal bones to make the force of the triceps surae effective through the foot to the floor.

Anterior Group of Muscles

The anterior muscle group of the leg is located on the lateral side of the anterior margin of the tibia, the sharp, bony ridge that is palpable from the tibial tuberosity all the way down to the ankle. It is separated from the lateral group by an intermuscular septum but appears, on palpation, to be continuous with it. The muscles of the anterior group include the tibialis anterior, extensor hallucis longus, extensor digitorum longus, and peroneus tertius. These muscles are also collectively referred to as **pretibial muscles** and are described in Table 11–4.

Tibialis Anterior

The tibialis anterior is responsible for the roundness of the leg anteriorly. When this muscle is paralyzed, a flatness or even slight concavity of this region results, so that the anterior margin of the tibia becomes even

TABLE 11–4 | ANTERIOR MUSCLES

Figure	Muscle	Proximal insertion	Distal insertion	Innervation	Action	Palpation
Tibialis anterior	Tibialis anterior	Lateral condyle and proximal half of the shaft of tibia, interosseous membrane, and fascia of the leg	Medial and inferior surfaces of medial cuneiform and base of the first metatarsal bone	A branch from the common peroneal nerve and a branch from the deep peroneal nerve (L_4–S_1)	Ankle dorsiflexion	The muscular portion is palpated proximally, on the lateral side of the anterior margin of the tibia when the foot is dorsiflexed. Its tendon is observed and palpated as it passes over the ankle, where it rises considerably when the foot is dorsiflexed.
Extensor hallucis longus	Extensor hallucis longus	Middle portion of shaft of the fibula and interosseous membrane	Base of distal phalanx of great toe	A branch from the deep peroneal nerve (L_4–S_1)	Extension of the first MTP and IP joints and ankle dorsiflexion	By resisting dorsiflexion of the great toe, the course of the tendon of EHL over the dorsum of the foot may be observed.
Extensor digitorum longus tendons	Extensor digitorum longus and Peroneus tertius	The EDL attaches to the upper portion of the tibia and fibula, interosseous membrane, and intermuscular septa and fascia. The peroneus tertius attaches to the distal portion of the fibula and to the interosseous membrane.	Four tendons of EDL go to the bases of the middle and distal phalanges of the four lesser toes. The peroneus tertius tendon goes to the dorsum of the fifth metatarsal bone.	A branch from the deep peroneal nerve (L_4–S_1)	Extension of MTP and IP joints of the four lesser toes and dorsiflexion and eversion of the ankle	To better see and palpate the tendons of the toe extensors without simultaneous contraction of the tibialis anterior, have the subject sit on a chair and lift the toes off the floor while maintaining the sole on the floor. If resistance is given to the four lesser toes, the individual tendons stand out better The tendon of the peroneus tertius, when present, is seen lateral to the tendon going to the fifth toe.

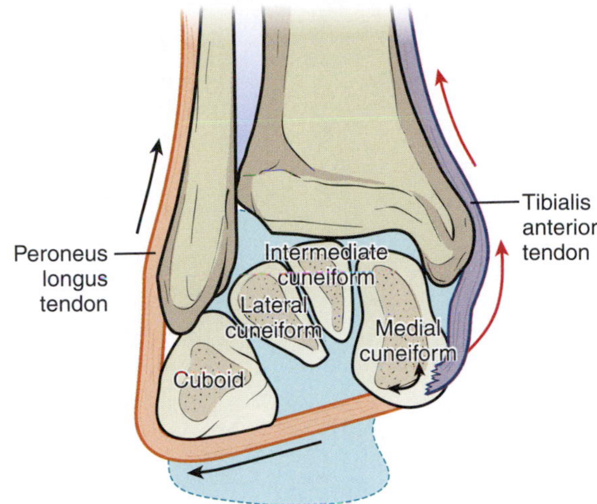

Figure 11.23 Peroneus tendon and tibialis anterior tendon work together to provide stability to the first ray and maintain foot arches. The tibialis anterior also controls the lowering of the arch through an eccentric contraction immediately after heel contact during gait.

more prominent than normal. The muscle becomes tendinous well above the ankle, and its tendon passes over the dorsum of the ankle. The tibialis anterior tendon is held down as it passes over the anterior ankle by the transverse and cruciate ligaments.

Because the muscle is superficial throughout its course, it may be readily observed and palpated all the way from proximal attachment to distal attachment (Fig. 11.24). In the photo, the subject dorsiflexes and inverts the ankle complex while he flexes the toes so that the tibialis anterior stands out while the extensor hallucis longus tendon, which lies just laterally to the tibialis anterior tendon, does not contract.

Extensor Hallucis Longus

In its upper portion, the extensor hallucis longus (EHL) is covered by the tibialis anterior and by the extensor digitorum longus. The tendon of the EHL passes over the dorsum of the ankle and immediately laterally to the tendon of the tibialis anterior (Fig. 11.25). Similar to the tibialis anterior, this tendon is held in place as it crosses the ankle by the transverse and cruciate ligaments. The muscular portion may be palpated in the distal half of the leg, but because it is almost entirely covered by the tibialis anterior and the extensor digitorum longus, it is not easily distinguished from these muscles.

Extensor Digitorum Longus and Peroneus Tertius

The extensor digitorum longus (EDL) and peroneus tertius muscles are described together because they are usually difficult to delineate from one another in their upper portions. The peroneus tertius is the most lateral part of the EDL but is sometimes described as a separate muscle. The EDL is superficial, sitting between the peroneal muscles on its lateral border and the extensor hallucis longus and tibialis anterior on its medial border. The extensor digitorum longus and peroneus tertius form a common tendon that passes on the dorsum of the ankle, and, like the other tendon in this region, it is held down by the transverse and cruciate ligaments. Once distal to the ankle, the tendon divides into five slips, of which the most lateral is the tendon of the peroneus tertius (Fig. 11.26). The peroneus tertius is not always present; cadaveric studies have demonstrated its absence anywhere from 5%[76] to 10.5%[77] of the time.

Function of the Pretibial Group

The tibialis anterior is the primary dorsiflexor of the ankle. It has good leverage, a straight line of pull, acts only on the ankle joint, and has twice the cross-sectional area of the toe extensors combined.[67,69] The extensor hallucis longus and the extensor digitorum longus extend the toes first, so, based on length-tension relationships, they lose their effectiveness to also act to dorsiflex the ankle. When the tibialis anterior is very weak or nonfunctioning, a limited range of dorsiflexion of the ankle is produced as the toe extensors attempt to take over the task. When the extensor digitorum longus acts in isolation, a strong eversion of the ankle also occurs because of its lateral position relative to the subtalar axis.

Since the tibialis anterior is also an inverter of the foot, it plays an important role during the stance phase of gait. When the foot contacts the ground, the longitudinal arch collapses to absorb impact forces. The tibialis anterior controls the rate of descent of the arch during this maneuver (Fig 11.23). The tibialis anterior along with the toe extensors also control the descent of the foot to the floor to provide a smooth landing after the heel makes contact. If these muscles fail to control foot motion to the floor, the foot slaps to the floor with a distinct sound that identifies inappropriate foot control with each step.

The pretibial group also moves the foot and toes in many important open chain motions. During the swing phase of gait, these muscles keep the foot and toes dorsiflexed to prevent the toes from scraping the ground. They move the foot from the car's accelerator to the brake, keep time with music, and wiggle toes that are crammed into uncomfortable shoes. Open chain motions of the foot require little muscle force

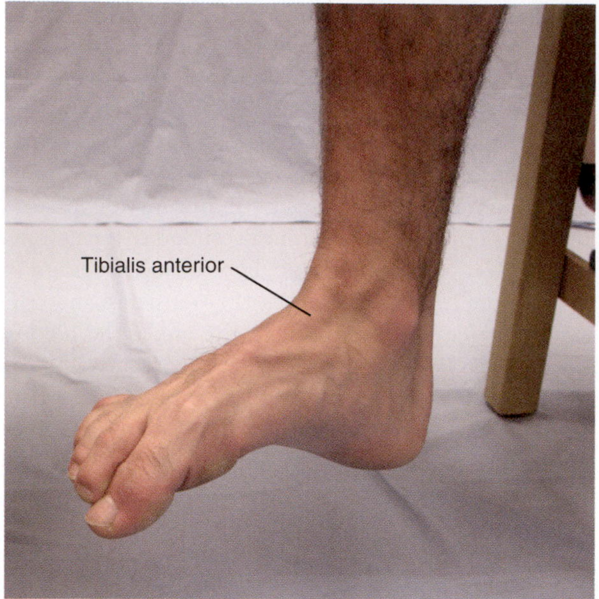

Figure 11.24 Tibialis anterior. This muscle and its tendon are superficial and may be identified and palpated from its proximal insertion to its distal attachment.

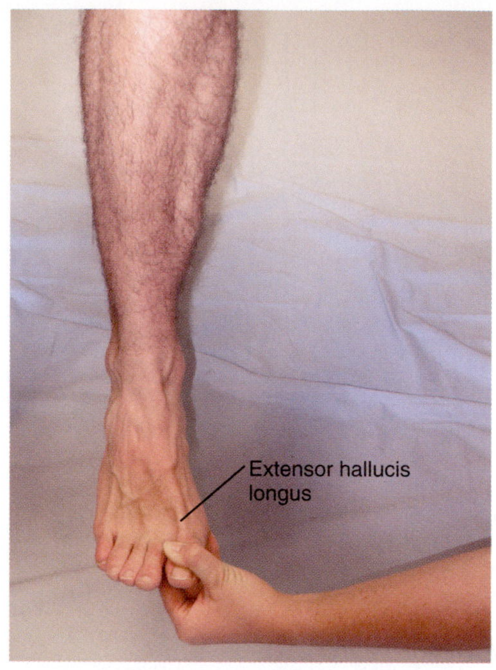

Figure 11.25 Extensor hallucis longus. Its tendon is observed when the great toe dorsiflexes against resistance. It lies just lateral to the tibialis anterior tendon at the ankle.

because the foot weighs only about 2 lb and the muscles have good leverage. Stronger contractions can be seen and palpated when a subject is standing on one foot in closed chain motion. Here a constant interplay can be found between all of the muscles of the foot to keep the center of gravity within its small base of support.

Intrinsic Muscles of the Foot

The foot has the same intrinsic muscles as the hand, except it lacks an opposition muscle. In spite of this deficiency, individuals with congenital amputations of the upper extremities, particularly if the entire limbs are missing, have been shown to develop and perform skilled sensorimotor tasks. These individuals learn to use their feet in an extraordinarily skilled manner and are capable of doing practically everything with their feet that able-bodied individuals do with their hands.

Most individuals, however, do not have these capabilities. Although the intrinsic muscles of the foot have names similar to those of muscles in the hand, they are more commonly used for vastly different functions than their counterparts in the hand. Four layers of intrinsic muscles are on the plantar surface of the foot. Descriptions of these muscles are given in Table 11–5. With the exception of the abductor hallucis (Fig. 11.27) and some of the other very superficial muscles (Fig. 11.28), these muscles are difficult to palpate because they are deep to a thick plantar fascia, are small, and are arranged in four layers on the

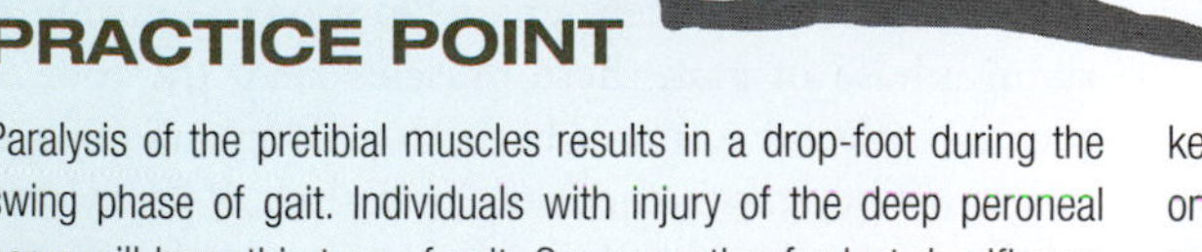

PRACTICE POINT

Paralysis of the pretibial muscles results in a drop-foot during the swing phase of gait. Individuals with injury of the deep peroneal nerve will have this type of gait. Compensation for lost dorsiflexors requires excessive hip and knee flexion during the swing phase to keep from tripping or dragging the toes on the floor. An ankle-foot orthosis designed to provide dorsiflexion during nonweight-bearing moves the ankle into dorsiflexion to eliminate the need for such active substitution of inadequate dorsiflexors.

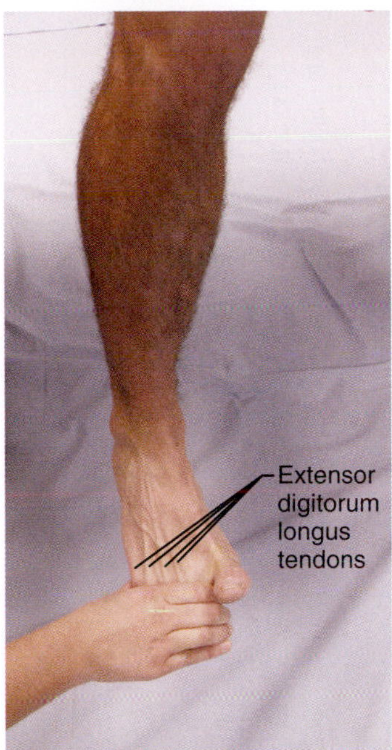

Figure 11.26 Extensor digitorum longus and peroneus tertius. Resistance to extension of the four lateral toes reveals the tendons on the dorsum of the foot.

plantar foot. Those palpable muscles are shown in photographs whereas those that are difficult to palpate are shown in illustrations (Figs. 11.29 through 11.32). In addition to bony attachments, these muscles have extensive connections with the plantar aponeurosis, ligaments, and tendons of the foot. These tissues form strong couplings of the static and dynamic structures of the foot.

Although the intrinsic muscles can perform motions such as abduction, adduction, and flexion of the toes, their major functions do not include these motions. Rather than acting individually as they do in the hand, these foot muscles tend to act more as a group.[78] The intrinsic muscles are used mainly for stability or balance and for providing support and assistance to the foot during activity. The intrinsic muscles play an important role in stability of the transverse tarsal arch and are, in fact, the major active contributors to the support of this arch.[78] The abductor hallucis has a major role in providing support to the medial longitudinal arch.[79] The abductor hallucis is very active during the last part of the stance phase of gait as the foot transforms to a rigid lever in preparation for propulsion of the body forward. In order to become a rigid lever, the longitudinal arch must elevate to tighten the foot joints; the abductor hallucis is active to assist in this positioning. In short, the intrinsic muscles, especially the abductor hallucis, flexor digitorum brevis, flexor hallucis brevis, and flexor digiti minimi, are active in their support of the arches during walking and running and in supplementing the force of the long toe flexors whereas the interossei and lumbricals stabilize the MTP joints and maintain the toes in extension for the forceful pull of the flexors at push-off.[78]

The extensor digitorum brevis and extensor hallucis brevis are the only intrinsic muscles on the dorsum of the foot (Fig. 11.33). The muscle belly appears as a small, round knob about the size of a dollar coin on the dorsal aspect of the foot. It may appear slightly bluish in color and becomes readily apparent when the toes are actively extended. The main function of the extensor intrinsic muscles is to assist their extrinsic counterparts in toe extension.

When pathology is present, the most noticeable change is observed in gait. Toe extension is an important function during gait. If the toes are not maintained in extension, they curl and the intrinsic muscles are unable to provide their normal assistance during push-off in the terminal stance phase of gait. In these cases, the force for push-off is ineffective and is noticeable with a resulting shortened stride. If a foot pronates for a longer than normal time during gait because of either muscle weakness or structural deficiency in the foot arches, the intrinsic muscles of the foot are required to work harder and longer throughout the gait cycle.[78] This causes the intrinsic foot muscles to sweat excessively; like other muscles in the body, intrinsic foot muscles that sweat produce an odor, which is a frequent reason for "smelly feet."

Function of Leg and Foot Muscles and Joints

The lower extremities have major functional requirements in high-energy closed chain motion. For example, it is impossible to move one leg in an open chain motion to kick a ball or even take a step unless the person can stand and support body weight on the opposite leg in closed chain motion. Muscles of the leg and foot are responsible for static and dynamic control, dynamic propulsion, and force absorption. If they are unable to perform their functions, notable deficiencies in activities from standing balance to jumping and running performance occur. Joint structure and function throughout the foot and ankle are complex and interdependent. Function of the foot and ankle joints is highly dependent upon not only their structure but also the muscles that cross them. Many muscles cross several joints, so more than one joint

(text continues on page 516)

TABLE 11-5 | INTRINSIC MUSCLES

Figure	Group	Muscle	Proximal insertion	Distal insertion	Innervation	Action
Abductor hallucis Extensor hallucis longus	Plantar, Layer 1	Abductor hallucis	Medial tubercle of plantar calcaneus, flexor retinaculum, and plantar aponeurosis	Medial aspect of base of #1 proximal phalange	Medial plantar nerve (S_2–S_3)	Abduction and flexion of great toe
Abductor hallucis Flexor digitorum brevis	Plantar, Layer 1	Flexor digitorum brevis	Medial tubercle of plantar calcaneus and plantar aponeurosis	Medial and lateral sides of middle phalanges of #2–5	Medial plantar nerve (S_2–S_3)	Flexion of toes #2–5
Abductor hallicus Abductor digiti minimi Flexor digitorum brevis	Plantar, Layer 1	Abductor digiti minimi	Calcaneal tuberosity, plantar aponeurosis, and intermuscular septum	Lateral base of proximal phalange of #5	Lateral plantar nerve (2 and S_3)	Abduction and flexion of #5

	Plantar, Layer 2	Quadratus plantae	Concave surface of calcaneus	Flexor digitorum longus tendons	Lateral plantar nerve (S_2 and S_3)	Assists the FDL in flexion of #2–5 toes
	Plantar, Layer 2	Lumbricals	Tendons of the flexor digitorum longus	Medial aspect of the extensor hood of MCP joints #2–5	#2: medial plantar nerve (S_2–S_3) #3–5: Lateral plantar nerve (S_2–S_3)	Flexion of proximal phalanges and extension of middle and distal phalanges of #2–5
	Plantar, Layer 3	Flexor hallucis brevis	Plantar aspect of cuboid and lateral cuneiform	Base of proximal phalange of the great toe	Medial plantar nerve (S_2–S_3)	Flexion of proximal phalanx of great toe

Continued

TABLE 11–5 | INTRINSIC MUSCLES—cont'd

Figure	Group	Muscle	Proximal insertion	Distal insertion	Innervation	Action
Flexor hallucis brevis; Adductor hallucis; Flexor digiti minimi brevis	Plantar, Layer 3	Adductor hallucis	Oblique head: Bases of #2–4 metatarsals Transverse head: plantar ligaments of MTP joints	Lateral base of proximal phalanx of the great toe	Deep branch of lateral plantar nerve (S_2–S_3)	Adduction of great toe. Provides assistance to maintenance of the transverse metatarsal arch
	Plantar, Layer 3	Flexor digiti minimi brevis	Base of 5th metatarsal	Base of proximal phalange of #5	Superficial branch of lateral plantar nerve (S_2–S_3)	Flexion of #5 toe
Plantar Interosseous; Dorsal Interosseous	Plantar, Layer 4	Dorsal interossei	Adjacent sides of all metatarsals	Extensor hood of MCP joints #2–4	Lateral plantar nerve (S_2–S_3)	Abduction of #2–4 and MTP flexion

	Plantar, Layer 4	Plantar interossei	Medial sides and bases of #3–5 metatarsals	Extensor hood of MCP joints #3–5	Lateral plantar nerve (S_2–S_3)	Adduction of #2–4 and MTP flexion
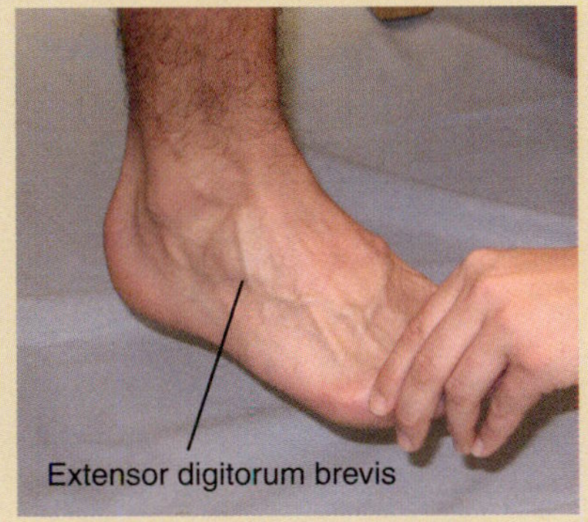 Extensor digitorum brevis	Dorsum	Extensor digitorum brevis and extensor hallucis brevis	Dorsolateral aspect of the foot distal to the sinus tarsi	Bases of proximal phalanges of #1–4	Lateral terminal branch of the deep peroneal nerve (S_1–S_2)	Assists in extension of toes #1–4

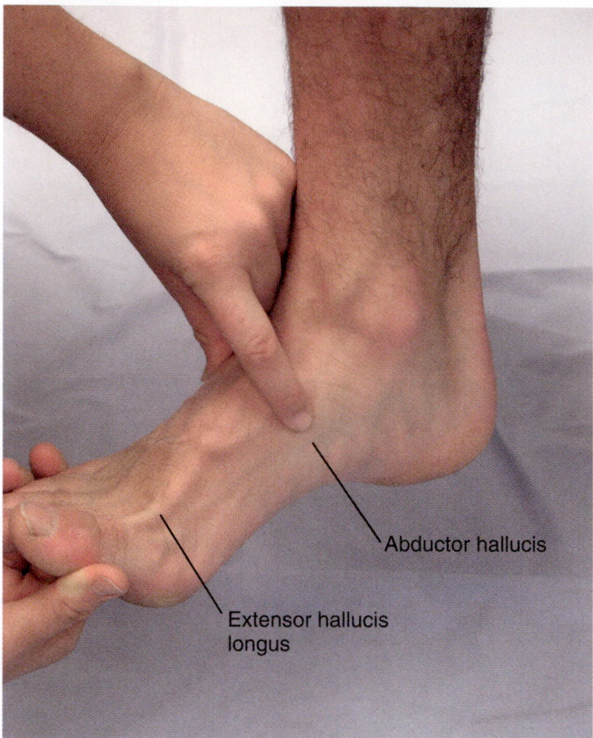

Figure 11.27 Abductor hallucis. This intrinsic muscle is palpated inferior to and slightly anterior to the navicular tubercle. The examiner passively positions the great toe in hallux valgus and has the subject attempt to actively move the toe into abduction. The muscle is felt contracting below the palpating finger.

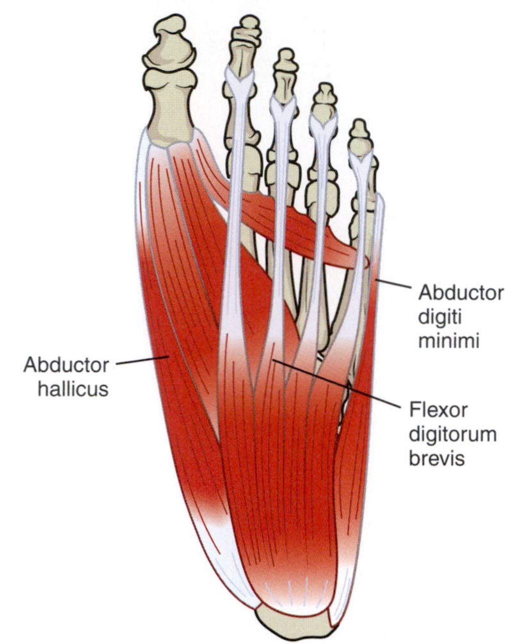

Figure 11.29 Plantar surface, first layer of intrinsic muscles. The first layer includes the abductor hallucis, flexor digitorum brevis, and abductor digiti minimi.

may be affected if a muscle is unable to function normally. In effect, the potential for a cascade of dysfunction of the foot exists if only one joint or one muscle fails to perform as it should. Since the foot plays a vital role in force absorption and transmission for the

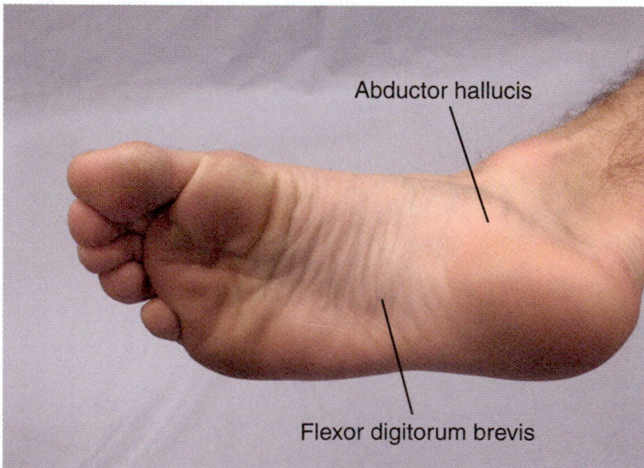

Figure 11.28 Flexor digitorum brevis. Some of the bellies of this muscle in the first layer of intrinsic muscles may be palpated in the middle of the longitudinal arch as the subject lightly flexes the toes.

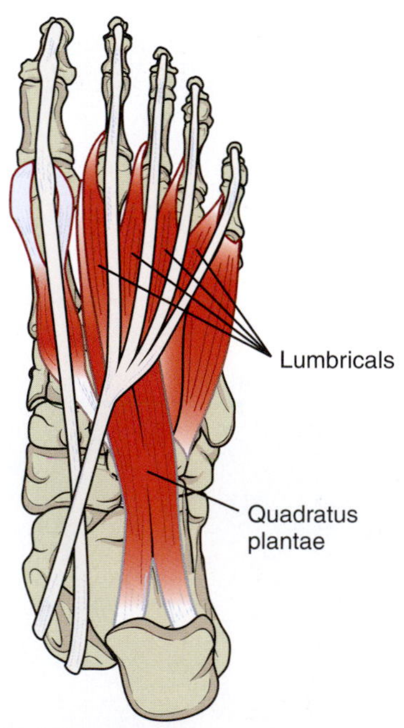

Figure 11.30 Plantar surface, second layer of intrinsic muscles. The second layer includes the quadratus plantae and lumbricals.

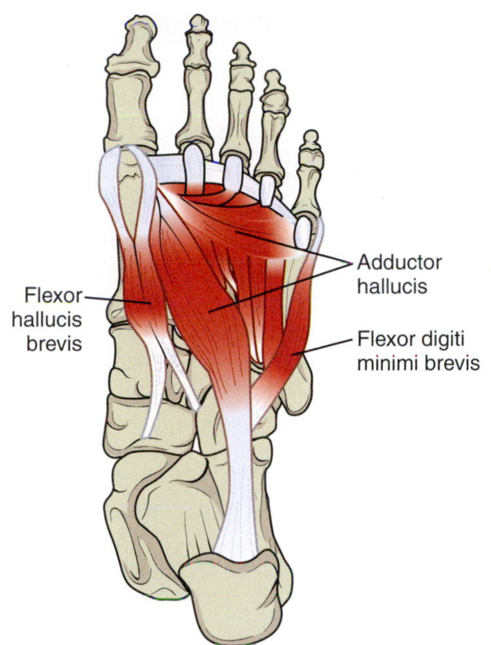

Figure 11.31 Plantar surface, third layer of intrinsic muscles. The third layer includes the flexor hallucis brevis, adductor hallucis, and flexor digiti minimi brevis.

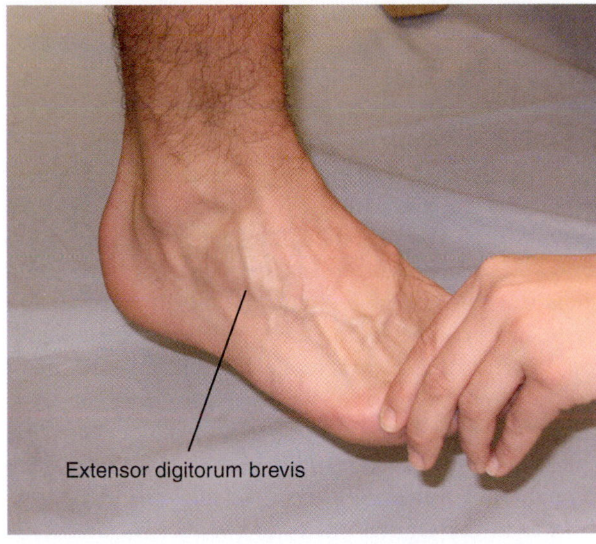

Figure 11.33 Extensor digitorum brevis and extensor hallucis brevis. These muscles are often merged as one muscle. The muscle belly appears as a small rounded knob on the dorsum of the foot just distal to the sinus tarsi. It is often bluish and about the size of a silver dollar. The tendons become evident when resistance is offered to toe extension. Occasionally, a tendon may be seen going to the great toe just lateral to the extensor hallucis longus tendon; this is the extensor hallucis brevis tendon.

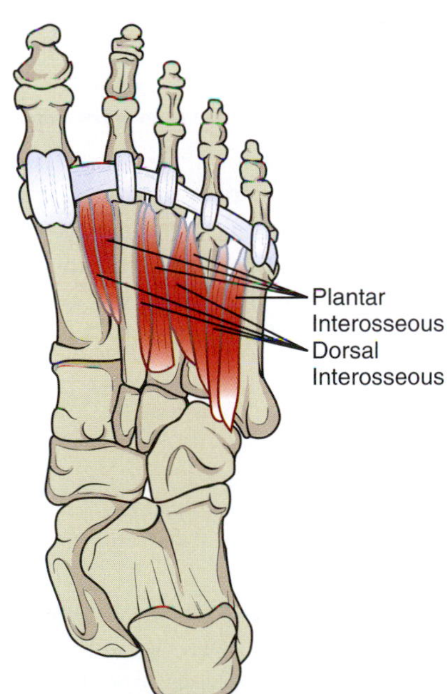

Figure 11.32 Plantar surface, fourth layer of intrinsic muscles. The fourth layer includes the plantar and dorsal interosseous muscles.

entire body, deficiencies here may affect other segments up the kinetic chain.

Within any one joint of the foot and ankle, relatively little range of motion occurs. The multijoint structure of the foot and ankle complex, however, involves many joints. These joints work together to produce a greater amount of mobility than is possible with only one joint. This arrangement also allows the foot to adapt and conform on many different surface structures and objects. In a closed chain activity, all of the toes want to be in contact with the surface on which the foot is standing. The multijoint system of the foot and ankle complex allows them to do just that. This segment pulls together the information from the previous segments (see page 511) of this chapter to create an understanding of the interrelationships that exist within the foot and ankle.

Pronation and Supination

Supination and pronation are important motions that the foot and ankle provide during static and dynamic activities and in both open and closed chain functions. These are the motions that allow the foot to adapt on many varied surfaces and still maintain good standing balance. These motions, however, involve many joints.

At the Subtalar Joint

It is important to realize that although the talocrural joint and subtalar joint are closely interrelated in function, pronation and supination occurs at the subtalar joint and are motions also involving the relationship between the talus and calcaneus. In the earlier discussion of terminology, it was mentioned that in an open kinetic chain, supination includes the motions of inversion, adduction, and plantarflexion, and pronation includes eversion, abduction, and dorsiflexion. In an open chain condition, the more proximal talus is stabilized in the subtalar joint as it sits within the mortise of the talocrural joint, and the distal calcaneus is free to move. Because of the subtalar joint's oblique axis, the calcaneus movement is triplanar. For example, during pronation the calcaneus everts in the frontal plane, dorsiflexes in the sagittal plane, and abducts in the transverse plane. As the calcaneus moves on the talus in the open chain in supination, it inverts in the frontal plane, plantarflexes in the sagittal plane, and adducts in the transverse plane.[39] You can see these motions in the three planes occurring with your own foot when you either maximally supinate or maximally pronate your foot with it off the floor.

When the foot is weight-bearing, the calcaneus is still able to move freely in the frontal plane, but it no longer moves freely in the sagittal and transverse planes. It is now fixed to the floor in these two planes by the force of the body weight on top of the foot. Therefore, pronation and supination still occur in the subtalar joint, but the bone that moves is the talus, not the calcaneus (Table 11–6). Therefore, in closed chain pronation motion, the calcaneus is still able to evert in the frontal plane, but now the talus plantarflexes and adducts on the calcaneus.[8] In closed kinetic chain supination, the calcaneus inverts in the frontal plane and the talus dorsiflexes on the calcaneus in the sagittal plane and abducts on the calcaneus in the transverse plane.[8] Since the body's line of gravity is medial to the axis of motion of the calcaneus in pronation and lateral to it in supination, the calcaneus moves to inversion during pronation and to eversion during supination. The coupled motions that go along with calcaneal inversion and eversion during pronation and supination

TABLE 11–6 | OPEN AND CLOSED KINETIC CHAIN MOVEMENTS OF PRONATION AND SUPINATION AT THE TALOCRURAL AND SUBTALAR JOINTS

Motion	Open Chain	Closed Chain
Supination	**Plantarflexion:** Calcaneus on talus **Adduction:** Calcaneus on talus **Inversion:** Calcaneus in frontal plane	**Dorsiflexion:** Talus on calcaneus **Abduction:** Talus on calcaneus **Inversion:** Calcaneus in frontal plane Transverse tarsal joint supination Tibiofibular lateral rotation Femoral lateral rotation
Pronation	**Dorsiflexion:** Calcaneus on talus **Abduction:** Calcaneus on talus **Eversion:** Calcaneus in frontal plane	**Plantarflexion:** Talus on calcaneus **Adduction:** Talus on calcaneus **Eversion:** Calcaneus in frontal plane Transverse tarsal joint supination or pronation, depending on forefoot needs Tibiofibular medial rotation Femoral medial rotation

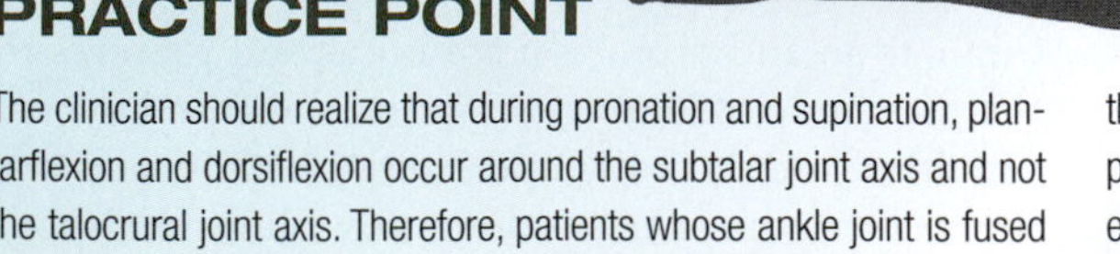

PRACTICE POINT

The clinician should realize that during pronation and supination, plantarflexion and dorsiflexion occur around the subtalar joint axis and not the talocrural joint axis. Therefore, patients whose ankle joint is fused because of arthritis or trauma will still have dorsiflexion and plantarflexion motion available to them in the subtalar joint. Similarly, since the talocrural joint is a triplanar joint with motion available in all three planes, when patients undergo an arthrodesis of the subtalar joint or even a triple arthrodesis (fusion of subtalar, calcaneocuboid, and talonavicular joints), they will still have some degree of inversion-eversion, dorsiflexion-plantarflexion, and abduction-adduction motions.[8]

now occur at the talus in weight-bearing. Specifically, with the body weight securing the calcaneus in the sagittal and transverse planes, the talus adducts towards its medial border in the transverse plane and the head of the talus plantarflexes in the sagittal plane in weight-bearing pronation. In weight-bearing supination, the opposite occurs: The calcaneus inverts and the talus rolls laterally, and the head of the talus elevates to produce talar abduction and dorsiflexion on the calcaneus. Rather than the calcaneus moving on the talus as it does during open chain motion, the talus moves on the calcaneus during weight-bearing, so the motions occurring are different, but the relative end positions of the subtalar joint are the same in either an open or closed kinetic chain. For example, if the calcaneus moves on the talus, its convex surface slides on the talus's concave surface to move into abduction; however, if the concave talus surface moves on the convex calcaneus surface, the movement of the talus is adduction. Whether the foot moves in an open chain or a closed chain, the relative end positions of the two bones are the same. Figures 11.34 and 11.35 illustrate how the open and closed kinetic chain conditions change to produce these different motions.

Other Joints

The talocrural and subtalar joints are not the only ones involved in closed chain supination and pronation. All of the joints of the foot participate in these motions.[48] Of these other joints, the most important one is the transverse tarsal joint. Within this joint, the talonavicular joint produces the most movement in supination and pronation.[48] Motion at the transverse tarsal joint is vital to maintaining the foot in contact with the ground, particularly on uneven surfaces. This joint has the ability to either pronate or supinate. When the rearfoot supinates, the transverse tarsal joint also supinates, moved into position by the joint's proximal bones—the talus and calcaneus. In the supinated position, the transverse tarsal joint, like the rearfoot joints, are locked into position (Fig. 11.16).

However, when the rearfoot is in any degree of pronation, the transverse tarsal joint is able to move into supination or pronation. Since the transverse tarsal joint serves as a transition between the forefoot and rearfoot, which position it takes depends upon the forefoot needs. Recall that the toes want to maintain contact with the ground. Therefore, if the rearfoot is pronated, the lateral toes would tend to lift off the ground if the rest of the foot followed the rearfoot. In this example, however, the transverse tarsal joint moves into supination to lower the lateral toes to the ground (Fig. 11.8).

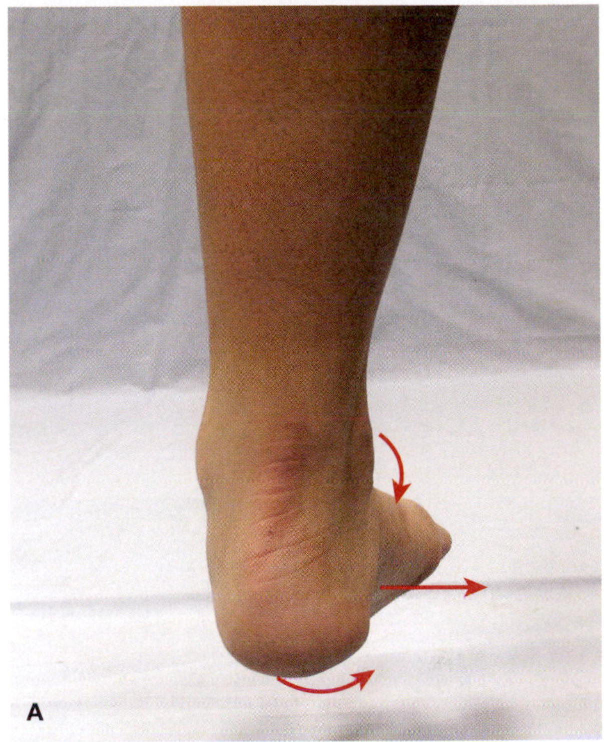

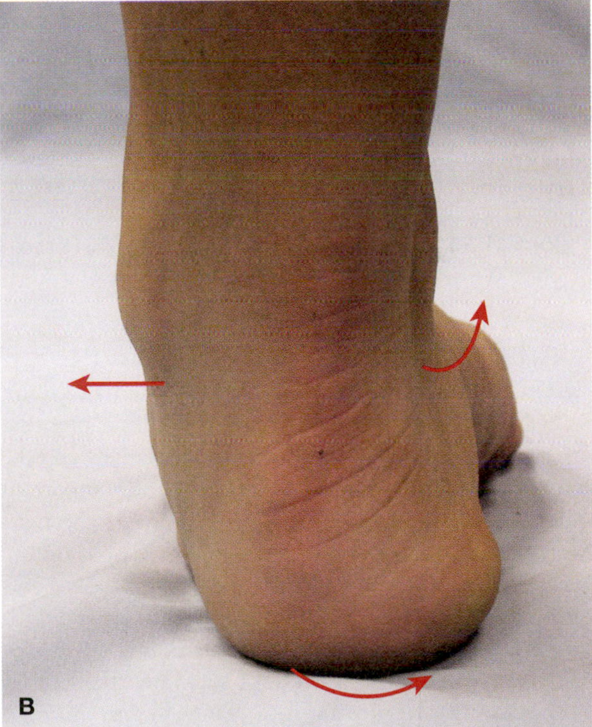

Figure 11.34 Supination in: **A)** open kinetic chain; **B)** closed kinetic chain.

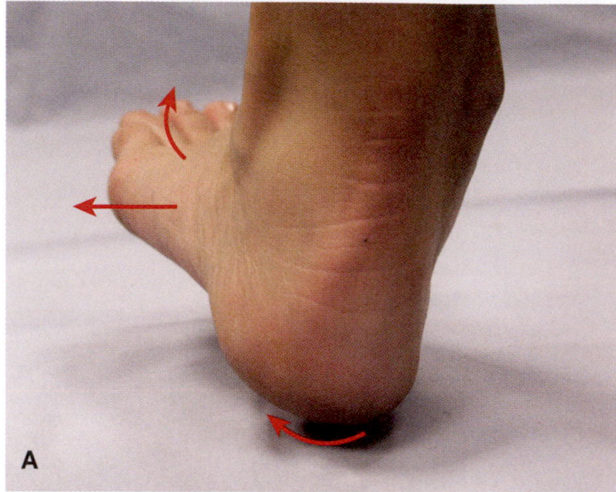

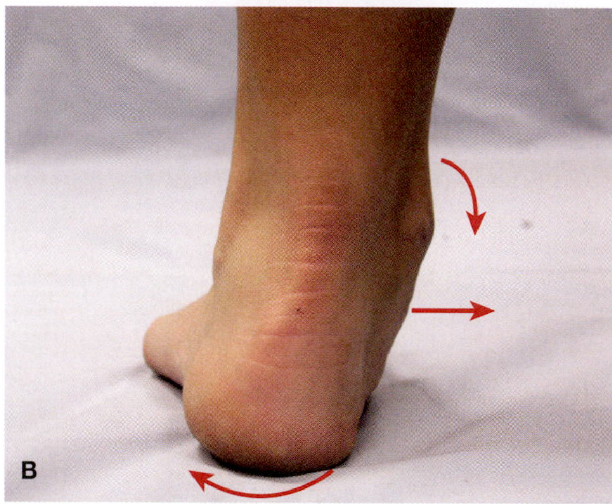

Figure 11.35 Pronation in: **A)** open kinetic chain; **B)** closed kinetic chain.

Additional compensation occurs at the tarsometatarsal joints when the transverse midtarsal joint is unable to do so. Recall from earlier in the chapter that the most flexible digits are the first ray medially and the fourth and fifth rays laterally. This becomes important when the rearfoot moves into supination. As the rearfoot supinates, the transverse tarsal joint is obligated to also supinate. With these joints in supination, the medial toes would have difficulty touching the ground were it not for mobility of the first, fourth, and fifth rays. When the rearfoot and midfoot supinate, the first ray pushes downward moving into plantarflexion until the toe reaches the floor. This plantarflexion motion of the first ray is counterbalanced by a dorsiflexion movement of the fourth and fifth rays to maintain the lateral toes on the ground.

Not only are joints distal to the subtalar and talocrural joints responsive to weight-bearing forces during pronation and supination, but the more proximal joints up the kinetic chain also move in response to these motions. As we have discussed, weight-bearing supination of the foot and ankle results in abduction of the talus. Because the joint axis is oblique, talus lateral rotation also occurs with abduction. This causes a chain reaction of lateral rotation of adjacent structures, the tibia and fibula. Similarly, when the talus adducts during closed chain pronation, it also rotates, but this time it medially rotates and subsequently leads to medial rotation of the tibia and fibula. Since adjacent joints are impacted during closed chain movements, tibial rotation is accompanied by corresponding femoral rotation; supination and lateral tibial rotation are accompanied by lateral femoral rotation whereas medial tibial and femoral rotation complement each other during pronation (Fig. 11.36A, B).

Arches of the Foot

The arches of the foot provide important functions: to allow the foot to adapt to various surfaces, absorb the forces imparted to the foot during closed chain activities, provide a weight-bearing surface and base of support for the body, and change the foot to a rigid lever for propulsion of the body. The ability of the foot to change from a flexible to a rigid structure within a single step is dependent upon the bony structure of the three arches of the foot, static ligament-fascial support, and dynamic muscle contraction. In closed chain motion, such as standing, the superincumbent body weight is distributed through the talus and calcaneal tuberosity posteriorly

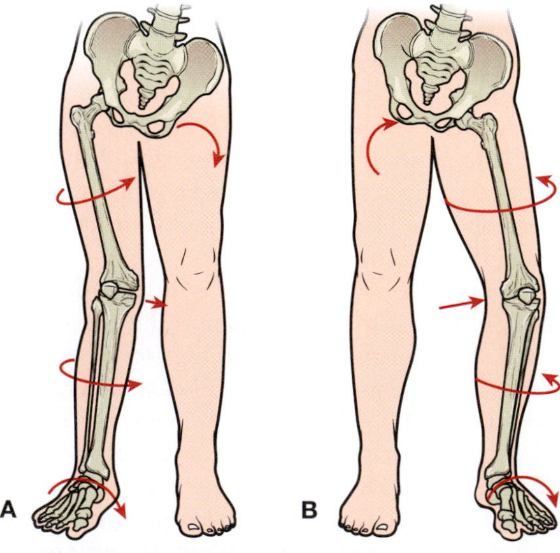

Figure 11.36 **A)** Pronation produces medial rotation of the tibia and femur. **B)** Supination produces lateral rotation of the tibia and femur.

and anteriorly to the heads of the metatarsal bones and the toes. Body weight is distributed to these points through the three arches.[80] The medial longitudinal arch is the longest and the highest. Its bony components include the calcaneus, talus, navicular, medial cuneiform, and first metatarsal bones. The lateral longitudinal arch is lower and composed of the calcaneus, cuboid, and fifth metatarsal. The transverse arch is concave in nonweight-bearing from medial to lateral in the midtarsal and tarsometatarsal areas. Distally to this arch, the heads of the metatarsal bones are flexible and conform to the contour of the ground.

Structurally, ligaments connect the tarsal and metatarsal bones on the dorsal and plantar surfaces to bind the bones of the arches into a structure with mechanical properties of a solid curved beam. Metatarsals are also curved to present a concave surface on the plantar aspect, reinforcing the curved-beam design. When loaded, the curved beam of the foot bends, compression forces occur on the top (convex side) and tension forces occur on the plantar surface (concave side).[81] Such a design allows acceptance of larger forces than if the structural design was a straight beam. Even larger forces can be supported by the beam if a tie-rod is placed across the base of the beam to serve as a truss to prevent the two ends from moving apart (Fig. 11.37A, B).[82] In the foot, the tie-rod is the plantar aponeurosis, which is actively reinforced by intrinsic and extrinsic foot muscles (Fig. 11.37C).[81]

The **plantar aponeurosis**, also referred to simply as the plantar fascia, is a strong series of fascial bands that support the sole and sides of the foot from the calcaneal tuberosity to the toes. The plantar aponeurosis is important to the integrity of all arches of the foot.[84] The aponeurosis is an attachment for intrinsic muscles of the foot such as the flexor digitorum brevis and is the fascial covering for others like the abductor hallucis. Tendon and neurovascular bundles perforate this aponeurosis on their way to the toes. Complex vertical septa (walls) and lateral mooring structures connect the longitudinal bands of the aponeurosis to deep structures, the skin, and each other. Distal attachments of the plantar aponeurosis are associated with the sheaths of the flexor tendons, plantar plates, and deep structures of the toes. These attachments are distal to the MTP joints, so when these joints hyperextend, tension is placed on the plantar aponeurosis. This tension prevents the displacement of the calcaneus from the metatarsal heads and the collapse of the arches.[81] Additionally, this tension compresses the tarsal and metatarsal bones to create a rigid structure. Such rigidity is required when standing on the toes and during the terminal stance phase of walking.

Mechanically, the MTP aponeurotic mechanism is similar to a **windlass mechanism.** A windlass is a horizontal cylinder that rotates with a crank to pull on a chain or rope that wraps around the cylinder; it is usually used to move heavy objects such as an anchor on a ship. When the MTP joints hyperextend, the aponeurosis becomes taut as it wraps around the metatarsophalangeal joints, so the metatarsal bone and tarsal bones pull together and are converted into a rigid structure, causing the longitudinal arch to rise.[84] The intrinsic and extrinsic muscles contract concentrically to add an active force to the passive plantar fascial force, creating a higher arch. This windlass mechanism can be observed when the first MTP joint is passively positioned in hyperextension (Fig. 11.38); the arches become rigid and the plantar aponeurosis becomes taut and easily palpated. When a person stands on his or her toes, an increase in the longitudinal arch's concavity can also be observed.

Both intrinsic muscles of the plantar foot and extrinsic muscles of the posterior leg play important roles in active support of the foot arches in weight-bearing activities.[74, 85] All of the extrinsic and most of the intrinsic muscles of the plantar foot cross under the arches. When these muscles contract in closed chain motion, the forces they produce tighten the arches. The

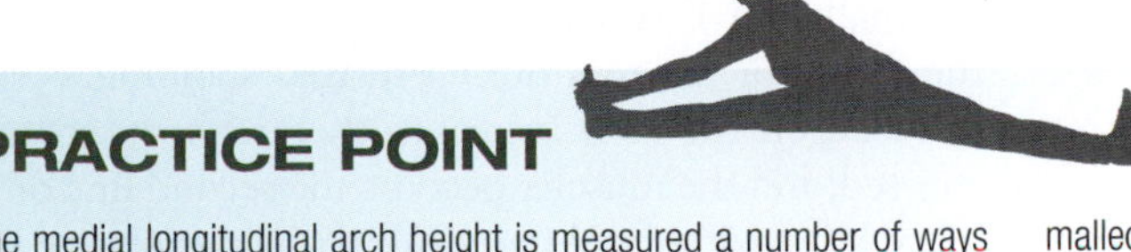

PRACTICE POINT

The medial longitudinal arch height is measured a number of ways to determine if it is of an appropriate height. One quick was is to evaluate the position of the navicular tubercle relative to the position of a line between the medial malleolus and first metatarsophalangeal joint. A line is drawn from the apex of the inferior medial malleolus to the plantar surface of the first MTP joint. If the medial longitudinal arch is normal height, the navicular tubercle sits on or close to this line.[83] If the arch is low, the navicular tubercle is below the line; if it is a high arch, the navicular tubercle is above the line. This line is known as "**Feiss' line.**"

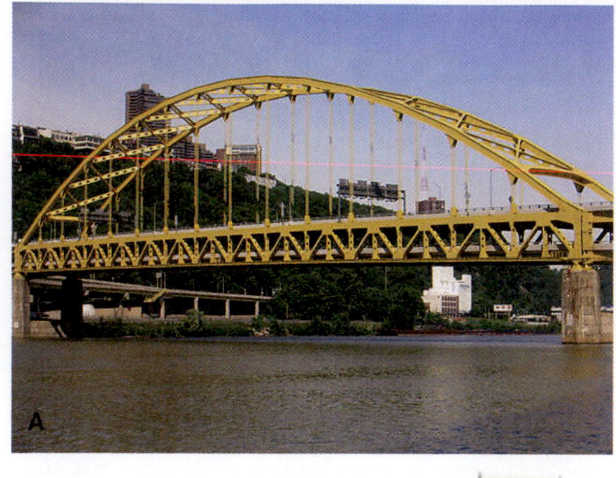

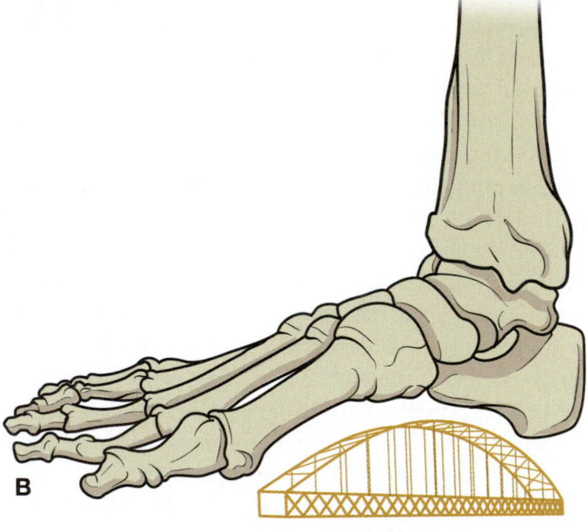

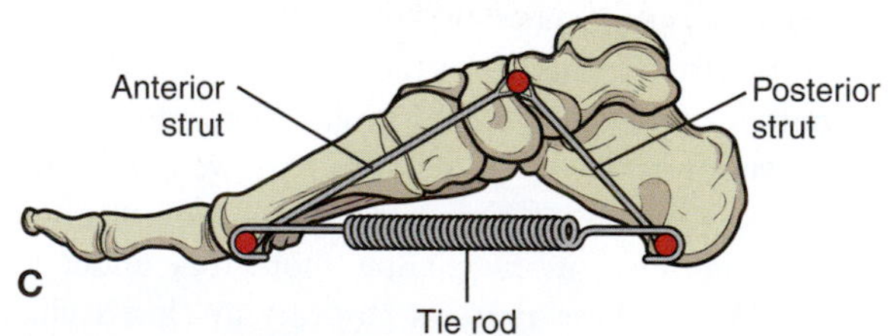

Figure 11.37 A & B) The curvature of the bones of the foot provide a structure able to absorb high forces. Similar to a bridge, the arch of the foot obtains its strength and support from its design to enable absorption of large, repetitive forces. C) Additionally, the supporting plantar aponeurosis along with active support from intrinsic and extrinsic muscles provide structural resilience by serving as a tie rod. *(Photo courtesy of Historicbridges.org)*

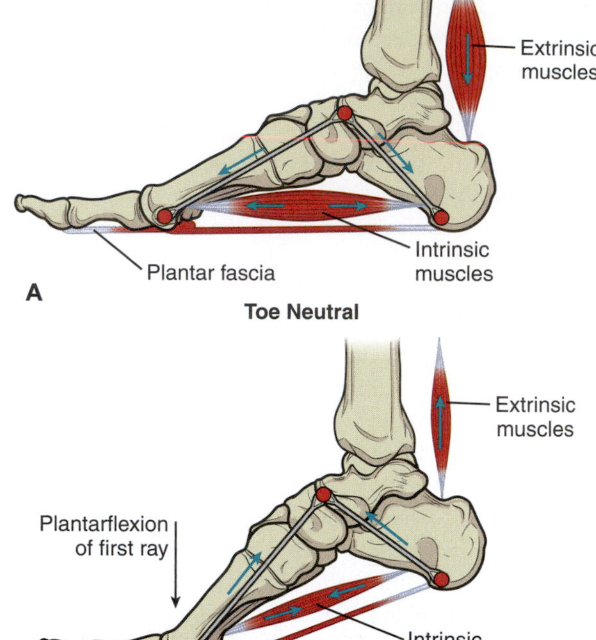

Figure 11.38 Windlass mechanism. A) The plantar aponeurosis along with the intrinsic muscles reinforce the longitudinal arch. B) When the individual raises onto the toes the fascial tension increases and intrinsic muscles contract. This locks the arch bones to provide a secure lever for the extrinsic muscles to produce the motion.

tibialis posterior and the peroneus longus with their extensive plantar attachments have a major impact on the transverse arch, and they also tighten both of the longitudinal arches.[74] The flexor hallucis longus and the abductor hallucis span the medial longitudinal arch, and the abductor digiti minimi runs the length of the lateral longitudinal arch, so these muscles affect the longitudinal arch during activity.[79] The flexor digitorum brevis, quadratus plantae, and flexor digitorum longus run the midplantar length and tighten the longitudinal arches. The adductor hallucis affects the transverse arch.

Unlike the muscles of the fingers, the toe muscles have little function or purpose during open chain motion. However, they have great importance in closed chain motions such as walking, running, and jumping. Normally, no EMG activity occurs in the muscles of the arches or the toes during relaxed standing.[85, 86] As the load on the arch increases, the arch's supports are stressed, and the muscles become the second line of stability. When a normal foot deals with an excessive load, the muscles supporting the foot arches are electromyographically active.[86] It has also been demonstrated that individuals with flat feet have activity of the tibialis anterior and tibialis posterior during standing.[87] When an individual has a lower than normal arch, the inert ligamentous structures are unable to provide normal structural stability, so the muscles increase their activity to compensate for this deficiency.

Loading of the Foot

Conventionally, weight distribution in standing is stated to be 50%–50% between the calcaneus and the metatarsal heads. Normal weight distribution of the metatarsal heads has the first metatarsal head absorbing twice the weight that each of the four lateral metatarsal heads supports in a proportion of 2:1:1:1:1.[81] There is, however, considerable variation in the distribution of pressure on the structures of the foot and a high degree of variability among subjects. Some have found more than half of the weight distributed to the heel[89] whereas others have found that younger adults tend to distribute more of their weight forward.[90] During gait, the heel and great toe encounter the greatest forces; these forces are ground reaction forces which occur as the foot either makes contact with the ground or pushes away from the ground. The relative amount of force applied to the heel or to the anterior foot is dependent upon the speed of gait.[91,92] The faster the speed of either walking or running, the greater the ground reaction forces. During varied walking speeds, the ground reaction force applied to the great toe and heel increase linearly with the great toe experiencing a greater load than the heel until the speed is increased to more than 2 m/sec (Fig. 11.39).[92] Fortunately, the heel pad has a thick fat pad that protects the calcaneus and distributes the forces imparted to it.[93] The anterior foot is also protected from these loading forces by the fascia and soft tissue that deflects forces from the bones.[94] In Chapter 12, additional information on ground reaction forces is presented in the kinetics of gait section.

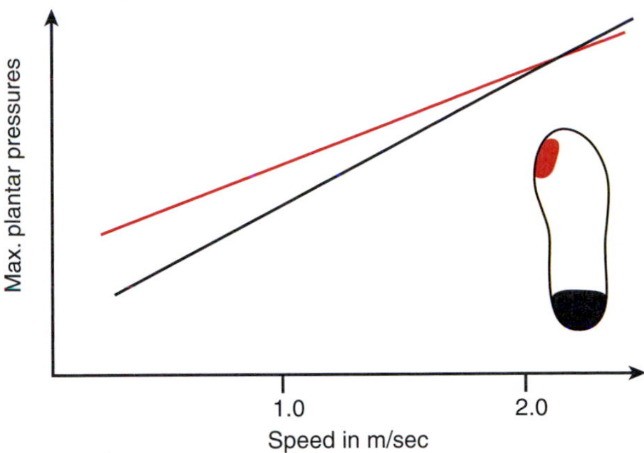

(Based on data from Segal, et al, 2004)

Figure 11.39 There is a linear increase in ground reaction force applied to the great toe and heel during progressive walking speeds. The great toe experiences greater forces applied to it until the walking speed approaches 2 m/s.

The foot's arches are loaded during activities such as walking, running, jumping, hopping, and going up on the toes. During these activities, muscle contraction and the windlass mechanism are recruited to provide the additional support required of the arches. EMG activity of the extrinsic and intrinsic muscles that support the arches begins shortly after the foot contacts the ground in the stance phase of walking and running and continues as the heel rises and the MTP joints hyperextend to tighten the plantar aponeurosis.[37] The muscle activity and the tension on the aponeurosis continue until the

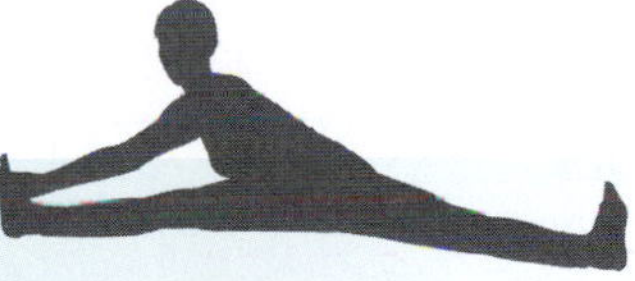

PRACTICE POINT

An example of a common sports-related injury of the arches of the foot is plantar fasciitis (*-itis,* inflammation). This problem has a high incidence in runners and aerobic dancers. Those with the problem complain of pain in the foot near the heel when they walk and that the pain becomes worse with jumping or running and after they have been sitting for awhile. A classic complaint is extreme pain in the morning when they first get out of bed. The pain can be reproduced by deep palpation at the proximal attachment of the plantar aponeurosis and simultaneously passively hyperextending the MTP joints to stretch the aponeurosis. This condition is usually multifactorial in its etiology and may include factors from the body or from the environment. Extraneous precipitating factors may include an increase in activity, changes in surfaces, or changes in shoe wear. Etiological factors from the body may include intrinsic muscle weakness, faulty alignment of the foot, reduced flexibility in the calf muscles, and excessive pronation of the foot. For example, an inverted calcaneus requires a pronation compensation at the calcaneotalonavicular joint to place the metatarsal heads parallel to the ground for weight-bearing.[88] Such malalignment, however, may never become a problem until the arches are overloaded as they are during running or jumping activities, and compensatory motions and muscle contractions fail to provide support. A careful history by the clinician usually reveals a marked increase in intensity of the activity or a change of running surfaces or shoes before the onset of pain.

toes leave the ground. These mechanisms can be observed and palpated on another person during standing and rising up on the toes. Note the marked supination of the longitudinal arch and inversion of the calcaneus when standing on the toes (Fig. 11.18).

Deformities of the Foot

Foot deformities may develop from a variety of causes. There may be congenital malformations of bones, muscular paralysis or spasticity, chronic stresses and strains in weight-bearing, poorly fitting shoes, or from a combination of several of these factors. In other words, these deformities may be either congenital or acquired. Since forces are transmitted up the extremity from the foot during ambulation, some of these deformities may influence other joints or body segments as changes occur to adapt to these deformities over time.

Pes Planus (Flat Foot)

This is a more or less permanent pronation of the foot, in which body weight acts to depress the medial longitudinal and transverse arches. This may be an acquired condition or congenital. In order for the foot to pronate, the calcaneus must roll into eversion. There is a natural tendency for the calcaneus to evert with weight-bearing since the line of gravity falls medial to the center of the calcaneus, but in people with pes planus, there are other deficiencies which lead to this problem. If it is not a congenital condition, the individual may have developed laxity in the foot ligaments, weakness in the muscles, or tightness in the extrinsic muscles. In a nonweight-bearing condition, the individual may have what appears to be a normal longitudinal arch, but when the person stands, the navicular bone drops towards the floor as the calcaneus is positioned in eversion. In its extreme condition, it is known as pes planus or a flatfoot (Fig. 11.40A). Pes planus may be either rigid or flexible. If it is rigid, the foot has no arch in either weight-bearing or nonweight-bearing and is often congenital. A flexible pes planus exhibits as a foot with an arch when nonweight-bearing, but the arch disappears in standing.

Standing with the calcaneus in eversion is seen frequently throughout the population to varying degrees, but the excessively flat foot is not as common. Individuals with a flexible flat foot have difficulty transferring the foot into a rigid lever during the last half of the stance phase of gait. Such a condition transfers forces created during push-off to the lateral foot while the foot is abducted.[35] Such a position produces excessive forces on the medial great toe, and over time, a bunion, or hallux valgus (see below), occurs.

With the midfoot rotated to the ground, a flat foot also stresses the tendons that are attached to the medial foot. The muscles that seem most susceptible to stresses are the peroneus longus and the tibialis posterior. In a foot which is perpetually pronated, these muscles and their tendons are placed on continual stress as they work unsuccessfully to perform their tasks during weight-bearing. These repetitive stresses that occur in these structures often

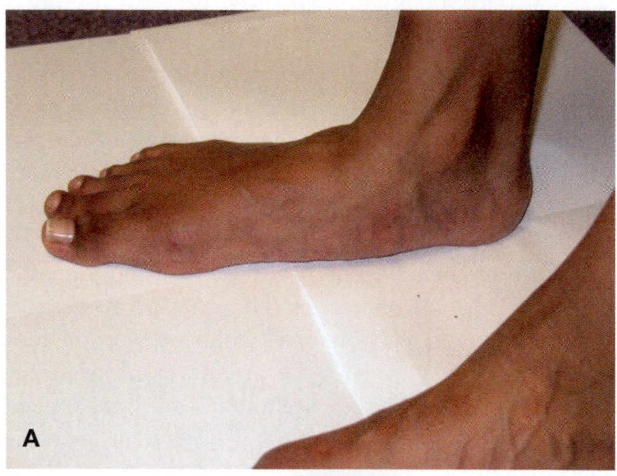

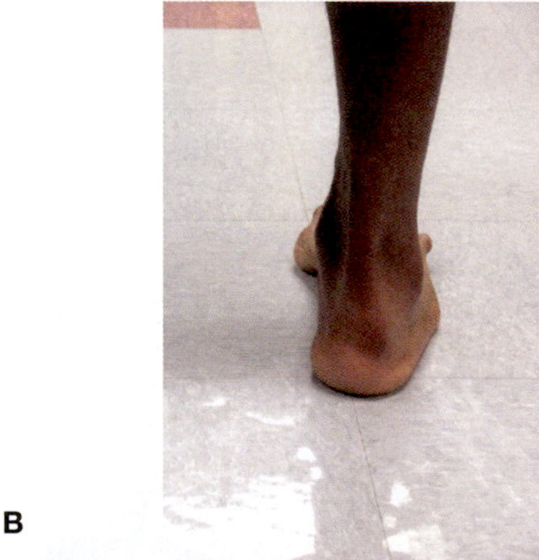

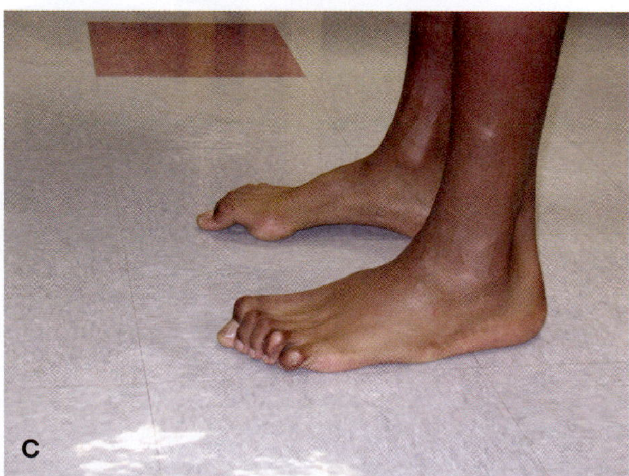

Figure 11.40 Structural deformities of the foot. **A)** Pes planus. **B &C)** Pes cavus.

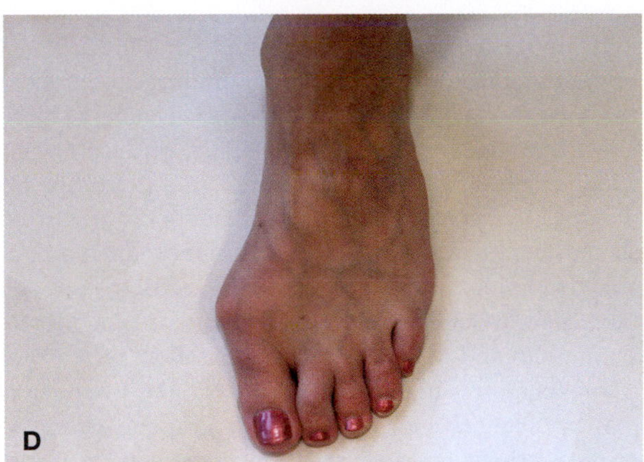

Figure 11.40—cont'd D) Hallux valgus.

develop conditions of tendinopathy, especially in feet that are not totally flat but have some arch to them.

When an individual is weight-bearing and the foot is pronated, other joints up the closed chain must respond to this position. As has been mentioned, the tibia medially rotates when the foot pronates. If the tibia medially rotates, the knee flexes and moves into a valgus position. This knee position, in turn, causes the thigh to adduct and medially rotate and the hip to flex (Fig. 11.36A). Although you may not have natural pronation of your feet when you stand, if you place your feet in a pronated position, you will see what happens up your kinetic chain.

Pes Cavus (Club Foot)

Pes cavus is a condition of a high medial longitudinal arch that occurs with inversion of the calcaneus. This is usually a rigid foot structure of a congenital nature. The calcaneal position causes the foot to move into a supination-inversion position so the body weight is transferred to the outside of the foot and, in extreme cases, the medial border of the foot is off the ground. Extreme cases are known as club foot.

Individuals with pes varus have little movement between the bones within the foot, so the foot acts as a rigid lever throughout the gait cycle. Therefore, the foot is unable to absorb the impact forces of walking and running. As a result, these individuals often suffer stress fractures either in the foot or up the extremity chain with proximal transmission of the unabsorbed forces. A high medial arch also causes the distal joints to change their alignment; the metatarsophalangeal joints eventually become hyperextended, causing the proximal interphalangeal joints to hyperflex and the distal interphalangeal joint to either hyperextend or remain in neutral so the toes are still able to touch the ground (Fig. 11.40C).

As with pronated feet, if the feet are supinated, as they are in pes cavus, the other joints up the chain will align accordingly when the individual is in a standing position. Individuals with supinated feet also find that they have lateral tibial rotation, the knees are in a varus position and in extension, the thighs abduct and laterally rotate, and the hips tend to be extended (Fig. 11.36B). Once again, if you move your feet into supination when standing, you will see your lower extremities assume a similar alignment.

Hallux Valgus

Hallux valgus is a lateral deviation of the great toe at the MTP joint. This condition is often accompanied by an inflammation of the bursa on the medial side of the toe joint. When it is irritated, it is very painful and difficult for the individual to wear shoes which rub against it.

As mentioned, a common cause of hallux valgus is pes planus or overly pronated feet. Because the foot pushes off from the medial part of the foot rather than the distal toes, the foot is in more abduction than normal. Since the great toe is in contact with the ground, it receives repetitive forces applied to its medial border with the MTP joint becoming the joint which suffers the results of this stress. Over time, the great toe becomes angled towards the lateral toes (Fig. 11.40D).

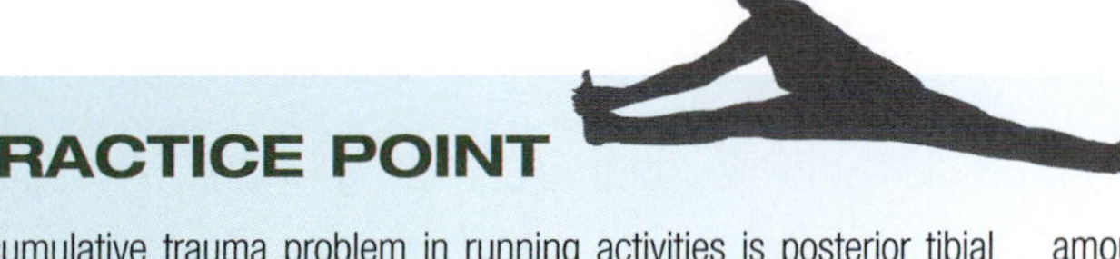

PRACTICE POINT

A cumulative trauma problem in running activities is posterior tibial shin splint, which causes pain with contraction or stretch of the muscle. The clinician is able to reproduce this pain by palpating the proximal attachment of the muscle along the inner posterior edge of the shin along its length. This problem is usually associated with overpronation, which requires more work from the tibialis posterior to support the longitudinal arch in activity. DeLacerda[95] measured the amount of depression of the navicular tuberosity before subjects started a running program. He found that those who later developed shin splints had an average depression of the navicular tuberosity of 9 mm between sitting and standing, whereas those who did not develop problems had a depression averaging 6 mm. Clinicians with patients diagnosed with shin splints should investigate their patients for possible overpronation as well as tightness of the posterior calf muscles.

Summary

The foot and ankle are a complicated structure. The ankle includes the distal tibia and fibula with the talus. The rearfoot includes the talus and calcaneus, the midfoot is comprised of the other tarsal bones, and the forefoot includes the metatarsals and phalanges. The rearfoot has a profound influence on the joints of the rest of the foot, especially during weight-bearing activities. Bones within the foot and ankle change their relative alignment during weight-bearing activities as the function of the foot and ankle change. The foot changes from a mobile adaptor during weight acceptance and weight-bearing to a rigid lever that propels the body forward at the end of the stance phase of walking and running. The arches of the foot are maintained by the joints, ligaments, fascia, and muscles. They assist in absorbing forces of impact. The toes want to be in contact with the ground, so the foot joints move to accommodate them. If a joint lacks its normal mobility, other joints will compensate to allow the toes to touch the floor. In these instances, these joints may undergo additional stresses because of this added responsibility. Muscles of the ankle and foot are divided into extrinsic and intrinsic muscles. The extrinsic muscles provide the power and motion for foot and ankle function whereas the intrinsic muscles provide more stability and adaptability of the foot. The intrinsic muscles and ligaments of the foot allow the foot to adapt to most surfaces, regardless of how irregular it may be. The calf muscles are the largest and strongest of the extrinsic muscles; they provide power for push-off and flexion of the ankle, foot, and toes. The arches of the foot along with the intrinsic and intrinsic muscles and fascia supporting the arches provide a windlass mechanism that allows for a strong base of the foot during activities when the heel is off the ground.

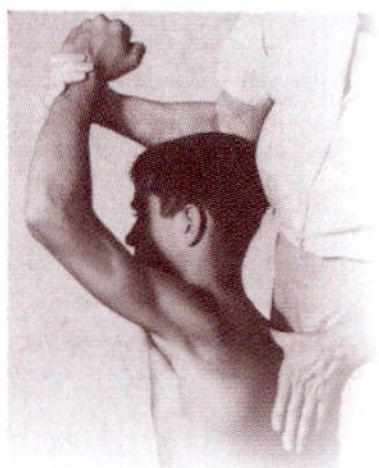

CLINICAL SCENARIO SOLUTION

As he prepares a mental list of things to include in his examination of his new patient, Chaz Michaels knows that he will have to examine the rearfoot and forefoot relationship of his patient. He also will have to examine the patient for intrinsic muscle strength, extrinsic muscle flexibility, and possible gait deviations. Chaz knows that excessive pronation is a common problem in people with plantar fasciitis, so he wants to see if this is present in his patient as well. When he reproduces the patient's pain, he suspects already that he will get a positive response when he performs a deep palpation over the medial calcaneal tubercle. He is prepared to ask all the pertinent history questions as well. He knows that plantar fasciitis is a multifactorial condition, so he suspects that his patient has probably increased her activity recently or changed shoes or surfaces on which she exercises, so he will ask her questions on these topics when he sees her. He is confident as he completes his mental list that he is ready to see this patient for the first time. He is also confident that his clinical skills will produce a good outcome for this patient.

Discussion Questions

1. List the joints that are formed by the bones involved in the ankle, foot, and toes. Identify how the foot is divided into segments and the bones of each of these three segments.
2. Identify the muscles of the anterior, lateral, superficial posterior, and deep posterior muscles. Identify the muscles that have similar distal insertion locations on the foot.
3. Explain how the rearfoot determines and controls the position of the rest of the foot during weight-bearing.
4. What happens to the rest of the foot if the calcaneus inverts when standing?
5. Explain in your own words what happens to the foot when a person lands on the heel when he walks and then moves his body over the leg, as in taking a step. Why is this process necessary?
6. If the arch of the foot is supinated until the foot hits the ground during walking, and then the foot moves into pronation, explain the activity of the peroneus longus during this part of the gait cycle.

7. Explain the activity of the tibialis posterior during the activity described in #5.
8. You are on a hike and decide to climb over a large boulder. This large boulder is big enough to stand on and walk over, but the surface of it is uneven. You notice as you stand at the top of this large boulder that your right foot is positioned at an angle in pronation while your left foot is positioned in supination. Describe the positions of the talocrural, subtalar, and transverse tarsal joints of your feet.
9. Describe how the windlass mechanism of the foot works. Identify three activities in which we use it.
10. Explain how a ballerina is able to make her ankle appear to be horizontal with her leg. If the ankle is able to plantarflex even 60°, this is still not close to 90°.

Lab Activities

1. On the skeleton, identify the following bones and bony landmarks. Locate on yourself and on a subject those that are palpable:

tibia	cuboid
fibula	three cuneiform bones
medial and lateral malleoli	metatarsal bones (heads, bases, shafts)
tuberosity of navicular	phalanges
talus	tuberosity of fifth metatarsal
calcaneus	sustentaculum tali

2. With disarticulated bones of the tibia, fibula, and foot, observe the articulating surfaces and simulate the motions of the:
   a. Talocrural joint
   b. Talocalcaneal joint (subtalar)
   c. Talonavicular and calcaneocuboid joints, which form the transverse tarsal joint
   d. Tarsometatarsal joints
   e. MTP joints
   f. Interphalangeal (IP) joints
3. Perform passive motion of the joints above on your partner's foot and describe the range of motion, the end feels, and the limiting structures. Your partner's leg and foot must be relaxed throughout the examination.
4. Measure the amount of active dorsiflexion that occurs when the knee is flexed to 90°, and compare it to the amount possible when the knee is extended. What structure limits dorsiflexion when the knee is extended?
5. Palpate the sole of your partner's relaxed foot between the calcaneus and the metatarsal heads. Then passively hyperextend the MTP joints and palpate to feel the tightening of the plantar aponeurosis (windlass mechanism). When in the range of MTP hyperextension does tightening begin? How far are you able to hyperextend the toe? Describe the palpation sensation you have of the sole before and at the end of the stretch.
6. Palpate around the head of the fibula to feel fibular motion as the subject actively dorsiflexes the ankle. Place your fingers on each malleolus and feel the slight spreading that occurs with dorsiflexion. Now hold the malleoli together and have your partner actively dorsiflex the ankle. What happens?
7. Grasp around the calcaneus and hold it in eversion (subtalar motion) and move the transverse tarsal joint in pronation and supination. Then hold the calcaneus in inversion and move the transverse tarsal joint. What is the difference in movement with the calcaneus in the two different positions? What is the importance of these two states of the transverse tarsal joint?

8. Measure the height of the navicular tuberosity when your partner is sitting with feet resting on the floor and in standing. Mark the tuberosity of the navicular and measure the distance to the surface. Have the subject stand and measure the distance again. Compare results with others. How does it change? What is your explanation?
9. Measure the amount of tibial torsion present and compare angles with other subjects:
   a. Have your subject sit in a chair with feet on the floor and with the patellae pointing straight ahead. Place a piece of paper under the foot. Passively lift the relaxed leg and foot up and set it down on the paper. Identify the knee axis (x axis) running through the medial and lateral epicondyles of the femur and project it to the paper (draw the line of the knee axis on the paper).
   b. Trace around the outline of the foot and mark projections of the medial and lateral malleoli on the paper. Remove the paper and draw a line through the projections for the malleoli to represent the axis of the talocrural joint.
   c. With a goniometer, measure the angle formed by the two axes (angle of tibial torsion). Compare with measurements on other subjects. What is the range of angles you measured? Do they fall within the normal range of tibial torsion?
10. On a subject, palpate ankle muscles and tendons from their proximal to distal insertions following descriptions in the muscle tables:

    gastrocnemius peroneus longus
    soleus peroneus brevis
    tibialis posterior
    flexor digitorum longus
    flexor hallucis longus
    extensor digitorum brevis
    tibialis anterior
    extensor hallucis longus
    extensor digitorum longus

11. Analyze by first observing and then palpating the synergistic muscle actions in weight-bearing (make sure that the subject is standing upright and looking straight ahead):
    a. Normal comfortable standing.
    b. Sway forward slightly from the ankles; observe first, then palpate, including the longitudinal arch and placing your finger(s) under the toes.
    c. Sway backward slightly from the ankles. Why is it possible to sway farther forward than backward?
    d. Rise up on the toes. Observe from behind and note the supination of the calcaneus occurring with plantarflexion.
    e. Stand on heels. Why is balance so poor compared to standing on toes?
    f. Stand on one foot. How long can your subject stand on one leg?
       1) What implications does this have for an individual with an amputation of one leg?
       2) If you had a patient with a history of multiple right ankle sprains, what would you expect his or her ability to be to stand on the right foot compared to the left foot? Can you explain why?
    g. Deep knee bend, keeping heels on floor and then letting heels rise.
12. Analyze jumping up. What muscles in the lower extremity are stretched in preparation for the jump? What muscles are the prime movers for the jump? What type of contraction is made? Analyze landing, identifying what muscles in the lower extremity are used and the type of contraction made.
13. Have a standing subject perform open chain rotation of the lower limb with the knee extended. Determine by palpation at which joints (in the lower extremity) motion is occurring. Then have the subject perform closed chain rotation with the knee extended and analyze where motion is occurring.

References

1. Stauffer RN, Chao EYS, Brewster RC. Force and motion analysis of the normal, diseased, and prosthetic ankle joint. *Clinical Orthopaedics and Related Research* 127:189–196, 1977.
2. Seber S, Hazer B, Köse N, Göktürk E, Günal I, Turgut A. Rotational profile of the lower extremity and foot progression angle: Computerized tomographic examination of 50 adult male adults. *Archives of Orthopaedic and Traumatic Surgery* 120(5–6):255–258, 2000.
3. Kristiansen LP, Gunderson RB, Steen H, O. R. The normal development of tibial torsion. *Skeletal Radiology* 30(9):519–522, 2001.
4. Clementz BG. Tibial torsion measured in normal adults. *Acta Orthopaedica Scandinavica* 59(4):441–442, 1988.
5. Moore K. *Clinically Oriented Anatomy*. Baltimore: Williams & Wilkins, 2004.
6. Bronner S, Noivella T, Becica L. Management of delayed-union sesamoid fracture in a dancer. *Journal of Orthopaedic and Sports Physical Therapy* 37(9):529–540, 2007.
7. Cohen BE. Hallux sesamoid disorders. *Foot and Ankle Clinics* 14(1):91–104, 2009.
8. McPoil TJ, Brocato RS. The foot and ankle: Biomechanical evaluation and treatment. In Gould JA, Davies GJ (eds): *Orthopedic and Sports Physical Therapy*, St. Louis: CV Mosby, 1985.
9. Helfet AJ. *Disorders of the Knee*. Philadelphia: JB Lippincott, 1974.
10. Radakovich M, Malone TR. The superior tibiofibular joint: The forgotten joint. *Journal of Orthopaedic and Sports Physical Therapy* 3(3):129–132, 1982.
11. Inman VT. *The Joints of the Ankle*. Baltimore: Williams & Wilkins, 1976.
12. Kapandji IA. *The Physiology of the Joints, Vol 2, Lower Limb*, ed 5. Edinburgh: Churchill Livingstone, 1987.
13. Milner CE, Soarnes RW. A comparison of four in vivo methods of measuring tibial torsion. *Journal of Anatomy* 193:139–144, 1998.
14. Güven M, Akman B, Unay K, Ozturan EK, Cakici H, Eren A. A new radiographic measurement method of evaluation of tibial torsion: A pilot study in adults. *Clinical Orthopaedics and Related Research* 467(7):1807–1812, 2009.
15. Davids JR, Davis RB. Tibial torsion: Significance and measurement. *Gait & Posture* 26(2):169–171, 2007.
16. Lang LM, Volpe RG. Measurement of tibial torsion. *Journal of the American Podiatric Medical Association* 88(4): 160–165, 1998.
17. Stuberg W, Temme J, Kaplan P, Clarke A, Fuchs R. Measurement of tibial torsion and thigh-foot angle using goniometry and computed tomography. *Clinical Orthopaedics and Related Research* 272:208–212, 1991.
18. Harper MC. Deltoid ligament: An anatomical evaluation of function. *Foot & Ankle* 8(1):19–22, 1987.
19. Lundberg A, Goldie I, Kalin B, Selvik G. Kinematics of the ankle/foot complex: Plantarflexion and dorsiflexion. *Foot & Ankle* 9(4):194–200, 1989.
20. Wong Y, Kim W, Ying N. Passive motion characteristics of the talocrural and the subtalar joint by dual Euler angles. *Journal of Biomechanics* 38(12):2480–2485, 2005.
21. Ying N, Kim W, Wong Y, Kam BH. Analysis of passive motion characteristics of the ankle joint complex using dual Euler angle parameters. *Clinical Biomechanics* 19(2):153–160, 2004.
22. Greene WB, Heckman JD, eds. *The Clinical Measurement of Joint Motion*. Rosemont, IL: American Academy of Orthopaedic Surgeons, 1994.
23. Hoppenfeld S. *Physical examination of the spine and extremities*. East Norwalk, CT: Appleton-Century-Crofts, 1976.
24. Boone DC, Azen SP. Normal range of motion of joints in male subjects. *Journal of Bone and Joint Surgery Am* 61(5):756–759, 1979.
25. Roaas A, Andersson GB. Normal range of motion of the hip, knee, and ankle joints in male subjects, 30–40 years of age. *Acta Orthopaedica Scandinavica* 53(2):205–208, 1982.
26. Grimston SK, Nigg BM, Hanley DA, Engsberg JR. Differences in ankle joint complex range of motion as a function of age. *Foot & Ankle* 14(4):215–222, 1993.
27. Engsberg JR, Allinger TL. A function of the talocalcaneal joint during running support. *Foot & Ankle* 11(2):93–96, 1990.
28. Valenti V. Proprioception. In Helal B, Wilson D (eds): *The Foot, Vol I*, New York: Churchill Livingstone, 1988.
29. van der Wees PJ, Lenssen AF, Hendriks EJ, Stomp DJ, Dekker J, de Bie RA. Effectiveness of exercise therapy and manual mobilisation in ankle sprain and functional instability: A systematic review. *Australian Journal of Physiotherapy* 52(1):27–37, 2006.
30. Willems T, Witvrouw E, Verstuyft J, Vaes P, De Clercq D. Proprioception and muscle strength in subjects with a history of ankle sprains and chronic instability. *Journal of Athletic Training* 37(4):487–493, 2002.

31. Konradsen L. Factors contributing to chronic ankle instability: Kinesthesia and joint position sense. *Journal of Athletic Training* 37(4):381–385, 2002.

32. Lephart SM, Pincivero DM, Rozzi SL. Proprioception of the ankle and knee. *Sports Medicine* 25(3):149–155, 1998.

33. Goto A, Moritomo H, Itohara T, Watanabe T, Sugamoto K. Three-dimensional in vivo kinematics of the subtalar joint during dorsi-plantarflexion and inversion-eversion. *Foot & Ankle International* 30(5):432–438, 2009.

34. Elftman H. The transverse tarsal joint and its control. *Clinical Orthopaedics* 16:41–61, 1960.

35. Hicks JH. The mechanics of the foot. I. The joints. *Journal of Anatomy* 87(4):345–357, 1953.

36. Manter JT. Movements of the subtalar and transverse tarsal joints. *Anatomical Record* 80:397, 1941.

37. Sarrafian SK. *Anatomy of the Foot and Ankle*. Philadelphia: JB Lippincott, 1983.

38. Stagni R, Leardini A, O'Connor JJ, Giannini S. Role of passive structures in the mobility and stability of the human subtalar joint: A literature review. *Foot & Ankle International* 24(5):402–409, 2003.

39. Leardini A, Stagni R, O'Connor JJ. Mobility of the subtalar joint in the intact ankle complex. *Journal of Biomechanics* 34(6):805–809, 2001.

40. Ball P, Johnson GR. Technique for the measurement of hindfoot inversion and eversion and its use to study a normal population. *Clinical Biomechanics* 11(3):165–169, 1996.

41. Donatelli RA. Normal biomechanics of the foot and ankle. *Journal of Orthopaedic and Sports Physical Therapy* 7(3):91–95, 1985.

42. McPoil TG, Cornwall MW. The relationship between static lower extremity measurements and rearfoot motion during walking. *Journal of Orthopaedic and Sports Physical Therapy* 24(5):309–314, 1996.

43. Rochar PA, Jr. The subtalar joint: Anatomy and joint motion. *Journal of Orthopaedic and Sports Physical Therapy* 21(6):361–372, 1995.

44. Close JR, Inman VT, Poor PM, Todd FN. The function of the subtalar joint. *Clinical Orthopaedics and Related Research* 50:159–179, 1967.

45. Root ML, Orien WP, Weed JH. *Clinical Biomechanics. Volume II. Normal and Abnormal Function of the Foot.* Los Angeles: Clinical Biomechanics, 1977.

46. Davis WH, Sobel M, DiCarlo EF, et al. Gross, histological, and microvascular anatomy and biomechanical testing of the spring ligament complex. *Foot & Ankle International* 17(2):95–102, 1996.

47. Sammarco VJ. The talonavicular and calcaneocuboid joints: Anatomy, biomechanics, and clinical management of the transverse tarsal joint. *Foot and Ankle Clinics* 9(1):127–145, 2004.

48. Lundberg A, Svensson OK, Bylund C, Goldie I, Selvik G. Kinematics of the ankle/foot complex: Part 2. Pronation and supination. *Foot & Ankle* 9(5):248–253, 1989.

49. Kaltenborn FM. *Manual Mobilization of the Joints. The Kaltenborn Method of Joint Examination and Treatment*, ed 6. Oslo, Norway: Olaf N Orlis Bokhandel, 2002.

50. Lakin RC, DeGnore LT, Pienkowski D. Contact mechanics of normal tarsometatarsal joints. *Journal of Bone and Joint Surgery Am* 83(4):520–528, 2001.

51. Ouzounian T, Shereff M. In vitro determination of midfoot motion. *Foot & Ankle* 10(3):140–146, 1989.

52. Glasoe WM, Yack HJ, Saltzman CL. Anatomy and biomechanics of the first ray. *Physical Therapy* 79(9):854–859, 1999.

53. Williams PL, Warwick R, Dyson M, Bannister LH, eds. *Gray's Anatomy,* ed 38. New York: Churchill Livingstone, 1999.

54. Incavo SJ, Alvarez RG, Trevino SG. Occurrence of the plantaris tendon in patients sustaining subcutaneous rupture of the Achilles tendon. *Foot & Ankle* 8(2):110–111, 1987.

55. Vanderhooft E. The frequency of and relationship between the palmaris longus and plantaris tendons. *American Journal of Orthopedics* 25(1):38–41, 1996.

56. Murray MP, Guten GN, Baldwin JM, Gardner GM. A comparison of plantar flexion torque with and without the triceps surae. *Acta Orthopaedica Scandinavica* 47(1):122–124, 1976.

57. Backlund L, Nordgren L. A new method of testing isometric muscle strength under standardized conditions. *Scandinavian Journal of Clinical and Laboratory Investigation* 21:33–41, 1968.

58. Beasley WC. *Ontogenetics and Biomechanics of Ankle Plantar Flexion Force*. Philadelphia: American Congress of Physical Medicine and Rehabilitation, 1958.

59. Beasley WC. Quantitative muscle testing: Principles and applications to research and clinical services. *Archives of Physical Medicine and Rehabilitation* 42:398–425, 1961.

60. Haxton HA. Absolute muscle force in the ankle flexors of man. *Journal of Physiology* 103(3):267–273, 1944.

61. Bernard BA. *Maximum Isometric Torque of the Plantar Flexors in the Sitting Position.* Denton, TX: Texas Woman's University, 1979.

62. Belnap B. *Maximum Isometric Torque of the Plantar Flexors.* Denton, TX: Texas Woman's University, 1978.

63. Moss CL. Comparison of the histochemical and contractile properties of human gastrocnemius muscle. *Journal of Orthopaedic and Sports Physical Therapy* 13(6):322–328, 1991.

64. Rice CL, Cunningham DA, Taylor AW, Paterson DH. Comparison of the histochemical and contractile properties of human triceps surae. *European Journal of Applied Physiology and Occupational Physiology* 58(1–2):165–170, 1988.

65. Joseph J. *Man's Posture: Electromyographic Studies*. Springfield, IL: Charles C Thomas, 1960.

66. Kaye RA, Jahss MH. Tibialis posterior: A review of anatomy and biomechanics in relation to support of the medial longitudinal arch. *Foot & Ankle* 11(4):244–247, 1991.

67. Wickiewicz TL, Roy RR, Powell PL, Edgerton VR. Muscle architecture of the human lower limb. *Clinical Orthopaedics and Related Research* 179:275–283, 1983.

68. Gans C, Gaunt AS. Muscle architecture in relation to function. *Journal of Biomechanics* 24(Suppl 1):53–65, 1991.

69. Brand RA, Pedersen DR, Friederich JA. The sensitivity of muscle force predictions to changes in physiologic cross-sectional area. *Journal of Biomechanics* 19(8):589–596, 1986.

70. Klein P, Mattys S, Rooze M. Moment arm length variations of selected muscles acting on talocrural and subtalar joints during movement: an in vitro study. *Journal of Biomechanics* 29(1):21–30, 1996.

71. Johnson CH, Christensen JC. Biomechanics of the first ray: Part I. The effects of peroneus longus function: a three-dimensional kinematic study on a cadaver model. *Journal of Foot and Ankle Surgery* 38(5):313–321, 1999.

72. Sutherland DH. The role of the ankle plantar flexors in normal walking. *Journal of Bone and Joint Surgery Am* 62:354–363, 1980.

73. Fujita M. Role of the metatarsophalangeal (MTP) joints of the foot in level walking. *Nippon Seikeigeka Gakkai Zasshi* 59(11):985–997, 1985.

74. Rattanaprasert U, Smith R, Sullivan M, Gilleard W. Three-dimensional kinematics of the forefoot, rearfoot, and leg without the function of tibialis posterior in comparison with normals during stance phase of walking. *Clinical Biomechanics* 14(1):14–23, 1999.

75. Cornwall MW, McPoil TG, Fishco WD, O'Donnell D, Hunt L, Lane C. The influence of first ray mobility on forefoot plantar pressure and hindfoot kinematics during walking. *Foot & Ankle International* 27(7):539–547, 2006.

76. Stevens K, Platt A, Ellis H. A cadaveric study of the peroneus tertius muscle. *Clinical Anatomy* 6(2):106–110, 1993.

77. Joshi SD, Joshi SS, Athavale SA. Morphology of peroneus tertius muscle. *Clinical Anatomy* 19(7):611–614, 2006.

78. Mann R, Inman VT. Phasic activity of intrinsic muscles of the foot. *Journal of Bone and Joint Surgery Am* 46:469, 1964.

79. Wong YS. Influence of the abductor hallucis muscle on the medial arch of the foot: A kinematic and anatomical cadaver study. *Foot & Ankle International* 28(5):617–620, 2007.

80. Caravaggi P, Pataky T, Goulermas JY, Savage R, Crompton R. A dynamic model of the windlass mechanism of the foot: Evidence for early stance phase preloading of the plantar aponeurosis. *Journal of Experimental Biology* 212:2491–2499, 2009.

81. Sarrafian SK. Functional characteristics of the foot and plantar aponeurosis under tibiotalar loading. *Foot & Ankle* 8(1):4–18, 1987.

82. Lapidus PW. Kinesiology and mechanical anatomy of the tarsal joints. *Clinical Orthopaedics and Related Research* 30:20–36, 1963.

83. Magee DJ. *Orthopedic Physical Assessment*, ed 5. St. Louis: Saunders Elsevier; 2008.

84. Wearing S, Smeathers J, Sullivan P, Yates B, Urry S, Dubois P. Plantar fasciitis: Are pain and fascial thickness associated with arch shape and loading? *Physical Therapy* 87(8):1002–1008, 2007.

85. Fiolkowski P, Brunt D, Bishop M, Woo R, Horodyski M. Intrinsic pedal musculature support of the medial longitudinal arch: An electromyography study. *Journal of Foot and Ankle Surgery* 42(6):327–333, 2003.

86. Basmajian JV. *Muscles Alive: Their Function Revealed by Electromyography*, ed 4. Baltimore: Williams & Wilkins, 1978.

87. Gray ER. The role of leg muscles in variations of the arches in normal and flat feet. *Physical Therapy* 49(10):1084–1088, 1969.

88. Tiberio D. Pathomechanics of structural foot deformities. *Physical Therapy* 68(12):1840–1849, 1988.

89. Cavanagh PR, Rodgers MM, Iiboshi A. Pressure distribution under symptom-free feet during barefoot standing. *Foot & Ankle* 7(5):262–276, 1987.

90. Martínez-Nova A, Pascual Huerta J, Sánchez-Rodríguez R. Cadence, age, and weight as determinants of forefoot plantar pressures using the Biofoot in-shoe system. *Journal of the American Podiatric Medical Association* 98(4):302–310, 2008.

91. Queen RM, Gross MT, Liu H-Y. Repeatability of lower extremity kinetics and kinematics for standardized and self-selected running speeds. *Gait & Posture* 23:282–287, 2006.

92. Segal A, Rohr E, Orendurff M, Shofer J, O'Brien M, Sangeorzan B. The effect of walking speed on peak plantar pressure. *Foot & Ankle International* 25(12):926–933, 2004.

93. Chi KJ, Schmitt D. Mechanical energy and effective foot mass during impact loading of walking and running. *Journal of Biomechanics* 38(7):1387–1395, 2005.

94. Weijers RE, Walenkamp GH, van Mameren H, Kessels AG. The relationship of the position of the metatarsal heads and peak plantar pressure. *Foot & Ankle International* 24(4):349–353, 2003.

95. DeLacerda FG. The relationship of foot pronation, foot position, and electromyography of the anterior tibialis muscle in three subjects with different histories of shin splints. *Journal of Orthopaedic and Sports Physical Therapy* 2(2):60–64, 1980.

INTRODUCTION TO

Unit 4 : Functional Activities

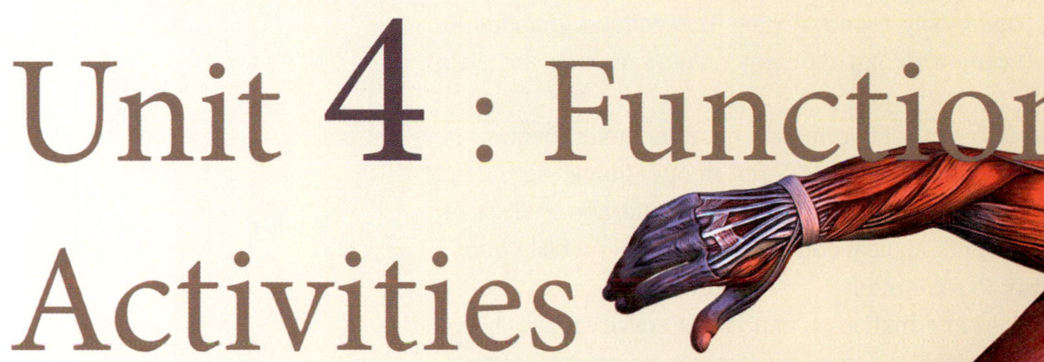

Now that the essentials of kinesiology have been established, this unit presents the functional applications of kinesiology from a clinical perspective. These chapters offer a fitting conclusion to this text on kinesiology as we apply all of the concepts and functional anatomy described in the preceding chapters to the performance of daily and functional activities. As was mentioned in the introduction of this text, this is the part of kinesiology that clinicians enjoy and appreciate the most. The chapters in this section are important for their application and the assistance that novices in the field are provided regarding what to look for in patient task execution and how to recognize the patient's deficiencies. Realizing that these factors are the first step in designing and providing a clinical plan to permit the patient's improved performance of functional tasks is crucial to any clinician's education.

Chapter 12 begins with posture analysis, postural control elements, and postural sway issues. The majority of this chapter involves investigation of gait. Differences in gait terminology are presented along with the determinants of gait, the kinematic and kinetic issues of gait for all the involved joints, challenges to gait efficiency, and ambulation with assistive devices. Additionally, gait as it changes over the life cycle is discussed along with pathologies commonly found in gait. The various changes in demands of joint motion during different running speeds are also presented.

Chapter 13 presents clinical information on ergonomics involved in common tasks in both household and occupational activities. Ergonomics as it affects the clinician is also presented. An analysis of functions involved in pathological conditions including mobility transfers is also a part of this chapter.

Chapter 14 provides information on analysis of activities of daily living with emphasis on requirements of the upper extremities. Common daily activities are investigated for their requirements of joint mobility, muscle activity, and sequencing.

Chapter 15 is the final chapter. This chapter identifies common sports and leisure activities and analyzes them for their kinesiological requirements. Activities that are commonly seen by clinicians are used as examples in this chapter.

Chapters 13 through 15 are here to help you begin to analyze motion in a variety of settings from daily activities each of us is required to perform to specialized activities that may be unique to different settings, environments, and populations. These chapters do not include all activities within the categories of each chapter but provide for you examples of motion analysis. All clinicians are required to know the demands of the activities of their patients so that appropriate rehabilitation programs will provide those patients with an optimal ability to perform their required activities. To that end, clinicians must understand the kinesiological requirements of each task and translate those requirements into the rehabilitation programs they provide for their patients. After completing these chapters, you should have an understanding of how to approach these and other activities.

CHAPTER 12

Stance and Gait

"The ultimate measure of a man is not where he stands in moments of comfort and convenience, but where he stands at times of challenge and controversy."
Martin Luther King, Jr., 1929–1968.
American pastor, activist, and leader in the African-American Civil Rights Movement

CHAPTER OUTLINE

Learning Outcomes
Clinical Scenario
Introduction
Stance Posture
- *Forces Required to Maintain Stance*
- *Postural Sway*
- *Balance of Forces Occurring in Symmetric Stance: Functional Applications*
- *Recovery Strategies*

Walking Gait
- *Gait Terminology*
- *Functional Tasks of Gait*
- *Kinematics of Gait*
- *Kinetics of Gait*
- *Muscles of Gait*
- *Gait Analysis*

Developmental Aspects of Gait: Life Span Changes
- *Immature Walking*
- *Mature Walking*
- *Gait Changes in the Older Adult*

Gait Efficiency
- *Determinants of Gait*
- *Challenges to Gait Efficiency*

Running Gait
- *Phases*
- *Kinematics*
- *Changes at Different Speeds*
- *Muscle Activity at the Hip, Knee, and Ankle in Running*
- *Kinetics of Running*

Summary
Clinical Scenario Solution
Discussion Questions
Lab Activities
References

LEARNING OUTCOMES

This chapter provides a descriptive analysis of upright stance control and gait. By completion of this chapter, the reader should be able to:

- ❑ Indicate the typical alignment seen in upright stance posture and summarize the mechanisms that preserve upright postural control;
- ❑ Use gait terminology fluently when describing or analyzing human gait;
- ❑ Describe gait by using the kinematic spatial and temporal descriptors seen in walking;
- ❑ Summarize the main functional tasks associated with gait;
- ❑ Identify the phases of the gait cycle and the main functional tasks associated with each phase;
- ❑ Summarize the basic angular joint displacements at the pelvis, hip, knee, and ankle that occur during the gait cycle and translate these into the functional minimal range of motion requirements for gait;
- ❑ Explain the muscular activation patterns at the trunk, pelvis, and lower extremities that occur during the gait cycle;
- ❑ Summarize the age-related differences seen in the gait characteristics of children, mature and older adults;
- ❑ Illustrate common methods of gait analysis;
- ❑ Explain gait efficiency and the factors that contribute to this efficiency;
- ❑ Describe the functional consequence on locomotion of commonly encountered pathological conditions;
- ❑ Contrast and compare walking to running.

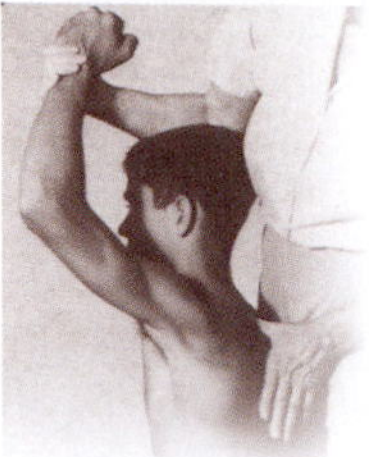

CLINICAL SCENARIO

Morgan is working with Cody, a distance runner who injured his right knee while downhill skiing during his vacation. The knee was placed in a brace, and Cody was limited to nonweight-bearing on the limb for three weeks. Now that he has progressed to full weight-bearing as tolerated, it is Morgan's responsibility to advance him from walking to running again. The first day Cody put weight on the right limb, he was unable to walk normally. Morgan expected this and is prepared to instruct Cody in the proper technique.

Introduction

This first chapter in Unit 4 describes and summarizes the two most common functional tasks we engage in throughout our day: controlling our posture and walking. It is amazing how smoothly these two daily tasks are performed and how efficiently our bodies orchestrate them without conscious effort. When is the last time you ever really paid any attention to what muscles you were using, for example, as you stood in line to buy your books or buy a ticket to a game or show? Do you realize that when you walk, more than 1,000 muscles synchronize to move more than 200 bones around 100 joints?[1] Your study of kinesiology in the preceding chapters has prepared you well for delving into the next step of clinical kinesiology: analysis of human movements. It is easier and most logical to begin with a static activity such as posture and move on to what is arguably the most common activity we perform on a daily basis—walking.

This chapter is divided into three main sections: The first section assesses proper upright stance posture; the second section analyzes walking gait; and the final section investigates running gait. As we have done throughout this text, the most important first step for us will be to define and describe the unique terminology of these activities so we all communicate using a common language.

In contrast to our four-legged friends, human beings are **bipedal** (L., *bi,* two, plus *pes,* foot). In most cases, we attain the independent ability to stand and walk within the first year or so of life. Moving from one place to another is broadly defined as **locomotion** (L., *locus,* place, plus *movere,* to move; in this case, moving from one place to another) and includes many forms of movement, including examples such as rolling, crawling and creeping, walking, running, and even hopping and skipping. Locomotion specifically in the *upright* bipedal form occurs along a sequential progression that begins with standing and advances to walking, then running. These activities require skills such as starting, stopping, changing direction, and altering speed.[2] **Gait** is upright locomotion in the particular manner of moving on foot, which may be a walk, jog, or run. **Walking** is a particular form of gait and the most common of human locomotor patterns. **Ambulation** (L., *ambulare,* to move about) is defined in a broad sense as a type of locomotion and is more often used in the clinical sense of describing whether or not someone can walk freely or with the assistance of some device.

Stance Posture

Posture is a general term that is defined as an alignment of body segments, a position or attitude of the body, the relative arrangement of body parts for a specific activity, or a characteristic manner of bearing one's body. Posture and movement are intimately related; movement begins from a posture and may end in a different posture in the same location or the same posture but a different location, such as when a person is in a sitting position and then moves to a standing position or when a standing person walks across the street.

Postural adjustments are rapid and automatic in normal function. This postural control requires multiple-system interactions such as the proprioceptive, visual, and vestibular sensory systems networking with the musculoskeletal system (see Chapter 3). A complete presentation of posture includes a description of standing posture, sitting posture, and the myriad complexities of postural control. Since this chapter deals primarily with gait, we will limit our discussion to stance and the kinesiological concepts related to maintaining an effective and efficient upright standing posture as a preparation to gait. Refer to other texts for an in-depth discussion and additional information on postural control.

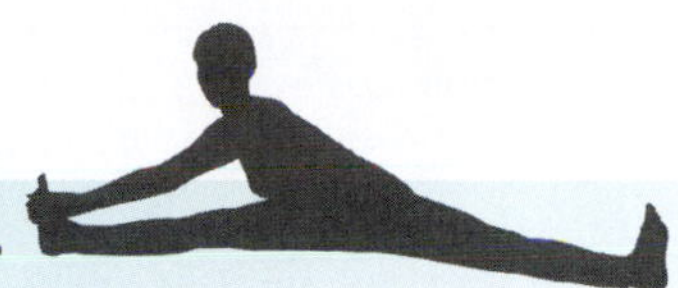

PRACTICE POINT

The body can assume a multitude of postures that are comfortable for long periods, and many postures accomplish the same purposes. In many cultures, for example, people do not sit in chairs but instead use a variety of floor-sitting postures such as crossed legs, side sitting, or a deep squat. A standing posture also has many individual variations, depending on the functional task and situation. For example, if standing must be maintained for any length of time, an individual has a variety of options. A common choice is to stand with the weight on one limb and periodically shift to the other leg; the contralateral foot is on the ground but bears little weight. Another common standing posture is with weight distributed over both feet in a wide base, the knees and hips in extension. Arm postures are also quite variable and may be held with hands at sides, behind the back, on hips, in pockets, or folded across the chest. When discomfort occurs as a result of joint compression, ligamentous tension, continuous muscle contraction, or circulatory restriction, the body commonly assumes a new posture. The need to change position is more frequently a result of vascular insufficiency in compressed joint cartilage and tense ligaments rather than from muscle fatigue. For example, a person standing still or at attention for a time and not performing isometric contractions of the calf and thigh muscles may experience pooling of venous blood in the extremities which causes an inadequate venous return that leads to an insufficient cardiac output to the brain and results in fainting. If a joint has been in one position for an extended time, the able-bodied person moves and stretches the joint and muscles. Habitual postures without positional changes may eventually lead to tissue adaptations, motion limitations, or postural deformity. Individuals with sensory deficiencies may fail to perceive the discomfort of vascular occlusion. If these occlusive pressures are not relieved by changing positions periodically, tissues become ischemic and break down; these episodes commonly result in *pressure sores*. Additionally, if the joints are not moved through their ranges of motion either passively or actively, the muscles and soft tissues surrounding joints adaptively shorten, resulting in a contracture and motion loss. It is important for clinicians working with patients with neurological or orthopedic disorders to maintain good tissue length and joint mobility in their patients.

Appreciation of the biomechanical principles of an upright standing posture is basic to understanding and correcting the abnormal postures clinicians often encounter in the individuals they treat. Normal stance posture is somewhat variable among individuals and is influenced by size, age, sex, and body type. In spite of these variations, standing static posture in all of us has some common characteristics. Although it is clinically important to appreciate postural variations, we can use these common characteristics to serve as guidelines in performing an individual's postural assessment.

Evaluation of normal postural alignment is best performed with the individual in relaxed standing with the feet positioned at approximately the width of the hips, the arms relaxed at the sides, and the eyes directed forward. Alignment of the head, shoulders, trunk, hips, knees, and ankles are assessed from anterior, posterior, and sagittal views (Fig. 12.1A, B, C). It is helpful to use a **plumb line** as a reference for the body's line of gravity. The muscles that support upright posture in a standing anatomical position are called **antigravity muscles**. These muscle groups primarily include the neck and back extensors, hip and knee extensors, and to a lesser degree, the neck and trunk flexors and hip abductors and adductors (see shaded areas in Fig. 12.1C).

Forces Required to Maintain Stance

As you can see from the sagittal view in Figure 12.1C, the line of gravity falls though the acromion process, anterior to the thoracic kyphotic curve, through the greater trochanter just posterior to the hip joint axis, anterior to the knee joint but posterior to the patella, and anterior to the ankle joint. Recall from our discussion in Chapter 2 that if the line of gravity falls through the joint axis, little or no torque is created to rotate the segment. On the other hand, if the line of gravity falls anterior or posterior to the joint axis, gravity creates a moment arm that applies a rotational force to the joint. For example, the line of gravity falls anterior to the ankle joint, so gravity exerts a torque that pulls the tibia anteriorly on the ankle (Fig. 12.2). This gravitational pull provides an external moment pulling the leg forward so a counterbalance force must be exerted by the posterior calf muscles to maintain the leg in its static and upright position. We see a similar situation at the knee with the line of gravity anterior to the knee joint's axis, but at the hip, the line of gravity falls posterior to the joint. As we continue to follow the line of

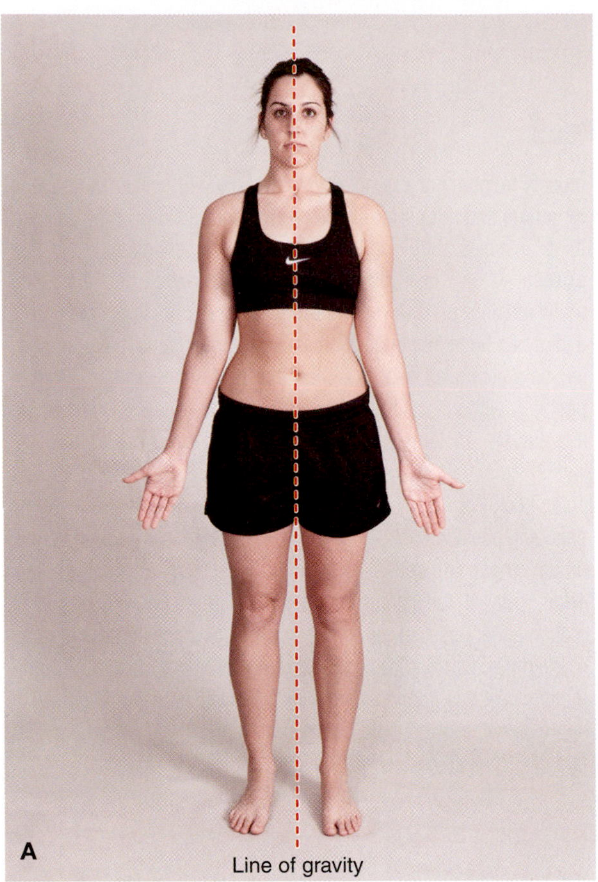

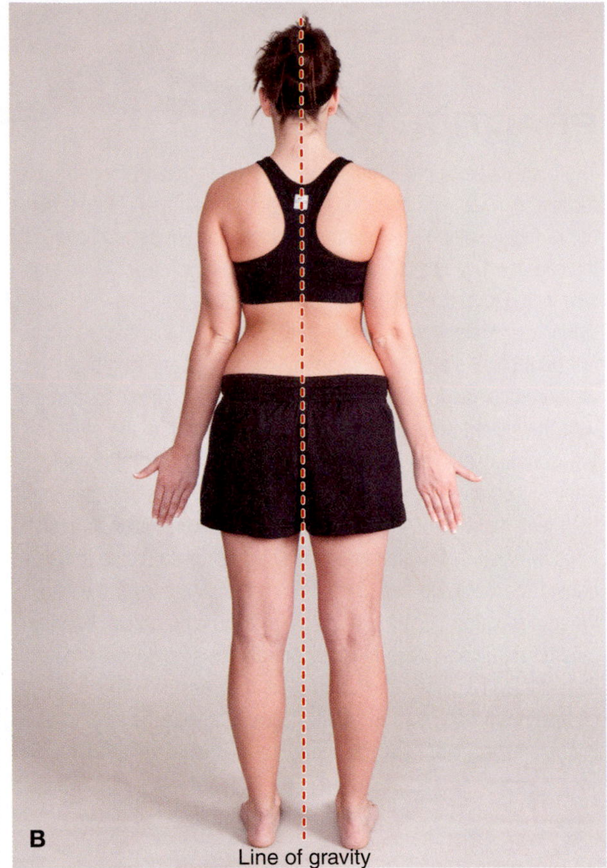

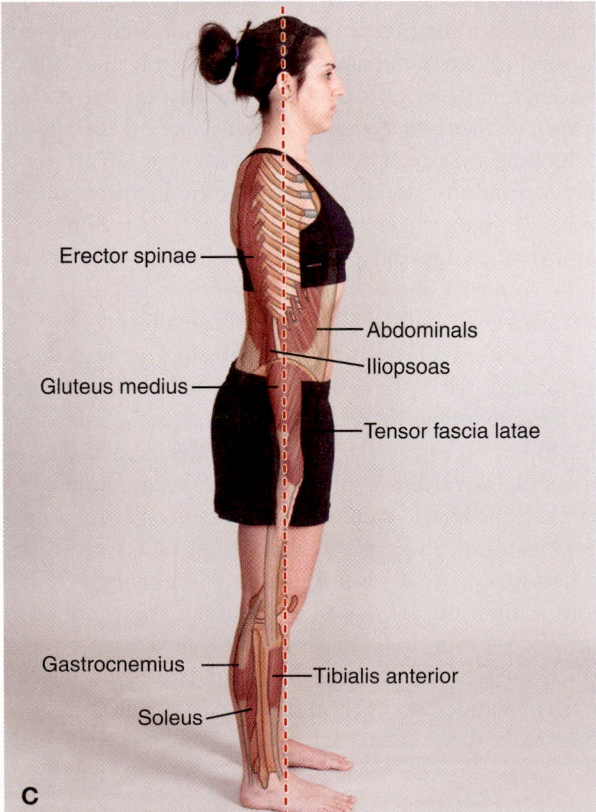

Figure 12.1 Gravitational line as it falls in **A)** anterior, **B)** posterior, and **C)** sagittal views. In the relaxed, standing posture, the gravitational force line through the center of mass falls behind the hip joint, in front of the knee joint, and in front of the ankle joint. In **C,** the location of muscles considered as *antigravity muscles* are depicted as shaded. Note that in the lower limbs, active muscle contraction for balance is required, but primarily in the gastrocnemius-soleus muscles and, to a lesser degree, the tibialis anterior muscle.

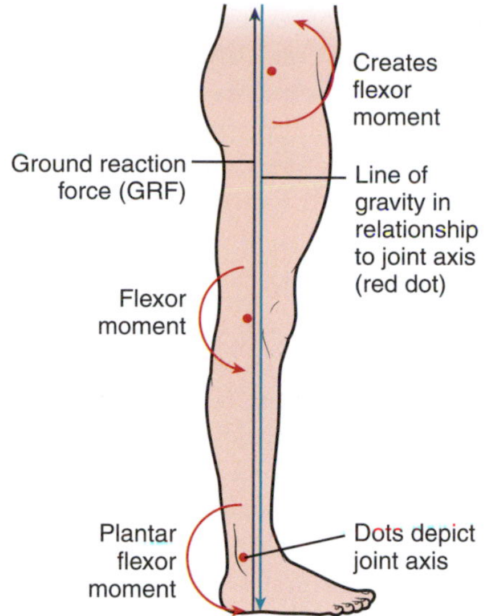

Figure 12.2 Drawing depicts how the line of gravity exerts a torque force that needs to be counteracted by an internal reaction force on the opposite side of the joint.

gravity up the body, we see that it falls on the concave side of each vertebral curvature, requiring a counteractive force on the convex side. In the trunk region, the erector spinae counteract the anterior gravitational pull on the thoracic spine, whereas the anterior head and neck musculature and the abdominals provide counterbalance at the cervical and lumbar areas, respectively. At body regions in which the line of gravity falls directly through a joint axis, there is no external moment applied, so the body is not required to produce a counteractive force at those joints to maintain the joint's position.

Postural Sway

To maintain a standing position, the body's relatively high center of gravity (COG) or center of mass (COM) at S_2 must remain within its relatively small base of support. The body is unable to maintain a perfectly stationary posture during standing. Ongoing organ functions such as respiration and cardiac contractions and ongoing neural adjustments cause small motions, so the body automatically and continually seeks and reestablishes equilibrium; this is called **postural sway** (Fig. 12.3). Postural sway

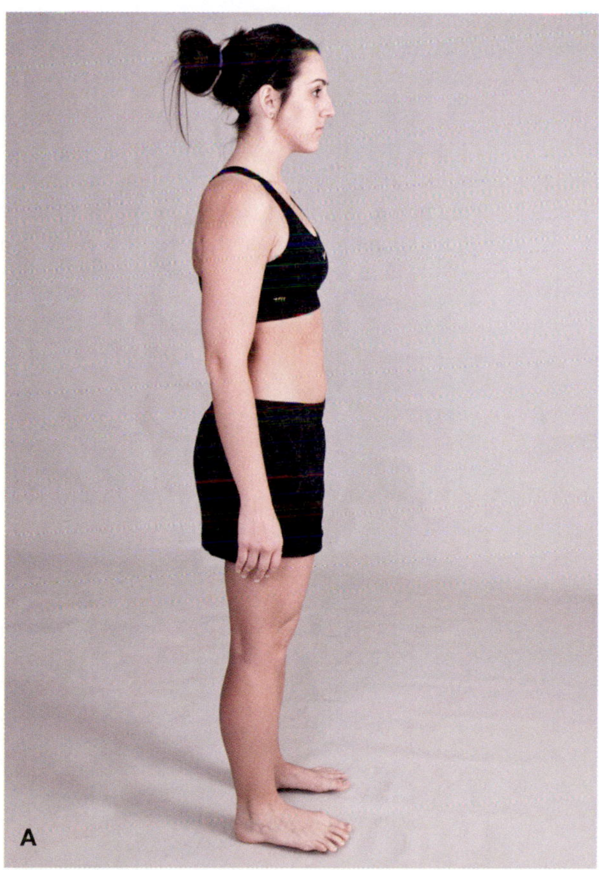

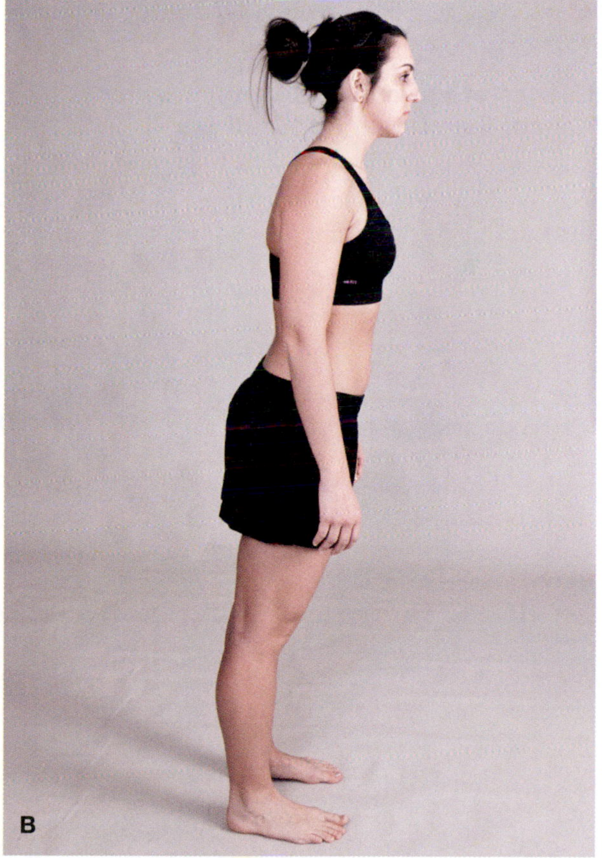

Figure 12.3 Postural sway is characterized by automatic adjustments, primarily at the ankle, to retain upright balance. **A)** Posterior. **B)** Anterior. Typical values as measured on a balance platform: mean amplitude of sway in inches = .13 × .15 Y; length of path = 32.2; velocity = .54 inch/sec. When balance is disturbed, an ankle strategy is used to reestablish equilibrium: **A)** disturbance posteriorly activates the anterior tibialis and **B)** disturbance anteriorly activates the soleus muscle.

is the motion of an upright body that is characterized by constant, minute displacements and corrections to maintain the COM over the body's base of support (BOS). The body sways in an anterior-posterior direction as well as side-to-side.[3] This sway occurs primarily at the ankle-foot segment, as evidenced by low-level alternating contractions in antagonistic ankle muscles, principally the anterior tibialis and soleus.

Standing posture is most stable in adults from about 20 to 60 years of age, whereas those in younger and older age groups have increased mean values and variability for all measurements of the center of pressure in the base of support (where the body weight is distributed in the plantar foot) in terms of size of the area of balance used, length of path of the COM moving within the BOS, velocity in how rapidly adjustments are made, and maximum amplitude of sway.[4] Both younger and older age groups also have slowed reaction time of muscle activity to disturbances of posture as compared with the adult age group.[5] Children approach adult values of postural stability by ages 12 to 15 but display a high variability until adulthood.[6] Increase in postural sway in the elderly has a high relationship to incidence of falls.[7]

Balance of Forces Occurring in Symmetric Stance: Functional Applications

In normal posture, gravity stresses are minimal since body segment alignment is optimal. How the body counteracts gravity is addressed in this section. When postural abnormalities are present, additional stresses are placed on different body segments. Which body segment receives the increased stress is dependent upon the postural abnormality. The Practice Points in this section identifies these abnormalities and the body's mechanisms for adjustment to them.

Functional Stance Control at the Ankle Joint

As we have just identified, the line of gravity of the body falls anterior to the ankle joint, setting up a rotary force to dorsiflex the tibia on the talus. Fortunately, the calf muscles oppose this movement with an equal counterforce to maintain a standing position. The soleus muscle is responsible for this equilibration, although the gastrocnemius also is active.[10] During postural sway, the body weight seldom, if ever, passes behind the axes of the ankle joints; consequently, the calf muscles remain continuously active to varying degrees during stance.[11] No additional muscular activity has been identified during quiet bilateral stance.

Functional Stance Control at the Knee Joint

The body mass above the knee joints consists of the head, arms, trunk (HAT), and thighs. The body's line of gravity falls slightly anterior to the knee joint's medial-lateral axis (Fig. 12.1C). Gravity creates a rotary force that produces an extensor moment at the knees. The necessary counterbalance force against gravity occurs at the posterior knee and is provided by a combination of passive resistance in the posterior

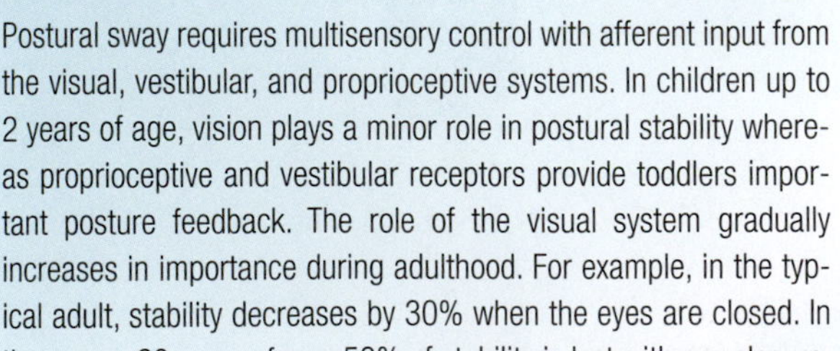

PRACTICE POINT

Postural sway requires multisensory control with afferent input from the visual, vestibular, and proprioceptive systems. In children up to 2 years of age, vision plays a minor role in postural stability whereas proprioceptive and vestibular receptors provide toddlers important posture feedback. The role of the visual system gradually increases in importance during adulthood. For example, in the typical adult, stability decreases by 30% when the eyes are closed. In those over 60 years of age, 50% of stability is lost with eye closure, thus making vision a major factor in balance of the elderly.[8] Poor visual acuity in people averaging 82 years of age was found to have a significant correlation with both increased postural sway on soft surfaces and incidence of falls.[9] Clinicians must keep these variations in posture mechanisms in mind when working with both young and older individuals.

Clinically, instructions in environmental adjustments should be provided to patients and family members to reduce the risk of fall, especially for the elderly and other individuals with balance deficiencies. Removal of scatter rugs, correction of uneven surfaces, and enhanced lighting are modifications that may assist in reducing falls.

extra-articular tissues (primarily the joint capsule) and active resistance of the hamstring muscles.[11] During postural sway, this line of gravity may occasionally, though rarely, move behind the axis of the knee joints. If this occurs during postural sway, a short burst of quadriceps activity occurs to realign the body.[12, 13] In most subjects, however, no electromyographic activity is detected in the quadriceps during bilateral standing.[14]

Functional Stance Control at the Hip Joint

Relaxed stance is usually characterized by incomplete extension at the hip, varying from 2° to 15° of hip flexion.[12] Although there is some variation in the literature regarding the location of the line of gravity with respect to the hip axis, it is most often agreed that the line of gravity runs posterior to the hip joint, so slight activity of the iliacus is required to counteract gravity's moment to move the body posteriorly.[14]

Functional Stance Control at the Head and Trunk

In standing, the line of gravity falls on the concave side each vertebral curve. Anterior to the thoracic kyphosis, it creates a tendency for the trunk to flex, thereby requiring tonic activity of the primary extensors—the erector spinae—to counteract that force. The rectus abdominis is essentially inactive with only slight activity occasionally recorded from the internal abdominal oblique muscles.[14] The head's center of mass is located about 1 inch (2.5 cm) above the transverse axis of the atlanto-occipital joints so that the

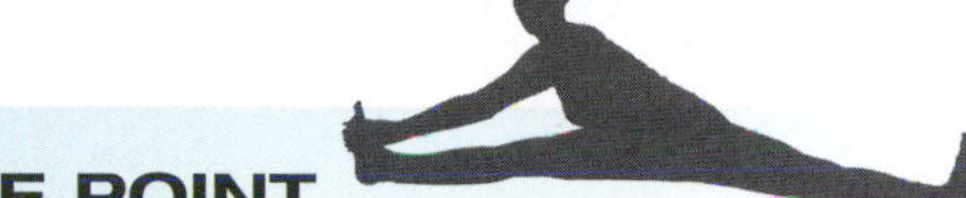

PRACTICE POINT

An individual with weak calf muscles may compensate for this insufficient strength by keeping his or her line of gravity over the axes of the talocrural joints. Such a position requires less activity from the calf muscles. When the body's line of gravity passes posteriorly to the talotibial joint, the ankle dorsiflexors counteract the now posterior moment arm of gravity; however, the safe range of this backward sway is extremely limited. Since reliance on the ankle dorsiflexors is difficult and awkward, the more likely observed compensations for calf muscle weakness include: (1) using a broader base of support; (2) holding on to nearby objects for stability; or (3) continual movement from one foot to the other.

Clinically, rehabilitation of injured or disabled individuals requires careful evaluation of the individual's stability and mobility. For example, positioning a prosthetic foot in neutral dorsiflexion in an above-knee prosthesis improves knee stability, although allowing dorsiflexion beyond neutral (0°) causes the knee to become unstable since it places a flexion torque on the knee. However, a young, active individual with excessive tightness of the Achilles may use a hip flexion posture so the line of gravity falls in front of the ankle.

Patients who cannot actively control the lower limbs compensate by moving the COM of the head, arms, and trunk posterior to the hip joint. For example, a person with paraplegia stands using his orthoses to lock the knees and actively positions his trunk posterior to the hips; such a position places the line of gravity posterior to the hips so the anterior hip ligaments provide counterbalance force against gravity, allowing him to maintain an upright posture (see Fig. 9.13). The upright posture of this patient standing in bilateral knee-ankle-foot orthoses (KAFO) is supported at the hips by the iliofemoral (Y) ligaments. If the ligaments are tight or if hip flexor spasticity exists, the patient will be unable to position his hips in extension; patients with these conditions may demonstrate increased lumbar lordosis in an attempt to maintain an erect position.

head is in unstable equilibrium. The atlanto-occipital joint is a first class lever, similar to a seesaw. The head's line of gravity falls a little anterior to the transverse axis for flexion and extension in normal posture (Fig. 12.4A). Therefore, in ordinary standing and sitting, the posterior neck muscles are moderately active to prevent the head from dropping forward. If the neck is flexed forward, such as commonly occurs while an individual is reading or writing, the demand on these muscles increases (Fig. 12.4B). When the head moves forward, however, the ligamentum nuchae becomes taut, and muscular activity is no longer needed. If the head is tipped backward, the line of gravity falls posterior to the transverse axis (Fig. 12.4C), and the neck flexors spring into action to stop or control the motion.

Recovery Strategies

As the body adjusts to maintain postural control, different movement strategies may be used. Although each strategy is different, they are common and match the direction and degree of the challenge given;[15] the greater the perturbation to posture, the greater the body must work to maintain its desired posture.[16] These postural adjustments serve to maintain the center of gravity within its base of support to allow safe and efficient voluntary movement.[16] These recovery strategies are categorized as ankle, hip, and stepping or reaching strategies.

Ankle strategy

Postural control initiated from the ankles and feet is called an **ankle strategy.** This is the most common automatic adjustment to anterior-posterior sway[17] (Fig. 12.3 A, B). Use of this strategy results in the head and body moving as a unit over the feet with minimal hip and knee movement.[18] Typically, this is the preference when the challenge is small, slow, and remains near the body's midline.[15] Originally, it was believed that ankle triggers provided input to

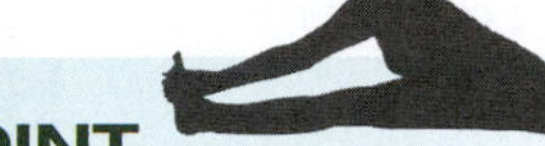

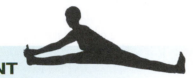

PRACTICE POINT

It is clinically important to remember that the cervical muscles, especially the posterior muscles, work continually when an individual is sitting or standing; the only time they rest is when the person is in a recumbent position. When treating patients with cervical sprains, they should be instructed to recline throughout the day when they experience increasing cervical muscle pain, especially in the early phase of treatment; it may be that the injured muscles are unable to tolerate the normal stress of holding the head in a proper posture because they are weakened by the injury.

Individuals with a forward head posture increase the normal energy expenditure requirements of the anterior and posterior cervical muscles. Gravity's moment arm becomes exaggerated with such a posture to not only add to muscle activity requirements but also increase stresses to the cervical discs and vertebrae.

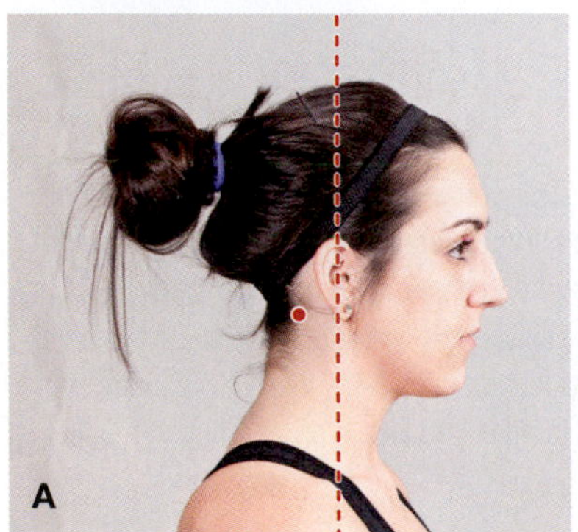

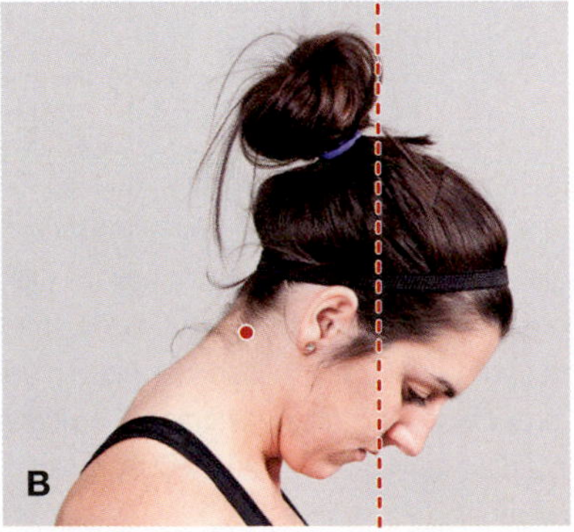

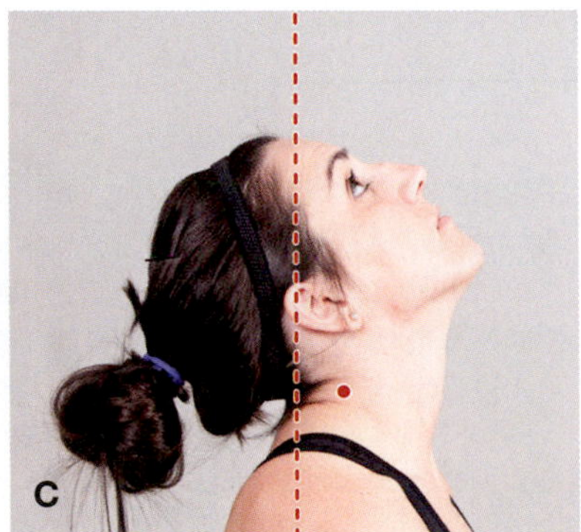

Figure 12.4 Relation of the center-of-gravity line of the head to the axis of the atlanto-occipital joints in different head positions. **A)** Head erect, center of gravity slightly anterior to axis, posterior neck muscles moderately active. **B)** Head forward, increased activity of posterior neck muscles. **C)** Head backward, center of gravity posterior to axis, anterior neck muscles active.

produce responses in leg muscles causing the distal-to-proximal balance corrections seen with the ankle strategy. However, research has now shown that triggers in the trunk and neck occur simultaneously with the ankle triggers, suggesting that a variety of other proprioceptive input contributes to postural responses.[19]

Hip strategy

Control of posture that comes from the hip, pelvis, and trunk is called a **hip strategy.** When the body is challenged to maintain posture because of large shifts in the body's line of gravity, the ankle strategy is insufficient to make the needed correction. Hip strategy is preferred when the postural challenge is large, fast, or if the support surface is too small to accommodate the ankle forces mentioned previously. Increasingly, the importance of trunk and hip input contributing to upright posture and its role in shaping balance strategy is being realized.[19] Its full role is yet to be understood.

Stepping or Reaching Strategies

Stepping or **reaching strategies** are used for very large or very fast changes and result in realignment of the COM within the base of support using steps, hops, or reaches in the direction of the change.[17] It is readily apparent that these strategies are required with sudden changes in body position to avoid instances such as collision with another body or object, adjustment to an overpowering force, or a change in position required because of an unanticipated need.

Walking Gait

Gait is the method by which land mammals move from one location to another. It may also be referred to in general terms as *locomotion*, but locomotion may include any method of movement from one location to another. The term used synonymously with gait is *ambulation.* Although we each develop our own specific style of gait, there are normal parameters within which we all move to provide an efficient method of transport. It is interesting to realize that people are often easily recognized by their gait, yet normal gait is amazingly similar from one individual to another. When abnormalities in anatomy or pathology in function occur, gait modifications must follow in order for ambulation to occur. This section provides information on normal and abnormal gait. How gait changes as the body moves through the life span is also covered. Gait includes both walking and running; this unit will delve first into walking gait and then into running gait.

Gait Terminology

Gait is defined as the manner or style of walking. Gait is discussed and investigated by its most fundamental unit, the gait cycle. One **gait cycle** is the time from when the heel of one foot touches the ground to the time it touches the ground again. The gait cycle is also known as a **stride.** The gait cycle is divided into two phases: stance (Fig. 12.5A) and swing (Fig. 12.5B). Stance phase and swing phase are subdivided and described in various ways. You will encounter some differences when reading different authors and their

PRACTICE POINT

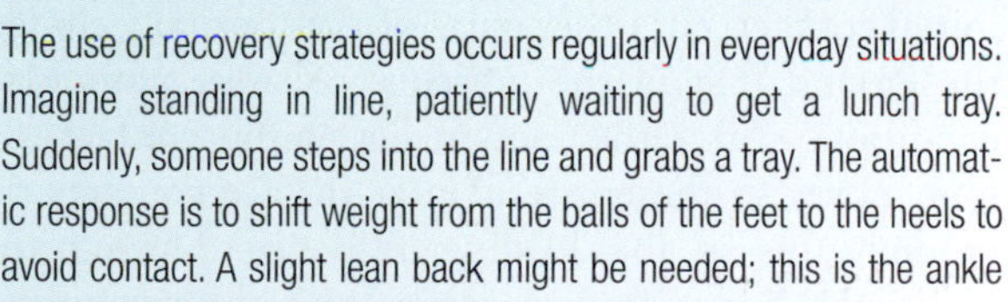

The use of recovery strategies occurs regularly in everyday situations. Imagine standing in line, patiently waiting to get a lunch tray. Suddenly, someone steps into the line and grabs a tray. The automatic response is to shift weight from the balls of the feet to the heels to avoid contact. A slight lean back might be needed; this is the ankle strategy at work to keep the body balanced and to avoid a fall.

Use of hip and stepping or reaching strategies may occur during body motion or when the body is statically positioned. An example of an adjustment when moving is an individual climbing back to his seat on the bleachers for the second half of an exciting basketball playoff. Trying not to spill soda onto the people already seated, a weight shift at the hips is used. The upper body moves forward and back to hold the handheld objects stable as the individual finds his footing because of the limited space between seats. Imagining the ongoing activities within the stadium, the hip strategy may have just saved another person from tumbling down the steps as the individual turns to see why the crowd is suddenly cheering and begins to lose their balance.

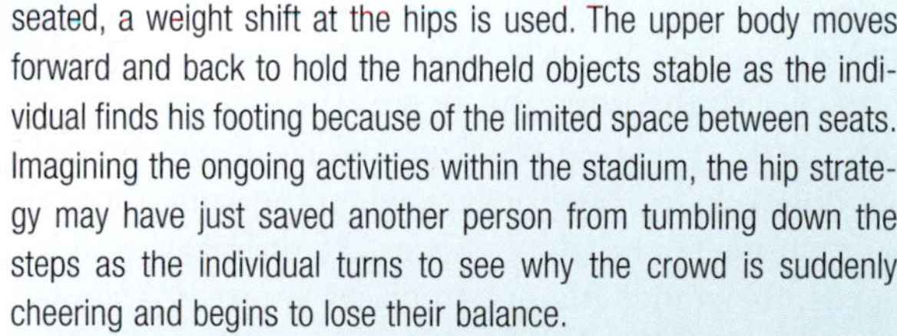

Finally, a stepping and reaching strategy protects another spectator from falling when the individual fails to realize he has one more step before he reaches the floor and flails his arms and legs as he struggles to regain postural control and balance.[18]

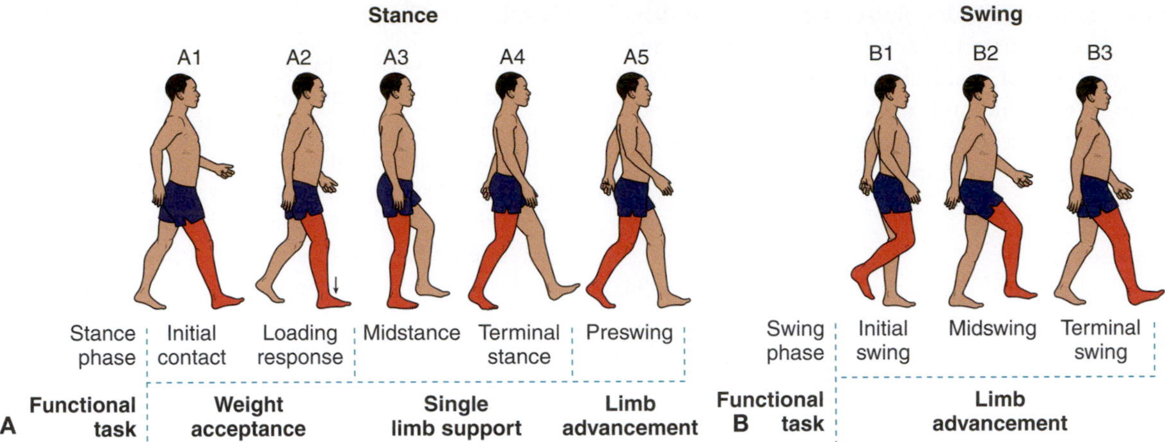

Figure 12.5 Gait Cycle Phases and Timing. **A)** Stance Phases: 1. Initial Contact; 2. Loading Response; 3. Midstance; 4. Terminal Stance; 5. Preswing. **B)** Swing Phases: 1. Initial Swing; 2. Midswing; 3. Terminal Swing.

use of slightly varying terminology systems. The traditional terminology system was developed first and describes the components of the gait cycle by naming the event or the critical action associated within each phase, such as heel strike, foot flat, heel off, or toe off. The second system is the Rancho Los Amigos (RLA) terminology, developed by Jacquelin Perry, a prominent gait researcher from this premier gait analysis center in California, which emphasizes the functional task associated within each phase.[20] Institutions around the country may use either RLA terminology or traditional terminology, depending on regional preferences. Since many experienced clinicians often interchange the terminology systems, therefore, it is advantageous for learners to become familiar with both systems.

We will use the RLA terminology system in this text (Table 12–1). This system divides the stance phase into five subphases and the swing phase into three.[20] Since walking may be performed at different speeds, one complete gait cycle is identified as 100% with the phases and subphases signified by percentages of the whole cycle. When the foot first makes contact with the floor, this begins the gait cycle, so the start of the cycle is at 0% time and continues on until one full cycle to 100% occurs, when the same foot initially contacts the floor again. At ordinary walking speeds, the stance phase comprises approximately the first 60% (62%) and the swing phase includes the last 40% (38%) of a single gait cycle, so the very end of the swing phase occurs at 100% of the cycle. At normal adult walking speeds, one cycle lasts 1 second and has a length of 1.4 meters.[20, 21] Figure 12.5 depicts a full gait cycle for the left and right lower extremities. Note that the right limb is shaded in the figure and is the reference leg throughout this chapter. It is important to also note that there are two times within the gait cycle when both feet are in contact with the ground, totaling about 20% (22%) of a gait cycle—10% at the beginning and 10% at the end of the stance phase. This time when both feet are in stance is called **double support.** During the middle 40% of its stance, the lower extremity is in **single limb support.** The duration of double support varies inversely with the speed of walking. In slow walking, this time is comparatively long in relation to the swing phase; but as the speed increases, double support time decreases.

As mentioned, each phase of the gait cycle is divided into subphases. Stance phase includes the subphases of initial contact, loading response, midstance, terminal stance, and preswing. The stance phase begins when the foot first makes contact with the ground. The heel is usually the foot section that makes **initial contact**, but other parts of the foot may contact the ground first in the presence of some pathologic conditions. After the foot makes initial contact, the foot moves so the entire plantar surface contacts the ground; this is the loading response. During this phase, the body's impact forces with the ground are absorbed. As the stance phase continues, the body's COM moves directly over the foot; this is **midstance**. As the body continues its forward movement and the heel lifts off the floor, the stance phase progresses into **terminal stance**. Stance ends at **preswing** when the toes leaves the ground. Swing phase includes initial

TABLE 12–1 | PHASES AND SUBPHASES OF THE GAIT CYCLE: DEFINITION AND TIMING

Phase	Definition and Description	Contralateral Limb
Stance Phase 60% gait cycle: 0%–60%		
Initial Contact 0%–2%	Floor contact, typically with heel. This is the initial period of double support.	End terminal stance
Loading Response 2%–10%	Body weight transferring to limb and foot lowering to floor **Double support continues.*	Preswing
Midstance 10%–30%	Begins at onset unilateral stance when opposite foot is lifted through to when HAT is aligned over single limb **Unilateral stance*	Midswing
Terminal Stance 30%–50%	Heel rises or "heel off," limb advances over forefoot and trunk moves ahead of support limb with the limb now trailing in extension	Terminal swing
Preswing 50%–60%	Floor contact is onto metatarsal heads coinciding with opposite foot making contact; ends with toe-off **Onset of second period of double support*	Initial contact-Loading
Swing Phase 40% gait cycle: 60%–100%		
Initial Swing 60%–73%	Foot lifted, and knee flexes to shorten limb and meet demand to accelerate	Early midstance
Midswing 73%–87%	Limb now under and then anterior to HAT and positioned almost directly opposite contralateral stance limb; maximum knee flexion	Late midstance
Terminal Swing 87%–100%	Begins with tibia perpendicular to floor through full limb advancement forward as limb decelerates for initial contact	Terminal stance

swing, midswing, and terminal swing. Swing begins at the point the foot is no longer in contact with the floor with **initial swing**. When the tibia is perpendicular to the floor and during the middle part of the swing, it is in the **midswing** phase. **Terminal swing** is the third and final portion of the swing phase; the leg prepares to make initial contact again with the ground during terminal swing. The moment the foot makes contact with the ground, the swing phase ends and stance phase begins again. Since Figure 12.5 shows both right and left limbs, a comparison of timing during stance of one limb and swing of the contralateral limb may be observed (see Table 12-1). Keep in mind that, in the presence of pathology, some of these subphases may not occur or may occur with altered timing. These subphases are presented in more detail in the successive sections.

Functional Tasks of Gait

From a functional perspective, there are three fundamental tasks associated with human gait: weight acceptance, single limb support, and limb advancement.[22] The stance phase plays a role in all three of these basic tasks, each of its subphases contributing to varying degrees.[23] Initial contact and loading response are the two subphases primarily responsible for weight acceptance. Single limb stance occurs at midstance and is the time when balance during ambulation is most precarious. The body's center of mass has shifted laterally and is centered over only one supporting limb at this time. Limb advancement creates forward motion of the body and includes the stance subphases of terminal stance and preswing; these subphases provide propulsive forces to move the limb forward and thereby move the body forward. The stance subphases utilize effective force absorption and efficient energy expenditure to accomplish these tasks.[24]

The swing phase is concerned with only one of the three fundamental tasks: limb advancement. Limb advancement during the swing phase requires sufficient clearance of the foot from the floor. The limb performs this activity during the first half of swing and prepares for initial contact during the latter half of swing. During the first two subphases of the swing phase, initial swing and midswing, the limb flexes at the hip, knee, and ankle to functionally shorten the limb so the foot clears the floor. The knee then begins rapid extension in terminal swing to lengthen the limb; this motion increases step length and forms a rigid limb in preparation for stability at initial contact.[24] Table 12–2 summarizes the requirements of gait, the purpose of each subphase and the ranges of motion and the primary muscular requirements of each subphase's activity.

Kinematics of Gait

A kinematic study of gait includes describing gait in terms of its spatial and temporal characteristics (how and when the foot hits the ground) and how the entire body and its segments move through space. The following section describes normal gait from a kinematic perspective.

Spatial and Temporal Characteristics of Gait

Spatial characteristics are those variables that are easily visualized by looking at the feet as they make a walking pattern on the ground, such as when visible footprints are produced during a walk on the beach. These characteristics include: step length, stride length, step width, and angle of progression (Fig. 12.6). **Step length** is the distance between the initial contact (measured at the midpoint of the heel) of one foot to the initial contact of the opposite foot. In other words, as you step forward with your right foot, your right step length is from where your left foot contacted the ground (usually at the heel) to the corresponding point where your right foot contacts the

TABLE 12–2 | FUNCTIONAL REQUIREMENTS OF SUBPHASES OF GAIT

Phase	Functional Task	Joint Angle Requirement	Prime Muscular Force
Initial Contact	Makes contact with surface Weight acceptance	Ankle: 0° Knee: 3°–5° flexion Hip: 25°–30° flexion	Tibialis anterior Quadriceps Gluteus maximus and medius
Loading	Weight acceptance Shock absorption	Ankle: 15° plantarflexion Knee: up to 15° flexion Hip: 25°–30° flexion	Tibialis anterior Quadriceps Gluteus maximus
Midstance	Single limb support	Ankle: from 15° plantarflexion to 15° dorsiflexion Knee: 5° flexion Hip: full extension	Gastrocnemius and soleus Gluteus maximus, gluteus medius minimus, and TFL
Terminal Stance	Single limb support Propulsion	Ankle: 15° dorsiflexion to 20° plantarflexion Knee: moves into full extension Hip: 10° extension	Gastrocnemius
Preswing	Propulsion	Ankle: 20° plantarflexion Knee: 40° flexion Hip: 10° extension	Gastrocnemius Hip adductors Rectus femoris
Initial Swing	Limb shortening for foot clearance	Ankle: to neutral dorsiflexion Knee: 40°–60° flexion Hip: from extension to 25°–30° flexion	Tibialis anterior Hamstrings Iliopsoas
Midswing	Limb shortening for foot clearance Generation of momentum	Ankle: neutral Knee: 60° flexion Hip: 25°–30° flexion	Tibialis anterior Iliopsoas
Terminal Swing	Limb advancement Preparation for initial contact Deceleration	Ankle: neutral Knee: to full extension Hip: 25°–30° flexion	Tibialis anterior Gluteus maximus and hamstrings

Adapted from: Bertoti DB. *Functional Neurorehabilitation through the Life Span.* Philadelphia; FA Davis Company, 2004.

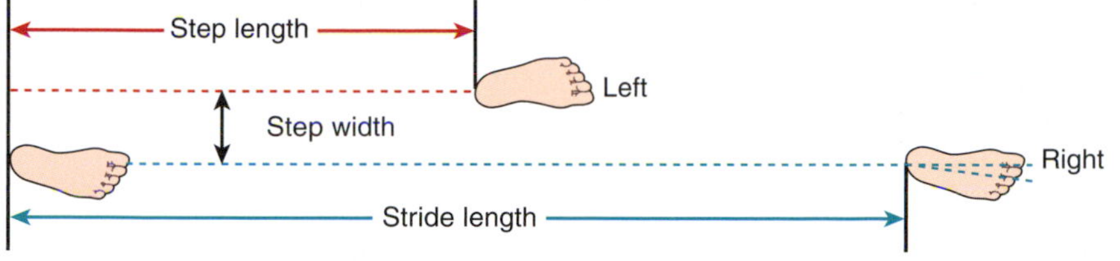

Figure 12.6 Spatial characteristics of gait: step length, stride length, step width, angle of progression.

ground (Fig. 12.6). **Stride length** is the distance between initial contact of one foot and initial contact of that same foot again. Stride length is synonymous with the combination of one right and one left step length. Typically, your step lengths are equal except during fast walking when the dominant leg has a little longer step because of its greater propulsive force.[25] In pathological conditions, step lengths may be significantly different between the involved and uninvolved extremities.[26, 27] **Step width** is the horizontal distance between the two feet, measured from the midpoint of one heel to the midpoint of the next heel contact. Step width measures typically between 2 to 4 inches (5 to 10 cm) for adults; again, this standard does not hold true in some pathological conditions. The **angle of progression** is the angle formed between the line of progression in a straight line and a line that bisects the foot at the heel's midpoint and runs between the second and third toes. Out-toeing of about 7° is typical in mature adults.[28]

Temporal characteristics are those variables that describe any characteristic that has to do with time, such as **velocity, step duration,** and **cadence. Velocity** is the distance covered over a unit of time such as meters per second or miles per hour. The number of steps completed per unit of time, usually given in steps per minute, is called **cadence.**[29] Normal walking velocity includes a wide latitude of speeds. Since there is such variation in walking speed, a description of an individual's gait pattern ordinarily includes velocity or cadence. Typical adult walking ranges from about 50 to 120–130 steps per minute. Calculated differently, average normal walking speed is about 80 m/min.[30] It is interesting to note that the optimal speed for most efficient walking individuals of average height is also at this speed.[30] Speeds lower or higher than this require more muscle effort and energy production.

Walking speed is important in a complete gait analysis since changes in speed impact other factors such as time and distance measurements, energy expenditure, and muscle activity. Normal subjects have the ability to alter their speed of walking from a stroll to a fast walk and into a run, thus making comparisons difficult. Each person, however, has a free or comfortable walking speed on a smooth, level surface that is most energy efficient for that individual. Part of the variability between individuals seen in walking speed is dependent on stride length, which is due to leg length. Free walking speed is often used in gait studies because it represents optimal efficiency for each individual, and the able-bodied subject reproduces the same values if the walking surface and the footwear remain the same.[30] In a study by Perry,[20] stride length averaged 1.4 m and the mean cadence was 113 steps per minute. The mean velocity of adults walking a free pace is 82 m/min, or approximately 3 miles per hour.[20] Men walked faster and had a longer stride length and a slower cadence than women (Table 12–3). Typical walking speed for men is 100 to 120 steps per minute; for women, it is 105 to 125 steps per minute.[20] Rates above or below these values are classified as fast or slow walking speeds.

Changes in walking speed are made by altering stride length or cadence, with the normal individual usually changing both parameters. Increased speed results in diminished duration of all of the component phases of the gait cycle: stance, swing, and double

TABLE 12–3 | MEAN STRIDE VALUES IN NORMAL ADULTS 20 TO 80 YEARS OF AGE WALKING AT FREE OR CUSTOMARY WALKING SPEED ON A SMOOTH LEVEL SURFACE[20]

	Males	Females	Total
Number of subjects	135	158	293
Velocity (meters per minute)	86	77	82*
Stride length (meters)	1.46	1.28	1.41*
Cadence (steps per minute)	111	117	113*

* Averages
Source: Data from Perry, J. *Gait Analysis: Normal and Pathological Function.* Thoroughfare, NJ: Slack, 1992.

PRACTICE POINT

Although no minimum standards for community-based living activities have been proposed, the World Health Organization (WHO), through its International Classification of Functioning, Disability and Health (ICF),[31] and rehabilitation investigators are in the process of identifying functional community needs for patients returning to their normal environments. Two major concerns are safety and functional distances for ambulation. Safety in ambulation involves stability during gait within the community as well as the ability to walk fast enough to cross a street. It is known that this safety speed requirement is 30 m/min.[32] In addition to velocity, ambulation distances must be sufficient for an individual to conduct basic and normal functions within the community such as grocery and department store shopping, banking, physician office visits, and other common functions. The distance that has been determined to be a functional level for community ambulation is 342 meters;[32] this is the distance required for an individual to walk from the parking lot, through a supermarket, and return to the car. Unfortunately, many clinicians do not require their patients to ambulate this distance during their rehabilitation program; it has been determined that the average distance achieved during rehabilitation treatment and care is 200 feet, only a fraction of what is needed to be functionally independent in the community.[32] Clinicians would provide the individuals they treat a much better service if they advanced them to ambulating community distances before they were discharged from care.

In addition to establishing ambulation distance, it is important to identify walking speed if an individual is to function in the community. An individual's average walking speed, stride length, and cadence can be determined by timing the subject walking across a measured distance of at least 15 m and then count the number of steps taken.[33]

support, with the double support phase decreasing toward zero and the swing phase decreasing the least.[20]

Angular Joint Displacements

The kinematics, or "geometry," of walking has been studied and recorded, looking at the angular movements of each body segment in all three planes. Advances in photographic techniques and computer technology have permitted more accurate study from a three-dimensional perspective. Since the sagittal plane motions are the largest and easiest to track, they have been most often investigated, so there is a general consensus regarding these values. On the other hand, displacement in the frontal and transverse planes is smaller and more difficult to measure; therefore, results are less accurate and reliable and more divergent and inconsistent. In spite of variations in the precise values in the literature, the patterns and sequence of joint motions during gait are highly consistent. The following sections summarize joint motions in all three planes at each body segment during normal gait (Fig. 12.7A, B, C).

As the body walks, its center of motion oscillates in the sagittal and frontal planes of motion. In the sagittal plane, the COM moves up and down twice during one gait cycle while it moves once from left to right in the frontal plane. These motions of the body's COM as well as movements at each of the joints during the gait cycle are presented as each of the body's three planes of motion during walking is discussed.

Sagittal Plane Motion

In the sagittal plane, the two vertical oscillations of the body's COM follow a smooth sinusoidal curve. The curve's highest point occurs at midstance for each foot while the lowest segment of the sinusoidal curve is at double support. Actual vertical displacement of the COM varies from 2 to 5 cm, depending on stride length and walking speed. Angular motions of flexion and extension occur at the hip, knee, and ankle in the sagittal plane (Fig. 12.7A).

PELVIS

The pelvis must multifunction during gait, providing both stability and mobility to upper and lower extremities. The pelvis offers a stable base of support for the lower limb and HAT but it also must allow for the contributions of thoracic and lumbar spine motions. Additionally, the pelvis must be stable enough to transmit weight as it transfers from one limb to the other, and it also needs to move the acetabulum in a favorable position for hip motion. In the sagittal plane, the pelvis remains relatively level, demonstrating an average anterior-posterior tilt excursion of only about 3° during the gait cycle. Although small, this motion is an important complementary companion to hip and lower limb motion. Two full cycles of sinusoidal motion occur with each step; immediately after initial contact the pelvis rotates first into a posterior tilt, then

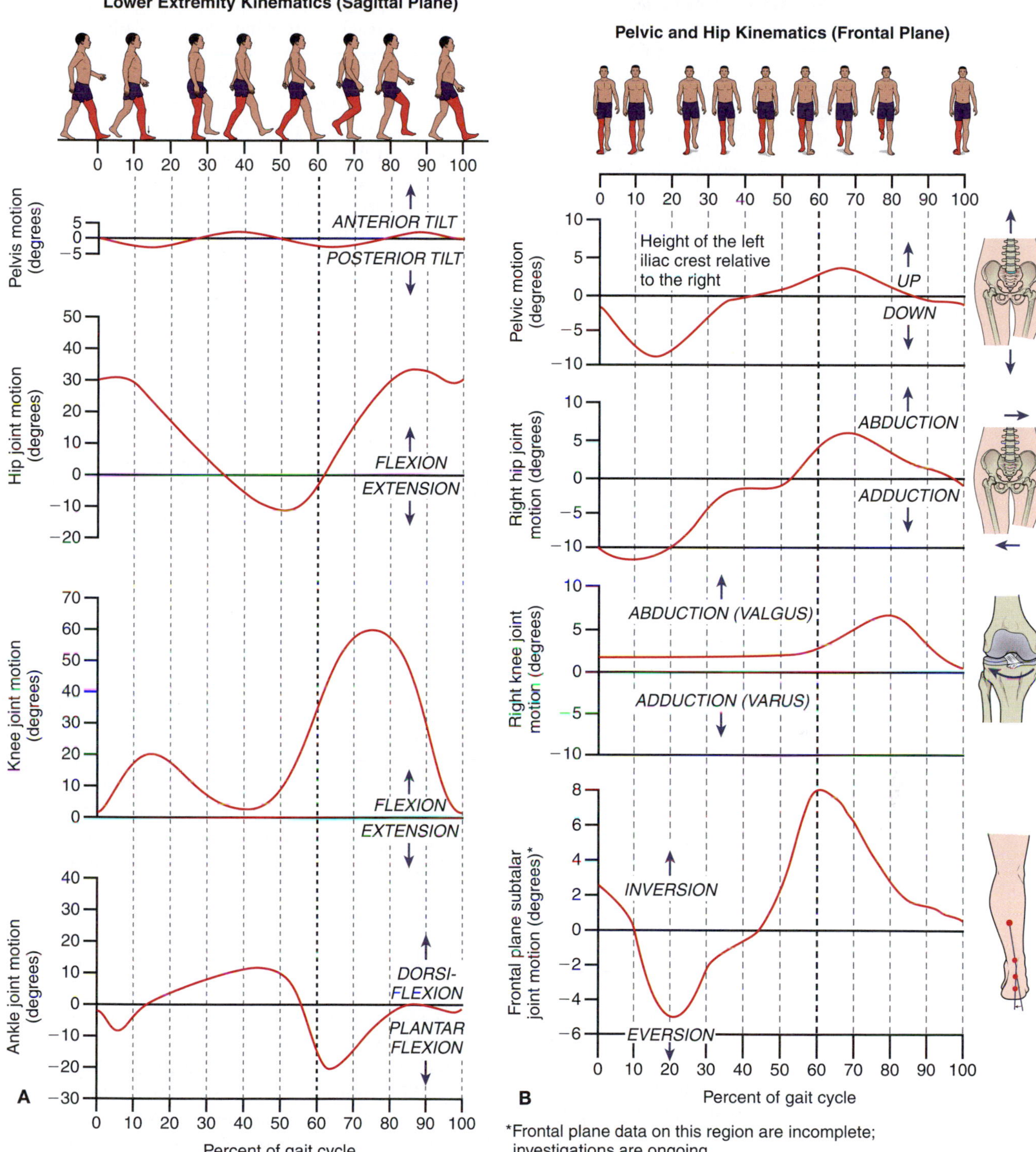

Figure 12.7 Angular joint displacement at hip, knee, and ankle during gait. A) Sagittal plane. B) Frontal plane. Adapted from Neumann;[33] modified from multiple sources.

Continued

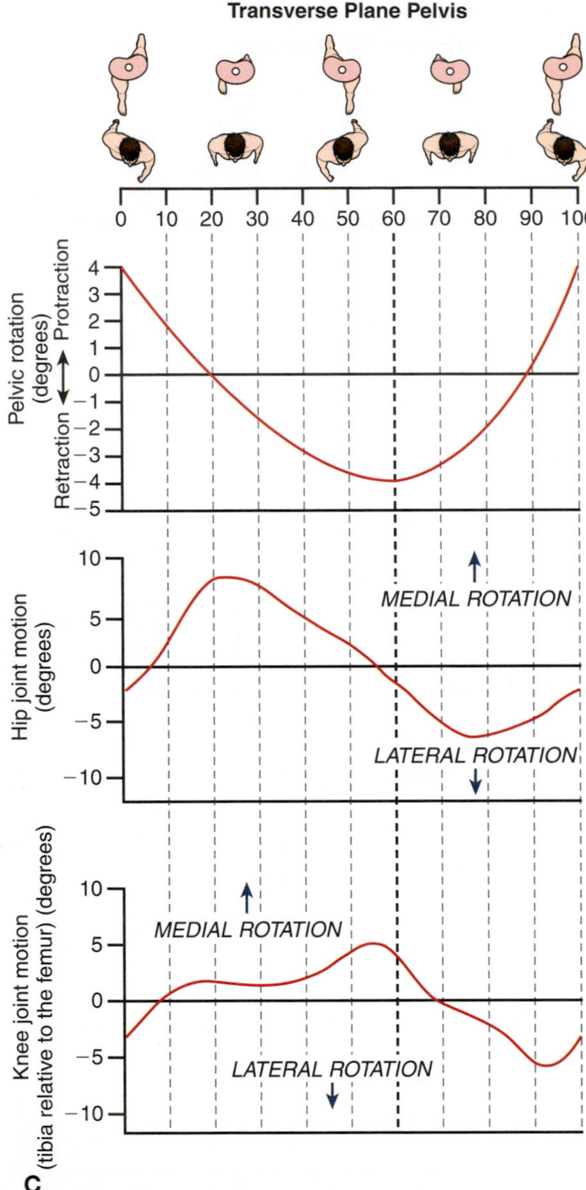

*See 12-7B for foot motion. Transverse plane data on this region are incomplete; investigations are ongoing.

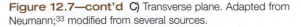

Figure 12.7—cont'd C) Transverse plane. Adapted from Neumann;[33] modified from several sources.

an anterior tilt, and half way through its second posterior tilt, the limb begins the swing phase, and the pelvis ends its swing phase as it moves through its last anterior tilt.[33] Looking more precisely at the subphases of the gait cycle, the pelvis reaches initial contact in a near-neutral position and moves through midstance in a slightly posteriorly tilted position. By the end of midstance when the hip begins moving into extension, the pelvis tilts anteriorly just slightly. By the time the limb reaches preswing, the pelvis tilts posteriorly again. During swing, the pelvis first completes its posterior tilt and then tilts anteriorly from initial to midswing, and in terminal swing it moves toward a posterior tilt in preparation for landing once again. There is a fluid rhythm that occurs as the pelvis tilting motions complement the hip flexion and extension that is described below. Companion tilting of the pelvis occurs to provide the additional motion that is required at the hip during ambulation. Specifically, an anterior pelvic tilt accompanies hip extension as the hip hyperextends after midstance and into preswing.

The amount of pelvic anterior and posterior tilt is dependent upon the region's soft tissue mobility and the walking speed. The amount of mobility in the hip joint's capsule and the flexibility of the hip and pelvic muscles determine the degree of anterior and posterior tilt while walking. Assuming normal soft tissue mobility, as walking speed increases, the amount of pelvic tilt increases to provide a functional lengthening of the limb to increase the size of the step length.

HIP

The hip joint moves through 40° of sagittal motion in a single gait cycle. At initial contact, the hip is flexed at 25° to 30°. As the stance phase continues, the hip progressively moves into extension, reaching its maximum extension at 10° of hyperextension by terminal stance. From initial contact to midstance, the trunk moves forward over the foot and continues its forward movement to advance in front of the foot immediately after midstance. Hip hyperextension at terminal stance is accompanied by extension of the lumbar vertebrae and an anterior pelvic tilt. Once the hip reaches maximum extension at terminal stance, the hip begins movement towards flexion during preswing as it prepares to lift the limb off the ground; by the end of stance, the hip is near neutral, and as the limb begins into the swing phase, the hip continues a steady increase into flexion until midswing when the hip is slightly more than 30° of flexion. After midswing, its flexion decreases slightly and is maintained until terminal swing when it starts to move towards extension in preparation for initial contact. These typical sagittal plane excursions from 10° of hyperextension to 30° of flexion occur during normal walking speed but are slightly higher in fast walking.[34]

KNEE

The knee joint moves through two cycles of flexion and extension during the gait cycle. At initial contact, the knee is near full extension (about 3° to 5° of flexion). Immediately following initial contact, the knee flexes during loading response. This flexion movement provides shock absorption of compression forces that occur when the body weight impacts the ground, and it also assists in weight transfer as the body begins to move toward a single leg support stance. By the end of the loading response phase, the knee is flexed 15° to 20°. The knee then moves towards extension during midstance; this motion minimizes muscular effort required during single limb weight-bearing. Maximum extension at the knee occurs during terminal stance. Immediately after achieving full extension, the knee starts to flex to achieve its maximal stance-phase flexion at 35° to 40° by preswing. During initial and midswing, the knee flexes to shorten the limb and clear the foot from the floor. Maximum knee flexion of the entire gait cycle occurs during midswing, with the knee at 60° to 65° of flexion. At midswing, the tibia is perpendicular to the floor. During terminal swing, the knee extends to nearly full extension so it is able to assist the other limb joints in achieving an adequate step length, advancing the limb, and preparing for initial contact once again.[20,21,33]

ANKLE AND FOOT

The ankle plantarflexes and dorsiflexes twice during the gait cycle. At the moment of initial contact, the ankle joint is in sagittal plane neutral. During loading response, the ankle rapidly plantarflexes so the entire plantar foot surface contacts the floor. After loading response, the tibia advances forward over the fixed foot into midstance, so by the end of midstance the ankle is in about 10° of dorsiflexion. Ten degrees of ankle dorsiflexion is the close-packed position of the ankle and provides maximal talocrural joint congruency. As the heel rises off the floor during terminal stance, a second wave of plantarflexion occurs, peaking at about 20° by preswing. This plantarflexion motion propels the limb into swing phase. The foot dorsiflexes to neutral or slight dorsiflexion to clear the toes from the floor and maintains this position throughout the swing phase.

More plantarflexion than dorsiflexion occurs during the gait cycle in the sagittal plane motion; the range of plantarflexion is 0° to 20° whereas the dorsiflexion range is 0° to 10°. The greatest amount of plantarflexion and dorsiflexion both occur during the stance phase.

An essential but often overlooked sagittal plane motion occurs in the metatarsophalangeal joints (MTP) during the stance phase after midstance to preswing. During loading response, the MTP joints are in a neutral position. The MTP joints hyperextend as the body's COM moves forward of the weight-bearing limb and the

PRACTICE POINT

Since the iliopsoas originates on the lumbar spine and the ilium, tightness in these hip flexors also affects the pelvis and lumbar spine during ambulation. During stance, hip flexor tightness is demonstrated with an exaggerated anterior pelvic tilt and lumbar lordosis. From terminal stance to initial swing, an even greater exaggeration of these pathologies may be observed by the clinician in individuals with extreme tightness.

Orthopedic pathologies such as restricted knee extension mobility or patellofemoral pain syndrome demonstrate two very different pathological gaits. The individual with reduced knee extension secondary to injury or surgery is unable to fully extend the knee sufficiently during terminal swing or initial contact. This individual may have a shorter stride length and ambulate without ever achieving knee extension. On the other hand, the individual with patellofemoral pain syndrome (PFPS) will be reluctant to place the knee in flexion because of pain with increased patellofemoral compression and/or weakness of the quadriceps. A typical gait with patellofemoral pain syndrome includes prolonged knee extension from initial contact throughout the stance phase. In extreme PFPS cases, the hip may flex to move the body's COM anterior to the knee to further reduce demands on the joint during the stance phase.

ankle starts to plantarflex. Extension becomes most apparent during terminal stance until the MTPs reach their maximum motion, 55° to 60°, by the end of preswing (Fig. 12.7). During the swing phase, hyperextension of the MTP joints is maintained at about 30° to 40°[35] for toe clearance but gradually decreases to 25° by the time of initial contact. The MTPs remain in neutral once the limb moves into loading response until right before terminal swing. Pain or restriction of motion of the MTP joints can have devastating effects on the ability to walk.

Frontal Plane Motion

As mentioned earlier, sinusoidal motion of the body's COM moves through only one full cycle in the frontal plane as the body goes through one complete gait cycle with each limb. This lateral movement allows the COM to be continually placed over the base of support. Not only does the pelvis shift, but the HAT also shifts laterally as the position of the base of support changes during ambulation (Fig. 12.7B). Maximum lateral displacement occurs during unilateral stance and is about 2 cm to the left and to the right. When visualized in both the sagittal and frontal planes during walking, the body's COM is at its highest in the sagittal plane and its most lateral position in the frontal plane at the same time, during unilateral stance in midstance (e.g., of the right leg). During normal ambulation, the COM moves lower and to the midline at double support during the last 10% of stance of the weight-bearing limb (right leg) and the first 10% of the weight-accepting limb (e.g., left leg), and it moves high and lateral toward the ipsilateral stance phase limb (left leg).

PELVIS

The pelvis tilts laterally in the frontal plane about 8° on each side. In unilateral stance, the pelvis of the swing leg tilts laterally downward about 8°.[36] This lateral drop occurs on the swing leg since the stance leg adducts. This small but important motion serves two purposes: It puts the hip abductor muscles of the stance leg on a slight stretch, thereby putting them at an improved length-tension advantage, and it reduces the rise of the center of mass of the swing leg. This reduction in the limb's COM elevation was initially thought to be important in decreasing energy expenditure.[37] However, this theory advanced by Saunders and associates[37] has not been demonstrated; and although the motion occurs, the importance of it in terms of reducing energy costs of ambulation has been recently questioned using mechanical models.[38] This point is presented in more detail later in this chapter under "gait efficiency."

HIP

As seen above, hip motions in the frontal plane directly impact pelvic motion. Frontal plane hip motions offer crucial contributions to stability and efficiency during gait. At initial contact, the hip is adducted to about 10° and continues to adduct another 5° during loading response, serving to puts the gluteus medius on the stance side on slight stretch. As mentioned in the pelvis section above, this position places the gluteus medius on

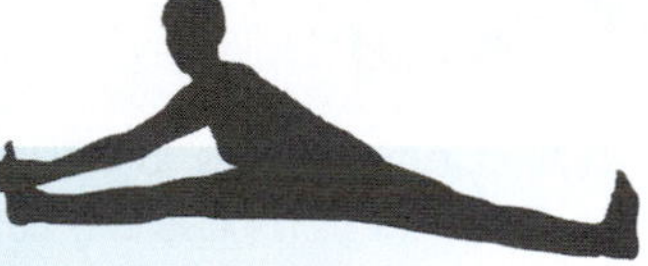

PRACTICE POINT

Because the ankle moves through 30° of motion within a very brief time during stance, if an ankle lacks normal mobility, a very characteristic "lurching" gait results. Clinicians readily recognize this type of gait since the individual lacks the mobility for rapid motion changes that is required of the ankle for a smooth gait. To compensate for this motion loss, the individual ambulates using a very brief stance phase on the affected limb and demonstrates a rapid transfer of weight-bearing to the contralateral extremity.

Individuals with gout or a "turf toe" (sprained #1MTP joint) are reluctant to dorsiflex (hyperextend) the toe during terminal stance and preswing. The clinician is able to easily observe pathological gait in these individuals because they are likely to ambulate with the limb laterally rotated to reduce the amount of hyperextension required at the MTP joint or they may fail to exhibit terminal stance and preswing but prematurely lift the limb off the ground after midstance to avoid hyperextension of the joint.

stretch so it may generate the forces needed to stabilize and hold the contralateral pelvis level during unilateral stance. From midstance through terminal stance, the thigh moves into a relatively neutral position. The hip abducts about 5° during swing phase to assist in clearing the foot from the floor and returns to neutral as it approaches the end of terminal swing.

KNEE

Total abduction-adduction motion of the knee is minimal because of the stable collateral ligaments supporting the joint. At initial contact the knee is in slight abduction and moves to its maximum of about 3° of abduction during loading response. During the swing phase, the knee moves into more abduction to a maximum of about 8° when it is at the height of its sagittal plane flexion.[20, 33]

Ankle and Foot

Although the talocrural joint is the primary ankle joint for sagittal plane movement, the subtalar and midtarsal joints functions are multiplanar, so they will be discussed together here.[39] All of the joints within the foot and ankle play a role in foot mechanics during ambulation.

Subtalar Joint

Subtalar joint motions of inversion and eversion occur during gait. The subtalar joint is in slight inversion at initial contact and immediately moves into eversion after making contact with the ground. The subtalar joint rapidly moves through to its maximum range of eversion, about 5°,[40] after loading response and by the time the limb is in early midstance. At midstance, the subtalar joint begins moving toward inversion. By preswing, it is at its maximum inversion position, approximately 8°[40] to 11°.[39] During the swing phase, the subtalar joint returns to neutral and is in slight inversion by the time the limb is in terminal swing.

Midtarsal Joint

As does the rest of the foot, the midtarsal joint follows the motions of the subtalar joint during all phases of ambulation. The two joints comprising the midtarsal joint, the talonavicular and calcaneocuboid joints, each have approximately 11° to 15° of total motion in the frontal plane during normal ambulation.[41] Immediately after initial contact, the midtarsal joint flattens to absorb impact forces and to allow the entire foot to touch the ground. Once in midstance, the arch elevates, following the inversion movements of the midtarsal and subtalar joints, to move the forefoot joints into more congruent positions in preparation of terminal stance and preswing.

Toes

The most important joint of the toes is the metatarsophalangeal joint. Its primary motion has already been discussed during sagittal plane movements. Investigations have not focused on frontal plane motion of the first metatarsophalangeal joint, but it may be assumed that motion of the joint in this plane is likely to be minimal in normal gait.

Transverse Plane Motion

Rotations within the transverse plane, around vertical axes occur at the vertebrae, pelvis, hips, knees, and ankle and feet. These rotations are observed during walking with the smooth reciprocal motions observed of the trunk and extremities. Transverse plane motions include the reciprocal motions of the shoulders and pelvis as the right arm and opposite left leg swing forward. (Fig. 12.7C) The upper vertebrae and shoulders rotate counterclockwise as the left leg swings forward and then reverses to clockwise as the right leg swings forward. This complementary rotation increases with walking speed, with the point of minimal rotation located near the seventh thoracic vertebra.[34]

PELVIS

Pelvic rotation in the transverse plane involves either protraction or retraction. Similar to the scapula, pelvic protraction (anterior rotation) moves the anterior pelvis forward as the pelvis rotates around a vertical axis as retraction moves the anterior pelvis backward as it rotates. If one hemipelvis rotates in protraction, the contralateral hemipelvis rotates in retraction. Since hip flexion and pelvic lateral rotation work cooperatively during transverse plane rotation, the pelvis will rotate anteriorly or forward with hip flexion and lateral rotation. The pelvis rotates anteriorly, or protracts, on the swing side 4° and rotates posteriorly, or retracts, on the stance side another 4°—producing a total of 8° of pelvic movement in the transverse plane. The magnitude of this pelvic rotation increases 10° to 20° with increased speed.[30] As described above, the pelvis also tilts laterally in the frontal plane about 5°. All of these pelvic motions occur to minimize movement of the body's COM and provide smooth reciprocal movement during ambulation. Maximum amount of anterior pelvic rotation occurs at initial contact in concert with maximum hip flexion (30°); these motions work cooperatively to provide a longer stride.

HIP

During each stride, the limb moves through an arc of both medial and lateral rotation in the transverse plane.

At initial contact, the hip is in slight lateral rotation, supported by the protracted position of the pelvis. Immediately after loading response, however, the hip medially rotates and maintains a medially rotated position through loading response and midstance until the hip moves into extension. From midstance to terminal stance, the hip moves to neutral rotation and continues into lateral rotation at preswing. During initial swing, the hip is in lateral rotation and oscillates between medial and lateral rotation until it returns to slight medial rotation as the limb prepares for ground contact. Peak hip medial rotation occurs at the end of loading response and maximum lateral rotation occurs at the end of preswing. Studies have shown that the total hip rotation ranges between 8° and 14° for normal adults.[20, 30]

KNEE

Throughout the entire gait cycle, the knee rotates a total of about 10° to 20°.[20, 30] Of this total rotation, the femur rotates on the tibia 6° to 7° medially, and laterally and the tibia rotates 8° to 9° in each direction.[33, 42] At initial contact, the knee is in slight lateral rotation (tibia relative to the femur) but then medially rotates as the limb accepts the weight. As the foot pronates during loading response, the tibia medially rotates about 8°, allowing the knee to flex. After midstance, the femur and tibia begin to rotate laterally in the transverse plane through preswing. When body weight is shifted to the other leg in preswing, the tibia is led into lateral rotation by the supinated foot and the limb moves into swing. During swing, the thigh, knee, and leg move toward and into medial rotation until terminal swing, when they laterally rotate in preparation for initial contact.[42]

Combined Ankle and Foot

Tibial rotation during weight-bearing is actually initiated by the joint between the talus and calcaneus; likewise, the more distal joints of the foot are also influenced by the subtalar joint. When the talus everts on the weight-bearing calcaneus, the tibia is forced to medially rotate through its connection to the ankle joint. Eversion at the subtalar joint causes the foot to rotate into pronation. Movement at the subtalar joint also causes the axes of the talonavicular and the calcaneocuboid joints to become parallel to one another; this parallel arrangement increases transverse tarsal joint flexibility and lowers the longitudinal arch. This midfoot rotation in the early part of the stance phase is essential for shock absorption and allows the foot to adapt to uneven surfaces as the foot moves into loading response. At midstance, the tarsal joints rotate into supination to transform the foot to a rigid lever that permits propulsion of the body forward as the foot pushes against the ground. This transformation occurs as the subtalar joint inverts to move the distal foot joints in their maximum congruency. The subtalar inversion causes the axes of the talonavicular and calcaneocuboid joints to diverge, resulting in a locking or rigidity of the transverse tarsal joint. Along with subtalar inversion, the tibia rolls toward lateral rotation.

As the heel moves off the ground during terminal stance, the MTP joints are passively forced into hyperextension; this MTP movement into hyperextension creates a "windlass" effect, causing the plantar aponeurosis to become taut, which further increases supination and promotes foot rigidity (Chapter 11). Although the intertarsal joint motions are small, they are a critical part of the gait cycle. If the motions in these joints are excessive, diminished, or occur at the wrong phase in the gait cycle, pain and dysfunction result, not only occurring in the foot but also producing symptoms up the entire kinetic chain. For example, with prolonged pronation, the leg and thigh have excess medial rotation after initial contact when they should be in neutral rotation. This pathological sequence places excessive stresses on structures, eventually becoming apparent as knee pain or patellofemoral tracking dysfunction.

Range of Motion Requirements of Normal Gait

For functional movement, the minimum range of motion requirements at each joint is as follows:

- Pelvis: 5° to 8° lateral tilt in the frontal plane, 3° anterior and posterior tilt in the sagittal plane, and a total of 8° protraction and retraction in the transverse plane.
- Hip: 10° extension to 25°–30° flexion in the sagittal plane; 15° adduction to 5° abduction in the frontal plane; and 8° to 14° in the transverse plane.
- Knee: full extension to 60° flexion in the sagittal plane; 3° to 8° in the frontal plane; 10° to 20° in the transverse plane.
- Ankle and foot: 10° dorsiflexion to 20° plantarflexion in the sagittal plane; 5°–8° inversion and eversion.[20]

If there is any limitation in range of motion at any of these body segments, a compensatory gait pattern occurs resulting in inefficiency overall and increased stress in other body segments.

Kinetics of Gait

As applied to the study of gait, kinetics includes an analysis of the main internal forces that produce ambulation as well as the main external force resisting the body every time we take a step. The external forces we

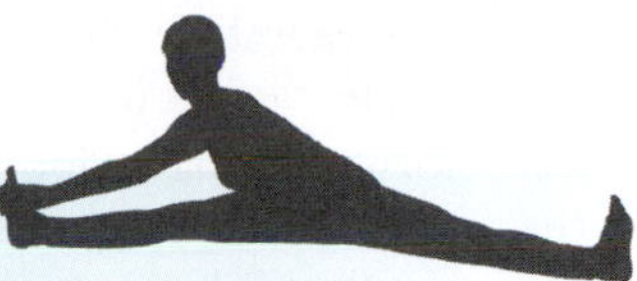

PRACTICE POINT

One of the first questions active individuals ask their clinicians is, "When can I start running?" Although running is presented later in this chapter, it is important for the clinician to put the individual's condition in perspective. To do this, the clinician should know what normal motions are required for ambulation and realize that even greater motion is necessary for running activities. Therefore, if an individual has less than 60° of knee flexion, for example, it should be made clear to the individual that it is essential to first have enough motion to walk before considerations for running is possible.

face include inertia, gravity, and friction, and the internal forces include muscle forces and passive tension from connective tissue structures such as ligaments, tendons, and joint capsules.

Ground Reaction Forces

Forces imparted by and on the body abide by Newton's Third Law of Motion: For every action, there is an opposite and equal reaction (Chapter 2). When the body takes a step, it imparts a force to the ground and the ground produces an equal reactive force in the opposite direction. This is **ground reaction force (GRF).** As with other forces, GRF is a resultant force, so it has magnitude and direction. Since the body functions three dimensionally, forces are imparted in a three-dimensional manner. These three different directions are vertical, anterior-posterior, and medial-lateral. Since the foot is the point of contact with the ground, the GRF between the ground and foot impacts at this location, as illustrated in Figure 12.8. The largest of these components is the vertical force (Y) directed perpendicular to the floor toward the earth. This force represents an acceleration or deceleration force to the body's forward motion. It is greatest at two specific points of the stance phase: at initial contact as the supporting limb lands on the ground and at preswing when the body mass accelerates to propel the leg and body forward. This component force exceeds body weight. The decrease in force that occurs between these two peaks to below body weight at midstance is due to elevation of the COM; since the COM moves up during this time of stance, the downward forces diminish.

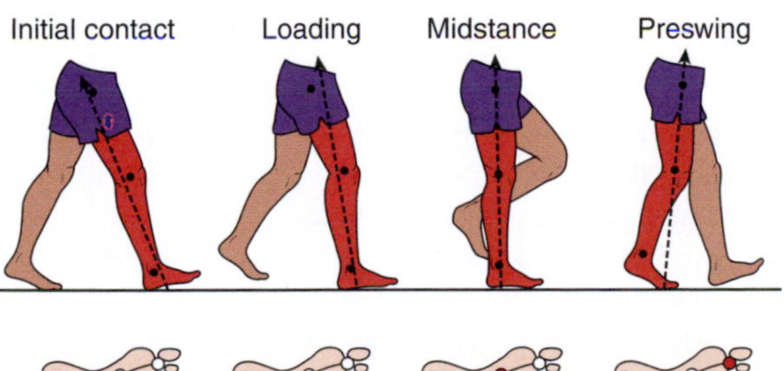

Figure 12.8 Relationship of the ground reaction force (GRF) and joint axes during stance phase. Note how the center of pressure (CoP) pathway moves from the heel at initial contact through the foot and to the great toe at the end of stance.

The Z-vector represents anterior-posterior forces directed at the foot during initial contact and preswing; these are shear forces. The anterior force of the foot occurring at initial contact is counteracted by the posterior force of the ground, producing friction to prevent the foot from slipping forward. The direction of these two forces switches at preswing so the foot produces a posterior force while the ground creates an anterior force; the friction created at this time provides the traction needed to advance the COM forward. In addition to allowing friction to secure a foothold, the AP force at initial contact primarily provides a deceleration of the limb, slowing the leg as it transitions from nonweight-bearing to weight-bearing. At the other end of the stance phase, the AP force becomes an accelerator of the limb as the force produced during preswing converts from friction to propulsion of the limb forward when it becomes non-weight-bearing. As one limb decelerates, the other accelerates, providing a smooth transition from one limb to the other throughout gait. During normal walking speeds, this anterior-posterior force is about 20% of the body's weight.[43] As the step length increases, the force magnitudes at initial contact and preswing also increase.

The X-force component is the medial-lateral shear between the foot and the ground. This force is the smallest of the three component forces making up ground reaction forces. This component is dependent upon the lateral movement of the body's COM as the body moves from one lower extremity to the other; since the amount of this lateral movement is variable and dependent upon factors such as the individual's size, weight, step width, and lateral hip muscle strength, there is a lot of variation in shear forces among individuals. As the foot makes initial contact with the ground, there is a lateral-to-medial force application of the heel since the lateral side of the heel first contacts the ground. This medially directed motion of the extremity is counteracted by a laterally directed ground reaction force. As the limb moves into single leg stance, both the COM and the ground reaction force move medially. At preswing, the foot is supinated and on its toes, so the forces are slightly laterally directed.[33]

Understanding the influences and applications of GRF is helpful in comprehending the complex muscle activity that occurs in gait. At initial contact, GRF is posterior to the ankle axis; this position creates a plantarflexion torque, which is controlled by eccentric contraction of the dorsiflexor muscles. Since the GRF runs through the axis of the knee at initial contact, no torque by the GRF is applied to the knee. However, the ground reaction force line of application is anterior to the hip, creating a flexion torque that is counterbalanced by the hip extensors. As the limb moves into loading response, the GRF becomes posterior to the knee, so the quadriceps activates eccentrically to control knee motion. At midstance, the GRF is well ahead of the ankle axis; the dorsiflexion torque created by the ground reaction force at this time is controlled by the gastrocnemius and soleus muscles.

Ground reaction forces are measured in a laboratory using a force platform that records a number of forces including postural sway and ground reaction forces. The location within the foot where the ground reaction forces are applied is the **center of pressure (CoP).** The center of pressure moves along a path through the foot from the heel to the toes throughout the stance phase as is depicted in Figure 12.8. At initial contact, the CoP is just lateral to the midpoint of the heel. As the body weight moves over the foot, the CoP also continues its forward progression to a near-center location in the midfoot at midstance then shifts more medially in the forefoot to between the metatarsal heads of the first and second toes at terminal stance and preswing.

Muscles of Gait

Gait is characterized by a recurring pattern of muscle activity followed by periods of muscle rest. The energy expenditure by the body during ambulation is kept relatively small through a minimum of motion requirements that are produced through efficient muscle function and an effective mechanical system of joint levers. These are some of the reasons why individuals are able to ambulate long distances.

Muscular Activation Patterns

Electromyography (EMG) detects when muscles are contracting or not during the gait cycle. The most valuable data gained from an EMG study is information related to the *timing* of muscle contraction and *points of peak forces*, rather than quantitative information about muscle force or tension. Electromyography records only the electrical activity of muscle fiber contraction.[44] In spite of its limitations, EMG is a valuable tool for providing an understanding of muscle function during gait. Electromyographic studies consistently demonstrate that peak muscle activity occurs during the stance phase, particularly around initial contact, with minimal muscle activity during the swing phase.[20, 45, 46]

Muscles perform a number of functions during gait. Muscles may act as stabilizers, accelerators, or decelerators. When muscles provide stabilization, they often work isometrically to position one joint or segment

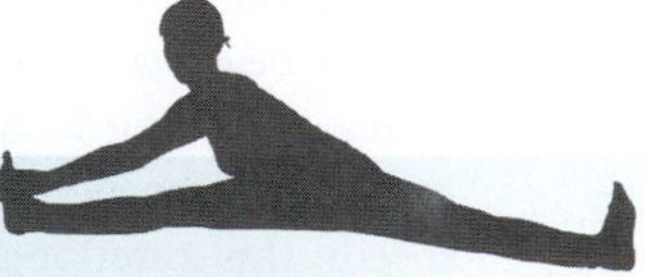

PRACTICE POINT

Ground reaction forces can be good or bad. We notice their absence, especially the medial-lateral and forward-backward forces, during the winter when we walk on ice; taking too large a step forward will cause us to lose traction since the forward force is greater than the ground's ability to produce a backward friction force. Likewise, if we push off the ice with too large a step length, the ice prevents the ground from providing adequate forward shear force, we find that our foot loses traction. On the good side, clinicians are able to identify problems associated with GRF and diagnose a problem based on an individual's report of where in the foot pain is located and within what part of the stance phase it occurs. For example, if an individual indicates pain on the ball of the foot from terminal stance through preswing, it is likely that the metatarsal heads are unable to tolerate the impact stresses of the vertical ground reaction forces; the clinician may instruct the individual to take a smaller step to reduce the forces or wear a shoe with a thicker or firmer sole so the stresses are absorbed by the shoe.

while another joint or segment moves. If muscles work as accelerators, they usually contract concentrically to move a segment forward. If they work as decelerators, they are eccentrically contracting to slow a movement or absorb forces produced by a motion. To gauge the participation of muscles in gait, we need to be able to visualize not only the limb movement in terms of its acceleration but also what happens as the limb decelerates.

Summary of Muscular Activation Patterns through the Gait Cycle

Muscles are recruited in a consistent, predictable pattern during a normal gait cycle. The muscular activation patterns recruited during human gait provide sequences with periods when a muscle works and periods when it rests, choreographing the timing of muscles to create a sequence that is remarkably smooth and efficient.[24] There are many instances during gait when a muscle switches its function from eccentric to concentric within fractions of a second whereas other muscles may perform only one type of activity. Muscle function during normal walking requires a surprisingly small amount of total force. Muscle activity is required over a relatively short time during a gait cycle, and there are large intervals within the gait cycle when the limb is actually carried forward by its own inertia.[47] Additional muscular forces are required during fast walking and traversing on surfaces such as uneven terrain, inclines, or stairs. Throughout the stance phase, muscles work to provide weight acceptance, limb stabilization, energy absorption, and propulsion of the limb into swing phase. In this section, we will look at muscle activity as it provides these functions within each phase of gait.

Initial Contact

During initial contact the limb is positioned to accept weight. The tibialis anterior and gastrocnemius-soleus muscles cocontract to maintain a stable neutral ankle. The hamstring muscles, having been activated during the last half of swing phase, exert a deceleration force to slow the knee as the limb prepares to land. The quadriceps muscles are firing to cocontract with the hamstrings to prepare and position the knee for landing. Although the hip is in flexion at initial contact, it is actively stabilized by the gluteus medius and maximus muscles.

Loading Response

Loading response provides a smooth transition from nonweight-bearing to weight-bearing. Deceleration of the limb occurs during this phase which immediately follows initial contact. Because there is a rapid change from nonweight-bearing to weight-bearing, stabilizers are also recruited to make the transition secure. Since the primary activity of muscles at this time is deceleration, most muscles function eccentrically. The tibialis anterior works eccentrically to control the rate at which the foot is lowered to the floor. As the knee moves into some flexion, shock absorption and weight acceptance at the knee occur with eccentric control of the quadriceps with slight cocontraction assistance from the hamstrings. Gluteus maximus muscle activity increases to provide hip stabilization during loading response as the body weight transfers onto the limb. Activity of the gluteus maximus also prevents the trunk from flexing.

Midstance

Since midstance is the time of single limb stance, it is the most precarious phase of stance, requiring significant effort of the calf and hip muscle groups. Stability is the primary requirement during this phase. The gastrocnemius and soleus maintain the ankle in a stable upright position during midstance. Although the quadriceps is fairly inactive at this time, knee control is provided by the gastrocnemius as it restrains forward movement of the tibia on the femur, thereby providing stable stance at the knee. The hip abductor muscles—especially the gluteus medius, gluteus minimus, and TFL—work in concert to stabilize the pelvis in the frontal plane during this time of unilateral support. Hip adductors also play a role, cocontracting with the abductors to aide in stabilizing the hip to maintain the COM over the single support limb.

Terminal Stance and Preswing

Force generation occurs in preparation for forward-limb propulsion in terminal stance. This force generation occurs primarily through concentric muscle activity. Most of this force is supplied by the gastrocnemius muscle, plantarflexing the ankle as the heel rises off of the floor. Propulsion force continues during preswing with additional contributions from the soleus, hip adductors, and iliopsoas.[48] In these two phases of stance, knee flexion results passively from the combined motions of hip flexion and ankle plantarflexion.

Swing Phases

Throughout the swing phase, muscles work to control momentum, advance the limb, and prepare the limb for stance. There are fewer muscles working during the swing phase than the stance phase. During the first half of the swing phase, the working muscles are primarily functioning as accelerators; in the last half of swing, muscles decelerate to slow the limb as it prepares to make contact with the ground. The iliopsoas and rectus femoris at the hip and tibialis anterior at the ankle contract concentrically during initial swing and midswing to flex the hip and dorsiflex the ankle, respectively, to clear the floor without stubbing the toe. Forward acceleration of the extremity during initial swing is also the responsibility of the iliopsoas and rectus femoris. Maximum knee flexion occurs by midswing to effectively clear the limb from the floor, but this motion is largely accomplished through pendular momentum rather than by active muscular contraction. By midswing, the iliopsoas and rectus femoris are inactive since their earlier activity provides a swinging momentum to continue forward motion of the limb. After midswing, the gluteus maximus and hamstrings fire eccentrically to decelerate the forward motion at the hip and knee. In terminal swing, the quadriceps also fires, working with the hamstrings to prepare the knee for weight acceptance as well as to lengthen the step. The tibialis anterior maintains a stable ankle position of neutral dorsiflexion in preparation for floor contact. Table 12–2 summarizes these functional requirements of gait, phase by phase.[24]

Function	Muscles	Gait Phase
Shock absorbers (Eccentric activity)	Quadriceps Dorsiflexors	Initial contact Loading
Stabilizers (Isometric activity)	Gluteus maximus, gluteus medius, and gluteus minimus Tensor fascia lata Erector spinae Ankle everters Tibialis posterior	Stance
Propulsion (Concentric activity)	Gastrocnemius Toe flexors and Soleus	Terminal stance Preswing
Accelerators (Concentric activity)	Adductor longus and magnus Sartorius Iliopsoas Rectus femoris	Preswing Initial swing
Foot control (Isometric activity)	Tibialis anterior	Swing
Decelerators (Eccentric activity)	Hamstrings Dorsiflexors	Terminal swing to Initial contact

Identification of Muscular Activation Patterns by Body Segment

This section approaches muscle activity from a segmental perspective rather than by gait cycles as the previous section did. The information here also expands on the activity summaries of the previous section. Efficient gait requires activation of muscles within specific phases of the gait cycle. It may be surprising to realize that gait requires activation of more than just the lower extremity muscles. Identifying the contributions of the upper extremities, trunk, and lower extremities is included in this section.

Upper Extremity Muscles

Although a lot of analysis and investigation exists of the lower extremities in ambulation, significantly less information is available on upper extremity activity during gait.[49, 50] Once thought to be a passive ballistic movement produced by lower extremity and trunk motions, reciprocal motion of the arms is now realized to be under muscular control.[51] Arm swing contributes to gait by assisting in stabilizing the body and reducing the lateral motion of the body's COM.[52] Electromyographic studies of the arms of unimpaired adults demonstrate moderate activity in the posterior and middle deltoid, beginning slightly before the arm starts its backward swing and continues through completion of the backward swing; no activity of the shoulder flexors occurs when the shoulder and elbow are flexing.[51, 53] Although the latissimus dorsi and teres major are active as shoulder extensors, forward arm swing at low walking speeds is the result of passive joint structures reacting to stretch during shoulder extension motion and gravity. With increased walking speeds, slight to moderate activity of the triceps brachii occurs. The posterior muscles accelerate the backward swing and decelerate the forward swing.

Trunk Muscles

The transversospinal, erector spinae, and quadratus lumborum muscles are active during the gait cycle especially initial contact.[20, 36, 51, 53] These muscles counterbalance the trunk flexion torque that occurs during

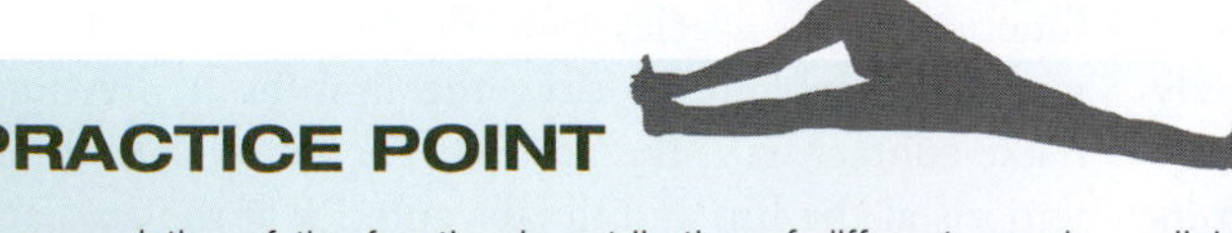

PRACTICE POINT

An appreciation of the functional contribution of different muscle groups to walking tasks offers an immediate translation into the clinical dilemmas encountered by patients with an impairment affecting those muscles or that functional task.

deceleration as the foot contacts the ground.[54] Electromyographic activity recorded in the rectus abdominis, external abdominal oblique, and internal abdominal oblique muscles is variable and appears to be dependent on walking speed. As walking speed increases, a consistently increasing recruitment of abdominal musculature throughout the gait cycle occurs.[20, 55, 56] The internal and external obliques demonstrate continuous, low phasic activity at terminal swing during both comfortable and fast walking speeds.[20]

One of the functions of the trunk muscles is to minimize head movement as the body changes from acceleration to deceleration throughout gait. Keeping the head motion minimal provides a stable platform for the eyes to maintain reliable vision during body motion.[57] The pelvis also assists in this function as it moves up and down, shifts side to side, tilts anteriorly and posteriorly, and rotates to each side as it smoothes excursions of the COM in all planes during gait. How well the pelvis accomplishes this goal is realized by the fact that although the HAT makes up 60% of the body weight, the average trunk angle in the sagittal plane varies only 2° to 5° over the course of one stride.[57, 58]

Lower Extremity Muscles

The upper extremity and trunk muscles provide important contributions to an efficient system of ambulation. The lower extremity muscles, however, provide the lion's share of effort that propels individuals from one location to another. Each segment works with the others to make gait efficient. Timing of muscle activity with periods of activity followed by periods of rest throughout the gait cycle permit persons to ambulate for long distances without fatigue. When these timing sequences are dysfunctional, gait requires greater effort and increased energy expenditure.

HIP FLEXORS

The primary hip flexors—the iliopsoas, rectus femoris, sartorius, and tensor fasciae latae—are active from late stance through the early part of swing. These muscles move the hip from maximum extension which occurs at terminal stance into flexion as the limb begins to move forward of the trunk. This muscle activity advances the limb forward as it lifts the limb to clear the foot from the floor.[20, 30, 57–59]

HIP EXTENSORS

The gluteus maximus, hamstrings, and posterior portion of the adductor magnus begin working eccentrically in terminal swing to decelerate the limb. These muscles continue firing during initial contact and loading response but switch to a concentric contraction to extend the hip and keep the trunk upright on the weight-bearing limb. The gluteus maximus is most active during loading response. Through its attachment on the iliotibial tract, the gluteus maximus also contributes to hip adduction deceleration, providing limb stabilization during early stance.[20]

HIP ABDUCTORS

The gluteus medius and minimus and tensor fasciae latae stabilize the pelvis in the frontal plane during unilateral stance. Gluteus medius activity begins during terminal swing and rises sharply to peak at midstance when the extremity is in unilateral stance; the gluteus medius exerts its force to minimize the drop of the contralateral pelvis in the frontal plane. During midstance, the weight-bearing hip adducts about 5°, and the gluteus medius contracts to limit the contralateral pelvic drop that results from this hip adduction. The muscle becomes inactive at terminal stance once the heel leaves the ground and both limbs share the body weight's load.

The tensor fasciae lata is composed of anteromedial and posterolateral fibers that are independently active and have different functions.[59] The posterolateral fibers become active at initial contact, whereas the anteromedial fibers are relatively inactive at this time. It has been suggested that the posterolateral fibers stabilize the

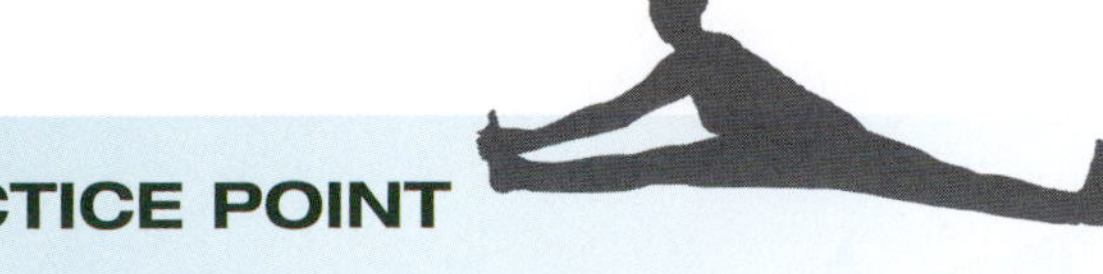

PRACTICE POINT

With profound hip extensor weakness, a gait deviation known as a *backward lurch* is likely to occur. At initial contact, the person leans the trunk backward at the hip, to place the COM posteriorly to the hip joint; such a move prevents the trunk from falling forward. This compensation relieves the deficient hip extensors of their responsibility of holding the trunk upright and uses passive tension of the strong iliofemoral ligament to stabilize the trunk as the limb accepts the body's weight. An alternative compensation in cases of less significant hip extensor weakness is a forward lean of the trunk at initial contact and loading response; in these cases, the hip extensors are functioning but have inadequate strength to maintain the proper trunk alignment.

iliotibial band against the contraction of the gluteus maximus at initial contact.[30] With increased walking speeds, the anteromedial fibers become active in initial swing, contributing to hip flexion and medial rotation.[30]

HIP ADDUCTORS

The adductors have two peaks of activity that occur in early and late stance. They cocontract with the gluteus maximus and the abductors, lending support to frontal plane pelvic and hip stability. Their early peak activity is almost synchronous with the peaks of the quadriceps, hamstrings, abductors, and gluteus maximus when deceleration and transfer of body weight occur.

Looking at some of the adductor muscles individually, we see some individual functional and timing differences. The adductor magnus is active in early stance, performing its role as a hip extensor; the adductor longus is most active in late stance; and the gracilis' primary activity occurs in initial swing.[20, 60] Individual interpretation of the function of each of the adductors in gait is difficult because their leverage changes throughout the limb's range of motion and the multiple actions these muscles produce. Because this group is a large muscle mass that can exert significant force, their role is more important in more vigorous activities such as running, jumping, climbing, and skiing.

KNEE EXTENSORS

Although the quadriceps is primarily active during stance, it also contracts during the late swing phase. In terminal swing, the quadriceps initiates activity to prepare the limb for contact. From initial contact and through the first 15% of the stance phase when the knee reaches about 15° of flexion, eccentric quadriceps activity is most evident.[20] This eccentric activity provides shock absorption to reduce impact forces occurring with ground contact, controls the rate of flexion during early stance, and maintains control of a slightly flexed knee so the knee does not buckle.[20] Following this knee flexion, knee extension occurs passively secondary to biomechanical changes in the hip and ankle joints. Additionally, since the body's COM remains anterior to the knee joint after this hip and ankle motion, active knee control is not necessary from midstance through midswing.

The quadriceps activity recorded in preswing is primarily the rectus femoris acting at the hip to assist in hip flexion. The knee motion occurring during early swing and midswing is produced by momentum rather than from muscle activity.

KNEE FLEXORS

Hamstring activity begins in late midswing before the quadriceps initiates its activity and peaks at initial contact. Hamstring activity during swing is eccentric at both the knee and hip; during the latter half of swing, the knee extends up to 70° as the hip flexes 25° to 35°.[20] This hamstring activity decelerates motions of hip flexion and the rapidly swinging leg. During initial contact, the hamstrings assists the gluteus maximus in maintaining hip extension.[30] Hamstring activity ceases by the time of loading response and remains relaxed throughout the remainder of the stance phase and in the swing phase during initial swing and midswing.[61]

ANKLE DORSIFLEXORS

The tibialis anterior, assisted by the extensor hallucis longus and extensor digitorum longus, is isometrically active throughout the swing phase to hold the ankle and toes in neutral so they clear the floor. Peak activity in this group occurs in stance phase just after initial contact. These muscles contract eccentrically during loading response to control the rate at which the foot lowers to the ground. This activity also provides shock absorption. Additionally, the tibialis anterior, which has distal attachments on the medial cuneiform and the first metatarsal, decelerating foot pronation during loading response.

ANKLE PLANTARFLEXORS

Gastrocnemius and soleus activity begins at loading response, becoming progressively greater throughout the rest of the stance phase until the last third of stance when they reach their peak output. Until the body's COM moves anterior to the ankle in

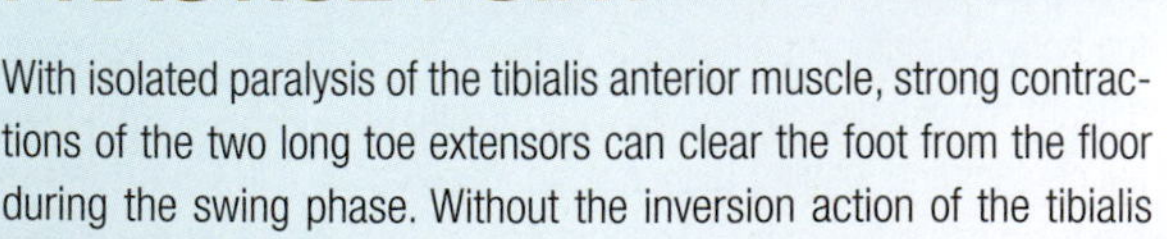

PRACTICE POINT

With isolated paralysis of the tibialis anterior muscle, strong contractions of the two long toe extensors can clear the foot from the floor during the swing phase. Without the inversion action of the tibialis anterior, however, the subtalar joint will evert. If the deep peroneal nerve to the anterior leg is paralyzed, foot clearance from the floor occurs by excessive hip flexion during swing and is followed by a characteristic foot slap during loading response since the ankle and foot lack eccentric control after initial contact.

midstance, calf muscle activity is primarily eccentric, providing control for smooth progression of the tibia over the foot. During initial contact and loading response, the soleus works at the ankle as the gastrocnemius functions to assist knee control. From loading response to midstance, the tibia advances rapidly into dorsiflexion as the knee continues to flex, requiring considerable effort from both the gastrocnemius and quadriceps muscles for a smooth motion. Peak activity of the gastrocnemius and soleus muscles occurs just after terminal stance when the heel lifts off the ground. Although controversial, some investigators indicate that the function of the gastrocnemius and soleus is to provide a burst of force to push off the limb from the floor and propel the body forward.[62] On the other hand, others specify that heel lift occurring during terminal stance places the body weight on the balls of the feet, requiring increased output of the gastrocsoleus as more effort is required to be on the toes; these investigators specify that actual forward advancement of the COM occurs from a combination of inertia and a rolling off the foot rather than a propulsion from the gastrocnemius and soleus.[20]

Although classified as plantarflexors, the tibialis posterior, flexor digitorum longus, and flexor hallucis longus contribute little in that role because of their small size and poor leverage, generating only about 10% of the plantarflexion torque of the soleus.[20] However, they have important activity at the tarsal joints and toes. The tibialis posterior has two peaks of activity, in early stance during loading response and towards the end of stance just after the heel leaves the ground. The tibialis posterior is inactive throughout the swing phase.[20,63] It acts eccentrically in loading response to provide a smooth midfoot deceleration into pronation and adjusts the foot to the ground's contour. From midstance to preswing, the tibialis posterior concentrically contracts to supinate the foot and thereby stabilize the tarsal joints. The flexor digitorum longus and the flexor hallucis longus activate after loading response, peak in terminal stance, and are then inactive throughout the swing phase. These long toe flexor muscles support the longitudinal arch as it flattens and elevates in pronation and supination, respectively, and help to stabilize the toes on the ground.

PERONEALS

The peroneus brevis and longus demonstrate phasic activity similar to the gastrocnemius-soleus muscles with contraction beginning early in the stance phase after loading response and peaking after terminal stance when body weight is on the metatarsal heads and toes.[30] These muscles, along with the tibialis posterior, provide control of the tarsal joints and the arches of the foot; this control allows foot adjustment to the ground's contour and mediolateral ankle stability. With its distal attachments on the plantar surface of the foot, the peroneus longus is the main muscular support of the three foot arches and stabilizes the first metatarsal head on the ground to convert it a rigid lever during the final moments of stance once the heel is off the ground.[60]

INTRINSIC MUSCLES OF THE FOOT

The intrinsic muscles of the foot (abductor digiti minimi, abductor hallucis, extensor digiti brevis, flexor digitorum brevis, flexor hallucis brevis, and interossei) demonstrate activity during the last half of the stance phase with no activity during swing or stance prior to midstance.[64] Intrinsic activity occurs when the flexible foot transitions to a rigid lever. The plantar intrinsic muscles and the extrinsic toe flexors supplement the plantar fascia in this function.

Gait Analysis

Gait is analyzed from two different perspectives: research and clinical. Before clinicians could compare their patient's ambulation to "normal" gait, research had to identify aspects of gait that could be used for this reference of comparison. Knowing what is typical allows the clinician to identify pathological gait. In this section, we provide you with a little history of that science and evolution of gait analysis. We feel this information is important since it will expand the depth and breadth of your understanding of gait analysis. At the end of this section, clinical applications are described to guide you through a systematic gait analysis.

Advances in Laboratory Gait Analysis

Gait analysis has evolved and developed as scientific knowledge and available technology have developed and improved over time. Although Giovanni Borelli, (1608–1679), a Renaissance Italian physiologist, physicist, and mathematician, and Aristotle (384–322 BC), a Greek philosopher long before Borelli, theorized about the manner in which humans walked, technology was not yet available to either man to offer any significant recordable measurement. However, their drawings and mathematical equations are still insightful and basically correct. It wasn't until the late 1800s, about 200 years after Borelli, that enough advances in photographic technology allowed for initial development of measurement technology. These early steps were pioneered in 1836 by the Weber brothers in Germany (Wilhelm Eduard Weber, 1804–1891 and Ernst Heinrich Weber, 1795–1878), Étienne-Jules Marey in Paris (1830–1904), and Eadweard Muybridge in America (1830–1904). Marey, an eminent French physiologist, recorded locomotion photographically beginning in 1890 with methods that eventually led to the development of motion pictures and the film industry. Marey's method consisted of making a series of exposures of a moving subject on a photographic plate. By means of a rotating shutter, exposures were made at 0.1 second intervals. Because superimposition of several pictures on one another gave a confused record, "geometric chronophotography" evolved. For this process, the subject was dressed in black. Brilliant metal buttons and shining bands were attached to the clothing to represent joints and bony segments (Fig. 12.9A). The subject was photographed as he or she walked in front of a black screen. Only the dots and lines appeared on the photographic plate because the rest of the body did not show against the black background (Fig. 12.9B).[65] In 1887, Muybridge published remarkable photographs of humans walking, running, jumping, climbing, and lifting; gait patterns of over 30 animals; and flight sequences of birds (Fig. 12.10). He used 48 electrophotographic cameras arranged in three batteries that made simultaneous lateral, anterior-posterior, and oblique exposures of the moving subject using camera speeds ranging up to 1/6000 of a second. Over 4,000 photographs of his work on humans and 4,000 photos of birds and animals have since been reprinted.[66, 67]

Because of the results of his brilliant photography, Eadweard Muybridge is considered to be the father of modern gait analysis. An interesting story illustrates how the techniques he developed for use in photography were then adapted for application to the study of human motion. Muybridge was hired by his friend, Leland Stanford to settle a dispute. Stanford, an industrialist and enthusiastic racehorse owner, was the founder of Stanford University. He insisted that there is a moment in a racehorse's gait when all four feet are off the ground. His friends and associates vehemently disagreed and a huge dispute ensued. Stanford hired Muybridge to help prove his assertion and settle what actually became a national debate and a friendly but rather steep monetary wager. Muybridge came up with a way to record the motion of Stanford's racehorse,

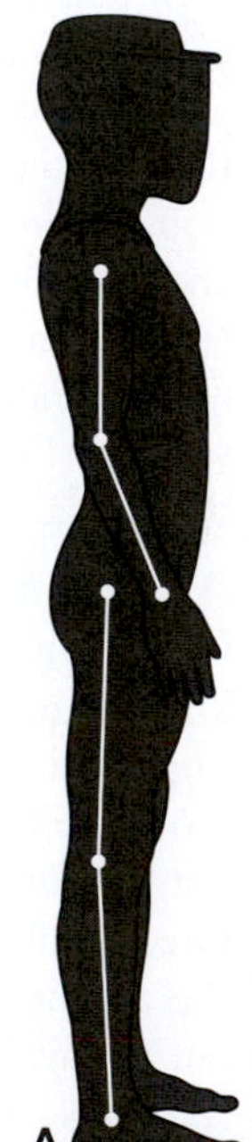

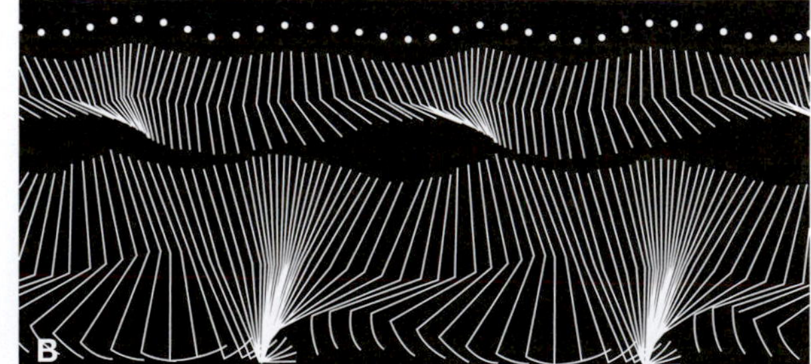

Figure 12.9 A) Artist depiction of the type of black suit worn by subjects in early chronophotography. The silver buttons and bands allowed easier identification of motion. B) As the subject moved in front of a black screen, pictures were taken using a rotating shutter with exposures taken at 0.1 second intervals.

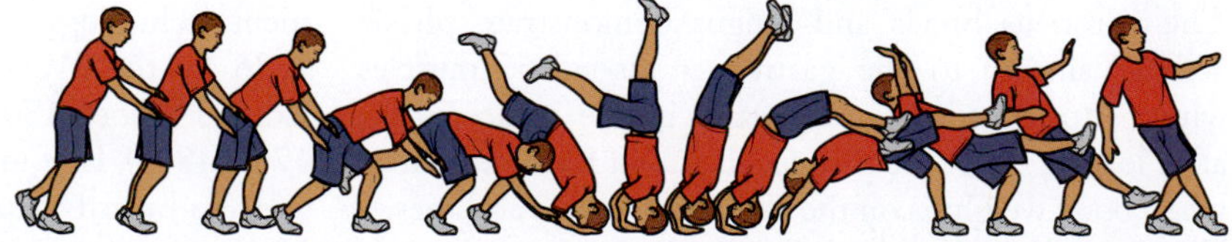

Figure 12.10 Artist depiction of the type of result created by use of early geometric chronophotography, similar to an image created by Marey known as the "pole vaulter" in 1883.

using multiple cameras, photographic emulsions, and trip wires to track and record the motions of all four of the racehorse's limbs during instants in time. He proved Stanford to be right, and modern day gait analysis was born out of his photographic ingenuity. His success was the beginning of not only modern motion analysis, but the motion picture industry as well.[68–70]

In the early 1900s, a German mathematician, Otto Fischer, together with Wilhelm Braune, an anatomist, calculated the trajectories, velocities, accelerations, forces, and torques of joints and segments of the body in 31 phases of the gait cycle to establish the scientific basis of the kinematics and kinetics of human gait. Among their many findings were calculations proving that the swinging leg was not only a pendular motion (as was the thinking up until this time) but a motion that required muscle forces for movement. Although this monumental work was originally published between 1890 and 1907, it is still cited in the literature.[71–73]

Major developments in gait analysis using three-dimensional motion analysis occurred after World War II with advances pioneered by Dr. Vern Inman, a professor of orthopedics at the University of California at Berkley, and later by his two residents, Dr. Jacquelin Perry and Dr. David Sutherland. The literature abounds with articles, books, and contributions from these three world-renowned rehabilitation scientists.

Early 20th century equipment included automated video-computerized digital systems recording the position of reflective markers placed on segments and joint centers of the body.[74] Two or more cameras were needed to record the three planes, and marker placement required great precision for accurate results. Multiple problems occurred due to difficulty in identifying landmarks, obesity, skin motion, and resolution difficulties because of short distances between markers.[20] Electrogoniometry later emerged as a technique to allow for continuous recording of joint motion, and triaxial parallelogram goniometers were developed for recording joint motion in three planes.[20] Advances in technology in the latter half of the 20th century allowed for the integration of cinematography with EMG and force plate data and the digitization of all of this data into what has now become known as a *motion analysis system* (Fig. 12.11).

Currently, modern gait analysis includes several components, available in a broad range of complexity and expense. The basic components of current clinical laboratory gait analysis usually consist of five key elements: videotape examination, measurement of general temporal and spatial gait parameters, kinematic analysis, kinetic measurement, and kinesiological EMG (KEMG). The kinematic analysis component requires the use of external markers that are representative of the joint centers so that angular kinematics can be measured and studied by a three-dimensional motion analysis system. There are more than thirty motion analysis systems in existence today, such as the Vicon System (VICON 512 System, Oxford, UK) or the Peak Performance System (Peak Performance Technologies, Englewood, CO). The kinetic analysis component employs the use of force plates to determine ground reaction force while EMG (specifically KEMG) records phasic muscle activity. All of this information is combined with anthropometric data such as limb length and girth, and interactive software then produces a detailed analysis.[68, 75, 76] For a detailed discussion of motion analysis, you are referred to other sources.[69, 75, 77–82] As technology continues to develop, ongoing advances will continue to improve human movement analysis methods, including gait. It is anticipated that video-based kinematic tools will become more readily available and increasingly useful in clinical settings.[77,81] One example of emerging technology is telerehabilitation software that captures video sequences of a person walking directly from a videoconferencing link, permitting online gait evaluation from a remote site.[78] It is also likely that three-dimensional video gait analysis will be commonly used in the near future.

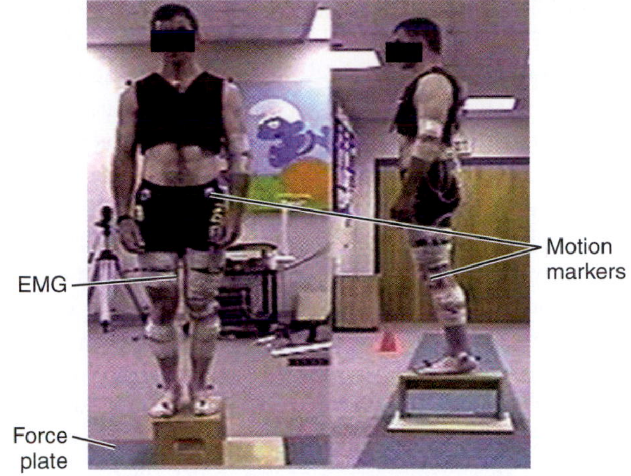

Figure 12.11 Example of a Motion Analysis System.

Observational Gait Analysis in the Clinic Setting

Although research laboratories have sophisticated equipment and technology to analyze gait, the cost of such equipment and technology is usually prohibitive in a clinical setting. Gait is routinely analyzed in clinical settings through systematic and methodical visual observations by the clinician. Basic to performing gait analysis is the clinician's appreciation of the components of gait and the timing, requirements, and functions of those components. Such an appreciation guides the clinician so that the observation, analysis, and subsequent treatment/intervention can be effective, accurate, and meaningful.

Analysis of an individual's gait is performed by carefully assessing the elements within each subphase of gait. Careful observation and analysis of one joint at a time and one motion at a time reveals impairments and allows logical advancement to a clinical management plan.

Gait analysis requires a global and a specific investigation. The global investigation involves overall observations. These general observations allow the clinician to obtain an initial impression of the individual's gait and includes assessment of stride length, stride width, cadence, arm swing, head and trunk alignment, and muscle atrophy or asymmetry. The specific investigation of gait analysis may occur one of two ways—either by joint assessment or by gait subphase assessment. In other words, the clinician may choose to focus on one joint throughout the gait cycle and then move on to another joint, or the clinician may wish to observe what each joint does at initial contact and then observe each joint at loading response and so forth throughout the entire gait cycle. Either method produces the same end results: identification of gait deviations. These findings are then followed by tests to confirm specific deficiencies observed during gait assessment. Table 12–4 provides an example of an observational gait analysis strategy.

TABLE 12–4 | OBSERVATIONAL GAIT ANALYSIS[24]

Body Segment	Guiding Questions
Sagittal Plane Analysis: Perform by viewing both right and left sides.	
Head, Trunk, and Arms	Does the head maintain an erect posture in a neutral position? Do the UEs swing rhythmically with the opposite LEs? Does the trunk rotate forward and backward with the swinging arm? Is there any excessive lean of the trunk either forward or backward, especially during early stance phase when weight is accepted?
Pelvis and Hips	Does the pelvis rotate forward on the swinging side and backward with the stance side? As weight is accepted over the stance limb, does the hip continue to extend in support of the limb and in preparation for stability and then propulsion? During swing, does the hip flex smoothly forward in preparation for initial contact?
Knees	Is movement of the knee smooth or jerky as it moves through flexion, extension, and then flexion again during stance? Does the knee appear to be stable as it accepts and loads weight? During swing, does the knee flex adequately for limb clearance?
Feet and Ankles	What does initial contact look like? Is it onto a heel strike or a foot flat? Is it quiet? During swing, does the foot dorsiflex adequately so that the foot clears the floor?
Frontal Plane Analysis: Perform by viewing both an anterior and posterior view.	
Head and Trunk	Does the head face the frontal plane in the midline? Is the trunk aligned in the midline from the fontal plane or is there any obvious asymmetry? Are the shoulder girdles retracted or protracted, elevated or depressed? Are the elbows relaxed or flexed?
Pelvis and Hips	Does the pelvis tilt down only slightly on the swinging side? Does there appear to be any excessive vertical displacement of the pelvis or hip? Is there excessive hip abduction or adduction? Does hip extension stability appear to be adequate for weight acceptance and then propulsion? During swing, what does the path of the limb look like? Is there any excessive medial or lateral rotation, or any sign of circumduction?
Knees	Is there any sign of excessive varus or valgus at the knees? Do the patellae face forward during the stance phase?
Feet and Ankles	Does the foot and ankle complex appear to be stable during weight-bearing? Is normal foot alignment maintained or is it positioned in excessive or prolonged supination or pronation? What is the stance width between the right and left feet? From a posterior view, do you see the same number of toes lateral to each foot?

Summarize your findings.
Reprinted with permission: Bertoti DB. *Functional Neurorehabilitation through the Life Span.* Philadelphia: FA Davis Company, 2004.

An ideal method of gait analysis is the use of a video camera that allows changes in film speed. Slowing the film may provide the clinician with opportunities to observe motions that occur rapidly during the gait cycle. During a normal gait speed of once cycle per second, the leg swings through at the rate of 20 to 30 mph. Additionally, the rapid changes from neutral to plantarflexion to dorsiflexion and to plantarflexion within about 0.6 of a second make it difficult to visualize movements. Since treadmill walking and overground walking reveal similar gait patterns,[83, 84] using a treadmill may allow sufficient gait analysis if video equipment is unavailable. If neither of these options is available, the clinician may have to resort to repetitive trips of the individual within a 10–15 foot runway as a way of observing his or her gait. Regardless of the technique used to obtain gait analysis, the clinician's systematic acquisition of first global and then specific information holds true.

Developmental Aspects of Gait: Life Span Changes

Although gait is not something we have to think about to perform, it is an extremely complex function. The mere fact that it took us several years before we were able to move from standing unsteadily as a 1-year-old to walking maturely as a 7-year-old and that it is one of the most frequent causes of falls in older individuals tells us that walking is no easy task. The changes that occur in ambulation as we age are presented here.

Immature Walking

The gait pattern of children (Fig. 12.12A) is very different from that of a mature adult (Fig. 12.12B). The average age of independent walking typically ranges from 11 to 15 months of age.[82] Children have a wide-based gait, with stepping initiated primarily at the hips while the knees remain fairly stiff. Initial contact is typically made with the entire foot with marked lateral rotation at the hip. Steps are short with an exaggerated time of double support compared to adults. When children first begin walking, the upper extremities are essential for balance. Several investigators[85–88] have identified an immature gait pattern in all children up until age 3, which includes these characteristics:

1. Uneven step length.
2. Swing phase includes excessive hip and knee flexion, hip abduction, and lateral rotation.
3. Stance phase includes initial contact with foot flat rather than with heel contact, knee hyperextension throughout stance, loading response and midstance weight-bearing onto a pronated foot.
4. Base of support is wider than the lateral dimensions of the trunk.
5. Upper extremities in a high-, medium-, and then low-guard position (Fig. 12.12A). The transition from high **on-guard position** to a beginning **reciprocal arm swing** starts to occur 4–5 months after the onset of walking.
6. Lack of pelvic mobility such as tilt or rotation.
7. Stride length is reduced and cadence is increased.[21, 24, 46]

In order to increase speed as needed, a child must increase cadence, since stride length is limited by leg length and limited pelvic mobility. By about 2 years of age, initial contact now occurs at the heel and the first wave of knee flexion in stance appears, the arms are lower, most toddlers at this age show reciprocal arm swing, lateral rotation of the hips decreases, and the base of support narrows. Motions at the joints resemble the adult pattern by age 3 and mature patterns are well established by the age of 7. Table 12–5 highlights the main functional gait changes that occur during childhood.

Mature Walking

According to Gage,[69] there are five major attributes of normal mature gait:

1. Stability in stance.
2. Sufficient foot clearance in swing.
3. Appropriate prepositioning of the foot during swing for initial contact.
4. Adequate step length.
5. Efficient energy expenditure.

It is important to appreciate that these mature attributes do not magically appear, but rather develop over the course of several years, beginning with the first movements in infancy, changing through the early toddler years, and finally culminating in the demonstration of a mature adult walking pattern by age 7. The development of mature gait with these attributes is very dependent on first having normal gait prerequisites: adequate motor control and CNS maturation (which implies an intact neurologic system), adequate ROM, strength, appropriate bone structure and composition, and intact sensation.[24] In addition to Gage's attributes, Burnett and Johnson[85, 86] identify key components necessary for mature gait:

1. Pelvic tilt and rotation.
2. Initial contact with a heel strike.
3. Knee flexion at midstance.
4. A mature relationship between mechanisms at the hip, knee, and ankle.
5. A mature base of support.
6. Reciprocal arm swing (Fig. 12.12B).

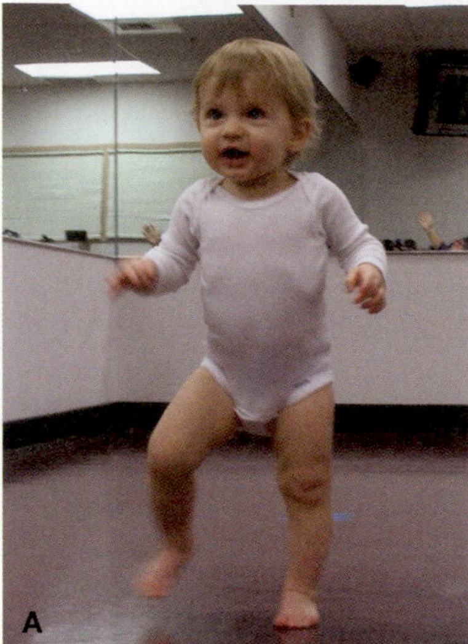

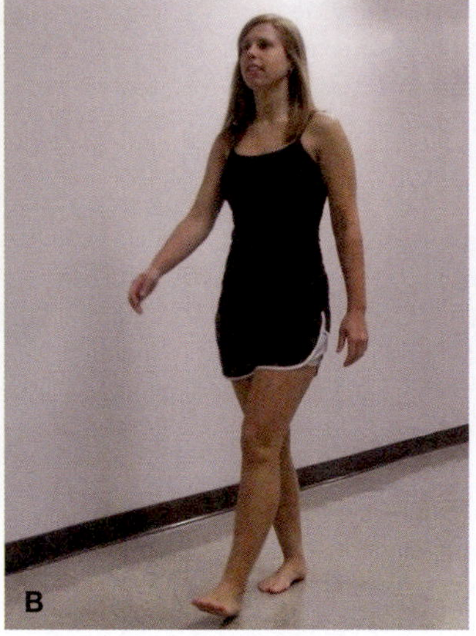

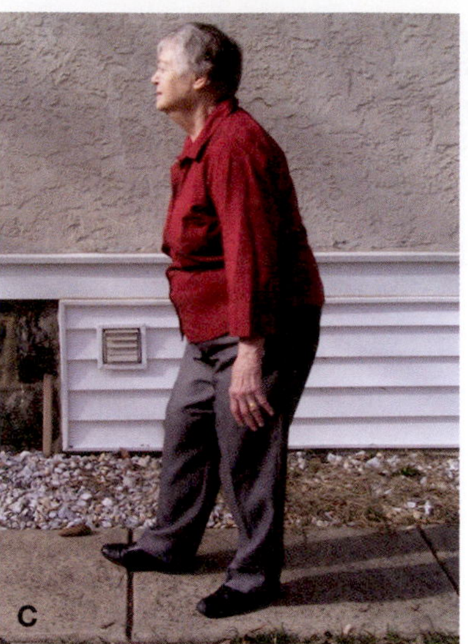

Figure 12.12 Gait as it changes over the life span. A) Gait during early childhood. B) Typical adult gait. C) Gait in an older adult.

TABLE 12-5 | GAIT CHANGES OVER THE LIFE SPAN[28, 70, 85-87, 89, 91, 151–161]

Age	Gait Changes
18 months	Heel strike emerges as point of initial contact
	Reciprocal arm swing emerging
	Most children can voluntarily increase walking speed for functional goal
2 years	Knee flexion more consistently present during stance
3 years	Gait pattern maturing: all adult components present except for increased cadence and decreased step length
	Running (with a non support phase) is emerging
42 months	BOS equal to or less than pelvic span
4 years	Reciprocal arm swing firmly established
6–7 years	Mature gait pattern
	Stride length will continue to increase as function of increasing leg length
Mature adult gait	Pelvic tilt and rotation
	Initial contact with a heel strike
	Slight knee flexion at midstance
	A mature relationship between mechanisms at the hip, knee, and ankle
	A mature base of support
	Reciprocal arm swing
	Refined muscle activation patterns
	Optimal energy efficiency
Older Adult (60–80)	Decreased velocity and slower cadence
	Decreased step and stride length
	Increased stride width and BOS
	Increased time in stance phase and in double support
	Decreased arm swing
	Decreased hip, knee, and ankle flexion
	Increased incidence of foot flat on initial contact
	Decreased dynamic stability during stance
	Re-emergence of muscular coactivation patterns

Reprinted with permission: Bertoti DB. *Functional Neurorehabilitation through the Life Span.* Philadelphia; FA Davis Company, 2004.

Free-walking velocity increases with age until adolescence, then plateaus until senescence. With maturity, muscle activation patterns become more refined and energy efficiency improves. Table 12–5 summarizes the characteristics of a mature adult gait pattern.

Gait Changes in the Older Adult

Balance ability, changes in leg muscle strength, flexibility and range of motion, and sensory information alter gait characteristics of older adults. Cognitive factors may also be an important contributor to alterations in gait.[24] Healthy older adults walk slower with shorter strides and shorter step lengths than young adults. Anticipatory locomotor abilities also change with age as older adults take more time to monitor the visual environment and step more cautiously to avoid obstacles.[89]

The gait characteristics of the very young and the very old have several similarities. Both show a shorter duration of single limb stance and an increase in support time. In both groups, this has been interpreted as an indication of balance deficiencies.[88, 90, 91] The gait of young walkers has a wide base of support as required for balance, a characteristic of the elderly as well. The muscular activation patterns in young children and older adults show coactivation of agonist and antagonist muscle groups during gait. This may be an adaptive mechanism to increase muscle stiffness, which helps with balance control.[92, 93]

Gait characteristics common to older adults include a wider base of support, decreased reciprocal arm swing, and slower cadence (Fig. 12.12C). Stride length decreases and time in double support increases. These gait changes are due to a combination of musculoskeletal age-related changes and a decline in the neurosensory system. Gait adaptations in the older adult may be associated with a general decrease in muscle strength due to loss of motor neurons, muscle fibers, and aerobic capacity.[94] Research indicates that the changes seen in locomotor patterns of aging adults is most commonly characterized by a decreased step length and increased time spent in double support.[95] In older adults, there is evidence of a return to agonist and antagonist coactivation patterns, as originally seen in toddlers. This coactivation pattern may be an adaptive strategy to compensate for decreased postural control and balance deficits.[93]

Gait changes in older adults compared to those under the age of 60 are highlighted in Table 12–5 and summarized as follows:

Temporal Characteristics

1. Decreased velocity
2. Increased time in stance phase
3. Increased time in double support
4. Decreased time in swing phase

Spatial Characteristics

1. Decreased step length
2. Decreased stride length
3. Increased stride width

Kinematic Changes

1. Decreased vertical movement of the center of gravity
2. Decreased arm swing
3. Decreased hip, knee, and ankle flexion
4. Increased incidence of foot flat on initial contact
5. Decreased dynamic stability during stance

Investigations on gait of senior citizens have failed thus far to present a clear-cut picture of the time of age changes because of the many other variables affecting gait (i.e., speed, leg length), the difficulty of excluding individuals with pathologies affecting gait, and differing research methodologies. Slight changes start to appear in some subjects after 60 to 65 years of age, but there is variability among and between individuals.

Gait Efficiency

Gait efficiency includes both the mechanics of walking as well as the energy expenditure required to walk. The body provides any number of adjustments in how it propels itself from one location to another, and the efficiency with which it performs this activity is dependent upon several factors. These factors include joint function, muscle strength, neurological control, and energy sources. Although energy expenditure is briefly mentioned here, since this is a kinesiology and not a physiology text, the focus on this section regards the mechanical efficiency of walking.

Determinants of Gait

Saunders, Inman, and Eberhart[37] first described six major features, called "determinants of gait," that were theorized to minimize energy expenditure during walking by reducing displacement of the center of gravity and abrupt changes in its direction. Although recent advances in biomechanical analysis have led to the abandonment of crediting these factors as "determinants" in minimizing energy expenditure,[96–98] they continue to be helpful in identifying how the body's biomechanical functions are synchronized during gait.[96, 99] These factors demonstrate how cooperatively the trunk, pelvis, and lower extremities work together throughout the gait cycle.[100] In alignment with the current literature, we present the list of specific determinants of

Saunders and associates to demonstrate this cooperativeness of the body segments during gait.

Pelvis and Hip Determinants

The pelvis maintains its relative stability in the frontal plane by the action of the erector spine on the swing leg side coupled with the action of the gluteus medius on the stance side to effectively minimize pelvic lateral tilt in the frontal plane. This muscular effort minimizes the rise of the COM by providing a downward tilt of the pelvis of approximately 5° on the swing side.

In addition to this frontal plane motion of the pelvis is its transverse plane motion of approximately 8°. This vertical axis of rotation provides crucial pelvic and limb movement during gait. Specifically, this transverse rotation moves the pelvis on the swing side forward, making the limb segment effectively longer and thereby preventing the COM from dropping as the heel moves to the ground. Likewise, the pelvis's backward rotation on the stance leg allows that limb to functionally "lengthen," providing a longer stride length.

Hip, Knee, Ankle, and Foot Determinants

Small but vital transverse plane motions in the hip, knee, ankle, and foot change what would be an otherwise abrupt arc of motion of the sagittal plane to a smooth sinusoidal curve. Knee motion in the sagittal plane, 15° to 20° of flexion, during loading response helps absorb the forces delivered during impact and also lower the COM. Imagine the jarring your body would feel when the foot impacted the ground if the knee did not flex to absorb the forces.

The adducted femur, the tibiofemoral angle, and the 125° femoral angle of inclination in the frontal plane all decrease the magnitude of the COM's lateral excursions. If the neck-shaft angle is less (coxa vara), wide lateral trunk shifts occur to place the COM over the supporting feet. If these angles were not present, the excursion of the COM during gait would be a total of 6 inches.[37]

Overall Effect of Determinants

As mentioned, determinants demonstrate the cooperative motions of the pelvis, hips, knees, ankles, and feet to minimize COM movement during gait. As a result, normal walking occurs with minimal vertical and horizontal displacements of the body's COM. The total displacement of the COM is limited to about 2 inches (5 cm) in vertical motions and about the same in its lateral movements.

Challenges to Gait Efficiency

Under normal conditions, our motor control systems develop and become very adept at automatically permitting an individual to walk without conscious effort. Disease or injury of the neural or musculoskeletal system can disrupt the normal gait pattern. When such a disruption occurs, a variety of compensatory mechanisms is recruited to maintain functional ambulation. These compensations manifest themselves as abnormal patterns of walking and are inefficient methods of gait.

The human body has extraordinary compensatory ability to walk in the presence of range of abnormalities ranging from joint sprains to paralysis or amputation. Regardless of the compensation used, a price is paid through increased energy expenditure and exaggerated stresses on other segments. Normal human walking is so energy efficient that any gait abnormality, be it minor or major, increases energy expenditure for the same speed or distance.[101–104] Energy expenditure increases in the presence of compensation because: (1) abnormal gait produces excessive displacements of the body's COM; (2) muscles may have to act at higher intensities and for prolonged periods in the gait cycle; or (3) additional muscles may be recruited to help in gait. Joint dysfunction and pain are often due to repetitive microtrauma from long-term abnormal alignment, resulting in overstretching of ligaments and wearing of cartilage.

Impaired Gait in Common Pathological Neurologic Conditions

Pathomechanics occurring in gait may be divided into two major types based on their source of pathology—neurological or orthopedic. This section briefly describes some of the more common pathological gaits within each category. The orthopedically compromised gaits are usually not as complicated or as difficult to analyze as the neurologically compromised gaits since there are not as many elements of gait affected. Likewise, gait dysfunctions caused by orthopedic pathology are not as difficult to correct. Figs. 12.13 through 12.14 demonstrate various gaits displayed by individuals with neurological impairment.

Neurological Gait: Cerebral Palsy

Individuals with cerebral palsy (CP) often display several pathokinematic differences in gait, including abnormalities in amplitude, timing, and phasing of muscular activity. Movement, including gait, is characterized by coactivation or reciprocal excitation of muscle groups rather than by reciprocal inhibition and smooth muscle phasing.[105, 106] The main deficiencies in the gait of persons with CP are as follows:

1. From a kinematic perspective, joint motion patterns during gait show more hip adduction, flexion, and medial rotation; exaggerated knee flexion

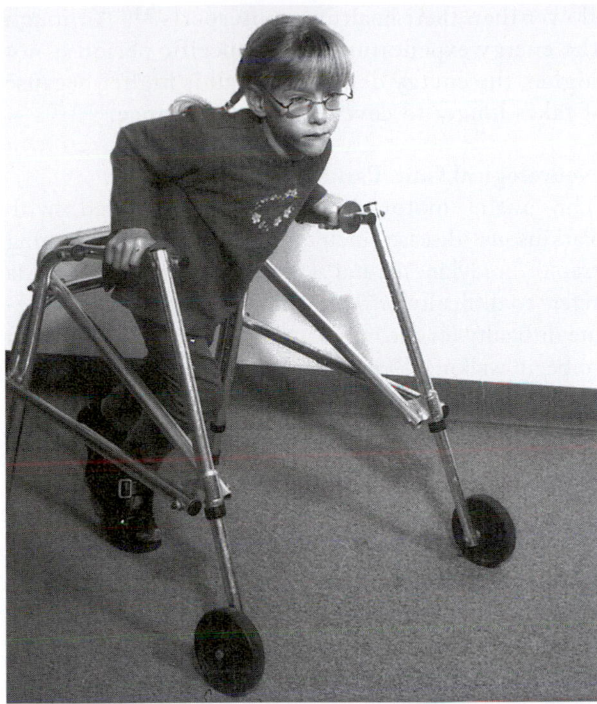

Figure 12.13 Example of gait pattern commonly seen in children with cerebral palsy: crouch gait.

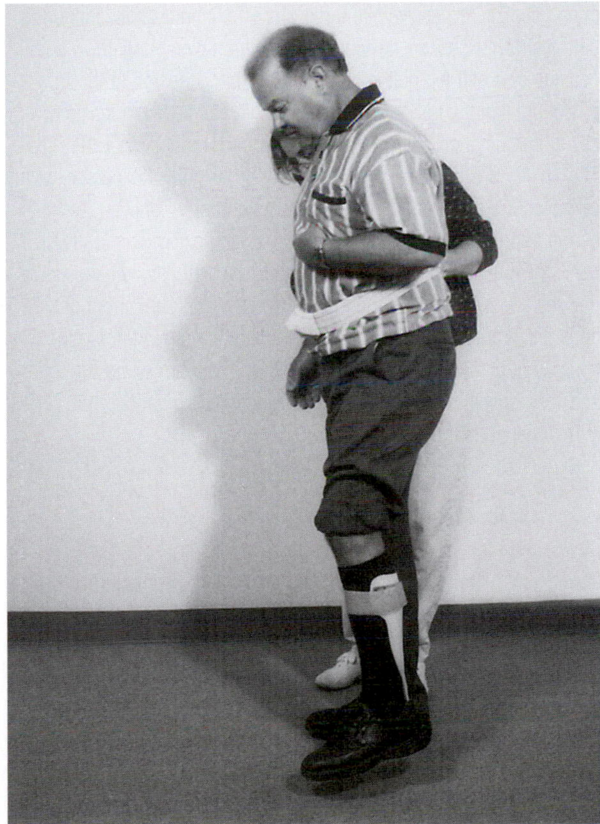

Figure 12.14 Gait commonly seen in an adult with hemiplegia.

during stance; and a forefoot strike pattern. Initial contact is often made with the knee in significant flexion and then either extension or excessive knee flexion throughout stance.[107] A weak gastrocnemius is not able to effectively restrain the forward movement of the tibia in stance, causing the knee to stay in flexion. Lack of dorsiflexion at the ankle frequently impairs the smooth movement of the tibia over the talus and may act to halt the forward movement of the trunk. This may cause either knee hyperextension or the individual to move onto the toes with a flexed hip and knee.

2. From a muscle output perspective, weakness is present throughout the lower extremities. Weakness is frequently seen in the gluteus maximus, gluteus medius, quadriceps, gastrocnemius, and anterior tibialis muscles. Inadequate force production creates stance instability and ineffective propulsion forward from terminal stance through preswing.

The energy cost of ambulation for individuals with CP is higher than for individuals without impairment.[107, 109–111] Generally, individuals with CP ambulate at about half the speed of individuals without CP with an energy demand estimated to be triple the demand for people without a neurological impairment.[112, 113] Energy cost is high due to the following factors: unnecessary levels of muscle activity that do not result in movement; erratic muscular activation and firing patterns; and the inability to efficiently transfer weight to the stance limb.[107]

Neurological Gait: Cerebrovascular Accident and Adult Hemiplegia

The causes of gait dysfunction in patients with hemiplegia are due to disordered motor control, a lack of voluntary muscle control and weakness, interference from abnormal muscle tone and muscle stiffness, and a disorganized postural control mechanism.[114] The gait of persons with hemiplegia is asymmetrical between the involved and uninvolved extremities and has several common characteristics (Fig. 12.14). During swing, atypical muscle firing, inappropriate initiation patterns, and the inability to sustain appropriate firing are more noticeable. Forward momentum is often lost, resulting in a choppy, inefficient gait. If the pelvis is retracted, initiation of swing phase often occurs with pelvic elevation and shortening of the trunk. Step length is shorter with the involved leg. Stance phase is characterized by increased double support time, reflecting increased time on the involved limb. Kinetic data show a loss of the normal phasing and modulation of muscle activity throughout the gait cycle. Although there are individual variations, three fairly distinct patterns have been identified:

1. A tendency for the flexor muscles to be active primarily during swing and the extensor muscles to be active primarily during stance in patients who demonstrate pattern-only motor control;[20]
2. A tendency for premature and continued activity of the stance muscles;
3. A tendency for cocontraction and coactivation patterns.[115]

Velocity following a stroke is decreased. Individuals affected by hemiplegic paralysis walk more than 50% slower than their healthy counterparts.[116] Although the energy expenditure in any specific period is not higher, the energy demand overall is higher because it takes longer to cover the same distance.[20, 117]

Neurological Gait: Parkinson's Disease

The main motor impairments associated with Parkinson's disease include muscle rigidity, resting tremor, bradykinesia, and akinesia (Chapter 3). Akinesia refers to difficulty *initiating* movement, which will create difficulty for the individual in initiating weight shift to begin walking. Bradykinesia refers to slowness or difficulty *maintaining* movement, once initiated. The impairment of rigidity and voluntary muscle weakness

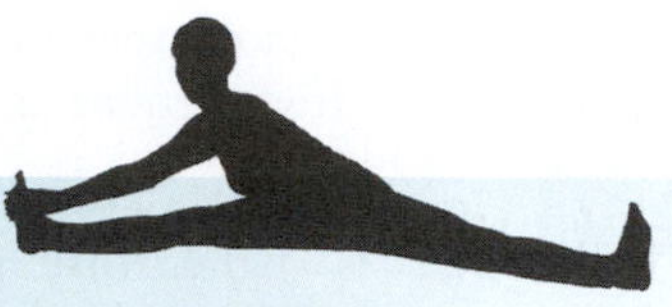

PRACTICE POINT

Clinically, four common characteristic gait patterns are observed in individuals with CP: a crouch gait, a gait characterized with genu recurvatum, a stiff leg gait, or a gait typical of hemiplegia.[20, 108] The most common, **crouch gait,** is a bilateral impairment characterized by excessive hip and knee flexion, dorsiflexion, and usually an anterior tilt of the pelvis (Fig. 12.13). Excessive hip and knee flexion is probably caused by a combination of overactivity of hip and knee flexors with weakness of antigravity hip and knee extensors. Poor control of the gastrocnemius muscle is thought to be the main impairment in a crouch gait. The weak gastrocnemius muscle does not effectively restrain the forward movement of the tibia in stance, causing the knee to remain flexed. Weakness of the quadriceps muscle is not considered to be a main contributing factor in stance control in a crouch gait, but rather contributes more to an ineffective step length by not extending the limb sufficiently at terminal swing.

Genu recurvatum presents the opposite clinical picture. The knee assumes a position of hyperextension during stance and the ankle often goes into excessive plantarflexion. The hip may still continue to demonstrate excessive flexion, as the trunk moves forward to compensate.[20] A **stiff leg gait** is characterized by extension at the trunk, posterior tilt of the pelvis, and excessive hip and knee extension usually in combination with medial rotation and adduction of the hips. The ankles are typically plantarflexed.[105] The gait of a person with hemiplegic CP is characterized by asymmetry, uneven weight-bearing and step length, hip retraction, knee flexion, and ineffective heel strike, usually with a plantarflexed ankle. Orthoses and assistive devices are prescribed as needed to assist in the attainment of safe ambulation. Intervention includes activities to improve force generation and functional strength, management of abnormal muscle tone, and task-specific training to reduce functional limitations and promote independent mobility.

Clinically, intervention for correction of gait in hemiplegia focuses on increasing hip extension in conjunction with trunk extension control to maintain alignment over the pelvis, initiation of the weight shift from the lower extremity in a forward direction, and the reestablishment of ankle, knee, and hip control. It is during single limb support that individuals with hemiplegia often experience the greatest risk of instability because the COM is at its highest point in midstance. Various approaches are possible to improve control during ambulation: (1) At the hip, intervention is directed to shift and move forward without excessive lateral trunk movement; (2) intervention at the knee focuses on retraining and strengthening the musculature around the knee for isometric, concentric, and eccentric control; and (3) at the ankle, intervention is directed at increasing concentric and eccentric dorsiflexor control during the appropriate phases throughout the gait cycle.

will also affect functional use of the lower extremities and locomotor skills. Individuals with Parkinson's disease encounter difficulty with all three of the subtasks of gait: weight acceptance, single limb support, and limb advancement. These functional limitations are caused by the constellation of impairments and symptoms that trouble the patient with Parkinson's disease: weakness, rigidity, abnormal muscular activation and sequencing, loss in flexibility, deformity and contracture formation, and impaired movement coordination. In the lower extremities, contractures commonly develop in the hip and knee flexors, hip adductors, and plantarflexors. These changes have a negative effect on the ability to properly load the lower extremity, a function that requires hip extension, knee control, and ankle dorsiflexion to at least neutral. A forward flexed trunk leads commonly to a kyphotic deformity, which eventually compromises trunk mobility and antigravity strength of both flexor and extensor muscle groups.

Because of these changes along with the symptoms of akinesia and bradykinesia, the gait pattern of a patient with Parkinson's disease has several unique clinical characteristics. Hip, knee, and ankle motions are reduced with a generalized lack of extension at the hip and knee, and dorsiflexion at the ankle. Trunk and pelvic motions are diminished, resulting in lack of reciprocal arm swing, limited rotation and dissociation, and inability of pelvic motion to contribute effectively to the gait cycle, limiting rotation, diminishing momentum, and reducing limb advancement. Stride length is greatly decreased so the patient walks with small, shuffling steps. The abnormally stooped posture contributes to the development of a **festinating gait,** characterized by a progressive increase in speed with a shortening in stride length.[118] The gait takes on an accelerating quality, called a **propulsive gait,** sometimes requiring that the patient come in contact with an object or a wall in order to stop. Patients with Parkinson's disease have great difficulty turning and changing direction when walking. Overall velocity may be decreased but cadence is increased, contributing to inefficiency. Heel strike at initial contact does not occur, with either a flatfooted or toe-heel progression seen instead. The trunk may be stooped, flexed, and rigidly limited in rotation. As mentioned, patients with Parkinson's disease frequently do not demonstrate a reciprocal arm swing, consistent with inflexibility and lack of trunk rotation.[24, 89, 118]

Neurological Gait: Ataxia

Evidence of dysmetria, movement decomposition, dysdiadochokinesia, and abnormal timing of multijoint movements frequently characterize ataxia (Chapter 3). As a symptom of disordered motor control, ataxia can accompany many neurological disorders, including multiple sclerosis, cerebellar, midbrain, or spinal disease, Friedreich's ataxia, chronic alcoholism, and in some types of CP. Ataxia is very common in multiple sclerosis (MS).

Ataxic gait is one in which step length is uneven, width is irregular, rhythm is absent, and the feet are often lifted too high. The normal relationship between

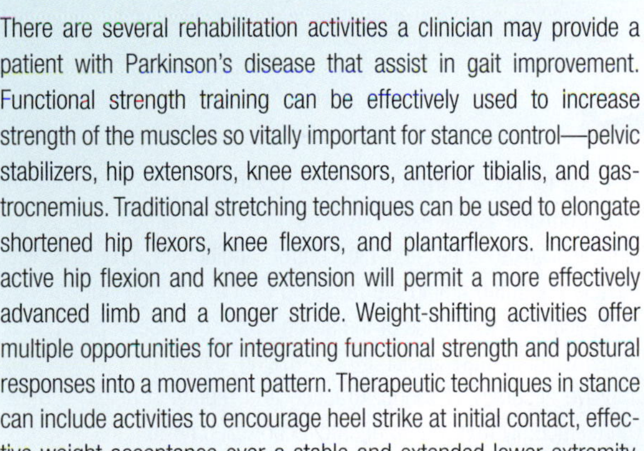

PRACTICE POINT

There are several rehabilitation activities a clinician may provide a patient with Parkinson's disease that assist in gait improvement. Functional strength training can be effectively used to increase strength of the muscles so vitally important for stance control—pelvic stabilizers, hip extensors, knee extensors, anterior tibialis, and gastrocnemius. Traditional stretching techniques can be used to elongate shortened hip flexors, knee flexors, and plantarflexors. Increasing active hip flexion and knee extension will permit a more effectively advanced limb and a longer stride. Weight-shifting activities offer multiple opportunities for integrating functional strength and postural responses into a movement pattern. Therapeutic techniques in stance can include activities to encourage heel strike at initial contact, effective weight acceptance over a stable and extended lower extremity, and weight shifting over one limb and onto the other extremity. Activities that encourage smooth control of the momentum force generated at the end of stance will offer the client the opportunity to control the advancing limb. Functional task training that includes clearing obstacles, negotiating uneven terrain, and changing speeds can be practiced in varying environments. Individuals with Parkinson's may require a focus on eccentric strength training so that increased voluntary control can be channeled into the deceleration tasks of muscles that naturally elongate during gait—hip extensors, hamstrings and quadriceps, and ankle plantarflexors and dorsiflexors. Attention to gait initiation should occur during smooth practice of both stance and swing phase, to take advantage of the natural momentum that occurs during the gait cycle.[23, 119]

stance and swing phases of gait is altered and arm swing is typically absent.[120] Movement is typically wide-based with evidence of poor proximal stability at the shoulders and pelvis. Motion during gait is also disturbed secondary to incorrect force generation, timing abnormalities, and an inability to regulate posture. Stance function can be impaired by interference from numerous constraints such as weakness especially in the hip and knee extensors, contracture, sensory impairment, and interference from abnormally low tone or uncoordinated movement. During swing, atypical muscle firing, inappropriate initiation patterns, and the inability to sustain appropriate muscle activation are more noticeable. Forward advancement of the limb is often demonstrated as a wide-based, abducted advancement of the limb, with evidence of dysmetria resulting in poor positioning of the limb for placement during stance. Momentum is often absent, resulting in a very jerky, ineffective swing.

Impaired Gait in Common Pathological Orthopedic Conditions

As you can see, most neurological pathologic conditions affect gait at several levels. Orthopedic pathologic conditions, however, are more local in their effects. That is not to say that only one joint is affected by an orthopedic condition. Since the lower extremity works in a closed chain system for the majority of the walking cycle, other joints may be affected, but the extensiveness of the impact of an orthopedic injury on gait is not as global as is seen with neurologic pathologies.

Orthopedic Gait: Quadriceps Weakness

Quadriceps weakness is a common occurrence following acute or chronic injury to the knee, surgery, pain, edema, and nonweight-bearing.[121, 122] Quadriceps weakness affects gait[123] (Fig. 12.15). Individuals with quadriceps weakness have characteristic gait alterations that compensate for the weakness and still allow ambulation. The quadriceps muscle works most from the very end of swing to control knee positioning through the first half of the stance phase by eccentrically controlling the knee so impact forces are absorbed. An individual with quadriceps weakness places the knee in extension or hyperextension. During terminal swing, knee extension is controlled by the upper gluteus maximus through its iliotibial band insertion on the anterolateral tibia.[20] A fast swing into hip flexion is followed by a rapid hip extension as the gluteus maximus contracts to move the femur posteriorly as the tibia continues its movement forward by momentum.[20] At initial contact and during loading response, the knee extends by one of two methods. If the hip extensors are used to keep the hip extended and the ankle plantarflexors move the ankle into plantarflexion, the knee is forced into extension. The alternative method of maintaining knee extension occurs when the individual moves into trunk flexion after initial contact, placing the body's COM in front of the knee to force the joint into extension. As the body's mass continues to move forward, the gastrocnemius pull on the posterior knee assists in maintaining knee extension. A longer stride length also encourages prolonged passive knee hyperextension during stance. If the individual moves the body's COM forward of the weight-bearing limb, the gait may appear as a pitch of the body over the limb with a forward lean of the trunk during the first half of stance on the affected extremity.

Orthopedic Gait: Knee Motion Restriction

Following a knee injury such as acute sprains and strains or surgery involving any procedure from arthroscopic debridement to total joint replacement, loss of

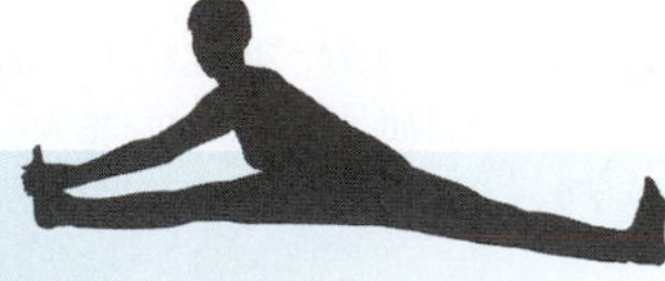

PRACTICE POINT

Clinicians who deal with patients displaying ataxic gait may use a variety of rehabilitation strategies that are specific to the particular gait deficit. Standing and walking activities should stress adequate weight transfer with trunk rotation, and retraining to re-establish a reciprocal arm swing, however limited. Intervention must establish compatible proximal and distal movement control. Proximal movement control goals focus on increasing hip extension in conjunction with trunk extension control to maintain alignment over the pelvis, with adequate postural control. The clinician intervenes to correct and cue for correct trunk and pelvic position, to initiate the weight shift from the lower extremity in a forward direction, and to re-establish ankle, knee, and hip control. Additionally, problems with muscle firing and timing are retrained with the stance limb forward to replicate the demands of the swing cycle. The use of proximal or distal weights may assist in decreasing ataxic movements and improve accuracy of swing. Practice and repetition helps to move more smoothly from preswing into a controlled flexion and advancement of the moving limb.

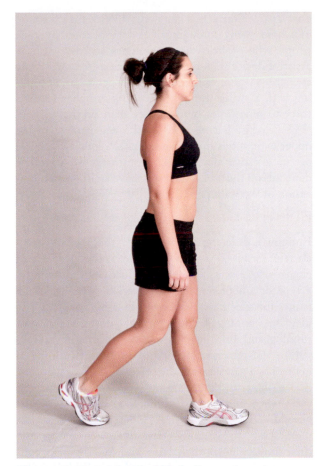

Figure 12.15 Gait in an individual with an orthopedic impairment; in this example—left quadriceps weakness.

motion is always a concern. Individuals whose knee is immobilized for extended periods following trauma are at even greater risk of losing joint motion. If the individual is unable to fully extend the knee because of either tightness within the knee joint or loss of flexibility in the hamstrings, initial contact does not occur at the heel but more towards the midfoot region. Since the knee is unable to fully extend during terminal swing, there is a shortened stride length because of a reduced swing excursion, perhaps providing a noticeable uneven cadence with a longer stride of the unaffected limb. The knee does not reach normal extension at initial contact, midstance, or terminal stance and remains in flexion throughout the stance phase. The gait may appear as a rolling gait with a lowered COM during stance on the affected limb along with increased hip flexion and increased ankle dorsiflexion of the limb. The pelvis may have a noticeable drop in the frontal and transverse planes during terminal swing and initial contact since the knee is unable to fully extend to reach the ground.

Orthopedic Gait: Ankle Motion Restriction

Reduced ankle motion following ankle sprains is very common. Dorsiflexion is the common motion that may lack several degrees to subsequently create a very typical pathological gait. When dorsiflexion motion is restricted, the greatest gait deviation occurs during midstance. Normally, the ankle is plantarflexed from loading response and moves quickly into dorsiflexion by midstance, but if dorsiflexion motion is lacking, the individual lurches forward, lifting the heel off the ground and moving rapidly into terminal stance. During stance, the individual may also position the hip in lateral rotation to permit midstance to occur with less lurching since this position will allow the midtarsal joints to collapse, compensating for reduced ankle dorsiflexion. Depending on how much dorsiflexion is lacking, the toes may be unable to clear the ground sufficiently if the ankle is unable to dorsiflex to neutral; in this case, the individual will clear the foot during swing by either increasing hip and knee flexion or circumducting the limb during swing.

Orthopedic Gait: Gluteus Medius Weakness

Gluteus medius weakness may occur as either a frank injury to the gluteus medius or secondarily following an injury to another aspect of the limb. The typical gait seen with the presence of gluteus medius weakness is a **Trendelenburg gait** (see Fig 9.28C). As you recall from discussions of the hip in Chapter 9, deficiency of the gluteus medius produces a drop of the contralateral pelvis during single limb weight-bearing. During the midstance phase of gait, the limb is in a single limb weight-bearing position, so the opposite hip and pelvis drops during this phase if the gluteus medius has insufficient strength to hold the pelvis level. For example, if the right gluteus medius is weak, when the individual is in midstance on the right, the left hip and pelvis drops. This is a Trendelenburg gait.

Another way an individual may compensate for a gluteus medius deficiency is to lean the trunk laterally towards the ipsilateral side of weakness during midstance. Moving the HAT directly over the limb reduces the force arm of the HAT so the weak gluteus medius is not required to exert as much force; this movement of the COM lowers the total torque required of the gluteus medius.

Regardless of the type of gait used with gluteus medius weakness, an assistive device is usually recommended to enable a more normal gait. A cane or crutch is commonly used. The device in the contralateral hand provides a force platform through which the pelvis remains level (see Fig. 9.28D). During ambulation, the assistive device and weakened lower extremity bear weight at the same time The upward force transmitted from the floor though the assistive device, onto the upper extremity, and then through the trunk assist in maintaining a level pelvis on the nonweight-bearing side. Even a small upward force from the cane or crutch provides significant reduction in the forces required by the gluteus medius. Such a force reduction is possible because the force arm of the cane is applied at a relatively long distance from the axis of motion compared to the body's COM. The force arm between the cane and the center of gravity is 4 to 5 times longer than the lever arm between the center of gravity and hip joint.[30] Such a long moment arm necessitates as little as 2% to 10% of equivalent body weight through the cane to provide adequate support[30] (see Fig. 9.28E).

Effect of an Assistive Device on the Functional Tasks and Efficiency of Gait

Use of an assistive device changes the nature of the walking task. The gait of an individual using an assistive device will demonstrate different characteristics than that of a typical gait cycle. An assistive device is appropriately prescribed to enhance stability in upright, widen the base of support, and allow for functional mobility in the face of significant limitations or constraints. When an individual uses an assistive device that requires the simultaneous engagement of both upper extremities, the upper extremities function differently during gait than during unaided walking. In this case, the upper extremities no longer engage in a reciprocal arm swing, the demands on the trunk consequently change, the ability of the trunk to freely rotate decreases, and the arms, pushing through an assistive device, are now a part of the actual gait cycle.[24] With the exception of a rapid, swing-through gait as demonstrated by some people who proficiently use crutches, walking with an assistive device is slower and in all cases, requires more energy.[124, 125] For example, energy expenditure of walking with a swing-through gait using crutches requires three to nine times more energy than normal gait.[102, 126, 127] Energy is consumed by the engagement of the upper extremities in this closed chain activity. The use of an assistive device also requires more cognitive demands on the user, which may have an impact on execution of the walking task itself.[128]

Running Gait

Running is different than walking in that the body travels at an increased velocity. However, as the speed of gait changes, so does its kinetics and kinematics. Running is a type of ambulation that has variable speeds, which makes the specific variables within running difficult to identify. Running includes jogging, slow running, fast running, and sprinting—each of these forms of gait falls within the general category of running. **Running** is defined as a gait wherein the swing phase is longer than stance phase, and there are two periods within the gait cycle when neither lower limb is in contact with the ground.

Walking and running have their differences and their similarities. Both walking and running gaits contain a stance and a swing phase and periods of single leg stance. They both propel the body forward in a linear direction. During walking, however, the body moves similar to an inverted pendulum producing a sinusoidal motion of the COM, but running causes the COM to

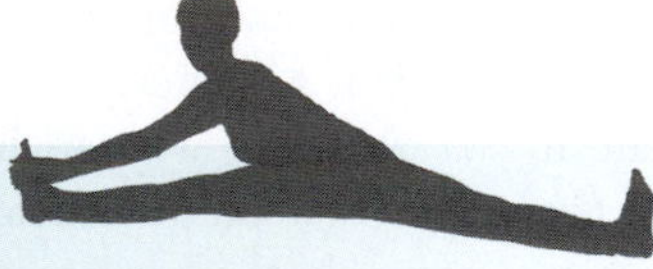

PRACTICE POINT

As mentioned, correction of an orthopedic pathological gait is less complicated than correcting a neurologic abnormal gait. Once a gait deviation is observed, it is the clinician's responsibility to realize the source of that deviation. Once this reason has been determined, the clinician is able to design a rehabilitation program to correct the orthopedic pathology or minimize the effect of the neurological impairment. It is common in rehabilitation that the clinician not only correct or minimize the pathology but also provide the patient with gait training to develop "new" habits of ambulation following an injury or dysfunction that has led to the gait pathology. In the case of orthopedic problems, sometimes one problem is producing more than one gait deviation and correcting it will eliminate a number of gait deviations, whereas at other times, several problems are creating the individual's abnormal gait. For example, if the patient has only joint tightness in the knee, the gait will have several pathological characteristics including increased hip flexion, increased ankle dorsiflexion, no knee extension at initial contact and terminal stance, shortened swing phase, asymmetrical cadence, increased pelvic drop on the ipsilateral side, and increased forward pelvic rotation at initial contract. The clinician must be able to recognize all deviations from normal gait and understand possible causes for these deviations before he or she corrects them.

move more like a bouncing ball or pogo stick, using muscle stiffness to provide elastic energy release to propel the body forward.[129] As the body transitions from walking to running, changes occur in the spatial and temporal variables of gait; the spatial variable of step length increases as do the temporal factors of velocity and cadence when step duration decreases. Ground reactions forces also increase with running. In walking, forward momentum is provided during the stance phase, but in running, movement of the arms and legs provides the momentum during the swing phase. Walking gait has a longer stance phase and a shorter swing phase, but running has the reverse, a longer swing phase and shorter stance phase. In walking, the time of overlap activity between the two lower limbs occurs in stance, but in running, this overlapping activity occurs during the swing phase. Finally, running gait is unique compared to walking in that running requires a greater range of motion of all the lower extremity joints, there is more eccentric activity of the muscles during running, the COM is lowered throughout the running cycle, there is no double support phase in running, and there is a time of no contact with the ground with either limb during running.

Running is defined by speed. The confounding factor in clearly defining different running categories is related to the fact that various investigators use their own definitions for jogging, running, and sprinting. Although the average walking pace is about 1.4 m/sec or 1.5 yd/sec, a running pace may likely vary anywhere from 2.2 to 5 times walking speed.[130] Running speeds examined have a wide range of variability with a range including these examples: 2.74 m/sec[131], 6 mph for jogging, and 12 mph for running [35]; 1.96 m/sec [132], and 10 to 15 km/hr.[133] In an attempt to standardize results and provide greater control of conditions, investigators have subjects run on treadmills to collect data.[133] Acceptable running speed determined for running studies is between 1.5 m/sec (3.36 mph) and 6 m/sec (13.42 mph) with an average speed at about 4 m/sec (8.95 mph).[134]

In contrast to running, **sprinting** is more simply defined: running as fast as possible for short distances.[135] The two main factors influencing any running speed are stride length and stride frequency or cadence.[136] Therefore, even sprinting may have various speeds, depending on how long the individual's stride is and how quickly that person is able to move the limbs. In our discussion here of running, we will compare and contrast the differences between walking, running, and sprinting. These three categories are used since the greatest differences in kinetics and kinematics occur when the body moves from walking to running and from running to sprinting. There are less noticeable differences within the different speeds under the category of running just as there are nominal differences in the different walking speeds; therefore, clinicians are not as concerned about the differences in, say, slow running and jogging as they are in the contrasts between running and sprinting. Tables 12–6 through 12–9 display comparisons of key kinematic and kinetic features of walking, running, and sprinting at the trunk and pelvis (Table 12-6), the hip (Table 12–7), the knee (Table 12–8), and the foot and ankle (Table 12–9), to be discussed further in the following section.

Phases

As mentioned, running and sprinting have stance and swing phases, similar to walking. Running and sprinting are divided into similar phases, so in this section we will discuss running and sprinting as essentially one category. The stance phase in running is divided into two subphases, absorption and propulsion, which are separated at midstance; the swing phase also has two phases, initial swing and terminal swing, which are delineated at midswing.[137] Midstance and midswing during walking are specific periods within the gait cycle where activity and motion occur, but in the running gait, these serve only as points of separation to delineate between the two halves of stance and swing phases, respectively. At the beginning of initial swing and the end of terminal swing, there is a period when neither limb is in contact with the ground; this time is called **double float** (Fig. 12.16) or simply, the **float phase**. This double float time creates more time during swing and less time during stance. The faster an individual runs, the more swing phase time there is along with a concomitant reduction in time during stance phase.

Stance Phase: Absorption

The absorption phase of stance is the time from initial contact of the foot to the time of midstance. When the foot makes contact with the ground during running, as in walking, the lateral heel contacts first with the foot in a slightly supinated position.[138] About 80% of runners make initial contact on the heel; the remaining 20% land on the midfoot.[139] Initial impact occurs very rapidly, and the limb moves immediately into a foot flat position, just as in walking although at a much faster rate. As the name of this phase implies, its purpose is to absorb the forces of the foot impacting with the ground. Therefore, this phase ends when the body begins preparations to move or propel the body forward.

Stance Phase: Propulsion

As the body's COM moves over the weight-bearing foot at midstance, the opposite limb is swinging forward. In

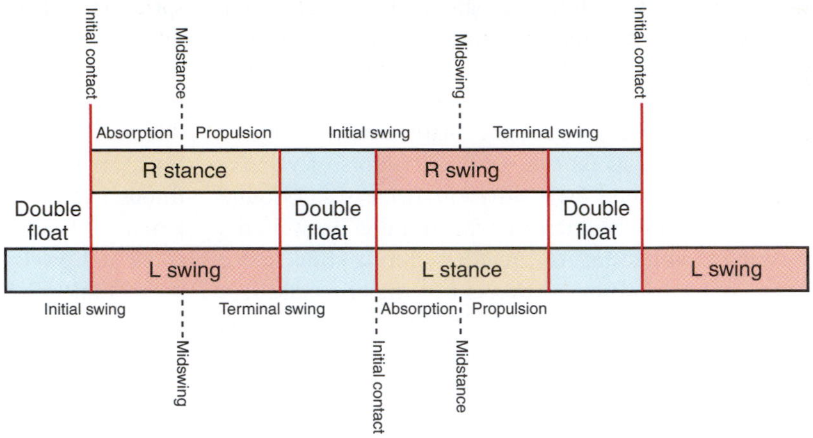

Figure 12.16 Phases of running. The stance phase is shorter than the swing phase. The swing phase contains a double float phase.

the early part of this phase, the heel of the stance leg lifts off the ground. While the stance heel is moving off the ground as it initiates its forward propulsion, the swing leg continues its forward advancement and begins preparations for stance. Once the foot leaves the ground, the stance phase ends, and the limb moves into the first double float phase.

Swing Phase: Initial Swing

The first half of initial swing is the first double float phase when both limbs are off the ground. The swing leg is moving forward and toward the ground in preparation for weight acceptance and the stance leg is moving upward and forward to advance the limb and entire body forward. During the second half of initial swing, the other limb makes contact with the ground and begins its own initial contact and weight-bearing cycle. The swing limb accelerates forward via the momentum produced by the force of pushing off the ground and swinging the limb forward.

In the early phase of initial swing, the limb is abducted in response to pelvic rotation. This pelvic rotation also impacts the contralateral limb that soon becomes the stance limb by rolling it into lateral rotation and supination. The ankle is held in dorsiflexion throughout the swing phase. Knee and hip flexion are also increasing during this time.

Swing Phase: Terminal Swing

The second half of the swing phase is marked by a change from acceleration to deceleration in preparation for initial contact. As the stance leg moves past toe-off, the last half of terminal swing begins. It is during this time that the second double float phase occurs. The limb joints move in preparation for initial contact.

Kinematics

As you recall, kinematics deals with movement without consideration of the forces that cause that movement. We will identify the movements that occur during the running phases, but the quantity of motions are not presented since the degrees of movement varies greatly, depending on an individual's speed, size, and training.[139]

Sagittal Plane Motion

More investigations of running have identified sagittal plane motions rather than frontal or transverse plane motions. This may be because there is more motion occurring during running in the sagittal plane than the other planes of motion. Sagittal plane motion of the joints is also most important since it is what produces forward motion of the body during walking, running, and sprinting.

Trunk and Pelvis

The faster a person moves, the more the center of mass is lowered; the COM is highest during walking and lowest when sprinting. Along with a lowered COM, there is a progressive forward lean of the trunk and an anterior pelvic tilt with an increase in speed of gait from walking to running to jogging. The forward tilt of the pelvis and trunk keep the ground reaction force forward of the COM so forward acceleration of the body is possible.[139] During the absorption phase of stance, the pelvis is slightly posteriorly tilted to reach a position of minimum anterior tilt.[140] After the pelvis reaches this position, it reverses directions, moving anterior to achieve its maximum anterior pelvic tilt just prior to the foot leaving the ground. During initial swing, the pelvis moves slightly posteriorly and then anteriorly during terminal swing; this posterior then anterior tilt is the result of the forces directed through the pelvis by the contralateral limb.[140]

Hip

Hip motion in the sagittal plane in running is similar to that during walking, except extension occurs slightly later, at the time of toe-off rather than heel lift.[139] In the last part of terminal swing, the hip moves towards extension, so the COM is not too far behind the foot at initial contact. Placing the COM behind the point of contact will serve to decelerate forward motion. When the foot hits the ground, the hip moves into slight flexion to absorb the impact forces.[138] Following this brief period of flexion, the hip moves towards extension for the remainder of stance until, as mentioned, maximum extension occurs either at the end of stance or immediately after the foot leaves the ground.[140] The hip reaches its maximum flexion during the beginning of terminal swing, and then during the last half of terminal swing, the hip moves towards extension as the limb begins preparation for stance. Maximum hip flexion of the swing leg occurs about the same time as toe-off on the contralateral limb.[140]

Knee

As with the hip, the pattern of motion in the sagittal plane is similar in walking and various running speeds, but the extremes of motion are profoundly different.[139] During the stance phase in running, the knee moves from about 45° during the absorption phase to its greatest extension of 20° at the end of the propulsion phase of stance.[139] After the knee reaches this maximum extension and the foot leaves the ground, the knee moves progressively into flexion, achieving its maximum flexion at about midswing. At this time, the knee may flex as much as 90° to 130°.[139] After midswing, the knee moves towards extension in preparation for landing.

Ankle and Foot

The foot hits the ground in dorsiflexion and the tibia moves forward after initial contact, causing more dorsiflexion to assist in force absorption. The ankle reaches maximum dorsiflexion of 20° just before midstance.[138] The propulsion phase begins ankle plantarflexion as the gastrocnemius and soleus prepare to propel the limb and body forward. Active contraction of the gastrocnemius and soleus muscles accelerates the stance leg during this last segment of the stance phase. Since the foot continues its advancement in supination, the foot provides a rigid lever from which the gastrocnemius-soleus group propels the body forward. As the foot leaves the ground, hip and knee extensor muscle groups provide additional thrust to allow the body to move into the float phase. Immediately after toe-off the ankle continues to move into plantarflexion as the momentum of the gastrocnemius and soleus force continues its effect. By mid initial swing, the ankle begins moving into dorsiflexion. Dorsiflexion continues until the last half of terminal swing when the ankle reduces its dorsiflexed position as it prepares to land.

Frontal Plane Motion

Motion in the frontal plane is not as great as in the sagittal plane for either walking or running. Investigations of frontal plane motion during running are primarily limited to the trunk, pelvis, and hips. Minimal significant information is available for other joint movements within this plane during any running activities.

Trunk and Pelvis

In the frontal plane, the trunk leans towards the weight-bearing leg during running: When the individual's right limb moves to early stance, the trunk leans laterally to the right and then reverses to the left during early stance on the left.[139]

Pelvic tilt in the frontal plane begins at initial contact with the pelvis slightly higher on the stance leg and slightly lower on the swing leg. By the time the limb reaches midstance, the pelvis has moved downward on the stance leg and upward on the swing leg so it is level. After midstance, the swing-leg pelvis continues its upward rotation as the stance limb pelvis rotates downward, achieving its maximum downward position at the time of toe-off.[140] When the limb moves into its initial swing, the ipsilateral pelvis rotates upward to move the limb off the ground while the contralateral pelvis rotates downward in preparation for initial contact. During midswing and through terminal swing the pelvis continues to move upward on the swing-leg side until it reaches its maximum upward rotation during the last half of terminal swing.[140]

Hip

The hip motion essentially mirrors pelvic motion.[139] The hip is adducted at initial contact during running to place the base of support under the body's COM. As forces are absorbed immediately after initial contact, the hip adducts slightly more. By the time the limb is at midstance, the hip is preparing for the propulsive phase of stance and is moving toward abduction until it achieves a position of slight abduction by toe-off. Abduction continues into initial swing until maximum abduction occurs about midswing. The hip then moves towards adduction in terminal swing in preparation for initial contact. It is thought that hip abduction occurs during toe-off and initial swing to assist the contralateral swinging limb to clear the foot from the ground.[140] Likewise, hip adduction during the last portion of terminal swing may function to better position the limb for a stable landing.[141]

Knee

When the foot hits the ground, the knee is slightly abducted and then moves into about 12° of adduction by midstance.[142] During the propulsive phase, the knee moves towards abduction although it stays in slight relative adduction throughout the cycle.[142]

Ankle and Foot

Since the talocrural joint moves only in the sagittal plane, the subtalar joint is that part of the ankle complex that moves in the frontal plane. The subtalar joint makes initial contact in about 10° of inversion and immediately moves into eversion.[143] This movement into eversion assists hip and knee flexion in force absorption. The rearfoot and midfoot then continue at a slower rate to move into pronation throughout the first half of the stance phase. As the limb moves through the propulsion phase, the subtalar joint rotates into inversion.

Transverse Plane Motion

Since these motions are very difficult to see without sophisticated and expensive three-dimensional laboratory equipment, there is little information currently available on transverse plane motion during running activities. Once again, the pelvis and hip have received the most attention of investigators; the available information is presented here.

Trunk and Pelvis

Trunk motion in the transverse plane is divided into opposite motions between the upper and lower spine. The lower spine rotates backward in coordination with extension of the trailing leg as the upper spine simultaneously rotates forward in synchrony with the arm on the ipsilateral side, so equilibrium and balance occur during running.[140]

As mentioned previously, forward pelvic rotation occurs when a side of the pelvis (hemipelvis) moves anteriorly, and backward pelvic rotation is when a side of the pelvis moves posteriorly; when one side of the pelvis moves into forward rotation, the opposite side moves into backward rotation. Pelvic motion during running is different than in walking.[139] In fact, pelvic motions during running are opposite to those in walking. At initial contact the pelvis is in slight backward rotation and continues to move in this direction until midstance.[140] During stance of the limb, the opposite limb is swinging forward. Pelvic rotation occurring from the motion of the swing limb causes lateral rotation torque of the stance limb. After midstance and throughout the propulsion phase of stance, the pelvis moves towards forward rotation, so by the time the limb is at the end of toe-off, the pelvis is in neutral rotation. The pelvis continues its movement into forward rotation until midswing when it reaches its maximum forward rotation.[140] During terminal swing the pelvis begins its movement toward backward rotation as it prepares for initial contact. It is believed that the pelvis moves in this pattern during running to provide for energy efficiency by reducing the posterior component of ground reaction force at initial contact.[140]

Hip

The hip is medially rotated during the absorption phase of stance; however, after midstance, the hip begins to laterally rotate so that it reaches a neutral position by toe-off.[139] As the hip moves through the swing phase, it maintains a position of minimal medial rotation.[141]

Knee

At initial contact the knee is in slight lateral rotation and immediately moves into medial rotation throughout the absorption phase.[142] Medial tibial rotation leads to talus abduction and, consequently, pronation.[142] During the propulsion phase of stance, the knee laterally rotates and continues to do so until toe-off.[142] By the time the foot is ready for initial contact, the tibia has returned to a position of slight lateral rotation.

Ankle and Foot

As mentioned, the weight-bearing talus adducts, causing the tibia to medially rotate. Consequently, the subtalar joint pronates when the foot is loaded in the absorption phase. At the very end of absorption, immediately before midstance, maximum foot pronation occurs as a result of the transverse tarsal joint axes becoming parallel; this position allows maximum mobility of the foot to accommodate to any surface on which the foot stands. This point of maximum pronation marks the end of the absorptive phase in stance.[138] It is during the propulsion phase when the subtalar joint inverts that the subtalar joint and midtarsal joints then move into supination. As the opposite limb swings forward ahead of the stance limb, this realignment of the weight-bearing subtalar joint locks the transverse tarsal joint axes to reduce their mobility and provide a rigid lever to propel the limb off the ground. During initial swing, the foot is in pronation as it is relaxed, but it moves to supination during terminal swing[141] and remains in supination throughout the swing phase.[144]

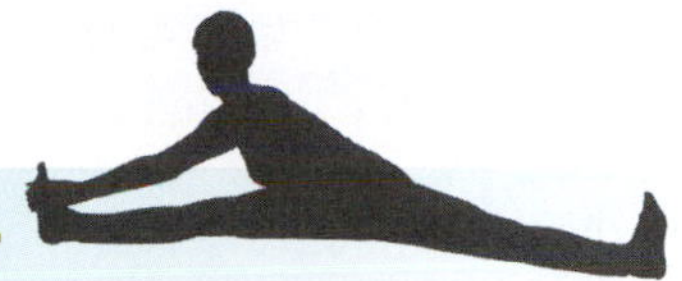

PRACTICE POINT

Injured athletes are often anxious to return to running following their injury. One of the most common questions clinicians encounter during the first treatment session following an injury is: "When can I start running?" Before a patient is able to return to running, not only must the injury be resolved, but the patient must also have sufficient range of motion in the lower extremity joints. How much motion is required at each joint depends upon the individual's running speed. Sprinters require significantly more motion than joggers and runners. Although only 60° of knee flexion is required to walk normally, a runner must have 90° of knee flexion to run, and sprinters require even more. These are requirements the clinician must realize and include in establishing goals for treatment.

Changes at Different Speeds

As the rate of locomotion changes from walking to running to sprinting, there are some differences that occur in motion requirements, timing of activity, and other parameters. General observations of changes seen with each progressive increase in speed include a lowered center of mass, a longer stride, faster cadence, shorter time during stance and longer time during swing, and increased ranges of motions in almost all joints. As has been mentioned, walking includes two periods of double support whereas running incorporates two periods of double float within a stride. There are additional specific changes that occur in each segment as well. Tables 12–6, 12–7, 12–8, and 12–9 below highlight the

TABLE 12–6 | TRUNK AND PELVIS COMPARISONS

Gait Phase	Walking	Running	Sprinting
Stance phase	Trunk remains erect throughout. Pelvis remains in near neutral throughout.	Slight forward lean of the trunk at initial contact. Pelvis has an anterior tilt.	Greater forward lean of the trunk at initial contact. Pelvis has an anterior tilt greater than during running.
Swing phase	Trunk remains erect throughout.	Forward lean of trunk.	Slight forward lean of trunk.

TABLE 12–7 | HIP COMPARISONS

Gait Phase	Walking	Running	Sprinting
Stance phase	Reaches maximum extension at heel-off.	Maximum extension occurs after toe-off.	Hip is never moved into full extension. Significantly more output of gluteus maximus occurs than in either walking or running.
Swing phase	Maximum hip flexion occurs at late swing into initial contact and is 30°.	Maximum hip flexion occurs after midswing and before the last half of terminal swing. The hip flexes about 20° more in running than in walking.[162]	Maximum hip flexion may be greater than 80°.[162] Significantly more output of hip flexors occurs than in either walking or running.

TABLE 12-8 | KNEE COMPARISONS

Gait Phase	Walking	Running	Sprinting
Stance phase	Knee extension nearly fully at initial contact and full at heel-off.	Knee extension never occurs.	Knee extension never occurs.
Swing phase	Maximum flexion is 60°.	Maximum flexion is about 90°.	Maximum flexion is about 130°.

TABLE 12-9 | ANKLE AND FOOT COMPARISONS

Gait Phase	Walking	Running	Sprinting
Stance phase	Initial contact is made at the heel. Rapid plantarflexion follows initial contact. Burst of calf activity occurs at end of stance. Impact absorption after initial contact of quads and calf occur at different times.	Initial contact is made at the posterolateral foot or midfoot. Rapid dorsiflexion follows initial contact. Rapid motion at initial contact from inversion to eversion occurs 5 times faster than in walking.[42] Nearly simultaneous bursts of energy absorption and production of calf and quads occur after initial contact and at end of stance.	Initial contact is made by at the toes. Dorsiflexion after initial contact and the heel may not touch the ground.
Swing phase	Ankle dorsiflexes to clear foot from floor.	Ankle dorsiflexes but knee and hip flexion provide foot clearance.	Ankle dorsiflexes, but knee and hip flexion provide foot clearance.

primary changes that occur in each of the segments during the three types of locomotion. Figure 12.17 demonstrates the ranges of motions of the joints during walking, running, and sprinting.

Muscle Activity at the Hip, Knee, and Ankle in Running

We have previously mentioned that impact forces are absorbed by the various segments at initial impact, so you may have already surmised that the muscles of these segments are working eccentrically to absorb energy created at this time of the running cycle. This time of absorption is followed by a generation of power as the segments prepare to propel the body forward. For this reason, as with walking activities, running activities produce the greatest amount of muscle activity immediately after initial contact, during the last half of stance (propulsion phase), and in the last portion of terminal swing. The major difference is that, with very few exceptions, the onset timing of muscle activity is a little sooner and the intensity of that activity is greater in running than in walking; this case of onset timing occurs even more quickly with greater muscle activity in sprinting (Fig. 12.18).

Hip Muscle Groups

The gluteus maximus output and timing of function is the same in both walking and running, regardless of the running speed.[145] Right before and right after initial contact, the hip extensors are active. The hip extensors are reversing hip motion, reducing the amount of hip flexion in preparation for landing before initial contact and then acting to absorb impact forces by controlling hip motion after contact. On the other hand, the gluteus medius activity timing is the same in walking and running, but as the running speed increases, so does the muscle's output amplitude.[145]

The hip flexors propel the hip into flexion as the limb leaves the ground, moving into the initial swing phase. Peak hip flexion occurs during the middle portion of swing for both running and sprinting.[139] During the latter portion of stance, the hip flexors decelerate hip extension as the limb prepares for the swing phase.

Adductor muscle activity is different in running than it is in walking. As has already been presented, the adductors are active at initial contact and toe-off to help stabilize the thigh during these phases in walking. On the other hand, the adductors are continually active during stance in running to stabilize and resist pelvic motion produced by the contralateral swing leg.[138] Peak periods of adductor activity in running occur during midstance, midswing, and the end of terminal swing.[145] With the limb in an adducted position during stance,

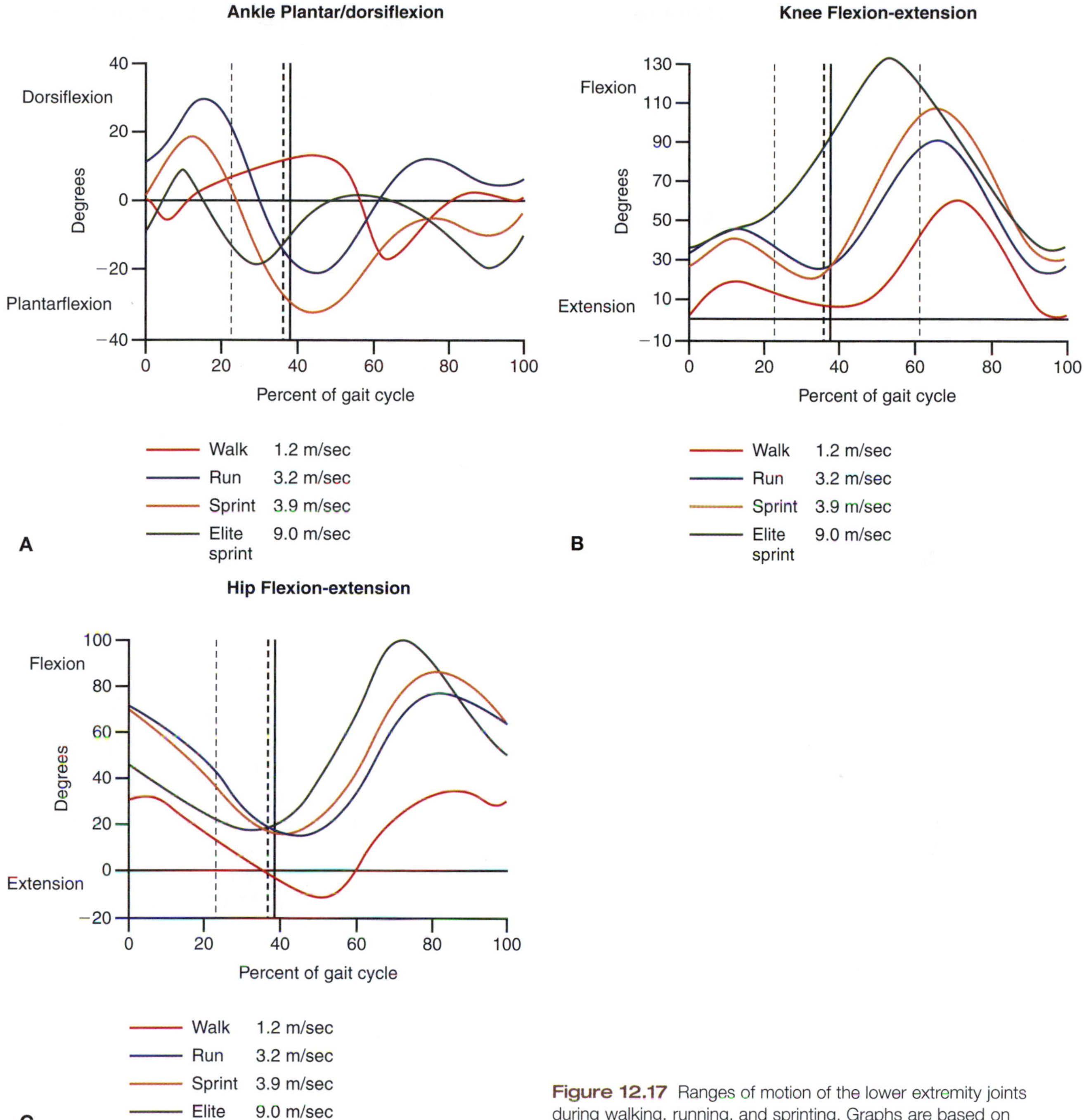

Figure 12.17 Ranges of motion of the lower extremity joints during walking, running, and sprinting. Graphs are based on Mann and Inman.[64]

the adductors work eccentrically to stabilize the body over the limb as the contralateral limb is swinging past the stance limb. During midswing, the limb begins to adduct as, in the final moments of swing, it positions the limb for an adducted landing to bring the base of support under the body's COM. The hip adductors are also active during the swing phase in running, working concentrically to move the femur toward the midline; essentially, these muscles are active throughout the entire running gait cycle.[138] The hip abductors are active during initial contact and immediately thereafter to help stabilize the hip when the foot strikes the ground.[138]

It is thought that the hamstrings' primary function during running occurs at the hip.[138] The gluteus

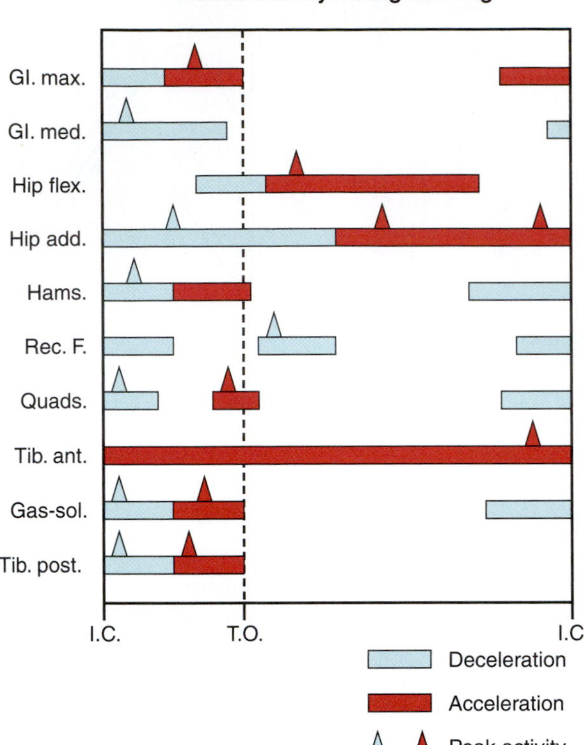

Figure 12.18 Muscle activity during running. Based on investigations of Kunz and Kaufmann,[136] Thordarson,[137] Dugan and Bhat,[138] Novachek,[139] McClay and Manuel,[142] and Gazendam and Huf.[145]

maximus and hamstrings are active in hip extension during terminal swing concentrically to provide an extensor thrust for propulsion and, in the first portion of absorption, working eccentrically to absorb the impact forces immediately after initial contact.[139] The hamstrings are active throughout the stance phase in running, acting eccentrically in the first half (absorption) and concentrically at the hip in the second half (propulsion).[138]

Knee Muscle Groups

Timing of quadriceps activity is longer in running than it is during walking. In walking, the quadriceps are active in the last 10% of the swing phase until about 15% into the stance phase at the end of loading response, whereas in running, the quads function from the last 20% of swing phase until the end of absorption phase.[137] An even greater duration of quadriceps activity occurs in sprinting with this muscle group remaining active during 80% of stance and the entire terminal swing phase.[137] The quadriceps peaks twice during running gait. The first activity burst occurs eccentrically at the start of the absorption phase and the second begins at the end of propulsion after toe-off, continuing into initial swing.[48] It is believed that the quadriceps provides more negative (absorption) work than positive (propulsion) work.[142] Since it is most active during the first half of stance, this is a likely conclusion.

The rectus femoris portion of the quadriceps has a dual responsibility during the first phase of stance during running. One role is to flex the hip to control the height of the body's COM, and the other role is to eccentrically control the amount of knee flexion when the COM is posterior to the knee joint.[138]

Although the hamstrings work concentrically as a hip extensor during propulsion phase, it is also active at the knee. The hamstrings assist the quadriceps in knee stabilization during the absorption phase of running, and they continue in this responsibility, cocontracting with the quadriceps as the COM moves forward of the knee joint.[138]

Ankle and Foot Muscle Groups

Of all the muscle groups involved in walking and running, the greatest changes in output and responsibility occur in the ankle muscle groups. These muscles are divided into anterior and posterior or calf compartment muscle groups. The calf group is active during the last half of stance during walking, but during running this group is active during the first 80% of stance until toe-off and the last 25% of swing.[137] During the propulsive phase of stance, the calf muscles generate an equivalent tension of up to 250% of body weight.[137] During the absorption phase immediately after initial contact, the posterior calf muscle group works eccentrically to provide ankle stability and control forward progression of the tibia that is produced by momentum and possible anterior compartment activity.[138] Once the limb moves into the propulsion phase, the posterior muscles concentrically contract to provide the power needed to move the leg and body forward. If the runner is sprinting on the toes, the intrinsic muscles will also be active to stabilize the foot during this phase.[146] As soon as the foot leaves the ground, the posterior muscles stop working and the anterior muscles take over. In contrast with the quadriceps, the gastrocnemius-soleus is thought to produce more positive than negative work.[142] Since it produces forces equivalent to 250% of the body's weight during the propulsive phase, this is a reasonable conclusion. During walking, the role of the posterior muscles appears to be to move the body horizontally but during running, there is more vertical propulsion.

The anterior compartment muscle group also changes its timing and responsibility from walking to running. During walking these muscles work concentrically from preswing and throughout swing to initial contact when it fires eccentrically to control the foot descent to the floor. However, during running, they work concentrically at the ankle following initial contact to stabilize the foot and possibly accelerate the tibia over the fixed foot to maintain or increase velocity.[138] Once the limb is in swing, the ankle remains in dorsiflexion throughout the swing phase by concentric contraction of the anterior muscles; in essence, the tibialis anterior remains active throughout the running cycle.

Since the limb is in an adducted position relative to the body's COM at initial contact, the subtalar joint moves from its initial position of inversion immediately to eversion when the foot hits the ground. The subtalar joint's change of position occurs passively because of the relationship between the point of contact with the ground and the body's COM; however, this eversion movement is controlled by an eccentric contraction of the tibialis posterior[142] and assisted by the gastrocnemius-soleus.[138]

Kinetics of Running

Kinetics involves the study of the forces that cause motion. There are internal and external forces produced when an individual runs. The internal forces are those produced by the body and its muscles and inert tissues such as ligaments and tendons; the external force we are primarily concerned about is gravity. Because of gravity, whether walking or running, ground reaction forces occur. Internal and ground reaction forces are briefly presented here.

Internal Forces

The purpose of running is to move the body quickly from one point to another. Since we are dealing with time as a factor relative to gait, power is the force element involved. Based on Novacheck,[139] the primary power sources used to produce forward propulsion in running include:

1. Hip extensor muscles working during late swing and early stance;
2. Hip flexors working after toe off; and
3. Quadriceps, gluteus medius, and plantarflexors working throughout stance.

In other words, the most important muscle groups producing power for running comprise the hip flexors, extensors, abductors, knee extensors, and gastrocnemius-soleus groups. Each of them is responsible for providing power at specific times within the gait cycle to allow an individual to run. During the first part of stance when the COM is behind the foot, the gluteus maximus and hamstrings must extend the hip to move the body forward. Once the COM moves over and past the foot, the quadriceps extends the knee and calf muscles plantarflex the ankle to continue to propel the body forward by pushing it ahead. The hip abductors may provide additional efficiency by keeping the pelvis stabilized laterally and perhaps provide additional lift.[139] The hip flexors then accelerate the hip forward and into the swing phase. As speed increases, the power produced by these muscles also increases.

Propelling the body like a spring utilizes the stretch reflex and provides additional energy during tendon and muscle recoil.[139] When a muscle stretches as it does during eccentric activity, most of the energy is absorbed by the tendons, so when the motion is reversed and the musculotendinous unit shortens, the tendon produces the majority of the work. In essence, there is absorption of potential energy during the eccentric phase and release of the energy as power during the concentric phase. You can liken the musculotendinous unit working to a spring: When the musculotendinous unit is stretched (like the Achilles during the absorption phase), it gains energy and then suddenly releases it during the propulsion phase as the ankle moves into rapid plantarflexion. A spring that is compressed and a tendon that is stretched both gain energy, and they each use that energy to add to their desired motion to create a stronger, more powerful effect.

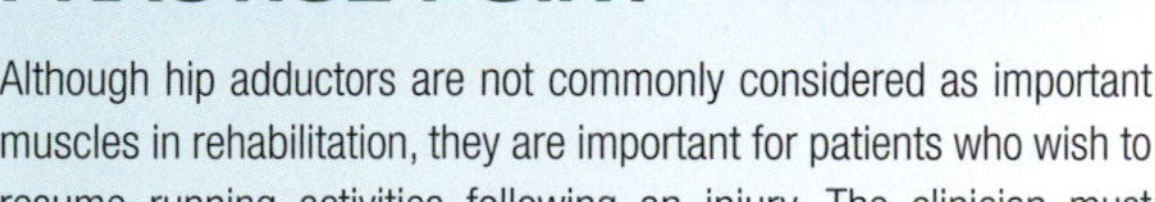

PRACTICE POINT

Although hip adductors are not commonly considered as important muscles in rehabilitation, they are important for patients who wish to resume running activities following an injury. The clinician must understand both the important role hip adductors play in the running cycle and the continuous activity requirements throughout the running cycle of this muscle group.

It should be noted that the contributions of the upper limbs to running have not been addressed in this unit. There is very little information available on the upper extremity role in running, and the information that is available is neither conclusive nor concordant. Some investigators indicate that the arms provide lift during running whereas others state that they provide a more constant horizontal velocity by counterbalancing rotation of the lower extremities.[139] Unfortunately, the data are not yet available to provide any significant information.

Ground Reaction Forces

When the foot contacts the ground, the body adheres to the Newton's Third Law of Motion regarding the forces of action and reaction: For every action, there is an opposite and equal reaction. Therefore, when the foot impacts with the ground, the ground pushes back with an equal force in every direction exactly opposite to those forces imparted to the ground by the foot. The greatest force imparted to the ground by the foot is a downward or vertical force. Similar to initial contact in walking as discussed earlier in this chapter, there is also a lateral-medial force and a fore-aft force applied during running. There is considerably more vertical ground reaction force applied during running than there is during walking because the body leaves the ground in running to create a type of bouncing contact with the ground at initial impact.[147]

You may recall from the earlier walking section that the ground reaction force (GRF) during walking creates a double bump configuration in the vertical forces applied to the body. There is also a double bump pattern seen in running GRFs, but the shape is different. There is a small impact force peak associated with initial contact within the first 20% of stance, and this is followed by a larger and longer impact during the propulsion phase.[138] The propulsive phase has a greater vertical force than the first vertical GRF impact; this greater impact force is created by the significantly greater forces generated for propulsion than for absorption. The magnitudes are also different between running and walking. The walking impact forces range from 1.3 to 1.5 times the body weight whereas the peak impact forces during running may increase to 2 to 3 times body weight.[141] Figure 12.19 compares the vertical ground reaction forces of walking and running.

Medial-lateral ground reaction forces and fore-aft ground reaction forces also occur during running. As during walking, the magnitude of these forces are minimal compared to the vertical ground reaction force. These GRFs in both fore-aft and medial-lateral directions are also comparable in magnitude to those forces created during walking.[141]

Summary

This chapter describes our most common functional movements: maintaining a stable stance posture, walking, and running. First, stance is defined and described in terms of how the body segments are balanced and efficiently counteract the ever-present force of gravity. The automatic minute postural adjustments that we make in order to stay standing are summarized. Gait terminology is then reviewed at length. In keeping with the organizational framework of this text, gait, as a functional movement, is described in both kinematic and kinetic terms. Changes in gait over the course of a life span are discussed. Challenges to gait efficiency and the functional consequences of impaired gait are described. The kinematics of running and sprinting are described and contrasted with walking.

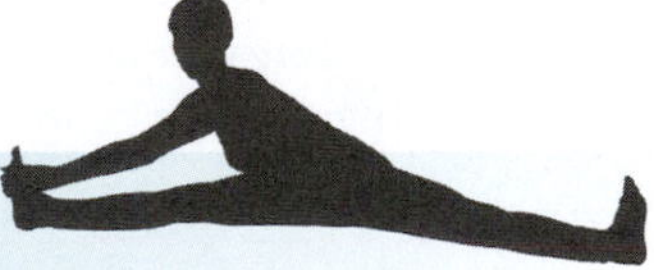

PRACTICE POINT

Ground reaction forces encountered by runners can be modified by shoe wear. Careful selection of proper shoes for the specific foot of the runner, his or her running style, and the running surface must all be taken into consideration when selecting a running shoe. Shoe wear will also alter ground reaction forces impacted on the body. Shoes that are worn out and no longer provide adequate support or are unable to withstand impact forces of running may be a source of injury for the runner. Although proper shoe selection is beyond the scope of this text, several other sources are available to guide and instruct in this pursuit.[148–150]

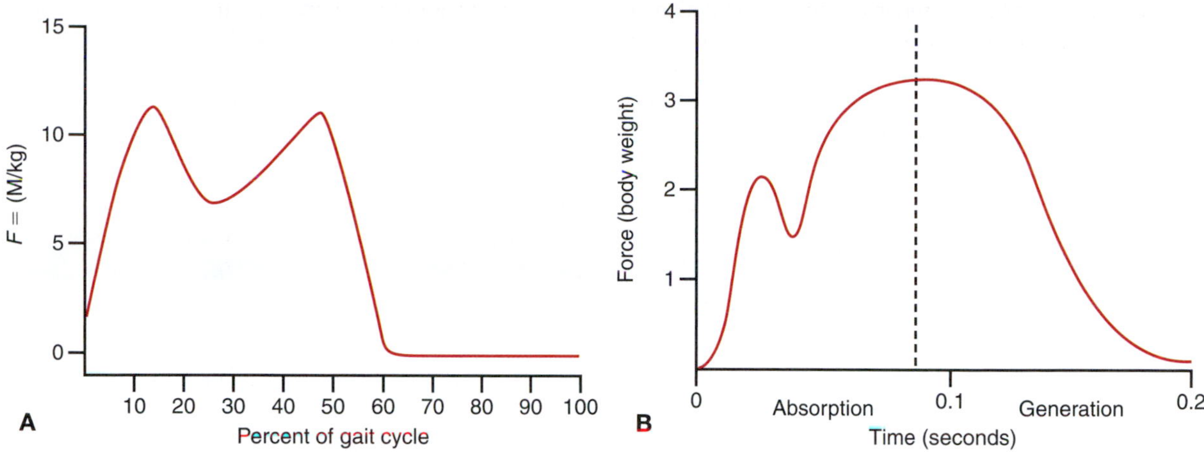

Figure 12.19 Comparison of vertical ground reaction forces in A) walking and B) running.

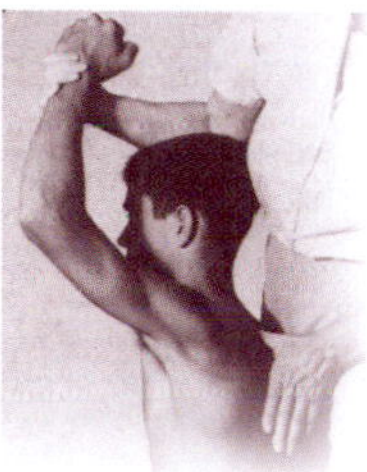

CLINICAL SCENARIO SOLUTION

Morgan's experience tells her that she must use specific key cues that will help Cody resume a normal walking gait. She also knows the maximum ranges of motion that each lower limb joint must have to ambulate normally, so before she instructs him in normal gait she must assess his hip, ankle, and knee joints for their mobility. Cody is anxious to resume running, so Morgan must explain to him the qualities he must have in his walking gait and the amount of additional motion his joints must have before he is able to advance to running.

Discussion Questions

1. How does the balance of forces around each body segment contribute to an effective but efficient control of stance posture?
2. How does the use of conventional gait terminology contribute to clinical gait analysis and intervention with clients?
3. How would you compare and contrast traditional gait terminology and RLA terminology? What are the unique benefits of each?
4. What are the main functional tasks associated with each phase of gait?
5. In what main ways does gait change over the course of the life span?
6. How do common impairments affect the functional efficiency of the daily task of walking?
7. Explain how the body propels itself during running. How do the key factors producing power provide the desired results of running?
8. What muscles are active throughout the running gait? Identify their functions.
9. What muscle groups perform similarly during walking, running, and sprinting? What differences do they display between the three different types of gait?
10. When during the running cycle do muscles perform most of their activity? What type of muscle activity is generally demonstrated during these phases and why?

11. Based on the clinical scenario and the solution presented, identify what ranges of motion are required for the ankle, knee, and hip joints for normal gait. If Cody is a distance runner who runs at an 8-minute mile, estimate what motions these joints must have for him to resume running. If Cody had sufficient strength and motions but was apprehensive about bearing weight on the right lower limb when he walked without crutches, how would his gait appear? How would his gait appear if he had knee motion that measured 10° to 45°?

Lab Activities

1. Using Figure 12.1, perform a postural analysis, viewing your lab partner from an anterior, posterior, and sagittal view and using a plumb line to represent the line of gravity.
2. When walking as slowly as possible, name the eight subphases of the gait cycle as you go though one cycle. Concentrate on the functional task associated with that subphase and the range of motion and muscular requirements needed to accomplish the needed task.
3. Observational Gait Analysis: Using Table 12–4, the following approach will offer you an opportunity to practice and refine an observational gait analysis strategy. First of all, observational analysis of any movement must be performed in a well-lit area devoid of obstacles, on a flat flooring surface, with the observed either in bare feet or wearing comfortable shoes.
   The following guidelines are offered:
   a. Observe the individual walking in a well-lit area devoid of obstacles, either in bare feet or wearing comfortable shoes and using an assistive device, if prescribed;
   b. Observation should be of several strides, a distance of several meters with the observer standing at the middle of this distance in order to focus on typical walking and not on either the acceleration or deceleration portions of the walk;
   c. Observe from a sagittal view and a frontal view, right and left sides, anterior and posterior;
   d. Observe in a systematic fashion starting at the head and neck, and moving to the trunk, the upper extremities, the pelvis, the hip, knee, and ankle/foot, as described in Table 12–4, using the series of questions as a guide in performing an observational gait analysis.
4. Analysis of the motions of normal walking and identification of abnormal gait deviations require the development of skill in selectively focusing on one joint or segment at a time in a rapid manner to cover all extremities and trunk. This skill can be also be practiced by watching a subject walking on a treadmill. Workings in groups of three to five, analyze each person's gait in the group. For each analysis, the observers should view from the side, in the sagittal plane, and from behind in the frontal plane. If a suitable overhead platform is available, the subject may be observed from above in the transverse plane. Observe and list all the gait deviations you see, even if they are subtle. Focus on the following parts of the body:
   a. Top of the head to see the vertical and lateral oscillations.
   b. In the sagittal plane, observe the near side hip motions, then the knee, then the ankle, and then the toes.
   c. Go to the opposite side of the treadmill to view the motions of the other leg.
   d. In the frontal plane, viewing from the back, observe the normal hip drop during the period of single limb support and then observe pronation and supination of the foot.
   e. Rotations of the hip and knee are best viewed from the front but are often obscured by the treadmill.
   f. Have the subject remove their shoes and walk on the treadmill.
5. Keeping the same groups as in #4, have each person run on a treadmill, with and without shoes. Make observations similar to those listed in #4. Identify deviations in running patterns and compare those to the ones found when the subject was walking. Do the deviations found in walking become diminished or exaggerated when the subject runs? Have the group rationalize why this is the case.
6. Toward the end of the class session, each group presents a case study of a member of the group to the class, identifying gait deviations and when they occur during the gait cycle in walking and running. It may be that more than one subject from each group has a deviation that should be identified to the class.

References

1. Clark JE. Dynamical systems perspective on gait. In Craik RB, Oatis CA (eds): *Gait Analysis: Theory and Application*. St. Louis: Mosby, 1995, pp 79–86.
2. DeLisa JA. Gait Analysis in the Science of Rehabilitation. Washington, DC: Veterans Health Administration/Diane Publishing, 1998.
3. Danis CG, Krebs DE, Gill-Body KM, Sahrmann SA. Relationship between standing posture and stability. *Physical Therapy* 78(5):502–517, 1998.
4. Hytönen M, Pyykkö I, Aalto H, Starck J. Postural control and age. *Acta Oto-Laryngologica* 113(1–2):119–122, 1993.
5. Woollacott MH. Posture and gait from newborn to elderly. In Amblard B, Berthoz G, Clarac F (eds): *Posture and Gait*. Amsterdam: Excerpta Medica, 1988, pp 3–13.
6. Taguchi K, Tada C. Change of body sway with growth in children. In Amblard B, Berthoz G, Clarac F (eds): *Posture and Gait*. Amsterdam: Excerpta Medica, 1988, pp 177–186.
7. Crilly RG, Delaquerrière Richardson L, Roth JH, Vandervoort AA, Hayes KC, Mackenzie RA. Postural stability and Colles' fracture. *Age and Aging* 16(3):133–138, 1987.
8. Pyykkö I, Jäntti P, Aalto H. Postural control in elderly subjects. *Age and Aging* 19(3):215–221. 1990.
9. Lord SF, Clark RD, Webster OW. Visual acuity and contrast sensitivity in relation to falls in an elderly population. *Age and Aging* 20:175, 1991.
10. Joseph J. *Man's Posture: Electromyographic Studies*. Springfield, IL: Charles C Thomas, 1960.
11. Smith JW. The forces operating at the human ankle joint during standing. *Journal of Anatomy* 91(4):545–564, 1957.
12. Åkerblom B. *Standing and Sitting Posture*. Stockholm: Nordiska Bokhandeln, 1948.
13. Joseph J, Nightingale A. Electromyography of muscles of posture: Thigh muscles in males. *Journal of Physiology* 126(1):81–85, 1954.
14. Basmajian JV. *Muscles Alive: Their Function Revealed by Electromyography*, ed 4. Baltimore: Williams & Wilkins, 1978.
15. Umphred D. *Neurological Rehabilitation*, ed 4. St. Louis: Mosby, 2001.
16. Frank J, Earl M. Coordination of posture and movement. *Physical Therapy* 70(12):855–863, 1990.
17. Horak F. Clinical measurement of postural control in adults. *Physical Therapy* 67(12):1881–1885, 1987.
18. Emery C. Management disorders of postural control and balance. In Bertoti DB (eds): *Functional Neurorehabilitation Through the Life Span*. Philadelphia: F A Davis, 2004, pp 267–294.
19. Allum JH, Bloem B, Carpenter MG, Hullinger M, Hadders-Algra M. Proprioceptive control of posture: A review of new concepts. *Gait & Posture* 8(3):214–242, 1998.
20. Perry J. *Gait Analysis: Normal and Pathological Function*. Thorofare, NJ: Slack, Inc, 1992.
21. Winter DA. *Biomechanics and Motor Control of Human Gait*, ed 2. Waterloo, ON, Canada: University of Waterloo Press, 1991.
22. Craik RB, Oatis CA (eds). *Gait Analysis: Theory and Application*. St. Louis: Mosby, 1995.
23. Carr R, Shepherd J. *Neurological Rehabilitation: Optimizing Motor Performance*. Oxford: Butterworth Heinemann, 1998.
24. Bertoti DB. *Functional Neurorehabilitation through the Life Span*. Philadelphia: FA Davis, 2004.
25. Seeley MK, Umberger BR, Shapiro R. A test of the functional asymmetry hypothesis in walking. *Gait & Posture* 28(1):24–28, 2008.
26. Archer KR, Castillo RC, Mackenzie EJ, Bosse MJ. Gait symmetry and walking speed analysis following lower-extremity trauma. *Physical Therapy* 86(12):1630–1640, 2006.
27. Lin C, Gross MT, Weinhold P. Ankle syndesmosis injuries: Anatomy, biomechanics, mechanism of injury, and clinical guidelines for diagnosis and intervention. *Journal of Orthopaedic and Sports Physical Therapy* 36:372–384, 2006.
28. Murray MP. Gait as a total pattern of movement. *American Journal of Physical Medicine* 46(1):290–333, 1967.
29. Larsson LE, Odenrick P, Sandlund B, Weitz P, Oberg PA. The phases of the stride and their interaction in human gait. *Scandinavian Journal of Rehabilitation Medicine* 12(3):107–112, 1980.
30. Inman VT, Ralston HJ, Todd F. *Human Walking*. Baltimore: Williams & Wilkins, 1981.
31. Ustün TB, Chatterji S, Bickenbach J, Kostanjsek N, Schneider M. The International Classification of Functioning, Disability and Health: A new tool for understanding disability and health. *Disability and Rehabilitation* 25:565–571, 2003.
32. Robinett CS, Vondran MA. Functional ambulation velocity and distance requirements in rural and urban communities: A clinical report. *Physical Therapy* 68(9):1371–1373, 1988.
33. Neumann DA. *Kinesiology of the Musculoskeletal System: Foundations for Physical Rehabilitation.* St. Louis: Mosby, 2002.

34. Smidt GL. Hip motion and related factors in walking. *Physical Therapy* 51(1):9–22, 1971.

35. Mann RA, Hagy JL. The function of the toes in walking, jogging, and running. *Clinical Orthopaedics and Related Research* 142:24–29, 1979.

36. Eberhart HD, Inman VT, Bresler B. The principle elements in human locomotion. In Klopsteg PE, Wilson PD (eds): *Human Limbs and Their Substitutes*. New York: McGraw-Hill, 1954, pp 437–471.

37. Saunders JB, Inman VT, Eberhart HD. The major determinants in normal and pathological gait. *Journal of Bone and Joint Surgery Am* 35(3):543–558, 1953.

38. Kuo AD. The six determinants of gait and the inverted pendulum analogy: A dynamic walking perspective. *Human Movement Science* 26(4):617–656, 2007.

39. deAsla RJ, Wan L, Rubash HE, Li G. Six DOF in vivo kinematics of the ankle joint complex: Application of a combined dual-orthogonal fluoroscopic and magnetic resonance imaging technique. *Journal of Orthopaedic Research* 24(5):1019–1027, 2006.

40. Arndt A, Westblad P, Winson I, Hashimoto T, Lundberg A. Ankle and subtalar kinematics measured with intracortical pins during the stance phase of walking. *Foot & Ankle International* 25(5):357–364, 2004.

41. Lundgren P, Nester C, Liu A, et al. Invasive in vivo measurement of rear-, mid- and forefoot motions during walking. *Gait & Posture* 28(1):93–100, 2008.

42. Chan CW, Rudins A. Foot biomechanics during walking and running. *Mayo Clinic Proceedings* 69(5):448–461, 1994.

43. Elftman H. Measurement of external force in walking. *Science* 88(2276):152–153, 1938.

44. Basmajian JV, DeLuca CJ. *Muscles Alive: Their Functions Revealed by Electromyography,* ed 5. Baltimore: Williams & Wilkins, 1985.

45. Chang WN, Lipton JS, Tsirikos AI, Miller F. Kinesiological surface electromyography in normal children: Range of normal activity and pattern. *Journal of Electromyography and Kinesiology* 17(4):437–445, 2007.

46. Sutherland DH. The evolution of clinical gait analysis. Part I: Kinesiological EMG. *Gait & Posture* 14(1):61–70, 2001.

47. Winter DA. Concerning the scientific basis for the diagnosis of pathological gait and for rehabilitation protocols. *Physiotherapy Canada* 37:245–252, 1985.

48. Ounpuu S. The biomechanics of walking and running. *Clinics in Sports Medicine* 13(4):843–863, 1994.

49. Cimolin V, Galli M, Romkes J, et al. Quantification of upper limb movements during gait in healthy subjects and in patients with cerebral palsy. *Gait & Posture* 24S:S242–S244, 2006.

50. Lee D. *The Pelvic Girdle*. Edinburgh: Churchill Livingstone, 1989.

51. Hinrichs RN. Whole body movement: Coordination of arms and legs in walking and running. In Winters JM, Woo SL (eds): *Multiple Muscle Systems*. New York: Springer-Verlag, 1990, pp 694–705.

52. Ortega JD, Fehlman LA, Farley CT. Effects of aging and arm swing on the metabolic cost of stability in human walking. *Journal of Biomechanics* 41(16):3303–3308, 2008.

53. Hogue RE. Upper extremity muscular activity at different cadences and inclines during normal gait. *Physical Therapy* 49(9):963–972, 1969.

54. Anderson GBJ, Winters JM. Role of muscle in postural tasks: Spinal loading response and postural stability. In Winters JM, Woo SL (eds): *Multiple Muscle Systems*. New York: Springer-Verlag, 1990, pp 377–395.

55. Sheffield FJ. Electromyographic study of the abdominal muscles in walking and other movements. *American Journal of Sports Medicine* 41:142–147, 1962.

56. Waters RL, Morris JM. Electrical activity of muscles of the trunk during walking. *Journal of Anatomy* 111:191–199, 1962.

57. Winter D, Ruder GK, MacKinnon DC. Control of balance of upper body during gait. In Winters JM, Woo SL (eds): *Multiple Muscle Systems*. New York: Springer-Verlag, 1990, pp 534–541.

58. Krebs DE, Wong D, Jevsevar D, Riley PO, Hodge WA. Trunk kinematics during locomotor activities. *Physical Therapy* 72:505–514, 1992.

59. Paré EB, Stern JT, Jr., Swartz JM. Functional differentiation within the tensor fasciae latae. *Journal of Bone and Joint Surgery Am* 63(9):1457–1471, 1981.

60. Kapandji IA. *The Physiology of the Joints, Vol 2, Lower Limb*, ed 5. Edinburgh: Churchill Livingstone, 1987.

61. Knutson LM, Soderberg GL. EMG: Use and interpretation in gait. In Craik RL, Oatis CA (eds): *Gait Analysis: Theory and Application*. St. Louis: Mosby, 1995.

62. Gottschall JS, Kram R. Energy cost and muscular activity required for propulsion during walking. *Journal of Applied Physiology* 94(5):1766–1772, 2003.

63. Kaye RA, Jahss MH. Tibialis posterior: A review of anatomy and biomechanics in relation to support of the medial longitudinal arch. *Foot & Ankle* 11(4):244–247, 1991.

64. Mann R, Inman VT. Phasic activity of intrinsic muscles of the foot. *Journal of Bone and Joint Surgery Am* 46:469, 1964.

65. Marey EJ. *Animal Mechanism: A Treatise on Terrestrial and Aerial Locomotion*. New York: D Appleton and Co, 1890.

66. Muybridge E. *The Human Figure in Motion*. New York: Dover Publications, 1955.

67. Muybridge E. *Animals in Motion*. New York: Dover Publications, 1957.

68. Baker R. The history of gait analysis before the advent of modern computers. *Gait & Posture* 26(3):331–342, 2007.

69. Gage JR. *Gait Analysis in Cerebral Palsy*. London: MacKeith Press, 1991.

70. Gage JR. The clinical use of kinetics for evaluation of pathologic gait in cerebral palsy. *Instructional Course Lectures* 44:507–515, 1995.

71. Barrack RL, Lund PJ, Skinner HB. Knee joint proprioception revisited. *Journal of Sport Rehabilitation* 3:18–42, 1994.

72. Braune W, Fischer O. *On the Centre of Gravity of the Human Body*. Berlin: Springer-Verlag, 1984.

73. Braune W, Fischer O. *The Human Gait*. Berlin: Springer-Verlag, 1987.

74. Kadaba MP, Ramakrishnan HK, Wootten ME. Measurement of lower extremity kinematics during level walking. *Journal of Orthopaedic Research* 8(3):383–392, 1990.

75. Sutherland DH. The evolution of clinical gait analysis. Part III: Kinetics and energy assessment. *Gait & Posture* 21:447–461, 2005.

76. Vaughan CL, Davis BL, O'Connor JC. *Dynamics of Human Gait*, ed 2. Cape Town, South Africa: Kiboho Publishers, 1999.

77. Churchill AJ, Halligan PW, Wade DT. RIVCAM: A simple video-based kinematic analysis for clinical disorders of gait. *Computer Methods and Programs in Biomedicine* 69(3):197–209, 2002.

78. Russell TG, Jull GA, Wootton R. The diagnostic reliability of internet-based observational kinematic gait analysis. *Journal of Telemedicine and Telecare* 9(Suppl 2):S48–S51, 2003.

79. Sutherland DH. The role of the ankle plantar flexors in normal walking. *Journal of Bone and Joint Surgery Am* 62:354–363, 1980.

80. Sutherland DH. The evolution of clinical gait analysis. Part III—Kinetics and energy assessment. *Gait & Posture,* 21(4):447–461, 2005.

81. Watelain E, Froger J, Rousseaux M, et al. Variability of video-based clinical gait analysis in hemiplegia as performed by practitioners in diverse specialties. *Journal of Rehabilitation Medicine* 37(5):317–324, 2005.

82. Wyatt MP. Gait in children. In Smidt G (ed): *Gait in Rehabilitation*. New York: Churchill Livingstone, 1990.

83. Nymark JR, Balmer SJ, Melis EH, Lemaire ED, S. M. Electromyographic and kinematic nondisabled gait differences at extremely slow overground and treadmill walking speeds. *Journal of Rehabilitation Research and Development* 42(4):523–534, 2005.

84. Riley PO, Dicharry J, Franz J, Croce UD, Wilder RP, Kerrigan DC. A kinematics and kinetic comparison of overground and treadmill running. *Medicine & Science in Sport & Exercise* 40(6):1093–1100, 2008.

85. Burnett CN, Johnson EW. Development of gait in childhood. II. *Developmental Medicine and Child Neurology* 13(2):207–215, 1971.

86. Burnett CN, Johnson EW. Development of gait in childhood. I. Method. *Developmental Medicine and Child Neurology* 13(2):196–206, 1971.

87. Sutherland DH, Olshen R, Cooper L, Woo SL. The development of mature gait. *Journal of Bone and Joint Surgery* 62:336–353, 1980.

88. Sutherland DH, Olshen RA, Biden EN, Wyatt MP. *The Development of Mature Walking*. Philadelphia: JB Lippincott, 1988.

89. Shumway-Cook A, Woollancott MH. *Motor Control: Translating Research into Clinical Practice*, ed 3. Philadelphia: Lippincott, Williams & Wilkins, 2007.

90. Bril B, Breniere Y. Posture and independent locomotion in childhood: Learning to walk or learning dynamic posture control? In Savelsbergh GJP (ed): *The Development of Coordination in Infancy*. Amsterdam: North Holland, 1993, pp 337–358.

91. Gabell A, Nayak US. The effect of age on variability in gait. *Journal of Gerontology* 39(6):662–666, 1984.

92. Winter DA, Patla AE, Rietdyk S, Ishac MG. Ankle muscle stiffness in the control of balance during quiet standing. *Journal of Neurophysiology* 85(6):2630–2633, 2001.

93. Woollancott M. Gait and postural control in the aging adult. In Savelsbergh GJP (ed): *The Development of Coordination in Infancy*. Amsterdam: North Holland, 1993 pp 327–336.

94. Bendall MJ, Bassey EJ, Pearson MB. Factors affecting walking speed of elderly people. *Age and Aging* 18(5):327–332, 1989.

95. Hausdorff JM, Nelson ME, Kaliton D, et al. Etiology and modification of gait instability in older adults: A randomized controlled trial of exercise. *Journal of Applied Physiology* 90(6):2117–2129, 2001.

96. Gard SA, Childress DS. What determines the vertical displacement of the body during normal walking? *Journal of Prosthetics and Orthotics* 13(3):64–69, 2001.

97. Kerrigan DC, Croce UD, Marciello M, Riley PO. A refined view of the determinants of gait: Significance of heel rise. *Archives of Physical Medicine and Rehabilitation* 81(8):1077–1080, 2000.

98. Whittle MW. *Gait Analysis*, ed 4. Philadelphia: Elsevier, 2007.

99. Gard SA, Childress DS. The influence of stance-phase knee flexion on the vertical displacement of the trunk during normal walking. *Archives of Physical Medicine and Rehabilitation* 80(1):26–32, 1999.

100. Crosbie J, Vachalathiti R. Synchrony of pelvic and hip joint motion during walking. *Gait & Posture* 6(3):237–248, 1997.

101. Waters R, Campbell J, Thomas L, Hugos L, Davis P. Energy costs of walking in lower-extremity plaster casts. *Journal of Bone and Joint Surgery* 64A(6):896–899, 1982.

102. Waters RL, Lunsford BR. Energy cost of paraplegic locomotion. *Journal of Bone and Joint Surgery Am* 67(8):1245–1250, 1985.

103. Waters RL, Mulroy S. The energy expenditure of normal and pathologic gait. *Gait & Posture* 9:207–231, 1999.

104. Waters RL, Perry J, Antonelli D, Hislop H. The energy cost of walking of amputees: The influence of level of amputation. *Journal of Bone and Joint Surgery Am* 58(1):42–46, 1976.

105. Cowan MM, Stilling DS, Naumann S, Colborne GR. Quantification of antagonist muscle coactivation in children with spastic diplegia. *Clinical Anatomy* 11(5):314–319, 1998.

106. Mykelbust BM. A review of myotatic reflexes and the development of motor control and gait in infants and children: A special communication. *Physical Therapy* 70(3):188–203, 1990.

107. Olney SJ. *Topics in pediatrics: Lesson 1.* Alexandria, VA: American Physical Therapy Association, 1989.

108. O'Byrne JM, Jenkinson A, O'Brien TM. Quantitative analysis and classification of gait patterns in cerebral palsy using a three-dimensional motion analyzer. *Journal of Child Neurology* 13(3):101–108, 1998.

109. Olney SJ, Costigan PA, Hedden DM. Mechanical energy patterns in gait of cerebral palsied children with hemiplegia. *Physical Therapy* 67(9):1348–1354, 1987.

110. Olney SJ, MacPhail HE, Hedden DM, Boyce WF. Work and power in hemiplegic cerebral palsy gait. *Physical Therapy* 70(7):431–438, 1990.

111. Rose SJ, Gamble JG, Medeiros J, Burgos A, Haskell WL. Energy cost of walking in normal children and in those with cerebral palsy: Comparison of heart rate and oxygen uptake. *Journal of Pediatric Orthopedics* 9(3):276–279, 1989.

112. Campbell J, Ball J. Energetics of walking in cerebral palsy. *Orthopaedic Clinics of North America* 9(2):374–377, 1978.

113. Mossberg KA, Linton KA, Friske K. Ankle-foot orthoses: Effect on energy expenditure of gait in spastic diplegic children. *Archives of Physical Medicine and Rehabilitation* 71(7):490–494, 1990.

114. Mauritz KH. Gait training in hemiplegia. *European Journal of Neurology* 9(Suppl 1):23–29, 2002.

115. Montgomery J. Assessment and treatment of locomotor deficits in stroke. In Duncan P, Badke MB (eds): *Stroke Rehabilitation: The Recovery of Motor Control*. Chicago: Year Book, 1987, pp 223–266.

116. Waters RL, Hislop HJ, Perry J, Antonelli D. Energetics: Application to the study and management of locomotor disabilities. Energy cost of normal and pathological gait. *Orthopaedic Clinics of North America* 9(2):351–356, 1978.

117. Gersten JW, Orr W. External work of walking in hemiparetic patients. *Scandinavian Journal of Rehabilitation Medicine* 3(1):85–88, 1971.

118. O'Sullivan SB, Schmitz TJ (eds). *Physical Rehabilitation,* ed 5. Philadelphia: F.A. Davis, 2007.

119. Halliday SE, Winter DA, Frank JS, Patla AE, Prince F. The initiation of gait in young, elderly, and Parkinson's disease subjects. *Gait & Posture* 8(1):8–14, 1998.

120. Melnick ME, Oremland B. Movement dysfunction associated with cerebellar problems. In Umphred DA (ed): *Neurological Rehabilitation*, ed 4. St. Louis: Mosby, 2001, pp 717–740.

121. Mohr KJ, Kvitne RS, Pink MM, Fideler B, Perry J. Electromyography of the quadriceps in patellofemoral pain with patellar subluxation. *Clinical Orthopaedics and Related Research* 415:261–271, 2003.

122. Young A, Stokes M, Iles JF. Effects of joint pathology on muscle. *Clinical Orthopaedics* 219:21–27, 1987.

123. Powers CM, Perry J, Hsu A, Hislop HJ. Are patellofemoral pain and quadriceps femoris muscle torque associated with locomotor function? *Physical Therapy* 77:1063–1078, 1997.

124. Foley MP, Prax B, Crowell R, Boone T. Effects of assistive devices on cardiorespiratory demands in older adults. *Physical Therapy* 76(12):1313–1319, 1996.

125. Franks CA, Palisano RJ, Darbee JC. The effect of walking with an assistive device and using a wheelchair on school performance in students with myelomeningocele. *Physical Therapy* 71(8):570–577, 1991.

126. Clinkingbeard JR, Gersten JW, Hoehn D. Energy cost of ambulation in the traumatic paraplegic. *American Journal of Physical Medicine* 43:157–165, 1964.

127. Gordon EE, Vanderwalde H. Energy requirements in paraplegic ambulation. *Archives of Physical Medicine and Rehabilitation* 37(5):276–285, 1956.

128. Wright DL, Kemp TL. The dual-task methodology and assessing the attentional demands of ambulation with walking. *Physical Therapy* 72(4):306–312, 1992.

129. Diedrich FJ, Warren WH, Jr. Why change gaits? Dynamics of the walk-run transition. *Journal of Experimental Psychology: Human Perception and Performance* 21(1):183–202, 1995.

130. Perry J. Gait analysis in sports medicine. *Instructional Course Lectures* 39:319–324, 1990.

131. Ishikawa M, Pakaslahti J, Komi PV. Medial gastrocnemius muscle behavior during human walking and running. *Gait & Posture* 25:380–384, 2007.

132. Sasaki K, Neptune RR. Differences in muscle function during walking and running at the same speed. *Journal of Biomechanics* 39(11):2005–2013, 2006.

133. Paróczai R, Kocsis L. Analysis of human walking and running parameters as a function of speed. *Technology and Health Care* 14(4–5):251–260, 2006.

134. Queen RM, Gross MT, Liu H-Y. Repeatability of lower extremity kinetics and kinematics for standardized and self-selected running speeds. *Gait & Posture* 23:282–287, 2006.

135. *Webster's II New College Dictionary,* ed 3. Boston: Houghton Mifflin, 2001.

136. Kunz H, Kaufmann DA. Biomechanical analysis of sprinting: Decathletes versus champions. *British Journal of Sports Medicine* 15(3):177–181, 1981.

137. Thordarson DB. Running biomechanics. *Clinics in Sports Medicine* 16(2):239–247, 1997.

138. Dugan SA, Bhat KP. Biomechanics and analysis of running gait. *Physical Medicine and Rehabilitation Clinics of North America* 16(3):603–621, 2005.

139. Novacheck TF. The biomechanics of running. *Gait & Posture* 7(1):77–95, 1998.

140. Schache AG, Bennell KL, Blanch PD, Wrigley TV. The coordinated movement of the lumbo-pelvic-hip complex during running: A literature review. *Gait & Posture* 10(1):30–47, 1999.

141. Ounpuu S. The biomechanics of running: A kinematic and kinetic analysis. *Instructional Course Lectures* 39:305–318, 1990.

142. McClay I, Manal K. A comparison of three-dimensional lower extremity kinematics during running between excessive pronators and normals. *Clinical Biomechanics* 13(3):195–203, 1998.

143. Cavanagh PR. The biomechanics of lower extremity action in distance running. *Foot & Ankle* 7(4):197–217, 1987.

144. Rodgers MM. Dynamic biomechanics of the normal foot and ankle during walking and running. *Physical Therapy* 68:1822–1830, 1988.

145. Gazendam MGJ, Hof AL. Averaged EMG profiles in jogging and running at different speeds. *Gait & Posture* 25:604–614, 2007.

146. Mann RV. A kinetic analysis of sprinting. *Medicine & Science in Sport & Exercise* 13(5):325–328, 1981.

147. Farley CT, Ferris DP. Biomechanics of walking and running: Center of mass movements to muscle action. *Exercise and Sport Sciences Reviews* 26:253–285, 1998.

148. Enke RC, Laskowski ER, Thomsen KM. Running shoe selection criteria among adolescent cross-country runners. *PM & R: The Journal of Injury, Function, and Rehabilitation* 1(9):816–819, 2009.

149. Heckman B. Selection of a running shoe: If the shoe fits—run. *Journal of Orthopaedic and Sports Physical Therapy* 2(2):65–68, 1980.

150. Yamashita MH. Evaluation and selection of shoe wear and orthoses for the runner. *Physical Medicine and Rehabilitation Clinics of North America* 16(3):801–829, 2005.

151. Blanke DJ, Hageman PA. Comparison of gait of young men and elderly men. *Physical Therapy* 69:144–148, 1988.

152. Hageman PA, Blanke DJ. Comparison of gait of young women and elderly women. *Physical Therapy* 66(9):1382–1387, 1986.

153. Leiper CI, Craik RL. Relationships between physical activity and temporal-distance characteristics of walking in elderly women. *Physical Therapy* 71(11):791–803, 1991.

154. Murray MP, Clarkson BH. The vertical pathways of the foot during level walking. II. Clinical examples of distorted pathways. *Physical Therapy* 46(6):590–599, 1966.

155. Murray MP, Drought AB, Kory RC. Walking patterns of normal men. *Journal of Bone and Joint Surgery Am* 46:335–360, 1964.

156. Murray MP, Kory RC, Clarkson BH. Walking patterns in healthy old men. *Journal of Gerontology.* 1969;24(2):169-178.

157. Murray MP, Kory RC, Sepic SB. Walking patterns of normal women. *Archives of Physical Medicine and Rehabilitation* 51(11):637–650, 1970.

158. Prince F, Corriveau H, Hébert R, Winter DA. Gait in the elderly. *Gait & Posture* 5(2):128–135, 1997.

159. Smidt GL. Aging in gait. In Smidt GL (ed). *Gait in Rehabilitation*. New York: Churchill Livingstone, 1990.

160. Wilder PA. *Developmental changes in the gait patterns of women: A search for control parameters*. Madison, WI: University of Wisconsin, 1992.

161. Winter DA, Patala AE, Frank JS, Walt SE. Biomechanical walking pattern changes in the fit and healthy elderly. *Physical Therapy* 70:340, 1990.

162. Mann RA, Hagy J. Biomechanics of walking, running, and sprinting. *American Journal of Sports Medicine* 8(3): 345–350, 1980.

CHAPTER 13

Kinesiology Applications in Daily Functional Activities

"What we can or cannot do, what we consider possible or impossible, is rarely a function of our true capability. It is more likely a function of our beliefs about who we are."
Anthony Robbins, American author and presenter

CHAPTER OUTLINE

Learning Outcomes
Clinical Scenario
Introduction
Mobility
Floor Mobility: Rolling and Floor-to-Stand
Sit-to-Stand Transfer
Occupational and Daily Activities
Lifting Tasks
Household Tasks
Occupational Tasks
Clinician Activities
Patient Protective Measures: Spotting during Ambulation
Clinician Ergonomics: Manual Resistance
Summary
Clinical Scenario Solution
Discussion Questions
Lab Activities
References

LEARNING OUTCOMES

By the end of this chapter, you should be able to:

- ❑ Perform a kinematic analysis of common functional movements;
- ❑ Describe the kinematics of floor mobility such as rolling and moving to a standing position;
- ❑ Describe the kinematics of a sit-to-stand transfer task;
- ❑ Describe the kinematics of common occupational daily activity such as lifting;
- ❑ Describe the kinematics performed during common household activities such as vacuuming;
- ❑ Describe the kinematics of common work activities such as working at a computer station or working on an assembly line;
- ❑ Describe the kinematics relevant to performing common client protective measures such as spotting during ambulation assistance;
- ❑ Describe the kinematics relevant to the performance of routine clinical activities such as the application of manual resistance.

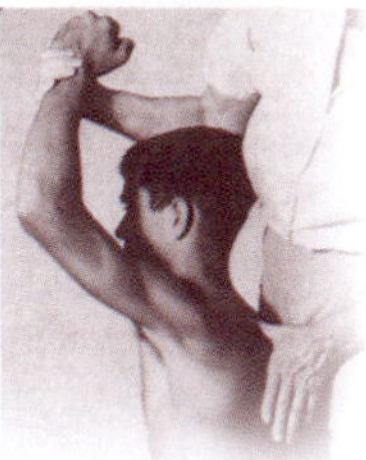

CLINICAL SCENARIO

Juan, a college student, has been working part time in the university library to help pay for his education. He works 20 hours a week, inputting information on a computer for the electronic library. Over the past two weeks, he has been spending a lot of extra hours on his own computer, completing three major reports that are soon due for two courses he is taking this semester. He has noticed that his wrist has recently started hurting after about 30 minutes at the computer. His neck also aches by the end of the day. He cannot afford to either cut back on his work hours or stop doing his homework. He thinks he is doing something wrong either at work or at home but he is not sure. He just knows that he has to fix the problem, whatever it is, before it gets worse.

Introduction

This chapter will describe the kinematics of everyday functional activities. It is provided to guide you in thinking through a kinematic analysis, using and applying your newly acquired kinesiology knowledge to analyze common movements. This chapter does not intend to give you an exhaustive list of the many different daily activities in which all of us engage, but rather offers a few examples to illustrate the process involved in a kinesiological analysis of common activities. By reading through and studying the examples illustrated, you will gain insight into the joint motions and muscle activity requirements needed to produce a movement safely and successfully. Once you develop these skills, you should be able to generalize this skill to any and all activities that you will encounter within your own daily life and to those of the individuals that you will work with in the clinical arena.

Each of these skill analyses will break down the activity into three elements. The first element identifies the sequence of activities performed from the start to the completion of the activity. The second element presents a description of the joint movements throughout the activity. The third and final element distinguishes the muscles and how they function to produce the joint movements to successfully perform the activity.

Mobility

Mobility is important in the ability to move from one position to another and to move the body into positions that permit desired functions. Mobility is basic to function. Without our ability to mobilize the body and its segments, function is extremely limited. In this section, we present basic types of mobility and changes in body position.

Floor Mobility: Rolling and Floor-to-Stand

One of the first mobility activities infants learn is rolling. It is shortly after they acquire that ability that infants learn to crawl and creep, and only a few months from those activities before they progress to standing and then to walking. The progression that humans make in mobility is relatively slow compared to other mammals; however, the activities humans acquire during their progression through the mobility phases are often used throughout the life cycle. Of these activities, rolling and moving to a standing position are the two most frequently used mobility tasks; they are examined in this section.

Rolling

During the development of locomotion, rolling is the earliest pattern used for floor mobility, and it remains a useful mobility skill throughout an individual's lifetime. **Rolling** is defined as moving from supine to prone or from prone to supine, usually involving some amount of trunk rotation. Rolling is a refinement of the righting reaction because as the head rotates, the rest of the body rotates to become realigned with the head. Rolling is an important early locomotor pattern that is used throughout the stages of life because of its obvious relevance to everyday activities such bed mobility and getting up from the floor. Therefore, throughout life, rolling is a meaningful and functional locomotor skill.

During infancy, the development of a mature rolling pattern closely follows the emergence and development of functional movement components. Rolling patterns develop, change, and become refined as the infant exhibits increasing mastery in antigravity extensor and flexor strength. Rolling progresses from a spontaneous motion to a voluntary motion as an infant masters this fundamental movement skill. When rolling first begins, the motion initiates primarily from the head and neck and occurs nonsegmentally using the whole body as one (Fig. 13.1A), but with practice, it becomes a fluid segmental movement pattern with a separation of motions between the pelvis and shoulders[1] (Fig. 13.1B).

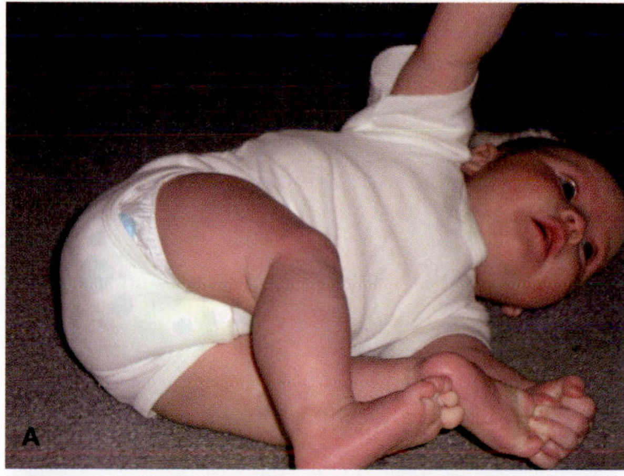

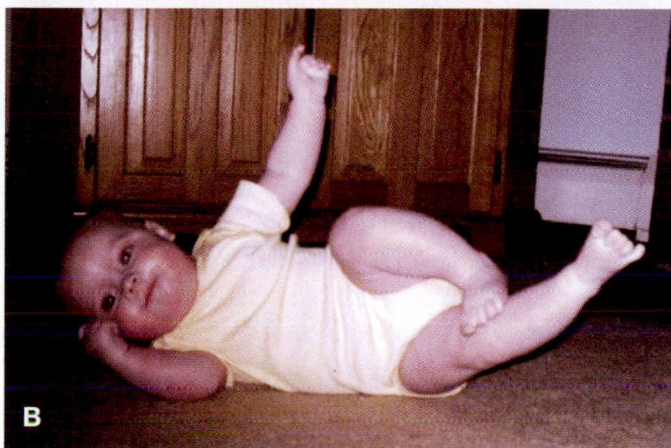

Figure 13.1 Rolling during infancy. A) Nonsegmental. B) Segmental.

During adulthood, rolling patterns are slightly different than they were during infancy and childhood. The most significant differences in adult versus childhood rolling patterns is that during adulthood, rotation and dissociation between the body segments continue to be evident, but the specific pattern used by adults may differ among them, depending on upper body strength versus lower body strength, abdominal and trunk strength, and whether the individual has any limitation in flexibility. Rolling patterns change over the course of adulthood.[2] For example, an age-related change is likely to occur if an individual develops degenerative joint disease with secondary joint pain and inflexibility; in this case, the patient may find it easier to roll like an infant, using a nonsegmental or total body rolling pattern. Variations in the initiation of rolling patterns allow an individual to perform functionally meaningful activities, such as moving to answer the phone or retrieve a glass of water from a bedside table. The ability to roll allows an individual to change position and transfer from supine to sitting on the edge of the bed.

A typical adult rolling pattern from supine to prone is described in the following section. For the sake of ease in reading and consistency, we describe rolling from right to left, although rolling may obviously be performed to either direction. After you study this analysis, you may want to analyze yourself or someone rolling from prone to supine.

Supine to Prone

Of the two movements, rolling supine to prone is more difficult than rolling prone to supine. Although there may be a variety of ways this motion occurs, we will look at only one method. You may choose to explore other possible ways of rolling supine to prone once you have completed this section.

SEQUENCE OF MOVEMENT

There is individual variation in rolling, especially in the initiation of the motion. In this example, we will describe a rolling pattern primarily initiated by the motion of the upper extremity (Fig. 13.2A, B). Other patterns of initiation include the initiation of the motion from the head and neck or from the hip. The rolling sequence to the right starts with the left upper extremity reaching across the body with movement initiated by the humerus and scapula and is immediately followed by the left elbow, wrist, and hand motions. Arm movement is followed by head motion, rotating to the right to look in the direction of motion. Head motion is immediately followed by trunk rotation to the right side. As the trunk rotates, the left hip begins its motion. Just before the body weight moves over the right upper extremity, this limb tucks next to the body to allow the body's rolling to continue unimpeded. Once full rotation to the prone position occurs, body weight rolls towards the left arm as the right upper extremity moves from beneath the body to align into a comfortable position.

JOINT MOTION

The left arm leads by scapular protraction and shoulder flexion and horizontal adduction to move the arm across the anterior trunk. Immediately after the left shoulder complex begins its activity, the left elbow moves toward extension, the forearm pronates with the wrist in neutral, and the fingers and thumb extend and abduct to extend the arm's reach across the body. The right arm prepares to move out of the way of the body roll, so the arm is positioned next to the side; the right shoulder extends next to the side with scapular retraction, the elbow extends with the forearm in midposition, and the wrist and fingers extend. The head turns to the right, the neck rotates and laterally flexes to the right, and the trunk flexes slightly and rotates to the right. As the motion continues, the neck and trunk both move into added

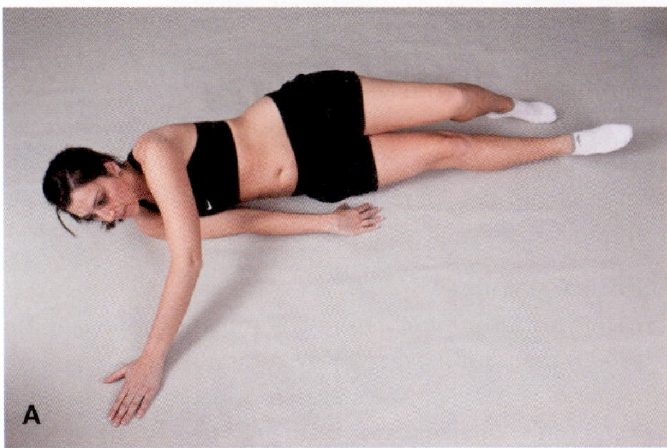

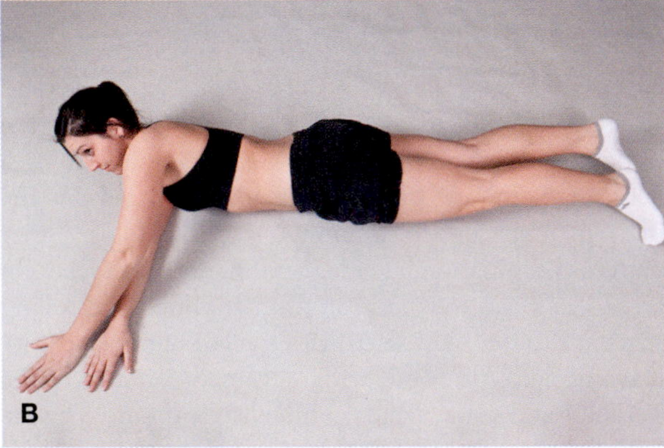

Figure 13.2 Adult rolling from supine to prone.

flexion, rotation and lateral flexion. The left side of the pelvis rotates forward, the left hip flexes and adducts, the knee flexes, and the ankle and foot is either held in neutral or assists by pushing off the floor in neutral or in slight plantarflexion (Fig.13.2A). The right lower limb is in extension throughout the motion. Once the body weight passes over the right arm, the right shoulder moves into flexion accompanied by scapular upward rotation, elbow flexion, and forearm pronation; the wrist and hand assist in controlling the rate of the roll if needed by pushing into the floor in an extended position. Once in side-lying, the left shoulder continues to flex as the neck and upper trunk simultaneously extend to begin to allow the right arm to be cleared and the weight to shift to both upper extremities. The lower extremities follow and the neck and trunk flex with eccentric control into a comfortable prone position (Fig. 13.2B). The neck and back extend to shift the body weight before settling into a relaxed prone position.

MUSCLE ACTIVITY

The left scapula protracts via action of the serratus anterior, upper trapezius, and lower trapezius muscles whereas the glenohumeral joint is flexed by the anterior deltoid, clavicular portion of pectoralis major, and coracobrachialis. As in all upper extremity motions, the rotator cuff muscles work to stabilize the head of the humerus in the glenoid fossa during arm motion. The humerus is also simultaneously horizontally adducted toward the right side by concentric contraction of the anterior deltoid and pectoralis major until the arm passes the body's midline, at which time the posterior deltoid controls the horizontally adducting shoulder by exerting an eccentric contraction against gravity. The elbow extends through action of the triceps and the forearm pronates through the combined efforts of pronator quadratus and pronator teres. The wrist is in slight extension through the efforts of extensor carpi radialis longus and brevis and extensor carpi ulnaris. The fingers are extended by the extensor digitorum and abducted by the dorsal interossei. The thumb extends through the action of extensor pollicis.

The head turns to the right as the neck rotates and laterally flexes to that side through the actions of the left sternocleidomastoid muscle and the right scalene muscles. The trunk flexes against gravity using the power provided by the rectus abdominus and rotates to the right using the right internal abdominal oblique and the left external abdominal oblique. Once the body weight is shifted beyond side-lying, in preparation to accept the body weight, the left shoulder flexes powered by the anterior deltoid, clavicular portion of pectoralis major, and coracobrachialis as the scapula is protracted by the serratus anterior, upper trapezius, and lower trapezius. The elbow and forearm are extended and pronated by the pronator muscles already identified, and the wrist, fingers, and thumb are moved into extension by the extensor carpi ulnaris, extensor carpi radialis longus and brevis, extensor digitorum, and extensor pollicis as the extremity is positioned into a prone prop position to accept the body weight. The fingers are abducted by the dorsal interossei. To complete the motion, the neck and upper trunk are first extended by a concentric contraction of the splenius capitus, splenius cervicus and upper erector spinae. Once the upper extremities are in position, these same muscles contract eccentrically to help settle the neck and back into the prone position with controlled stability.

Floor-to-Stand

The ability to get from the floor to standing requires joint motion and muscle action from the entire body. Just as with rolling, this skill undergoes several changes over the course of the lifespan.[3–6] For example, an infant first accomplishes the task by using the arms to hold on to furniture and pull his or her body up with the arms, first moving to kneeling and then to half-kneeling before moving to full standing. As development continues, the individual rises from the floor to a standing position without using the arms. In our older years, there is often a return to increased need for support. The example here describes the typical sequence that many individuals such as able-bodied college students use to stand up from a seated position on the floor. You may choose to perform the activity as we describe the movement. Let's assume that the starting position is sitting cross-legged on the floor and that the movement to stand is toward the right side.

Sequence of Movement

From a seated position on the floor, the head and trunk stay erect as the lower extremities prepare and the movement is set up; the arms are unengaged. The knees extend in front and the hips stay flexed as the individual assumes a long-sitting position (Fig. 13.3A). As weight is shifted over to the right hip, the right arm supports part of the trunk weight with the hand on the floor as both sets of knees and hips flex with the left leg on top of the right leg in a side-sitting position. This position results in some rotation of the trunk and pelvis (Fig. 13.3B). From this position, the trunk and pelvis rotate further to move both arms into a weight-bearing position and the knees are moved underneath the body to bear the body weight in a quadruped position (Fig. 13.3C). From here, the individual extends the hips, moving to a kneeling position (Fig. 13.3D, E). From kneeling, the weight is shifted to the right knee to place the left foot flat on the floor (Fig. 13.3F, G). The trunk flexes over the left thigh as the left limb extends to lift the body to an erect standing position (Fig. 13.3H, I).

Joint Motion

Throughout the motion, the head and trunk are aligned with each other. From a seated position on the floor, the head and trunk stay upright in neutral as the lower extremities are positioned with the hips flexed at 90° and the knees extended in a long-sitting position (Fig. 13.3A). To initiate the movement sequence, first the weight shifts over the right buttocks as the right arm is placed in extension, medial rotation and some abduction at the right side. The right elbow, wrist, fingers, and thumb are all extended to allow weight-bearing on the extremity. The neck and trunk rotate and laterally flex to the right. The hips may flex a little more and the knees flex to move the body into a side-sitting position. In this position, the left leg is on top of the right leg with the right hip slightly abducted and laterally rotated whereas the left hip is adducted and medially rotated (Fig. 13.3B).

From side-sitting, the trunk rotates over the lower extremities and the body shifts into quadruped with the hips, shoulders, and knees flexed at 90°, the scapula and pelvis stabilized, and the elbows, wrist, fingers, and thumbs all extended (Fig. 13.3C). From quadruped, the

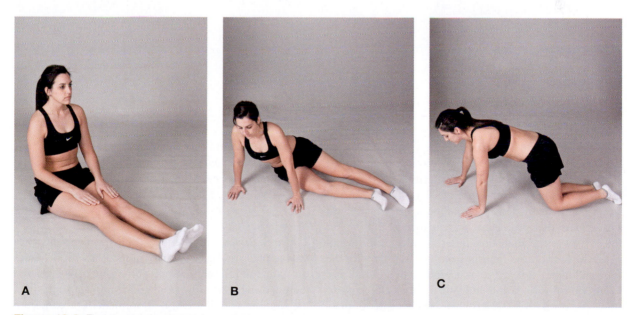

Figure 13.3 Floor-to-stand movement sequence.

Continued

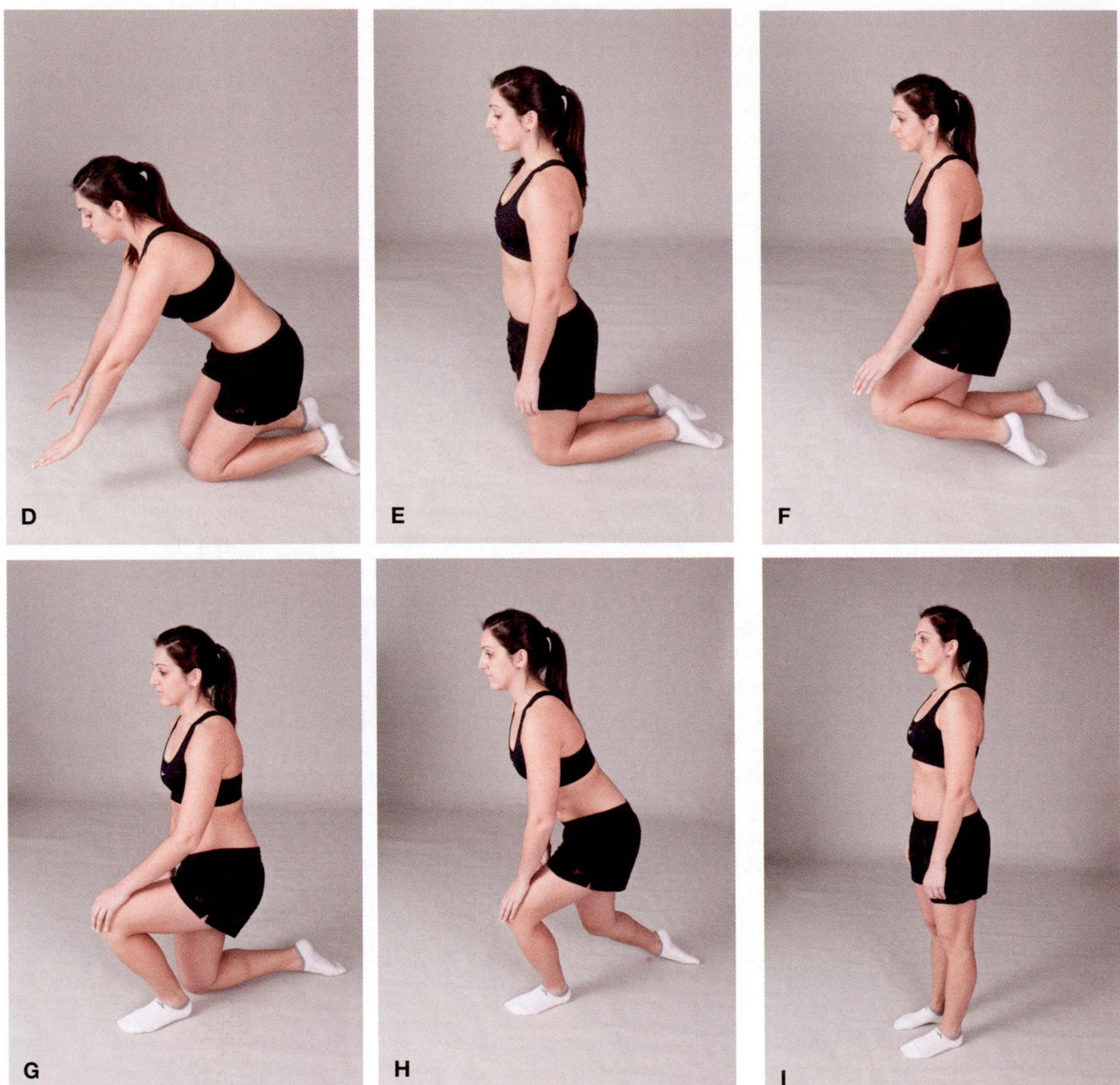

Figure 13.3—cont'd

hips extend as the back remains straight to move the trunk into an upright kneeling position. (Fig. 13.3D, E) When kneeling, the body weight shifts to the right knee, maintaining right hip extension. The neck and trunk are maintained in erect midline alignment. The left hip abducts, then flexes and laterally rotates, and the left knee flexes as the ankle dorsiflexes to move the limb and place the foot on the floor in front of the body with the knee and hip each flexed to or beyond 90° (Fig. 13.3F, G). From this position, the individual flexes the hips to move the trunk over the left knee. As the center of mass moves forward and over the left lower extremity, the left hip and knee extend to lift the body upward and the right hip and knee extend as the body moves to a standing position (Fig. 13.3H, I).

Muscle Activity

The neck flexors and extensors (SCM, scalene and splenius capitus and cervicus) in conjunction with the erector spinae and the abdominals at the trunk cocontract to maintain stability of the head and trunk when sitting in preparation to initiate the movement. Once motion begins to move to side-sitting, the right scapula retracts and depresses through concentric contraction of the rhomboids and middle and lower trapezius. Muscles producing humeral extension, abduction, and medial rotation include latissimus dorsi, teres major, posterior deltoid, middle deltoid, supraspinatus, subscapularis, pectoralis major, teres minor, and infraspinatus. The rotator cuff actively stabilizes the humeral head within the glenoid fossa. The elbow is extended to support the arm via the triceps and the wrist, thumb and fingers extend through action of the extensor carpi ulnaris, extensor carpi radialis longus and brevis, extensor digitorum, and extensor pollicis muscles. The neck laterally flexes a little to the right by the SCM and scalenes as the trunk and pelvis are laterally flexed and rotated to the right by the abdominal muscles and the eccentric contraction of the left quadratus lumborum and left gluteus medius. Hip flexors, mainly the iliopsoas, rectus femoris, and pectineus, flex the hips a bit more as the hamstrings flex the knees. The left hip gluteal muscles continue to work eccentrically to lower the thigh into adduction against gravity.

When moving from side-sitting to a quadruped position, the trunk rotates to the right, powered by the left external and right internal obliques until the left arm is brought all the way across to prop next to the right arm. Left arm motion occurs as a result of the left serratus anterior and pectoralis minor protracting the scapula, and glenohumeral motion of forward reaching and adduction occur from activity of the pectoralis major and anterior deltoid with joint stabilization from the rotator cuff. The left elbow extends with the forearm in pronation, controlled by a contraction of both the pronator teres and quadratus. The wrist, fingers, and thumb all reach in extension though activation of extensor carpi ulnaris, extensor carpi radialis longus and brevis, extensor digitorum, and extensor pollicis. The right arm maintains positions of the elbow, wrist, thumb, and fingers by isometric contraction of the previously identified muscles.

When performed correctly, movement from the quadruped to the kneeling position actually comes from the hips rather than the back. Rather than using the back to extend as many people incorrectly do, motion should be from the hips, going from about 90° of flexion first to increased flexion (Fig. 13.3D) via concentric contraction of the hamstrings at the knees and eccentric gluteal contractions. The erector spinae and abdominal muscles contract isometrically to maintain a straight spine during the hip and knee motion.

From upright kneeling to half kneeling (Fig. 13.3G), the right gluteus maximus maintains right hip extension; the pelvic stabilizers on both the left and right (gluteus medius and minimus), abdominals, and erector spinae all fire to support the body's weight shift to the right knee as the left thigh abducts and the trunk laterally flexes to move the center of mass over the right limb. Once the left knee is unweighted, the left hip abducts through the actions of gluteus medius, minimus, and TFL. Further motion into abduction with hip flexion and lateral rotation is attained through the action of the sartorius muscle (Fig. 13.3F). The iliopsoas flexes the hip, and the deep lateral rotators work with the sartorius to laterally flex the hip through asufficient range of motion to lift the extremity off the floor. The thigh is then rotated into adduction to align the left foot with the left hip. The knee, flexing to or beyond 90° from the kneeling position, first flexes using hamstring power to ensure clearance between the trunk and floor. Once clear, the knee may extend slightly, using the quadriceps to attain a 90° angle at the knee. The ankle is held in neutral through the concentric action of the anterior tibialis to ensure foot clearance from the floor. Once placed onto the floor into a left foot forward half kneeling position, the ankle is stabilized by cocontraction of the gastrocnemius-soleus with the tibialis anterior (Fig. 13.3G).

Moving to a standing position, the erector spinae eccentrically control a straight spine during forward motion of the trunk as the center of mass is shifted forward over the left hip and knee. The gluteus maximus and hamstrings are engaged eccentrically on the left to control the amount and speed of this forward shift over a hip flexing to about 70° as the right knee is becoming unweighted. The left ankle maintains its stable position through eccentric control by the gastrocnemius as the tibia advances over the foot and the COM moves anterior to the ankle. Once the left leg is stabilized in this forward position, the right hip extends through the action of the gluteus maximus and the hamstrings, the knee is extended by the quadriceps, and the right foot pushes off the floor from a plantarflexed ankle, propelled by the force of the gastrocnemius. As the foot pushes off the floor, the left knee simultaneously extends via concentric contraction of the quadriceps, the left hip extends using the gluteus maximus, and the foot is stabilized on the floor by the gastrocnemius and other posterior calf muscles.

Sit-to-Stand Transfer

A **transfer** refers to movement from one surface or position to another and may be accomplished independently or with assistance. The movement goal of a transfer is to change the center of gravity of the body from sitting on one surface to standing or sitting upon another surface. There are many different types of transfer tasks. The specific method of transfer selected depends upon the individual's ability and function as well as the assistive devices available, when the individual requires assistance. Since it is the most commonly executed transfer task, the sit-to-stand transfer will be discussed here. Advanced discussion of varying types of transfer tasks is typically discussed in a rehabilitation course, and you can apply the kinematic analysis strategy learned here to those other types of transfers. Let's analyze the sit-to-stand movement.

To stand up from a sitting position, the individual must be able to control the trunk and lower extremities and have dynamic balance. The center of mass changes from having a relatively larger base of support (hips, thighs, and feet) to having a small base of support (the feet) as the body moves from sitting to standing. This is a difficult activity if balance and strength are inadequate to manage it.

The actual sit-to-stand task requires force generation in many muscles spanning the lower extremities and the trunk. A review of the literature demonstrates that this task has the following common elements:

1. Tibialis anterior muscle—activated for preparatory placement of foot backward and tibial stabilization.
2. Simultaneous onset of activity in the hip extensors (gluteus maximus and biceps hamstrings) and knee extensors (rectus femoris, vastus lateralis and medialis muscles). Activity of these extensors peaks when the thighs are lifted off the seat, and to varying degrees, the gastrocnemius and soleus muscles play a role in postural control.[7–9]
3. Although moving through sit-to-stand and then returning to sitting from standing appear to be fundamentally the same task in reverse, these two tasks have different muscular demands. The joint excursions at the hip, knee, and ankle are similar, but in retuning to a seated position, the muscles of the lower extremities act eccentrically. The same muscles activate in the sit-to-stand, but act concentrically. There is some evidence that the trunk is of less importance in this aspect of the transfer task, whereas the greatest demands occur at the knee.[9,10]
4. How older individuals perform this task frequently reflects the normal aging changes seen in the musculoskeletal system. Arthritis in weight-bearing joints and the vertebral column or weakness in the lower extremities and back extensor muscles require that older adults develop an adaptive strategy when they transfer between sitting and standing.

Sit-to-Stand from a Seated Position using the Arms of a Chair

People of all ages often use their arms to assist in rising up from a chair (Fig. 13.4A). Individuals with lower extremity injuries or poor balance or elderly individuals may require the assistance of chair arms whenever they stand from a seated position.[7,8,11]

Sequence of Movement

Prior to standing, the body is positioned so the lower extremities are prepared to accept the body weight. The hips move to the edge of the seat and the body leans forward to place the trunk's center of mass over the legs. The hands are on the arms of the chair. As force is directed down on the hands, the center of mass moves forward over the feet as the lower limbs simultaneously extend. As the lower extremities reach their end extension position, the trunk moves upright to place the body's center of mass over the feet, and the hands move to rest by the lateral thighs.

Joint Motion

In preparation for rising out of a chair, the hips are moved forward in the chair either by "walking the hips forward" or by pushing the back against the back of the chair. In walking the hips forward, the body weight moves from one side of the pelvis to the other as the nonweight-bearing pelvis rotates forward until the hips are on the edge of the seat. If the individual moves forward by pushing against the back of the chair, the back extends into the chair to allow the hips to slide forward, then the trunk moves to an upright position when the hips are at the edge of the seat. Also in preparation, the hands are placed on the arms of the chair with the elbows flexed at about 90° (depending upon the height of the arm rests and the individual's trunk and arm length), the shoulders are hyperextended with the elbows behind the trunk, and the hips are flexed to position the trunk forward over the thighs. The knees are flexed beyond 90° to move the feet under the hips, and the ankles are dorsiflexed. The individual should look forward to keep the back straight. The forearm position depends on how the arms of the chair are grasped; they may be in either pronation or neutral midposition.[8–10] The wrists are in extension and the fingers and thumbs are flexed, grasping the arms of the chair.

As movement to standing begins, the shoulders move from hyperextension to either slight hyperextension or neutral extension, the elbows extend, and the wrists move toward neutral as the hands come off the chair arms. The neck moves from hyperextension to align with the trunk in neutral as the hips and knees extend.

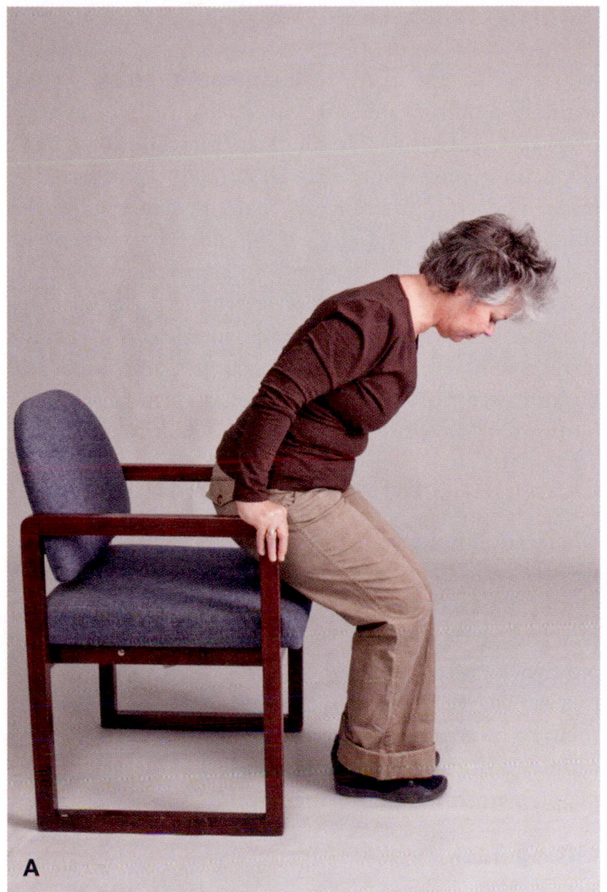

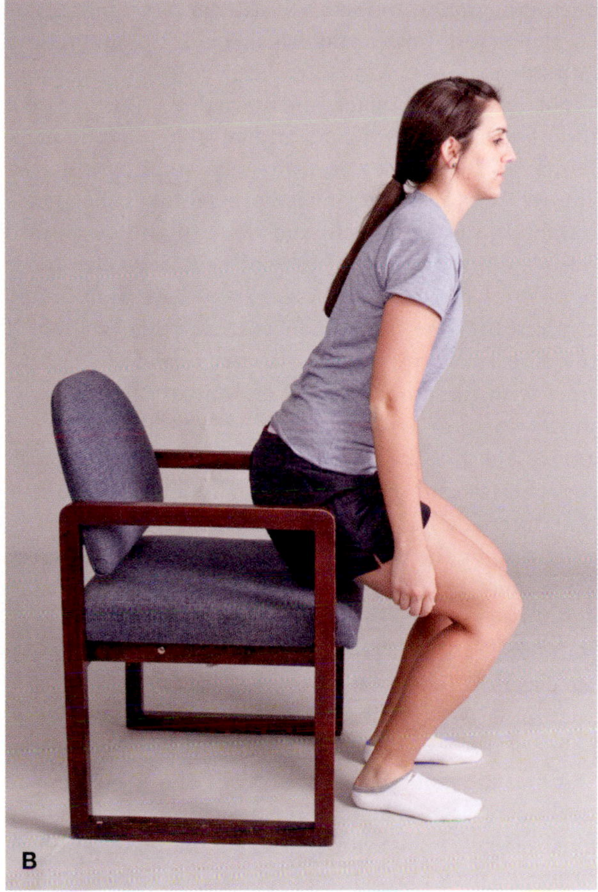

Figure 13.4 Sit-to-stand transfer. A) Using arms of a chair. B) Without using arms.

Before the hips extend to move the body upright, the head must move ahead of the feet so the center of mass is positioned over the feet (Fig. 13.4A). If this does not occur, the individual is likely to have difficulty rising without assistance. The feet stay firmly planted on the floor but the ankles move from dorsiflexion to a neutral position. As the motion continues and the body's weight is fully accepted by the lower extremities, the hands release their grasp on the chair arms, and the thumb and fingers move to a resting position.

Muscle Activity

Preparation occurs with low level activity of the trunk and lower extremity muscles. The upper extremity muscles also perform minimal activity to position the arms during the preparatory phase. If the individual walks the hips forward, the quadratus lumborum and gluteus medius and minimus on the elevated hip lift and rotate the pelvis forward as the contralateral weight-bearing side elongates. If the back is pushed against the back of the chair to move the hips forward, the back extensors contract concentrically to slide the hips forward. The abdominal muscles (rectus abdominus, internal, and external obliques) then flex to move the trunk to an erect position. The hamstrings contract to increase knee flexion so that the feet slide under the chair. The gastrocnemius assists in knee flexion and also contracts to stabilize the feet on the floor whereas the ankles are dorsiflexed primarily by the tibialis anterior. The posterior deltoid, latissimus dorsi, and teres major move the shoulder into extension as the downward scapular rotators (rhomboids and levator scapulae) position the scapula. The elbow and wrist are passively positioned through the shoulder's motions and placement of the hand on the chair arm.

Trunk muscles, especially the erector spinae, contract isometrically to stabilize the trunk throughout most of the activity. The scapular muscles also work isometrically to stabilize the scapula; specifically, these muscles include the downward rotators (rhomboids, pectoralis minor, and levator scapulae) and the scapular depressors (lower trapezius, pectoralis minor, and latissimus dorsi). Moderate activity from the latissimus dorsi, teres major, and sternal head of the pectoralis major extend and adduct the glenohumeral joints, and later they work as arm stabilizers as the elbows extend.[12] The rotator cuff stabilizes the glenohumeral joint to prevent the force of the downward push from moving the humeral head into the upper portion of the glenoid fossa. Elbow extension occurs as a result of the triceps concentrically contracting. If the forearm is in midposition, the supinators cocontract with the pronator teres and quadratus; however, if the forearm is fully pronated, the pronators act alone. The fingers are flexed by the flexor digitorum superficialis and profundus and adducted by the palmar interossei. The wrist is passively maintained in extension by the weight of the body on the hands, but there may be some coactivation of the flexor and extensor carpi muscles as they work synergistically to stabilize the wrist. The trunk is held over the hips by an eccentric contraction of the erector spinae. The abdominals and multifidus stabilize the low back and pelvis.

Once the motion begins, the neck and trunk isometrically contract to maintain spinal position using the splenius cervicus and erector spinae. As the body continues rising, the neck moves from hyperextension to neutral by eccentric contraction of the cervical extensors (cervical erector spinae and upper trapezius) and slight cocontraction of the cervical flexors (scalenes, SCM) once the trunk is upright. The shoulders continue to be extended and adducted by the latissimus dorsi, teres major, and sternal portion of the pectoralis major, with the scapula continually stabilized in downward rotation and scapular depression as described above. The rotator cuff muscles support the glenohumeral joints at all times. The elbow is further extended by the triceps; the forearm continues to be stabilized either in midposition or pronation; the wrist, fingers, and thumb continue the actions described above. Once the buttocks are lifted from the chair, the hips extend via concentric contraction of the gluteus maximus and hamstrings. The knees extend by quadriceps concentric contraction, and the gastrocnemius eccentrically assists in control of knee extension and ankle motion to neutral. As the hands are released from the chair arms, the hand further opens with slight finger abduction, supplied by the dorsal interossei and thumb extension (extensor polis longus and brevis), and abduction (abductor pollicis). These muscles along with all other upper extremity muscles move the arms into a relaxed position with the arms at the sides.

Sit-to-Stand from a Seated Position without using the Arms on a Chair

Many of us rise from a seated position in a chair without requiring the use of our arms to push up (Fig. 13.4B). In this case, all of the joint motions, muscle actions, and sequences described above are the same. The only difference is that the arms will either simply be resting quietly at the sides or perhaps be holding an object as the stand-up task occurs. Without assistance from the upper extremities, the lower extremity muscles must provide more power for the motion. Therefore, their sequence and activation will be similar to what has already been presented, but their output will be greater.

Occupational and Daily Activities

There are hundreds of tasks each of us do throughout the day without even thinking about the demands made on our bodies to perform them. Some of them are simple, and some are more complex, but each of them requires a specific sequence of events performed with a precise degree of movement and muscle tension for them to be completed successfully. Presented here are a couple examples of common daily activities that most people perform at home or at work.

Lifting Tasks

Lifting is a common activity performed both at work and at home. It is also an activity that is often performed incorrectly. Individuals who lift frequently are at risk of a cumulative injury if they perform lifting tasks repeatedly incorrectly. One of the main elements of a safe lifting task is the importance of proper body mechanics. Proper body mechanics will ensure that the back is well protected and that the motions required at the contributing body segments are not only effective, but efficient. Safety should be maximized and energy expenditure minimized during lifting. As an illustration of these concepts, let's analyze lifting a large box off the floor (Fig. 13.5).

Sequence of Movement

The movement begins with an active postural "set" by the head, trunk, and pelvis. The individual holds his or her head and trunk in their midline alignment and stabilizes the lumbar spine by moving the pelvis into its neutral position. At no time during the activity should the individual flex the spine; it should remain in its properly aligned position, using the hips to move the torso rather than the back. Prior to lifting, the individual tests the object to be lifted to get an idea of its weight. The individual then establishes a wide base of support standing close to the object as he or she prepares to lift it. To move into a squat, the hips laterally rotate to about 45° and flex to about to 90°. The ankles move into dorsiflexion as the tibia moves forward over the foot, and the knees flex to lower the body so the hands are able to grasp the box. The hip position of abduction and lateral rotation is maintained throughout the preparation phase. As the squat brings the individual's hands closer to the box, the hips flex to move the torso over the box, keeping the back straight and in its neutral position. As the squat lowers the individual close to the box, the upper extremities move forward into shoulder flexion with extended elbows to reach and obtain a firm grasp of the object (Fig. 13.5A).

To begin to lift the box, the hands obtain a secure grasp on it in finger flexion with the shoulder girdle, elbow, and wrist muscles "set" to accept the weight. The box is then moved closer to the body; with the trunk erect, the individual moves to stand up (Fig. 13.5B). Once the box is secured, the standing motion is accomplished from the power in the lower extremities. The standing motion is initiated by the hips and knees. As the individual stands, the box remains close to the body, the trunk maintains its neutral position, and the feet maintain a wide base of support (Fig. 13.5C).

Joint Motion

The movement begins by positioning the head, trunk, and pelvis. These segments are "set" by cocontraction of the anterior and posterior muscles to maintain their stable positions throughout the lift. The upper extremities move to perform the lifting task while the body and lower extremities are stabilized.

To begin to lift the box, the scapular rotators (upward and downward) cocontract to stabilize the scapula as the shoulders move to about 60° of flexion, adducted near the trunk with the shoulders midway between medial and lateral rotation. The elbows and forearms are in extension and midposition to reach for the box and grasp it. The wrists extend into functional position and the thumb and fingers move first into full extension and abduction to reach the box and then into flexion and adduction to grasp it. The shoulders are adducted toward the trunk, and the scapulae are stabilized against the thorax. Once the box is secured and moved closer to the trunk, the hips and knees move into extension, maintaining a wide base of support with the hips in some abduction and lateral rotation.

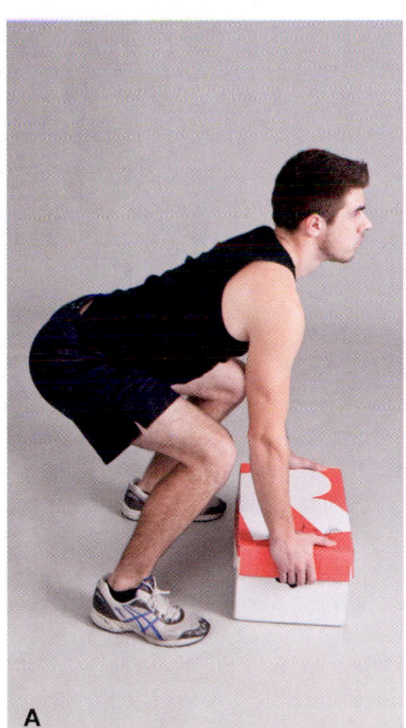

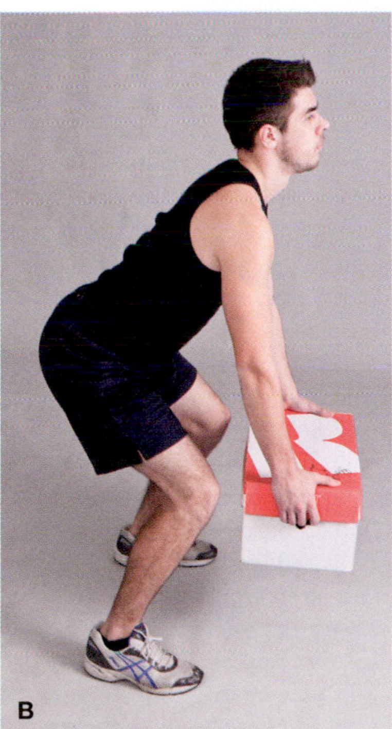

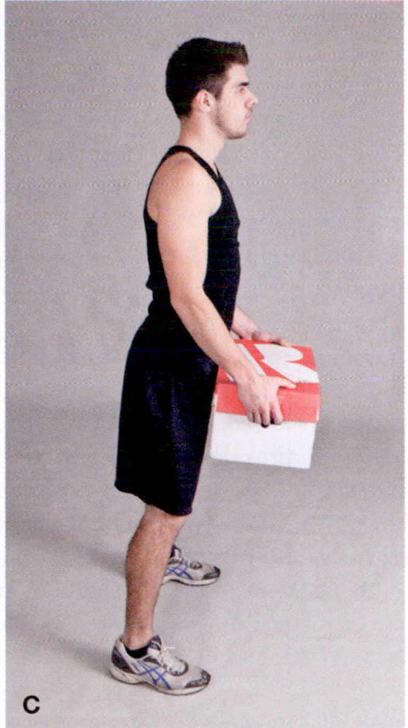

Figure 13.5 Lifting a box. **A)** Squat in proximity of box to begin lift. **B)** Box is lifted and brought to chest. **C)** Box is lifted and held in stance.

Muscle Activity

The postural "set" to stabilize the body for this movement requires activation of all of the postural control muscles: neck flexors (SCM and scalenes) and extensors (spleneii). The erector spinae and abdominals contract to stabilize the trunk. The pelvis and lumbar spine maintain their neutral position by cocontraction of the transverse abdominus and multifidus muscles. The wide base of support in hip abduction is accomplished by contractions of the gluteus medius and minimus, TFL, and the sartorius. The hips are laterally rotated by the gluteus maximus and deep lateral rotators, with contributions from the sartorius. Moving into a squat, the erector spinae muscles isometrically contract to maintain proper spinal position and the abdominals provide lumbar stabilization. The hips and knees flex using eccentric contractions of the gluteus maximus and hamstrings at the hip and quadriceps at the knee. As the squat deepens, the deep lateral rotators, gluteus maximus, and sartorius continue to maintain the hips in lateral rotation. The gastrocnemius-soleus muscles stabilize the ankles in this closed chain position on the floor. Additionally, the gastrocnemius fires eccentrically to control the tibia moving forward over the foot into dorsiflexion. As the squat brings the individual closer to the box, the hip extensors eccentrically control the required amount of trunk motion forward to reach toward the box; during this part of the preparation phase, the erector spinae maintains the "set" spinal position through an isometric contraction. In order to execute the lift, the upper extremities will now be engaged to perform the lifting task as the body and lower extremities stay stabilized in position.

As the box is lifted, the shoulders move into flexion by the clavicular portion of pectoralis major, anterior deltoid, and coracobrachialis, and are adducted alongside the trunk by the pectoralis major, latissimus dorsi, and teres major, midway between medial and lateral rotation by the subscapularis, anterior deltoid, infraspinatus, and teres minor muscles. Since the shoulders are not elevated much during this motion, the scapulae maintain their positions with cocontraction of upward and downward rotators to provide a stable base for the humeral head. The elbows are maintained in extension by cocontraction of the triceps and elbow flexors (biceps brachii, brachialis, and brachioradialis). The wrists are stabilized in functional position by cocontraction of wrist extensors (extensor carpi radialis longus and brevis and extensor carpi ulnaris) and finger flexors (flexor digitorum superficialis and profundus); the fingers are also adducted by the palmar interossei. The thumb is adducted and flexed by the flexor pollicis and adductor pollicis to hold the sides of the box. Once the box is firmly secured, all of these muscles maintain an isometric contraction to grasp and hold the box in place. When the individual is ready to lift the box, the knees and hips extend through concentric contraction of the gluteus maximus and hamstrings at the hip and quadriceps at the knee. The base of support stays wide in hip abduction; lateral rotation is provided by the gluteus medius, gluteus minimus, sartorius, gluteus maximus, and deep lateral rotators to stand up holding the box.

Household Tasks

There are many household tasks from which to select for movement analysis. We have selected one as an example: vacuuming. Using the movement analysis modeled in the chapter, you could analyze others such as sweeping, snow shoveling, and doing laundry, to name a few.

Vacuuming

Using a vacuum cleaner to is a good example of performing a push-pull activity using the upper extremities to serve as the deliverer of lower extremity forces. Figure 13.6 depicts the motion described here. Note that the individual is in a tandem stance with the right hip ahead of the left one and flexed so the right foot is positioned forward and the right upper extremity is positioned so the right hand grasps the vacuum cleaner handle. The left arm is unengaged at the side.

Sequence of Movement

The motion begins with the individual in a tandem stance with one leg ahead of the other; the head and trunk are maintained in their neutral positions with the trunk aligned with the hips. The right hip is flexed with the knee extended and ankle plantarflexed. The left hip and knee are extended and the ankle is in neutral with the body weight primarily on this back leg. Both hips are in lateral rotation and slightly abducted. The right scapula is slightly protracted because the shoulder is flexed; the forearm is in midposition and the hand grasps the handle in a power grasp (Fig. 13.6A). The elbow alternately extends with some additional shoulder flexion to push the vacuum cleaner forward and then flexes with shoulder hyperextension to pull it back across the carpet.

Although this vacuuming motion occurs to some degree in the shoulder and elbow, the thrust of the force is delivered from the legs as weight is transferred back and forth between the back and the front lower limbs. As the shoulder moves into flexion with elbow extension, the weight transfers to the front leg, pushing off from the back leg, (Fig. 13.6B), and when the shoulder moves into extension with elbow flexion, the weight is

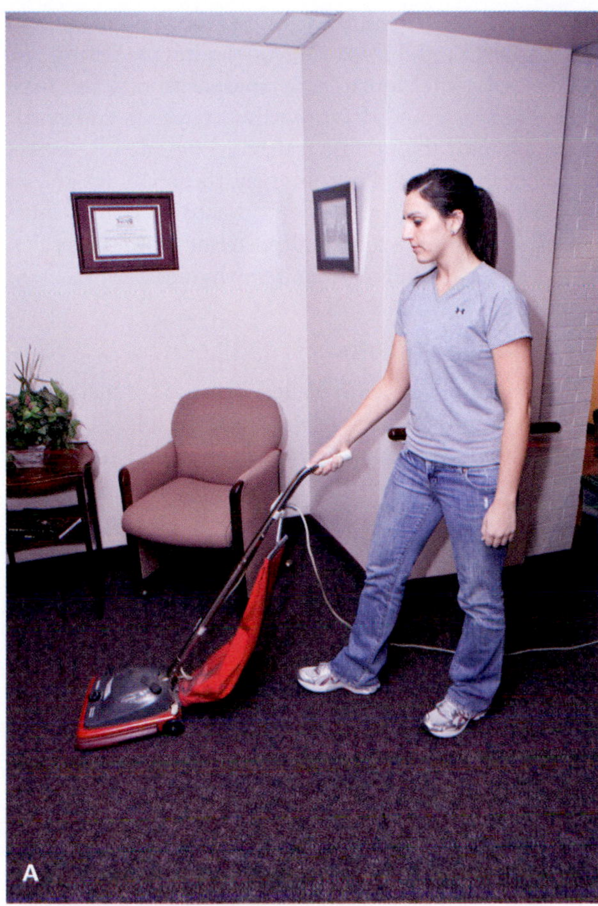

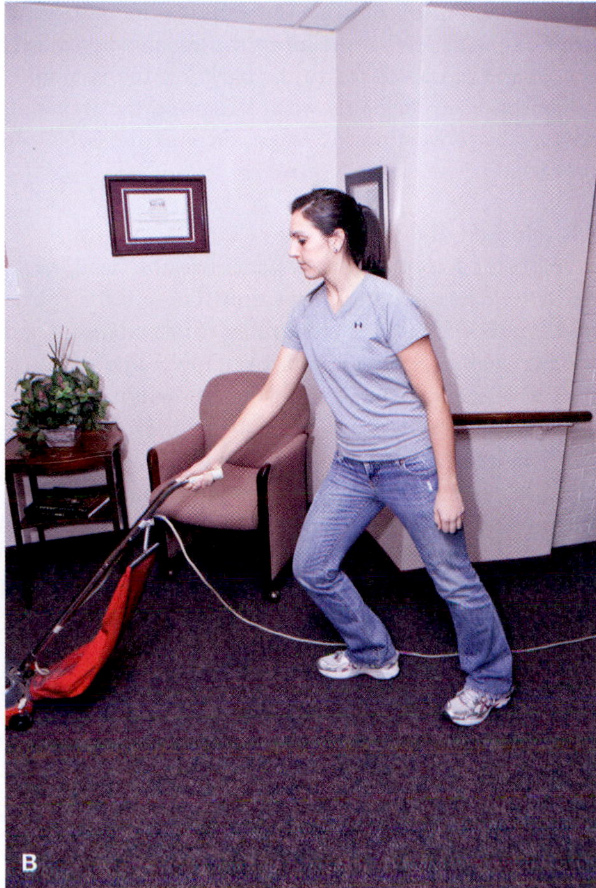

Figure 13.6 Vacuuming movement sequence.

pushed from the front leg to the back leg. As the front leg accepts the body weight, its knee flexes a little more than the back knee does, and then it moves into extension as weight is transferred again to the back limb. The left upper extremity is unengaged in a resting position at the side. It may provide some balance as the motion is performed. As the vacuuming proceeds across the floor, the individual steps forward, leading with the right lower extremity and then stepping forward with the left lower extremity to reach a new area to clean.

Joint Motion

The head, neck, trunk, and pelvis maintain their neutral positions in proper alignment throughout this activity. The front leg—in this example, the right leg—is forward of the left leg with the hip in about 20° of flexion, with lateral rotation and abduction in a forward stance position (similar to a fencer). The right knee is extended with the ankle in about 10° of planter flexion. The left hip is in some abduction and lateral rotation with the body weight primarily on this leg. The left knee is extended and the ankle is in neutral with the foot flat on the floor.

The right scapula is protracted and slightly upwardly rotated since the shoulder is flexed. When pushing forward, the elbow moves from partial flexion to full extension with the forearm in midposition. The hand grasps the vacuum cleaner handle in a power grip with thumb opposing the fingers and the fingers flexed and adducted. The wrist is in extension. To pull the vacuum cleaner back toward the body, the forearm, wrist and hand stay in position but the elbow flexes and the shoulder moves toward extension. Humeral extension and then hyperextension is accompanied by scapular tilt, downward rotation, and retraction. Throughout the action, the shoulder is maintained midway between lateral and medial rotation. Power for movement of the vacuum is provided by weight transfer between the back and front legs. As the vacuum cleaner is pushed forward, the individual pushes the body weight from the back leg to the front leg, so the right hip moves toward flexion, the knee flexes, and the tibia moves forward over the planted foot into ankle dorsiflexion as the left (or trailing limb) extends and abducts at the hip as the left ankle everts. As the weight is transferred to the back leg, the vacuum is pulled back. During this weight transfer, the right hip will again move towards extension and the sequence repeats.

Muscle Activity

The postural control muscles stabilize the head, neck, and trunk in the upright position. The erector spinae and the abdominals are controlling trunk extension and lumbar stabilization in upright stance. The trunk is rotated slightly to the right by the left external abdominal obliques and right internal abdominal obliques. Both gluteus medius muscles are actively engaged to control a level pelvis and shift weight from one leg to the other. The right hip adductor group works eccentrically and concentrically when the body weight moves forward and backward, respectively. The left hip abductors work concentrically to move the hip into abduction when the body weight moves forward, and they work eccentrically to adduct the hip against gravity as the body weight is transferred back to the left leg. When pushing the vacuum forward, the right hip flexes through eccentric effort of the gluteus maximus, and the ankle moves into dorsiflexion, eccentrically controlled by the gastrocnemius. Knee extension and flexion of both knees are achieved through the action of the quadriceps group, and the ankle is plantarflexed by gastrocnemius-soleus. The peroneus longus and brevis evert the left ankle.

At all times, the head of the humerus is depressed within the glenoid fossa by the rotator cuff muscles to maintain humeral stability. The right scapula protracts by activity from the serratus anterior, and it upwardly rotates through the force couple actions of upper and lower trapezius and serratus anterior. The shoulder is flexed by the anterior deltoid, clavicular portion of pectoralis major, and coracobrachialis. The forearm is maintained in midposition through the combined actions of the supinator and pronator teres and quadratus. To accompany the push forward, the elbow extends by the triceps. The opponens pollicis opposes the thumb, and the flexor digitorum superficialis and profundus and the palmar interossei flex and adduct the fingers to grasp the handle. This grasp is synergistically accompanied by the extensor carpi ulnaris and extensor carpi radialis longus and brevis extending the wrist. The shoulder is positioned midway between lateral and medial rotation, stabilized by subscapularis, infraspinatus, and teres minor.

To pull the vacuum backward, the brachialis, brachioradialis, and biceps all contribute to flexing the elbow with the forearm in midposition. The right scapula retracts and downwardly rotates via concentric contraction of the middle trapezius, rhomboids, levator scapula, and pectoralis minor as the shoulder moves towards extension by concentric activity of the latissimus dorsi, teres major, and posterior deltoid muscles. The scapula is tilted to accompany humeral hyperextension by the pectoralis minor.

Occupational Tasks

Clinicians are frequently called upon to evaluate work tasks, especially when they work with an injured worker. At other times, clinicians may be required to provide suggestions and work station assessments to optimize work environments and prevent injuries. One of the common elements that lead to injury in occupational settings is the repetitive nature of work activities. Since many occupational injuries treated by clinicians involve repetitive activities, we have selected two common repetitive work tasks. We will kinematically analyze and describe a repetitive task performed in sitting—working at a computer station—and one performed in standing—working on a factory assembly line.

Computer Stations

Many people spend hours every day performing tasks at a computer station. The most obvious task, perhaps the one that consumes most of an individual's time at the computer, is using the keyboard (Figure 13.7).

Before we are able to analyze the task, we need to identify the proper position to assume when working at a computer. The first element is selecting the proper chair. The chair should fit the individual. The chair is the proper size if the individual is able to sit in the chair with the hips all the way to the back of the chair and has about a 2-inch space between the end of the chair and the posterior knee. The correct height of the seat allows the individual's feet to be flat on the floor with the hips and knees each at 90°. With the shoulders relaxed, the forearms should rest comfortably near the sides (not with the shoulders abducted) on the arm rests. Ideally, there should be a lumbar roll in the chair back to support the lumbar spine. In a properly seated position, the individual's head and shoulders are directly over the ischial tuberosities with the head and spine in neutral alignment. The height of the back of the chair should be no lower than the inferior angle of the scapula. Some chair backs come to the top of the shoulder and others may be high enough to support the head; these chairs usually

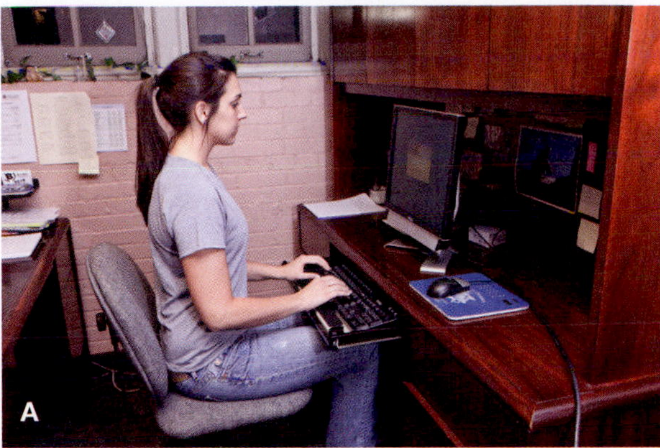

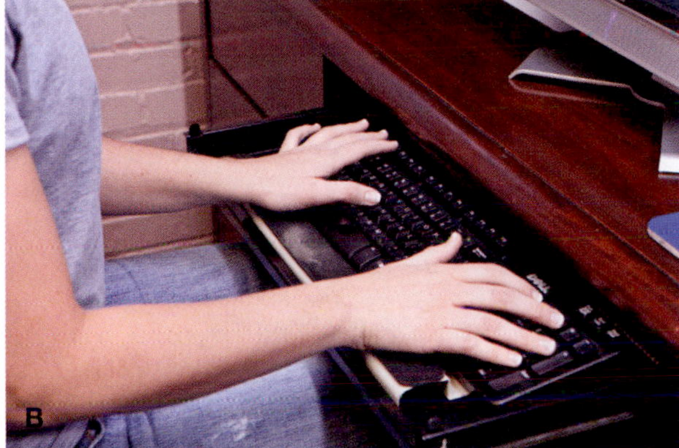

Figure 13.7 Working at a computer station.

recline. With the person properly seated in the chair, the keys of the computer keyboard are reached by the fingers with the elbows flexed at 90° or slightly more, the wrists in neutral, and the fingers flexed at the IP joints. The computer screen should be at the same level as the eyes (Fig. 13.7A).

Sequence of Movement and Joint Motions

Since there is little movement occurring during computer typing, both the sequence of movement and the joint motions are presented in this section together. The motion used in typing involves primarily the wrist and digits with some assistance from the elbows.

The task begins with the individual properly seated in a chair: head, neck, and trunk are maintained in their neutral positions. The shoulders are stabilized in either 0° extension or very slight flexion to allow the fingers to reach the keyboard. The elbows are close to 90°, and the forearms are pronated. The wrists are in their functional position of slight extension, and the thumb and finger metacarpal joints are in 0° extension and slight abduction with the IP joints in some flexion until the keys are reached (Fig. 13.7A). During keyboarding, although there is some motion required of the shoulder complex, the keyboard task is predominately executed by the actions of the elbow, wrist, and fingers and thumb as the forearm stays pronated. Searching for the keys is typically accomplished by wrist radial and ulnar deviation motions along with the required finger flexion and extension and abduction and adduction movements (Fig. 13.7B).

Muscle Activity

The postural control muscles at the neck (neck flexors—SCM, scalenes; extensors—spleneii) and trunk (erector spinae and abdominals) have a minimal but continual level of contraction to maintain a proper sitting position. If the individual leans forward, motion occurs at the hips through eccentric contraction of the gluteus maximus and hamstrings as the erector spinae contract to maintain correct spinal alignment. The lower extremities are otherwise relaxed in the sitting position, anchored between the floor and the chair.

The shoulders are either by the sides or slightly flexed. They may also be in slight medial rotation through effort of the subscapularis, although this is variable and depends on the individual's size and the size of the keyboard. The humerus is stabilized by the rotator cuff muscles and the scapula remains stabilized by its rotator muscles. The elbows maintain flexion through contraction of the brachialis and pronator teres, with the forearm pronated by both pronators. In proper alignment, if the chair has arms, the arm rests can be used to support the elbows so the upper trapezius is not overstressed. The wrists hold a neutral or slightly extended functional position through the efforts of cocontraction of the five carpi muscles. The thumb and finger are in extension and abduction at the MCP joints, powered by the extensor digitorum, extensor pollicis, and dorsal interossei. Although there is minimal motion required of the proximal upper extremity muscles to reach for keys, the keyboard task itself is predominately executed by actions from the wrist and digits with stabilization for these joints provided by the more proximal joint muscles. Moving across the keys is typically accomplished by medial and lateral rotators of the shoulder and the rotator cuff muscles (subscapularis for medial rotation; teres minor and infraspinatus for lateral rotation). Wrist radial and ulnar deviation actions are supplied by either the flexor carpi radialis and extensor carpi radialis longus for radial deviation or the flexor carpi ulnaris and extensor carpi ulnaris muscles for ulnar deviation. The required wrist, finger, and thumb actions will move from flexion or extension as needed, powered by the long finger flexors or extensors.

Assembly Line Workers

Let's analyze the motions performed by an individual who runs a drill press on an assembly line. In our example, the task requires the individual to reach to a conveyor in front and to the right of the worker, pick up a piece of metal and place it under the drill press. She then presses down the drill press handle to drill the hole and replaces the drilled bar onto the conveyor at her left side. The photographs and movement sequence demonstrate that this experienced factory worker uses an economy of body movement such that the bar is retrieved, drilled, and replaced onto the conveyor without large joint excursions and without the need to step out of a stable stance position. She uses good body mechanics by keeping her pelvis in neutral to minimize low back strain, and she retrieves and replaces the bar onto the conveyor by simply shifting her weight rather than stepping or rotating her trunk.

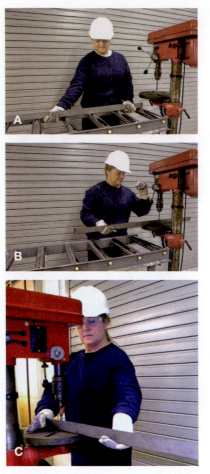

Figure 13.8 Working on an assembly line movement sequence.

Sequence of Movement

The individual is in a side-to-side stance, facing the conveyor. The head, neck, and trunk are erect in neutral alignment. The task movement begins as the individual reaches with the right arm for the metal bar approaching her on the conveyor. When the right upper extremity grasps the metal bar, the left arm moves into flexion to assist in lifting the bar (Fig. 13.8A). The bar is then removed from the moving belt using a firm grasp with both hands. The grasp is synergistically supported by wrist extension. Both forearms are in supination and the elbows flex to lift the bar off of the belt. Throughout the bar retrieval, the arms are stabilized against the trunk.

The metal bar is placed under the drill press. The worker holds the bar in place with her right hand as she reaches and grasps the drill handle with her left hand, and then presses it to drill the bar. The drill press is at a level that does not require the worker to lift the metal bar more than a few inches and keeps the bar below shoulder level for ease of drill press operation (Fig.13.8B).

Once the bar is drilled, the worker slides the bar across the press plate with her right hand as her left hand guides the metal bar onto the conveyer to redeposit it at her left side (Fig.13.8C).

Joint Motion

The individual stands facing the conveyor belt. The trunk is in neutral alignment and maintained in this position throughout the activity. The task movement begins as the individual reaches to the right with the right arm moving into abduction and lateral rotation. Assisting in this movement, the scapula is stabilized by its rotators. The right elbow extends with the forearm in supination; the wrist extends to a neutral position or slight extension as the fingers and thumb flex and adduct to grasp the bar. As the right hand makes contact with the bar, the left arm assists in the retrieval of the bar by flexing the elbow in supination with wrist extension, and finger and thumb flexion and adduction. The left shoulder remains adducted against the trunk.

Once the bar is placed under the drill press, she holds the bar level with her right hand with the hand positioned in a comfortable grasp as most of the task of holding the bar is accomplished with the elbow flexed at 90° in supination and the shoulder laterally rotated, adducted, and extended against the trunk. In order to run the drill with the left hand, the worker flexes (in slight abduction) her left shoulder as she flexes the elbow in midposition, grasps the press handle, and pushes it down to make the hole in the metal bar.

Once the bar is drilled, the worker uses her right hand to slide the drilled bar across the press plate by horizontally adducting her shoulder and extending her elbow. Rather than step to the left, she simply shifts her weight to the left and guides the bar with her left arm. The left shoulder abducts in lateral rotation, and the elbow extends with forearm supination, lowering the drilled bar back onto the conveyer at her left side.

Muscle Activity

The postural control muscles at the neck (flexors—SCM, scalenes and extensors, spleneii) and trunk (erector spinae and abdominals) maintain the worker in correct posture throughout the task. The pelvic muscles and lower extremities maintaining proper alignment of these segments primarily include the abdominals, gluteus maximus, gluteus medius and minimus, and the gastrocnemius-soleus muscles.[17] The reach with the right arm to the right is executed by the middle deltoid, supraspinatus, infraspinatus, and teres minor, which work together to abduct and laterally rotate the glenohumeral joint. These glenohumeral motions are supported by active stabilization of the scapular stabilizers: serratus anterior and upper and lower trapezius (upward rotators), and the middle trapezius and rhomboids (retractors). The right elbow extends to reach the metal bar by eccentric contraction of the elbow flexors (biceps, brachialis, and brachioradialis). The supinator supinates the forearm. The wrist is synergistically extended by the extensor carpi ulnaris and extensor carpi radialis longus and brevis, whereas the fingers and thumb flex and adduct to grasp the bar using flexor digitorum superficialis, profundus, palmar interossei, flexor pollicis longus, and adductor pollicis. Instants later, the left arm assists in retrieval of the bar by moving the elbow into flexion with supination using the biceps brachii, brachialis, and supinator as the humerus stays stabilized in adduction and extension against the trunk (pectoralis major, latissimus dorsi, teres major, and the rotator cuff). These muscles along with the downward rotators and retractors (levator scapula, pectoralis minor, rhomboids, and middle trapezius) stabilize the scapula. The left extremity reach is adjusted for proper distance by the elbow flexors. The prime movers involved in grasp include the wrist, finger, and thumb muscles named previously.

Once the metal bar is placed under the drill press, the right hand continues to hold a grasp position through the synergistic actions of the wrist extensors (extensor carpi radialis longus and brevis, extensor carpi ulnaris) and the finger flexors (flexor digitorum superficialis and profundus) as the more demanding task of holding the bar is accomplished by the biceps brachii, brachialis, and supinator, holding the elbow flexed at 90° in supination. The shoulder is adducted, extended, and laterally rotated against the trunk through the actions of pectoralis major, latissimus dorsi, teres major, infraspinatus, and teres major with the scapula stabilized in downward rotation and retraction (levator scapula, pectoralis minor, rhomboids, and middle trapezius). The rotator cuff muscles of each shoulder are active, stabilizing the head of the humerus in the glenoid fossa. In order to run the drill, the worker flexes the left shoulder (in slight abduction) using the clavicular portion of pectoralis major, anterior deltoid, and coracobrachialis, accompanied by scapular downward rotation for stabilization (levator scapula, pectoralis minor, rhomboids). She flexes the elbow in midposition with the brachioradialis, brachialis, and cocontraction of both pronators and the supinator as the left hand grasps the press knob. Grasp is executed as described previously.

After the bar is drilled, the worker horizontally adducts her right shoulder (pectoralis major and anterior deltoid), as the scapula is protracted by the serratus anterior, and she extends her right elbow using the triceps to slide the drilled bar across the press plate. Rather than step to the left, she simply shifts her weight to the left and uses minimal muscle force as the weight of the bar is guided toward the conveyer by her left arm. The left shoulder is abducted in lateral rotation by middle deltoid, supraspinatus, infraspinatus, and teres minor, whereas the scapula is positioned and stabilized by upper and lower trapezius, serratus anterior, middle trapezius, and rhomboids. The elbow extends with eccentric control exerted by biceps brachii with forearm supination (supinator), lowering the drilled bar back onto the conveyer at her left side.

Clinician Activities

The following section discusses a kinesiological perspective of activities that clinicians commonly perform. Clinical work requires utilization of proper body mechanics to effectively and efficiently perform daily skills. Not only does a clinician risk injury if proper techniques are not used, but fatigue because of inefficient execution of those skills serves to wear and tear on the clinician physically. Before we look at a couple of examples of kinesiological application to clinical tasks, a review of some physical concepts that make the body more efficient is warranted.

As you may recall from Chapter 2, the basic physical concepts related to body movement and positioning include the following:

- To be stable, the body's center of mass must fall within its base of support. Since a clinician must be stable so that movement to either assist or resist a patient is performed safely, the clinician must have a base of support of sufficient size to provide adequate stability. If the clinician intends to receive a large force or requires his or her body to produce a large force, it may be necessary to increase the size of the base of support.

- Stability during dynamic activity requires that the feet be placed in the direction of forces applied. If the clinician is moving a patient from left to right, the clinician's feet should be placed in a side-to-side position. On the other hand, if the clinician is providing resistance in a forward-backward motion, then the feet should be placed in a front-to-back position.
- Further stability occurs if the center of mass is lowered. Therefore, if the clinician is to provide or resist a force, it will be better achieved if the body moves into a partial squat to lower the center of mass and improve stability.
- A "straight" spine provides the greatest stability for the back and the most efficient transfer of forces from the legs to the arms. In other words, the clinician should maintain a neutral spine throughout all activities. If delivering manual resistance, it is a good idea to maintain a neutral spine so the forces from the legs may be utilized through the transfer of forces to the upper extremities where the force is applied.
- In that same vein, to maximize effectiveness and preserve the smaller joints, it is advantageous to use the powerful leg muscles to provide the clinician with the leverage and power while minimizing repeated large stresses to smaller and weaker upper body segments.

Patient Protective Measures: Spotting during Ambulation

Instruction in ambulation either with or without assistive devices is a common clinical activity. Patients who require assistance place additional demands on the clinician. Specific techniques are used to protect the patient as well as the clinician during ambulation instruction and progression to independence. We will assume that the patient has advanced from ambulation instruction in the parallel bars to ambulation instruction with crutches, and the clinician has already provided the patient with instructions and demonstration so the patient is now ready to begin ambulation. This patient is partial weight-bearing on the left lower extremity. The technique is outlined here.

Sequence of Movement

A gait belt is secured around the patient, and the patient is standing, ready to walk with the crutches (Fig. 13.9A). The clinician stands behind and slightly to the side of the patient and grasps the gait belt with the hand closest to the patient. The other hand is placed on the front of the patient's ipsilateral shoulder. The clinician may stand on either the patient's involved or uninvolved side.[18] Some experienced clinicians prefer to stand on the involved side, assuming that if the patient falls, he will fall to that side; other clinicians prefer to stand on the uninvolved side, anticipating more control of the patient should he require sudden assistance. A gait belt is required for safety; relying on the patient's clothing is never a good idea since it may give way when there is a need to grasp the patient.

In our example, the clinician stands on the patient's uninvolved side, behind and to the right of the patient. Therefore, the clinician's right foot is positioned behind the patient and aligned patient's right crutch and right leg, and the clinician's left foot is behind and between the patient's two feet (Fig.13.9A). The clinician's right leg is ahead of the back leg in a forward-backward straddle position, aligned in the direction of movement. As the patient moves the crutches forward, the clinician moves her right foot forward (Fig. 13.9B), and when the patient takes a step, the clinician moves her left foot forward. It is important that the clinician maintain a forward-backward straddle when the patient ambulates so she is able to control his movements if it is suddenly necessary to either prevent a fall or allow for a safe fall.

If the patient loses balance and begins to flex at the trunk, the clinician pulls on the shoulder to extend the trunk and pushes on the hips at the belt to move the pelvis forward and place his center of mass over his base of support (Fig. 13.9C). However, if it is apparent that the patient is going to fall, the clinician pulls the patient towards her to aid in a safe movement to the floor.

JOINT MOTION

Since the clinician is in a forward-backward straddle position with the lower extremities, the right hip is in slight flexion with partial flexion of the knee and slight plantarflexion of the ankle. The clinician begins with most of her weight on the left lower extremity; the hip, knee, and ankle are all close to neutral in the sagittal plane. The left hip is slightly laterally rotated. The head, neck, and trunk are in alignment over the pelvis.

The clinician's left upper extremity is positioned with the shoulder in slight flexion; the elbow is flexed to about 90° (the actual amount of flexion depends on the clinician's and patient's heights); the forearm is supinated; the wrist is in its power position of slight extension; and the hand is in a power grasp around the belt behind the patient. The clinician's right upper extremity is in shoulder flexion with upward rotation of the scapula (the actual amount of glenohumeral flexion and scapular rotation depends on the patient's height); the elbow is in some flexion; the forearm is pronated; the wrist is in slight flexion; and the fingers are in slight flexion to make contact with the patient's anterior shoulder.

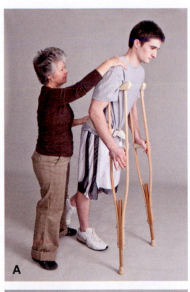

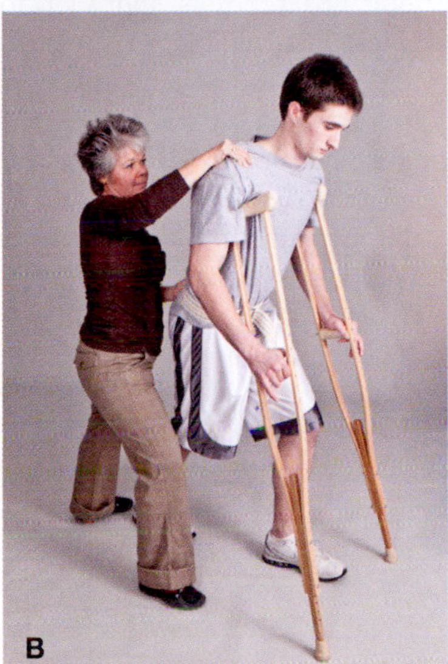

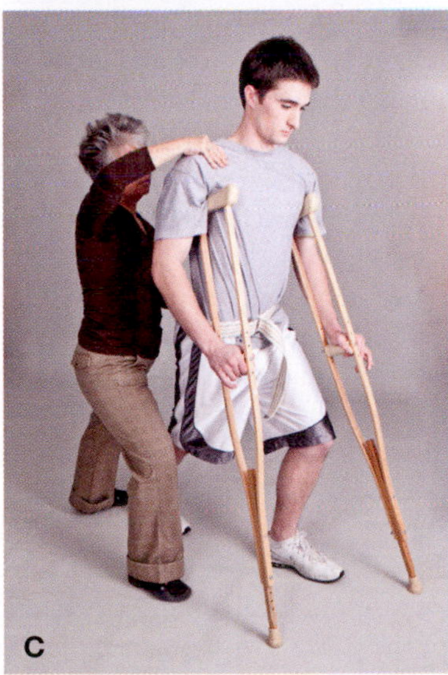

Figure 13.9 Spotting during ambulation assistance.

When the patient moves the crutches forward, the clinician moves the right leg forward to place it more in front of her body, flexing the hip and knee slightly and plantarflexing the ankle. Both shoulders move into more flexion as the elbows move into more extension to maintain their hand positions on the patient. When the patient moves his body forward, the clinician transfers all of her body weight to the right lower extremity, moving the hip and knee towards extension and the ankle towards dorsiflexion. The left lower extremity's hip and knee move into flexion as the ankle dorsiflexes to lift the limb from the floor and take a small step forward. Simultaneously, the shoulders and elbows move towards their starting position as the clinician moves closer to the patient.

If the patient begins to lose his balance as his trunk moves into flexion, perhaps lacking control of the momentum created by his body motion forward, the clinician abducts her hips and slightly flexes her knees to increase her base of support and lower her center of gravity for increased stability as she simultaneously moves to pull his shoulder toward her, flexing her left shoulder to move his pelvis forward. As the right shoulder is stabilized to control the patient's forward trunk movement, the right elbow flexes; when the left shoulder flexes, the left elbow moves towards extension to push the patient's hips beneath him (Fig. 13.9C).

MUSCLE ACTIVITY

To move her body into position, the lower extremities are positioned first. The right lower extremity is positioned using the iliopsoas and rectus femoris to move the hip into slight flexion as the gluteal muscles laterally rotate and stabilize it. The knee's position is produced by the quadriceps, and the body's center of mass position over the back leg moves the right ankle into slight plantarflexion as cocontraction of the gastrocnemius-soleus and anterior tibialis maintain the ankle in its sagittal plane position. The left lower extremity is maintained in a near neutral, sagittal plane position primarily by eccentric contraction of the gluteus maximus at the hip, quadriceps at the knee, and gastrocnemius-soleus at the ankle. The hip is in lateral rotation through the efforts of the six small rotators, assisted by the gluteals. Trunk position is maintained throughout the activity by the stabilizers (abdominals, multifidus). The erector spinae provides eccentric control of the trunk when the body moves forward and the abdominals provide concentric contraction during upper extremity motions.

The upper extremities move into position in preparation for the activity by the upward rotators of the scapula of the right shoulder complex (upper and lower trapezius and serratus anterior) and the humerus of both shoulders elevate through function of their pectoralis major and anterior deltoid. Since the left shoulder has minimal elevation, the scapula is stabilized through cocontraction of its rotators. Both elbows are positioned via eccentric contraction of their elbow flexors (biceps, brachialis, and brachioradialis). The left forearm supinates via action of the supinators and biceps brachii, and the right forearm pronates through eccentric contraction of the supinators cocontracting with both pronators. The right wrist is flexed using eccentric contraction of the wrist extensors (extensor carpi radialis longus and brevis and extensor carpi ulnaris). The fingers are positioned in slight flexion to rest on the top and anterior right shoulder of the patient through eccentric contraction of the extensor digitorum longus. The left wrist is in slight extension and maintained in this position through activity of the extensor carpi radialis and ulnaris as the fingers grasp the belt through concentric contraction of the flexor digitorum superficialis and profundus. The thumb opposes the hand in a power grip utilizing the opponens pollicis and flexor pollicis.

As the patient moves the crutches forward, the clinician's hands maintain their positions on the patient, now actively engaging the finger flexors to grasp the patient's shoulder and the gait belt. The clinician's right, hip flexes to move the limb forward through concentric contraction of the iliopsoas and rectus femoris (Fig. 13.9B). The knee is controlled by the quadriceps, and the ankle plantarflexes passively by its position anterior to the line of gravity. The left hip gluteus maximus and medius accept the total body weight as the right limb moves forward, and the six lateral rotators aided by the gluteals maintain lateral rotation of the hip. The quadriceps and gastrocnemius-soleus maintain the knee and ankle in the sagittal plane as the limb accepts the body's weight. Flexion of the shoulders is controlled by the anterior deltoid and pectoralis major as the scapula is stabilized by its rotators (trapezius, serratus anterior, rhomboids, pectoralis minor, and levator scapulae). Elbow positions occur secondarily to maintain connection between the clinician's shoulder and the patient, so they move passively but are then maintained by slight cocontraction of the elbow flexors (biceps, brachialis, and brachioradialis) and triceps.

As the patient moves forward to bring his body to the crutches, the clinician transfers her body weight to the right lower extremity. In doing so, the right hip extends through active contraction of the gluteus maximus and medius as the knee extends by contraction of the quadriceps. The ankle moves towards dorsiflexion that occurs passively through transfer of her center of mass over the leg but is controlled by eccentric contraction of the gastrocnemius-soleus group. The left hip flexes through iliopsoas and rectus femoris contraction and lifts the limb off the floor. As the limb lifts, the quadriceps controls knee flexion and the ankle dorsiflexes through concentric contraction of the tibialis anterior. As the lower limbs alter their positions, the upper extremities—shoulders and elbows—return to their positions at the start of the motion.

If the patient loses his balance and requires assistance to remain upright by the clinician, she moves quickly in the following sequence. She abducts both hips using the gluteus medius and minimus and flexes the knees using eccentric contraction of the quadriceps to provide herself with a stable base as her right hand uses concentric contraction of the flexor digitorum profundus and superficialis along with concentric contraction of the elbow flexors (already listed) and shoulder extensors (latissimus dorsi, posterior deltoid, teres major) with scapular downward stabilizers (rotators) to pull the patient's shoulder towards her. At the same time, she uses her left hand to maintain a firm grasp on the gait belt with strong contraction of the long finger flexors and adductors (palmar interossei and lumbricals) along with isometric cocontraction of wrist flexors and extensors to stabilize the wrist as the triceps forcefully extends the elbow and the shoulder's anterior deltoid and pectoralis major supply some shoulder flexion. Since the shoulder does not elevate substantially during this maneuver, the scapular rotators work to stabilize the humerus in the glenoid. These motions by the clinician place the patient's center of mass over his feet to stabilize him and prevent him from falling.

Clinician Ergonomics: Manual Resistance

As mentioned earlier, it is vital that the clinician be aware of correct body mechanics and use his or her body safely and efficiently to both protect against injury and conserve energy. The general concepts involved in correct body mechanics were reviewed at the beginning of this section, but let us see how they are specifically put to use during some examples of providing manual resistance to a patient during a lower and an upper extremity exercise. To make the activities difficult, we will assume that the patient in each example has a grade of 4/5 strength in the muscles resisted. We will also assume that the patient is male and the clinician is female. The patient is familiar with the exercises presented, so the clinician is not required to provide instruction and demonstration prior to their execution. As the patient pushes against the clinician in each exercise, the clinician provides an equivalent force that allows for smooth movement through the entire range of motion.

Upper Extremity Resistance

If the patient is supine and the clinician provides manual resistance to shoulder abduction, the clinician stands at the side of the patient with one hand just proximal to the lateral wrist and the other hand just proximal to the lateral elbow. The clinician's forearms are supinated (supinator) with the wrists extended (eccentric activity of the flexor carpi muscles). The elbows are in slight flexion, controlled by cocontraction of the elbow flexors (biceps and brachialis) with the triceps. The thumbs are on the anterior surface of the patient's upper extremity whereas the fingers are on the posterior surface; the thumbs are placed in opposition to the fingers through activity of the opponens pollicis. The fingers and thumbs are not required to grasp the extremity, so they may be relaxed, in partial flexion. Both shoulders are in slight flexion via contraction of the anterior deltoid and pectoralis major with stabilization of the scapula provided by the scapular rotators (trapezius, serratus anterior, and rhomboids). As the patient abducts the shoulder, the clinician resists the movement with isometric contraction of these muscles just mentioned (Fig. 13.10). As the arm moves through the motion into full abduction, the clinician uses the power of the legs to control the speed of shoulder abduction. The gluteal muscles and hamstrings control hip extension motion, the quadriceps controls knee motion, and the gastrocnemius and soleus control tibial motion over the ankle as the clinician walks toward the head of the table as the patient moves his shoulder through full abduction. When each foot is raised off the floor, the tibialis anterior provide ankle dorsiflexion to clear the foot from the floor. The clinician's trunk must remain in neutral throughout the activity so the forces from her legs may be transferred and used in her upper extremities. Her arm positions remain unchanged throughout the patient's range of motion. At the completion of one repetition, the clinician maintains control of the patient's arm and walks to return to the patient's side, ready for another repetition.

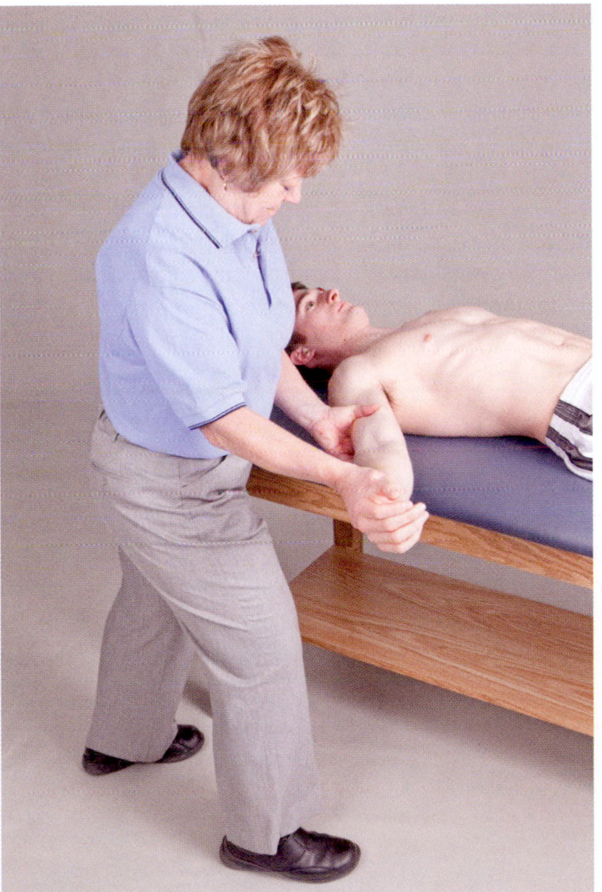

Figure 13.10 Clinician offering manual resistance to upper extremity.

Lower Extremity Resistance

In this example, the patient is to receive manual resistance to knee extension. The patient is sitting over the side of a treatment table with the knees just off the edge and the legs hanging down. A rolled towel is placed under the distal thigh to level the thigh with the table. The knee to receive the exercise is the patient's right knee.

The clinician faces the patient, in front of and slightly to the right of his right knee. She kneels down on her right knee and maintains good spinal alignment. The left leg is flexed at the hip and knee with the foot flat on the floor and ahead of the right knee. She places her right hand at the anterior ankle. In this position, the clinician's right hip is extended (gluteal muscles and hamstrings) while the left one is flexed (iliopsoas and rectus femoris) (Fig. 13.11). Both of her knees are flexed to about 90° (hamstrings). As the clinician leans forward from the hips, her right gluteus maximus and hamstrings eccentrically control the amount of motion. Her right hand is positioned with the thumb opposing the other fingers (opponens pollicis) and all the digits are in some flexion (flexor

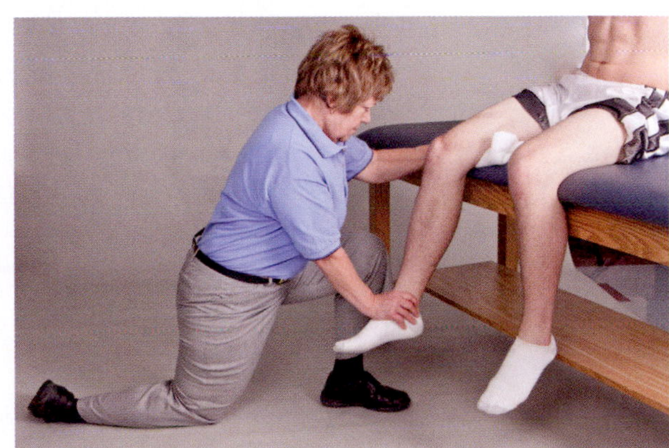

Figure 13.11 Clinician offering manual resistance to lower extremity.

digitorum longus and brevis, flexor pollicis longus and brevis). The wrist is in extension and radial deviation (extensor carpi radialis longus and brevis and flexor carpi radialis). The elbow is initially positioned into some flexion by the elbow flexors (biceps, brachialis, and brachioradialis) but once the motion begins, the triceps and these muscles cocontract to hold the elbow in position. The shoulder moves into some flexion through effort from the anterior deltoid, coracobrachialis, and pectoralis major. Since the shoulder motion is less than 60°, the scapula is maintained in a stabilized position by its rotators, as has been previously mentioned. If the patient is strong, the clinician may choose to anchor her body by placing her left hand on top of the table surface. If this is done, then the left shoulder elevates forward; the muscles used to achieve this are the same as for the right shoulder girdle except the scapular upward rotators (serratus anterior and upper and lower trapezius) rotate the scapula to achieve the desired shoulder elevation. The elbow is near extension and the forearm is pronated with the palm of the hand in contact with the table top. To achieve this position, the triceps moves the elbow towards extension as the pronator quadratus and teres pronate the forearm. The fingers move into extension and abduction (extensor digitorum and pollicis longus and dorsal interossei) so the palmar surface is in contact with the table top.

As the patient's quadriceps contract to extend his knee, the clinician provides a resistance that provides a steady motion throughout the knee's entire range of motion. With her body in front of her arm, she initially transfers her weight from the front foot to the back leg, and as the patient's knee continues to extend, she moves to a standing position so her right upper extremity does not change its position relative to the patient's limb. As she provides resistance, the scapular, shoulder, elbow, and wrist muscles contract isometrically, similar to the upper extremity resistance example. The back is maintained in a neutral and stable position whereas the strength of the hips and thighs is used to control the resistance applied to the patient.

Summary

This chapter demonstrated how to perform a kinematic analysis and how to kinesiologically describe the movement sequence, joint motions, and muscle activity that occur during common functional movements. The strategy that was used included the description and analysis of movement by carefully studying a movement, and then describing it in the following steps: description of the sequence of the motion, the joint motions, and finally the muscle activity used in the performance of the activity. Common examples of daily activities, work tasks, and clinical skill applications were provided to assist in understanding how kinesiological analysis occurs and why it is necessary. Once you have identified the activities involved in a task, you are able to make a rehabilitation program for an individual more meaningful and appropriate. Now that you have acquired an idea of how kinesiological analysis of an activity occurs, we will get into more specific applications. The next two chapters expand on analysis and look at upper extremity involvement in activities of daily living (Chapter 14) and total body involvement in sports and leisure activities (Chapter 15).

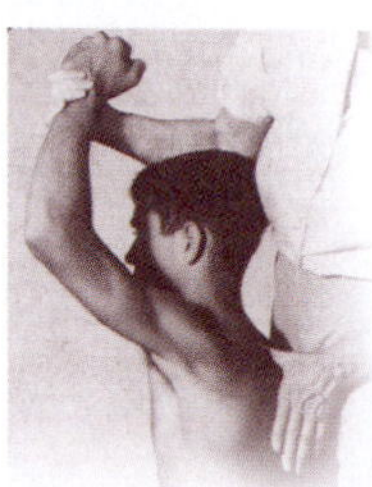

CLINICAL SCENARIO SOLUTION

Juan realizes that neither computer station he uses at home or at the library is set up properly for him. At the library, he sits with his body leaning forward and his back rounded with his elbows below his hands and his wrists in hyperextension. At home, his chair is too high for him, so he sits with his back arched as he tries to reach the floor with his feet. His computer screen at home requires him to move his head up whenever he looks at the screen. His goal is to have both work stations in proper order before the end of today. He is looking forward to fixing them so he does not continue to have problems with his neck and wrist.

Discussion Questions

1. Review each of the kinematic analyses described in this chapter and answer the following questions based on your understanding of that review:
   a. Of the joint segments involved, on which is the demand the highest? The lowest?
   b. Of the joints involved in performing the task, which segment or joint is at risk for impairment over time either because of repetitive motion or impingement?
2. Identify the problems in Juan's work station and his computer set up at home. List the changes you would suggest to correct them.
3. Based on the kinesiology descriptions of how to manually resist a patient during shoulder abduction and knee extension exercises, how would you describe the clinician's position and movement if the movement that is resisted is hip flexion with the patient in supine?
4. Now that you understand the motion and activities involved in using a vacuum cleaner, how would you explain the requirements to sweep a floor with a broom?
5. Describe the motion requirements for an individual to move a box from waist level to head level. What concerns should you have regarding the safety of this task?
6. Using good body mechanics, describe how you would help push a car that is stuck in the mud. How do you transfer the force from your hips and legs to your arms?
7. Do you think it is easier to pull a heavy object or push it? Explain your answer. Describe how to do it most kinesiologically correctly.
8. If you stand on a moving bus, how should you place your lower extremities? Explain your answer.

Lab Activities

1. Working with a partner or in a small group, review each of the kinematic analyses described in this chapter and offer a modification of that activity, given some constraints that you would anticipate seeing in the clinical environment.
2. Using the kinematic analysis model provided in this chapter—sequence of motion, joint motion, and muscle activity—practice analyzing the following additional common functional activities:
   a. Washing and drying dishes;
   b. Loading a top loading washing machine;
   c. Folding laundry;
   d. Emptying a front loading clothes dryer;
   e. Using a blow drier and hairbrush;
   f. Taking a shower;
   g. Donning a winter coat;
   h. Donning a pullover sweater;
   i. Pulling up a zipper;
   j. Tying your shoes;
   k. Shoveling snow;
   l. Using a computer mouse to scroll and search the internet;
   m. Performing jumping jacks in aerobics class; and
   n. Dancing (you pick the dance!).

Feel free to challenge yourself and your classmates by coming up with more examples. Have fun!

References

1. McGraw MB. *The Neuromuscular Maturation of the Human Infant*. New York: Haffner Press, 1945.
2. Richter RR, VanSant AF, Newton RA. Description of adult rolling movements and hypothesis of developmental sequences. *Physical Therapy* 69:63–71, 1989.
3. Bertoti DB. *Functional Neurorehabilitation through the Life Span*. Philadelphia: F A Davis Company, 2004.
4. Cech DJ, Martin S. *Functional Movement Development across the Life Span*. Philadelphia: WB Saunders, 2002.
5. Shumway-Cook A, Woollacott MH. *Motor Control: Translating Research into Clinical Practice*, ed 3. Philadelphia: Lippincott, Williams & Wilkins, 2007.
6. Van Sant A. Rising from a supine position to erect stance. *Physical Therapy* 68:185, 1988.
7. Kelley DL, Dainis A, Wood GK. Mechanics and muscular dynamics of rising from a seated position. In Komi PV (ed): *Biomechanics*, Baltimore: University Park Press, 1976, pp 127–134.
8. Millington PJ, Myklebust BM, Shambes GM. Biomechanical analysis of the sit-to-stand motion in elderly persons. *Archives of Physical Medicine and Rehabilitation* 73:609–617, 1992.
9. Richards CL. EMG activity level comparisons in quadriceps and hamstrings in five dynamic activities. In Winter DA, Norman RP, Wells RP (eds): *International series on biomechanics IX-A*, Champaign, IL: Human Kinetics Publishers, 1985, pp 313-317.
10. Carr R, Shepherd J. *Neurological Rehabilitation: Optimizing Motor Performance*. Oxford: Butterworth Heinemann, 1998.
11. Janssen W, Bussmann H, Stam H. Determinants of the sit-to-stand movement: A review. *Physical Therapy* 82:866–879, 2002.
12. Magermans DJ, Chadwick EKJ, Veeger, HEJ, van der Helm FCT. Requirements for upper extremity motions during activities of daily living. *Clinical Biomechanics* 20(6):591–599, 2005.
13. Cools A, Witvrouw E, Declercq G, Danneels L, Cambier D. Scapular muscle recruitment patterns: Trapezius muscle latency with and without impingement symptoms. *American Journal of Sports Medicine* 31(4):542–549, 2003.
14. Tyler AE, Karst GM. Timing of muscle activity during reaching while standing: Systematic changes with target distance. *Gait & Posture* 20(2):126–133, 2004.
15. Haugstvedt JR, Berger RJ, Berglund LJ. A mechanical study of the moment-forces of the supinators and pronators of the forearm. *Acta Orthopaedica Scandinavica* 72(6):629–634, 2001.
16. Nachemson A. Lumbar intradiscal pressure. *Acta Orthopaedica Scandinavica* 43:1–104, 1960.
17. Archambault P, Pigeon P, Feldman AG, Levin MF. Recruitment and sequencing of different degrees of freedom during pointing movements involving the trunk in healthy and hemiparetic individuals. *Experimental Brain Research* 126(1):55–67, 1999.
18. Pierson FM, Fairchild SL. *Principles & Techniques of Patient Care*, ed 3. Philadelphia: Saunders, 2002.

Kinesiology Applications of Upper Extremity Activities of Daily Living

Ingrid Provident, EdD, OTR/L, and Peggy A. Houglum, PhD, PT, ATC

"Sometimes creativity just means the daily work of helping others to see a problem in a different way."

—Joseph L. Badaracco, John Shad Professor of Business Ethics at Harvard Business School

CHAPTER OUTLINE

Learning Outcomes
Clinical Scenario
Introduction
Functional Applications
- *Activities Requiring Primarily Shoulder Complex Movement*
- *Activities Requiring Primarily Elbow Movement*
- *Activities Requiring Primarily Forearm Movement*
- *Activities Requiring Primarily Wrist Movement*

Summary
Clinical Scenario Solution
Discussion Questions
Lab Activities
References

LEARNING OUTCOMES

By the end of this chapter, you should be able to:

- ❑ List muscles that are prime movers in common activities of daily living (ADL);
- ❑ Name muscle groups that function to position and move the upper extremity in specific functional activities;
- ❑ Identify prehension patterns of the hand used during common daily activities;
- ❑ Present a systematic model for activity analysis;
- ❑ Perform your own analysis of ADL activities.

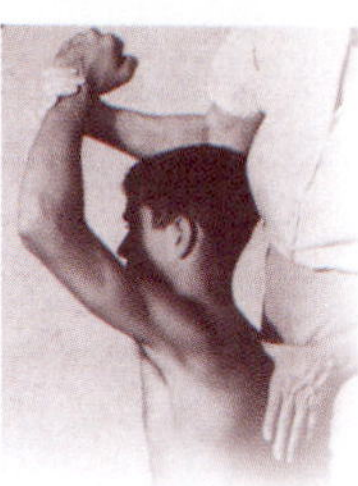

CLINICAL SCENARIO

Sam has treated Nathaniel for the past month to rehabilitate an elbow injury that was sustained when Nathaniel was working in interior remodeling and new construction. Nathaniel is now ready to return to work, but before he does, Sam is meeting Nathaniel at his work site this afternoon to assess his job and performance requirements. Sam wants to make sure that he has properly prepared Nathaniel to return to work to perform his job skills safely and effectively.

Introduction

Every day, human beings carry out simple and complex movements involved in activities of daily living, activities involved in taking care of themselves, performing work related tasks, and enjoying leisure or recreation activities. Every individual carries out these tasks in a unique manner unto themselves; therefore, there is high variability in the way muscles are recruited and used during similar activities. For example, you may get out of bed in the morning differently than your brother or sister, and your routine of getting dressed and ready for school may be different than your roommate's or friend's routine. Before a clinician is able to assist a patient in adapting activities to overcome movement disorders, an understanding of normal movement must first be achieved. For this reason, the examples provided within the chapter assume normal movement. The descriptions of movement included in this chapter do not include all muscles involved in the tasks but only the major contributing muscles. The activities described within this chapter are organized in a proximal to distal direction, citing examples that utilize mostly shoulder movement first, then moving on to activities that require more elbow movement, and finally, activities that require more movement of the hand and fingers are discussed.

Functional Applications

Functional applications in this chapter include only those activities and muscles of the upper extremity. If a person is standing while performing the upper extremity activity, then muscles of the lower extremity are also involved in the task, as are the trunk muscles. To prevent this chapter from becoming unwieldy in its content, however, focus will remain only on functions of the upper limb. It would be, of course, impossible to include all activities of the upper extremity that are involved in all activities of daily living and daily function in one chapter. One of the purposes of this chapter is to provide you with examples of some of the more common upper limb activities so that you may grasp the general concepts of functional movement analysis. Once you are able to appreciate these general methods of movement analysis, then you may progress to assimilating your own movement analysis of other functional activities you will encounter in patients you will treat. Additional study in your professional curriculum will build upon these basic kinesiological functional application examples.

Each of the activities described will follow a presentation sequence of the information so that it will be easier to understand and compare. First, the sequence in which movements or muscle activity occurs is presented. Then the joints and motions of the joints involved in the upper limb will be identified. Lastly, the muscles for each of the joints and their functions will then be presented to provide a full picture of the activity.

Activities Requiring Primarily Shoulder Complex Movement

As you recall from previous chapters, the role of the shoulder is to position the hand so it can be used for function. Since the shoulder complex often initiates upper limb movement during daily activities, it is presented first in this chapter's sequence. There are five types of activities involving the shoulder presented in this section.

Reaching Overhead and Forward

To carry out many activities of daily living such as reaching to a high shelf in a closet to get a book, or hanging up a jacket on a hanger in the closet, the shoulder requires a varying but optimal range of motion (Fig. 14.1A, B). Before a clinician is able to identify a patient's functional abilities, the clinician must realize what requirements must be present for activities to be performed adequately.

Sequence of Movement

Before the shoulder moves, the trunk muscles must first prepare the body for this movement.[5] The upper trapezius and serratus anterior then stabilize the scapula as the humerus begins elevation.[5] When humeral elevation

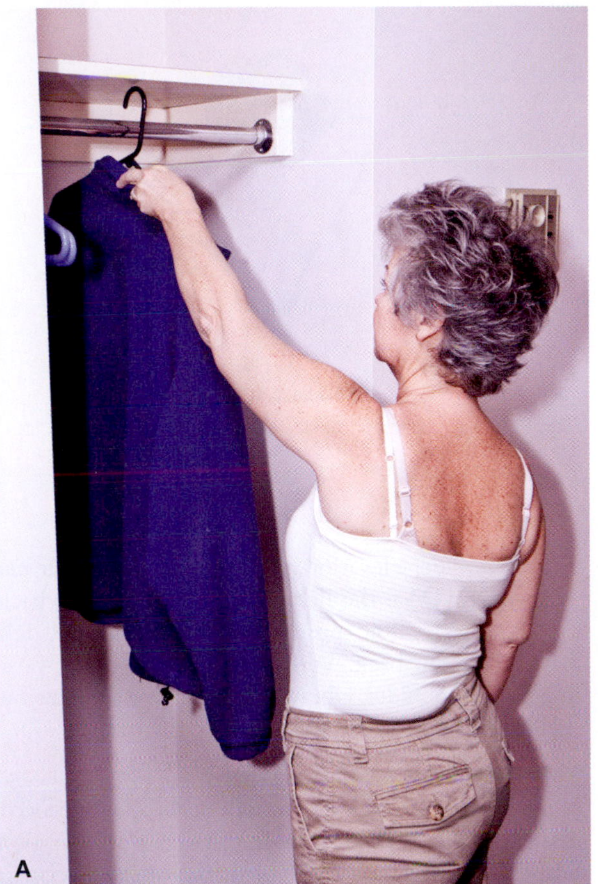

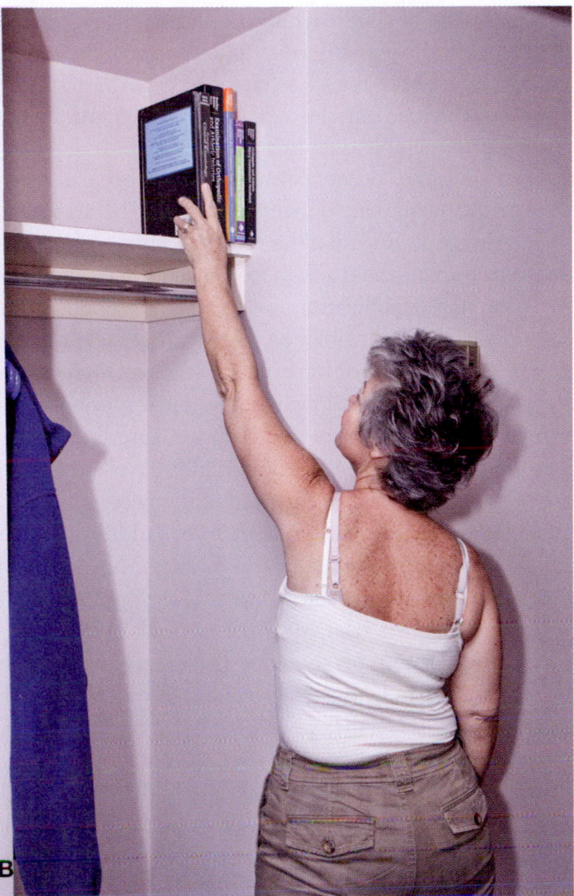

Figure 14.1 A) Hanging a hanger in a closet or B) Reaching a high shelf requires shoulder, elbow, wrist, and hand movements.

begins, the rotator cuff stabilizes the humeral head in the glenoid. As the reach goes higher, the scapular muscles begin to also produce upward rotation and protraction of the scapula, and the rotator cuff muscles continue to stabilize the humeral head in the glenoid fossa. As the extremity elevates more, elbow extension progressively occurs to accurately position the hand to grasp the object. As the hand approaches its target—the book or hanger—the fingers extend and fine tune their position (by the finger extensors) to match the size of the object. Once the object is in the hand, the fingers flex to conform the hand to the book or hanger, and the wrist extensors synergistically fire to stabilize the wrist in slight extension. As the object is grasped, isometric activity of the stabilizing muscles of the scapula, glenohumeral joint, elbow flexors and extensors, and wrist flexors and extensors occurs to allow the individual to pick up the object before glenohumeral muscles elevate the humerus to lift the object off the shelf or closet rod.

Joint Motion

The daily activities which require the largest ranges of motion in glenohumeral elevation include overhead reaching and combing hair.[1] Joints and motions involved in overhead shoulder complex activities include scapular upward rotation and protraction, glenohumeral flexion, and elbow extension. When the person is facing the shelf or closet and performing true shoulder flexion, the motion of the shoulder and elbow occurs in the sagittal plane on a frontal axis. Forearm motion will depend upon the specific requirement of hand placement and may include either supination or pronation. The wrist is in slight extension whereas the fingers are in some degree of flexion for grasping or maintaining a grasp.

Muscle Activity

As with most activities, the muscles farther away from the site of activity activate prior to the muscles performing the activity. In the case of reaching, the muscles that fire first include the tibialis anterior, followed quickly by the quadriceps.[2] These muscles function as body stabilizers. The erector spinae muscles actually begin activity after the tibialis anterior and quadriceps; this delayed activity of this muscle group occurs because the erector spinae controls trunk movement during reaching activities.[2] Once body stability occurs, shoulder motion begins with postural stabilization of the trunk in a balanced stance and proximal scapular stabilization of the glenohumeral joint. Once the trunk is stabilized, the arm is then elevated against gravity by a combination of scapular rotation and protraction and humeral flexion.[3] Scapular motion is performed by the trapezius and serratus anterior whereas glenohumeral motion is predominantly produced by the large movers—the clavicular head of the pectoralis major, coracobrachialis, and anterior deltoid. Additionally, the rotator cuff works to stabilize the humeral head into the lower glenoid socket as the humerus is elevated. The exact height of the shelf relative to the person's height determines the amount of shoulder flexion needed for the reach. As the arm begins its elevation, the triceps initially contract to extend the elbow; as the extremity moves higher, the elbow flexors take over to control the elbow.[4] When the arm is overhead, although the elbow is in extension, the antigravity elbow force is provided by the biceps and brachialis working eccentrically to position the elbow to allow the hand to grasp the object. The position of the hand is also determined by the amount of forearm pronation or supination and the degree of wrist flexion or extension needed to position the hand correctly so the object may be manipulated as desired. The wrist is positioned as needed and is then stabilized by cocontraction of the wrist flexors and extensors (flexor carpi ulnaris, extensor carpi radialis longus and brevis, and extensor carpi ulnaris). The hand assumes a spherical grasp to take the book from the shelf. If it is a hanger that is being placed on a closet rod, the hand will assume a hook grasp around the hanger until it is released onto the rod.

Reaching Overhead and Backward

Reaching up and around to scratch your back between the scapulae is an activity that also requires a maximal amount of shoulder motion (Fig. 14.2). This hand placement incorporates shoulder elevation in more than one plane of motion.

Sequence of Movement

The scapula is stabilized when shoulder activity begins. Shoulder flexion initiates humeral elevation movement, but the movement changes to shoulder abduction before the end of elevation. As the shoulder elevates, the shoulder laterally rotates and the elbow flexes until the end of shoulder elevation, when both are at their end when range. Once the hand is behind the upper back, the posterior deltoid positions the hand in the right location of the back. With the hand correctly positioned, the shoulder, elbow, and wrist are stabilized as the fingers flex and extend to relieve the itch.

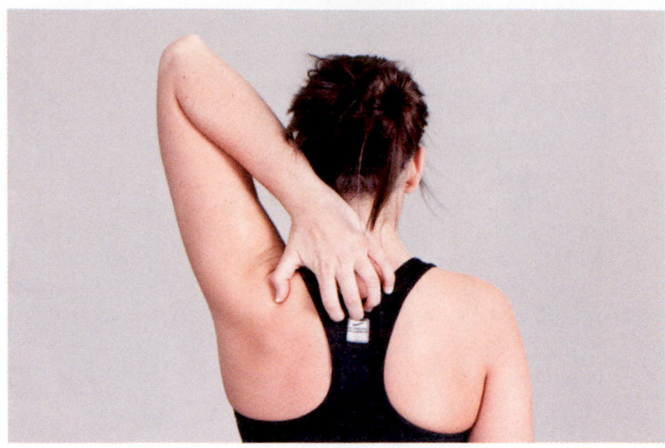

Figure 14.2 Reaching behind the back to the midback to scratch an itch.

Joint Motion

Shoulder flexion, lateral rotation, and abduction occur in the glenohumeral joint during this tri-planar motion. Scapular upward rotation and retraction also occur in the shoulder complex. Elbow flexion, forearm supination, and finger flexion and extension occur as the wrist remains in a static neutral position.

Muscle Activity

Scapular upward rotation is performed by the upper and lower trapezius and serratus anterior. The scapula also retracts via activity of the rhomboids and middle trapezius. Shoulder flexion motion is performed by the clavicular head of the pectoralis major and anterior deltoid. Shoulder abduction occurs through activity of the supraspinatus and middle deltoid as the other rotator cuff muscles stabilize the humeral head in the inferior glenoid fossa. The posterior deltoid also plays a role in positioning the hand behind the upper back by moving the humerus in the desired position above the head. Lateral rotation of the humerus is the result of activity from the infraspinatus and teres minor. The elbow joint is initially flexed by concentric contraction of the biceps and the forearm rotates into full supination by the supinator's concentric activity so the hand is correctly positioned between the scapulas to scratch the back. Once the hand is overhead, the triceps eccentrically control the lowering of the hand to the back. The wrist is stabilized in neutral by coactivation of the wrist flexors and extensors to allow the finger flexors and extensors to flex and extend the fingers, respectively, to scratch the area of the back that itches.

Hobby or Work Activity: Sanding Wood

A common upper extremity work activity performed by individuals both at work and at home is sanding wood (Fig. 14.3). Many people have work responsibilities, recreational hobbies, or perform home projects which require this type of action. For this reason, this activity is selected as a work activity for analysis here. Specifically, we will use sanding the top of a large piece of furniture for refinishing.

Sequence of Movement

The trunk muscles contract to maintain trunk stability prior to beginning shoulder activity and throughout the activity. The scapular rotators stabilize the scapula throughout the activity. Scapular retraction occurs with glenohumeral horizontal abduction and scapular protraction occurs with glenohumeral horizontal adduction. The wrist remains statically positioned by isometric contraction of its muscles throughout the activity. The finger flexors also work statically to maintain a grasp on the sandpaper. If a sandpaper sheet is used, the individual may use a lateral pinch grip. As depicted in the photograph, when a sandpaper block is used, the grip may be a hook or a cylinder grasp.

It should be noted that the sequence of firing within the shoulder complex may change with differences in speed of activity. Investigators have found that slow and fast speeds alter the firing sequence between the deltoid and scapular muscles[6] and when the subject is unable to anticipate motion.[5] When motion is anticipated, the upper trapezius and serratus anterior fire before glenohumeral muscles.[4] However, if the movement becomes rapid or the demand of the activity occurring is unpredictable, the scapular muscles fire immediately after the deltoid muscle begins glenohumeral motion.[6]

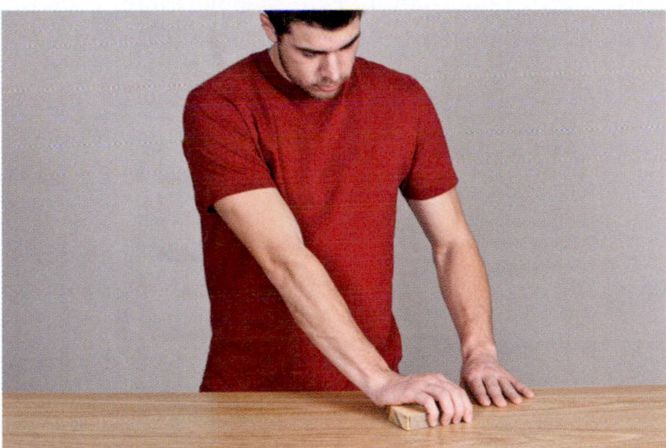

Figure 14.3 Work activities such as sanding require both stabilization and contraction of upper extremity muscles, especially those of the shoulder complex.

Joint Motion

Such a project requires shoulder motions of horizontal abduction and adduction and a minimal level of shoulder elevation. Along with these shoulder motions are scapular protraction and retraction, elbow extension and flexion, wrist extension, and finger flexion.

Muscle Activity

Trunk and hip muscles work throughout the activity to stabilize the trunk and lower limbs during upper extremity movement. Consistent with other examples in this chapter, only the upper extremity, and specifically in this section, the shoulder, are presented for analysis. The person initially engages the scapular rotators to act as stabilizers and the glenohumeral flexors (clavicular head of the pectoralis major and anterior deltoid) and extensors (latissimus dorsi and teres major) to stabilize the upper extremity at the correct height in the sagittal plane. Scapular retraction is the responsibility of the rhomboids and middle trapezius contracting concentrically, and scapular protraction occurs from concentric contraction of the serratus anterior and pectoralis minor. Horizontal abduction occurs from concentric contraction of the posterior deltoid as it moves the arm across the surface and laterally from the body. Returning to the original spot of sanding (Fig. 14.3) occurs with horizontal adduction as the pectoralis major, coracobrachialis, and the anterior deltoid muscles contract concentrically. The wrist is positioned in slight extension by the cocontraction of the wrist flexor and extensor muscles (extensor carpi radialis longus and brevis, extensor carpi ulnaris, and flexor carpi radialis and ulnaris). Fingers maintain their cylinder grasp on the sandpaper block with flexion and adduction of the flexor digitorum superficialis and profundus and the interossei muscles. The thumb maintains its grasp via contraction of the flexor pollicis longus and brevis and adductor pollicis.

Hygiene Activity: Oral Care

Activities of daily living (ADL) certainly include hygiene. The routine of morning and evening hygiene typically consists of brushing one's teeth (Fig. 14.4). Since this is an activity all individuals perform, it is analyzed here as an example of a typical ADL.

Sequence of Movement

Once the trunk and scapula are stabilized, the shoulder is elevated so the glenohumeral joint is at about 80° of

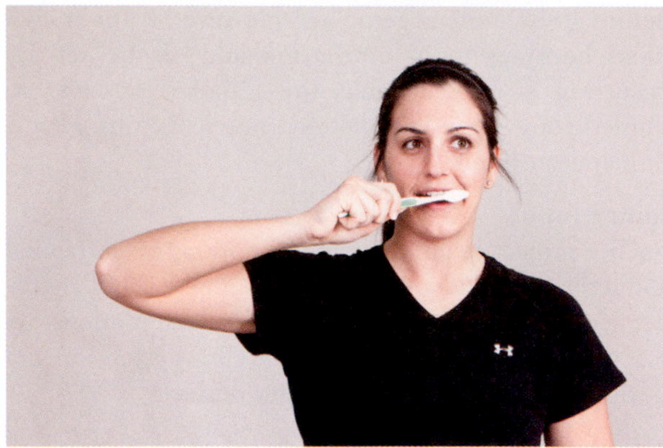

Figure 14.4 Tooth brushing is an activity of daily living we all perform. The activity is much more complicated than it appears and requires cooperative movements of all upper extremity joints.

elevation, close to the scapular plane. The elbow is then flexed by the biceps to bring the toothbrush to the mouth, and the forearm is pronated to place the toothbrush on the teeth. Once the toothbrush is properly positioned, small motions of the entire upper extremity's joints provide the tooth brushing activity; the elbow, wrist, and hand grip muscles along with the shoulder complex muscles make small adjustments as the toothbrush is moved to various parts of the mouth and the toothbrush is oscillated over the teeth to clean them.

Joint Motion

This activity of daily living uses a great deal of glenohumeral joint motion, namely flexion, abduction, horizontal abduction, and horizontal adduction. Scapular rotation with protraction and retraction accompany these glenohumeral motions. The elbow slightly flexes and extends. The forearm maintains pronation, but the wrist alternates between small radial and ulnar deviation movements with slight flexion and extension while brushing the teeth.

Muscle Activity

This relatively "simple" activity requires a lot of muscles working cooperatively to produce the desired results. Once again, trunk muscles stabilize the trunk as the upper extremity performs the task. The scapula muscles have more than one function: The upward rotators (upper and lower trapezius and serratus anterior) position the scapula in some upward rotation and then act as stabilizers to maintain the scapular position during the tooth brushing activity. The scapular protractors (serratus anterior and pectoralis minor) and the scapular retractors (rhomboids and middle trapezius) work concentrically in conjunction with the glenohumeral horizontal adductors (pectoralis major, anterior deltoid, and coracobrachialis) and the horizontal abductor (posterior deltoid), respectively. Maintaining the arm in an elevated position throughout the activity requires continual effort of the deltoid and rotator cuff working as a force couple at the glenohumeral joint to hold this position of glenohumeral abduction and elevation. Since elbow motion occurs as the forearm and arm maintain a horizontal alignment to the ground at shoulder level, the small amount of elbow flexion is controlled by concentric activity of the brachialis and biceps brachii and elbow extension results from triceps concentric contraction. The hand assumes a modified hook grasp of the toothbrush with a lateral pinch to control the stability of the toothbrush. The teeth are brushed by back and forth motions coming from contractions of agonist and antagonist muscles controlling glenohumeral horizontal abduction and adduction with scapular retraction and protraction. Short excursions of the elbow occur during the activity in flexion and extension; these motions are controlled by alternating contractions of the elbow flexors and extensors. Although motions are small, wrist flexors and extensors along with radial and ulnar flexors play a very important role in the positioning of the toothbrush and angling it to reach all of the teeth.

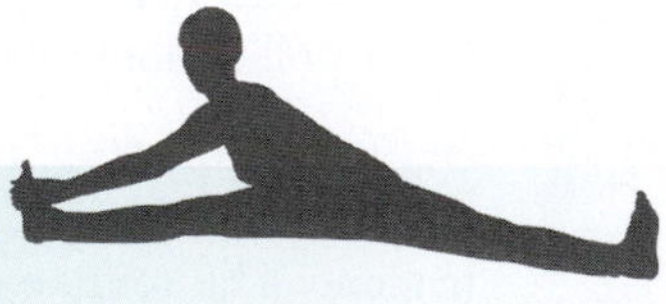

PRACTICE POINT

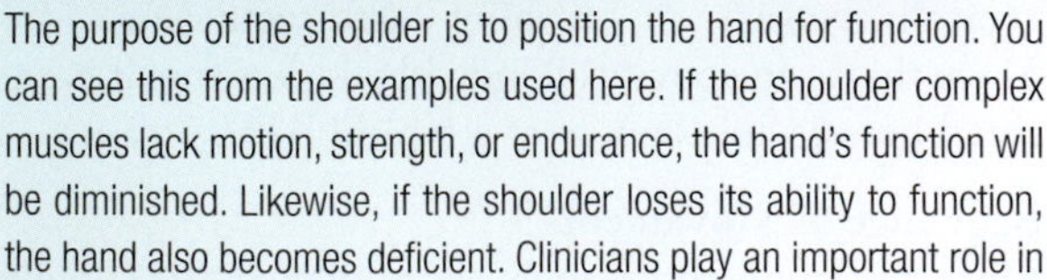

The purpose of the shoulder is to position the hand for function. You can see this from the examples used here. If the shoulder complex muscles lack motion, strength, or endurance, the hand's function will be diminished. Likewise, if the shoulder loses its ability to function, the hand also becomes deficient. Clinicians play an important role in identifying deficits in both the glenohumeral and scapulothoracic regions of the shoulder complex and in providing restoration of those deficits. If complete restoration is not possible, then the clinician must devise alternative methods for successful completion of daily and work tasks.

Activities Requiring Primarily Elbow Movement

As you have no doubt noticed, the activities just discussed place the majority of effort requirements on the shoulder complex. There are several activities of daily living that require less effort of shoulder complex muscles and more effort of the muscles which control the elbow. The primary responsibility of the elbow is to position the hand relative to the body, either closer to or farther away from it. Two of these functional activities which position the hand for use are presented here.

Feeding

Feeding is an activity that requires synchronization of several upper extremity joint motions including shoulder flexion, elbow flexion, and forearm supination.[7] Utensils used in eating require primarily stabilization activities of the shoulder, wrist, and hand, whereas the elbow is the joint which moves the most (Fig. 14.5A, B). Its muscles are responsible for controlling the amount and direction of motion and the amount of force required to complete the task successfully.

Sequence of Movement

As in most other functional activities, stabilizing muscles contract immediately when the motion begins. Therefore, the scapular and glenohumeral stabilizers contract when the finger flexors grasp the spoon or fork. The forearm pronates to pick up the food (Fig. 14.5A), and then there is a simultaneous movement of the forearm into supination and the elbow into flexion as the food is brought toward the mouth (Fig.14.5B). If any elevation of the shoulder is required, it is during this part of the activity that it occurs to assist in moving the utensil to the mouth. The motions occur in reverse order when the individual returns the fork or spoon to the plate or bowl for more food.

Joint Motion

Feeding oneself is an activity that requires considerable range of motion at the elbow joint.[1] The act of bringing the hand to the mouth requires that a person maintain the appropriate grasp on the utensil. The grasp used is typically a three-jaw chuck grasp using the thumb, index, and middle fingers (Fig. 14.5A). The elbow flexes to bring the hand to the mouth for food consumption. The elbow moves towards extension but requires the elbow to move to approximately 30° of flexion when the individual returns the utensil to pick up another bite of food from the plate. During this elbow excursion, subtle hand and utensil positioning is often required to reach the food or keep a spoon level when delivering soup to the mouth. These movements typically include some forearm pronation in positioning the hand to pick up the food and forearm supination to bring the utensil to the mouth. The shoulder is usually maintained in a scapular plane slightly away from the body throughout the activity.

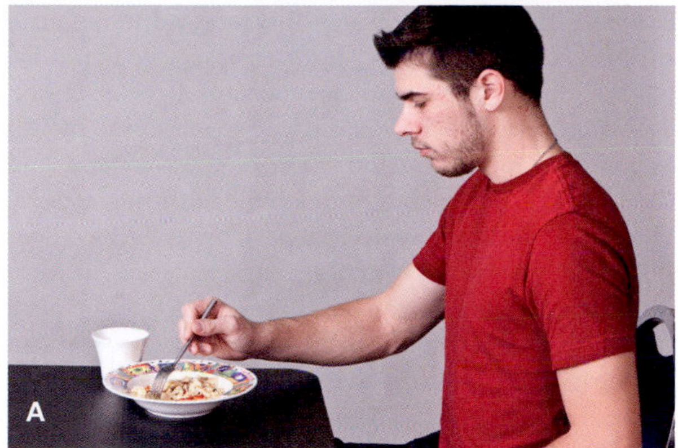

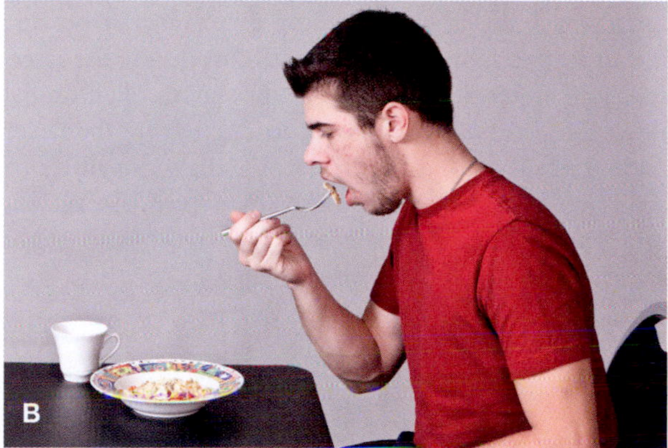

Figure 14.5 A) The most common grasp for eating is a three-jaw chuck grasp. B) As the elbow flexes, the forearm supinates to move the food to the mouth.

Muscle Activity

Scapular and glenohumeral stabilizers provide for proximal stability of the extremity during elbow motions through isometric contractions. Scapular stabilizers include the upward (trapezius and serratus anterior) and downward (rhomboids, levator scapulae, and pectoralis minor) rotators whereas the glenohumeral stabilizers include the rotator cuff and deltoid, which maintain the humeral head in the fossa. There may be minimal activity of the large muscles to elevate the arm when the fork or spoon approaches the mouth. If this glenohumeral elevation is needed, the anterior deltoid and pectoralis major activate concentrically; these same muscles work eccentrically to lower the arm as the individual returns for more food. As the utensil is brought to the mouth, the biceps brachii and brachialis control the elbow flexion concentrically. When the utensil is returned to the plate or bowl, the same elbow flexors contract eccentrically, controlling the speed and direction of elbow extension against gravity. Moving the fork or spoon to the mouth requires a concentric contraction of the supinator and biceps brachii supinating to rotate the forearm anteriorly to keep the utensil in an upright position so the food does not fall off before it gets to the mouth. Rotating the forearm into pronation as the utensil is returned to the plate or bowl for more food, such as soup, occurs with an eccentric contraction of these same muscles. Isometric contraction of wrist flexors (flexor carpi radialis and ulnaris) and wrist extensors (extensor carpi radialis longus and brevis and extensor carpi ulnaris) provide cocontraction to maintain wrist stability during the activity. As the utensil is brought to the mouth, slight radial deviation occurs through concentric activity of the flexor carpi radialis and extensor carpi radialis longus. The finger and thumb flexors (flexor digitorum superficialis and profundus and flexor pollicis longus) with slight contraction of the adductor pollicis maintain an isometrically flexed position of the first three digits to maintain a grasp of the utensil.

Donning Socks or Pants

Although they may not sound similar, in terms of motion and muscle activity required of the upper extremities, putting on a pair of socks or a pair of pants are very similar to each other (Fig. 14.6, Fig 14.7). These functions require active use of the elbow muscles and some activity by muscles of the other upper limb joints.

Sequence of Movement

Motion begins once the individual bends over to bring the sock to the foot (Fig.14.6A). As trunk flexion is controlled by eccentric contraction of the erector spinae muscles, the shoulders elevate to meet the foot. With the fingers grasping the sock, the sock is placed over the toes and then pulled up the foot, around the ankle and heel, and up the leg. As the sock is pulled over the foot, the elbows flex (Fig.14.6B). If pants are being pulled up

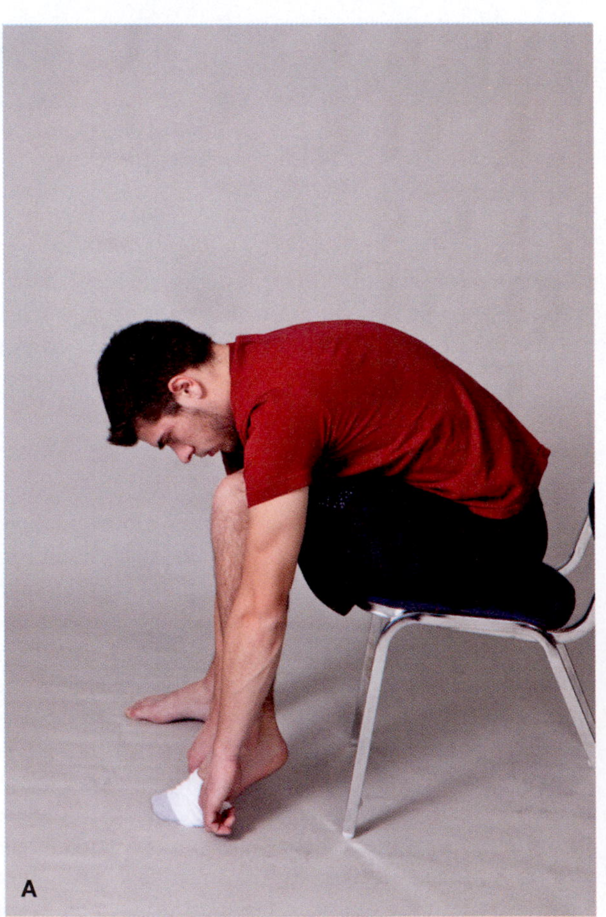

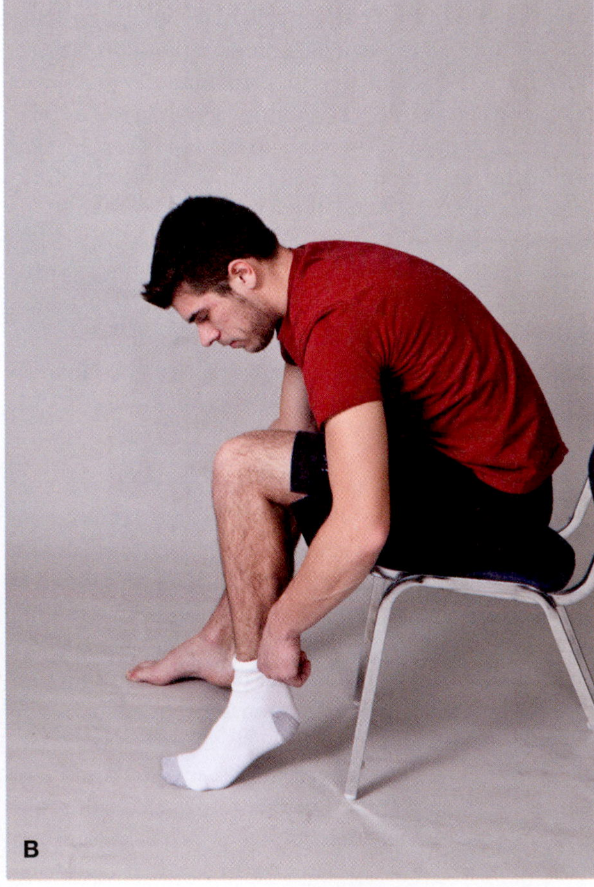

Figure 14.6 As the socks are put on, the elbows increase their flexion angle until the socks are fully on the foot.

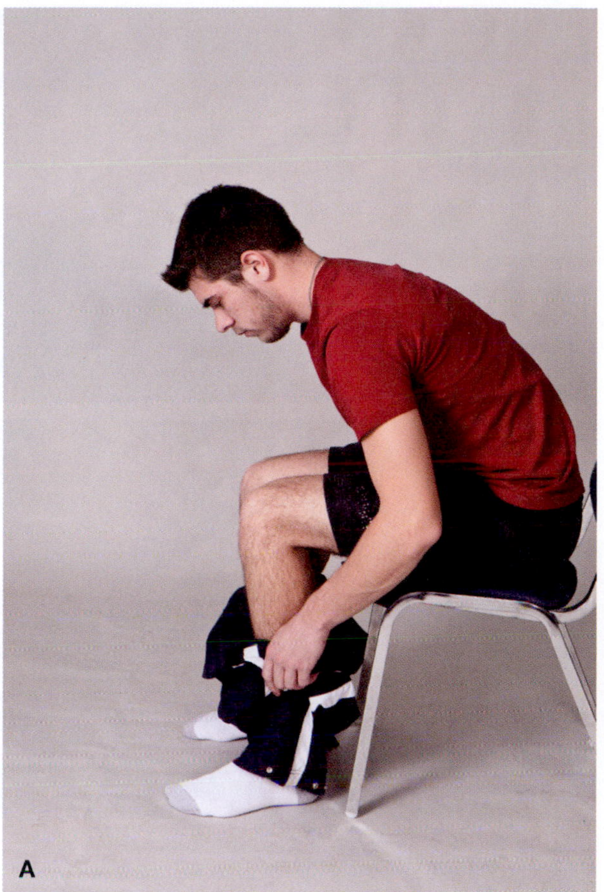

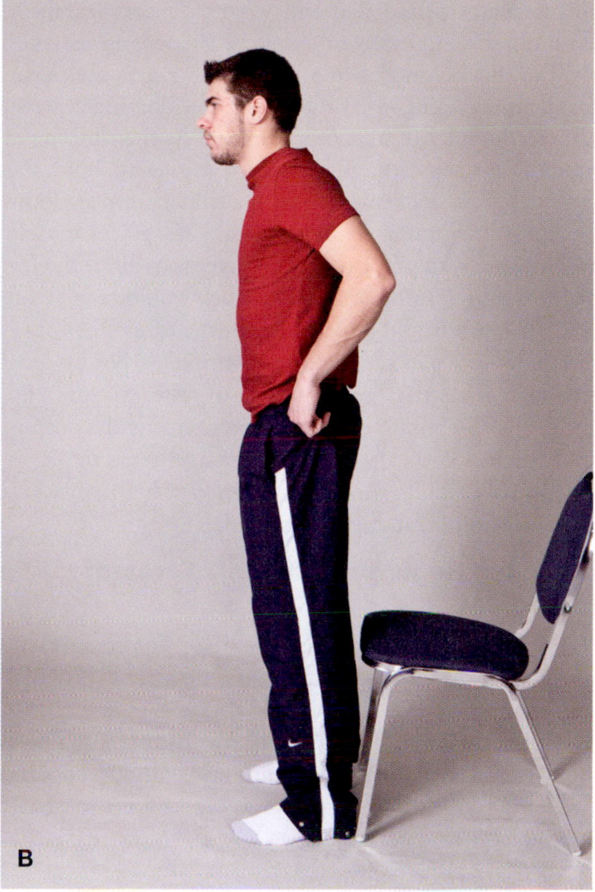

Figure 14.7 A) Donning pants also requires upper limb activities similar to donning socks. B) Once the pants are pulled up the lower leg, the person stands to pull the pants all the way up and, unlike donning socks, must use greater elbow flexion and shoulder hyperextension to complete the task.

(Fig. 14.7A), once they have reached the thighs, the individual stands (Fig. 14.7B). With the wrists stabilizing the hand to maintain a grasp on the pants, the elbows continue to flex as the shoulders move into hyperextension and the scapulae downwardly rotate.

Joint Motion

The person begins in the seated position for this ADL. At the start of the activity, the shoulders are flexed and the elbows are fully extended. The wrists begin in a functional position, slightly extended, and the hands assume a lateral pinch grasp. Once the motion initiates, the wrists flex. The elbows move from near extension into flexion throughout the activity until the socks are pulled up the calf. If the individual is putting on a pair of pants, he or she continues the movement by placing the leg into the other pant leg before transferring to a standing position to pull the pants completely up and over the upper legs and hips; this movement requires continued flexion of the elbows. During this process, the glenohumeral joints move from the initial position of slight flexion to hyperextension and the scapulae rotate downwardly. If the individual has balance difficulties, the pants are pulled up to the knees while in the sitting position, and the individual then lies on the bed with the hips and knees flexed and performs a bridge to lift the hips up so the pants may be pulled over the hips.

Muscle Activity

Trunk balance and control are required for the individual to lean forward to begin putting on socks. Eccentric contraction of the erector spinae controls the trunk's flexion to allow the hands to reach the feet. Scapular and glenohumeral stabilizers, as mentioned in previous activities, are active to stabilize the scapula on the thorax and the humeral head in the glenoid fossa, respectively. Shoulder flexors, including the pectoralis major and anterior deltoid, are active to move the shoulders into flexion at 90°. The wrist begins in a functional position by cocontraction of the wrist flexors (flexor carpi ulnaris and flexor carpi radialis) and wrist extensors (extensor carpi ulnaris and extensor carpi radialis longus and brevis) but quickly moves to a flexed position as the flexor carpi radialis and ulnaris become the dominant wrist muscles to pull the sock over the foot. As the clothing is brought up the legs, the hands continue to hold the material of the sock or pants with a lateral grasp as elbow flexion is predominately controlled by the biceps muscle and brachialis to pull the sock up over the calf of the leg or the pant leg to the thigh. The sock would now be on and the grasp would be released. In the case of continuing to don the pants, the elbows continue to flex by continued concentric contraction of the biceps and brachialis. Glenohumeral extension occurs with concentric activity of the latissimus dorsi and teres major as downward scapular rotation is controlled by rhomboids, pectoralis minor, and levator scapulae.

Activities Requiring Primarily Forearm Movement

Many activities throughout the day require forearm movement. Pronation and supination may not seem like important motions, but without them, even something as simple as starting your car becomes difficult. There are three activities described here, and without a doubt, you will be able to identify several others after you have completed this section.

Driving

Driving a vehicle is a complex activity that requires many body segments functioning at one time and the brain operating at several different levels simultaneously. For our purposes here, we will focus on the forearm function during operation of the steering wheel (Fig. 14.8A, B). In this example, we will focus on the action of using the arms to turn to the right while driving.

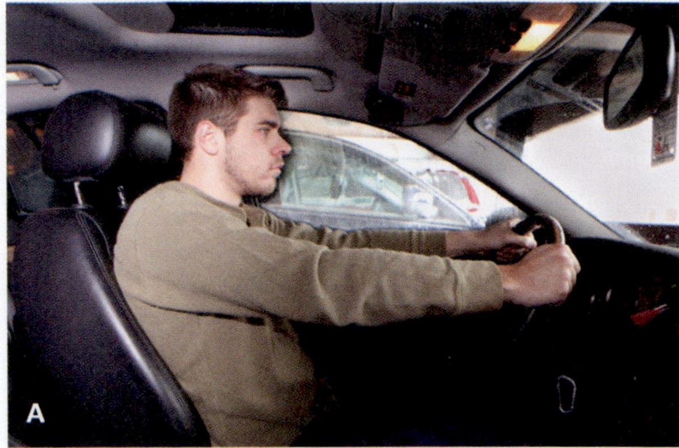

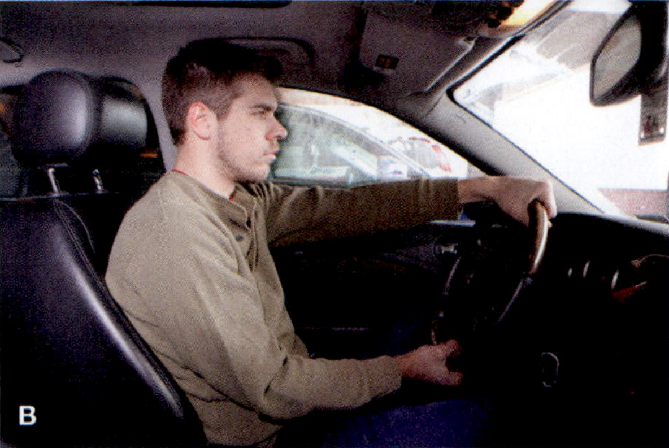

Figure 14.8 A) From the start position with the hands positioned on the steering wheel at the 10 and 2 o'clock position. B) When the steering wheel is turned, motion of the forearms and shoulders is required.

Sequence of Movement

Simultaneous supination of the near forearm (direction of the turn) and pronation of the far forearm (away from the direction of the turn) occur with simultaneous lateral rotation of the near shoulder and medial rotation of the far shoulder. Cocontraction of the wrist, finger, and scapular muscles occur as the shoulder and forearm muscles move the steering wheel.

Joint Motion

Driving a vehicle requires a person to have active forearm movement to turn the steering wheel. Maintaining the hands on the steering wheel occurs with a hook grasp.

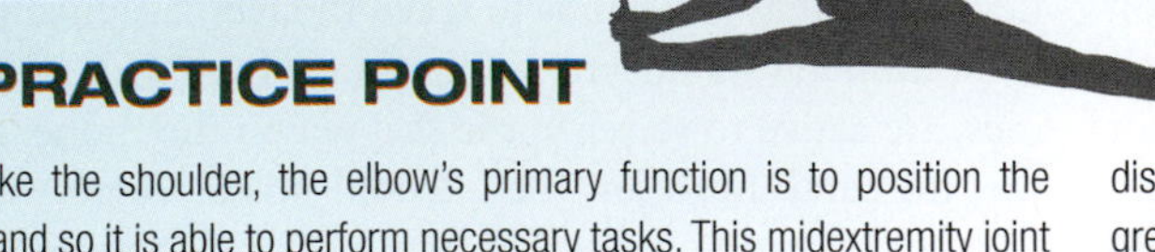

PRACTICE POINT

Like the shoulder, the elbow's primary function is to position the hand so it is able to perform necessary tasks. This midextremity joint allows adjustments of the limb in both distance and position so the hand may be more exactly positioned for its function. If injury or disability prevents either full strength or full motion, the individual is greatly impeded in the ability to reach and position the limb for functional activities. Compensation must occur either from the trunk or other joints of the upper extremity.

With the hands placed in the recommended 10 o'clock and 2 o'clock positions, there is slight pronation of the forearms (Fig. 14.8A). Turning the steering wheel requires forearm supination and pronation (Fig.14.8B). The elbows and shoulders are held in a relatively fixed position with the elbow at an approximate 60° to 90° angle, depending on the seat position relative to the steering wheel. Similarly, the shoulders are in slight flexion, depending upon the steering wheel position.

When the driver turns the wheel, the primary moving segments include the forearm and the shoulders. If the driver uses a hand-over-hand technique to rotate the steering wheel, the upper extremity closest to the direction to which the car is turning moves into some shoulder lateral rotation with forearm supination as the extremity farthest from the direction of the turn medially rotates at the shoulder with slight horizontal adduction and pronates at the forearm (Fig. 14.8B).

Muscle Activity

Once the hands are placed on the steering wheel and rest on it, the shoulder girdle and elbow muscles have little activity. If the hands hold the wheel tightly, then muscles throughout the upper limb cocontract isometrically to stabilize their joint to permit function of a more distal joint.

If the steering wheel is turned to the right, the right glenohumeral lateral rotators (infraspinatus and teres minor) concentrically contract as the other rotator cuff and deltoid muscles stabilize the humerus in the glenoid fossa. The left subscapularis medially rotates the left shoulder as the pectoralis major and anterior deltoid activate to horizontally adduct the shoulder during extremity movement to the 12 o'clock position as the steering wheel is turned. Since there is relatively no elevation of the shoulder, the scapular rotators stabilize the scapula to permit glenohumeral motion to occur. The elbow flexors and extensors of both extremities cocontract to stabilize the elbow whereas the right forearm supinator and biceps brachii supinate the forearm. Wrists of both extremities remain in a functional position through cocontraction of the extensors and flexors and the long fingers flexors maintain a grasp on the steering wheel. If the turn is not complete at the end of these movements, the right hand is lifted over and across the steering wheel to grasp the wheel on the other side of the left hand as the left hand is repositioned to the left side of the right hand on the wheel, and the procedure occurs again. For this repositioning to occur, the fingers must extend to release their grasp and the shoulders elevate slightly to lift the hands off the wheel and then lowers the shoulders to reposition the hands on the wheel. Slight horizontal adduction of the right shoulder and slight horizontal abduction of the left shoulder occur during this hand-repositioning maneuver.

Pouring

Another common everyday activity that requires forearm pronation is pouring coffee into a cup (Fig. 14.9A, B, C). Other fluids such as orange juice, tea, water, or milk may be poured to start your day, but regardless of what is poured, the elements of the activity are the same. The major difference is determined by the shape of the container from which the liquid is poured; this will alter the grip, but other components are essentially the same.

Sequence of Movement

As the coffee pot or container is grasped by the hand, the wrist, elbow, and shoulder girdle muscles contract to stabilize their respective joints. Forearm pronation then occurs as these muscles control the other upper extremity joints as the coffee or other liquid is poured into a cup or glass.

Joint Motion

The coffee pot is held with a hook grasp with the forearm initially positioned in a neutral alignment, midway between pronation and supination. The person typically positions the arm next to the body with the elbow at 90° of flexion. The coffee is poured with the glenohumeral joint moving into the scapular plane and the forearm moving into pronation until the cup is full; then the limb resumes its former position with the forearm in neutral. In some cases, this movement may be combined with shoulder abduction. (Note: In pathologic situations, shoulder abduction is a common substitution movement for forearm pronation.)

Muscle Activity

Scapular muscles, glenohumeral muscles, and elbow muscles cocontract to stabilize the shoulder and elbow so the forearm is able to pronate. If shoulder elevation is used in the maneuver, the pectoralis major and the anterior deltoid perform that motion. Wrist muscles stabilize the hand and the long finger flexors grasp the container (Fig.14.9A). Forearm pronation occurs via eccentric contraction of the supinator and biceps brachii (Fig. 14.9B). As the container is placed back to its original position, the forearm supinates back to its neutral position through concentric activity of the supinator and biceps (Fig 14.9C).

Turning a Key

Turning a key in a lock is another example of a motion requiring predominately forearm movement. Whether

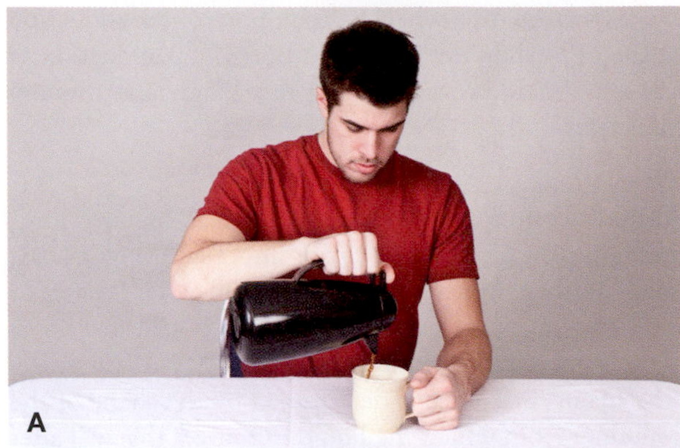

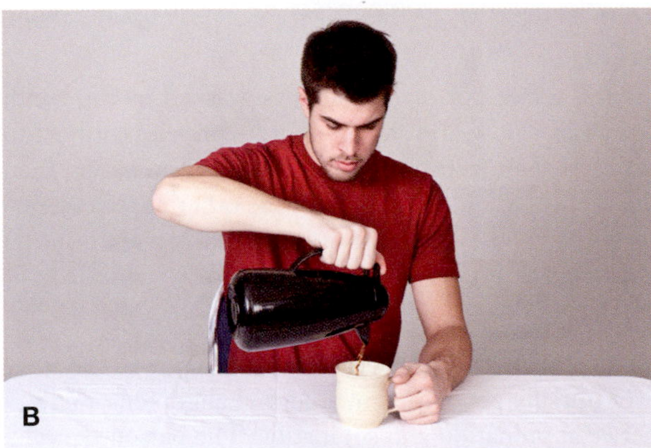

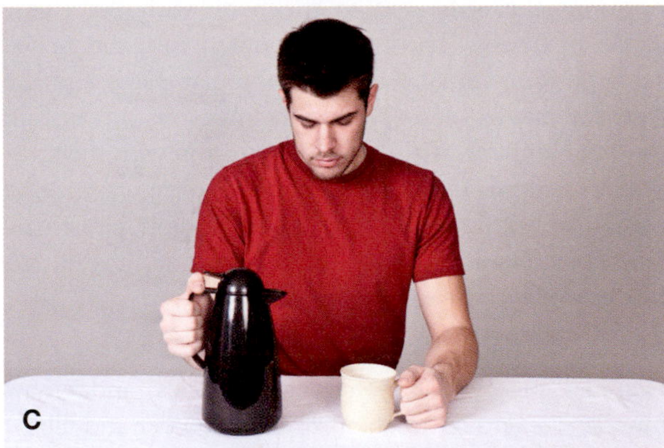

Figure 14.9 Pouring coffee into a mug requires forearm and shoulder motion as other muscles maintain an isometric contraction. Note the change in forearm position from A & B in pronation to C in midposition.

the lock is on the door of your home or apartment, your locker, or your car, if a key is used to access it, the motion is similar for all situations.

Sequence of Movement

The key is grasped in the hand. As the individual approaches the lock, the elbow is flexed to the level of the target (key hole) with its position at the side maintained by humeral and scapular muscles (Fig. 14.10A). Slight forward flexion of the shoulder may be required to place the key in the lock (Fig. 14.10B). Once the key enters the lock, the supinator, aided by the biceps brachii, rotates the key to open the lock (Fig. 14.10C).

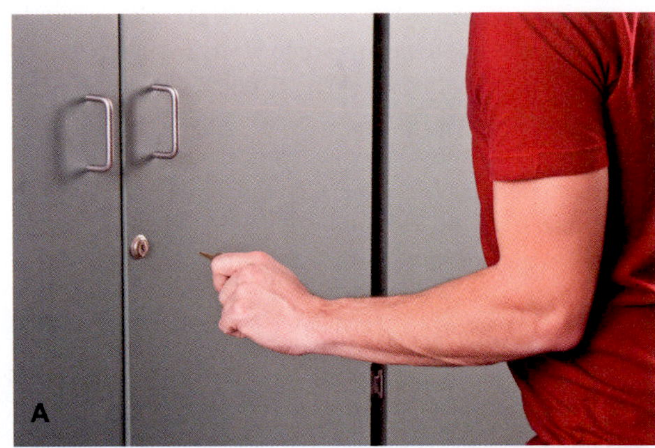

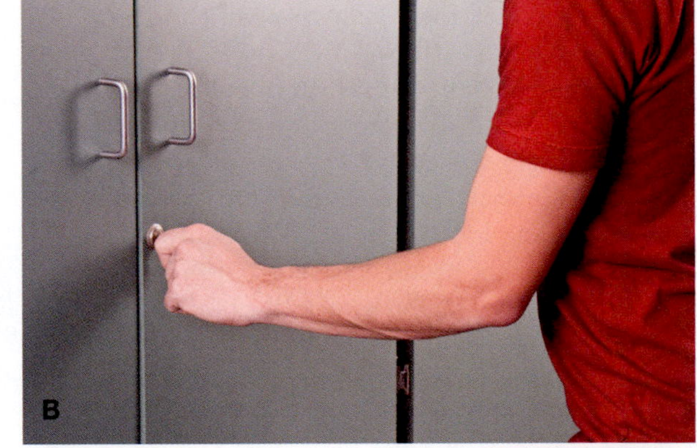

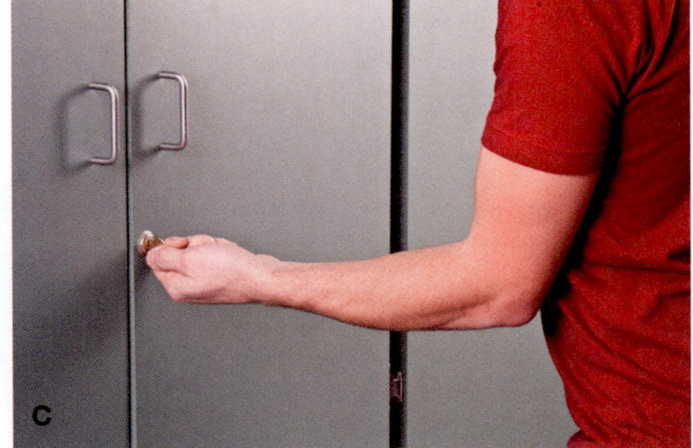

Figure 14.10 Turning a key to unlock a lock is predominantly performed by forearm supinators as other muscles maintain and isometric contraction.

Joint Motion

The key is turned to unlock a lock usually by rotating the key either clockwise or counterclockwise. In the photo in Figure 14.10, the left hand grasps the key and places it in the key hole and the forearm supinates, rotating toward the ceiling. Most locks are designed to be opened with supination since supination is a stronger motion than pronation.[8]

Little motion of other joints occurs during this activity. Slight flexion of the shoulder joint may be required to advance the key into the lock. The amount of elbow flexion required depends on the height of the lock relative to the individual's height. The key is held in the hand with a lateral prehension grasp. Once the extremity is positioned with the arm at or near the side and the elbow flexed to ~90° with the wrist in slight extension and the fingers partially flexed and the thumb adducted in a lateral pinch, essentially the only motion occurring is forearm supination.

Muscle Activity

Unlocking a lock requires only stabilization efforts of almost all the other upper extremity segments except the forearm. The scapula rotators stabilize the scapula as the humerus is held at the side. If slight glenohumeral elevation is required to bring the key to the keyhole, stabilization by the rotator cuff occurs as slight activity of the anterior deltoid and pectoralis major advance the arm forward. The biceps brachii and brachialis move and maintain the elbow at the appropriate degree of flexion required for matching the height of the hand to that of the lock, and the wrist flexors and extensors cocontract to maintain the wrist in its functional position of slight extension. Rotating the key is performed by the supinator and biceps brachii. Although the supinator is recruited during slow, unresisted supination, the biceps is recruited for fast and resisted supination activities, so how difficult the key is to turn and how fast the individual performs the motion will depend upon the specific recruitment of each of these muscles.[9]

Since the key is held in the hand with a prehension grasp, intrinsic muscles are used. These muscles include the opponens pollicis, adductor pollicis, and lumbricals, which work isometrically to maintain this lateral grasp. The long finger flexors (flexor digitorum superficialis and profundus) contract isometrically, which holds the digits in a partially flexed position.

Activities Requiring Primarily Wrist Movement

Wrist muscles are often used as stabilizers of the wrist to allow the hand to perform its functions. However, many daily activities also require specific wrist motion beyond being a stabile platform for finger and hand activities.

Using a Hammer

Hammering a nail is both a common work and home activity. At first glance, this activity may seem to require the more frequently incorporated wrist activity of stabilization for hand and finger function, but a closer look at this activity shows the importance of wrist movement in hammering a nail.

Sequence of Movement

The hand grasps the hammer and then muscles of the shoulder complex position the extremity (Fig. 14.11A). The degree of humeral elevation depends on the level at which the nail is in relation to the rest of the body. Once the shoulder is positioned, the elbow flexes and the wrist radially deviates to "windup" for the downward motion of the hammer to the nail (Fig. 14.11B). The hammer blow to the nail initiates at the shoulder and rapidly unwinds the extremity, moving first to the elbow and then to the wrist. This timing produces a summation of forces so the nail is impacted with a force greater than just that delivered by the hand and weight of the hammer.

Joint Motion

Hand tool use often requires movements of the wrist in ulnar and radial deviation as well as flexion and

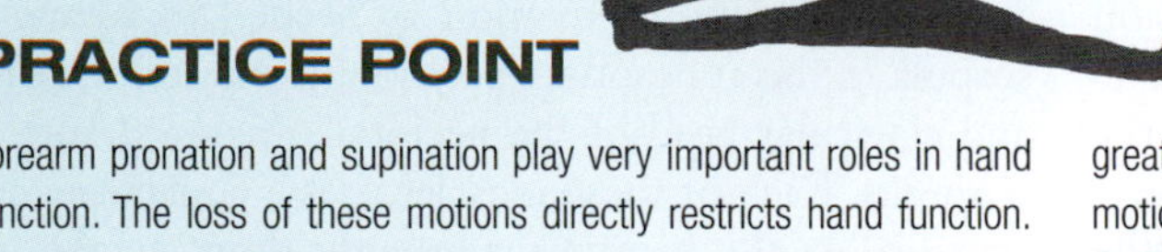

PRACTICE POINT

Forearm pronation and supination play very important roles in hand function. The loss of these motions directly restricts hand function. For example, an individual whose wrist is immobilized following a Colles' fracture is impeded in performing even the most basic tasks of brushing teeth, combing hair, and feeding. Substitutions, including greater use of the shoulder and elbow during restricted forearm motion, are often necessary while the wrist is immobilized but are difficult habits to break once the mobility returns. Clinicians must be aware of these substitutions and create exercises that promote and re-educate correct activity execution.

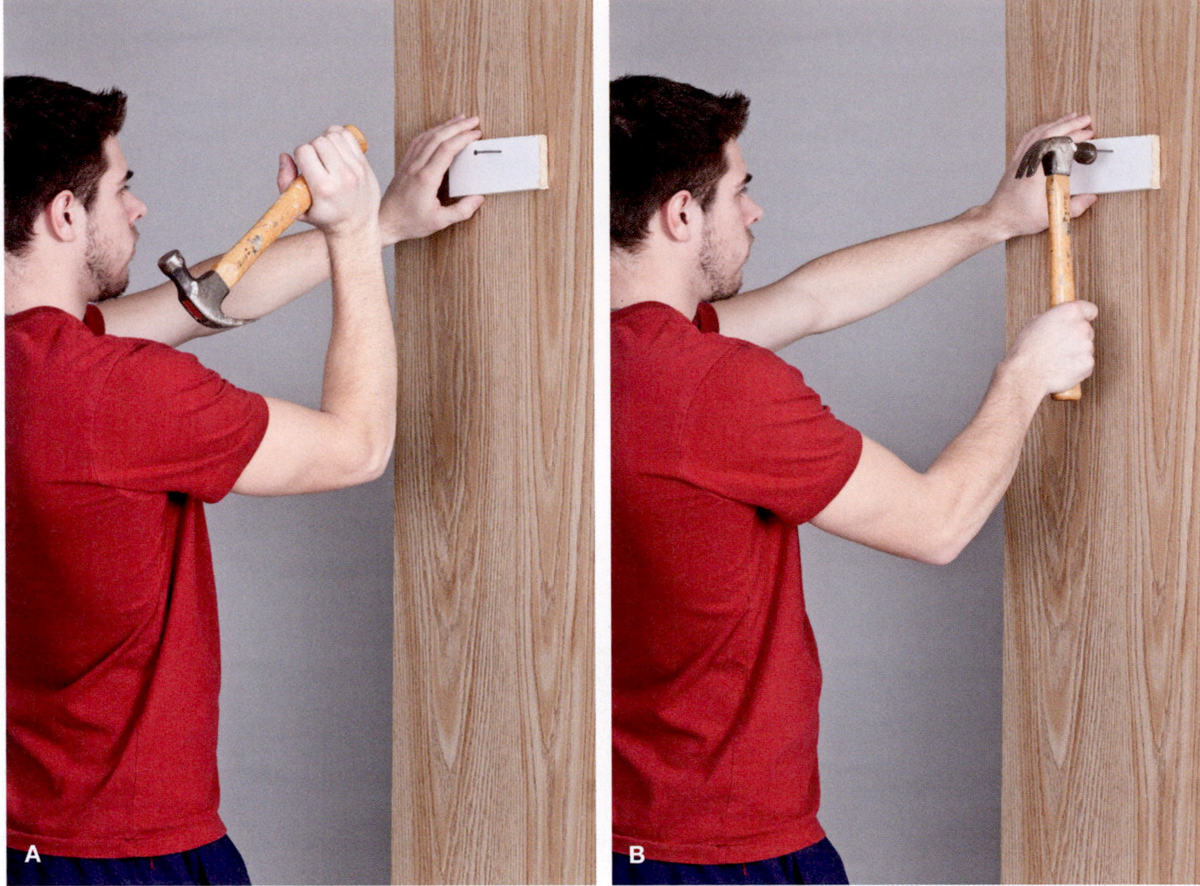

Figure 14.11 Hammering a nail requires timing of forces delivered by the upper extremity. Note the change in wrist position from **A)** radial deviation to **B)** ulnar deviation.

extension. Using a hammer to drive a nail into wood requires a person to position the upper extremity at a height above the wood and nail. Glenohumeral flexion is required for this activity; how much flexion is necessary depends on the level of the surface at which the nail is to be imbedded and the height of the individual doing the hammering. For example, if the nail is hammered into the wall to hang a picture, the shoulder may be elevated higher than 90°, but if the nail is going into a floor board, less shoulder flexion is used. The shoulder is moved into flexion to swing the hammer upward, and then moves towards extension as the hammer blow is delivered to the nail. The elbow also moves from flexion to extension during the wind-up motion, but the amount of movement required is usually greater at the elbow than at the shoulder. Neither joint usually achieves full extension during the movement. Although the wrist is maintained in the sagittal plane in its functional position of slight extension, it moves from radial deviation to ulnar deviation from the start to the end of the motion, respectively. The fingers maintain a firm cylinder grasp of the hammer throughout the activity.

Muscle Activity

Since the amount of scapular upward rotation is dependent upon the amount of humerus elevation, if the shoulder is not elevated above 30°, these muscles work primarily to stabilize rather than move the scapula. If the humerus is positioned above 60°, the upward rotators (trapezius and serratus anterior) move the scapula into upward rotation as needed to rotate the scapula to the appropriate position; the anterior deltoid and clavicular head of the pectoralis major elevate the humerus. Each of these muscles uses a concentric contraction. As the hammer is brought down to the nail, these muscles contract eccentrically to lower the hammer, but when the hammer hits the nail of the head, the downward scapular rotators including rhomboids, levator scapulae, and pectoralis minor contract

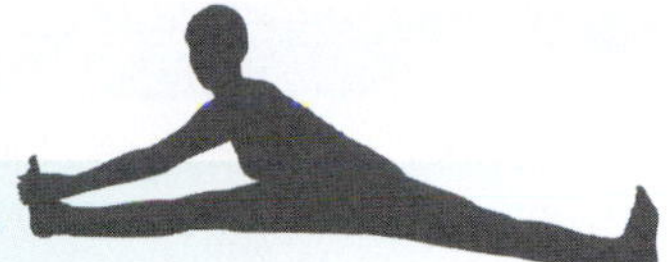

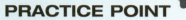

PRACTICE POINT

Injuries to the hand or fingers usually also result in either loss of wrist motion or muscle weakness and greatly inhibit use of the wrist. The wrist is often stabilized as the hand functions, but if injury to the hand or fingers occurs, wrist weakness also occurs since its function is reduced as the hand or fingers recover from injury. Such deficits of the wrist create instability during hand and finger activities. Therefore, it is important for clinicians to include wrist strengthening and motion exercises whenever rehabilitating hand or finger injuries.

concentrically to deliver the force. Likewise, the anterior deltoid and clavicular head of the pectoralis major use eccentric movement to control the speed of descent of the hammer, but the latissimus dorsi, teres major, and posterior deltoid contract when the hammer hits the nail. Don't forget that the deltoid and rotator cuff muscles work synchronously as a force couple to position the humeral head in the glenoid fossa.

The position in which the arm is readied for the activity determines which muscles move the elbow into flexion. If the shoulder is positioned below the level of the head, the biceps brachii and brachialis flex the elbow using concentric motion, but if the arm is overhead, the triceps works eccentrically against gravity to control elbow flexion. When the hammer moves towards the nail, whichever muscle(s) initially positioned the elbow is/are the muscle(s) performing the motion now contracting eccentrically if it initially contracted concentrically and vice versa. Once contact is made with the nail, the triceps concentrically contracts to deliver the power.

Wrist flexors and extensors cocontract to maintain the functional position of wrist extension. If the hammer is below the level of the individual's head, the simultaneous concentric contraction of the flexor carpi radialis longus and brevis and extensor carpi ulnaris move the wrist toward the radius in radial deviation. These same muscles contract eccentrically as the hammer is lowered to the nail; when the hammer impacts the nail, the flexor carpi ulnaris and extensor carpi ulnaris deliver the force to pound in the nail.

Throughout the motion, the hand maintains a cylinder grasp on the hammer shaft. The flexor digitorum superficialis and profundus, flexor pollicis longus and brevis, and opponens pollicis maintain this grasp. The heavier the hammer and the more force applied with the hammer, the greater the recruitment of additional motor units is required of these muscles and all of the limb muscles.

Summary

Activities of daily living are complex movements carried out by several upper extremity muscles and guided by visual and sensory information. In this chapter, the movements of the upper extremity were analyzed, much as they would be by occupational therapists observing persons involved in their everyday activities of daily living. Understanding these common movements can serve as a helpful guide to therapeutic intervention as clinicians often ask patients to engage in familiar activities to practice motor movements and practice normal range of motion.

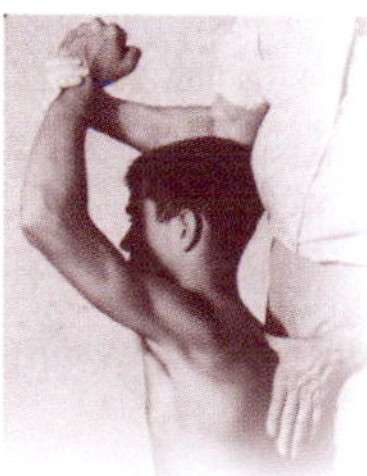

CLINICAL SCENARIO SOLUTION

Nathaniel works in construction. As part of his responsibility, he erects walls in new homes that are being built. His responsibilities include many tasks such as lifting and carrying heavy 4 ft × 8 ft wall board, pounding nails, mudding, and sanding. Since each of these tasks requires different muscle recruitment strategies and ranges of motion, Sam decides the best way to approach this analysis is to look at the requirements of each task individually. As Nathaniel explains each task, Sam identifies the motions, muscle activity, and motion sequence of each of them. Sam realizes that when he breaks each task down, his ability to perform his analysis becomes less overwhelming to him. Sam successfully identifies the requirements of Nathaniel's job. Based on his physical examination of Nathaniel and his analysis of Nathaniel's tasks, Sam's assessment is that Nathaniel is ready to return to work. Are you able to identify, as Sam did, the motion and muscle activity requirements of Nathaniel's tasks?

Discussion Questions

Think about the concepts presented throughout this text related to the degrees of freedom at each joint and how they contribute to functional movement of the entire segment. Discuss how injury would change the degrees of freedom at each of the contributing joints—scapula, glenohumeral joint, elbow joint, radioulnar joint, wrist, fingers, or thumb—and how might that alter the sample motions described in this chapter:

- Reaching overhead and forward
- Reaching overhead and backward
- Pushing to stand from a seated position
- Sanding wood
- Brushing your teeth
- Feeding yourself
- Donning socks or pants
- Driving
- Pouring
- Turning a key
- Using a hammer

1. As a clinician, think about the clinical decision-making process that you might engage in when faced with such a situation and the issues related to assisting your client by either intervening to remediate the impairment or teaching your client an appropriate movement compensation or adaptation.
2. Refer to the opening scenario of this chapter. What information should Sam have before he is able to assess Nathaniel's work station? Given that Nathaniel suffered an elbow injury, what should Sam be particularly interested in regarding Nathaniel's work requirements in order to determine Nathaniel's readiness to return to work?

Lab Activities

1. For the following 10 activities, perform the activity with a partner and list the movements of the upper body (shoulder, elbow, and hand) used to perform these normally. List the major muscles involved in initially positioning the extremity (if applicable), and then list the muscles involved in carrying out the task.
   a. Catching a ball thrown above your head
   b. Pulling a roller suitcase behind you
   c. Putting on a coat
   d. Buttoning a shirt
   e. Turning a doorknob
   f. Taking off a jacket
   g. Applying suntan lotion to your lower back
   h. Grabbing the handle of a pot
   i. Brushing your hair
   j. Turning on the ignition of your car
2. Think about the upper extremity by joint, proximally to distally. Beginning with the shoulder complex and moving sequentially to the fingers, list at least five functional activities that require predominantly:
   a. Shoulder flexion
   b. Shoulder extension
   c. Shoulder horizontal abduction and adduction
   d. Shoulder internal and external rotation
   e. Elbow flexion

   f. Elbow extension
   g. Forearm supination
   h. Forearm pronation
   i. Wrist flexion
   j. Wrist extension
   k. Finger flexion (making a fist)
   l. Lateral pinch
   m. Three-jaw chuck (pinch)
   n. Tip-to-tip prehension (pinch)

3. Identify five ADLs that you do each day and analyze them for their motions and muscle activities. List the movements of the upper limb (shoulder, elbow, and hand) that you use to perform these normally. List the major muscles involved in initially positioning the extremity (if applicable), and then list the muscles involved in carrying out the task.

4. Explain why it is important to identify areas of weakness in joints other than one that is affected by injury. For example, if you are treating a wrist sprain in a patient who works as a plumber, why should you also examine his shoulder girdle, elbow, and hand?

References

1. Magermans DJ, Chadwick EK, Veeger HE, van der Helm FC. Requirements for upper extremity motions during activities of daily living. *Clinical Biomechanics* 20(6):591–599, 2005.
2. Tyler AE, Karst GM. Timing of muscle activity during reaching while standing: Systematic changes with target distance. *Gait & Posture* 20(2):126–133, 2004.
3. Cools A, Witvrouw E, Declercq G, Danneels L, Cambier D. Scapular muscle recruitment patterns: Trapezius muscle latency with and without impingement symptoms. *American Journal of Sports Medicine* 31(4):542–549, 2003.
4. Gabriel DA. Shoulder and elbow muscle activity in goal-directed arm movements. *Experimental Brain Research* 116(2):359–366, 1997.
5. Archambault P, Pigeon P, Feldman AG, Levin MF. Recruitment and sequencing of different degrees of freedom during pointing movements involving the trunk in healthy and hemiparetic individuals. *Experimental Brain Research* 126(1):55–67, 1999.
6. Cools AM, Witvrouw EE, De Clercq GA, et al. Scapular muscle recruitment pattern: Electromyographic response of the trapezius muscle to sudden shoulder movement before and after a fatiguing exercise. *Journal of Orthopaedic and Sports Physical Therapy* 32(5):221–229, 2004.
7. Engen TJ, Spencer WA. Method of kinematic study of normal upper extremity movements. *Archives of Physical Medicine and Rehabilitation* 49(1):9–12, 1968.
8. Askew LJ, An KN, Morrey BF, Chao EY. Isometric elbow strength in normal individuals. *Clinical Orthopaedics and Related Research* 222:261–266, 1987.
9. Haugstvedt JR, Berger RA, Berglund LJ. A mechanical study of the moment-forces of the supinators and pronators of the forearm. *Acta Orthopaedica Scandinavica* 72(6):629–634, 2001.

CHAPTER 15

Sports and Recreation

"A happy person is not a person in a certain set of circumstances, but rather a person with a certain set of attitudes."

—Hugh Downs

American broadcaster, television host, producer, and author

CHAPTER OUTLINE

Learning Outcomes
Clinical Scenario
Introduction
Sports Activities
- *Baseball Pitching*
- *Fast Pitch Softball Pitching*
- *Soccer Instep Kick*
- *Freestyle Swimming*

Leisure Activities
- *Golf Swing*
- *Tennis Serve*
- *Cycling*

Summary
Clinical Scenario Solution
Discussion Questions
Lab Activities
References

LEARNING OUTCOMES

By the end of this chapter, you should be able to:

- ❑ Perform a kinesiologic analysis of common sports activities;
- ❑ Describe the joint motions and muscle activity of a baseball pitch;
- ❑ Describe the joint motions and muscle activity of a soccer instep kick;
- ❑ Describe the joint motions and muscle activity of a softball fast pitch;
- ❑ Describe the joint motions and muscle activity of the freestyle swimming stroke;
- ❑ Describe the joint motions and muscle activity of a full golf swing;
- ❑ Describe the joint motions and muscle activity of a tennis serve;
- ❑ Describe the joint motions and muscle activity of the lower extremities in cycling.

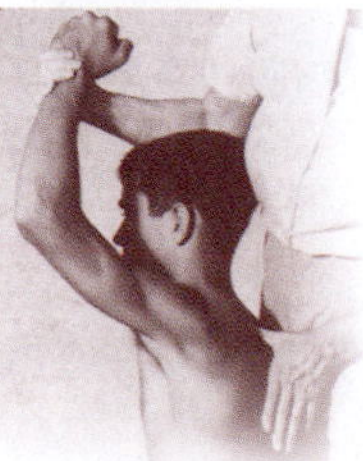

CLINICAL SCENARIO

Cody is a high jumper for the high school track team and in his last year at Bessemer High. About five weeks ago, he suffered an anterior cruciate ligament injury and subsequently had surgery two weeks ago to replace the ligament. Morgan is working with Cody in his rehabilitation program and knows that Cody wants to return to the high jump after he completes his rehabilitation. Morgan has been in contact with Cody's coach to understand the biomechanics and demands of the high jump and is ready to incorporate a progression of exercises that are geared to Cody's goal of returning to the high jump. Morgan is confident that the specific exercises that will be added to the program when they are appropriate will strengthen the muscles Cody will need so he may return to compete in his last year of high school track and field.

Introduction

As preventative medicine and modern medicine combine forces to produce healthier populations, longevity of life expectancy increases. By the year 2030, it is estimated that there will be 70 million people in the United States over the age of 65.[1] Because older people are now healthier than in past generations, they are more active as well.[1] Additionally, an increase in leisure time means that more people are able to participate in sport and recreational activities.[2] More children and adolescents participate in organized sport activity than in the last century. Club and interscholastic sports provide millions of preteen and teenaged youths opportunities for sports participation. Physicians advocate exercise for individuals of all ages, from young to old. More people participating in sport and recreational activities means that clinicians are likely to treat individuals who experience injuries in these activities. Not even accounting for older individuals receiving recreation and sport-related injuries, about 3 million youngsters are injured in organized sports each year in this country.[3] Most of these injured individuals, both young and old, will want to return to their sport or recreational activities.

Part of the treatment and rehabilitation programs used to manage these injuries will include the traditional methods used to deal with orthopedic injuries. However, for those patients wishing to return to recreational or sport activities, the clinician must have additional tools with which to accomplish this patient goal. Clinicians must be able to incorporate into the rehabilitation program activities that will provide for optimal function of patients in their sport or recreational pursuits. To do this, clinicians must understand the activity and know what physical demands these activities place on the body and the skills required to perform them. Clinical kinesiology utilizes this understanding of activity skills and the clinician's observation and analysis of movement to allow clinicians to provide patients who want to return to athletic activities the assistance to do so.

Before the clinician can provide a patient with assistance in reacquiring athletic skills, the clinician must have an idea of what the skill involves, what it looks like, the level of skill of the patient, and must be able to break the skill down into its component parts. In essence, what we do to understand the requirements of an activity is perform a **qualitative analysis** of the activity. We do not act as biomechanists, who use formulas and quantitative measurements to perform detailed analysis, but rather, we act as clinicians and primarily use investigations of others to know what is normal in terms of muscle and joint movement in conjunction with our own skills of observation to compare what is expected to what the individual does. By so doing, we may provide the individual with corrections and cues to improve his or her performance. Therefore, the information in this chapter presents reports of investigators who have identified muscle and joint motions throughout each of the selected activities. Once you have the information of what is "normal," it becomes easier to identify what aspects of the individual's performance require correction. Although the activities performed usually involve smooth and continuous motion, each activity is broken down into segments or phases so it is easier to both discuss the information and identify performance expectations. If the clinician is unfamiliar with a particular sport or activity, there are numerous resources available to obtain the necessary information to assist the patient. Some resources include local coaches, books, videos, and online resources.

To get you started in how to process and understand an activity, this chapter is divided into two sections. The first section addresses competitive sports that are common at high school, college, club, professional, and recreational levels; the second section addresses common lifetime activities that many people play either recreationally or competitively. One specific activity within each of these selections is analyzed for its skill and motion requirements. As stated earlier, these are merely examples to assist you in moving on to other activities and providing your own analysis of any other movement you may encounter.

Information in this chapter is presented a little differently than in the previous chapters on movement analysis in this unit. The previous chapters have prepared you to look at the timing of muscle sequencing, motion requirements, and muscle activity to understand and appreciate the necessary components of movement. Rather than separate these elements out in this chapter, we are now advancing to the next step: putting all of these elements together and looking at the entire body during an activity. Part of the learning process is taking apart an activity and dividing it into its elements, but once this is accomplished, it is also necessary to put them into their normal context. We will discuss the phases of each activity, identify the beginning and ending of each phase, look at the motions occurring with each phase, and then identify the muscles that produce those motions. The ability to appreciate the entire activity and its segments allows a clinician to obtain a full picture of not only the demands of the activity but how to select techniques within a full spectrum of possibilities to correctly instruct in performance of that activity.

Sports Activities

The sports activities that have been selected here for examples of motion analysis include movements from four sports that are commonly seen in many interscholastic, intercollegiate, club and recreational leagues. They have been selected because it is likely that clinicians will see injuries from these sports. It is beyond the scope of this chapter to provide analysis of all movement requirements within each sport, so only one movement has been selected for each sport.

Baseball Pitching

Of all the sports motions that have been biomechanically analyzed, the baseball pitch is probably one of the most commonly analyzed activities. To develop an understanding of the components of pitching, similar to gait analysis, it has been divided into different phases; some investigators have used anywhere from four phases[4] to six phases[5, 6] to describe the baseball pitch. To coincide with most investigators, we will divide the fast pitch into five phases. These phases include: 1) windup; 2) early cocking; 3) late cocking; 4) acceleration; and 5) follow-through (Fig. 15.1). Sometimes the early cocking phase is also called the "stride" phase, and sometimes the follow-through is delineated into deceleration and later follow-through.[6] Since most pitchers are right handed, the descriptions here are based on a right-handed pitcher. Since the majority of baseball pitchers are males, the gender referred to in this section is male.

Windup Phase

Standing with the hands together in front of the body, the glove hiding the ball from the batter, the pitcher begins the windup phase when motion begins. The windup ends when the ball separates from the glove.[7] Rather than grasping the ball in the palm, the pitcher uses the fingers to grasp the ball so he is able to maintain contact of the ball with the hand for as long as possible before it is released.

As you may expect, this is the quietest phase of the activity. It is during this time that the pitcher prepares to perform the pitch, so the entire body is at its most inactive state. The body is usually positioned in one of two positions.[8] One position is with the body fully facing the target, or batter, with both feet in contact with the pitching rubber; this is called the windup stance (Fig. 15.2A). The other common stance is with the glove-hand side facing the batter; this is called the stretch stance (Fig. 15.2B). The pitcher's back foot is parallel to and in contact with the front edge of the pitching rubber and must remain in contact with the rubber until the ball is released. The front foot, or the foot ipsilateral to the glove arm,[4] is the stride leg and the pivot foot is ipsilateral to the throwing arm—for a right-handed pitcher, the pivot leg is the right leg; the pivot leg is touching the pitching rubber with the pitcher's weight primarily on

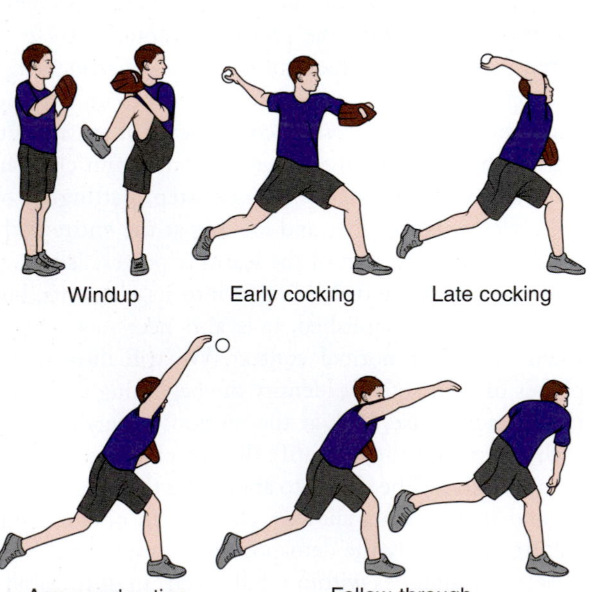

Figure 15.1 The phases of the baseball pitch.

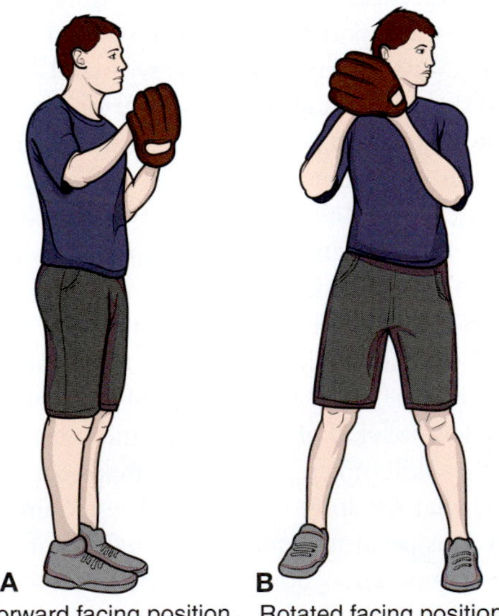

Figure 15.2 Alternative stance positions for the baseball windup. A) Forward facing the batter in a windup stance. B) A rotated position with the glove shoulder to the batter in a stretch stance.

that leg.[9] Pitchers and coaches believe that the stride stance provides a more rapid release of the ball, so they use this stance when runners are on bases. However, one study looking at these two stances found no differences in delivery times of the ball to the plate.[8] As the hands separate, the body weight begins to transfer from the front to the back leg. As the hands separate, the shoulders begin to move into flexion to bring the arms overhead. Beyond these procedures, the windup varies greatly from one pitcher to another, so a variety of poses may be observed in different pitchers.

Motions during the windup include a transfer of body weight from the front leg to the back leg and a winding up of the front lower extremity and trunk around the pivot leg. The front hip and knee are flexed to about 90° each.[10] As the arms are raised and the ball hand and glove separate, the front hip and knee flex and the back flexes to produce this winding up of the body.

In terms of muscle contractions, little activity occurs within the muscles during this phase.[4] As the weight moves from the front leg to the back leg, the front leg pushes the body weight backward onto the pivot leg. Muscles of the pivot leg acting to absorb the body weight are primarily the hip abductors, adductors, and extensors. The trunk movement into some flexion occurs with eccentric contraction of the back extensors with assistance from the hip extensors. When the weight is off of the front leg, the limb's hip flexors work concentrically to flex the hip and the knee extensors eccentrically control the amount of knee flexion that occurs (this is variable) during hip flexion. As the arms separate and move into flexion, there is concentric activity of the anterior deltoid and pectoralis major at the glenohumeral joint, and the upper trapezius, serratus anterior, and lower trapezius contract to produce upward scapular rotation. Abdominal muscles work to rotate and stabilize the trunk whereas the back extensors control the amount of trunk flexion that occurs with hip flexion. Table 15–1 indicates when the muscles are active at a high, moderate, or minimal level throughout the baseball pitch. As a rule, contraction of a muscle less than 30% of its maximum isometric contraction (MVIC) is at a minimal level; a level of output 35% to 65% of MVIC is a moderate level; and over 65% is a high level.

TABLE 15–1A | SHOULDER AND ELBOW MUSCLE ACTIVITY DURING THE BASEBALL PITCH*

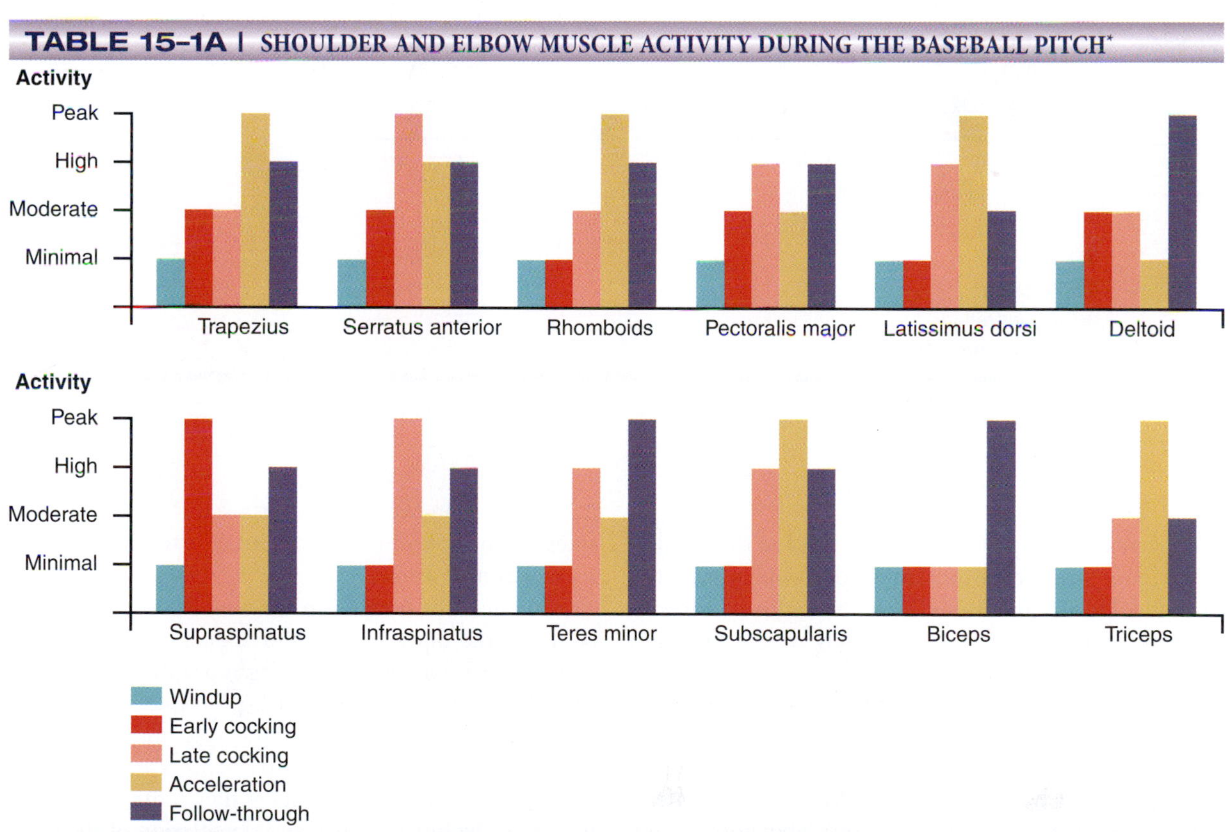

*Based on data from Moynes, et al;[4];Jobe, et al;[19] and Jobe, et al.[20]

TABLE 15–1B | FOREARM AND TRUNK MUSCLE ACTIVITY DURING THE BASEBALL PITCH*

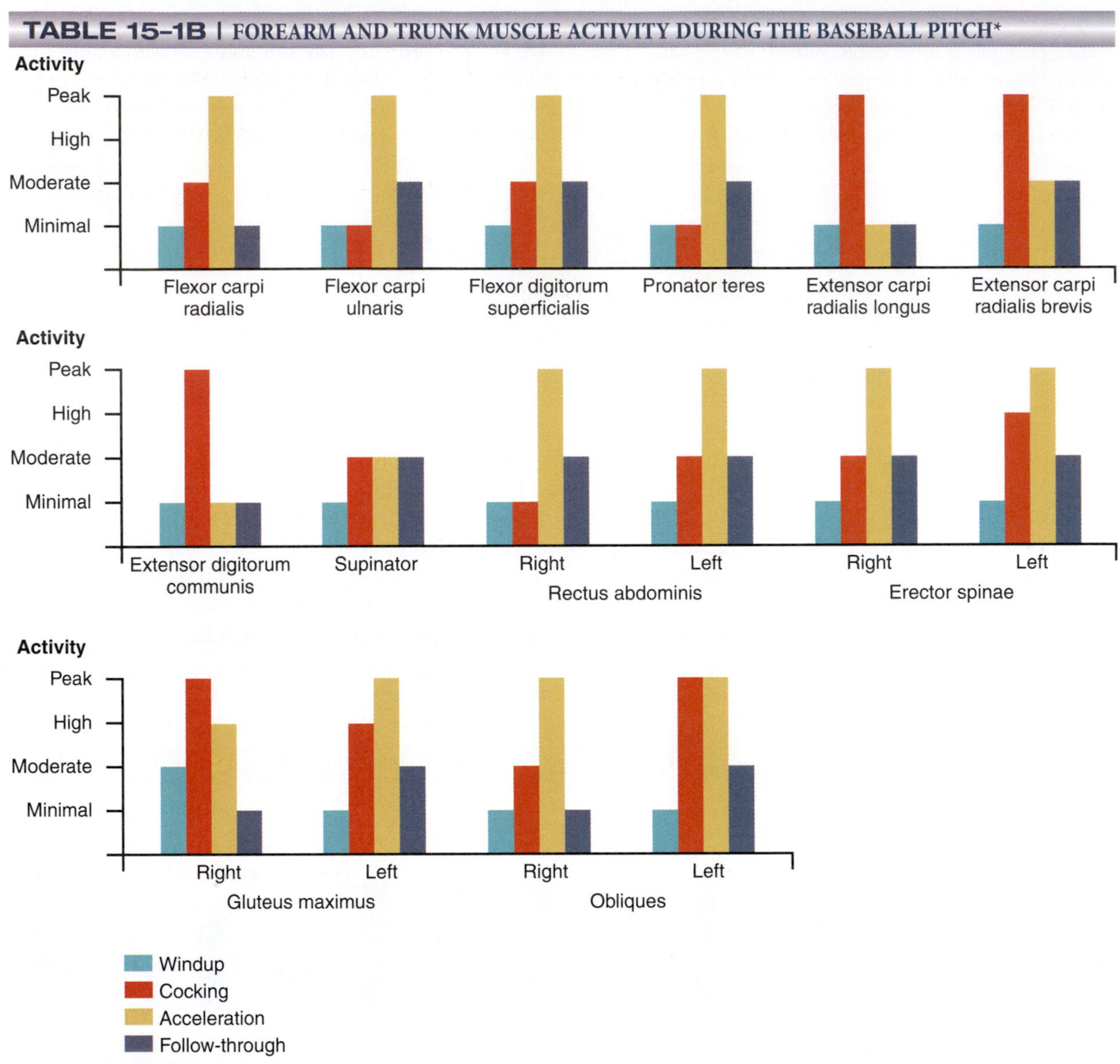

*Based on data from Watkins, et al;[18] and Hamilton, et al.[16]

Early Cocking (Stride) Phase

The early cocking phase is from the end of the windup to the time when the front, or stride, foot contacts the ground.[6] During this time the body begins its forward motion toward the target so the body weight moves to the front leg.

During this time, the pitcher moves the hand and ball away from the target as far as possible.[4] The scapula moves into a retracted position, the elbow becomes flexed, and the humerus moves into abduction, lateral rotation, and horizontal extension (abduction). The body begins to move forward, keeping the arm behind it. This position becomes important during acceleration since the body will propel the arm forward, increasing its acceleration speed.

Motion of the body from the back leg to the front leg occurs as the hip extensors and abductors, knee flexors, and plantarflexors of the back leg move the body weight onto the front leg.[11] The front leg muscles are accepting only some of the body's weight at this time, so there is some eccentric activity of the hip extensors and adductors, knee extensors, and calf muscles as they control the rate of flexion of the hip and knee and dorsiflexion of the ankle to lower the body's center of gravity.[10] The abdominal

TABLE 15–1C | LOWER EXTREMITY MUSCLE ACTIVITY DURING THE BASEBALL PITCH*

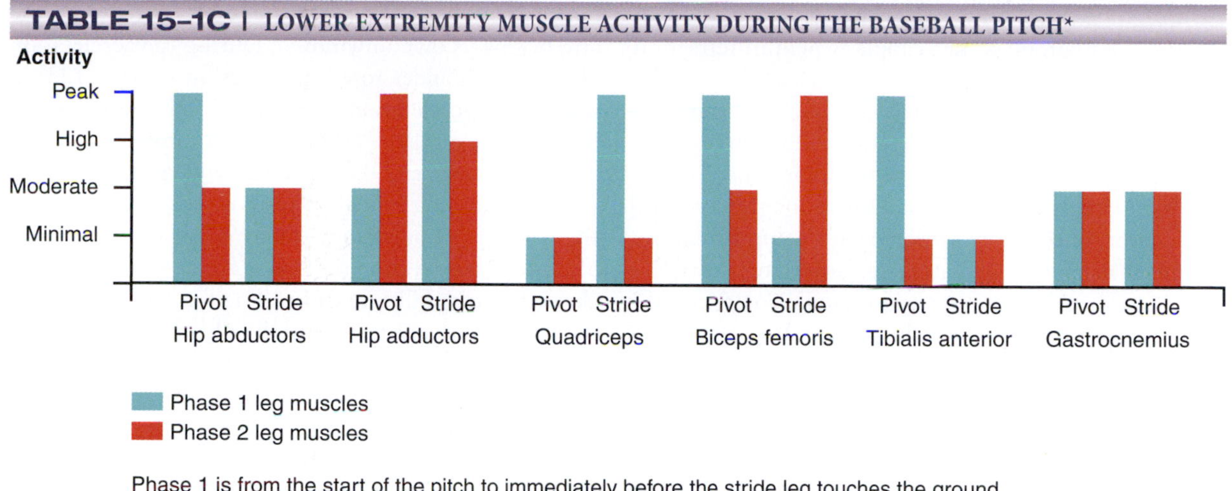

Phase 1 is from the start of the pitch to immediately before the stride leg touches the ground.
Phase 2 is from the time the stride leg touches the ground to the end of the pitch.

*Based on data from Yamanouchi.[11]

muscles provide a stable base for the shoulders and legs and the back extensor muscles keep the trunk upright. The scapular retractors position the scapula as the deltoid moves the humerus to elevate the elbow to shoulder level and horizontally extend the shoulder. In addition to the deltoid, the supraspinatus, infraspinatus, and teres minor work with the deltoid during elevation, and the infraspinatus and teres minor start movement of the humerus into lateral rotation. An eccentric activity of the glenohumeral medial rotators controls the humeral movement to the end of its lateral rotation. The biceps is somewhat active in early cocking.[4]

Late Cocking Phase

The late cocking phase begins when the front foot hits the ground and ends when the pitching shoulder achieves maximum lateral rotation.[6] Once the foot is on the ground, the stride foot faces the target with slight flexion of the pivot knee.[9] The stride foot of the right-handed pitcher is left of an imaginary line from home plate to the pitching rubber's center; this stride foot position will allow maximum rotation of the pelvis and trunk at the time when it is needed most—when the ball is released.[9, 10] In late cocking, the trunk is perpendicular to the target, facing the third base line (for the right handed). It is during this phase that the arm moves into its optimal position to propel the ball forward. As the stride leg becomes closest to the target, the hand becomes farthest from the target; this posture produces a maximal elongation of the body to allow a buildup of forces within it.[12] During the end of this phase, the upper extremity's position is finalized and prepared for the next phase.

Early cocking flows into late cocking as the pitching elbow elevates to about shoulder level in the scapular plane. In this position, the scapula is retracted, and the elbow flexed to 90° as the humerus abducts to about 90°, horizontally extends, and laterally rotates; the wrist is in neutral.[9] By the end of this phase, the humerus achieves its maximal lateral rotation of about 175°.[13] This is likely not pure glenohumeral rotation but a combination of glenohumeral rotation with scapulothoracic rotation and trunk extension.[9] It appears that 120° of lateral rotation is from the glenohumeral joint.[14] The wrist is in maximum extension and fully cocked by the end of this phase.[15]

During this phase, the hips, pelvis, and trunk transfer the energy their muscles are producing to the upper extremity. This provides more force available than would otherwise be produced if the arm muscles were the only force-generating mechanism. These larger muscles provide over 50% of the force for pitching, so they are an important part of the pitching motion.[16] With the stride foot anchored to the ground, the pelvis begins its rotation toward the home plate at about 600°/sec.[17]

There are several muscles throughout the body that are active during this time. The hip extensors, knee flexors, and calf muscles of the back leg continue to contract concentrically to transfer their forces up the kinetic chain. The abdominal muscles control trunk stability and rotation, and the back extensors maintain an upright posture with some lumbar extension.[18] In the shoulder complex, the scapula is held in retraction by the rhomboids and middle trapezius whereas the posterior deltoid, middle deltoid, and supraspinatus concentrically contract to elevate and horizontally extend the humerus.[4] As mentioned, the subscapularis controls lateral humeral rotation through eccentric contraction once the humerus passes neutral rotation; before that point, the lateral rotators concentrically contract to roll the humerus into lateral rotation until the subscapularis takes over the motion. It is during the cocking phase that the contralateral arm also elevates to about 90° abduction; this motion occurs through concentric activity of the deltoid and rotator cuff muscles. Both arms align in a straight line from left side to right side. The nonthrowing shoulder is in medial rotation. The wrist extensors (extensor carpi radialis longus and brevis and extensor carpi ulnaris) are at their most active as the wrist achieves maximum extension at the end of cocking.[15]

To summarize the muscle activity during late cocking, the muscles are active to position the hand for delivery of the ball during the next phase. These muscles perform this responsibility through high levels of activity during the cocking phase. These highly active muscles include the trapezius to move the scapula; the deltoid, supraspinatus, infraspinatus, and teres minor to move the glenohumeral joint; and the biceps to position the elbow.[4] These muscles become least active during the next phase, acceleration.[4]

Acceleration Phase

The acceleration phase begins right after the shoulder has achieved maximum lateral rotation and begins its forward movement toward the target and ends with release of the ball.[6] Momentum is produced as the body unwinds and propels its weight forward toward home plate.[9] This is the most explosive phase of the pitch and lasts about 1/20 of a second.[9] It is during this time that the energy produced by the unwinding hips, pelvis, and trunk add to the rotational forces occurring at the shoulder. The trunk achieves its greatest rotation speed as it rotates to face the batter when the acceleration phase begins.[9] Following pelvic rotation, the trunk rotates at about 1000°/sec, faster than the pelvis but not as fast as the shoulder will rotate once it begins its unwinding.[17] The shoulder is behind the trunk so this pelvis and trunk rotation provides a thrust to propel the upper extremity forward. In other words, this addition of torque forces from the pelvis and trunk acts like a whip, allowing the arm to move at a top speed of just under 9200°/sec and an average speed of over 6000°/sec during this phase.[9] As the trunk ends its rotation, the arm begins its own unwinding. During the acceleration phase, the shoulder rotation excursion is from 122° at the start of acceleration to 48° of lateral rotation when the ball is released.[9] The scapula protracts as the humerus rotates and moves toward extension.

Elbow motion in acceleration moves toward extension so its position changes from 90° of flexion to 120° of flexion. By the time the ball is released, the elbow is about 25° from full extension.[9] The forearm pronates as the elbow moves into extension. The wrist begins this phase in extension and ends it in a neutral position when the ball is released.[9] At the time the ball is released, the forearm is in full pronation.

With the trunk facing the batter by the end of acceleration, it is also flexed.[14] There are individual differences in the lateral position of the trunk; some will have a pronounced lateral flexion of the trunk and may even have the appearance of throwing a side-arm pitch whereas others may appear to throw over the top because of little lateral trunk flexion. The stride leg bears the majority of the body weight with its hip and knee each flexed close to 90°. The pivot leg is positioned with the hip in extension, the knee in flexion, and the ankle in plantarflexion.

Muscle activity during this time is primarily concentric in nature. The subscapularis along with assistance from the sternal head of the pectoralis major provide for medial glenohumeral rotation.[14] The serratus anterior is highly active during acceleration as the scapula protracts. The pectoralis major, latissimus dorsi, and triceps are also highly active during acceleration to move the shoulder and elbow toward extension and across the body.[4,19] Wrist and forearm muscles, including the flexor carpi radialis and ulnaris and the pronator teres, achieve their most active state during this phase as the wrist moves into flexion. The flexor digitorum superficialis is also most active during this time as it maintains a grasp on the ball prior to its release at the end of this phase.[15]

Follow-through (Deceleration) Phase

Follow-through is the period from the release of the ball to the end of all motion.[9] The first part of follow-through involves a large deceleration of the arm as the shoulder moves into full medial rotation; the second part of the follow-through ends with the arm adducted across the body.[6] During the deceleration portion of the follow-through, there are tremendous forces applied to the shoulder and elbow because the joints are suddenly changing from moving several thousand degrees per second to stopping. The muscles are "putting on the brakes," decelerating at a rate of ~500,000°/sec^2.[9]

The end of full shoulder medial rotation marks the end of the deceleration portion of the follow-through phase and is completed in less than 0.1 second.[4] The shoulder continues to adduct across the body as trunk rotation and scapular motion lessen.

The muscles acting are primarily functioning eccentrically as they are responsible for this deceleration. The serratus anterior, rhomboids, and trapezius decelerate the scapula's protraction motion; the subscapularis, pectoralis major, latissimus dorsi, and biceps decelerate the shoulder joint;[19, 20] and the triceps and biceps together control the elbow with much of the effort coming from eccentric contraction of the biceps.[4] As the deceleration process proceeds, the shoulder continues its movement into horizontal flexion (adduction) and medial rotation, the elbow flexes to about 45°, and the forearm pronates.[9] The trunk ends its flexion motion through eccentric contraction of the back extensors, and then during the later part of follow-through, a concentric contraction moves the trunk to a more upright position.[14] During the remaining follow-through phase, the rest of the body "catches up" with the arm, continuing a forward progression of the pivot leg so the pitcher is able to move into his field position to respond to the batter's swing. The pivot leg's hip flexors move the leg forward.

Fast Pitch Softball Pitching

Although not as extensively examined as the baseball pitch, some investigative research has gone into the mechanics and kinetics of the softball fast pitch. Although there are several fast pitch softball leagues throughout the country, there is also an abundance of interscholastic and intercollegiate leagues as well. Once again, there are many different styles of pitches used in fast pitch softball. One of the more common ones is the windmill pitch, so this is the pitch we will examine here. As with the baseball fast pitch, we will break down the activity into phases. The phases in the windmill pitch are divided into 6 phases: 1) windup; 2) 6 o'clock; 3) 3 o'clock; 4) 12 o'clock; 5) 9 o'clock; and 6) follow-through.[21] These clock phases are titled here based on the end of each phase, but with any phase, it is actually the motion that occurs between the end of the prior phase and the end of its own phase that is of primary interest. Once again, the actual motion is continuous but is divided into phases so it is easier to discuss the motion. Since most of the fast pitch softball pitchers are female, reference to the pitcher in this section is to a female.

The windmill pitch is so named for its circular pattern of shoulder movement. The pitching arm starts at the side with the shoulder in neutral extension. As the pitcher begins to pitch, the arm moves forward into flexion until it is fully flexed overhead (Fig. 15.3). The circular motion then continues with movement of the shoulder in an arc behind the body until the hand comes to the side and the ball is released. The total circular movement of the shoulder through one entire pitch encompasses about 450° to 500° of shoulder motion.[22]

Windup Phase

This phase begins when motion is initiated and ends when the pitching arm moves the ball to the 6 o'clock position.[23] There is a lot of variability in the windup phase. Most of the time, the body begins by facing the target. However, the amount of trunk lean, elbow flexion, and shoulder hyperextension relative to the sagittal plane of the body is individualized.[21] Pitchers often stand in a straddled tandem stance with the pivot foot on the pitching rubber and the stride leg behind the pivot foot. The weight begins on the back leg. As the pitcher begins arm motion, she pushes off from the pitching rubber with the pivot foot, and the body moves forward toward the batter.[22] Throughout most of the pitch, the wrist is stabilized in extension with a power grip with the fingers grasping the ball.

As occurs during the baseball pitch, there is relatively little muscle activity during this initial phase of motion. Albeit minimal activity, there are muscles that perform during this phase. As the body weight moves

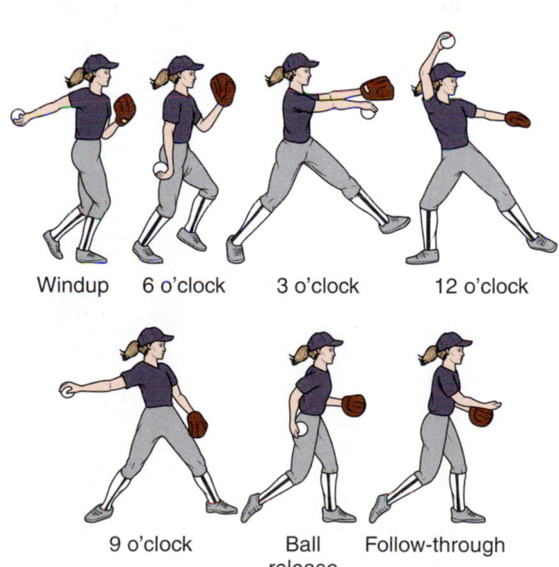

Figure 15.3 The phases of the fast-pitch windmill pitch in softball.

forward toward the batter, the back leg uses its hip and knee extensors and plantarflexors to provide transfer of the body weight toward the pivot foot which is in contact with the pitching rubber. The pivot leg accepts the body weight by eccentric contraction of the hip and knee extensors. The shoulder flexors (pectoralis major and anterior deltoid) move the shoulder to the 6 o'clock position. Since both arms and legs move during this activity, the core muscles work to maintain trunk stability for these extremities throughout the phases. Table 15–2 provides activity levels of muscles that have been investigated during the fast pitch windmill pitch.

6 o'clock Phase

The pitching arm moves from the 6 o'clock to the 3 o'clock position during this phase. The body's weight is on the leg ipsilateral to the pitching arm but shifting forward. The pitching arm medially rotates and elevates to about 90° so it is just anterior to the scapular plane.[23]

During this phase, the arm begins its movement toward an overhead position. Along with humeral elevation, the scapula begins to upwardly rotate. The elbow remains fairly straight throughout this motion until the hand is overhead. The rate of shoulder flexion is very fast during this phase; the fastest the shoulder moves in this phase is about 5000°/sec.[22] The trunk starts to rotate around the pitching arm (face third base).

The infraspinatus and supraspinatus produce their greatest output during this phase as they begin to accelerate the shoulder and elevate it overhead. The anterior deltoid and pectoralis major provide moderate levels of concentric force to move the shoulder upward. Upward rotation of the scapula occurs because of concentric activity of the trapezius and serratus anterior. The triceps maintain the elbow in relative extension and the wrist flexors and extensors cocontract to maintain the wrist in a functional position. Of course, the finger flexors maintain their grip on the ball. Since the body weight is shifting toward the pivot leg, the pivot leg hip extensors and knee extensors accept the weight and control these joints' flexion to maintain a near-extension position yet still absorb the impact forces. The back leg's hip and knee extensors and plantarflexors begin to push the body weight toward the front leg.

TABLE 15-2 | SHOULDER AND ELBOW MUSCLE ACTIVITY DURING THE SOFTBALL PITCH*

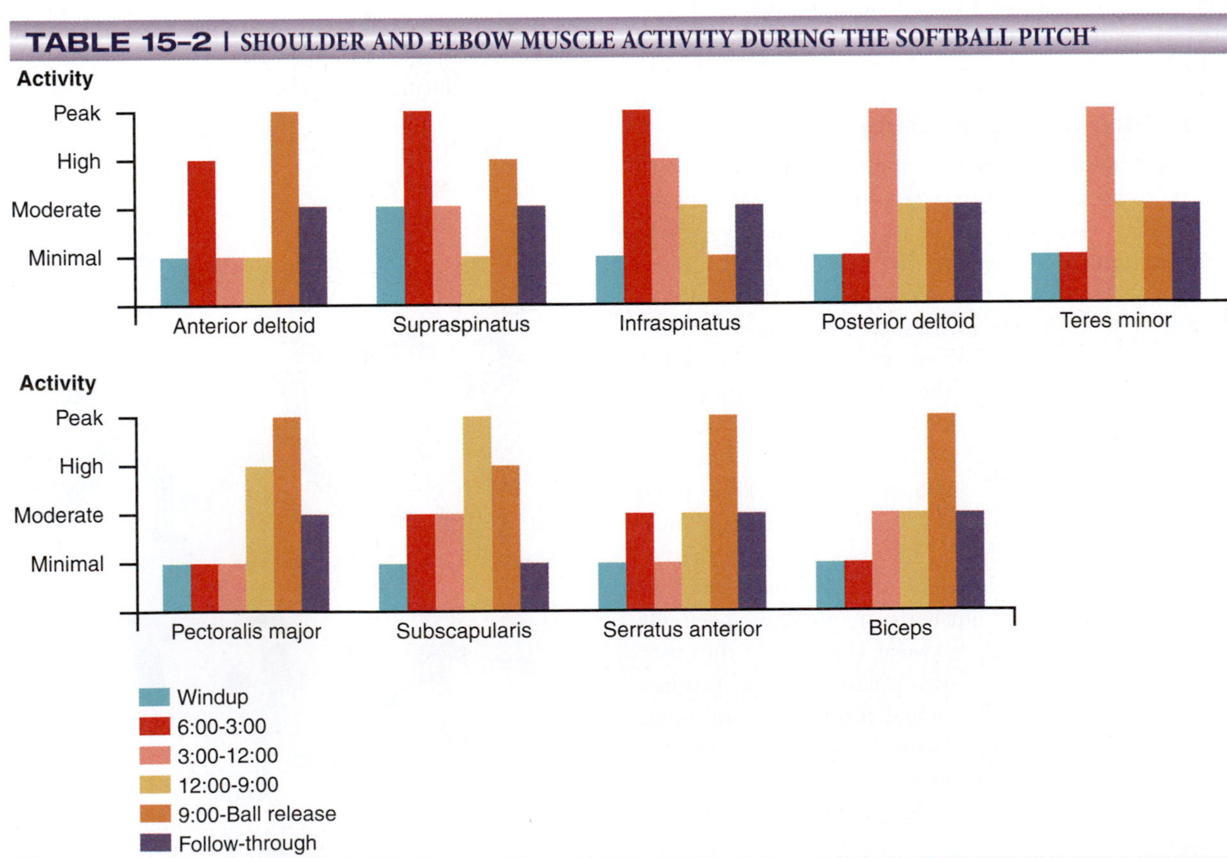

*Based on data from Maffet, et al[21] and Barrentine, et al.[22]

3 o'clock Phase

During this phase, as the arm moves from its 3 o'clock position, it completes its overhead motion and continues to gain acceleration. By the end of this phase, the shoulder is in 180° of abduction and flexion and in lateral rotation.[21] Also during this time, the body weight moves forward as the body rotates towards the pitching arm.[21] The stride leg moves forward to advance the pelvis forward. The foot is directed toward the target.[25]

Stabilization of the trunk and scapula are important during this phase. Pelvic and trunk stabilization provide for transfer of forces from the legs and hips to the upper extremities and scapular stabilization provide a stable base for the glenohumeral joint to be positioned overhead.[24] Therefore, core and hip muscles are active as are the scapular muscles.[23] The infraspinatus and teres minor muscles of the rotator cuff also reach their peak activation to move the glenohumeral joint into lateral rotation and stabilize against distracting forces on the shoulder joint.[24] The posterior deltoid is at its peak activity as the shoulder is moved posteriorly and rotated laterally overhead.[24] Since the supraspinatus muscle is used more to initiate elevation at lower positions, its activity dropped to almost half of its earlier levels during this phase; it appears to work to approximate the humeral head into the glenoid while the deltoid continues the elevation.[21] The biceps brachii continues to increase its activity to control elbow positioning as the upper extremity moves through the windmill motion. Triceps activity remains fairly constant throughout this early part of the pitch.

12 o'clock Phase

With the arm overhead and the body rotated around the pitching arm, the body weight begins to transfer to the contralateral foot. The pitching arm is adducted.[23]

This is the phase in which the shoulder begins its medial rotational acceleration as it prepares to deliver the ball. Moving the shoulder from lateral to medial rotation as the arm begins delivery is an important contributor to ball speed at the time of release.[24] The body begins to unwind, starting at the pelvis and then the trunk before the arm so that the rotational torque provides a summation of forces to increase ball delivery speed. The stride leg is far in front of the body with the body weight transferring strongly to it by a push from the pivot leg.

Because of the profound medial rotation, the subscapularis and pectoralis major are very active in this phase.[21] The subscapularis is active in this phase to serve as a stabilizer of the humeral head in the glenoid fossa. The serratus anterior is active as it attempts to stabilize the scapula so the glenoid is in its proper position as the humerus rotates rapidly into medial rotation.[25] Along with the serratus anterior, the trapezius contributes eccentrically to downward scapular rotation as the humerus is lowered from overhead. Transition from triceps to biceps activity occurs when the arm begins movement in this phase. The biceps contracts to control the elbow position and move it into some flexion during this phase. As the body weight translates forward onto the stride leg, the leg muscles complete their functions that began in the previous phase: hip flexors control the stride leg as hip extensors and knee extensors on the pivot leg push the body forward. Some lateral lean of the trunk to the pitching arm occurs because of eccentric contraction of the contralateral abdominal muscles.

9 o'clock Phase

As the body unwinds, the rotational force is transferred to the arm, maximizing the force delivered through the arm to the ball at ball release.[23] During this phase, the arm is laterally rotated and kept close to the body in the frontal plane. The elbow is in some flexion but extending until right before ball release.[26] The wrist moves into hyperextension until the ball is released. The pelvis moves to face forward, as does the trunk by the time the ball is released.

Several muscles are most active during this phase of the softball pitch. The greatest activity of the biceps brachii occurs during this time.[23] Overall, it is more active throughout the softball windmill pitch than during a baseball fastball pitch.[23] The serratus anterior produces its highest output during this phase as it stabilizes the scapula for the rapidly rotating humerus.[21] The trapezius works with the serratus anterior to control scapular motion. Before ball release, the pectoralis major adducts the shoulder to move it close to the body in the frontal plane. The subscapularis and pectoralis major also provide their greatest output as they work eccentrically to secure the glenohumeral joint from distracting forces after the ball is released.[27] The biceps continues to maintain slight elbow flexion, and wrist flexors snap the wrist into flexion at the time of ball release. Rotation of the pelvis and trunk occurs via hip rotators and abdominal obliques. The final push off from the pivot leg from hip and knee extensors and plantarflexors moves the entire body weight onto the stride leg.

Follow-through Phase

Once the ball leaves the hand, the follow-through phase begins. Immediately after ball release, the arm makes contact with the lateral hip and thigh, stopping forward motion of the arm.[23] Allowing the arm to collide with the hip and thigh allows the leg to absorb much of the deceleration forces.[21] The throwing arm continues its motion with the shoulder continuing into more and more flexion along with flexion of the elbow and wrist.[28] The pitcher's body continues to move forward until the body's center of mass is over the stride leg; the pivot leg may continue to move forward until it comes either up to the stride leg or past it.

The muscle activity of the upper extremity is relatively low compared to that of the baseball fast pitch. During this phase in the baseball pitch, many muscles are very active as they decelerate the upper extremity. However, the muscles produce relatively subdued activity during this time of the softball pitch. Elbow flexors continue to flex the elbow and shoulder flexors and adductors move the arm across and up the front of the body as the wrist continues to flex in its follow-through.[28] The stride leg now holds the entire body weight, so the hip and knee extensors are the primary muscles working along with the hip abductors and adductors to stabilize the body over the limb. Back and abdominal muscles work to maintain an upright position of the trunk. Hip flexors of the pivot leg lift the extremity upward and forward.

Soccer Instep Kick

Soccer is the most popular sport in the world.[29] It is played by literally millions of people of all ages. Although the sport is not as popular in the United States as it is in other parts of the world, it has an extensive following from youngsters in youth soccer league groups to interscholastic teams to young adults on intercollegiate teams and to older-adult club teams. Of all the skills involved in this sport, kicking is probably one of the most important. Of the v arious kicks in soccer, one of the most commonly used ones is the instep soccer kick.[30] This kick is analyzed here. As with other sports activities, the instep soccer kick is divided into phases: (1) backswing; (2) leg cocking; (3) acceleration; and (4) follow-through (Fig. 15.4).[31]

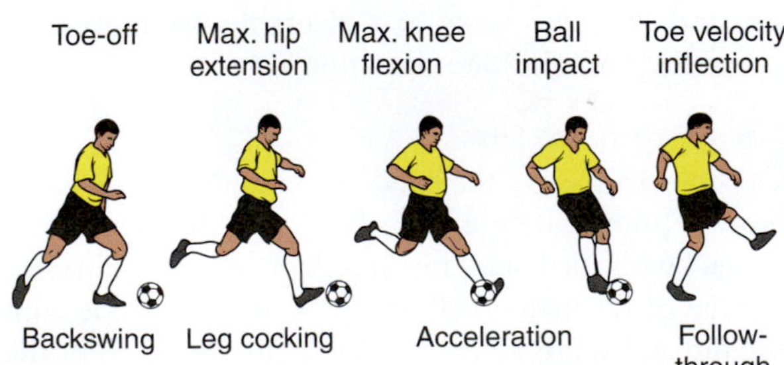

Figure 15.4 The phases of an instep soccer kick.

As with most other sports and sport skills, there is a difference in execution between unskilled and skilled players. Unskilled players generally have more motion involved in their motor execution with more poorly coordinated movements; in soccer, the kick predominantly involves the approach before the kick as more skilled players take longer strides and utilize their approach as part of the kick motion.[32] Skilled soccer players appear to have some common qualities in performance of an instep soccer kick. According to Shan and Westerhoff,[29] these include:

- A "tension arc" at the beginning of the kick that occurs as a combination of excessive extension-abduction of the hip and rotation of the trunk toward the nonkick side;
- A release of this tension arc by a whip-like motion of the kick leg toward the ball with a simultaneous rotation of the trunk toward the kick side; and
- A maximal distance between the kick-side hip and the nonkick side shoulder.

These investigators believe that these kinematic characteristics provide for optimal ball speeds following the kick.[29] As we have found in other sport motions, the winding up of the body and a sequential unwinding allows a transfer of forces through the body. Similar to a game of "crack the whip" (Chapter 1), the greatest motion of the distal segment occurs as the "whip" motion occurs rotationally, with each segment's force transferred to the people at the end of the chain. In the soccer kick, then, the idea is to wind both the limb and the trunk to allow the foot to hit the ball at its greatest speed, thereby producing its greatest force on the ball.

Throughout the kick, the upper extremities provide balance and assist in holding the center of mass over the supporting limb. The shoulders are primarily responsible for performing this function. Their muscles position the arms into some abduction away from the body and varying positions of horizontal flexion or horizontal extension to compensate for the kicking leg positions and still maintain the line of gravity over the support leg.

As the player approaches the ball, the ideal angle to the ball is 30° to 45°.[33] With an instep kick, the foot makes contact with the ball on the dorsum of the foot.[34] The player keeps his eye on the ball throughout the kick. In this discussion, the player will kick the ball with the right foot. We will assume the player is male for convenience of discussion.

Backswing Phase

The start of the soccer kick begins with the movement of the kicking limb backward, as the foot leaves the ground and the hip moves into maximum extension. The arms are elevated in abduction and the contralateral arm is in some horizontal extension as the kicking limb moves behind the line of gravity. Since the right arm is elevated slightly, the scapular rotators provide a stable base for the humerus to move into some abduction via the action of the deltoid and rotator cuff muscles. However, the left arm is elevated to about 90° of abduction and in horizontal extension. Therefore, the left scapula is retracted through contraction of the middle trapezius and rhomboids, and the humerus is elevated by concentric activity of the middle deltoid and rotator cuff. The posterior deltoid horizontally extends the humerus behind the trunk. The trunk is maintained in an erect position by cocontraction of anterior and posterior (abdominals and spinal muscles) trunk muscles, but the upper torso is rotated away from the kick leg with the horizontal extension of the contralateral arm.

As the player runs toward the ball, his support leg is moving forward as the kick leg moves behind him. Right before the support leg lands about a foot from the ball and even to it, the kick leg is moving through the backswing phase. During this time the right hip is moving into extension, medial rotation, and abduction as the pelvis tilts anteriorly. The knee moves into flexion as the ankle remains stable in neutral in the sagittal plane. The left hip is moving into some flexion as the leg prepares for the foot to touch the ground. The left knee is moving toward extension whereas the ankle is dorsiflexed to clear the ground. The shoulders are both elevated to some degree in abduction with the left arm (contralateral to the kick leg) near 90° of abduction and moving into horizontal extension.

With the kick leg, the gluteal hip extensors and hamstrings work as agonists to extend the hip.[31] The gluteus medius and minimus abduct the hip. The gluteus medius and minimus, gracilis, and TFL medially rotate the thigh. The hamstrings are also beginning to flex the knee, and the biceps femoris also rotates the tibia laterally. The tibialis anterior dorsiflexes and the peroneus longus and brevis evert the ankle. On the support leg, the hip is moving into flexion through action of the iliopsoas and rectus femoris as the quadriceps extends the knee and the tibialis anterior maintains the ankle in dorsiflexion. Table 15–3 identifies the muscles that have been investigated and their activity levels

TABLE 15–3A | LOWER EXTREMITY MUSCLE ACTIVITY DURING THE INSTEP SOCCER KICK, KICK LEG*

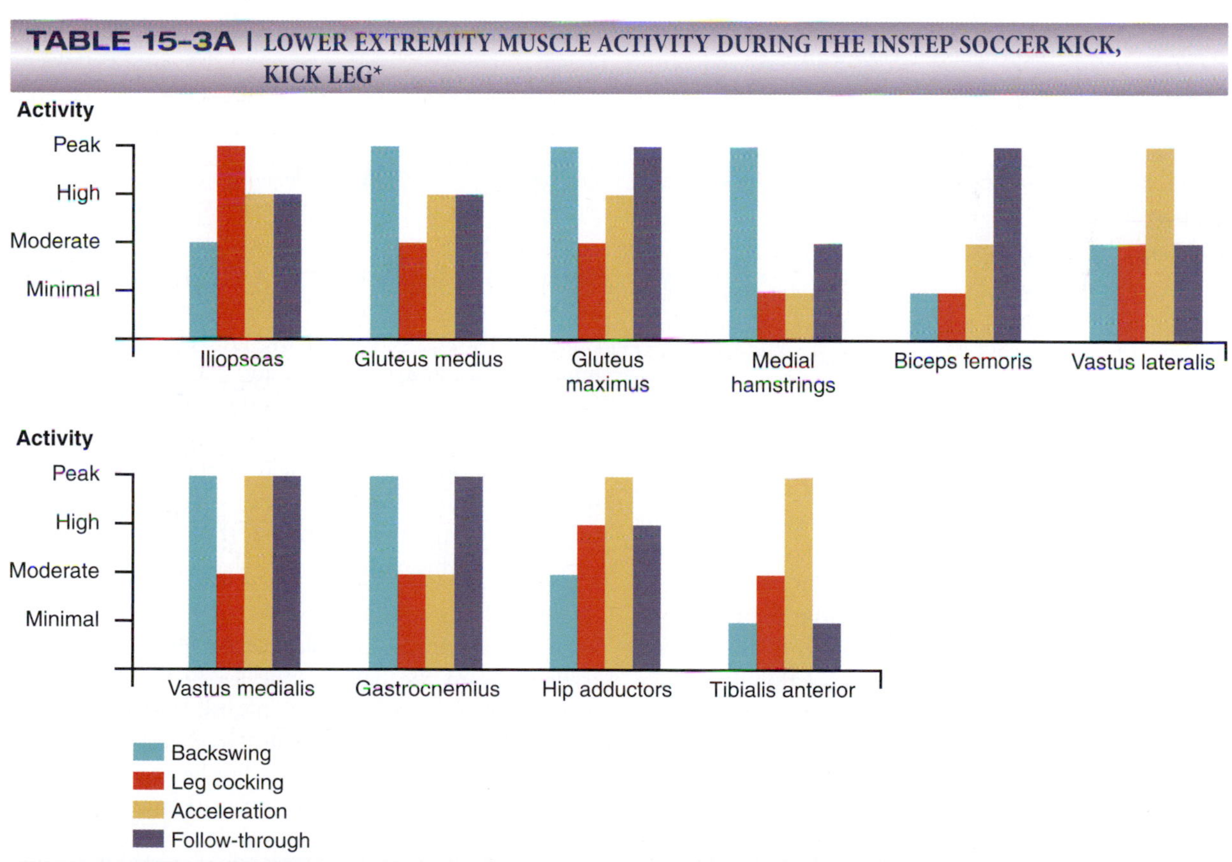

*Based on data from Brophy, et al;[34] Fields, et al;[31] and Kellis, et al.[35]

TABLE 15–3B | LOWER EXTREMITY MUSCLE ACTIVITY DURING THE INSTEP SOCCER KICK, SUPPORT LEG*

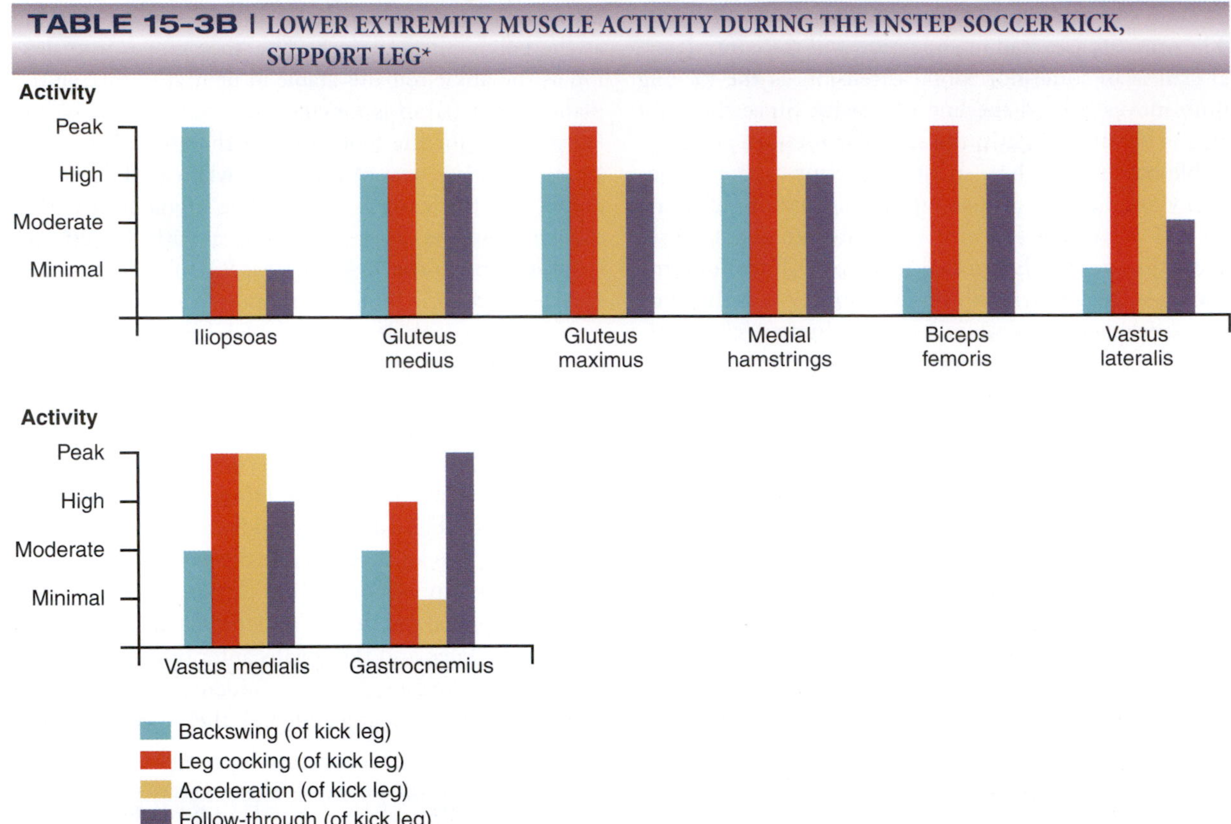

*Based on data from Brophy, et al;[34] Fields, et al;[31] and Kellis, et al.[35]

throughout the instep soccer kick for the kick and support legs.

Leg-Cocking Phase

Leg cocking begins when the knee moves into flexion to prepare to accelerate the leg to the ball, and the phase continues until the knee reaches maximum flexion.[31] The shoulders maintain their relative position of slight elevation of the ipsilateral arm with the contralateral arm in horizontal extension at about shoulder level through this phase. The upper torso is rotated toward the left arm and the pelvis is rotated toward the kicking leg moving the left arm and right leg away from each other to create torsion at the trunk. The pull of the left shoulder and right hip are responsible for this trunk position, but it is controlled eccentrically by the internal and external obliques. Eccentric contraction of the rectus abdominus provides slight extension of the trunk.

As the gluteals continue to extend the right hip, the hamstrings work aggressively to flex the knee.[31] The hip also maintains it medially rotated and abducted position, using the muscles already identified. The biceps femoris laterally rotates the knee as it moves into flexion. The foot is plantarflexed by contraction of the gastrocnemius and soleus.

At this point the center of mass is between the left and right feet but is moving forward toward the front left foot. This means that the left hip is becoming extended through effort of the gluteal muscles (maximus, medius, and minimus), and the left knee is also extended via concentric contraction of the quadriceps. Since the center of mass is behind the foot, the ankle is in plantarflexion and controlled by the gastrocnemius-soleus muscles. By the end of this phase, the foot is in full contact with the ground, so these muscles are all very active in this phase to move the body over the foot.

Acceleration Phase

Following maximum knee flexion, the limb begins accelerating toward the ball. As the leg begins its forward motion, the acceleration phase begins; it ends when the foot makes contact with the ball.[31] The kick knee is over the ball and the center of mass is just behind the support foot. The trunk is unwinding from its most open to a closed position to provide optimal force generation. The force of the kick is generated during this phase and continues to build until the foot makes ball contact.[31] Both shoulders are more elevated in this phase, and as the kicking limb advances forward, the contralateral arm moves into more elevation and horizontal flexion across the body, whereas the ipsilateral arm moves into extension. The left shoulder's pectoralis major and anterior deltoid move the humerus in front of the body as the scapular rotators stabilize it to provide the humerus with a stable base. The right shoulder's posterior deltoid, latissimus dorsi, and teres major extend the shoulder as the scapula's downward rotators (rhomboids, pectoralis minor, and levator scapula) position and stabilize the left scapula. The triceps of both arms hold the elbows in extension. Wrist motion is variable. The trunk is also rotating with the upper torso rotating toward the right and the pelvis rotating toward the left as the kick leg moves forward. Rotation occurs through concentric contraction of the left external abdominal obliques and right internal abdominal obliques. The trunk also moves into flexion through eccentric contraction of the erector spinae muscles.

The dominant kick-leg muscles in this phase include the hip flexors and quadriceps, working aggressively to flex the hip and simultaneously extend the knee.[35] The hip adductors are also active as the kick moves from abduction to adduction across the body. The hamstrings contract eccentrically right before ball contact to control contact with the ball and prevent the knee for hyperextending.[31] The tibialis anterior reaches its peak activity as it holds the foot in position to kick the ball.

Muscles of the support leg working most during this phase include the gluteus medius to maintain a single leg support and a stable pelvis as the center of mass is just behind the left foot during this time but advancing forward rapidly. The quadriceps are highly active during this time to keep the knee is slight flexion as the body's weight is anchored by the extremity as the ball is kicked by the other leg.

Follow-through Phase

Follow-through occurs from ball contact to completion of the activity. As with other activities, follow-through is important to reduce the risk of injury through dissipation of forces, and the longer the foot maintains contact with the ball the greater momentum will be applied to the ball.[32] During this phase, the contralateral shoulder and kick hip move toward each other as the trunk continues its rotation. In other words, the left shoulder moves into some horizontal flexion through contraction of the anterior deltoid and pectoralis major as its elbow flexes via activity of the biceps, brachialis, and brachioradialis. The right shoulder is in abduction and horizontal extension through contraction of the posterior deltoid, latissimus dorsi, and teres major with support from the downward rotators of the scapula (rhomboids, pectoralis minor, and levator scapulae). The triceps moves the elbow in extension. Wrist motions of both arms are variable. The trunk also continues to flex forward with the momentum of the kick leg whereas the erector spinae are active to control and decelerate trunk flexion. The kick leg moves across the body and into hip flexion and knee extension. The hamstrings are quite active as they "put the brakes" on knee extension. Gluteus maximus is also highly active as it decelerates hip flexion. The gastrocnemius is decelerating ankle dorsiflexion.

On the support leg, the gluteus medius works to maintain a level pelvis on the single-stance leg as the gluteus maximus continues to keep the hip in extension. The quadriceps hold the knee in extension and the gastrocnemius move the ankle into plantarflexion as the body's center of mass moves forward, ahead of the support limb.

Freestyle Swimming

Freestyle swimming, like soccer, is an activity that appeals to a wide range of age groups. However, unlike soccer, this activity may be performed as a member of a team or as an individual, either competitively or recreationally. We have chosen to place it here with other competitive sports since many injuries seen in this activity occur in individuals who are members of competitive teams. The freestyle stroke is selected because it is the swim stroke most people are familiar with and may be able to relate to in terms of their own swimming experiences. It is also the stroke common to many swimming shoulder injuries. The freestyle stroke is divided into two primary phases: pull-through and recovery.[36] The propulsion, or pull-through, phase is broken down into: 1) hand entry; 2) early pull-through; 3) middle pull-through; and 4) late pull-through. Although the recovery phase is sometimes approached as a two-step phase of early and late recovery, we will address it here as one phase (Fig. 15.5).

Most of the investigations into swimming look at either the physiology requirements or the upper extremities. Little research has identified two other important components of any swim stroke—the legs and the trunk. Before we analyze the freestyle stroke, it will be valuable to understanding the total body requirements if we address the legs in kicking and the trunk in rolling first.

Kicking

Although not as much research has been performed looking at the legs during swimming, they play an

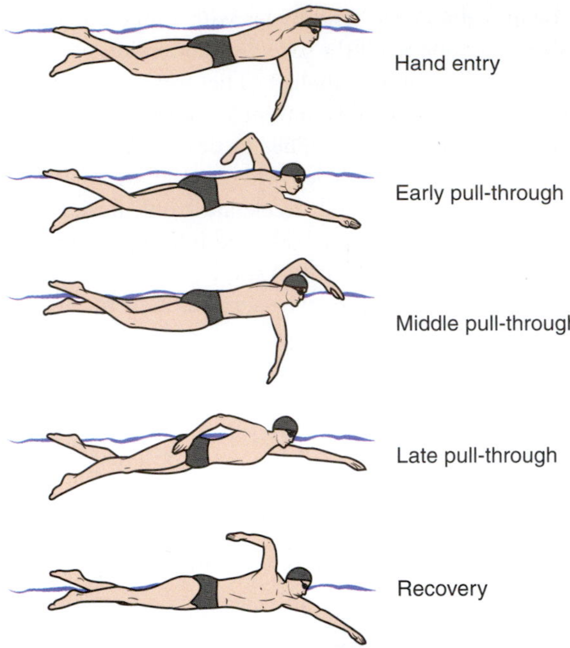

Figure 15.5 Phases of the freestyle swim stroke.

important role in any swim stroke.[37, 38] The legs contribute about 10% of the speed of the swimmer.[39] They also provide for a smooth stroke that would otherwise be jerky from the intermittent propelling surges of the arms.[40] The legs improve the efficiency of the body's movement in the water by keeping the body horizontal so there is less drag from water resistance. For every arm stroke, there are three leg kicks.[37] The leg produces a two-stroke cycle: a downbeat occurs when the extremity is pushed downward in the water, and an upbeat occurs when the extremity is moved upward in the water. The downbeat is the power phase and the upbeat is the recovery phase. Let's take a look at how the arms and legs are coordinated in an example to more easily realize this concept: Entry of the right arm into the water occurs at the same time as the downbeat of the right leg; as the arm moves to the pull-through phase, the left leg produces a downbeat in the water; and finally, as the arm moves into the late pull-through phase and begins moving upward in the water, another downbeat of the right leg occurs.[37] As a result, during one swim cycle of the arms, each leg moves through three of their cycles; this is sometimes referred to as a six-beat flutter kick.

Most of the motion of the legs occurs at the hips. The knees stay fairly extended but move similar to a whip, following the force propelled from the hips throughout the swimming cycle. The ankles remain plantarflexed. During the downbeat, the hip moves into some flexion. The knee maintains near extension and passes the downbeat force to the ankle, which stays in plantarflexion.

Muscles working in the lower extremities, then, are mainly hip muscles. The gluteal muscles and hamstrings provide hip extension motion whereas the iliopsoas and rectus femoris provide power for hip flexion. The knees move through transfer of forces from the hip and contraction of the quadriceps. The gastrocnemius and soleus are the primary muscles that maintain the ankle in its position of plantarflexion and provide some force during the kick.

Rolling

Roll of the body during the freestyle swim varies greatly among investigators. Some have found as little as 35°[41] whereas others have recorded from 60°[40] to about 80°[42] of rotation to one side during freestyle swimming. Body roll during the freestyle swim stroke is important for several reasons. Most obviously, it allows the swimmer's mouth to move above the water line so a breath may be taken while swimming. Less obviously, perhaps, it allows the arm to be taken out of the water with less stress to the shoulder; by rolling the body as the arm moves out of the water, less horizontal extension and less lateral rotation is necessary to lift the arm up, protecting the shoulder against impingement of soft tissues during shoulder elevation. If the body does not adequately roll, the shoulder undergoes stress and the hand is not correctly positioned for entry into the water, further adding stresses to the extremity.[40]

The body rolls as three units—the head, the upper trunk, and the pelvis. Whether the swimmer is selecting to breathe or not on a stroke depends on which unit rolls first. When the swimmer breathes, the head rolls first, followed by the upper trunk, which is immediately followed by the pelvis; however, if the swimmer does not breathe during the stroke, the pelvis rolls first and is followed by the upper trunk and head.[41] An investigation demonstrated, however, that the time difference between the initiations of motion between the pelvis and upper trunk for each group examined were not significant,[41] so in essence, the upper trunk and pelvis may be considered to roll at the same time.

Pull-through Phase

This part of the freestyle stroke begins when the hand first enters the water. It ends when the hand exits the water. This is the propulsive phase of the stroke. The body is propelled through the water using primarily the arms, but as mentioned, the trunk and legs also play important roles in this phase. The legs assist the arms during the swimming cycle by coordinating with the body roll to provide power during the pull-through phase.[42] The pull-through phase of the swimming cycle makes up about 65% of the entire stroke.[40] Both arms are in the water at the same time during a portion of one swim stroke.[40] As each arm moves through the water, the hand creates an S-shaped path of motion in the water. As the shoulder moves from some abduction when the hand enters the water and the elbow moves into flexion, moving the hand under the trunk, and then as the elbow extends and the shoulder abducts to move the hand away from the body before it exits the water, the hand makes a large "S" pattern in the water (Fig. 15.6).

Because the glenohumeral joint moves through large ranges of motion throughout the freestyle cycle, scapular stabilization is crucial from start to finish in providing a stable glenoid base from which the humerus moves through this large range of motion, allowing the glenohumeral muscles the platform they need to provide power to move the body through the water. These scapular muscles that are active include the levator scapulae, rhomboids, trapezius, and serratus anterior. Of course, the rotator cuff muscles also serve as important stabilizers for the glenohumeral joint of the shoulder complex. It is interesting to note that the flexor carpi ulnaris contracts significantly throughout most of the freestyle stroke with levels of force ranging between about 50% to 80% of its maximum isometric force.[43] This is a strenuous requirement for a muscle, especially when it is active throughout the pull and recovery cycles. It is not known if this high activity demand is because of the requirements made of the muscle at the wrist, the elbow, or both. Muscle activity occurring during the freestyle swim stroke is seen in Table 15–4.

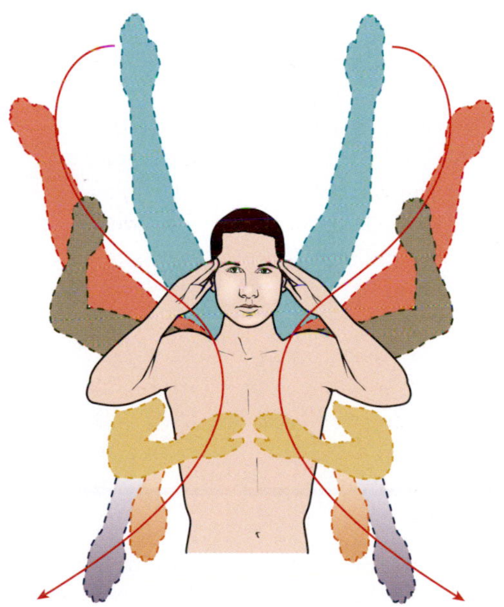

Figure 15.6 The S-path of the hand during the freestyle swimming stroke.

Hand-entry Phase

The first to enter the water is the fingertips. They enter the water in front of the head between the body's midline and the end of the shoulder.[42] The fingers are together and the hand is positioned with the thumb pointing down to reduce the amount of drag, or resistance.[42] The hand's entry into the water creates a "hole" through which the wrist and elbow also enter the water. Hand placement at entry is important since improper placement may lead to injury.[40] As the wrist and elbow enter the water, the hand reaches forward to extend the arm in front of the body.[42]

As you may expect, joint motions include scapular upward rotation along with shoulder elevation into abduction. The shoulder is also medially rotated. The elbow is partially flexed, moving into extension, whereas the wrist is already in extension and the fingers are adducted. Body roll begins in this phase. The first downbeat of the ipsilateral leg also occurs at this time.

Immediately after the hand touches the water, the triceps begin to extend the elbow. As previously mentioned, the scapular stabilizers are active as is the rotator cuff. The middle deltoid and supraspinatus work to abduct the shoulder, and the subscapularis begins to contract as the arm prepares to begin medial rotation after it hits the water. The serratus anterior and subscapularis are active at varying levels throughout the entire stroke.[44] It is during hand entry as the scapula moves through its greatest upward rotation that the serratus anterior is most active.[44]

Early Pull-through Phase

The early pull-through phase begins immediately after the arm is at its most extended point at the end of the hand-entry phase and continues until the arm is at its deepest point in the water.

At the start of this phase, the wrist flexes about 40° as the shoulder and forearm rotate to face the palm outward away from the body.[42] The hand moves outward away from the shoulder and downward in the water as the shoulder abducts, moves into extension, and rotates to a neutral position. The elbow is moving into slight flexion. The trunk rolls toward the arm about 60° to place the shoulder under water.[40] At the end of this phase, the hand is at its deepest point in the water and

TABLE 15–4 | SHOULDER AND ELBOW MUSCLE ACTIVITY DURING THE FREESTYLE SWIMMING STROKE*

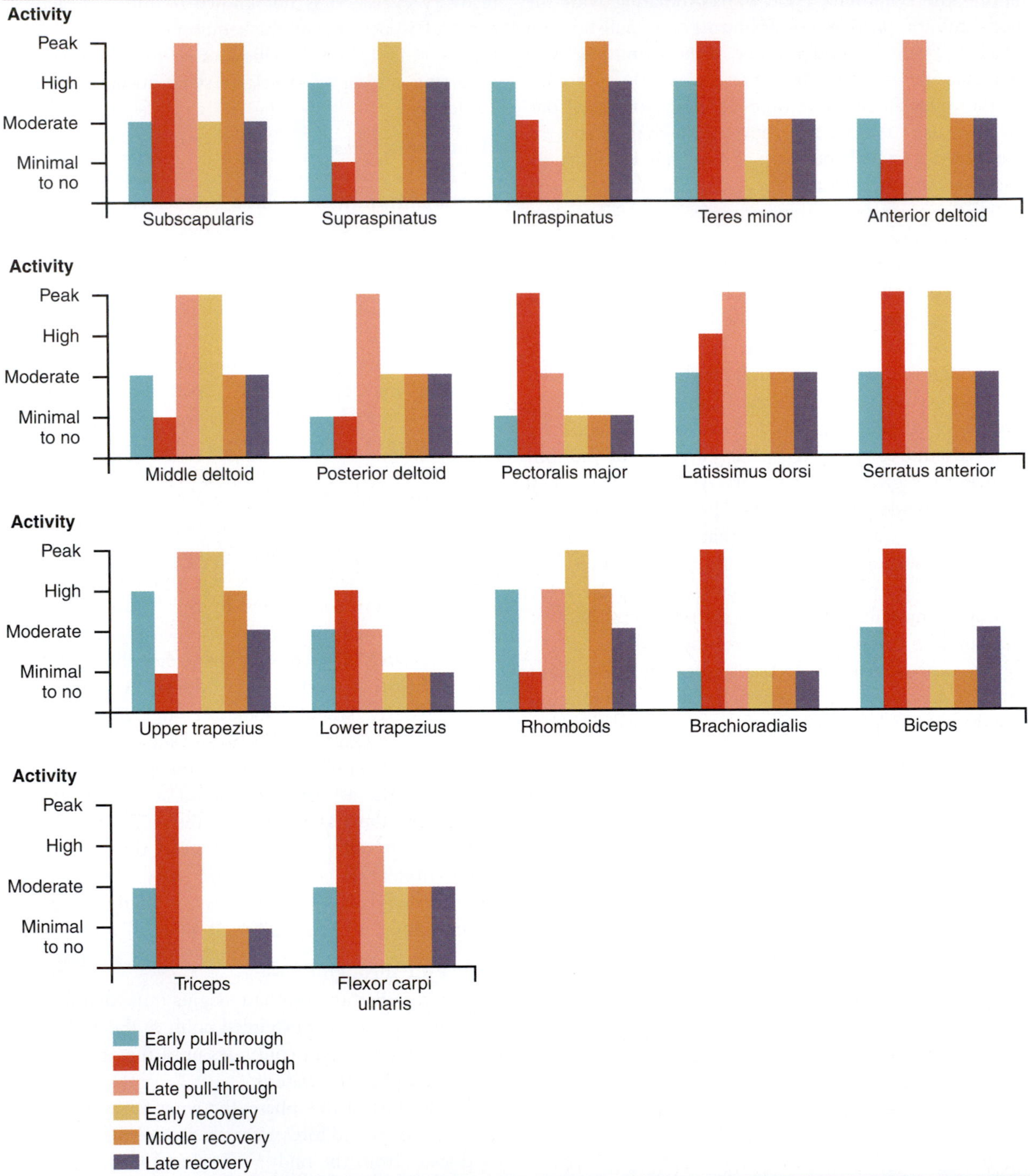

Activity

Peak
High
Moderate
Minimal to no

Subscapularis
Supraspinatus
Infraspinatus
Teres minor
Anterior deltoid

Activity

Peak
High
Moderate
Minimal to no

Middle deltoid
Posterior deltoid
Pectoralis major
Latissimus dorsi
Serratus anterior

Activity

Peak
High
Moderate
Minimal to no

Upper trapezius
Lower trapezius
Rhomboids
Brachioradialis
Biceps

Activity

Peak
High
Moderate
Minimal to no

Triceps
Flexor carpi ulnaris

Early pull-through
Middle pull-through
Late pull-through
Early recovery
Middle recovery
Late recovery

*Based on data from Moynes, et al;[4] Nuber, et al;[45] Scovazzo, et al;[45] Clarys and Rouard;[43] and Pink, et al.[44]

may be up to 1.5 ft below the water's surface for women and up to 2 ft for men.[42] The contralateral leg produces its downbeat right before the end of this phase and continues into the early part of the next phase.

The humeral muscles involved in the abduction and then extension movements here include the middle and posterior deltoids, teres major, and latissimus dorsi with the downward rotators of the scapula (rhomboids, levator scapulae, and pectoralis minor) coordinating scapular movement during shoulder motion.[45] Elbow muscles involved in activity include the biceps and brachialis cocontracting with the triceps to stabilize the elbow after the flexors have positioned it.[46] Wrist and hand stabilization occur also through cocontraction of their flexor and extensor muscles, as previously mentioned. Muscles involved in producing trunk roll have also been previously discussed, as have the lower extremity muscles producing leg motion.

Middle Pull-through Phase

The middle pull-through phase begins from the end of early pull-through and ends when the arm is under and perpendicular to the trunk. At the start of this phase, the palm rotates inward as the hand sweeps toward the swimmer's chest.[42] Other joint motions during this phase include downward rotation of the scapula, which is combined with adduction and continued extension of the humerus. The humerus also medially rotates. The elbow flexes during this phase to about 90° whereas the forearm supinates. The wrist maintains slight flexion as the fingers remain extended and adducted. At the very end of this phase, moving into the next, the ipsilateral leg produces its second downbeat. The body begins to roll back toward neutral at the end of this phase to prepare for entry of the other hand into the water.[36]

The latissimus dorsi and pectoralis major are at their most active as they pull against the water to move the body over the arm. The shoulder adducts and extends through their concentric activity; they also work with the subscapularis to medially rotate the humerus.[44] The downward rotators of the scapula (pectoralis minor, rhomboids, and levator scapula) concomitantly move the scapula. Biceps and coracobrachialis muscles provide forceful elbow flexion.[42] The brachioradialis provides its strongest output in this phase.[43] The extensor carpi ulnaris and flexor carpi ulnaris cocontract to maintain the wrist position.[47] Long finger flexors and extensors (flexor digitorum profundus and superficialis and extensor digitorum longus) and lumbricals hold the fingers in extension and adduction to form a paddle of the hand.

Late Pull-through Phase

This phase begins from where the arm is perpendicular to the body and ends when the hand moves out of the water.[42] During this time, the hand continues to sweep upward and backward toward the water's surface.[42] Additional joint motions include a continued downward rotation of the scapula on the thorax and extension with adduction and medial rotation of the shoulder so that of the fingers, the little finger comes out of the water first. Elbow extension occurs throughout this phase. The ipsilateral leg completes another downbeat in the early part of this phase.

During this phase the posterior deltoid activity is followed by activation of the middle and anterior deltoid as the hand moves out of the water.[44, 45] The latissimus dorsi and teres major continue their activity as the shoulder continues to extend. Scapular muscles also continue to fire through shoulder extension and then abduction as the body rolls. Elbow flexion is maintained through eccentric control of the triceps and then concentric activity as the elbow moves into extension.

Recovery Phase

The recovery phase is the remaining 35% of the freestyle swim stroke.[48] It begins with hand exit and continues until the hand moves into the water again. During this time, the elbow flexes and is high in the air, leaving the water first. The muscles act during this time to move the arm from behind the body to over the head, readying it for re-entry into the water. It is important that these muscles position the arm for optimal placement in the water to provide maximal propulsion.

Upper trunk rotation aids in removing the extremity from the water. The trunk rotates sufficiently to lift the shoulder out of the water.[42] Shoulder motions throughout the recovery phase start from glenohumeral joint positions of medial rotation, extension, and adduction. By the time the hand is ready for entry into the water again, the shoulder is elevated into flexion with slight abduction and medially rotated to place the index finger in the water first. The scapula moves from downward rotation at the start of the recovery to upward rotation at the end of recovery. The elbow is flexed throughout this phase until the very end when it moves toward extension. The body is rolled to the contralateral side when the hand comes out of the water and then rolls to a neutral position by the time the hand is ready to re-enter the water.

The large erector spinae muscles posteriorly and the oblique muscles anteriorly provide the upper torso roll out of the water and then return to a neutral position by the time the hand re-enters the water.[42] Hip flexors and extensors along with the ankle plantarflexors assist the roll by providing power through their kicking activity.[42] The muscles in the shoulder complex working during recovery include the upward rotators of the scapula (serratus anterior and trapezius), retractors (middle trapezius and rhomboids) along with all four of the rotator cuff muscles and deltoids to elevate and medially rotate the glenohumeral joint. The infraspinatus works eccentrically to medially rotate the shoulder as it prepares to re-enter the water.[44]

Leisure Activities

Three types of activities have been selected for analysis of leisure activities. These are common recreational activities in which many members of the general population engage throughout their life cycles. Since running was covered in Chapter 12, it is not included here, but it is certainly a common recreational activity in which many individuals participate. The three leisure activities in this section include golfing, cycling, and tennis. As with the sports activities, one aspect of each of these recreational activities will be identified and analyzed.

Golf Swing

Just as there are several different golf clubs that a golfer uses during a round of golf, there are also several types of swings a golfer uses. Therefore, we will analyze a full golf swing. The golf swing may be divided into four phases: 1) windup; 2) forward swing; 3) acceleration; and 4) follow-through[49] (Fig. 15.7).

So it is easier to discuss the left and right extremities during analysis of the golf swing, we will assume the golfer is right handed. Therefore, the left extremities are the lead extremities, the arm and leg facing the target, whereas the right extremities are the trail extremities, the arm and leg farthest from the target.

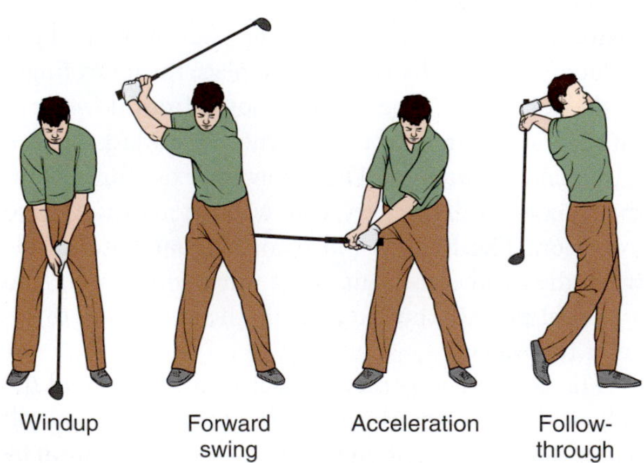

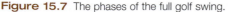

Figure 15.7 The phases of the full golf swing.

As with so many other activities in which it is necessary to transfer forces from the lower to the upper extremities, the back remains straight in the sagittal plane throughout the motion. The multifidus and transverse abdominus play important roles in maintaining this spinal alignment for a golfer.[50] Although these muscles will not be mentioned as we go through the swing motion, keep in mind that these muscles function throughout the majority of the activity. The abdominal obliques and erector spinae muscles assist in stabilizing the spine and rotating the trunk during the golf swing.[50,51] These larger trunk muscles are able to reduce stresses on the intervertebral joints by transmitting forces from the legs, spine, and pelvis to the arms through the thoracolumbar fascia.[50]

You may notice as we go through the golf swing that the deltoid is relatively quiet throughout the swing. This is unusual since the deltoid usually plays an important role in upper extremity function.[4] It is assumed that the reason the deltoid is relatively inactive during this activity is because the shoulder does not elevate substantially throughout any portion of the swing.[52]

Until the ball is hit, the head remains down so the golfer looks at the golf ball. During the windup, this means that the head is in essence rotated to the left. Once the ball is hit, the golfer follows the flight of the ball with his or her eyes, so the neck extends to neutral and the head is rotated toward the right. The muscles responsible for these movements include the erector spinae muscles as they work to position the head to look down as the contralateral SCM and ipsilateral upper trapezius rotate the head. Muscles and their activity levels that have been investigated during the golf swing are presented in Table 15–5.

Windup Phase

The windup phase begins with the club moving away from the ball and ends with the club at the top of the backswing. The windup phase is also sometimes referred to as either the backswing phase or the takeaway phase. In keeping with descriptions of other activities we have already presented, we will use the term windup phase.

Before the club is swung, the golfer moves into position. The hips are flexed about 45° with the knees flexed about 20° to 25°, with at least half of the body weight distributed over the back foot, and the right shoulder slightly laterally tilted downward from a right lateral bend of the spine.[53] Since the right hand is lower on the club shaft than the left, the right scapula is slightly depressed and downwardly rotated.[53] The hands grip the club with a power grip, using an interlocking of the

TABLE 15–5A | MUSCLE ACTIVITY OF THE LEAD EXTREMITIES (LEFT FOR A RIGHT-HANDED GOLFER) DURING THE GOLF SWING*

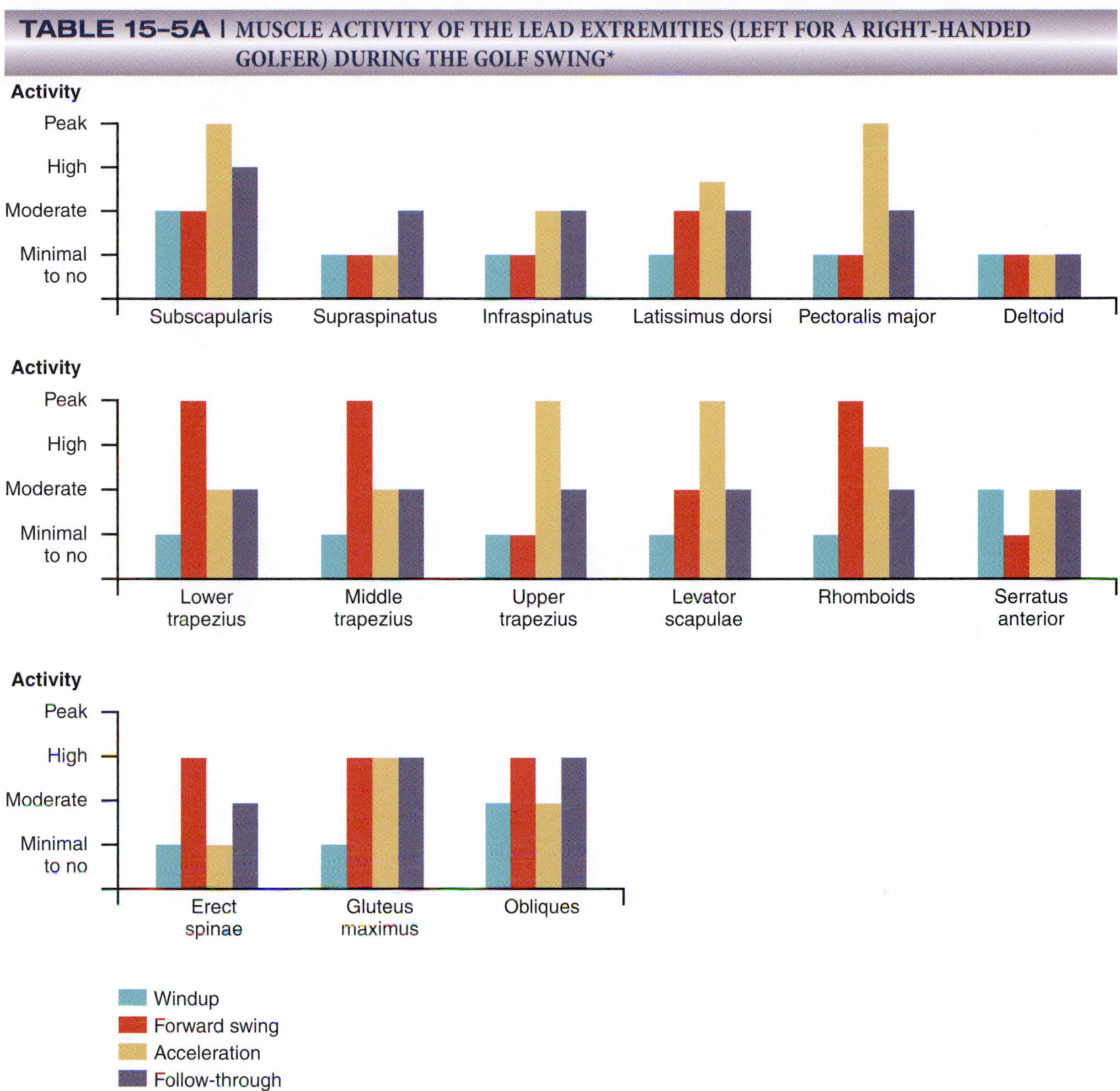

*Based on data from Jobe, et al;[58] Kao, et al;[59] Bulbulian, et al;[51] Watkins, et al;[54] and Pink, et al.[43]

left index finger around the right little finger and the right hand more distal on the handle than the left hand. Since both hands are rotated clockwise on the grip, the left hand's dorsum is visible when the golfer looks down on the grip. The hands are in slight wrist flexion and ulnar deviation.[54] The line of the body is parallel with the line from the ball to the target.

As the movement begins, about 60% of the body's weight transfers to the front and medial aspect of the trail leg,[53, 55] and the torso and pelvis rotate around the trail leg. The torso and shoulders rotate slightly more quickly than the pelvis although the pelvis motion is completed before shoulder rotation.[56] This causes the lead knee to flex more, and the left hip laterally rotates relative to pelvic alignment; this is important to realize since, at first glance, it may appear that the thigh medially rotates if the pelvis position is not taken into account. Movement of the body weight more to the trail leg with knee flexion causes the foot to move into eversion as it stays on the ground. As the hands move up and behind the golfer, the right arm abducts until it reaches about 75° to 90° of elevation and laterally

TABLE 15–5B | MUSCLE ACTIVITY OF THE TRAIL EXTREMITIES (RIGHT FOR A RIGHT-HANDED GOLFER) DURING THE GOLF SWING*

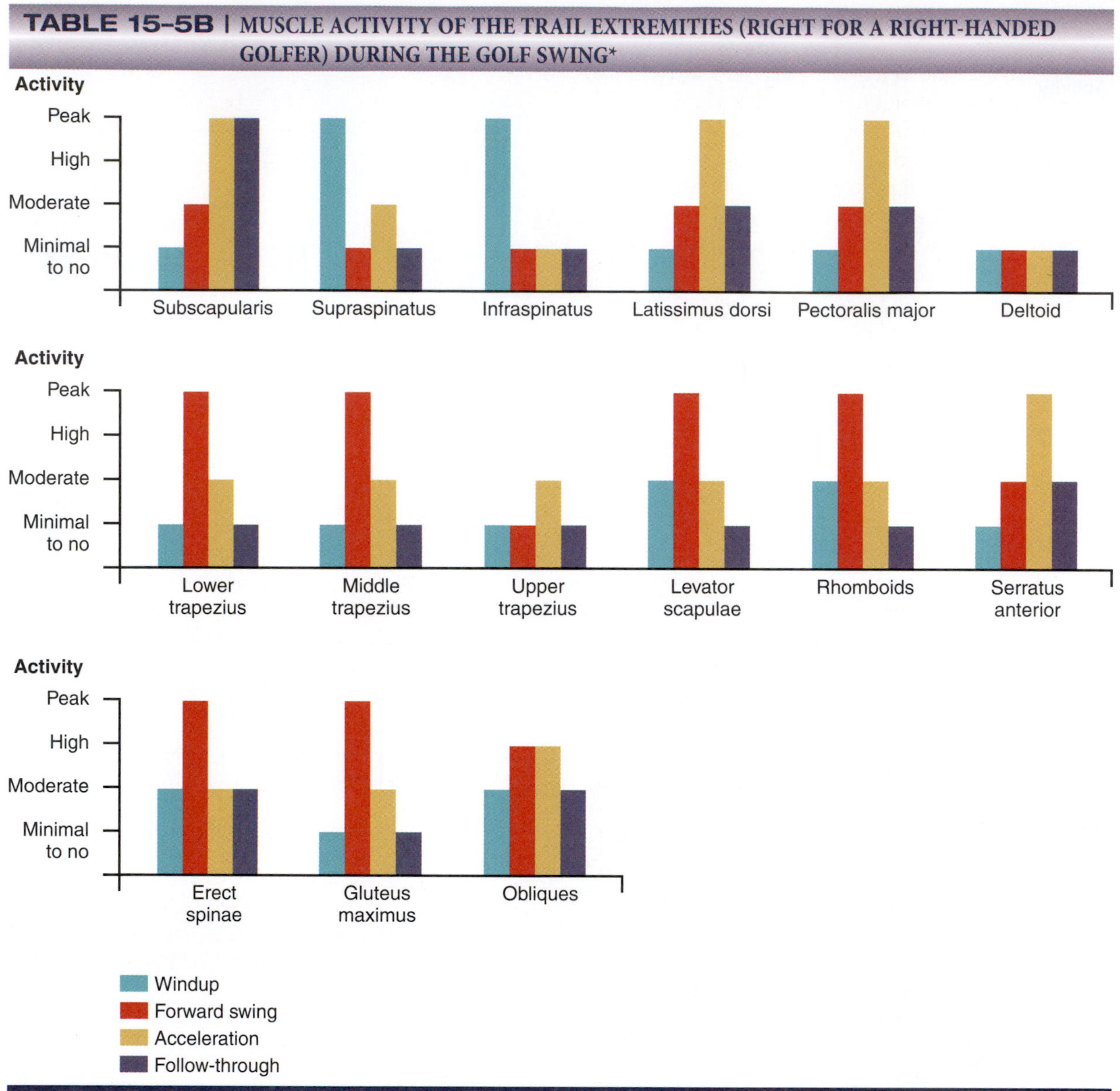

*Based on data from Jobe, et al;[55] Kao, et al;[56] Bulbulian, et al;[48] Watkins, et al;[54] and Pink, et al.[49]

rotates to about 90° as the right elbow flexes.[53] The left shoulder, on the other hand, adducts across the body and medially rotates with a nearly extended elbow.[53] By the top of the backswing, the left scapula is protracted and in slight upward rotation. The wrists are in a position of function, extension, and cocked in some radial deviation, although this is variable depending on the individual's strength and flexibility.[54, 55]

Although there is obviously some activity as the body moves the arms overhead and toward the trail side of the body, output of muscles throughout the body is relatively minor. The right erector spinae muscles and both oblique muscles are probably the most active, although only moderately so.[57] Since shoulder elevation is not significant during the backswing, the rotator cuff and deltoid muscles of both shoulders are relatively quiet as the arms are raised.[4] Although the supraspinatus and infraspinatus are active to only about 25% of their maximal output, this is the time of their greatest output during the golf swing.[25] The subscapularis of the lead arm shows the most activity of the rotator cuff as the shoulder moves into medial rotation during elevation behind the right shoulder.[58] The serratus anterior is also moderately active as the left scapula protracts and upwardly rotates.[59] Moderate activity of the trail arm's levator scapulae and rhomboids provide for retraction of the scapula. Cocontraction of the biceps and triceps hold the golf club at the top of the swing. Wrist flexors and extensors also cocontract to position the wrist as the long finger flexors grasp the club handle. The eccentric activity of the gluteal, hamstring, and quadriceps maintains the hip and knees in some flexion during the backswing. Weight-bearing on the limbs with rotation of the pelvis through activity from the deep lateral rotators provides for passive positioning of the lower extremities. Peroneals control eversion of the ankle, although the motion initiates with pelvis rotation.

Forward Swing Phase

This phase begins from the top of the backswing and ends when the club is horizontal to the ground.[58] During this phase, the muscles begin more activity as the club is brought down to position to move into acceleration. Muscles generally have the most amount of activity in either this phase or the acceleration phase.

The pelvis initiates an unwinding motion before the upper torso ends its windup motion; however, the upper torso accelerates at a greater rate during this unwinding, as it did during the windup phase. Simultaneously, the left ankle supinates and the left hip laterally rotates as the trunk maintains its sagittal position but begins to rotate to the left.[53] Weight begins its transfer from the trail leg to the lead leg. During the forward swing, the left shoulder laterally rotates as it moves toward the body's midline. The right shoulder medially rotates and adducts as its elbow moves into extension.[53] The wrists maintain their cocked position through this phase but begin to uncock, moving into ulnar deviation as the body enters the acceleration phase.

The hip extensors (gluteus maximus) and abductors (gluteus medius and minimus, TFL) of the right hip and the adductors (adductor magnus especially) of the left hip initiate pelvic motion as this phase begins. This is the time of peak activity of the right gluteus maximus muscle as it begins the power drive into acceleration of the club.[57] The left gluteus maximus is very active in this phase and the acceleration phase, as it stabilizes the body during transition of body weight from primarily the right to the primarily the left lower extremity.[50] The erector spinae perform eccentrically to maintain upright trunk alignment.[57] During this phase, the left external abdominal oblique and the right internal abdominal oblique are at their greatest activity. The rhomboids of both scapulae are at their most active as the scapulae move into downward rotation, accompanying efforts by each shoulder's latissimus dorsi and pectoralis major as they move the arms toward extension.[58, 59] The left triceps maintains its elbow position in near extension as the right triceps moves the elbow toward extension.

Acceleration Phase

Acceleration begins when the club is horizontal to the ground and ends with ball contact.[58] During this time, the club speed increases through transfer of forces from the unwinding of the hips, pelvis, and trunk to the arms. Weight transfers to the lead leg and the movement of the arms follows the direction of weight transfer. As the club hits the ball, the club's face should be pointed toward the target.

The pelvis and trunk continue their unwinding at an accelerated pace until right after ball strike; they are moving the fastest as they approach near neutral in the transverse plane by the time the ball is hit.[56] As the pelvis rotates to the left, the right hip adducts, the right knee flexes, and the foot everts to push the weight from the medial foot. The shoulders are moving into extension with the right arm adducting as the left arm abducts. The right shoulder is also medially rotating as the left shoulder moves toward lateral rotation. As the right shoulder medially rotates, the forearm is pronating so the ball is hit with the dorsal hand facing the target. The left shoulder is in some lateral rotation with the forearm supinated.

This is the phase of greatest muscle activity throughout the body. As the body continues this rotation during acceleration, spinal muscle control moves from the right erector spinae and obliques eccentrically controlling posture to the left erector spinae and oblique muscles as they become more active as the body moves to the left side.[53] The pelvis rotates through efforts from the right hip adductors and left hip lateral rotators (deep rotators). Right knee flexion is controlled by eccentric activity of the quadriceps. The right ankle evertors (peroneals) and gastrocnemius-soleus group provide push off from the right foot to assist in transferring the body's weight to the left extremity. The left pectoralis major and latissimus dorsi achieve their greatest output during this phase. As the right shoulder medially rotates, the subscapularis increases its activity during this phase to its greatest activity level of the swing. The left triceps is active as the elbow moves into extension at the time of contact with the ball. The right forearm pronators (pronator quadratus and teres) and left forearm supinators (supinator and biceps) provide for forearm movement and positioning in this phase. The wrists uncock from radial to ulnar deviation immediately before the club hits the ball, adding to ball propulsion. The flexor and extensor carpi ulnaris muscles provide this motion. Cocontraction of the wrist stabilizers maintains a functional position of the wrists as the long finger flexors maintain their grasp on the club.

Follow-through Phase

Follow-through begins at ball contact and ends with the completion of the swing motion.[58] As with other follow-through movements in other activities, the muscles acting during this phase work primarily in eccentric functions to slow down the motion of the extremities. Most of the motion during this phase is the result of the momentum of the arms moving from a down position at the time of ball contact to the up position at the end of the stroke. The right lower extremity follows the path of motion as the body weight transfers from the right to the left leg.

By the completion of the follow-through phase, the trunk and pelvis are facing the target and in some lateral flexion. The body weight is primarily on the left leg. The right lower extremity is in neutral hip or slightly extended in the sagittal plane with some medial rotation, whereas the knee is partially flexed and the ankle is in plantarflexion. The lead leg is medially rotated at the hip and moves from some flexion to less flexion by the end of the phase. The left foot is on the ground in inversion. By the end of the swing, the left shoulder is abducted and laterally rotated with its scapula in retraction. The left elbow is flexed. On the other hand, the right shoulder is horizontally flexed, elevated a little above 90°, and medially rotated. The right elbow is in some flexion. Both wrists are in radial deviation.

The most active muscles in this phase include the left gluteus maximus, right subscapularis, and left abdominal obliques. The left gluteus maximus is holding the body upright as it controls body weight on top of the left lower extremity. As the right upper extremity remains in contact with the club, its subscapularis follows the path of the club to reach up and around to the golfer's left upper quadrant region. The left abdominal oblique slows the arm movement down as the body comes to a stop. Hip medial rotation occurs through activity of the TFL, gluteus medius and minimus, and gracilis. Knee motion is controlled by the quadriceps. Left ankle inversion is controlled by the tibialis posterior. Right ankle plantarflexion is assisted by the gastrocnemius-soleus muscles. In the upper extremities, most of the muscles are relatively quiet. The left scapular muscles provide scapular positioning against the thorax and retraction (trapezius, rhomboids, serratus anterior, and levator scapulae) as the clavicular portion of the pectoralis major provides upper motion of the humerus. The right scapula's most active muscle, the serratus anterior, is at a moderate level of activity as the scapula retracts with humeral adduction across the body, which is provided by the sternal head of its pectoralis major. Right humeral medial rotation is provided by the latissimus dorsi and subscapularis. Elbow flexion occurs through cocontraction of the elbow flexors and extensors on the right and contraction of the elbow flexors on the left. Radial deviation initially occurs as a function of the extensor and flexor carpi radialis muscles, but once the wrists move overhead, the motion continues through eccentric contraction of the flexor and extensor carpi ulnaris muscles.

Tennis Serve

The tennis serve is a popular competitive or recreational activity. There are several types of tennis strokes and some of them may become very complicated with the addition of factors such as placing spin on the ball and producing excessive speed on a return. Of the strokes, we will analyze the flat serve. The serve is more complicated than a forehand or backhand groundstroke and the most rigorous of the tennis strokes.[60] Therefore, once we investigate the aspects of a serve, it may be easier to identify the elements involved in these other strokes. As with the other activities we have presented in this chapter, there is a wide range of skill levels in tennis. Likewise, there are also variations on how the ball may be served in tennis. We will present a standard approach to a serve. There are four phases of a tennis serve. These include: (1) windup; (2) cocking; (3) acceleration; and (4) follow-through (Fig. 15.8).[4]

As with many other sport activities, the tennis serve requires the "winding up" of the body to maximize the force transfer from the legs and trunk to the arms. The shoulder produces only 13% of the total energy expenditure in the tennis serve, so the output must come from other body segments.[12] The kinetic chain allows the

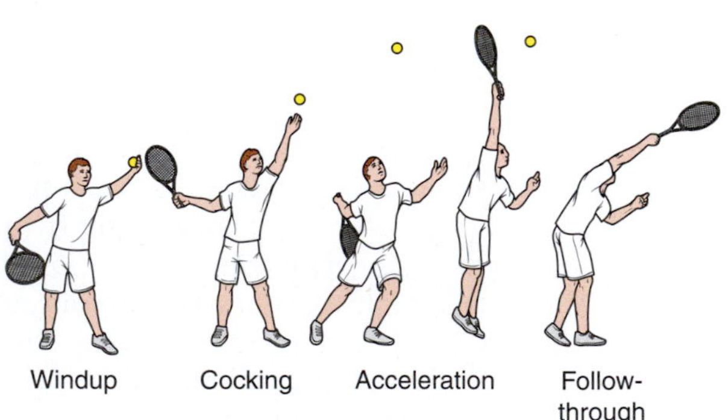

Figure 15.8 The tennis serve phases.

transfer of forces that are developed in the lower extremities and trunk to the hand and the racquet. The shoulder and elbow serve as a conduit to transmit both the forces coming from the trunk and legs and the forces they generate by their own motions. Sequential timing of activity, then, is important for this buildup and transfer of forces to where they are needed—in the hand—at the right time.

So it is easier to discuss, we will assume that our tennis player is right handed. Obviously, everything outlined here is reversed for left-handed players.

Windup Phase

Windup starts as the tennis player begins movement to toss the ball into the air. This phase ends when the ball is released from the hand.[4] During this phase, the player initiates motion by tossing the ball into the air above and in front of the body. Little activity outside the nonracquet (left for a right-handed player) arm occurs. The nonracquet arm's movement is primarily from the shoulder, moving into flexion to propel the ball into the air. The elbow is held in slight flexion with the forearm supinated. The wrist is in slight flexion as the fingers are flexed to maintain a light grasp on the ball. The right shoulder is in slight abduction away from the body.

The front leg, also the left foot for a right-handed player, points somewhere between the target and the sideline whereas the right thigh is rotated laterally and the foot faces between the sideline and behind the player. Weight begins more on the right leg and transfers to the left leg at the end of cocking; the hips and knees are partially flexed. The trunk remains in a neutral position with a forward trunk lean occurring from hip flexion. By the end of this phase, the trunk leans laterally to the right.

As with other activities, the core muscles (multifidus and transverse abdominus) contract to stabilize the spine. The left erector spinae eccentrically contract to a moderate level to control the trunk position toward the latter half of the phase as the trunk leans away from the left leg to the right.[61,62] Hip lateral rotators (deep rotators) of both hips position the hips in lateral rotation whereas the gluteals (maximus, medius, and minimus) eccentrically control hip flexion and stabilize the pelvis. The quadriceps holds the knees in partial flexion as the gastrocnemius and soleus of each lower limb maintain some dorsiflexion at the ankles. Scapular stabilizers of the right shoulder complex (all rotators) keep the scapula in position on the thorax as the deltoid and supraspinatus position the shoulder in slight abduction. Right triceps maintain elbow extension whereas the wrist and fingers are in flexion via activity from the wrist flexors (flexor carpi ulnaris and flexor carpi radialis) and finger flexors (flexor digitorum superficialis and profundus). The thumb is positioned in a power grip throughout the motion by thumb flexors and the opponens pollicis. As the left shoulder elevates via contraction of the anterior deltoid, supraspinatus, and pectoralis major, the other rotator cuff muscles (infraspinatus, teres minor, and subscapularis) maintain the humerus in the glenoid as the upward scapular rotators (serratus anterior, upper and lower trapezius) upwardly rotate and stabilize the scapula. As the scapula increases its upward rotation, it also retracts through effort of the rhomboids and middle trapezius. The left elbow is extended through eccentric activity of the elbow flexors (biceps, brachialis, and brachioradialis). The fingers extend as the ball is released through eccentric contraction of the finger flexors. Although these muscles are all activated, their output is relatively mild since there is no resistance to these motions except gravity.[4]

Cocking Phase

When the ball leaves the hand, this phase begins. The cocking phase continues until the racquet shoulder is in maximum lateral rotation.[4] During this phase, the body winds up in preparation for the acceleration phase when the body's forces convert from the potential energy it is creating in this phase to the kinetic energy it releases during acceleration.[60] This transfer of energy occurs as muscles are prestretched during the cocking phase and converted to concentric movement during the acceleration phase.[63]

The weight moves from the right leg to more onto the left leg as the trunk rotates, extends, and starts to lean to the left. The hips and knees are partially flexed until the end of this phase when they start to move into extension. The ankles also start movement into plantarflexion toward the end of this phase. The left shoulder reduces its elevation and may be around 90° of abduction by the end of this phase, although this height is variable. Right shoulder positioning in this phase is a key factor in determining the success of the acceleration phase. The right shoulder moves into abduction and lateral rotation, achieving its maximum lateral rotation at the end of this phase. The elbow becomes maximally flexed after the shoulder moves into its highest elevation.[60] The elbow is flexed to over 115° and the forearm is in some supination.[26]

Many muscles reach their peak activity during this phase (Tables 15–6A, B). The scapular muscles begin activity before the glenohumeral muscles.[64] The upward scapular rotators move the scapula into position of upward rotation up to 60° and maintain a stable platform

TABLE 15-6A | SHOULDER AND ELBOW MUSCLE ACTIVITY DURING THE TENNIS SERVE*

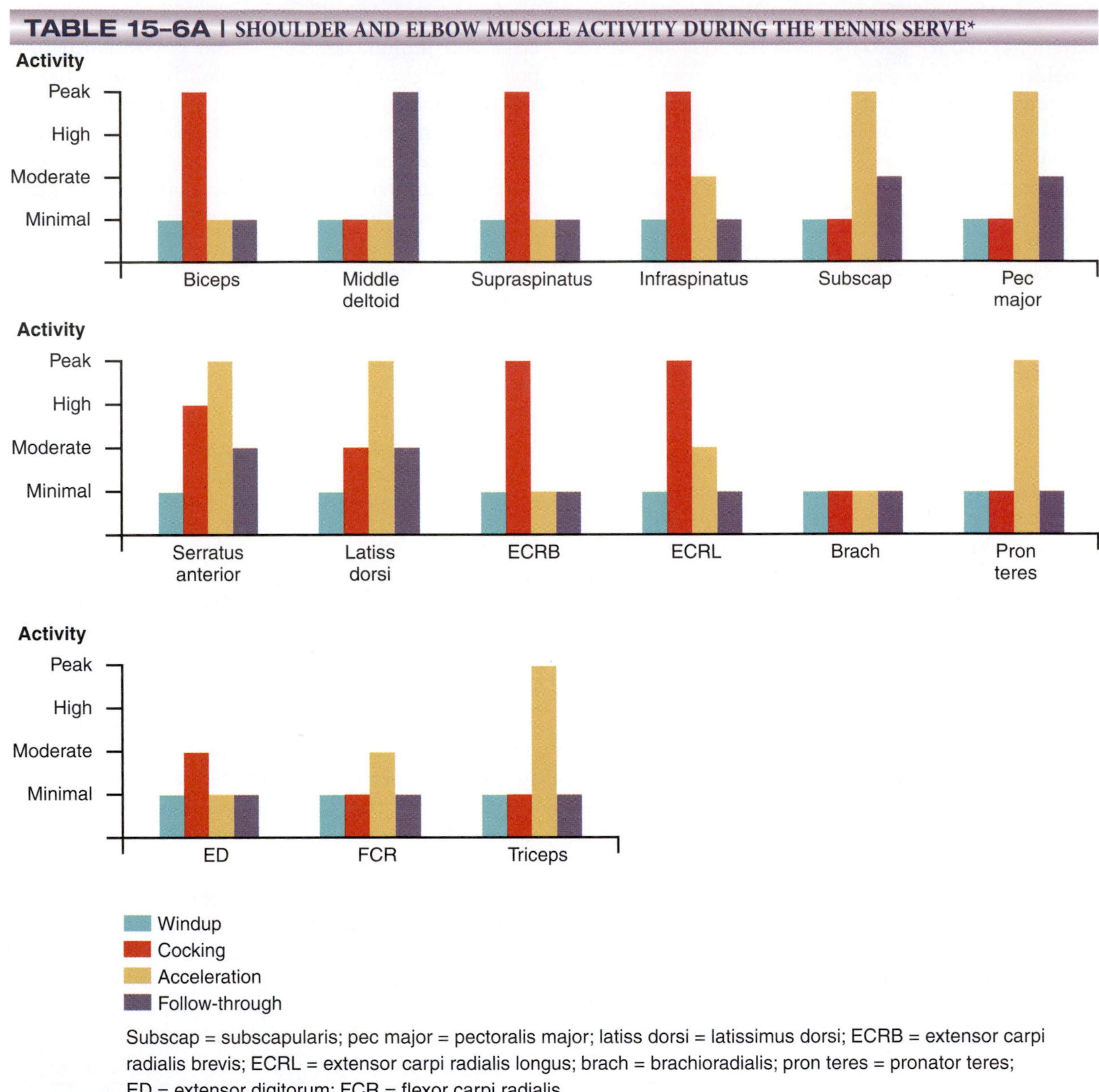

Subscap = subscapularis; pec major = pectoralis major; latiss dorsi = latissimus dorsi; ECRB = extensor carpi radialis brevis; ECRL = extensor carpi radialis longus; brach = brachioradialis; pron teres = pronator teres; ED = extensor digitorum; FCR = flexor carpi radialis.

*Based on data from Ryu, et al[61] and Morris, et al.[20]

from which the rotator cuff is activated.[64] Since the scapula is also retracted by the end of cocking, the middle trapezius and rhomboids aid in maintaining this position of stability. With the shoulder in lateral rotation and abduction, the rotator cuff muscles, especially the supraspinatus and infraspinatus, are active as they assist in humeral elevation and stabilize the humeral head in the glenoid fossa. Toward the end of this phase, the subscapularis becomes more active to decelerate the lateral rotation as the arm prepares for the acceleration phase.[4] Biceps activity is high during this phase as the elbow flexes. Wrist extension with radial deviation is produced by strong contraction of the extensor carpi radialis longus and brevis. The extensor digitorum contracts to a moderate level; this is likely because of its tenodesis affect on the fingers, adding to grip strength.

Toward the last half of this phase, the hips and knees begin extending to provide the progression of acceleration

TABLE 15-6B | TRUNK AND LOWER EXTREMITY MUSCLE ACTIVITY (FOR A RIGHT-HANDED PLAYER) DURING THE TENNIS SERVE*

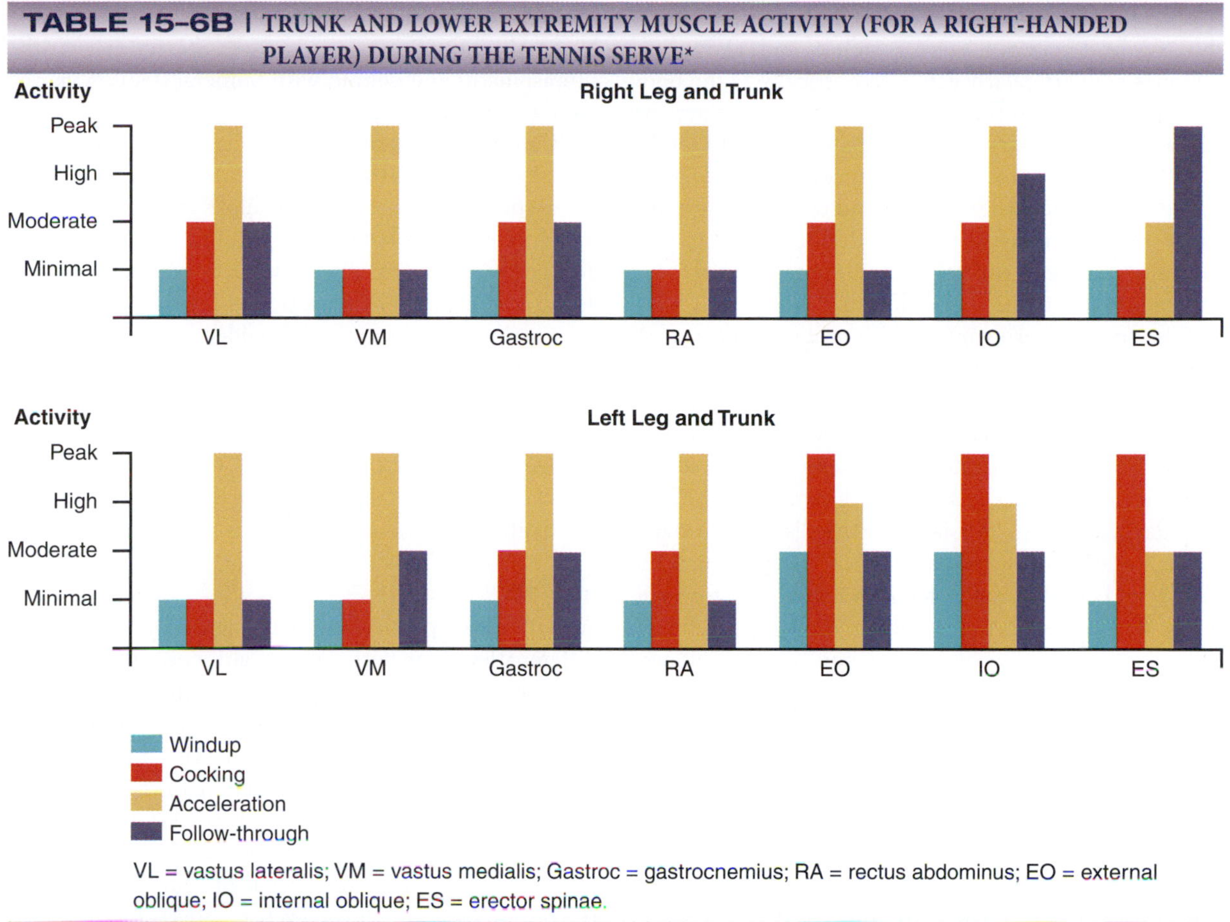

VL = vastus lateralis; VM = vastus medialis; Gastroc = gastrocnemius; RA = rectus abdominus; EO = external oblique; IO = internal oblique; ES = erector spinae.

*Based on data from Ryu, et al[62] and Chow, et al.[61, 65]

forces from the legs through the trunk and to the arm. The gluteal muscles, quadriceps, and gastrocnemius-soleus muscles all begin concentric activity during the end of this phase. As the trunk extends and leans to the right, it is stabilized by cocontraction of the erector spinae and abdominal oblique muscles.[65] The left rectus abdominus and external abdominal oblique muscles are especially active as they provide trunk rotation to the right.[65]

Acceleration Phase

As the racquet shoulder begins medial rotation, the acceleration phase begins and continues until the racquet hits the ball.[4] Although this is the shortest phase of the tennis serve, most muscles achieve their maximum output during this phase as the body unwinds, creating force to provide acceleration to the body and then to the ball.

Immediately after the shoulder achieves maximum lateral rotation, the body moves to hit the ball. The right shoulder flexes and abducts; this is followed by elbow extension, wrist ulnar deviation, medial rotation of the shoulder with pronation of the forearm, and wrist flexion.[60] Of these motions, shoulder medial rotation and wrist flexion contribute the most to the ball's velocity because of their rapid conversion from eccentric to concentric movement.[63] Powerful contributions from the triceps and pronator teres also aid in producing and determining ball velocity.[26] The power coming from the lower extremities actually cause the body to leave the ground before ball impact with the racquet.[63] The trunk rotates from right to left as it also flexes forward and laterally flexes to the left. Motion of the left upper extremity is variable, but moves toward shoulder extension as the trunk rotates from right to left.

Muscle activity is at its greatest in the lower extremities during this time. The gluteal muscles extend the hips as the quadriceps extends the knees, and the gastrocnemius-soleus group plantarflexes the ankles. All of the trunk muscles are active to control and stabilize the trunk. The right erector spinae and abdominal obliques are particularly active eccentrically as the body leans and rotates to the left. The erector spinae activity also assists the player in reaching a greater height on the ball.[65] The right erector spinae steadily increase their activity from the cocking phase and continue high levels of activity through the follow-through phase to provide rotation and control of the spine as the trunk moves into left rotation and flexion.[65]

The right upper extremity also produces most of its muscle activity during this phase. Immediately after the leg and trunk muscles have peaked in their output performance, the shoulder complex produces its burst of activity.[4] The serratus anterior produces its greatest output as it holds the scapula against the thorax.[4] The subscapularis, latissimus dorsi, and pectoralis major provide medial rotation of the shoulder as the triceps extend the elbow and the pronator teres pronates the forearm. Right before the racquet contacts the ball, the biceps contract to prevent hyperextension of the elbow.[4] Contraction of the wrist muscles, with more activity coming from the flexor carpi radialis, provides stability of the wrist at ball contact.

Follow-through Phase

Follow-through occurs from the time the ball is hit until the end of the serve motion.[4] As with other activities, the follow-through is the time of deceleration of movement. There is a moderate to high level of activity in many muscles as they work primarily eccentrically to slow joint and segment motions.

As the body continues to move forward after the ball has been hit, the trunk moves into forward flexion and left lateral flexion as it also unwinds from right to left. The lower extremities are landing on the ground, first on the left leg and then on the right as the body moves to receive the returned ball. To accept body weight, the lower extremities flex at the hips, knees, and ankles during the follow-through. The left upper extremity moves into shoulder abduction in response to rotational motion of the trunk and body.

The erector spinae and obliques cocontract to stabilize the spine as the right erector spinae and obliques also continue to decelerate trunk rotation to the left. The gluteal muscles and hamstrings are working eccentrically to control forward trunk motion and hip flexion as the lower limbs reach the ground. The knees and ankles are controlled eccentrically by the quadriceps and gastrocnemius-soleus group, respectively. Left shoulder motion occurs through stabilization of the scapula and abduction of the humerus. Scapular stabilization occurs through contraction of its rotators, whereas glenohumeral abduction occurs through action of the supraspinatus and deltoid with humeral stability via the remaining rotator cuff muscles.

Right upper extremity activity is primarily eccentric as it slows down its forward movement. The muscles of the right upper extremity are most active during the first half of the follow-through.[4] The latissimus dorsi and pectoralis major quickly reduce their activity level as the arm relaxes. The posterior and middle deltoid and teres major contract to slow shoulder motion as the serratus anterior maintains scapular position on the thorax; the subscapularis is moderately active to control shoulder medial rotation. The elbow is in slight flexion and the wrist is in slight extension as the elbow and wrist muscles relax after ball contact, letting gravity and momentum provide most of the motion.

Cycling

As with most sport activities, riding a bicycle has many different levels of performance abilities, ranging from recreational to professionally competitive. However, unlike most sports, cycling is an activity in which an individual is in continual contact with machine and both together determine the outcome of the activity.

Cycling has many styles and, within these styles, some aspects are universal regardless of the level of expertise or competition, the type of equipment used, or the terrain over which the cyclists moves. Cycling provides a linear progression of the individual and the machine through the circular motion of the pedal and gears. Within the cycling motion are two phases: the power phase and the recovery phase. The power phase is the downward stroke on the pedal whereas the recovery phase is the upward pedal stroke (Fig. 15.9).

There are many variables that could be considered in cycling. Variables that impact muscles used and muscle intensity include factors such as the type of bike that is used, the incline and type of terrain on which the bike is ridden, the level of experience and age of the individual, the type of handlebars and position of the rider using them, and the speed at which the individual is cycling.[66–68] There seems to be a lot of variability from one person to another in cycling;[69, 70] for the most part, however, investigators have come to a general consensus on the key points that will be made here. Of course, the most important muscles functioning during cycling are the lower extremity muscles. The trunk and upper extremity muscles are used to varying degrees and depend on a number of these factors. For the most part, the trunk remains in a neutral position with the pelvis tilted anteriorly. This allows the upper extremities to

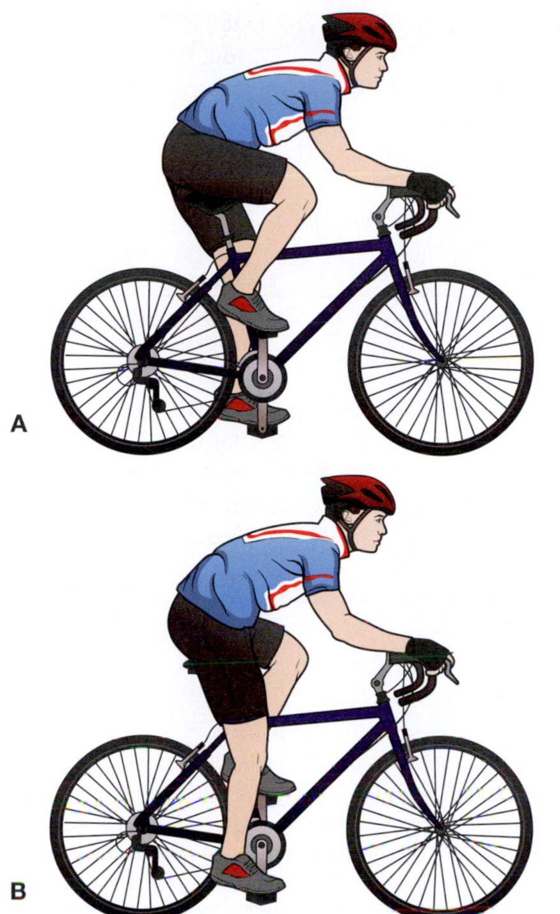

Figure 15.9 The phases of the leg during cycling. **A)** Power phase. **B)** Recovery phase.

provide stability as the lower extremities provide power during cycling. Rather than complicate the discussion of cycling, we will mention that the latissimus dorsi, biceps, and triceps play important roles during cycling, but we will only focus on the lower extremity muscles for now.

The assumptions we make for this activity are that the individual sits on the bike seat throughout the cycling motion, is riding on flat terrain, and is using shoe cleats. We also assume that the bike is correctly fitted for the cycler's size, the individual is a competent cyclist, and the individual's cycling rate is about 80 revolutions per minute.

Power Phase

Looking at the pedal crank on the bike, the power phase moves the pedal from the 12 o'clock position to the 6 o'clock position. However, cyclists and researchers usually refer to these two positions as 0° and 180°, respectively. Within the power phase are two segments that move the pedal on the crank—first from 0° to 90° and then from 90° to 180°. The downward motion of the crank provides the cyclists with power for forward propulsion of the bike.

As the leg begins at the top of the power phase, the hip and knee are both in flexion. The ankle begins in neutral at the start of the power phase. The limb stays in sagittal alignment throughout the motion.

The single joint muscles such as the gluteus maximus, vastus medialis and lateralis, tibialis anterior, and soleus are the primary force producers during the power phase.[69] On the other hand, the biarticular muscles seem to provide a transfer of energy between the joints during critical times of the cycle so the movement is smooth and powerful.[69] With the exception of the ankle muscles, the lower extremity muscles do not begin or end their activity at the start or end of the power or recovery phases. As the limb approaches the start of each phase, the muscles of the hip and knee begin to contract so they are able to provide their maximum output when it is needed.[71]

With the pedal at the top of the power phase, the gluteus maximus is most active as it initiates the motion to about 130° into the rotation.[70] During the middle portion of the power phase, the hamstrings joins efforts with the gluteus maximus to extend the hip.[72] As the limb approaches the 180° position at the end of the power stroke, the hamstrings are still working to extend the hip but the gluteus maximus relaxes. The hamstrings also begin transitioning to flex the knee in the recovery phase. Their firing sequence appears to compliment the vasti muscles and rectus femoris.[73] As the hamstrings begin their activity in the power phase, the quadriceps muscles relax, and later as the hamstrings relax toward the middle of the recovery phase, the rectus femoris contracts (Table 15–7).

At the knee, the rectus femoris begins activity before the vasti muscles prior to reaching the start of the power stroke, but they all cease activity by about 90°.[70] Although the hamstrings work as hip extensors in the first part of the power phase, they convert to working at the knee during the last part of this phase and into the recovery phase. It is during the second half of the power phase that the leg begins a sweeping-type motion, kind of like wiping the mud off the bottom of your shoe on a rug after you enter a building.[74] It is likely that the hamstrings provides this sweeping motion, and this is the reason for their high activity level, as the multi-joint muscles (semitendinosus and biceps femoris) provide a transfer of power from the hip to the knee.[75]

TABLE 15-7 | LOWER EXTREMITY MUSCLE ACTIVITY DURING ONE CYCLING PHASE*

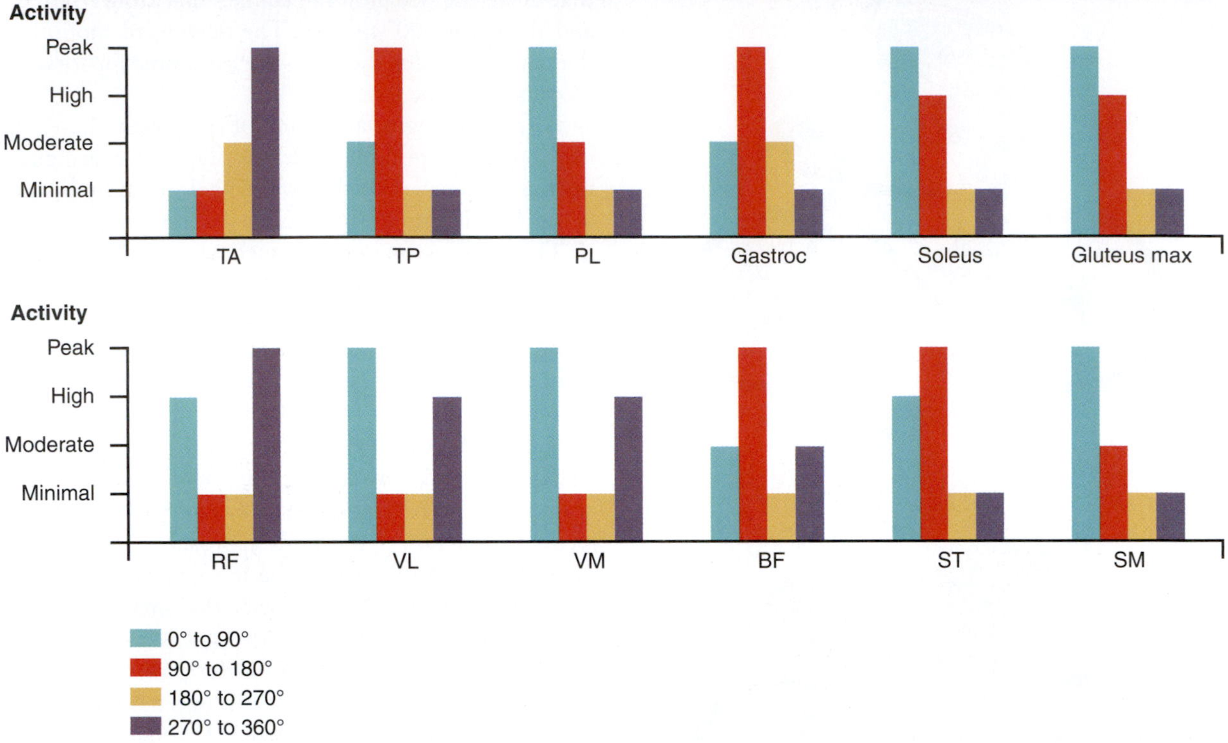

Activity

Peak
High
Moderate
Minimal

TA TP PL Gastroc Soleus Gluteus max

Activity

Peak
High
Moderate
Minimal

RF VL VM BF ST SM

0° to 90°
90° to 180°
180° to 270°
270° to 360°

TA = tibialis anterior; TP = tibialis posterior; PL = peroneus longus; gastroc = gastrocnemius; max = maximus; RF = rectus femoris; VL = vastus lateralis; VM = vastus medialis; BF = biceps femoris; ST = semitendinosus; SM = semimembranosus.

*Based on data from Baum & Li;[71] Chapman, et al;[67] Mohr, et al;[72] Hug, et al;[70] and Gregor, et al.[69]

Ankle motion during the power phase is movement from a neutral position into plantarflexion to add to the power of the downstroke. The soleus contracts before the gastrocnemius toward the end of the recovery phase, and it also relaxes before the gastrocnemius before the end of the power phase.[73] In fact, the gastrocnemius works throughout the majority of the entire cycle with its greatest output occurring during the second half of the power phase.[67] Maximum output of the soleus occurs in the first half of the power phase.[67] The tibialis posterior and peroneals are active during the same phase as the gastrocnemius and soleus; in all likelihood, these muscles work to stabilize the leg in the frontal plane through the powerful sagittal plane activity during the power phase.

Recovery Phase

The recovery phase moves the pedal on the crank from 180° to the start of the rotation at 0°, also referred to as the 360° position when discussing the end of the phase. Like the power phase, this phase is also divided into two 90° segments. The first one is from 180° to 270° and the second segment is from 270° to 360°, or the return to the start position of the power phase. Muscle effort during this phase serves to return the pedal and leg to the power position to begin propulsion in earnest at the top of the pedal position.

As the knee moves from maximum extension into flexion, the ankle moves from its position of some plantarflexion toward dorsiflexion. The first segment of the recovery phase is truly the greatest amount of recovery as most of the muscles are relaxed. The muscles most active during this time are the tibialis anterior and the gastrocnemius as they likely cocontract to stabilize the ankle before it moves into dorsiflexion. The gastrocnemius may also be assisting in flexing the knee to pull the pedal around.[75]

In the last half of the recovery cycle, muscle activity increases. The tibialis anterior is highly active, dorsiflexing the foot and pulling upward on the pedal to move it to its top position.[70] The other muscles working in this phase are preparing the limb for the power phase. The rectus femoris is highly active as it flexes the hip, and the vasti muscles are active, but not at their peak as the rectus femoris is, as they prepare to produce a powerful knee extension force after the limb reaches the top of the pedal position.

Summary

This chapter has brought the entire text's information to a useful conclusion in the analysis of a variety of sports activities from competitive to recreational. We have analyzed joint and muscle activity involved in events of competitive sports such as pitching in baseball and fast pitch softball, instep kicking in soccer, and freestyle swimming. Recreational or leisure sports activities we have analyzed include a full golf swing, a tennis serve, and cycling leg mechanics. The contents of this chapter advanced from delineating a sequencing of events from joint motions and muscle activity to combining them into a more clinical application, similar to what is expected in a clinical environment.

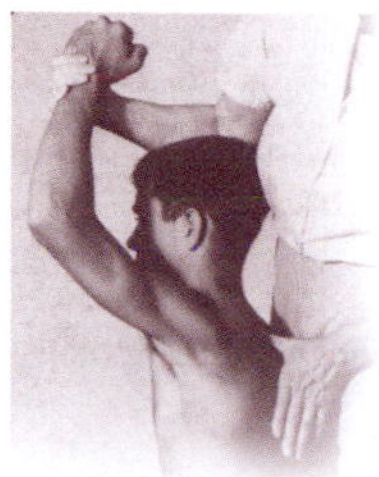

CLINICAL SCENARIO SOLUTION

Once Morgan understood the high jump and the flexibility, strength, coordination, and timing of events that occur in the activity, she was able to design a progression of rehabilitation exercises to match those demands. She has worked with many patients whose jobs and activities were foreign to her, but by contacting the appropriate supervisor or coach and finding additional resources in the library and online, she has been able to design programs to meet those patient's needs. Although she had never worked with a high jumper before, she followed the same process she has used before to acquire the knowledge she needed to design Cody's program. She knows that he must have strength and power in his quadriceps, gluteal muscles, gastrocnemius, and soleus to take off for the jump. She also knows that he will need to practice his approach and landing to become reacquainted with these activities after a prolonged time away from them. In fact, she has an entire progression of activities planned for him. Morgan knows that as the program progresses the activities will become more aggressive and challenging, but she also knows that Cody will be able to perform them since he has already shown that he is determined and dedicated to working hard to achieve his goals.

Discussion Questions

1. Identify the major muscle groups that Cody (in the clinical scenario) uses during his high jump activities. Based on these requirements, identify two exercises for each major muscle group you would include in his rehabilitation program.
2. Based on the information in this chapter, you should have realized that an activity is broken down into its segments based on changes in muscle function. For example, there is a windup phase of some type followed by an approach and/or an acceleration phase, and finally a follow-through phase. Using this model, identify what you think may be the phases for the following activities and list what changes in muscle function you anticipate occurring within each phase:
   - **a.** Punt in football
   - **b.** Tennis backhand volley
   - **c.** Volleyball serve
   - **d.** Basketball jump shot
   - **e.** Ice hockey pass
   - **f.** Long jump in track and field

3. A full golf swing was presented in this chapter. Looking at the muscle activity tables, identify what you think would be changes in these muscles' activity levels if the golfer performed a halfswing as in a short lob.
4. Now that you have completed this chapter, identify what upper extremity and trunk muscles you think will be active during cycling.
5. Think of the position an individual is in while cycling. Identify what you estimate are the maximum range of motion requirements for the hips, knees, and ankles.
6. Look at Table 15–1B and explain what the muscles that are at peak activity are doing and what the muscles that are at medium to high levels of activity are doing during the acceleration phase of the baseball pitch.
7. If you had a patient who is a fast-pitch softball pitcher, identify the upper extremity muscles that you will have to assure are strong before she resumes pitching.
8. Looking at Tables 15–3A and B of muscle activity during a soccer instep kick, explain why the stance leg seems to have more muscle activity requirements than the kick leg. Based on this information, how would you identify an individual's dominant leg using a ball-kicking skill?
9. Based on the information from Table 15–4, which muscles would you identify as the most important ones for a swimmer? Explain your rationale.
10. Based on the information in Tables 15–6A and B, identify the muscles you would include in a preseason workout program for a tennis player.

Lab Activities

1. Select one sport, perhaps a favorite of yours in which you participate or enjoy watching. Identify four different activities within that sport and list what you think are the muscles that are primarily responsible for producing each activity.
2. Analyze you lab partner's movement up and down a set of stairs. Identify the muscles involved in going up the stairs and those involved in going down the stairs.
3. Analyze the movement sequence, motion requirements, and muscles that are used to open an outside door and move from the outside to the inside of a building. After you have completed this task, have your partner perform the activity and verify if your answer is correct.
4. Push your lab table away from you, and then pull it toward you. Identify the shoulder and hip muscles that are used for each of these activities. Is it easier to push or pull the table? Why is this so?
5. If you have a patient who must walk nonweight-bearing on the right leg using crutches, which muscles must he or she use? List one exercise for each muscle that you would use to strengthen each muscle you have listed.

References

1. Best TM, Hart L. A growing concern: The older athlete. *Clinical Journal of Sports Medicine* 18(6):477–478, 2008.
2. Kallinen M, Markku A. Aging, physical activity and sports injuries: An overview of common sports injuries in the elderly. *Sports Medicine* 20(1):41–52, 1995.
3. Koester MC. Adolescent and youth sports medicine: A "growing" concern. *Athletic Therapy Today* 7(6):6–12, 2002.
4. Moynes DR, Perry J, Antonelli DJ, Jobe JW. Electromyography and motion analysis of the upper extremity in sports. *Physical Therapy* 66:1905–1911, 1986.
5. Escamilla RF, Fleisig GS, Barrentine SW, Zheng N, Andrews JR. Kinematic comparisons of throwing different types of baseball pitches. *Journal of Applied Biomechanics* 14(1):1–23, 1998.
6. Park S, Loebenberg M, Rokito A, Zuckerman J. The shoulder in baseball pitching: Biomechanics and related injuries. Part 2. *Bulletin of the Hospital for Joint Diseases* 61(1/2):80–88, 2002.

7. Park SS, Loebenberg ML, Rokito AS, Zuckerman JD. The shoulder in baseball pitching: Biomechanics and related injuries. Part 1. *Bulletin of the Hospital for Joint Diseases* 61(1/2):68–79, 2002.

8. Dun S, Kingsley D, Fleisig GS, Loftice J, Andrews JR. Biomechanical comparison of the fastball from wind-up and the fastball from stretch in professional baseball pitchers. *American Journal of Sports Medicine* 36(1):137–141, 2008.

9. Pappas AM, Zawacki RM, Sullivan TJ. Biomechanics of baseball pitching: A preliminary report. *American Journal of Sports Medicine* 13:216–222, 1985.

10. Hay J. *The biomechanics of sports techniques*, ed 4. Englewood Cliffs, NJ: Prentice-Hall, 1993.

11. Yamanouchi T. EMG analysis of the lower extremities during pitching in high-school baseball. *Kurume Medical Journal* 45(1):21–25, 1998.

12. Lintner D, Noonan TJ, Kibler WB. Injury patterns and biomechanics of the athlete's shoulder. *Clinics in Sports Medicine* 27(4):527–551, 2008.

13. Escamilla R, Barrentine S, Fleisig G, et al. Pitching biomechanics as a pitcher approaches muscular fatigue during a simulated baseball game. *American Journal of Sports Medicine* 35(1):23–33, 2007.

14. Perry J. Anatomy and biomechanics of the shoulder in throwing, swimming, gymnastics, and tennis. *Clinics in Sports Medicine* 2:247–270, 1983.

15. Hamilton CD, Glousman RE, Jobe FW, Brault J, Pink M, Perry J. Dynamic stability of the elbow: Electromyographic analysis of the flexor pronator group and the extensor group in pitchers with valgus instability. *Journal of Shoulder and Elbow Surgery* 5(5):347–354, 1996.

16. Mullaney MJ, McHugh MP, Donofrio TM, Nicholas SJ. Upper and lower extremity muscle fatigue after a baseball pitching performance. *American Journal of Sports Medicine* 33(1):108–113, 2005.

17. Fleisig G, Barrentine S, Escamilla R, Andrews J. Biomechanics of overhand throwing with implications for injuries. *Sports Medicine* 21(6):421–437, 1996.

18. Watkins RG, Dennis S, Dillin WH, et al. Dynamic EMG analysis of torque transfer in professional baseball pitchers. *Spine* 14(4):404–408, 1989.

19. Jobe FW, Moynes DR, Tibone JE, Perry J. An EMG analysis of the shoulder in pitching: A second report. *American Journal of Sports Medicine* 12(3):218–220, 1984.

20. Jobe FW, Tibone JE, Perry J, Moynes D. An EMG analysis of the shoulder in throwing and pitching: A preliminary report. *American Journal of Sports Medicine* 11(1):3–5, 1983.

21. Maffet MW, Jobe FW, Pink MM, Brault J, Mathiyakom W. Shoulder muscle firing patterns during the windmill softball pitch. *American Journal of Sports Medicine* 25(3):369–374, 1997.

22. Barrentine SW, Fleisig GS, Whiteside JA, Escamilla RF, Andrews JR. Biomechanics of windmill softball pitching with implications about injury mechanisms at the shoulder and elbow. *Journal of Orthopaedic and Sports Physical Therapy* 28(6):405–414, 1998.

23. Rojas IL, Provencher MT, Bhatia S, et al. Biceps activity during windmill softball pitching: Injury implications and comparison with overhand throwing. *American Journal of Sports Medicine* 37(3):558–565, 2009.

24. Werner SL, Guido JA, McNeice RP, Richardson JL, Delude NA, Stewart GW. Biomechanics of youth windmill softball pitching. *American Journal of Sports Medicine* 33:552–560, 2005.

25. Escamilla RF, Andrews JR. Shoulder muscle recruitment patterns and related biomechanics during upper extremity sports. *Sports Medicine* 39(7):569–590, 2009.

26. Loftice J, Fleisig GS, Zheng N, Andrews JR. Biomechanics of the elbow in sports. *Clinics in Sports Medicine* 23(4):519–530, 2004.

27. Werner SL, Fleisig GS, Dillman CJ, Andrews JR. Biomechanics of the elbow during baseball pitching. *Journal of Orthopaedic and Sports Physical Therapy* 17(6):274–278, 1993.

28. Read D. Checking the windmill. *Training & Conditioning* 16:7, 2006.

29. Shan G, Westerhoff P. Full-body kinematic characteristics of the maximal instep soccer kick by male soccer players and parameters related to kick quality. *Sports Biomechanics* 4(1):59–72, 2005.

30. Markovic G, Dizdar D, Jaric S. Evaluation of tests of maximum kicking performance. *Journal of Sports Medicine & Physical Fitness* 46(2):215–220, 2006.

31. Fields KB, Bloom OJ, Priebe D, Foreman B. Basic biomechanics of the lower extremity. *Primary Care: Clinics in Office Practice* 32:245–251, 2005.

32. Barfield WR. Biomechanics of kicking in soccer. *Clinics in Sports Medicine* 17(4):711–728, 1998.

33. Lees A, Nolan L. The biomechanics of soccer: A review. *Journal of Sport Sciences* 16(3):211–234, 1998.

34. Brophy RH, Backus SI, Pansy BS, Lyman S, Williams RJ. Lower extremity muscle activation and alignment during the soccer instep and side-foot kicks. *Journal of Orthopaedic and Sports Physical Therapy* 37(5):260–268, 2007.

35. Kellis E, Katis A. The relationship between isokinetic knee extension and flexion strength with soccer kick kinematics: An electromyographic evaluation. *Journal of Sports Medicine & Physical Fitness* 47(4):385–394, 2007.

36. Richardson AB, Jobe FW, Collins HR. The shoulder in competitive swimming. *American Journal of Sports Medicine* 8:159–163, 1980.

37. Siefert L, Choliet D, Allard P. Arm coordination symmetry and breathing effect in front crawl. *Human Movement Science* 24(2):234–256, 2005.

38. Chollet D, Chalies S, Chatard JC. A new index of coordination for the crawl; Description and usefulness. *International Journal of Sports Medicine* 21(1):54–59, 2000.

39. Deschodt VJ, Arsac LM, Rouard AH. Relative contribution of arms and legs in humans to propulsion in 25-m sprint front-crawl swimming. *European Journal of Applied Physiology* 80(3):192–199, 1999.

40. Murphy TC. Shoulder injuries in swimming. In Wilk KE (ed): *The Athlete's Shoulder*. New York, 1994, Churchill Livingstone, pp 411–424.

41. Lee J, Mellifont R, Winstanley J, Burkett B. Body roll in simulated freestyle swimming. *International Journal of Sports Medicine* 29(7):569–593, 2008.

42. Troup JP. The physiology and biomechanics of competitive swimming. *Clinics in Sports Medicine* 18(2):267–285, 1999.

43. Clarys JP, Rouard AH. The front crawl downsweep: Shoulder protection and/or performance inhibition. *Journal of Sports Medicine & Physical Fitness* 36(2):121–126, 1996.

44. Pink M, Perry J, Browne A, Scovazzo ML, Kerrigan J. The normal shoulder during freestyle swimming. *American Journal of Sports Medicine* 19:569–576, 1991.

45. Scovazzo ML, Browne A, Pink M, Jobe FW, Kerrigan J. The painful shoulder during freestyle swimming: An electromyographic cinematographic analysis of twelve muscles. *American Journal of Sports Medicine* 19(6):577–582, 1991.

46. Rouard AH, Billat RP. Influences of sex and level of performance on freestyle stroke: An electromyographic and kinematic study. *International Journal of Sports Medicine* 11(2):150–155, 1990.

47. Caty V, Aujouannet Y, Hintzy F, Bonifazi M, Clarys JP, Rouard AH. Wrist stabilisation and forearm muscle coactivation during freestyle swimming. *Journal of Electromyography and Kinesiology* 17(3):285–291, 2007.

48. Nuber GW, Jobe FW, Perry J, Moynes DR, Antonelli D. Fine wire electromyography analysis of muscles of the shoulder during swimming. *American Journal of Sports Medicine* 14:7–11, 1986.

49. McHardy A, Pollard H. Muscle activity during the golf swing. *British Journal of Sports Medicine* 39(11):799–804, 2005.

50. Gluck GS, Bendo JA, Spivak JM. The lumbar spine and low back pain in golf: A literature review of swing biomechanics and injury prevention. *Spine Journal* 8(5):778–788, 2008.

51. Bulbulian R, Ball KA, Seaman DR. The short golf backswing: Effects on performance and spinal health implications. *Journal of Manipulative & Physiological Therapeutics* 24(9):569–575, 2001.

52. Pink M, Jobe FW, Perry J. Electromyographic analysis of the shoulder during the golf swing. *American Journal of Sports Medicine* 18(2):137–140, 1990.

53. Hume PA, Keogh J, Reid D. The role of biomechanics in maximising distance and accuracy of golf shots. *Sports Medicine* 35(5):429–449, 2005.

54. Cahalan TD, Cooney WP, III, Tamai K, Chao EY. Biomechanics of the golf swing in players with pathologic conditions of the forearm, wrist and hand. *American Journal of Sports Medicine* 19(3):288–293, 1991.

55. Adlington GS. Proper swing technique and biomechanics of golf. *Clinics in Sports Medicine* 15(1):9–26, 1996.

56. Burden AM, Grimshaw PN, Wallace ES. Hip and shoulder rotations during the golf swing of sub-10 handicap players. *Journal of Sport Sciences* 16(2):165–176, 1998.

57. Watkins RG, Uppal GS, Perry J, Pink M, Dinsay JM. Dynamic electromyographic analysis of trunk musculature in professional golfers. *American Journal of Sports Medicine* 24(4):535–538, 1996.

58. Jobe FW, Moynes DR, Antonelli DJ. Rotator cuff function during a golf swing. *American Journal of Sports Medicine* 14:388–392, 1985.

59. Kao JT, Pink M, Jobe FW, Perry J. Electromyographic analysis of the scapular muscles during a golf swing. *American Journal of Sports Medicine* 23(1):19–23, 1995.

60. Elliott B, Fleisig G, Nicholls R, Escamilla R. Technique effects on upper limb loading in the tennis serve. *Journal of Science and Medicine in Sport* 6(1):76–87, 2003.

61. Chow JW, Shim JH, Lim YT. Lower trunk muscle activity during the tennis serve. *Journal of Science and Medicine in Sport* 6(4):512–518, 2003.

62. Ryu RKN, McCormick J, Jobe FW, Moynes DR, Antonelli DJ. An electromyographic analysis of shoulder function in tennis players. *American Journal of Sports Medicine* 16:481–485, 1988.

63. Girard O, Micallef JP, Millet GP. Lower-limb activity during the power serve in tennis: Effects of performance level. *Medicine & Science in Sport & Exercise* 37(6):1021–1029, 2005.

64. Kibler WB. Biomechanical analysis of the shoulder during tennis activities. *Clinics in Sports Medicine* 14:79–85, 1995.

65. Chow JW, Park SA, Tillman MD. Lower trunk kinematics and muscle activity during different types of tennis serves. *Sports Medicine, Arthroscopy, Rehabilitation, Therapy, & Technology* 13(1):24, 2009.

66. Li L, Caldwell GE. Muscle coordination in cycling: Effect of surface incline and posture. *Journal of Applied Physiology* 85(3):927–934, 1998.

67. Chapman AR, Vicenzino B, Blanch P, Hodges PW. Leg muscle recruitment during cycling is less developed in triathletes than cyclists despite matched cycling training loads. *Experimental Brain Research* 181:503–518, 2007.

68. Suzuki S, Watanabe S, Homma S. EMG activity and kinematics of human cycling movements at different constant velocities. *Brain Research* 240(2):245–258, 1982.

69. Gregor RJ, Broker JP, Ryan MM. The biomechanics of cycling. *Exercise and Sport Sciences Reviews* 19:127–169, 1991.

70. Hug F, Laplaud D, Lucia A, Grelot L. EMG threshold determination in eight lower limb muscles during cycling exercise: A pilot study. *International Journal of Sports Medicine* 27(6):458–462, 2006.

71. Baum BS, Li L. Lower extremity muscle activities during cycling are influenced by load and frequency. *Journal of Electromyography and Kinesiology* 13:181–190, 2003.

72. Mohr KJ, Kvitne RS, Pink MM, Fideler B, Perry J. Electromyography of the quadriceps in patellofemoral pain with patellar subluxation. *Clinical Orthopaedics and Related Research* 415:261–271, 2003.

73. Timmer CAW. Cycling biomechanics: A literature review. *Journal of Orthopaedic and Sports Physical Therapy* 14(3):106–113, 1991.

74. Olsen B. Bicycle biomechanics. www.wheelwerksbikes.com. Accessed 12 December 2009.

75. Mohr T, Allison JD, Patterson R. Electromyographic analysis of the lower extremity during pedaling. *Journal of Orthopaedic and Sports Physical Therapy* 2(4):163–170, 1981.

Glossary

A

Abduction *(Chapter 1, 11).* Position or frontal plane movement of the body segment away from the midline. In the foot, abduction occurs in a transverse plane around a vertical axis.

Acceleration *(Chapter 2).* A rate of increase in velocity.

Accessory motion *(Chapter 1).* Also known as component motions. Motions that take place at a joint as a natural smooth accompaniment to active range of motion.

Acetabular fossa *(Chapter 9).* Central area of acetabulum, devoid of hyaline cartilage, which houses fibroelastic fat pad and ligamentum teres.

Acetabulum *(Chapter 9).* The cup of the pelvis into which the head of the femur fits to form the hip joint, structurally comprised of portions from all three pelvic bones.

Actin *(Chapter 3, 4).* The thinner protein filament that contains troponin and tropomyosin, which control the binding between actin and myosin that occurs during muscle contraction.

Action potential *(Chapter 3).* Electrochemical signal propagated within nervous system whereby an excitable nerve or muscle cell is sufficiently depolarized then repolarized.

Active insufficiency *(Chapter 4).* When a muscle that crosses more than one joint is at its shortest position but the joint still has more motion available. The muscle's actin and myosin overlapping sites are used up, but the joint has not reached the end of its motion. This occurs in muscles that cross more than one joint; e.g., the hamstrings are used to fully extend the hip but are unable to fully flex the knee simultaneously.

Active tension *(Chapter 4).* Force produced by the muscle itself through crossbridge activation between the actin and myosin fibers of muscle tissue. Of all factors contributing to overall muscle force, active tension is the largest. See passive tension.

Adduction *(Chapter 1, 11).* Position or frontal plane movement of the body segment toward the midline. In the foot, adduction occurs in transverse plane around a vertical axis.

Adductor tubercle *(Chapter 9).* Projection proximal to the medial epicondyle at the distal femur, so named because the adductor magnus muscle attaches to it.

Aerobic metabolism *(Chapter 3).* Oxidative metabolism of fats, carbohydrates, and proteins for the production of energy within the muscle.

Afferent nerves *(Chapter 3).* Sensory nerves that send impulses into the central nervous system.

Agonist *(Chapter 4).* Muscle or muscle group that is primarily responsible for producing a motion.

Akinesia *(Chapter 3, 12).* Difficulty initiating movement. It is a condition that is seen typically in Parkinson's disease.

All-or-none law *(Chapter 3).* Principle in which all of the muscle fibers within a motor unit will contract maximally when the nerve is activated.

Alpha (α) motor neuron *(Chapter 3).* Large neuron that innervates skeletal muscle.

Ambulation *(Chapter 12).* Defined in a broad sense as a type of locomotion but is more often used in the clinical sense of describing whether or not someone can move about or walk freely or with the assistance of some device.

Amphiarthrosis *(Chapter 1).* Joint classification hallmarked by a cartilaginous structure with combinations of both fibrous and hyaline (or articular) cartilage and typically a disc between the bony partners, so that both a stability and mobility function can be achieved, such as seen at the intervertebral joints of the spine, the pubic symphysis, and the first sternocostal joint.

Anatomical position *(Chapter 1).* Reference position for the human body defined as standing erect with head, palms, and toes facing forward and the fingers extended.

Anaerobic metabolism *(Chapter 3).* Reactions that do not require the expenditure of oxygen as the energy source.

Angle of inclination *(Chapter 5, 8, 9).* The angle that is formed between either the humeral or femoral heads and their respective bony shafts. In the humerus, the angle of inclination is created by the lines running through the shaft of the humerus and the humeral head. Normal angle of inclination of the humerus is 130° to 150° with about 125° in the average adult. There is also an angle of inclination in the hip; this angle is formed between the shaft of the femur and the long axis of the femoral neck. The femoral angle of inclination is about 127°.

Angle of pelvic inclination *(Chapter 9).* The inclination in degrees of the amount of range of motion of anterior and posterior pelvic tilt, visualized by drawing a line representing an oblique plane through the PSIS and the foremost portion of the symphysis pubis, resulting in an angle of this plane with the transverse or horizontal plane.

Angle of progression *(Chapter 12).* This is the angle in gait that is formed between the line of progression in a straight line and a line that bisects the foot at the midpoint of the heel and runs between the second and third toes. An out-toeing of about 7° is typical in mature adults.

Angle of torsion *(Chapter 5, 9).* This is the angle formed between the plane of the humeral head and the plane of the humeral condyles. Normal angle of torsion is in 30° of retroversion. In the hip, it is the angle formed between the shaft and neck in the transverse plane, visualized by a line drawn bisecting the femoral head and neck and superimposing that line on a line running between the medial and lateral femoral condyles; this angle is reflective of the innate twist in the femur so that the head and neck are rotated anteriorly 13° to 15°.

Angular (rotary) motion *(Chapter 1).* Motion occurring around an axis or a pivot point. See rotary motion.

Ankle complex *(Chapter 11).* The talocrural joint and subtalar joints of the ankle and foot are often referred to as the ankle complex. Together, they function to provide mobility and adaptability of the foot and ankle, especially during closed chain activities.

Ankle strategy *(Chapter 12).* Posture control that is initiated from the ankles and feet.

Ankylosis *(Chapter 8).* Restriction of joint movement caused by pathology within the joint.

Annular ligament *(Chapter 6).* A fibrous ligament, lined with hyaline cartilage, which forms a ring around the head of the radius as a major support at the proximal radioulnar joint.

Antagonist *(Chapter 4).* Muscle or muscle group that is primarily responsible for producing motion that is directly opposite the desired or intended motion.

Antecubital *(Chapter 6).* The anterior aspect of the elbow; at the fold or bend of the elbow complex.

Anterior inferior iliac spine (AIIS) *(Chapter 9).* This is a landmark, not easily palpated, located inferior to the ASIS on the anterior aspect of the ilium of the pelvis.

Anterior radioulnar ligament *(Chapter 6).* Ligament that stabilizes the anterior aspect of the distal radioulnar joint.

Anterior superior iliac spine (ASIS) *(Chapter 9).* Easily palpable prominence is on the most anterior and superior aspect of the crest of the ilium of the pelvis.

Anterior tilting *(Chapter 5).* Rotation of the scapula around a medial-lateral axis so that the superior aspect of the scapula rotates forward or anteriorly. The motion occurs as the glenohumeral joint is hyperextended.

Anteversion *(Chapter 9).* An increase in the femoral angle of torsion, clinically presenting as intoeing, or "pigeon toes."

Antigravity muscles *(Chapters 3, 4, 12).* Postural muscles that maintain the body in an upright position against gravity. They have more type I muscle fibers than type II fibers. These muscles include primarily the neck and back extensors, hip and knee extensors, and to a lesser degree, the neck and trunk flexors and hip abductors and adductors.

Apophyseal plate *(Chapter 6).* The center of ossification or growth at the long end of a bone.

Apraxia *(Chapter 3).* Difficulty with planning a movement in which the individual's movements are typically slow and clumsy, with mild proximal weakness and loss of coordination around the proximal joints.

Areflexia *(Chapter 3).* Absent stretch reflexes; sign of a pathological condition.

Arthrokinematics *(Chapter 1).* Subdivision of kinematics, focused on a description of movement of the joint surfaces upon each other.

Arthrology *(Chapter 1).* (Gr. *arthron;* joint) The study of the classification, structure, and function of joints.

Association neuron *(Chapter 3).* Interneurons within the association cortexes of the CNS.

Ataxia *(Chapter 3).* Muscular incoordination that manifests when voluntary muscular movements are attempted, often seen as wide based movements; a common clinical symptom of cerebellar damage.

Athetosis *(Chapter 3).* Dystonic movement disturbance characterized by slow involuntary writhing or twisting, usually involving the upper extremities more than the lower extremities, whereby muscle tone appears to fluctuate in an unpredictable manner from low to high; most commonly manifested as a type of cerebral palsy.

Atrophy (*Chapter 4).* Decrease in a muscle's cell size, overall muscle girth, and strength secondary to injury, disuse, disease, or age.

Autogenic inhibition *(Chapter 3).* Mechanism of nonreciprocal inhibition mediated by GTO whereby activation of GTO by sufficient musculotendinous tension will cause inhibition of the agonist muscle and excitation of the antagonist (opposing) muscle.

Axial skeleton *(Chapter 8).* The part of the bony skeleton comprising vertebral column, skull, and ribs.

Axis *(Chapter 1, 2).* The point around which rotation occurs.

Axis of rotation *(Chapter 1, 2).* Pivot point for the angular motion at a joint, located within or near the surface of the joint.

B

Ball and socket joint *(Chapter 1).* Triaxial joint with a spherical type "ball" paired with a concave cup, such as seen at the hip and glenohumeral joint.

Base of support (BOS) *(Chapter 2).* The total surface area that supports a body or an object. It includes the area between and within the points of contact. The larger the base of support, the more stability the body or object it has.

Biaxial joint *(Chapter 1).* Joint that moves in two planes around two axes, having two degrees of freedom; includes three structural types: condyloid, ellipsoidal, and saddle.

Bipedal *(Chapter 12).* (L., *bi,* two, plus *pes,* foot) Walking on two extremities.

Biomechanics *(Chapter 1).* Application of the principles and analysis of mechanics to the living human body.

Bipennate *(Chapter 4).* Muscle fiber arrangement with two groups of parallel fibers running to the muscle's central tendon, similar to a feather's arrangement.

Bony (or hard) end feel *(Chapter 1).* Normal end feel felt when the motion is stopped by contact of bone on bone, as in elbow extension when the olecranon process of the ulna fits snugly into the olecranon fossa of the humerus.

Bradykinesia *(Chapter 3, 12).* Slowness or difficulty maintaining movement once it is initiated.

Bruxism *(Chapter 8).* Grinding of the teeth.

Bursa *(Chapter 1).* Fluid filled sac whose purpose is to decrease friction and offer some added protection or shock absorption between joint surfaces; can be natural or acquired.

C

Cadence *(Chapter 12).* A temporal characteristic of gait that is defined as the number of steps completed per unit of time such as steps per minute.

Capitulotrochlear groove *(Chapter 6).* A groove on the distal humerus between the capitulum and trochlea, within which the radius slides during elbow flexion.

Capitulum *(Chapter 6).* The distal bony prominence of humerus that articulates with the radius deep within elbow joint.

Capsular (firm or ligamentous) end feel *(Chapter 1).* A springy, normal end feel in which the limitation is from ligamentous, capsular, or muscle structures, such as in wrist flexion.

Cardinal planes *(Chapter 1).* Three-dimensional coordinate system used as frame of reference to describe and record location in space of human body and the motions at its joints.

Carrying angle *(Chapter 6).* This is anatomically known as the cubital angle, created between the humerus and forearm whereby the forearm deviates laterally in relation to the humerus because the axis for flexion and extension of the elbow is not fully perpendicular to the shaft of the humerus; this angle varies somewhat in individuals and is usually more pronounced in women than in men.

Catalyst *(Chapter 3).* A substance that acts to accelerate a chemical reaction but is not permanently changed by the chemical reaction.

Center of gravity (COG) *(Chapter 1, 2).* Center around which the mass is centered. It identifies the point at which gravity exerts its influence on an object or body's center of mass.

Center of mass (COM) *(Chapter 2).* The point around which the mass of an object or body is evenly distributed. Center of gravity for the human body, located just anterior to the second sacral vertebrae in humans. See center of gravity.

Center of pressure (COP) *(Chapter 12).* The location of the application point of the resultant ground reaction force within the foot.

Central nervous system (CNS) *(Chapter 3).* Composed of the brain and spinal cord.

Central pattern generators *(Chapter 3).* Complex patterns of muscle activation that produce purposeful movement through neural connections at a spinal level.

Cerebral Palsy *(Chapter 3).* A general term used to describe a group of motor disorders that generally results from damage to the developing brain.

Cerebral shock *(Chapter 3).* Time of profound depression of motor function in which all muscles of the affected body segments are involved, used to describe the temporary flaccid state in the muscles of the person following a brain injury when the nervous system is in a state of shock after a lesion of acute onset.

Chopart's joint *(Chapter 11).* This joint is the transverse tarsal joint, also known as the talonavicular joint of the midfoot. It is called Chopart's joint, named after French physician, François Chopart, who lived and practiced medicine in Paris during the 1700s.

Choreiform movements *(Chapter 3).* Type of dystonic movement characterized by quick, involuntary, jerky, rapid, or irregular movements whereby muscle tone appears to fluctuate in an unpredictable manner from low to high.

Circumduction *(Chapter 1, 7).* Movement performed during which the moving segment moves in a path similar to following the surface of a cone and the tip of the segment traces a circular path; typically seen in triaxial joints.

Clonus *(Chapter 3).* Spasmodic alterations of muscle contractions between antagonistic muscle groups, caused by hyperactive stretch reflexes; a symptom of CNS pathology.

Closed chain motion *(Chapter 1, 4).* When the distal portion of the segment is anchored or fixed, so movement of one part of the segment influences the other parts of the segment. These motions are typically used for force production rather than speed. Also referred to as closed kinematic chain.

Close-packed position (CKC) *(Chapter 1).* Joint position whereby the surfaces of the joint pairs match each other in maximum congruency (coinciding exactly) so that the maximum area of surface contact occurs, the attachments of the ligaments are farthest apart and under tension, the capsular structures are taut, and the joint is mechanically compressed and difficult to distract (separate).

Coactivation *(Chapter 6).* Muscle recruitment pattern whereby the agonist and antagonist both fire, often seen in new or unskilled movements.

Cogwheel rigidity *(Chapter 3).* Type of rigidity characterized by alternate episodes of resistance and relaxation, commonly seen in patients with Parkinson's disease.

Component vectors *(Chapter 2).* Forces whose combined magnitudes and directions produce a resultant vector.

Composition of forces *(Chapter 2).* Sum of all forces acting on a body or segment.

Concave-Convex principle *(Chapter 1).* Mechanical principle, but not a steadfast rule, that establishes that if the bone with the convex joint surface moves on the bone with the concavity, the convex joint surfaces move in the opposite direction to the bone segment, whereas if the bone with the concavity moves on the convex surface, the concave articular surface moves in the same direction as the bone segment.

Concurrent force system *(Chapter 2).* Two or more forces acting on a segment or body. The result of these forces creates a resultant force, and this resultant force is a combination of both original forces with its origin at the same site as the two original forces.

Concentric motion *(Chapter 4).* Muscle activation that produces shortening of the muscle as it moves the joint.

Conduction velocity *(Chapter 3).* Speed of transmission of an impulse along a nerve axon; related to the axon diameter and presence or absence of myelin.

Condyle *(Chapter 6).* Knob-like enlargements of long bones, such as the femur and humerus.

Condyloid joint *(Chapter 1).* Type of biaxial joint; a condyloid joint shape can be described as a spherical convex surface partnered with a shallow concave surface, as seen in the metacarpophalangeal joints of the hand (your knuckles) and foot.

Constraints *(Chapter 3).* Limitation or restriction imposed on the movement.

Contact pressure *(Chapter 10).* The ratio between the amount of joint reaction force and the area of contact. The larger the area of contact, the less stress applied to a structure.

Coronal (frontal) plane *(Chapter 1).* or XY plane, so named because it is parallel to the frontal bone along the coronal skull suture, dividing the body into front and back parts. It is the plane within which abduction and adduction movements occur.

Coronary ligament *(Chapter 10).* The ligament that connects the lateral rim of each meniscus to the tibia. This is a loose ligament that allows some movement of the menisci during knee motion. Also known at meniscotibial ligaments.

Coronoid fossa *(Chapter 6).* A cavity on the anterior aspect of distal humerus; receives coronoid process of ulna when elbow is in full flexion.

Coronoid process *(Chapter 6).* A distinctive bony process on anterior medial superior surface of the ulna.

Counternutation *(Chapter 8).* Movement of the sacrum by which the sacral promontory moves superiorly and posteriorly as the distal sacrum and coccyx move anteriorly. During counternutation, the iliac crests move apart and the ischial tuberosities move closer together.

Coupling motions *(Chapter 8).* Motions occurring in one plane that occurs with simultaneous motion(s) in another plane(s) because of the orientation of the planes of the joints. An example is lateral flexion of the spine and spinal rotation—it is not possible to isolate either lateral flexion or rotation of the spine.

Coxa valga *(Chapter 9).* A persisting increase in the neck-shaft angle whereby the angle of inclination is greater than 130°, resulting in several functional consequences: the limb will appear to be longer, placing the limb in an adducted position during weight-bearing, resulting in a functional increase of limb length.

Coxa vara *(Chapter 9).* A condition whereby the femoral neck-shaft angle is smaller than the typical 125° (approaching 90°), resulting in several functional consequences: a functional decrease in leg length; the limb appears to take on a more abducted position with a wide base of support.

Crawling *(Chapter 13).* The progression in the prone position in which the belly is in contact with the supporting surface, and the extremities are used in a reciprocal fashion to propel the body forward or backward.

Creep *(Chapter 4).* Elongation of tissue with the application of a low-level force over time.

Creeping *(Chapter 13).* A progression in quadruped in which the belly is lifted off of the supporting surface and the extremities move reciprocally to move the body forward or backward.

Crossbridges *(Chapter 3, 4).* Myosin "heads" extending from "arms" at angles from the myosin, whose function is to connect myosin to actin thereby providing muscle contraction.

Cubital *(Chapter 6).* (L., *cubitum*, elbow) Pertaining to the elbow or forearm.

Cubital angle *(Chapter 6).* The carrying angle. The angle created between the humerus and forearm with the elbow in full extension whereby the forearm deviates laterally in relation to the humerus because the axis for flexion and extension of the elbow is not fully perpendicular to the shaft of the humerus; this angle varies somewhat in individuals, usually being more pronounced in women than in men.

Curvilinear *(Chapter 1).* Subset of linear motion whereby the object travels in a curved path such as that seen when tossing a ball to a friend.

Cubitus valgus *(Chapter 6).* The lateral angulation of the forearm with respect to the humerus; also known as carrying angle when at about 15° or less. Term also can be used to signify excessive lateral angulation of the forearm with respect to the humerus.

Cubitus varus *(Chapter 6).* The medial angulation of the forearm with respect to the humerus.

D

Deceleration *(Chapter 2).* A rate of decrease in velocity.

Degrees of freedom *(Chapter 2, 3).* The number of planes through which a joint is able to move. For every degree of freedom, there is an axis of movement. In kinesiological terms, the number of independent planar movements permitted at a joint, functionally translate into how many movement options exist at that joint or body segment.

Delayed-onset muscle soreness (DOMS) *(Chapter 4).* Soreness that develops in muscles about 24 hours after exercise, especially eccentric activities.

Demifacet *(Chapter 8).* A notch on the superior and inferior posterior thoracic vertebral body (T1-T9) that articulates with the head of the rib.

Depolarization *(Chapter 3).* Rapid exchange of positive and negative ions across nerve or muscle cell membrane resulting in a movement of the membrane to a more positive charge.

Depression *(Chapter 5).* The scapular motion in which the scapula slides downward on the thorax relative to its resting position.

Diarthrosis *(Chapter 1).* Joints whose primary purpose is to provide mobility; structurally hallmarked by the presence of a synovial joint capsule; further subdivided into uniaxial, biaxial, and triaxial joints.

Dislocation (*Chapter 1).* The two bony partners at the joint are completely removed or disassociated from each other, usually meaning that some damage, even rupture of the capsule, has occurred.

Displacement *(Chapter 2).* When motion of a body or a body's segment occurs with application of a force.

Distal attachment *(Chapter 4).* The point at which a muscle inserts into bone. The distal attachment is also called the insertion (as opposed to its origin). This location is more distal from the body than the other end of the muscle attachment site. See proximal attachment.

Disuse atrophy *(Chapter 3).* Muscular atrophy, secondary to immobilization or bed rest.

Dorsal (posterior) radioulnar ligament *(Chapter 6).* Ligament that stabilizes posterior aspect of distal radioulnar joint.

Dorsiflexion *(Chapter 1, 11).* Near-sagittal plane flexion movement of the dorsum of the foot toward the anterior aspect of the tibia.

Double float phase *(Chapter 12).* The part of the gait cycle during running when neither lower limb is in contact with the ground. There are two double float phases, one at the beginning of initial swing and one at the end of terminal swing. Also called float phase.

Double-limb support *(Chapter 12).* The part of the gait cycle during walking in which both lower extremities are in contact with the ground. This occurs at the first and last 10% of each limb's stance phase.

Dynamic action system *(Chapter 3).* Any system that demonstrates change over time; used to describe the human motor control system.

Dynamic action system model *(Chapter 3).* Theoretical model that views movement as emerging from the dynamic cooperation of many subsystems in a task and environment specific context.

Dysmetria *(Chapter 3).* Inability to gauge distance in reaching or stepping; common clinical symptom of cerebellar damage.

Dystonia *(Chapter 3).* A syndrome dominated by sustained muscle contractions and disordered muscle tone, frequently causing abnormal postures, twisting, or writhing movements, and repetitive abnormal postures, often associated with basal ganglia disturbance.

E

Eccentric motion *(Chapter 4).* A muscle activation in which the muscle lengthens as it produces tension to control joint motion. Joint motion is produced by an outside force, and the muscle's force controls the rate of motion change.

Efferent nerves *(Chapter 3).* Nerves that send a response from the central nervous system to the muscles.

Elasticity *(Chapter 4).* The ability of tissue to succumb to an elongating force and then return to its normal length when the force is released.

Elevation *(Chapter 5).* The scapula slides upward on the thorax relative to its resting position.

Ellipsoidal joint *(Chapter 1).* Type of biaxial joint whereby the shape is spindle-like with one somewhat flattened convex surface articulating with a fairly deep concave surface such as seen at the radiocarpal joint at the wrist.

Electromyography (EMG) *(Chapter 8).* Used as a diagnostic tool in medicine or an investigative tool in research. It detects electrical activity of muscles and nerves. The three types of electrodes used to detect EMG include surface, wire, and needle. Needle electrodes are used in diagnostic techniques, whereas the surface and wire are more often used in research investigations to identify muscle activity.

Empty end feel *(Chapter 1).* A pathologic end feel denoting an abnormal absence of resistance on motion and sometimes, pain.

End feel *(Chapter 1).* Resistance to further motion felt by the examiner when a normal joint is moved passively to the end of its range of motion; also called the physiologic end feel; further clarified as firm (capsular or ligamentous) or hard (bony).

Endomysium *(Chapter 4).* The fascial layer surrounding individual muscle fibers.

Endoplasmic reticulum *(Chapter 3).* A system of interlaced tubes within the interior of a muscle fiber that plays a vital role in excitation and contraction comprised of the sarcoplasmic reticulum and the transverse tubules.

Endurance *(Chapter 3).* The ability to perform the same act repeatedly over a period of time. Loss of endurance may be a sign of cardiopulmonary, muscular, or neurological problems.

Epicondyle *(Chapter 6, 10).* A prominence or eminence superior to a condyle. The most noted ones are on the distal humerus and distal femur. They serve as locations for muscles and ligaments to attach.

Epimysium *(Chapter 4).* The fascial layer surrounding an entire muscle.

Eponym *(Chapter 11).* Something that is named after an individual, real or fictitious.

Equilibrium *(Chapter 2).* When a system is in balance, it is in equilibrium. One direction of forces equals the opposing direction of forces.

Eversion *(Chapter 1, 11).* Transverse plane motion at the subtalar joint of turning the foot outward.

Excitable *(Chapter 3).* A membrane or cell responding when a sufficient stimulus is applied to it.

Extensibility *(Chapter 4).* The ability to stretch, elongate, or expand.

Extension *(Chapter 1).* Straightening motion at a joint in which one bony partner moves away from the other and there is an increase in joint angle; occurring in the sagittal plane.

Extensor lag *(Chapter 10).* When a joint is unable to achieve full active extension but has full passive extension. It may be the result of weakness or pain.

Extensor mechanism *(Chapter 7).* The unique arrangement of the long extensor tendons of the digits and the attachments of the intrinsic muscles of the hand. Also known as extensor hood mechanism, extensor expansion, apparatus, aponeurosis, retinaculum, or hood.

External moment arm *(Chapter 2).* The perpendicular distance from the joint's axis to the external force.

External (lateral) rotation (Chapter 1). A transverse plane motion of turning toward the side or outward, sometimes used instead of lateral rotation; lateral rotation is the term preferred over external rotation since it more adequately indicates the motion.

Extrafusal muscle fibers *(Chapter 3).* Skeletal muscle fibers.

Extrapyramidal tract or system *(Chapter 3).* Efferent (UMN) tract containing axons that descend into the brainstem that synapse there outside of the medullary pyramids; distinctive from pyramidal or corticospinal tract.

Extrinsic muscles *(Chapter 7, 11).* Muscles of the hand or foot that originate more proximally on the limb and insert onto the hand or foot. These muscles are generally designed for power or force production. See intrinsic muscles.

F

Fascia *(Chapter 4).* Connective tissue, composed primarily of collagen, that surrounds tissue. It is a fibrous sheet that separates muscle cells, fascicles, and layers.

Fasciculus *(Chapter 3).* Term used to describe the organization of skeletal muscle fibers into bundles, each called a fasciculus.

Fast-twitch fiber *(Chapter 3).* Type II or phasic muscle fiber; uses a fast glycolytic metabolic process and fatigues easily.

Fatigue *(Chapter 3).* A failure to maintain the required or expected force of muscle contraction, due to any one of several physiologic mechanisms.

Fascicle *(Chapter 4).* A bundle of muscle fibers or a bundle of nerve fibers. If it is a muscle bundle, it is surrounded by perimysium. If it is a nerve bundle, it is surrounded by perineurium.

Feiss' line *(Chapter 11).* A line drawn from the apex of the medial malleolus to the plantar surface of the first MTP joint. If the medial longitudinal arch is normal, the navicular tubercle will fall on or close to this line.

Festinating gait *(Chapter 12).* A typical gait seen in Parkinson's patients that includes an acceleration of the shuffling gait with a shortening of the stride length.

Firm (or capsular or ligamentous) end feel *(Chapter 1).* A springy normal end feel in which the limitation is from ligamentous, capsular, or muscle structures, such as in wrist flexion.

First-order neuron *(Chapter 3).* Sensory neuron from the receptor which has an uninterrupted axon and enters the dorsal horn of the spinal cord; the main fiber usually ascends through the spinal cord to synapse on other neurons in the CNS.

Flaccid *(Chapter 3).* A complete loss of muscle tone with an absence of deep tendon reflexes. It may follow a lower motor neuron lesion or in the acute stage of an upper motor neuron lesion.

Flaccidity *(Chapter 3).* Pathological condition in which muscle tone is absent.

Float phase *(Chapter 12).* During running, at the beginning of initial swing and again at the end of terminal swing when neither limb is in contact with the ground; this provides more time during swing and less time during stance. Also called double-float.

Fusimotor neurons *(Chapter 3).* or gamma (γ) motor neurons; referred to as such because the neurons supply motor impulses to the intrafusal muscle spindle fibers.

Flexion *(Chapter 1).* Bending motion at a joint in which one bony partner moves toward the other and there is a decrease in joint angle; occurs in the sagittal plane.

Foramen of Weitbrecht *(Chapter 5).* Area between the middle and superior anterior glenohumeral ligaments that is a common site of anterior glenohumeral joint dislocations because of the capsule's weakness in the region.

Forefoot *(Chapter 11).* The forefoot is that part of the foot made up of all of the metatarsals and phalanges.

Force *(Chapter 2).* A push or pull that produces displacement. The mathematical formula for force is F = m x a, where F is the amount of force created, m is the mass of the object and a is the acceleration of the object.

Force arm *(Chapter 2).* Also called lever arm. The perpendicular distance from the force applied to produce motion to the axis of motion.

Force couple *(Chapter 5).* Rotation around an axis by two or more muscles that otherwise work opposite to one another.

Force feedback reflex *(Chapter 4).* This is an inhibitory reflex caused by muscle activity and occurs with activation of the Golgi tendon organs (GTO). Little is known about this reflex, but it is thought to play a role in coupling antigravity muscles that cross different joints during multijoint movements.

Force vector *(Chapter 2).* A force that is applied to a body has two dimensions—magnitude and direction.

Fovea *(Chapter 6, 7).* A concave depression at the base of the ulnar styloid process that provides attachment for the wrist's fibrocartilaginous disc. There is also a concave articulating fovea that serves as the articulating surface atop the radial head.

Free body diagram *(Chapter 2).* Simplified drawings of the body with the force vectors acting on the body or a segment.

Friction *(Chapter 2).* The resistance to movement between two surfaces or objects in contact with each other, typically in a horizontal direction.

Frontal (Coronal) plane: (XY plane) *(Chapter 1).* So named because it is parallel to the frontal bone along the coronal skull suture, dividing the body into front and back parts. It is the plane within which abduction and adduction movements occur.

Functional excursion (of a muscle) *(Chapter 4).* The distance a muscle is capable of shortening after it has been elongated as far as the joint(s) over which it passes allows.

Fundamental position *(Chapter 13).* This is similar to the anatomical position except the palms face the body; forearms are in neutral midposition.

Fusiform muscle *(Chapter 4).* Muscle fascicle arrangement that is parallel, creating a spindle-shaped muscle with tapered ends. Designed for speed of movement rather than force. Also known as strap muscle.

G

Gait *(Chapter 12).* The manner or style of walking.

Gait cycle *(Chapter 12).* The fundamental unit of human walking, described by studying the events associated with when the foot makes contact with the ground, swings through the air, and then makes contact with the ground again. The time from when one foot makes contact with the ground to the next time it makes contact again.

Gamma (γ) motor neurons *(Chapter 3).* Neurons that innervate the contractile element called the intrafusal (within the spindle) muscle fibers. Contractile element within the muscle spindle sensory receptor, composed of two types of fibers—nuclear bag and nuclear chain fibers.

Ganglia *(Chapter 3).* Aggregations of functionally and anatomically related neurons on the CNS; also called nuclei.

Genu valgus or genu valgum *(Chapter 10).* When the knee has an excessive Q angle and angles medially. Also called knock knee.

Genu Varus or genu varum *(Chapter 10).* or bowleg, when the knee has a diminished Q angle or the knee is laterally convex.

Gliding *(Chapter 1).* This term is synonymous with the basic joint motion of "sliding." See sliding.

Gluteus medius gait *(Chapter 9, 12).* or Trendelenburg gait, is a gait compensation seen in persons with significant hip abductor weakness might, demonstrated by lateral flexion of the trunk during the stance phase of gait over the stance limb. This maneuver will shift the center of gravity and the weight of HAT laterally over the hip joint axis, minimizing the torque demand on the weakened abductors.

Glycolysis *(Chapter 3).* Breakdown of glycogen from storage depots in muscles and liver for the purpose of supplying energy.

Golgi tendon organ (GTO) *(Chapter 3).* Sensory receptor located at musculotendinous junction that is receptive to tension stimulus.

Gomphosis joint *(Chapter 1).* The fit of a tooth in its socket; a type of synarthrodial joint.

Goniometer *(Chapter 1).* Measurement device which looks like a protractor with two arms hinged at a fulcrum. It is placed parallel to the two body segments to be measured and with the axis of the joint and the axis (fulcrum) of the goniometer superimposed so that the angle at the joint can be measured and recorded.

Goniometry *(Chapter 1).* An application of the coordinate system to a joint to measure the degrees of motion present in each plane of a joint.

Gunstock deformity *(Chapter 6).* Cubital varus, or a carrying angle of less than the normal 5° to 15° valgus angulation.

Gray matter *(Chapter 3).* Regions of CNS in which nerve cell bodies are concentrated; appears gray in color.

Greater sciatic notch *(Chapter 9).* An opening in the pelvic bone through which the sciatic nerve and piriformis muscle pass.

Greater trochanter *(Chapter 9).* Is easily palpated superior lateral prominence of the proximal femur; attachment site for the gluteus medius and lateral rotator muscles and an important landmark used in measuring leg length.

Ground reaction force (GRF) *(Chapter 12).* A resultant force comprised of reaction forces acting on the foot that occur in three different directions—vertical, anterior-posterior, and medial-lateral.

H

Hallux valgus *(Chapter 11).* A lateral deviation of the first MTP joint so the toe is at an angle toward the other toes. It is often a result occurring from excessive pronation.

Hard (or bony) end feel *(Chapter 1).* Normal end feel felt when the motion is stopped by contact of bone on bone, as in elbow extension when the olecranon process of the ulna fits snugly into the olecranon fossa of the humerus.

Head of the femur *(Chapter 9).* A large rounded proximal aspect of femur; articulates within the acetabulum as an articulating partner at the hip joint.

Head of the radius *(Chapter 6).* The superior prominence of the radius.

Heterarchy *(Chapter 3).* When the contributing systems are not arranged in a hierarchy; rather, all the contributing systems work parallel to each other.

Hierarchy *(Chapter 3).* When the contributing systems are arranged in a linear fashion, in which one is more important than the other and the lowest level is overseen by a higher level.

Hinge joint *(Chapter 1).* A type of uniaxial joint; e.g., the humeroulnar joint.

Hip strategy *(Chapter 12).* Control of posture that comes from adjustment movements produced at the hip, pelvis, and trunk.

Horizontal (Transverse) plane: (XZ plane) *(Chapter 1).* So named because it is parallel to the horizon and the floor, dividing the body into upper and lower parts, like a view from above. It is the plane within which rotational movements occur.

Hypermobile *(Chapter 1).* More joint motion than is expected or typical.

Hyperpolarization *(Chapter 3).* An increased negative potential (more negative than the resting potential) of the cell membrane.

Hyperreflexia (*Chapter 3).* Exaggerated stretch reflexes; sign of a pathological condition.

Hypertonia *(Chapter 3).* A motor disorder characterized by a velocity-dependent increase in the stretch reflex with exaggerated tendon jerks resulting from hyperexcitability. Common in upper motor neuron lesions.

Hypertrophy *(Chapter 4).* An increase in a muscle's cell size and overall muscle girth that accompanies gains in muscle strength.

Hypokinesis *(Chapter 3).* Decreased activity, often seen in the older adult.

Hypomobile *(Chapter 1).* Less joint motion than what is expected or typical.

Hyporeflexia *(Chapter 3).* Diminished stretch reflexes; a sign of a pathological condition.

Hypotonia *(Chapter 3).* A reduction of muscle stiffness characterized by low muscle tone, weakness, and a decreased ability to sustain muscle activation.

I

Iliac crest *(Chapter 9).* The very prominent and easily palpable superior bony border of the ilium of the pelvis, one on the right and one on the left side.

Iliac fossa *(Chapter 9).* A large concave well on the internal surface of the ilium, to which a portion of the large iliopsoas muscle attaches.

Ilium *(Chapter 9).* The more anterior and superior of the three pelvic bones; the bone that you feel when you "put your hands on your hips."

Impairments *(Chapter 3).* The typical consequences of disease or pathological processes indicated by signs and symptoms.

Inertia *(Chapter 2).* The reluctance of a body to change its current state of being, either stationary or in a uniform motion. Newton's First Law of Motion deals with this concept.

Inferior pubic ramus *(Chapter 9).* The bony aspect of inferior pubic bone; attachment site for most of the muscles that adduct the hip.

Initial contact *(Chapter 12).* The first subphase of the stance phase of gait during walking. During running, initial contact is not heel strike since most runners do not contact the ground with the heel first. Initial contact is when the foot makes contact with the ground. Also called heel strike.

Initial swing *(Chapter 12).* This is the first subphase of the swing phase of gait as the leg is off the ground and begins to swing forward. During this phase, the limb accelerates forward. Also called early swing.

Innervation ratio *(Chapter 3).* Average number of muscle fibers per motor unit in a given muscle.

Instant center of rotation (ICR) *(Chapter 10).* The theoretical axis of rotation of a joint that changes as the joint surface rolls and glides. Because of the joint's mechanics, the center of rotation, or its axis, changes as the joint moves through its range of motion.

Intention tremor *(Chapter 3).* Sometimes called an action tremor, a tremor evidenced upon purposeful movement of the body part, typically seen during reaching with the upper extremity, or stepping with the lower extremity, a symptom commonly seen in patients with cerebellar lesions.

Intercondylar fossa *(Chapter 10).* The distal femur's separation between the medial and lateral condyles that is evident at the bone's most distal aspect and posteriorly. This is the fossa through which the cruciate ligaments traverse between the tibia and femur.

Intercondylar groove *(Chapter 10).* A pulley-like furrow between the medial and lateral condyle of the distal femur. It is the femoral component of the patellofemoral joint. It is also known as the trochlear groove.

Internal moment arm *(Chapter 2).* The perpendicular distance from the joint's axis to the muscle.

Internal (medial) rotation *(Chapter 1).*Transverse plane movement of turning inward toward the midline, sometimes used instead of medial rotation; the more preferred term is medial rotation since it more accurately reflects the direction of motion.

Interneurons *(Chapter 3).* Neurons within the ventral horn and intermediate areas of the spinal cord that are essentially involved in the transmission to and regulation of movement via their action on alpha and gamma motor neurons.

Interosseous membrane *(Chapter 6, 11).* A strong, fibrous connective tissue located between the radius and ulna and between the tibia and fibula.

Intervertebral disc *(Chapter 8).* A fibrocartilaginous structure containing an annulus fibrosis outer section and a gelatinous-like nucleus pulposus. With the exception of the first and second cervical vertebrae and the sacrococcyx, an intervertebral disc sits between each vertebra of the spine. They allow motion and transfer weight between the vertebrae.

Intrafusal muscle fibers *(Chapter 3).* Literally means "within the fuse or spindle;" contractile element (two types—nuclear bag and nuclear chain fibers) within the muscle spindle sensory receptor, innervated by gamma (γ) motor neurons.

Intrinsic muscles *(Chapter 7, 11).* Muscles of the hand or foot that originate and insert on the hand or foot, respectively. They do not come from outside the hand or foot segment. These muscles are used for fine motions and stability of the hand or foot.

Inversion *(Chapter 1, 11).* Transverse plane motion at the subtalar joint of turning the foot inward.

In vivo *(Chapter 4).* Refers to the living body. This is usually contrasted with *in vitro* which is an experimental environment in which, for example, a muscle fiber, bone, or other tissue may be isolated and investigated in a lab without regard to its normal environment.

Irritable *(Chapter 3).* Capable of responding to a stimulus.

Ischial ramus *(Chapter 9).* A not easily palpable bony extension, medially connecting the body of the ischium to the ramus of the pubis; an attachment site for the adductor magnus and for some of the small lateral rotators of the hip.

Ischial tuberosity *(Chapter 9).* A notable large palpable feature on the most inferior aspect of the ischium of the pelvis; an important landmark because it is the weight-bearing prominence upon which you sit and serves as the common attachment for the hamstring muscles.

Isometric activation *(Chapter 4).* A muscle tenses, or produces force, without motion.

Isotonic activation *(Chapter 4).* A muscle produces force that produces the same tension throughout its motion. This occurs in the laboratory but not in the human body.

J

Joint play *(Chapter 1).* Amount of additional joint motion able to be discerned by the examiner; occurs only in response to external force. These slight passive translations that occur in most joints are described by defining the direction of the translation: anterior-posterior, medial-lateral, and superior-inferior.

Joint reaction force *(Chapter 2).* The amount of force either compressing or distracting the joint surfaces when forces such as muscle force and gravity are applied to a body segment. Also referred to as joint force.

Joint receptors *(Chapter 3).* Located within joint capsules and ligaments, they are afferent sensors; continually provide feedback to CNS by informing the nervous system of momentary angulation of joints and of the rate of movement of joints.

K

Kilograms *(Chapter 2).* Measurement of mass in the metric system; 1 kg = 0.031 slugs.

Kinematics *(Chapter 1).* Describing and measuring human movement by focusing on the type of motion, the direction, and the quantity of the motion without regard for the forces that may produce that movement; further subdivided into osteokinematics and arthrokinematics.

Kinematic chain *(Chapter 1).* Combination of several joints uniting successive segments, further clarified as open (distal segment free) or closed (distal segment fixed) kinematic chain.

Kinesthesia *(Chapter 3).* Awareness of dynamic joint motion.

Kinetics *(Chapter 1).* The science that deals with forces that produce, stop, or modify motion of bodies as a whole or of individual body segments. The study of forces acting on the body.

Krebs cycle *(Chapter 3).* Or tricarboxylic acid cycle is the process whereby the chemical energy reserves for muscle contraction are restored by oxidative metabolism of fats, carbohydrates, and proteins in the mitochondria of muscle fibers. Enzymes split the large molecules into smaller units that can be oxidized in a series of chemical reactions yielding reaction end products of carbon dioxide, water, and ATP, which are used for restoration and maintenance of energy stores or are released in respiration.

Kyphosis *(Chapter 8).* An exaggerated posterior convex curvature of the spine.

Kyphotic curve *(Chapter 12).* Considered functionally to be a *primary* curvature of the vertebral column because it is the first demonstrated curve of the column.

L

Lamina *(Chapter 8).* The part of a vertebra that is part of the neural arch and lies between the vertebra's transverse process and spinous process. This section of the vertebra is usually excised in a laminectomy.

Lateral epicondyles *(Chapter 6, 10).* A bony prominence that is superior to a lateral condyle and serves for a site of insertion for tendons and ligaments; e.g., there are lateral epicondyles in the elbow and knee.

Lateral femoral condyle *(Chapter 10).* A large knob-like lateral distal end of the femur, forming part of the femoral connection at the knee joint.

Lateral flexion *(Chapter 1).* Frontal plane motion of side-bending of the neck or trunk.

Lateral malleolus *(Chapter 11).* See malleolus.

Lateral (external) rotation *(Chapter 1).* A transverse plane motion of turning toward the side or outward. This term more accurately reflects the movement rather than the term "external rotation."

Lateral supracondylar ridge *(Chapter 6).* The bony ridge superior to the lateral epicondyle of the humerus; an attachment site for the brachioradialis muscle.

Lateral tilting *(Chapter 5).* Or lateral rotation of the scapula is the rotation of the scapula around a vertical axis to position the glenoid fossa away from the body. This motion occurs at the AC joint.

Lead pipe rigidity *(Chapter 3).* Type of rigidity characterized by a constant resistance to movement throughout the range of motion.

Length feedback reflex *(Chapter 4).* A reflex mechanism that is theorized to contribute to improved force output during plyometric activities. This reflex is triggered when a muscle is stretched and occurs at the same time of the muscle's stretch reflex. In addition to exciting the muscle to contract, it also excites the muscle's synergists while inhibiting the muscle's antagonists. This simultaneous excitation and inhibition is thought to improve the muscle's performance.

Lesser trochanter *(Chapter 9).* Prominence on proximal femur located medially and posteriorly to the greater trochanter, serving as an attachment site for the iliopsoas muscle.

Lever *(Chapter 2).* A simple machine consisting of a rigid bar that rotates around a fulcrum or axis.

Leverage factor *(Chapter 2).* A concept regarding muscle force production which states that the greater the perpendicular distance between the muscle's line of action and the joint's center (moment arm distance), the greater the rotational component produced by the muscle at that joint.

Ligamentum flavum *(Chapter 8).* A ligament primarily composed of elastic fibers that connects one lamina to the adjacent-level laminae throughout the spine.

Ligamentum interspinale *(Chapter 8).* The interspinous ligament. This ligament connects the spinous processes of adjacent vertebrae to each other.

Ligamentum intertransversarium *(Chapter 8).* The intertransverse ligament. This ligament connects the transverse processes of adjacent vertebrae to each other.

Ligamentum nuchae *(Chapter 8).* The nuchal ligament. A thick sagittal ligament band at the posterior neck that extends from the external occipital protuberance laterally to the posterior border of the foramen magnum and caudally to seventh cervical spinous process.

Ligamentum supraspinale *(Chapter 8).* The supraspinous ligament. This ligament is in the cervical region and attaches to the posterior edges of the spinous processes of the vertebrae in this area. It merges with the ligamentum flavum.

Linear (translatory) motion *(Chapter 1).* Motion whereby all points on the moving object travel the same distance, in the same direction with the same velocity and at the same time; further clarified as rectilinear if the movement is in a straight line or curvilinear if the motions travel in a curved path such as that seen when tossing a ball to a friend.

Linea aspera *(Chapter 9).* A prominent ridge running almost the entire length of the posterior femur; serves as an attachment for some of the adductor muscles.

Line of Gravity (LOG) *(Chapter 2).* The direction of pull of the force of gravity. It is perpendicular to the surface of the earth.

Lisfranc's joint *(Chapter 11).* The joints of the tarsometatarsals, named after French surgeon Jacques Lisfranc.

Lister's tubercle *(Chapter 7).* A tubercle on the distal dorsal surface of the radius that serves as a pulley to redirect the pull of the extensor pollicis longus.

Loading response *(Chapter 12).* Or flat foot is the second subphase of the stance phase of gait during walking. During this time the body absorbs the forces of impact and the foot is lowered to the ground.

Locomotion *(Chapter 12).* Moving from one place to another, including many forms of movement such as rolling, crawling and creeping, walking, running, hopping and skipping.

Loose-packed position (or open-packed) *(Chapter 1).* Joint position whereby the joint surfaces do not fit perfectly but are incongruent, the ligamentous and capsular structures are slack, and the joint surfaces may be distracted several millimeters.

Lordosis *(Chapter 8).* An anterior convexity (or posterior concavity) of the spine from a sagittal view. Normally seen in the lumbar and cervical vertebral regions. Lordosis may be either normal or excessive.

Lordotic curve *(Chapter 12).* Occurs first at the cervical spine as the baby develops head control in prone and then in the lumbar region as the infant sits and stands upright. These curves develop once the infant begins rolling and sitting. They are called secondary curves.

Lower motor neuron *(Chapter 3).* A motor (efferent) nerve whose cell body and axon originate in the ventral horn of the spinal cord and synapse directly onto skeletal muscle. This is often referred to as the *final common path* between the nervous system and the muscular system.

M

Malleolus *(Chapter 11).* The landmarks on the medial and lateral aspect of the ankle. The medial malleolus is formed by the distal projection of the tibia and the lateral malleolus is formed by the distal projection of the fibula.

Mass *(Chapter 2).* The amount of matter contained within an object. Measured in kilograms (kg) or slugs.

Medial epicondyle *(Chapter 6, 10).* A bony prominence that is superior to a medial condyle and serves for a site of insertion for tendons and ligaments; e.g. there are medial epicondyles in the elbow and knee.

Medial femoral condyle *(Chapter 10).* A large knob-like medial distal end of the femur, forming part of the femoral connection at the knee joint.

Medial femoral epicondyles *(Chapter 10).* A palpable superior aspect of medial femoral condyle.

Medial malleolus *(Chapter 11).* See malleolus.

Medial (internal) rotation *(Chapter 1).* Transverse plane movement of turning inward toward the midline. This term more accurately reflects the motion than does the term "internal rotation."

Medial tilting *(Chapter 5).* Rotation of the scapula around a vertical axis to rotate the glenoid fossa towards the midline of the body. Also called internal rotation of the scapula. This motion occurs at the AC joint.

Meniscotibial ligament *(Chapter 10).* See coronary ligament.

Meniscus *(Chapter 10).* A crescent-shaped fibrocartilaginous structure between the tibia and femur. The knee has a medial and lateral meniscus.

Metabolic equivalent (MET) *(Chapter 3).* The energy requirements of activities; based on the resting oxygen consumption of an individual whereby one MET is equal to 3.5 ml of oxygen per kilogram of body weight per minute.

Midfoot *(Chapter 11).* The midfoot is comprised of the navicular, cuboid, and three cuneiform bones.

Midstance *(Chapter 12).* The middle subphase of the stance phase of gait. During this time, the body's weight is entirely on the one limb. The COM is at its highest point.

Midswing *(Chapter 12).* The second and middle subphase of the swing phase of gait. It is the middle of the swing when the nonweight-bearing limb is moving under the trunk.

Mobility muscles *(Chapter 4).* Muscles with more fast-twitch fibers or type II fibers than type I fibers. They fatigue quickly but are able to produce force and power quickly. Also called nonpostural muscles.

Moment *(Chapter 2).* The shortened term for moment of force.

Moment arm *(Chapter 2).* The force arm, or lever arm, when discussing rotary forces. It is the perpendicular distance from the force vector to the axis of motion. See torque arm.

Moment of Force *(Chapter 2).* Torque created around an axis. It is the product of a force and its moment arm. In mathematical terms, a moment (M) is the product of this distance (d) and the force (F): $M = d \times F$.

Motion *(Chapter 2).* Displacement of a body or object from one place to another.

Motion segment *(Chapter 8).* This is most basic section of the spine that produces motion. One motion segment consists of two adjacent vertebrae, three intervertebral joints (the joint between the bodies of the vertebrae and the two facet joints), the soft tissues of the intervertebral disc, longitudinal and intersegmental ligaments, and the capsules of the facet joints.

Motor control *(Chapter 3).* A field of study directed at the study of movement as the result of a complex set of neurological, physical, and behavioral processes. Motor control is the ability of the individual to maintain and change posture and movement based on an interaction among the individual, task, and the environment.

Motor learning *(Chapter 3).* Area of study concerned mostly with how motor skills are acquired, made proficient, transferred, and retained.

Motor unit *(Chapter 3).* An individual motor neuron, together with its axon and all of the muscle fibers that are innervated by the motor neuron.

Movement system *(Chapter 3).* The functional interaction of several subsystems and structures that contribute to the act of moving. The contributing systems include the nervous, somatosensory, and musculoskeletal systems.

Multipennate muscles *(Chapter 4).* Muscles whose fibers have more than two pinnate groups attaching to more than one centralized tendon.

Muscle fibers *(Chapter 3).* Contractile tissue, made up of groups of myofibrils.

Muscle spindle *(Chapter 3).* A unique type of proprioceptor, located between the fibers of skeletal muscle, which has both sensory and motor properties. Detects change in muscle length (stretch) and rate of that change, and plays a role in setting resting muscle tone.

Muscle tone *(Chapter 3).* Steady state of alert or arousal of the muscular system for the task demands to be placed on it; determined by the level of excitability of the entire pool of motor neurons controlling a muscle, the intrinsic stiffness of the muscle itself, an intact CNS, and the level of sensitivity of many different reflexes.

Myofibril *(Chapter 4).* The contractile structures of skeletal muscle. It contains the myofilaments of actin and myosin.

Myofilaments *(Chapter 4).* The protein structures of skeletal muscle that provide muscle contraction. Myosin is the thicker protein filament that possesses the crossbridge heads (myosin heads) that connect to actin. Actin is the thinner protein filament that contains troponin and tropomyosin, which control the binding between actin and myosin which occurs during muscle contraction.

Myoneural junction *(Chapter 3).* Synaptic junction between nerve and muscle at motor end plate.

Myosin *(Chapter 3, 4).* This is the thicker protein filament that possesses the crossbridge heads (myosin heads) which connect to actin.

Myotatic reflex *(Chapter 3).* Or the stretch reflex is a monosynaptic simple reflex arc, mediated at the spinal cord level, whereby a change in muscle length (stretch) of a sufficient amount and at a sufficient rate, will activate the muscle spindle eliciting a reflex contraction of the agonist muscle undergoing the stretch.

N

Negative work *(Chapter 4).* See eccentric motion.

Neutral equilibrium *(Chapter 2).* When the center of gravity is displaced, it remains at the same level; i.e., it neither falls nor returns to its former position.

Neck of the femur *(Chapter 9).* Narrow area just inferior to the head of the femur, connecting to the femoral shaft.

Newton *(Chapter 2).* Force in the metric system. 9.8 N = 1 kilogram-force (kgf); 1 N = 0.225 lb.

Neural arch *(Chapter 8).* Sometimes called the posterior neural arch. It forms the vertebral canal through which the spinal cord travels.

Neurotransmitter *(Chapter 3).* Chemical released at a synapse.

Nonpostural muscles *(Chapter 4).* See mobility muscles.

Normal force vector *(Chapter 2).* In resultant vector configurations, this vector is the component that produces rotation around the axis of movement. At its greatest, it is applied 90° to the lever arm.

Nuclei *(Chapter 3).* Aggregations of functionally and anatomically related neurons on the CNS; also called ganglia.

Nutation *(Chapter 8).* Motion of the sacrum by which the sacral promontory moves inferiorly and anteriorly as the distal sacrum and coccyx move posteriorly. In this motion, the iliac crests move towards each other and the ischial tuberosities move apart.

O

Oblique cord *(Chapter 6).* A flat fascia band on ventral forearm running from radial notch of ulna to radial tuberosity; reinforces and stabilizes the proximal radioulnar joint.

Obturator foramen *(Chapter 9).* Opening in the pelvic bone through which several vessels and nerves pass toward the lower extremity.

Olecranon fossa *(Chapter 6).* A deep bony cavity on the posterior aspect of the distal humerus, providing a stable articulating surface for the superior ulna.

Olecranon process *(Chapter 6).* A distinctive bony prominence of the superior ulna on the posterior aspect.

On-guard position *(Chapter 12).* Posturing of the upper extremities during early walking in a high-, medium-, and then low-guard position.

Open kinematic chain (OKC) *(Chapter 1, 4).* Movement that occurs during nonweight-bearing when the distal portion of the segment is free to move and each part of the segment may move independently of the others. These motions are used for speed rather than force production. Also referred to as open chain motion.

Open-packed position. *(Chapter 1).* Or loose-packed position. Joint position whereby the joint surfaces do not fit perfectly but are incongruent, the ligamentous and capsular structures are slack, and the joint surfaces may be distracted several millimeters.

Opposition (Chapter 7). A rotation of the first metacarpal on the trapezium to place the pad of the thumb opposite the pads of the fingers.

Optimal sufficiency *(Chapter 4).* The result seen when an antagonist of a multijoint muscle or muscle group positions and stabilizes one joint to lengthen the multijoint muscle or group to allow improved function of the multijoint agonist at another joint; i.e., hip flexors position the hip in flexion (preventing hip extension) so the hamstrings can exert its force in knee flexion.

Osteokinematics *(Chapter 1).* A subdivision of kinematics, focused on a description of movement of the shafts of the bones on each other.

Osteophyte *(Chapter 8).* A bony growth that usually occurs around a joint.

Ovoid *(Chapter 1).* Egg-shaped joint surface type whereby the radius of curvature varies from point to point and the articular surfaces of the two bones form a convex-concave paired relationship, with this concave-convex joint relationship ranging from "nearly planar," as in the carpal and tarsal joints, to "nearly spheroid," as in the glenohumeral and hip joints.

P

Palmar radioulnar ligament *(Chapter 6).* Or anterior radioulnar ligament. The ligament that stabilizes the anterior aspect of distal radioulnar joint.

Parallel elastic component *(Chapter 4).* The connective tissues that surrounds or lies parallel to muscle.

Passive elastic component *(Chapter 4).* The fascia, or connective tissue, that surrounds muscle, from the entire muscle down to the smallest muscle component. When a muscle is stretched, the elastic component of the muscle's fascia provides additional muscle force as the muscle contracts.

Passive insufficiency *(Chapter 4).* When muscles become elongated over two or more joints simultaneously, they reach a length that does not allow further motion by the opposite muscle. This usually occurs in muscles crossing more than one joint and is the result of the muscle being stretched as far as possible but insufficiently to allow full motion of each joint it crosses; i.e., hamstrings are stretched in full knee extension, but the hip is unable to fully flex since the hamstrings have no more ability to lengthen.

Passive tension *(Chapter 4).* Tension developed in a muscle when it is elongated. This tension is the result of connective tissue surrounding the muscle (parallel elastic fibers) and the tendon (series elastic fibers) being stretched as slack is removed from the muscle during the stretch. See active tension.

Patellar groove *(Chapter 10).* A groove on the anterior distal femur between the two femoral condyles, providing a track for the underside of the patella at the patellar femoral joint.

Patellectomy *(Chapter 10).* Surgical removal of the patella.

Pathologic end feels *(Chapter 1).* These are normal end feels that occur at places in the range of motion or in joints other than what is expected, or it is an end feel that is not characteristic of the joint.

Pectineal line *(Chapter 9).* The small line located between the greater trochanter and the linea aspera on the posteromedial proximal femur so named because the pectineus muscle attached here.

Pedicle *(Chapter 8).* That part of the vertebrae that connects the transverse process to the body of the vertebrae.

Pelvic inclination *(Chapter 8).* Alignment of the pelvis when the ASIS and pubic symphysis do not align on the same vertical line. There is an increased, or forward, pelvic inclination when the ASIS are forward of the pubic symphysis and a posterior, or backward, pelvic inclination when the ASIS are backward of the pubic symphysis. In an anterior pelvic tilt, hip flexion increases; in posterior pelvic tilt, hip flexion decreases.

Pelvis *(Chapter 9).* Comprised of the two innominate bones, also called os coxae, formed by the fused ilium, ischium, and pubic bones, joined to the sacrum posteriorly.

Pennate muscle *(Chapter 4).* Muscle fascicle arrangement that is feather-like and oblique to the muscle's common tendon. More pennate muscles provide greater strength and fusiform muscles. Their pennate arrangement may be unipennate, bipennate, or multipennate. Designed for force rather than speed of motion.

Perimysium *(Chapter 4).* The fascial layer surrounding muscle fiber groups, or fascicles.

Peripheral nervous system *(Chapter 3).* Composed of receptors and effectors of the body, peripheral ganglia, and neuronal processes that connects the peripheral nervous system to the CNS.

Perseveration *(Chapter 3).* Repetitive speech or movement; symptom of a pathological condition.

Pes anserinus *(Chapter 9, 10).* The anterior proximal region of the medial tibia into which the sartorius, gracilis, and semitendinosus tendons insert. This region is called this because the insertion site appears similar to the foot of a goose.

Pes cavus *(Chapter 11).* A foot deformity that has a higher than normal medial longitudinal arch. This is usually a congenital condition. The foot joints are usually rigid, permitting little if any force absorption by the foot during weight-bearing activities. Known as club foot in its extreme condition.

Pes planus *(Chapter 11).* A foot deformity in which the joints of the foot are flexible and do not move into position as a rigid lever at the appropriate times during weight-bearing or during ambulation. This may be a congenital or acquired condition. Known as flat foot in its extreme condition.

Phasic *(Chapter 3).* Qualitative description given to a receptor or a muscle referring to the type of activity it generates; in this case, signifying a distinct stage or phase.

Pivot joint *(Chapter 1).* A type of uniaxial joint, such as the radioulnar joint.

Plafond *(Chapter 11).* Saddle-shaped structure on the inferior aspect of the tibia.

Plane of the scapula *(Chapter 5).* 30° to 45° forward of the frontal plane, so called because this is the angle at which the scapula lies on the posterior thorax when in its resting position. This is the plane in which the rotator cuff is best aligned to produce glenohumeral elevation.

Plantar aponeurosis *(Chapter 11).* Thick fascial covering of the plantar aspect of the foot. It consists of a series of fascial bands beginning about 2 to 3 cm proximal to the calcaneal tuberosity and ending distally on the toes. It provides the foot with a windlass mechanism that converts the tarsal and metatarsal bones of the foot to a rigid lever to permit rising on the toes. The arches are increased by this mechanism. This structure is also known as the plantar fascia.

Plantarflexion (*Chapter 1, 11).* Near-sagittal plane motion of the ankle in which the dorsum of the foot moves away from the anterior leg.

Plica *(Chapter 10).* Folds or seams in the synovial membrane.

Plumb line *(Chapter 12).* A vertical line used as a reference to assess posture. It is usually a string or cord with a weight at the bottom so the string is taut as it hangs freely.

Plyometrics or Plyometric exercise *(Chapter 4).* See stretch-shortening cycle.

Popliteal fossa *(Chapter 10).* The posterior region of the posterior knee. The fossa contains the popliteal artery, vein, and nerve.

Position sense *(Chapter 3).* The awareness of static position of one's joints.

Positive work *(Chapter 4).* See concentric motion.

Posterior inferior iliac spine (PIIS) *(Chapter 9).* Landmark, not easily palpated, located inferior to the PSIS on the posterior aspect of the ilium of the pelvis.

Posterior radioulnar ligament *(Chapter 6).* Also called the dorsal radioulnar ligament. A ligament that stabilizes posterior aspect of distal radioulnar joint.

Posterior superior iliac spine (PSIS) *(Chapter 9).* Prominence on the most posterior and superior aspect of the crest of the ilium of the pelvis.

Posterior tilting *(Chapter 5).* Rotation of the scapula around a medial-lateral axis so that the superior scapula rotates backward or posteriorly. The motion occurs as the scapula returns to the resting position from an anteriorly tilted position.

Postural muscles *(Chapter 4).* See antigravity muscles.

Postural tone *(Chapter 3).* Development of muscular tension, in particular muscles that are actively engaged in holding different parts of the skeleton in proper relationships to maintain particular postures.

Postural sway *(Chapter 12).* Small, automatic motions required as we continually seek and re-establish equilibrium because of body motions occurring secondary to respiration, heart beat, and metabolic functions.

Posture *(Chapter 12).* General term that is an alignment of body segments, a position or attitude of the body, the relative arrangement of body parts for a specific activity, or a characteristic manner of bearing one's body.

Pound *(Chapter 2).* Measurement of force in the US system. 1 pound = 4.448 N.

Power *(Chapter 3).* The rate at which physical work is performed.

Preswing *(Chapter 12).* The final subphase of the stance phase of gait. It is during this time that the foot moves from the lifted heel (terminal stance) to lifting the foot off the ground. Also called toe-off.

Pretibial muscles *(Chapter 11).* Muscles of the anterior leg (tibialis anterior, extensor digitorum longus, extensor hallucis longus, and peroneus tertius) are collectively referred to as pretibial muscles because of their position relative to the tibia.

Prime mover *(Chapter 4).* See agonist.

Promontory *(Chapter 8).* A ridge or protrusion. On the sacrum, it is the top of the body of the sacrum that is in contact with the lowest lumbar vertebra. It juts out anteriorly and serves as an important obstetrical landmark.

Pronation *(Chapter 1, 11).* Triplanar motion of the foot and ankle that occurs differently in the open kinetic chain than it does in the closed kinetic chain. In the open kinetic chain, the combined motions include eversion, abduction, and dorsiflexion. In the closed kinetic chain, the motions include plantarflexion, adduction, and eversion.

Proprioception *(Chapter 3).* Refers to the use of sensory input from receptors in muscle spindles, tendons, and joints to discriminate joint position and joint movement, including direction, amplitude, and speed, as well as relative tension within tendons.

Proprioceptors *(Chapter 3).* Class of receptors that gives sensory input about joint position, joint movement, and muscle length and tension; includes golgi tendon organs (GTO), several different types of joint receptors, and muscle spindles.

Propulsive gait *(Chapter 12).* A gait that takes on an accelerating characteristic, sometimes requiring that the patient come in contact with an object or a wall in order to stop.

Protraction *(Chapter 1, 5).* The lateral end of the clavicle and the scapula move anteriorly around the rib cage in curvilinear fashion, with the medial borders of the scapula moving away from the midline 5 to 6 inches (13 to 15 cm). This motion is also referred to as abduction of the scapula.

Proximal attachment *(Chapter 4).* The location at which one end of a muscle inserts into the bone. The proximal attachment site is the location closest to the center of the body. Formerly known as the muscle's origin. See distal attachment.

Pubic tubercle *(Chapter 9).* Small prominence on the most medial and superior aspect of the superior ramus of the pubis to which the inguinal ligament attaches.

Pyramidal tract *(Chapter 3).* Anatomically known as the corticospinal tract; referred to as such because many of the cell bodies located in the motor cortex are triangular in shape and have the appearance of small pyramids when a section of cortex is stained and viewed under a light microscope. Most of the corticospinal axons cross to the opposite side in the brainstem within the pyramid of the medulla.

Q

Quadrate ligament *(Chapter 6).* The ligament that arises from radial notch of ulna to neck of radius; it reinforces joint capsule and stabilizes the proximal radioulnar joint.

Qualitative analysis *(Chapter 15).* An analysis of a movement that breaks down the movement into segments and assesses the segments for its muscle and joint activity without quantifying the segments.

Q angle *(Chapter 10).* Quadriceps angle. The angle formed by the intersection of the line from the anterior superior iliac spine (ASIS) to the center of the patella and the line from the tibial tuberosity to the center of the patella. Normal is 170°.

R

Radial abduction *(Chapter 1, 7).* In the anatomic position, wrist movement in the frontal plane through an anterior-posterior axis that moves the hand away from the side of the body toward the thumb. Also known as radial flexion or radial deviation.

Radial collateral ligament *(Chapter 6).* The three-part stabilizing ligament located on the lateral side of the elbow region; contributes some stability in the frontal plane. Also called the lateral collateral ligament of the elbow.

Radial deviation *(Chapter 1, 7).* See radial abduction.

Radial fossa *(Chapter 6).* Cavity on distal anterior humerus superior to the capitulum; receives the radial head at full elbow flexion.

Radial fovea *(Chapter 6).* A deep concavity atop the radial head; articulates with the humeral capitulum.

Radial head *(Chapter 6).* Superior aspect of radius, just below the head.

Radial neck *(Chapter 6).* Narrowed area just inferior to radial head.

Radial notch *(Chapter 6).* Concave bony landmark on proximal lateral ulna, articulation between ulna and radius at proximal radioulnar joint.

Radial styloid process *(Chapter 7).* The distal process of the radius that extends somewhat more distally than the corresponding process of the ulna. The radial styloid process serves as the attachment site for the radial carpal collateral ligament and the brachioradialis muscle.

Radial tuberosity *(Chapter 6).* Bony landmark on anterior proximal radius just distal to radial head and neck; attachment site for biceps brachii muscle.

Range of movement or range of motion (ROM) *(Chapter 3).* Excursion of a joint through its arc of motion.

Ray *(Chapter 11).* A toe unit that is anterior to the midfoot and incorporates the cuneiform with its corresponding metatarsal in the case of the three medial rays and only the metatarsals in the case of the lateral two rays.

Reaching strategy *(Chapter 12).* See stepping or reaching strategy.

Reafference *(Chapter 3).* Property of the cerebellum giving it the ability to receive sensory feedback from receptors about the movements as the movement is occurring.

Rearfoot *(Chapter 11).* That part of the foot made up of the calcaneus and talus. The rearfoot guides the rest of the foot.

Reciprocal arm swing *(Chapter 12).* The manner of swinging the upper extremity rhythmically with the contralateral lower extremity during walking; e.g., the RUE swings forward into shoulder flexion when the LLE steps forward at initial contact.

Reciprocal innervation *(Chapter 3).* Spinal mechanism whereby antagonist muscles relax when agonist muscles are activated; allows for fluidity of human movement.

Recruitment *(Chapter 3).* Process whereby strength of muscle contraction occurs by increasing the number of motor units activated simultaneously.

Repolarization *(Chapter 3).* An active process of an excitable cell membrane, occurring immediately after depolarization, to re-establish the resting membrane potential.

Rectilinear *(Chapter 1).* A subset of linear motion whereby movement is in a straight line.

Reposition *(Chapter 7).* The opposite of thumb opposition or returning the thumb back into anatomical position from a position of opposition.

Resistance arm *(Chapter 2).* The perpendicular distance from the resistance force applied to a segment to the axis of motion.

Resting length *(Chapter 4).* A muscle's resting length is the point at which there are the most available actin-myosin crossbridges.

Resting position *(Chapter 1).* A position of a joint at which there is the least congruency and the most slack in the capsule and ligaments; this position is often near the joint's midrange.

Resting potential *(Chapter 3).* Charge across nerve or muscle membrane at equilibrium; ranges from –60 to –90 mV.

Resting tremor *(Chapter 3).* A tremor occurring in a body part that is not being voluntarily activated and is supported against gravity; a symptom of Parkinson's disease, secondary to basal ganglia dysfunction.

Resultant vector *(Chapter 2).* When two or more forces are applied to an object or body segment, a resultant force is created as a combination of these forces. The resultant force will have a direction and magnitude that reflects the combination of these forces and is the resultant vector.

Retinacular system *(Chapter 7).* This is a complex fascial and ligamentous arrangement that provide functions on both the palmar and dorsal hand. These functions include enclosing, compartmentalizing, and restraining the joints and tendons as well as the nerves, blood vessels, and skin.

Retraction *(Chapter 1, 5).* The lateral end of the clavicle and the scapula move posteriorly in a curvilinear fashion, and the medial borders of the scapula approach the midline. This motion is also called scapular adduction. At the sternoclavicular joint, the total range for protraction and retraction is approximately 25°.

Retroversion *(Chapter 5, 9).* Posterior rotation or a backward rotation. In the hip, it may clinically present as out-toeing (lateral rotation) during standing and walking.

Rigidity *(Chapter 3).* Heightened resistance to passive movement, but independent of the velocity of a stretch or movement. Associated with lesions of the basal ganglia, and appears to be the result of excessive supraspinal drive acting upon a normal spinal reflex mechanism. There are two types of rigidity, lead pipe and cogwheel. A constant resistance to movement throughout the range characterizes **lead pipe rigidity**, whereas **cogwheel rigidity** is characterized by alternate episodes of resistance and relaxation. Rigidity is frequently associated with lesions of the basal ganglia, commonly seen in Parkinson's disease.

Rocking *(Chapter 1).* A synonym for basic joint motion of "rolling." See rolling.

Rolling *(Chapter 1, 13).* When discussing joints, it is a rotary or angular type of basic joint motion whereby each subsequent point on one articulating surface contacts a new point on the other surface, such as in "rolling" a ball across the floor. Also called rocking. When discussing body movement, it is moving the body from supine to prone, or from prone to supine, usually involving some amount of trunk rotation.

Rotary motion *(Chapter 2).* Movement around an axis which occurs in an arc or circular movement. Also called angular displacement or angular motion. Joint movement is rotary motion.

Rotation *(Chapter 1).* Angular motion of a bony lever around an axis.

Running *(Chapter 12).* A gait wherein the swing phase is longer than the stance phase and there are two periods within one gait cycle when neither lower limb is in contact with the ground.

S

Saddle joint *(Chapter 1).* A type of biaxial joint in which each bony partner has a concave and convex surface oriented perpendicular to each other; like a rider in a saddle; such as seen in the carpometacarpal joint of the thumb.

Sagittal plane *(Chapter 1).* Or YZ plane, so named because it is parallel to the sagittal suture of the skull, dividing the body into right and left sides. It is the plane within which flexion and extension movements occur.

Sarcolemma *(Chapter 4).* Cell membrane surrounding a muscle fiber.

Sarcomere *(Chapter 3, 4).* Contractile unit of muscle fiber; made up of actin and myosin myofilaments.

Sarcoplasmic reticulum *(Chapter 3, 4).* A component of the endoplasmic reticulum of a muscle cell; involved in the storage and release of calcium ions during contractile process.

Scalar quantities *(Chapter 2).* Items that have only one dimension. It has magnitude but no direction; e.g., 5 horses, 3 shoes, 1 mile.

Scaption *(Chapter 5).* Shoulder elevation in the scapular plane. This term was first coined by Dr. J. Perry and has become a universally accepted term for this motion.

Scapulohumeral rhythm *(Chapter 5).* The synchronous motion between the scapula and humerus during glenohumeral elevation. Although not consistent throughout, there is roughly a 2:1 ratio of glenohumeral motion to scapular motion.

Scoliosis *(Chapter 8).* A postural deviation such that there is a lateral curvature of the vertebral column.

Screw home mechanism *(Chapter 10).* The terminal lateral rotation of the tibia on the femur that occurs in nonweight bearing because the lateral femoral condyle has completed its motion but the medial femoral condyle has not so the lateral condyles rotate as the medial condyles complete their motion. The motion in weight bearing is medial rotation of the femur on the tibia. Also called terminal rotation of the knee.

Second order neurons *(Chapter 3).* Sensory neurons that receive synaptic input from a peripheral sensory neuron (from a first order neuron) and conduct action potentials from the spinal cord or brainstem to sensory centers in the CNS.

Sellar joint *(Chapter 1).* Joint surface type so named because the surfaces resemble the matching of a rider in a saddle, both surfaces having convex and concave surfaces perpendicular to each other, such as seen in the carpometacarpal joint of the thumb and the ankle (talocrural joint).

Semilunar notch *(Chapter 6).* Also called the trochlear notch. Concave surface, shaped like a half moon, on proximal ulna that articulates with the trochlea of the humerus at the elbow joint.

Series elastic component *(Chapter 4).* The term given to a muscle's tendons because of the alignment of tendon–muscle–tendon. Force transmission is provided in series from the muscle to the tendon to the bone.

Sesamoid bone *(Chapter 10).* A small bone that lies within a tendon. It serves to protect the tendon and change the angle of pull of the tendon.

Shaft of the femur *(Chapter 9).* Bony body of the femoral bone.

Shoulder complex *(Chapter 5).* See shoulder girdle.

Shoulder girdle *(Chapter 5).* Combination of the scapula, clavicle, and manubrium, together with left and right components that form a girdle around the upper thorax.

Shoulder joint *(Chapter 5).* Connection between the glenoid fossa and the humeral head.

Sigma (Σ) *(Chapter 2).* Greek symbol used in formulas to signify sum or addition total.

Sigmoid notch *(Chapter 7).* See ulnar notch.

Single-limb support *(Chapter 12).* When only one lower extremity is in stance phase. This occurs during the middle 40% of the stance cycle.

Sinus tarsi *(Chapter 11).* Channel that runs between the articulations of the talus and the calcaneus, housing proprioceptors; it may be palpated slightly distal and lateral to the talar dome.

Sliding *(Chapter 1).* A translatory or linear type of basic joint motion whereby one point of reference contacts new points across the adjacent surface and the movement of one joint surface is parallel to the plane of the adjoining joint surface, such as when a figure skater "glides" across the ice. Also referred to as gliding.

Sliding filament theory *(Chapter 3).* Theoretical concept that actin and myosin filaments slide past each other during muscle contraction.

Slow-twitch fiber *(Chapter 3).* Type I or tonic muscle fibers; use a slow oxidative metabolic process and are resistant to fatigue.

Slug *(Chapter 2).* Term for mass in the US system. 1 slug = 14.59 kg. 1 pound = 0.031 slugs.

Soft end feel *(Chapter 1).* A feeling that is felt at the end of joint range when soft tissue, typically fleshy muscular bulk, approximates and stops further motion.

Somatosensory *(Chapter 3).* Pertaining to sensation.

Space diagram *(Chapter 2).* See free body diagram.

Spasticity *(Chapter 3).* A condition of increased muscular tone which produces involuntary and rapid contractions and relaxations and an associated hyperreflex response. See hypertonicity.

Spatial characteristics *(Chapter 12).* Those variables that are defined in terms of length, width, or depth. They identify characteristics that include space. In gait, they include items such as step width, step length, and stride length.

Speed *(Chapter 4).* The rate of motion.

Spinal shock *(Chapter 3).* Time of profound depression of motor function in which all muscles of the affected body segments are involved; used to describe the temporary flaccid state in the person with a spinal cord injury when the nervous system is in a state of shock after a lesion or acute onset.

Spinous process *(Chapter 8).* A process on the posterior aspect of vertebra that form the neural arch of the vertebra. The transverse processes are the other two processes along with the laminae that form the neural arch.

Spinning *(Chapter 1).* A rotary or angular basic joint motion whereby one point of contact on each surface remains in constant contact with a fixed location on the other surface, such as in "spinning" a top.

Spondylolisthesis *(Chapter 8).* A pathological condition usually seen in the lumbar spine in which the vertebral body of one segment slips forward of the one below it.

Sprinting *(Chapter 12).* Running as fast a possible for short distances.

Stable equilibrium *(Chapter 2).* When the center of gravity of a body is disturbed slightly and the body tends to return the center of gravity to its former position.

Stance phase *(Chapter 12).* The period of the gait cycle when the foot is in contact with the ground.

Step duration *(Chapter 12).* A temporal characteristic of gait defined as the amount of time the foot is in contact with the ground.

Step length *(Chapter 12).* The distance between the initial contact of one foot to the initial contact of the opposite foot.

Stepping or reaching strategies *(Chapter 12).* The use of steps, hops, or reaches to maintain the center of mass within the base of support. This strategy is usually used during fast changes of line of gravity and requires an adjustment of the COM position.

Step width *(Chapter 12).* The horizontal distance between the two feet measured from the midpoint of one heel to the midpoint of the next heel contact, typically from 2 to 4 inches (7–9 cm) for adults.

Stiff-leg gait *(Chapter 12).* Characterized by extension at the trunk, posterior tilt of the pelvis, and excessive hip and knee extension usually in combination with medial rotation and adduction of the hips.

Stiffness *(Chapter 3).* A change in the viscoelastic physical properties of the muscle accompanying hypertonicity, which contributes to the increased resistance to passive stretch.

Strain *(Chapter 4).* The body, segment, or muscle's ability to withstand a stress that is applied to it. The amount of deformation it is able to tolerate before it succumbs to the stress.

Stratum fibrosum *(Chapter 1).* Thick outer layer of joint capsule primarily comprised of dense irregular fibrous tissue, laden with joint receptors.

Stratum synovium *(Chapter 1).* The inner, highly vascular layer of the joint capsule; it produces and secretes synovial fluid.

Strength *(Chapter 4).* The ability of a muscle to develop or produce force or generate active tension.

Stress *(Chapter 4).* A load or force applied to a body, segment, or muscle.

Stress fracture *(Chapter 4).* Application of a repetitive force on a bone that causes breakdown of that bone; application of the stress-strain principle to bone.

Stress-strain curve *(Chapter 4).* The relationship between a structure's ability to absorb the forces applied to it. Every structure has its unique strain quality to deform as a stress is progressively applied to it, and every structure also has its breaking point at which no further stress is tolerated. Also referred to as stress-strain principle.

Stretch reflex *(Chapter 3).* Or myotatic reflex is a monosynaptic simple reflex arc, mediated at the spinal cord level whereby a change in muscle length (stretch) of a sufficient amount and at a sufficient rate, will activate the muscle spindle eliciting a reflex contraction of the agonist muscle undergoing the stretch.

Stretch-shortening cycle *(Chapter 4).* A type of activity that uses a rapid eccentric activity of a muscle followed quickly by a sudden and forceful concentric activity of the same muscle. It is also more commonly referred to as plyometrics or plyometric exercises and is used in many sports activities.

Stride length *(Chapter 12).* The distance between initial contact of one foot to initial contact of that same foot again; equivalent to one gait cycle.

Structure fatigue *(Chapter 4).* Fatigue of a structure that occurs with the application of repeated stresses so the accumulation of stresses causes failure of the structure.

Subluxation *(Chapter 1).* Abnormal condition that occurs when there is a separation of the two bony partners and the joint partners are partially disassociated from each other, but usually there is no rupture of the connecting tissue.

Superior pubic ramus *(Chapter 9).* Bony aspect of superior pubic bone; attachment site for most of the muscles that adduct the hip.

Supination *(Chapter 1, 11).* Triplanar motion of the foot and ankle that occurs differently in the open kinetic chain than it does in the closed kinetic chain. In the open kinetic chain, the combined motions include inversion, adduction, and plantarflexion. In the closed kinetic chain, the motions include dorsiflexion, abduction, and inversion.

Suprapatellar pouch *(Chapter 10).* A pouch formed by the proximal expansion of the synovial lining of the knee. It extends proximal to the patella and lies between the femur and quadriceps muscle. It provides an area within which the patella moves during knee flexion to ultimately provide an increased ability to flex the knee.

Supraspinatus outlet *(Chapter 5).* The area under the coracoacromial arch.

Sustentaculum tali *(Chapter 11).* A portion of the middle calcaneus that projects medially to serve as a shelf on which the talus sits.

Swing phase *(Chapter 12).* The period of the gait cycle when the foot is not in contact with the ground.

Symphysis *(Chapter 8).* The point of contact between two bones that is separated in early development or early life but becomes fused later in life.

Symphysis pubis *(Chapter 9).* Amphiarthrodial connection between the two pubic bones anteriorly.

Synarthrosis *(Chapter 1).* Joints whose primary purpose is to offer stability and are therefore largely fibrous in structure, such as seen in the sutures of the skull or the syndesmosis at the tibiofibular articulation.

Syndesmosis *(Chapter 1).* A subtype of synarthrodial joint, such as found longitudinally between the radius and ulna and between the tibia and fibula, where these pairs of bones are joined by a strong interosseous membrane in order to maintain a close relationship of the bones next to each with little or no mobility allowed.

Synergist *(Chapter 4).* The muscle or muscle group that assists the agonist to produce the desired motion.

Synergy *(Chapter 3).* Functional muscle groups that work together to produce motor behavior. In pathological conditions, synergy is also used to describe impaired motor control whereby muscles are activated as a bound unit.

Synovial fluid *(Chapter 1).* A pale, viscous fluid secreted by the capsule into the joint space, constantly nourishing and lubricating the joint surfaces.

Synovial joint *(Chapter 1).* A term used interchangeably with diarthrodial joint.

T

Tangential force vector *(Chapter 2).* In resultant vector configurations, this vector is the component that produces either a compressive or a distraction force to a segment moving around its axis. When the force vector is parallel to the lever arm, all of the force is either compressing or distracting the joint.

Temporal characteristics *(Chapter 12).* Variables that are defined by time; examples include velocity, acceleration, power, and cadence.

Tendinopathy *(Chapter 4).* Application of the stress-strain curve to a tendon; repetitive stress applied to a tendon that does not allow recovery sufficiently to restore tendon strength causes break down of that tendon.

Tenodesis *(Chapter 4, 7).* When passive tension of tendons produce movements of joints as the muscle is elongated over two or more joints. For example, extending the wrist places passive tension on the long finger flexors, allowing the fingers to grasp an object even though active finger flexion does not occur.

Terminal rotation of the knee *(Chapter 10).* See screw home mechanism.

Terminal stance *(Chapter 12).* The fourth subphase of the stance phase of gait. It is during this time that the heel is lifted off the ground.

Terminal swing *(Chapter 12).* Third and final subphase of the swing phase of gait. The extremity prepares to impact the ground.

Thoracic outlet syndrome *(Chapter 8).* Pathological condition producing pain and dysfunction. In this condition, the ventral nerve roots of cervical nerves and/or blood vessels become compressed secondary to anatomical anomalies, hypertrophy, spasm, or poor posture.

Tibial torsion *(Chapter 11).* Angle created between the alignment of the knee and the alignment of the ankle. It is caused by the tibia's longitudinal lateral rotation. Normal measurements are 15° to 40° in the adult.

Tonic *(Chapter 3).* Qualitative description given to a receptor or a muscle, referring to the type of activity it generates; in this case, signifying continuous activity.

Tract *(Chapter 3).* Axonal bundles of upper motor neurons with common origin, function, and termination.

Torque *(Chapter 2).* Force applied to produce rotation. It is the product of the force times the perpendicular distance from its line of action to the axis of motion. It is symbolized in formulas as τ.

Torque arm *(Chapter 2).* Moment arm (lever arm) of a rotational force.

Transfer *(Chapter 13).* Movement of the body from one surface or position to another. It may be accomplished independently, with assistance, or with supervision.

Translatory motion *(Chapter 2).* Motion in which all points on the moving object travel the same distance, in the same direction with the same velocity and at the same time; further clarified as being rectilinear if the movement is in a straight line or curvilinear in which motions travel in a curved path such as that seen when tossing a ball to a friend. Also called linear motion.

Transverse plane *(Chapter 1).* A plane of motion so named because it is parallel to the horizon and the floor, dividing the body into upper and lower parts, like a view from above. It is the plane within which rotational movements occur. Also called the XZ plane or the horizontal plane.

Transverse process *(Chapter 8).* There are two on each vertebra. They sit on either side of the spinous process, and with the spinous process and laminae, form the vertebral arch.

Transverse tubular system *(Chapter 3).* "T" system; a component of the endoplasmic reticulum of a muscle cell which speeds the transmission of a muscle action potential to all portions of the muscle fiber.

Tremor *(Chapter 3).* A rhythmical, involuntary, oscillatory movement of a body part, symptomatic of damage to the CNS.

Trendelenburg gait *(Chapter 9, 12).* Pathological gait caused by weakness of the gluteus medius. During stance phase, the contralateral hip drops since the gluteus medius is unable to hold the pelvis level.

Trendelenburg sign *(Chapter 9).* Clinical sign characterized by dropping of the pelvis on the unweighted side during unilateral stance; associated with a severely weakened or paralyzed gluteus medius on the stance limb.

Triangular fibrocartilage (TFCC) *(Chapter 7).* Name given to articular disc at the distal or inferior radioulnar joint, so named because of its shape.

Triaxial joint *(Chapter 1).* A joint that moves in three planes around three axes having three degrees of freedom, such as seen at the hip and glenohumeral joint.

Triceps surae *(Chapter 11).* The superficial posterior calf muscles of the medial and lateral gastrocnemius along with the soleus are called the triceps surae.

Triplanar axis *(Chapter 11).* A joint axis that is not perpendicular to the cardinal planes but intersects all three planes.

Trochlea *(Chapter 6).* Bony prominence that usually articulates with a concave surface such as a groove or notch. The distal humerus is an example of a trochlea.

Trochlear groove *(Chapter 11).* Groove that separates portions of the trochlea of the humerus. See intercondylar groove.

Trochlear notch *(Chapter 6).* Concave surface that interfaces with a trochlear notch. An example is the semilunar notch of the proximal ulna articulating with the trochlea of the humerus at the elbow joint.

Trochlear ridge *(Chapter 6).* Ridge that runs between trochlea. This is seen when a bone such as the humerus articulates with more than one bone—the radius and ulna—at its distal joint.

Type I fiber *(Chapter 3).* Also referred to as slow-twitch or slow-oxidative; contains large number of mitochondria and high concentration of myoglobin, uses oxidative enzymes and aerobic metabolism, and is fatigue-resistant.

Type II fiber *(Chapter 3).* Also referred to as fast-twitch or fast-glycolytic; contains few mitochondria and little myoglobin, uses glycolytic enzymes and anaerobic metabolism, and fatigues quickly.

U

Ulnar abduction *(Chapter 1, 7).* In the anatomic position, wrist movement in the frontal plane through an anterior-posterior axis that moves the hand toward the side of the body and the little finger. Also known as ulnar flexion or ulnar deviation.

Ulnar collateral ligament *(Chapter 6).* The three part stabilizing ligament located on the medial side of the elbow. It contributes the primary stability in the frontal plane. Also referred to as the medial collateral ligament of the elbow.

Ulnar deviation *(Chapter 1, 7).* See ulnar abduction.

Ulnar notch *(Chapter 7).* The distal ulnar notch on the radius that serves as the articulating surface for the distal radioulnar joint. Also called the sigmoid notch.

Ulnar styloid process *(Chapter 7).* Bony projection palpated, when the forearm is pronated, on the ulnar side of the wrist. It is the distal end of the ulna.

Ulnar tuberosity *(Chapter 6).* The bony landmark located on the anterior proximal ulna, inferior to the coronoid process; an attachment site for the brachialis muscle.

Uniaxial joint *(Chapter 1).* Joint that moves in one plane around one axis having one degree of freedom; including two types—hinge or pivot.

Unipennate muscles *(Chapter 4).* Muscles whose fibers have one parallel fiber arrangement.

Unstable equilibrium *(Chapter 2).* Center of gravity of a body is disturbed and the body does not to return the center of gravity to its former position and falls.

Upper motor neurons *(Chapter 3).* Neurons located within the CNS.

V

Valgus *(Chapter 10).* A condition in which the distal portion of a joint segment is positioned outward or away from the midline of the body. Also referred to as valgum.

Varus *(Chapter 10).* A condition in which the distal portion of a joint segment is positioned inward or towards the midline of the body. Also referred to as varum.

Vector quantity *(Chapter 2).* Physical quantity that has two dimensions—magnitude and direction. Forces are directional quantities.

Velocity *(Chapter 2, 12).* A temporal characteristic; the rate of motion in a specific direction. In gait, it is the distance covered in a unit of time such as meters per second or miles per hour.

Viscoelasticity *(Chapter 4).* A structure that has the characteristics of both viscosity and elasticity. Most tissue is viscoelastic; viscoelastic tissue has the ability to withstand forces or loads to resist changing shape, but if the force is sufficient, the structure's shape changes and does not return to its original shape.

Viscosity *(Chapter 4).* Resistance a structure has to an external force or load that causes a permanent deformation of the structure.

W

Walking *(Chapter 12).* Particular form of gait; the most common of human locomotor patterns.

Weakness *(Chapter 3).* Inability to generate normal levels of muscular force.

Weight *(Chapter 2).* Force of gravity acting on a mass; measured in pounds (lb) or Newtons (N).

White matter *(Chapter 3).* Term used to describe areas of CNS that contain predominantly nerve tracts and axons, covered in myelin.

Z

Zygapophyseal joints *(Chapter 8).* Also called facet joints or apophyseal joints. These joints are formed by the inferior articular processes of a superior vertebra and the superior articular processes of the immediately adjacent inferior vertebra. There is one inferior process and one superior process forming two zygapophyseal joints with its inferior and superior vertebrae on each side of the vertebra, respectively. Zygapophyseal joints are synovial joints.

Index

Note: Page numbers in *italic* type indicate figures, boxes, or tables.

A

A-bands, 94, 95
Abdominal oblique muscles, 347, *348*, *348–349*, *351*
Abduction, 9
- deltoid, 197
- finger, 302–303, *304*
- foot, 480, *481*
- glenohumeral joint, 180–182
- hip and pelvis, 385, *386–387*, 403–405, 412–414, *415*, 559–560
- scapular plane glenohumeral, 183

Abductor digiti minimi, 279, *282*, *512*
Abductor hallucis, 511, *512*, *516*
Abductor pollicis brevis, 279, *281*
Abductor pollicis longus, 274, 279
Abnormal muscle tone, 115
Absorption phase in running, 575
Acceleration phase, 31, 34
- baseball pitching, 640
- golf swing, 655–656
- soccer instep kick, 646–647
- tennis serve, 659–660

Accessory movements, 22
Acetabula fossa, 380
Acetabular anteversion angle, 378–379
Acetabular labrum, 381
Acetabulofemoral articulation, 380–381
Acetabulum, 372, 374
- biomechanical angulations of, 378–379
- hip joint, 380–381

Acetylcholine, 94–95
Achilles, 478
Acromioclavicular joint, 164, 166–168, 173–175
Acromion process, 163–164
Actin, 91–93, 94, *95*
Action potentials, 85
Action-reaction, 34–35
Activation, muscle, 127–128
Active excursion of muscles, 144–150
- leverage and length-tension interactions, 145–146
- open kinetic chain vs. closed kinetic chain, 149–150
- positive and negative work in, 146–149

Active insufficiency, 144–145
Active tension, 140–141
Adduction, 9
- deltoid, 197
- finger, 302–303, *304*
- foot, 480, *481*
- glenohumeral joint, 180
- hip and pelvis, 385, *386–387*, 402–403, 415, 417, 560

Adductor brevis, 390, 391, *395*, 402, *402*
Adductor hallucis, *514*
Adductor longus, 390, 391, *394*, 402, *402*
Adductor magnus, 390, 391, *395*, *402*, 402–403
Adductor pollicis, 280, *283*, *286*
Adductor tubercle, *376*
Adenosine diphosphate, 93, 95, 96
Adenosine triphosphate, 93, 95, 96, 148
ADP. *See* Adenosine diphosphate
Adult gait pattern, 565–567
Adult hemiplegia, 569–570
Afferent nerve fibers, 86, 88, 90
- muscle spindle as, 101–102

Afferent receptors, 84
Age and muscle strength, 141, *142*
Agonist muscles, 129
- elbow and forearm complex, 244

All-or-none law, 98
Alpha motor neurons, 98
Ambulation, 536
- spotting during, 610–612

Amphiarthrodial joints, *12*, *13*, 18
Anatomic activity, muscle, 128–129
Anatomic pulleys, 72–73
Anatomical position, 5–6
Anatomical snuff box, 256, *258*
Anconeus, 240, 247
Angle of inclination, 165, 375–377
Angle of progression, 547
Angle of torsion, 165, 377–378, *378*
Angle of Wiberg, 378
Angles
- cubital or carrying, 224
- forces acting at, 45–47, *48*, *49*
- laws of the right triangle and, 49–51

Angular joint displacements, 548
Angular motion, 10
Angular velocity, 59, *60*
Ankle and foot, 475, 526
- anterior muscles, 507–510
- arches, 477, 520–523
- base of support and, 56–57, *58*
- bones, 475–479
- calf muscles and, 504–505
- deformities, 524–525
- function of the pretibial group, 509–510
- function of the triceps surae, 502–503
- functional stance control at, 540
- hallux valgus, 525
- intrinsic muscles, 510–517, 561
- joints, 480–497
- lateral muscles, 505–507
- leg bones, 475–477
- ligaments, *484–488*
- loading, 523–524
- metatarsal bones, 479
- motion terminology, 480
- muscles, 497–525
- pain, 478
- pes cavus, *524*, 525
- pes planus, 524–525
- phalanges, 479
- plantarflexion, 456, 560–561
- posterior muscles, 497–505
- posture recovery strategies, 542–543
- pronation and supination, 480, *482*, 517–520
- running and, 568, 577, 578, 580–583
- tarsal bones, 477–479
- walking and, 551–552, 554, 568

Ankle and foot joints
- calcaneocuboid, 493–495
- functional stance control at, 540
- intermetatarsal, *488*, 496–497
- interphalangeal, 262–263, *488*, 497
- metatarsophalangeal, *488*, 497
- midtarsal, 553
- motion terminology and, 480
- pronation and supination and, 518–519
- subtalar, *484–486*, 489–492, *493*, 518–520, 553
- talocrural, 482–483, *484–485*, 489, 519–520
- talonavicular, *486*, 493
- tarsometatarsal, *487*, 495–496, 520
- tibiofibular, 480–482
- transverse tarsal, *486*, 492–495, *496*

Ankle and foot muscles
- abductor digiti minimi, *512*
- abductor hallucis, 511, *512*, *516*
- adductor hallucis, *514*
- anterior group, 507–510
- calf muscles and, 504–505
- dorsal interossei, *514*
- extensor digitorum brevis, 511, *515*, *517*
- extensor digitorum longus, *508*, 509, *511*
- extensor hallucis longus, *508*, 509, *510*
- flexor digiti minimi brevis, *514*
- flexor digitorum brevis, *512*, *516*

flexor digitorum longus, *499,* 503, 504–505
flexor hallucis brevis, 511, *513*
flexor hallucis longus, *500,* 503, 504–505
function of, 511, 516–525
function of the pretibial group, 509–510
function of the triceps surae, 502–503
gastrocnemius, 450, *498,* 501, 502
intrinsic, 510–511, 510–517, *512–515*
lateral group, 505–507
lumbricals, *513*
peroneus brevis, 505–507
peroneus longus, 505–507, 522
peroneus tertius, *508*
plantaris, *447,* 450, *498,* 501
posterior group, 497–505
quadratus plantae, *513*
running and, 568, 577, 578, 582–583
soleus, *498,* 501, 502
tibialis anterior, 507–509, *510*
tibialis posterior, *499,* 503, 504–505
Ankle strategy, 542–543
Annular ligament, *226,* 230, 231
Annulus fibrosus, 322
Antagonist muscles, 129–130
elbow and forearm complex, 244
synergistic muscle actions and, 203–204, *205*
Anteromedial band, 435
Anterior and lateral trunk muscles, 343, 347, 351
Anterior ankle and foot muscles, 507–510
Anterior cervical muscles, 336, *337–339,* 341
Anterior cruciate ligament (ACL), *431,* 434–435
injury, 462, 463
Anterior inferior iliac spine (AIIS), 372
Anterior longitudinal ligaments (ALL), 323
Anterior meniscofemoral ligament, *433*
Anterior pelvic tilt, 382
Anterior radioulnar ligament, *227,* 232
Anterior scalene muscles, 336, *338*
Anterior superior iliac spine (ASIS), 372
Anterior talofibular ligament, *484*
Anterior vertebral joint elements, 322–324
Anterior-posterior tilting of the scapula, 169–170
Anterolateral bundle, 435
Anteversion, 377–378
angle, acetabular, 378–379
Antigravity muscles, 104–105, 537
Apophyseal plate, 220
Application of resistances to the body, 69–70
Arches, foot, 477, 520–523
Arcuate ligament, *432*
Aristotle, 3
Arm(s)
external moment, 61, 63
force, 38, 40
golf swing and, 652–656
internal moment, 61, 63
lever, 32, 59
moment, 32, 45, 138–139, 205–206
pitching activities and, 636–644
resistance, 38, 40
tennis serve and, 656–660
Arthrokinematics, 5, 17–25. *See also* Kinematics
basic joint motions, 20–24
calcaneocuboid joint, 494–495
clinical applications, 24–25
close-packed and open-packed joint positions, 24
definition of, 17
finger motions, 290–291
foot, 489
glenohumeral joint, 182–183
humeroulnar and humeroradial joints, 223–224
joint axes in function, 23–24, *24*
joint shapes as they pertain to, 22–23, *23*
joint structure and, 18–20
patellofemoral joint, 441
pelvis and hip, 388
proximal radioulnar joint, 230
sternoclavicular joint, 172–173
subtalar joint, 492
tibiofemoral joint, 439
tibiofibular joint, 482
types of joints and, 17
wrist motions, 289–290
Arthrology, 18
Articularis genu, 449
Articulations, radioulnar, 229–232
Assembly line workers, 608–609
Association neurons, 90
Ataxia, 571–572
Athetosis, 119
Atlanto-axial joint, 326–327
ATP. *See* Adenosine triphosphate
ATPase activity, 95, 96
Atrophy, 135
disuse, 115
Attachments, muscle, 128–129
Attrition, 180
Axes of motion, 5–6
in function, 23–24
Axial rotation, 437–438
Axial skeleton, 162. *See also* Head, neck, and trunk region; Vertebral column
center of gravity, 315–316
components, 315
Axons, 88–89
corticospinal tract, 109–110
gamma, 101
reticulospinal tract, 109

B

Backswing phase, soccer instep kick, 644–646
Balance of forces occurring in symmetric stance, 540–542
Balance scale, 38–39
Balanced forces in normal hand function, 303–307
Ball-and-socket joints, 11, *12*
Basal ganglia, 110, 111–112
disorders, 119
Base of support, 56–57, *58*
Baseball pitching, 636–641
Bending and lifting, forward, 355–357
Biaxial joints, 11, *12, 13*
Biceps brachii, 195–196, 201, 232, 239, 246, 248, *249*
Biceps femoris, 390, *397,* 403, *445, 448,* 449
Biceps tendon, *195*
Bicipital aponeurosis, *233*
Bicipital groove, 183
Bifurcated ligament, *486*
Biomechanical angulations
of the acetabulum, 378–379
of the femur, 375–378
Biomechanics, 4
Bipedal movement, 536
Bipennate muscles, 136
Body
applying resistance to the, 69–70
base of support, 56–57, *58*
center of gravity and center of mass, 52–55
diagrams, free, 60–61, *63, 64, 67*
force applications to the, 51–52
motion and segment, 6, 30
muscles and levers and forces on the, 57–59, *60, 61*
neutral equilibrium, 55–56
stable equilibrium, 55–56
unstable equilibrium, 55–56
Bones, ankle and foot
leg bones, 475–477
metatarsal, 479
phalanges, 479
tarsal, 477–479
Bones, elbow and forearm complex
humerus, 219–220
radius, 221
ulna, 220–221
Bones, femur, 374–379
Bones, knee, 425–428
femur, 425–426
patella, *426,* 427–428
tibia, 426–427
Bones, pelvis, 371–374
Bones, shoulder complex
acromioclavicular joint, 164, 166–168, 173–175
clavicle, 163
glenohumeral joint, 163, 166–168
humerus, 165–166
manubrium, 163
scapula, 163–165
scapulothoracic joint, 167–168, 175–176
sternoclavicular joint, 170–173
Bones, vertebral column, 315–321

Bones, wrist and hand, 255–256
 carpal, 256–258
 distal radius, 256
 distal ulna, 256
 metacarpals, 258–259
 phalanges, 259
Bony end feel, 16
Borelli, Giovanni, 3
BOS. *See* Base of support
Boutonnière deformity, 305
Brachialis, 232, 246, 248, *249*
Brachioradialis, 239, *240,* 240–241, 248, *249*
Brainstem, 107, 109, 110
Breathing and coughing, 359
British units, 33
Bruxism, 362
Bursae, 180
 elbow complex, 228
Bursitis
 greater trochanteric, 389
 olecranon, 228

C

Cadence, 547
Calcaneocuboid joint, 493–495
Calcaneofibular ligament, *485*
Calcaneus, 478, 518–519, 524
Calcium, 95
Calculation
 of joint forces, 65–69
 of muscle forces, 61–65
Calf muscles, 504–505
Capitate bone, 256
 ligaments, 263–265
Capitulotrochlear groove, 220
Capitulum, lateral, 219
Capsular end feel, 16
Capsular reinforcement, glenohumeral joint, 177–180
Capsules, joint, 18–19
 foot, 483
 knee, 435–436
Cardinal planes, 5, *6*
Carpal bones, 256–258
Carpal tunnel syndrome, 310
Carpometacarpal (CMC) joint, 260, *261, 261–262,* 305
Carrying angle, 224
Cartilaginous plates, 322
Catalysts, 95
Cell(s)
 membranes, 84–85
 muscle, 90
Center edge angle, 378
Center of gravity, 52–55, 58, *62,* 542
 axial skeleton, 315–316
 stable, unstable, and neutral equilibrium and, 55–56
Center of mass, 52–55, 61, *62,* 539–540, 541, 548
 determinants of gait and, 567–568
 ground reaction forces and, 555–556
 orthopedic gait and, 572–574
 running and, 581–583
Center of motion, 56–57
Center of pressure, 556
Central nervous system, 86
 association neurons, 90
 cerebrovascular accident and, 119
 dynamic action system model, 108
 gray matter, 90
 motor control and, 107–108
 muscle weakness and, 113–115
 nerve fibers in, 89–90
 postural tone and, 105, *106*
 tremors and, 116
Cerebellum, 111
 disorders, 119
Cerebral motor centers, 109–110
Cerebral palsy, 118, 568–569
Cerebrovascular accident, 119
 gait and, 569–570
Cervical ligament, *486*
Cervical muscles
 anterior, 336, *337–339,* 341
 posterior, *340,* 341–342
Cervical vertebrae
 C-7 prominence, 320
 first and second, 318–319
 joints, 326–327
 third to sixth, 319–320
Cervical vertebral articulations, 327
Chains, kinematic, 16–17
Challenges to gait efficiency, 568–574
Change of motion, 31
Characteristics, muscle
 creep, 134
 elasticity and extensibility, 131, 133
 stress-strain, 133–134
 viscosity, 131
Children, gait pattern of, 565
Cholinesterase, 95
Chopart's joint, 492
Circumduction, 11
Classifications
 of motor and sensory nerve fibers on basis of axonal diameter in peripheral nervous system, 88–89
 nervous system, 86–87
 of sensory fibers on the basis of fiber origin within the peripheral nervous system, 89
Clavicle, 163
 absent, 172
 sternoclavicular joint and, 166–168, 170–173
Clinical applications
 of externally applied forces, 70–75
 neuromuscular impairments and, 113–116
Clinical goniometry, 11, 14
Clinician activities, 609–610
Closed kinematic chains (CKC), 16–17
 ankle and foot and, *518*
 elbow complex and, 247
Close-packed joint position, 24
Club foot, *524,* 525
CMC joint. *See* Carpometacarpal (CMC) joint
Coactivation, 115
Coccygeal joints, 335
Coccyx, 320–321
Cocking phase, tennis serve, 657–659
COG. *See* Center of gravity
Collagen, 136
Collateral ligaments, 430, *431, 488*
COM. *See* Center of mass; Center of motion
Component vectors, 45
Composition of forces, 36–37
Compression, joint, 69–70
 patellofemoral joint, 458–460
Computer stations, 606–607
Concentric muscle activity, 127
Concurrent force system, 46
Condyles
 knee, 425, 435
 mandible, 317–318, *319, 320*
Condyloid joints, 11, *12*
Constraints, movement, 108
Contraction, muscle, 94
 excitation-contraction coupling, 95
 gradation of strength of, 98–99
 sliding filament model, 94, 95–96
 speed of, 139–140
 synergistic, 244
Contralateral motor control, 110, 111
Control, motor, 107–108
 within the brainstem, 109
 cerebral motor centers, 109–110
 dynamic systems approach to understanding, 108
 integration to produce functional movement, 112–113
 intermediate control centers, 111–112
 at the spinal region, 108–109
Conversion factors, *32*
Convex-concave principle, 23
Coordination problems, 115–116
Coracoacromial arch, 179–180, 201
Coracoacromial ligament, 179
Coracobrachialis, *194,* 200
Coracohumeral ligament, 177–178
Coracoid process, 164
Coronal plane, 6
Coronary ligament, 429
Coronoid fossa, 220
Coronoid process, 220, *225, 233, 319*
Cortex, motor, 110
Corticospinal tract, 109
Cosine, 49–51
Costal joints, 327–329
Costoclavicular ligament, 171
Coughing and breathing, 359
Counternutation, 333
Coupling
 excitation-contraction, 95
 vertebral, 325–326

Coxa valga, 377, 378
Coxa vara, 377, 378
Creep, 134
Cricoid cartilage, *320*
Crossbridges, 93
  mechanisms differences, 148
Crouch gait, 570
Cruciate ligaments, *431,* 434–435
Crus, 482
Cubital angle, 224
Cubital valgus, 224
Cubitus varus, 224
Cuboid, 478, 479
Cuneiforms, three, 479
Curves, vertebral column, 315–316
Curvilinear motion, 10
Cycle, gait, 543–545
Cycling, 660–663
Cylindrical grip, 291, *293, 296*

D

Da Vinci, Leonardo, 3
Daily functional activities
  clinician activities, 609–614
  donning socks or pants, 624–626
  driving, 626–627
  feeding, 623–624
  household tasks, 604–606
  mobility, 594–602
  occupational and, 602–609
  occupational tasks, 606–609
  pouring, 627, *628*
  requiring primarily elbow movement, 623–626
  requiring primarily shoulder complex movement, 618–622
  turning a key, 627–629
  vacuuming, 604–606
Deceleration phase, baseball pitching, 640–641
Deep intrinsic (midpalm) muscles, 280, *283*
Deep tendon reflex, 102, *103, 104*
Deep transverse metatarsal ligament, *488*
Deficiency applications, shoulder complex, 208–209
Deformities of the foot, 524–525
Degenerative disc disease, 329
Degrees of freedom, 11, *12*
  elbow and forearm complex, 218
Delayed-onset muscle soreness, 151
Deltoid, 197, *198, 200,* 209
  ligament, *484*
  rotator cuff and, 201–203
Depolarization, 85, 95
Depression, shoulder girdle, 168, 174
Determinants
  of gait, 567–568
  of motions, 29–31
Developmental aspects of gait, 565–567
Deviation
  radial, 9
  ulnar, 9
Diagrams
  force vector, 35–36
  free body, 60–61, *63, 64, 67*
Diaphragm, *350,* 351
Diarthrodial joints, *12, 13,* 18–19
Digastric muscle, 361
Digits. *See* Fingers
Direction of motion, 30
Disc, lumbar, 323–324
Dislocation, joint, 21
  elbow, 228
Displacement, 31
Distal attachments, 128–129
Distal radioulnar joint, 230
Distal radius, 256
Distal ulna, 256
Distance, 30, *32*
Distracting component of muscle force, *46,* 48–49
Distraction injury, 231
Disuse atrophy, 115
DOMS. *See* Delayed-onset muscle soreness
Donning socks or pants, 624–626
Dorsal, plantar, and interosseous ligaments, *488*
Dorsal interossei, 280, *284, 285,* 287, 300, *514*
Dorsal ligaments, *487*
Dorsal radioulnar ligament, *227,* 232
Dorsal tubercle, 256
Dorsiflexion, 9
  ankle and foot, 480, *481,* 482, 489, *490,* 494–495, 496, 551
  gait and, 560
Double support, 544
Downward rotation, shoulder girdle, 168, 176
Driving, 626–627
Dynamic action system, 108
Dynamic alignment and patellofemoral static, 440–441
Dynamic stabilization of the glenohumeral joint, 201
Dysfunction, joint, 22
  temporomandibular, 361–362
Dystonia, 116

E

Early cocking phase, baseball pitching, 638–639
Eccentric muscle activity, 127, 146
Efferent motor nerve impulses, 84, 86–87, 102
Efficiency, gait, 567–574
Elastic forces of muscle, 148–149
Elastic range, 134
Elasticity, 131, 133
Elbow and forearm complex, 9
  activities requiring primarily movement of the, 623–629
  angular motion, 10–11
  bones, 219–221
  carrying angle, 224
  distal radioulnar joint, 230
  elbow extensors, *236–237,* 240
  elbow flexors, 232, *233–235,* 239–240, 246
  forearm pronators, 242–243
  forearm supinators, 240–242
  functional movement and muscles of, 243–247
  humeroradial joints, 221–228
  humeroulnar joints, 221–228
  humerus, 219–220
  introduction to, 218–219
  joints, 221–232
  leverage factor and, 73
  muscles, 232–247
  one-joint and multijoint muscles of, 245
  placing the hand behind the head motion and, 248
  proximal radioulnar joint, 230
  pulling motion and, 248–249
  radioulnar articulations, 229–232
  radius, 221
  soft tissue, 224, 228, 230–232
  supination and pronation, 229–230, 240–242, 246–247
  typical function, 245–247
  ulna, 220–221
Elbow and forearm complex joints
  humeroulnar and humeroradial, 221–228
  radioulnar articulations, 229–232
Elbow and forearm complex muscles
  activity during common functional movement, 248–249
  as agonists, antagonists, and/or synergists, 244
  elbow extensors, *236–237,* 240
  elbow flexors, 232, *233–235,* 239–240
  forearm pronators, 242–243
  forearm supination, *237,* 240–242
  one-joint and multijoint, 245
  selection in functional movement, 244
Elbow extensors, *236–237*
Elbow flexors, 232, *233–235,* 239–240
Electrical potential, 84
Electromyography, 126–127, *132, 133,* 146, 147
  elbow and forearm muscles, 245–247
Elevation, shoulder girdle, 168, 174
  glenohumeral joint, 181
Ellipsoidal joints, 11, *12*
EMG. *See* Electromyography
Empty end feel, 16
End feel, 14, 16
Endomysium, 136
Endoplasmic reticulum, 95
Endplates, vertebral, 322
Energy expenditure, 146–148, 244
Epicondyles, 219, 220
  knee, 425
Epimysium, 90, *92,* 136

Equilibrium
base of support and, 56–57, *58*
neutral, 55–56
postural, 107
stable, 55–56
state of, 31
static, 40
unstable, 55–56
Erector spinae muscles, 342, *344, 344–346, 353*
bending and lifting and, 356
breathing and, 359
Ergonomics, clinician, 612–614
Eversion, 9, 480, *481*
Excitable tissue, physiology of, 84–86
Excitation-contraction coupling, 95
Excursion of muscles
active, 144–150
passive, 141–143, *144*
Exercise-induced muscle injury, 151
Expenditure, energy, 146–148, 244
Extensibility, 131, 133
Extension, 9
glenohumeral joint, 181
hip, 385, *386–387,* 410–411, 559
humeroulnar joint, *239*
knee, 436–437, 442, *445,* 451–452, 454–456
triceps, 247
Extensor carpi radialis brevis, 266, *267,* 275–276, 277
Extensor carpi radialis longus, 266, *267, 274,* 276
Extensor carpi ulnaris, 266, *268, 274,* 277
Extensor digiti minimi, *271,* 277, 303
Extensor digitorum, 266, *270, 274,* 277
tendons, 285–287
Extensor digitorum brevis, 511, *515, 517*
Extensor digitorum longus, *508,* 509, *511*
Extensor hallucis brevis, *515*
Extensor hallucis longus, *508,* 509, *510*
Extensor hood, 287–288
Extensor indicis, *270,* 277, 287
Extensor lag, 460
Extensor pollicis brevis, *273,* 277
Extensor pollicis longus, *272,* 277
Extensor retinaculum, 277
Extensors, elbow, *236–237,* 240
Extensors, finger, *270–271,* 277
Extensors, hip, *396, 396–397,* 403
Extensors, knee, 442, 451–452, 454–455, 560
Extensors, thumb, 279
Extensors, wrist, 266–267, *267–268*
External abdominal oblique muscle, 347, *351*
External intercostal muscle, 347
External moment arms, 61, 63
External occipital protuberance, 317, *318, 319*
Externally applied resistances, 31, 33
clinical application of, 70–75
Extrafusal skeletal muscle, 89, 100
Extrinsic finger extensors, *270, 270–271,* 277
Extrinsic finger flexors, 277
Extrinsic thumb muscles, *272, 272–273*
Extrinsic wrist flexors, *271–272*

F

Facet joints, thoracic, 327, *328*
Failure range, 134
Fasciculi, 90, *92*
Fast glycolytic muscle fibers, 97
Fast oxidative glycolytic muscle fibers, 97
Fast pitch softball pitching, 641–644
Fast-twitch muscle fibers, 97
Feedback reflex, 149
Feeding, 623–624
Feiss' line, 521
Femur. *See also* Hip joint
angle of inclination, 375–377
angle of torsion, 377–378, *378*
biomechanical angulations of, 375–378
knee and, 425–426
shaft of, 375–376
structure, 374–375
FG. *See* Fast glycolytic muscle fibers
Fibers, muscle, 90–93
active tension and, 140–141
architecture, 135–136
types, 96–98, 129
Fibers, nerve, 87
afferent, 86, 88, 90
in the central nervous system, 89–90
in the peripheral nervous system, 88
types, *89*
Fibrocartilage, triangular, 231
Fibrocartilaginous disc, 265
Fibula, 476–477
Fingers, 255, 260–262. *See also* Thumbs; Wrist and hand complex
abduction and adduction, 302–303, *304*
balanced forces, 305
deformities, 305
extrinsic muscles, 277
grasping and, 300–302
ligaments, 265–266
motions, 290–291
muscles, *270–274,* 276–280
retinacular system, 287–288
strength of grip and, 293–297
synergic action of wrist muscles in movements of the thumb and little, 307
tendinous system, 285–287
Firm end feel, 16
First law of motion, 33–34, 35
First order neurons, 90
First-class levers, 38–39
torque and, 44–45
Fist grip, 291, *293, 297*
Flaccidity, 111, 115
Flat foot, 524–525
Flexion, 9
dorsi-, 9
elbow, 232, *233–235,* 239–240, 246
glenohumeral joint, 181–182
hip, 385, *386–387,* 390–391, *392–394,* 551, 559
humeroulnar joint, *239*
knee, 436–437, *447, 447–448,* 449–450, 452–453, 454–456, 461–462, 553, 560
lateral, 9
plantar-, 9
radial, 9
wrist, *268–269,* 274–276
Flexor carpi radialis, *269,* 274
Flexor carpi ulnaris, *269,* 274–275
Flexor digiti minimi, 279, *282,* 303
Flexor digiti minimi brevis, *514*
Flexor digitorum brevis, *512, 516*
Flexor digitorum longus, *499,* 503, 504–505
Flexor digitorum profundus, *272,* 274, 277, 278, 288, 310
Flexor digitorum superficialis, *271,* 274, 277, 288, 310
Flexor hallucis brevis, 511, *513*
Flexor hallucis longus, *500,* 503, 504–505
Flexor pollicis brevis, 279, *280, 282,* 303
Flexor pollicis longus, *273,* 274, 278
Floor mobility, 594–599
Floor-to-stand mobility, 596–599
Fluid, synovial, 18
FOG. *See* Fast oxidative glycolytic muscle fibers
Follow-through phase
baseball pitching, 640–641
fast pitch softball pitching, 643–644
golf swing, 656
soccer instep kick, 647
tennis serve, 660
Foot. *See* Ankle and foot
Foramen magnum, 317, *318*
Force applications to the body, 51–52
base of support, 56–57, *58*
calculation of joint forces and, 65–69
calculation of muscle forces and, 61–65
free body diagrams, 60–61
levers and muscle activity and, 57–59, *60, 61*
neutral equilibrium, 55–56
pulleys, 70–73
stable equilibrium and, 55–56
unstable equilibrium, 55–56
Force arm, 38, 40
mechanical advantage and, 39–40
Force couple, 203
Force feedback reflex, 149
Forces
acting at angles, 45–47, *48, 49*
affecting human movement, 4, *5*
clinical application of externally applied, 70–75
composition of, 36–37
concurrent system, 46

defined, 31
equilibrium, 31
externally applied resistances, 31
friction, 31
gravity, 31
ground reaction, 555–556, 584
joint reaction, 65–66
knee joint, 456–462
levers and, 37–40
magnitudes of, 35, *36,* 40
mechanical advantage and, 39–40
muscle, 31
Newton's laws of motion and, 33–35
patellofemoral joint, 458–460
points of peak, 556
pressure, 74–75
required to maintain stance, 537–539
resolution of, 45
running, 583–584
shoulder complex muscle, 205–206
stabilizing component of muscle, *46,* 48–49
static equilibrium, 40
stretching vs. joint mobilization, 73–74
tibiofemoral joint, 456–458
types of, 31–37
vectors and their considerations, 35–36, *62*

Forearms. *See* Elbow and forearm complex
Forefoot, 479
Forward bending and lifting, 355–357
Forward reaching, 618–620
Forward swing phase, golf swing, 655
Fovea, 221, 256
Free body diagrams, 60–61, *63, 64, 67*
Freestyle swimming, 647–652
Friction, 31
Frontal lobe, 110
Frontal plane motion, 6
and control at the hip and pelvis, 411–415
gait and, 552–553
running and, 577–578
Functional activity, muscle, 129–131
elbow and forearm complex, 243–247
extremities and trunk, 358–359
gait, 545–546
head, neck, and trunk, 351–359
hip, 406–417
interaction of muscles and ligaments in knee function, 462–464
leg and foot, 511, 516–525
shoulder complex and, 207–209
stance control, 540–542
wrist and hand, 291–303, 303–307
Functional excursion of muscles, 141–142
Fusiform muscles, 136
Fusimotor neurons, 104

G

Gait. *See also* Running; Stance; Walking
analysis, 561–565
cycle, 543–545
defined, 536, 543–544
determinants of, 567–568
developmental aspects of, 565–567
efficiency, 567–574
frontal plane motion and, 552–553
functional tasks of, 545–546
gluteus medius, 414
gluteus medius weakness and, 573–574
ground reaction forces and, 555–556
immature, 565
impaired, 568–574
mature, 565–567
muscles of, 556–561
neurological, 568–574
orthopedic, 572–574
Parkinson's disease, 570–571
peroneals and, 561
range of motion requirements of normal, 554
spatial and temporal characteristics, 546–548
stiff leg, 570
terminology, 543–545
Galen, Claudius, 3
Galileo, 3
Gamma axons, 101
Gamma motor neurons, 89
Ganglia, 88, 90
Gastrocnemius, *447,* 450, *498,* 501, 502
Gender
center of gravity and, 53, *62*
muscle strength and, 141, *142*
Generators, pattern, 109
Geniohyoid, 361
Genu articularis, *445*
Genu valgum, 441
Genu varum, 441
Girdle, shoulder, 162, 167–170
depression, 168, 174
downward rotation, 168, 176
elevation, 168, 174
protraction, 168, 176
retraction, 168, 176
scapulohumeral rhythm, 183–185
upward rotation, 168, 176
Glenohumeral joint, 163, 166–168
arthrokinematic motions, 182–183
bursae, 180
capsular reinforcement, 177–180
coracoacromial arch, 179–180
defined, 176–177
functional deficiency applications, 208–209
kinematics, 180–182
passive and dynamic stabilization of, 200–203
scapulohumeral rhythm, 183–185
Glenohumeral stabilizing muscles of the shoulder, 191–197
Glenoid fossa, 164–165, 318
Gliding motion, 21
Gluteus maximus, 390, 391, *396, 399,* 403
Gluteus medius, 390, 391, *398,* 404, 412, *416*
gait, 414
weakness, 573–574
Gluteus minimus, 390, 391, *398,* 404–405
Golf swing, 652–656
Golgi tendon organs, 89, 100, 149
Gomphosis joints, 18
Goniometry, clinical, 11, 14
Gracilis, 390, 391, *396, 402,* 403, *448,* 449–450, 452
Gradation of strength of muscle contractions, 98–99
Grasps/grips
grasping action, 295–302
role of intrinsic muscles in, 300–302
role of long finger flexors in, 300
role of wrist extensors in, 295–300
strength, 293–295
types of, 291–293
Gravity, 31
center of, 52–55, 58, *62,* 542
line of, 56, 537–539, 540
stable, unstable, and neutral equilibrium and center of, 55–56
Gray matter, 90
Greater trochanter, 374–375, *376,* 389, *398*
Greater tubercle, 165–166
Ground reaction forces, 555–556, 584
GTO. *See* Golgi tendon organs
Gunstock deformity, 224

H

Hallux valgus, 525
Hammering activity, 629–631
Hamstrings, 404, *445–446, 449,* 452–453
lateral, 403
to quadriceps torque ratio, 462
strain, 151–152
Hand. *See* Wrist and hand complex
Hand tools, 629–631
Hand-entry phase, freestyle swimming, 649
Hard end feel, 16
Hard palate, *319*
Head. *See* Skull
Head, arms, and trunk (HAT) center of gravity, 52–54
Head, femoral, 375
Head, neck, and trunk region
anterior and lateral trunk muscles, 343–351
anterior cervical muscles, 336, *337–339,* 341
anterior vertebral joint elements, 322–324
bones, 315–321
cervical region joints, 326–327
coccyx, 320–321
coupling motions, 325–326
first and second cervical vertebrae, 318–319
functional stance control at, 541–542
ligaments, 324–325

lumbar region joints, 329–330
muscles, 335–359
nonpalpable structures, 316–317, *318*
normal curves, 315–316
palpable structures, 317–321
posterior cervical muscles, *340,* 341–342
posterior thoracic and lumbar muscles, 342–343
posterior vertebral joint elements, 324–326
primary neck flexors, 336, 341
sacrum, 320–321, 331–335
sternum and, *320,* 321
temporomandibular joints, 317, *319,* 359–362
third to sixth cervical vertebrae, 319–320
thoracic and lumbar vertebrae, 320
thoracic region joints, 327–329
thorax and, 321
vertebral motions, 321
Head of the radius, 221, *226*
Headaches, tension, 341
Heel pain, 478
Hemiplegia, adult, 569–570
Heterarchy, 107
Hierarchy, 107
Hinge joints, 11, *12*
Hip extension function, 410–411
gait and, 559
knee extension combined with, 455–456
knee flexion combined with, 454
Hip flexion function, 409–410, 551
gait and, 559
knee extension combined with, 454–455
knee flexion combined with, 455
Hip joints, 380–381. *See also* Femur; Pelvis
arthrokinematics, 388
functional stance control at, 541
ligaments, 385, *386–387,* 388–389
motion on pelvis, 385, *386–387*
soft tissue at, 388–389
transverse plane motion, 415–417
walking and, 550, 553–554, 568
Hip muscles, 389–390. *See also* Pelvis
abduction, 403–405, 412–414, 559–560
adduction, 402–403, 415, 417, 560
adductor brevis, 391, *395,* 402
adductor longus, 391, *394,* 402
adductor magnus, 391, *395,* 402–403
analysis of activity, 408–417
biceps femoris, 391, *397*
extensors, 403
factors affecting roles of muscles of, 406–408
frontal plane motion and control at, 411–415, 552–553
gluteus maximus, 390, 391, *396, 399,* 403
gluteus medius, 391, *398,* 404, 412, *416*
gluteus minimus, 391, *398,* 404–405
gracilis, 391, *396, 402,* 403
hip flexion function, 409
iliopsoas, 390, 391, *392, 400*
lateral rotators, 405
line of pull and leverage, 407
medial rotators, 406
muscular sufficiency, 407–408
pectineus, 391, *394, 396,* 401, *402*
piriformis, *398–399*
rectus femoris, 390, 391, *393, 401*
running and, 568, 576–577, 580–581
sagittal plane motion, 408–411
sartorius, 390, 391, *393, 399, 401*
secondary flexors, 401–402
semimembranosus, 391, *397,* 403
semitendinosus, 391, *397,* 403
tensor fascia latae, 391, *394, 398,* 401, *402,* 405
transverse plane motion and, 415–417
weight-bearing and nonweight-bearing functions of, 408
Hip strategy, 543
Hippocrates, 3
Historical perspective of kinesiology, 3, *4*
Hobbies, 621
Hook grip, 292, *296*
Horizontal plane, 6
Horizontal plate of palatine bone, *319*
Household tasks, 604–606
Humeroradial joints
arthrokinematics, 223–224
osteokinematics, 221–223
soft tissue, 224, 228
Humeroulnar joints
arthrokinematics, 223–224
osteokinematics, 221–223
soft tissue, 224, 228
Humerus, 165–166, 219–220
ligaments, *225–227*
Hygiene activities, 621–622
Hyoid bone, *320*
Hyperextension, 9, 182
elbow, 223
Hypermobile joints, 24
Hyperpolarization, 86
Hypertonia, 105, 115
Hypertrophy, 135
Hypomobile joints, 24
Hypotenuse, 49, *50,* 51
Hypothenar muscle group, 279–280, *282*
Hypotonia, 105, 115
H-zone, 94

I

IFMF. *See* Intrafusal muscle fibers
Iliac crest, *320, 349, 351,* 372, *373*
Iliac fossa, 372
Iliocostalis cervicis, 342, *344*
Iliocostalis lumborum, *346*
Iliocostalis thoracis, 343, *346*
Iliofemoral ligament, *386*
Iliopsoas, 390, 391, *392, 400*
Ilium, 372
Immature walking, 565
Impaired gait, 568–574
Impairments, neuromuscular, 113–116
Impulses, nerve, 85
transmission from nerves to skeletal muscle fibers, 94–95
Inclination, angle of, 165, 376–377
pelvic, *383,* 384–385
Inertia, 33–34, 35
Inferior nuchal line, *319*
Inferior oblique muscles, *340,* 341
Inferior ramus, 374
Infrahyoid muscles, 341, 359
Infraspinatus, *192,* 195, *196*
Inhibition, reciprocal, 103
Initial swing, 545, 576
Injury
ankle, 491
anterior cruciate ligament, 462, 463
delayed-onset muscle soreness, 151
elbow and forearm distraction, 231
exercise-induced muscle, 151
hamstring, 151–152
peripheral nerve, 118, 308–310
posterior tibial shin splint, 525
Instantaneous center of rotation (ICR), 437
Insufficiency
active, 144–145
passive, 142, *143*
Integration of motor control to produce functional movement, 112–113
Intention tremor, 116
Intercarpal ligaments, 265
Intercondylar fossa, 425
Intercondylar groove, 425
Intermediate control centers, 111–112
Intermetatarsal joints, 496–497
ligaments, *488*
Internal abdominal oblique muscle, 347
Internal intercostal muscle, 347
Internal moment arms, 61, 63
International System of Units (SI), 33
Interneurons, 87, 90
Interossei
foot dorsal and plantar, *514, 515*
hand dorsal and palmar, 280, *284, 285,* 287, 300
Interosseous cuneometatarsal ligaments, *487*
Interosseous ligament, *485*
Interosseous membrane, 230, 231
Interphalangeal joints, 262–263, 497
ligaments, *488*
Interspinalis muscles, 342
Interspinous ligaments, 324–325
Interspinous muscles, *345*
Intertransversarii muscles, 342, *344*
Intertransverse ligaments, 325
Intrafusal muscle fibers, 89, 100–101
Intrinsic muscles of the foot, 510–517, 521–522
Intrinsic-minus position, 302
Intrinsic-plus position, 302
Inversion, 9, 480, *481*
Involuntary movements, 116

Ipsilateral motor control, 111
Irritability, 85
Ischial ramus, 373
Ischial tuberosity, 372–373
Ischiofemoral ligament, *387*
Ischium, 372–373
Isokinetic muscle activity, 128
Isometric muscle activity, 127, 137–138
Isotonic muscle activity, 127–128

J

Jaw. *See* Mandible
Joint motion
 clinician activities and, 610
 daily functional activities and, 595–596, 597–598, 600
 donning socks or pants, 625
 driving, 626–627
 feeding, 623
 household tasks and, 605–606
 occupational and daily activities, 603
 occupational tasks and, 607, 608–609
 oral care, 622
 pouring, 627
 reaching overhead and backward, 620
 reaching overhead and forward, 619
 turning a key, *628,* 629
 using a hammer, 629–630
 wood sanding activity, 621
Joints
 amphiarthrodial, *12, 13,* 18
 axes in function, 23–24
 ball-and-socket, 11, *12*
 biaxial, 11, *12, 13*
 calculation of forces, 65–69
 capsules, 18–19
 classification by structure and function, *13*
 compression, 69–70, 458–460
 degrees of freedom, 11, *12*
 diarthrodial, *12, 13,* 18–19
 dislocation vs. subluxation, 21
 dysfunction, 22, 361–362
 gomphosis, 18
 hypermobile, 24
 kinematic chains, 16–17
 materials found in synovial, 19–20
 mobilization vs. stretching, 73–74
 motion ranges, 14, *15*
 naming movements at, 6–9
 osteokinematics, 9–11, *12–13*
 play, 22
 positions, close-packed and open-packed, 24
 reaction force, 65–66
 receptors, 99–105
 shapes as they pertain to arthrokinematic motion, 22–23
 special cases, 9
 structure, *13,* 18–20
 surface motion, 17–25
 surfaces, 19, *20*
 synarthrodial, *12, 13,* 18
 syndesmosis, *12, 13,* 18
 synovial, 18, 19–20
 triaxial, 11, *12, 13*
 uniaxial, 11, *12, 13*
Joints, ankle and foot
 calcaneocuboid, 493–495
 functional stance control at, 540
 intermetatarsal, *488,* 496–497
 interphalangeal, 262–263, *488,* 497
 metatarsophalangeal, *488,* 497
 midtarsal, 553
 motion terminology and, 480
 pronation and supination and, 518–519
 subtalar, *484–486,* 489–492, *493,* 518–520, 553
 talocrural, 482–483, *484–485,* 489, 519
 talonavicular, *486,* 493
 tarsometatarsal, *487,* 495–496, 520
 tibiofibular, 480–482
 transverse tarsal, *486,* 492–495, *496*
Joints, elbow and forearm complex
 humeroulnar and humeroradial, 221–228
 radioulnar articulations, 229–232
Joints, hip, 380–381
 arthrokinematics, 388
 functional stance control at, 541
 gait and, 550, 553–554
 ligaments, 385, *386–387,* 388–389
 motion on pelvis, 385, *386–387*
 soft tissue at, 388–389
Joints, knee
 axes for flexion and extension, 436–437
 axial rotation, 437–438
 forces, 456–462
 functional stance control, 540–541
 gait and, 550–551, 553, 554
 muscles acting at the knee, 453–456
 patellofemoral, 439–441, 458–460
 Q angle, 441
 tibiofemoral, 428–430, *431,* 436–439, 456–458
Joints, pelvis, 379–380
 gait and, 548, 550, 553
Joints, shoulder complex, 166–167, 210
 acromioclavicular, 164, 166–168, 173–175
 definition of shoulder girdle movements and, 167–170
 glenohumeral, 176–183
 scapulothoracic, 167–168, 175–176
 sternoclavicular, 166–168, 170–173
Joints, temporomandibular, 317, *319,* 359–362
Joints, vertebral column
 anterior, 322–324
 cervical region, 326–327
 lumbar region, 329–330
 posterior, 324–326
 sacrum region, 331–335
Joints, wrist and hand complex
 carpometacarpal, 260, *261, 261–262,* 305
 finger motion and, 290–291
 interphalangeal, 262–263
 metacarpophalangeal, 260–262, 290–291, 300–302, 305
 midcarpal, 259
 radiocarpal, 259

K

Key, turning a, 627–629
Kicking
 freestyle swimming, 647–648
 soccer instep, 644–647
Kinematics, 5, 25, 29. *See also* Arthrokinematics; Osteokinematics
 acromioclavicular joint, 174–175
 calcaneocuboid joint, 494
 chains, 16–17
 gait, 546–554
 glenohumeral joint, 180–182
 patellofemoral joint, 440–441
 radioulnar joint, 229–230
 running, 576–578
 scapulothoracic, 173–174
 sternoclavicular joint, 171–172
 subtalar joint, 491–492
 tibiofemoral joint, 436–439
 tibiofibular joint, 481–482
 walking, 548, *549*
Kinesiology
 historical perspective of, 3, *4*
 introduction to, 3–4
 purpose of studying, 4
 terminology, 4–9
Kinesthesia, 105–106
Kinetic chain, open vs. closed, 149–150
Kinetics, 5, 29, 31
 gait, 554–556
 running, 583–584
Knee
 bones, 425–428
 capsule, 435–436
 cruciate ligaments, *431,* 434–435
 extensors, 442, 451–452, 454–455, 560
 femur and, 425–426
 flexion, *447–448,* 449–450, 452–453, 454–455, 461–462, 553, 560
 forward bending and lifting from the, 355–357
 functions of muscles of the, 451–456
 introduction, 424–425
 joints, 428–451
 kinematics, 436–439
 ligaments, 430, *431–433,* 434–435, 462–464
 menisci, 428, 429–430, 457
 motion restriction, 572–573
 muscles, 441–456
 one-joint and two-joint muscles acting on the, 453–456
 patella and, *426,* 427–428
 patellofemoral joint, 439–441
 Q angle, 441, 442
 running and, 568, 577, 578
 sensory innervation and reflexes of, 463

soft tissue structures, 435–436
terminal rotation of, 438–439
tibia and, 426–426
tibial rotators, 450–451
tibiofemoral joint, 428–430, 436–439
torque of muscles acting at the, 460–462
walking and, 550–551, 553, 554, 568
Knee joints
axes for flexion and extension, 436–437
axial rotation, 437–438
forces, 456–462
functional stance control, 540–541
gait and, 550–551, 553, 554
muscles acting at the knee, 453–456
patellofemoral, 439–441, 458–460
Q angle, 441
tibiofemoral, 428–430, *431,* 436–439, 456–458
Knee muscles, 441–442
biceps femoris, 390, *397,* 403, *445, 448,* 449, *449*
extensors, 442, *445,* 451–452, 454–455
flexor, *447–448,* 452–453, 454–455
functions of, 451–456
gastrocnemius, *447,* 449
genu articularis, *445*
gracilis, *448,* 449–450, 452
hamstrings, 151–152, 403, 404, *445, 445–446, 449,* 452–453
interaction of ligaments and, 462–464
one-joint and two-joint, 453–456
plantaris, *447,* 450
popliteus, *448,* 450, 453
protection of ligaments, 463–464
rectus femoris, *443, 449,* 452
running and, 582
sartorius, *448,* 449, 452
semimembranosus, *446*
semitendinosus, *446, 448,* 449–450
tensor fascia lata, *448*
tibial rotators, 450–451
torque of, 460–462
vastus intermedius, *444*
vastus lateralis, *443*
vastus medialis, *444*
Kyphosis, 315

L

Laboratory gait analysis, 561–563
Lag, extensor, 460
Lambdoid suture, *319*
Lamina, superficial and deep, 330
Large muscle movers of the shoulder, 197–200
Late cocking phase, baseball pitching, 639–640
Late pull-through phase, freestyle swimming, 651
Lateral, posterior, and medial talocalcaneal ligament, *485*
Lateral ankle and foot muscles, 505–507
Lateral calcaneonavicular ligament, *486*
Lateral capitulum, 219
Lateral collateral ligament (LCL), *226,* 228, 231, 430, *431,* 483
Lateral epicondyle, 219, 220, *226, 237*
Lateral flexion, 9
Lateral hamstring, 403
Lateral longitudinal arch, 477
Lateral malleolus, 476
Lateral pelvic tilt, 382, *383,* 384
Lateral pinch grip, *294, 298*
Lateral pterygoid muscle, 360–361
Lateral pterygoid plate, *319*
Lateral rotation, 9
hip, 385, *386–387*
Lateral supracondylar ridge, 219
Latissimus dorsi, 197, *199,* 359
Laws of motion, Newton's, 33–35
Laws of the right triangle, 49–51
Learning, motor, 112
Leg(s). *See also* Ankle and foot
bones, 475–477
cycling and, 660–663
foot arches and, 521–522
and foot muscle and joint function, 511, 516–525
freestyle swimming and, 647–648
raises, 409–410
soccer instep kick and, 644–647
Leg-cocking phase, soccer instep kick, 646
Leisure activities. *See also* Sports activities
cycling, 660–663
golf, 652–656
tennis, 656–660
Length-tension relationships, 137–138
leverage and, 145–146
Lesser trochanter, 375, *376*
Lesser tubercle, 165–166
Levator scapulae, *189,* 191
Lever arm, 32, 59
Levers, 37–40
muscle activity and, 57–59, *60, 61*
torque and, 44–45
Leverage
factor, 73
and length-tension interactions, 145–146
Life expectancy, 635
Life span changes and gait, 565–567
Lifting, *60,* 602–604
and bending, forward, 355–357
squat, 357, *358*
Ligament of Humphrey, *433*
Ligament of Wrisberg, *433*
Ligamenta flava, 324–325
Ligaments
acromioclavicular joint, 174
ankle and foot, *484–488*
coracoacromial, 179
coracohumeral, 177–178
hip joint, 385, *386–387,* 388–389
humeroulnar and humeroradial articulations, 224–228
knee, 430, *431–433,* 462–464
menisci, 429
radioulnar joint, *226,* 230, 231
sacrum, 333–334
sternoclavicular joint, 170–171
vertebral, 324–325
wrist, 263–265
Ligamentum nuchae, 317, *318,* 325
Ligamentum teres, *387,* 389
Line of gravity, 56, 537–539, 540
Linea alba, 343, *349, 351*
Linea aspera, 375, *376*
Linear distance, 30
Linear motion, 10
Lisfranc's joint, 496
Lister's tubercle, 256, *257,* 258
LMN. *See* Lower motor neurons
Loading
of the foot, 523–524
response, 557
Location of motion, 30
Locomotion, 536
LOG. *See* Line of gravity
Long plantar ligament, *487*
Longevity, 635
Longissimus capitis, 342, *344*
Longissimus cervicis, *344*
Longissimus lumborum, *346*
Longissimus thoracis, 343, *346*
Longitudinal ridge, 220
Longus capitis, 336, *337,* 362
Longus colli, 336, *338,* 362
"Loose" hinge joints, 222
Loose-packed joint position, 24
Lordosis, 315
Lower extremities
clinician ergonomics and, 613–614
muscles and gait, 559–561
Lower motor neurons, 90
Lumbar vertebrae, 320
joints, 329–330
Lumbricals, 280, *283, 286,* 300, 302, *513*
Lumbosacral junction, 329, *330*
Lunate, 257–258
ligaments, 263–265

M

Magnetic resonance imaging, 135
Magnitude of motion, 30
Magnitudes of forces, 35, *36,* 40
Mandible, 317. *See also* Temporomandibular joint (TMJ)
condyles of, 317–318, *319*
muscles, 360–361
Manual resistance and clinician ergonomics, 612–614
Manubrium, 163, *320*
Mass, 31–32
center of, 52–55, 61, *62,* 539–540, 541, 548, 555–556, 568
Mastoid process, 317, *319*

Mature walking, 565–567
Maximum isometric muscle force, 150–152, 206
MCP joint. *See* Metacarpophalangeal (MCP) joint
Mechanical advantage (MA), 39–40
Medial collateral ligament (MCL), *225,* 228, 430, *431, 484*
Medial epicondyle, 219, 220, *225*
Medial longitudinal arch, 477
Medial malleolus, 475
Medial pterygoid muscle, 360
Medial pterygoid plate, *319*
Medial rotation, 9
  hip, 385, *386–387*
Medial trochlea, 219
Medial-lateral tilting of the scapula, 170
Median nerve, *235, 238,* 307–310
Membrane, interosseous, 230, 231
Men
  center of gravity in, 53, *62*
  muscle strength in, 141
Menisci, 428, 429–430, 457
Meniscofemoral joint, *433*
Meniscotibial ligaments, 429
Meromysin, *92*
Metacarpals, 258–259
Metacarpophalangeal (MCP) joint, 259, 260–262, 305
  finger motions and, 290–291
  in grasping, 300–302
  ligaments, 263–265
Metatarsal bones, 479
Metatarsophalangeal joints, 497
  ligaments, *488*
Midcarpal joint, 259
Micrometers, 91
Middle pull-through phase, freestyle swimming, 651
Middle scalene muscles, 336, *339*
Midfoot, 477
Midpalm muscle group, 280, *283,* 300
Midstance, 544, 557
Midswing, 545
Midtarsal joint, 553
Mitochondria, 91, 147
Mobility
  floor, 594–599
  sit-to-stand transfer, 599–602
Mobilization, stretching vs. joint, 73–74
Modified hinge joint, 223
Moment arm, 32, 45, 138–139
  external, 61, 63
  internal, 61, 63
  shoulder complex muscle forces, 205–206
Motion. *See also* Movement
  acceleration and, 31, 34
  action-reaction and, 34–35
  angular, 10–11
  axes of, 5–6
  basic arthrokinematic joint, 20–24
  center of, 56–57
  center of gravity changes with, 55–56
  change of, 31
  determinants of, 29–31
  direction of, 30
  finger, 305
  inertia and, 33–34
  joint surface, 17–25
  location of, 30
  magnitude of, 30
  Newton's laws of, 33–35
  open-chain, 39
  osteokinematics and types of, 10–11
  planes of, 5–6
  range of, 23, 30
  ranges, joint, 14, *15*
  rate of, 31
  rolling or rocking, 21, *21*
  rotary, 10–11, 30
  segment and body, 6
  sliding or gliding, 21, *21*
  spinning, 21, *21*
  thumb, 306
  translatory, 10, *22,* 29–30
  types of, 29–30
Motion, vertebral column, 321
  anterior vertebral joint elements and, 322–324
  cervical region, 326–327
  coupling, 325–326
  sacrum region, 331–335
  thoracic region, 327–329
Motion, wrist and hand complex
  finger motions, 290–291
  wrist motions, 288–290
Motion segment of the spine, 321
Motor control, 107–108
  within the brainstem, 109
  cerebral motor centers, 109–110
  dynamic systems approach to understanding, 108
  integration to produce functional movement, 112–113
  intermediate control centers, 111–112
  at the spinal region, 108–109
Motor cortex, 110
Motor fibers, classification on basis of fiber destination, 89
Motor learning, 112
Motor neurons, 88–89
  alpha, 98
  gamma, 89
  lower, 90
  upper, 90
Motor units, 96, 98–99
Movable pulleys, 71–72
Movement. *See also* Motion
  control (*See* Motor control)
  forces affecting, 4, *5*
  kinetics and kinematics in, 5, 25
  naming movements at joints, 6–9
  neural physiology and, 83–84
  planes of motion and axes of motion in, 5–6
  segment and body motion, 6
  system, human, 84, 117–119
Multifidus muscles, *340,* 342, *345*
Multipennate muscles, 136
Muscle activity
  activation, 127–128
  anatomic, 128–129
  characteristics, 131–141
  clinician activities and, 611–612
  concentric, 127
  daily functional activities, 598–599, 601–602
  donning socks or pants, 625–626
  driving, 627
  eccentric, 127, 146
  feeding, 623–624
  functional, 129–131
  household tasks and, 606
  isokinetic, 128
  isometric, 127, 137–138
  isotonic, 127–128
  muscle attachments in, 128–129
  muscle strength and, 134–141
  occupational and daily activities, 604
  occupational tasks and, 607, 609
  oral care, 622
  pouring, 627
  reaching overhead and backward, 620–621
  reaching overhead and forward, 619–620
  recording, 126–127
  turning a key, 629
  using a hammer, 630–631
  viscosity and, 131
  wood sanding activity, 621
Muscle characteristics
  creep, 134
  elasticity and extensibility, 131, 133
  stress-strain, 133–134
  viscosity, 131
Muscle contraction, 94, 95–96
  speed, 139–140
Muscle fiber
  active tension and, 141
  architecture, 135–136
  structure, 90–93
  types, 96–98, 129
Muscle strength, 134–135
  active tension and, 140–141
  age and gender in, 141, *142*
  factors affecting maximum isometric muscle force and, 150–152
  fiber architecture and, 135–136
  moment arm and, 138–139
  passive components in, 136–137
  speed of contraction and, 139–140
Muscles, 31
  active excursion of, 144–150
  agonist, 129

all-or-none law, 98
antagonist, 129–130
antigravity, 104–105, 537
conduction of impulses to the interior of the muscle fiber, 95
coordination problems, 115–116
elastic forces of, 148–149
endoplasmic reticulum, 95
excitation-contraction coupling, 95
extrafusal skeletal, 89, 100
force, distracting component of, *46*, 48–49
force, stabilizing component of, *46*, 48–49
forces, calculation of, 61–65
fusiform, 136
intrafusal, 89, 100–101
involuntary movements, 116
jaw, 360–361
joint, tendon, and muscle receptors, 99–107
kinesthesia and proprioception, 106–107
leverage factor of, 73
and levers, forces on the body, 57–59, *60, 61*
mobility in daily functional activities and, 596–599
motor units, 96, 98–99
myoneural junction, 94–95
passive excursion of, 141–143, *144*
pennate, 136
receptors, 99
relaxation, 94, 96
resting length of, 137
scapular stabilizer, 185, 190–191
of the shoulder complex, 185–208
sliding filament model of contraction by, 94, 95–96
spindles, 89, 100–105
stiffness, 104
structure of skeletal, 90–96
synergist, 130
synergy, 107, 116
tendon action of, 143, *144*
tissue physiology, 84–86
tone, 104
tone, abnormal, 115
wasting, 114–115
weakness, 113–115
Muscles, ankle and foot
abductor digiti minimi, *512*
abductor hallucis, 511, *512, 516*
adductor hallucis, *514*
anterior group, 507–510
calf muscles and, 504–505
dorsal interossei, *514*
extensor digitorum brevis, 511, *515, 517*
extensor digitorum longus, *508*, 509, *511*
extensor hallucis longus, *508*, 509, *510*
flexor digiti minimi brevis, *514*
flexor digitorum brevis, *512, 516*
flexor digitorum longus, *499*, 503, 504–505
flexor hallucis brevis, 511, *513*
flexor hallucis longus, *500*, 503, 504–505
function of, 511, 516–525
function of the pretibial group, 509–510
function of the triceps surae, 502–503
gastrocnemius, 450, *498*, 501, 502
intrinsic, 510–517, 561
lateral group, 505–507
lumbricals, *513*
peroneus brevis, 505–507
peroneus longus, 505–507, 522
peroneus tertius, *508*
plantaris, *447*, 450, *498*, 501
posterior group, 497–505
quadratus plantae, *513*
running and, 568, 577, 578, 582–583
soleus, *498*, 501, 502
tibialis anterior, 507–509, *510*
tibialis posterior, *499*, 503, 504–505
walking and, 551–552, 554, 568
Muscles, anterior and lateral trunk, 343, 347, 351
Muscles, calf, 504–505
Muscles, cervical
anterior, 336, *337–339*, 341
posterior, *340*, 341–342
Muscles, elbow and forearm complex
activity during common functional movement, 248–249
as agonists, antagonists, and/or synergists, 244
elbow extensors, *236–237*, 240
elbow flexors, 232, *233–235*, 239–240
forearm pronators, 242–243
forearm supination, *237*, 240–242
one-joint and multijoint, 245
selection in functional movement, 244
Muscles, gait
identification of muscular activation patterns by body segment, 558–561
initial contact, 557
loading response, 557
midstance and, 557
muscular activation patterns and, 556–557
swing phases and, 557–558
terminal stance and preswing and, 557
upper extremity, 558
Muscles, head, neck, and trunk, 335–351
functions of, 351–359
Muscles, hip, 389–390. *See also* Pelvis
abduction, 403–405, 412–414, 559–560
adduction, 402–403, 415, 417, 560
adductor brevis, 391, *395*, 402
adductor longus, 391, *394*, 402
adductor magnus, 391, *395*, 402–403
analysis of activity, 408–417
biceps femoris, 391, *397*
extensors, 403
factors affecting roles of muscles of, 406–408
frontal plane motion and control at, 411–415, 552–553
gluteus maximus, 390, 391, *396, 399*, 403
gluteus medius, 391, *398*, 404, 412, *416*
gluteus minimus, 391, *398*, 404–405
gracilis, 391, *396, 402*, 403
hip flexion function, 409
iliopsoas, 390, 391, *392, 400*
lateral rotators, 405
line of pull and leverage, 407
medial rotators, 406
muscular sufficiency, 407–408
pectineus, 391, *394, 396*, 401, *402*
piriformis, *398–399*
rectus femoris, 390, 391, *393, 401*
running and, 568, 576–577, 580–581
sagittal plane motion, 408–411
sartorius, 390, 391, *393, 399, 401*
secondary flexors, 401–402
semimembranosus, 391, *397*, 403
semitendinosus, 391, *397*, 403
tensor fascia latae, 391, *394, 398*, 401, *402*, 405
transverse plane motion and, 415–417
weight-bearing and nonweight-bearing functions of, 408
Muscles, knee, 441–442
biceps femoris, 390, *397*, 403, *445, 448, 449*
extensors, 442, *445*, 451–452, 454–455
flexor, *447–448*, 452–453, 454–455
functions of, 451–456
gastrocnemius, *447*, 449
genu articularis, *445*
gracilis, *448*, 449–450, 452
hamstrings, 151–152, 403, 404, *445, 445–446, 449*, 452–453
interaction of ligaments and, 462–464
one-joint and two-joint, 453–456
plantaris, *447*, 450
popliteus, *448*, 450, 453
protection of ligaments, 463–464
rectus femoris, *443, 449*, 452
running and, 582
sartorius, *448*, 449, 452
semimembranosus, *446*
semitendinosus, *446, 448*, 449–450
tensor fascia lata, *448*
tibial rotators, 450–451
torque of, 460–462
vastus intermedius, *444*
vastus lateralis, *443*
vastus medialis, *444*
Muscles, lumbosacral, 331
Muscles, posterior lumbar, 342–343
Muscles, posterior thoracic, 342–343
Muscles, respiratory, *350*, 351, 359
Muscles, shoulder complex
function of, 200–208
glenohumeral stabilizing, 191–197
large muscle movers, 197–200
regions, 185, *186–189*
scapular stabilizer, 185–191

Muscles, wrist and hand complex, 266
finger, *270–274,* 276–280
midpalm, 280, *284,* 300
thumb, *272,* 277–280, *281–283*
wrist extensors, 266, *267–268, 274*
wrist flexors, *268–269,* 274–276
Musculocutaneous nerve, *233*
Myelin, 87, 88–89
Mylohyoid, 361
Myofibrils, 91, *92,* 135
Myofilaments, 91, *92*
Myoglobin, 96
Myoneural junction, 94–95
Myosin, *92,* 93, 94, *95,* 114
Myotatic reflex, 102, *103, 104*

N

Naming movements at joints, 6–9
Nasal septum, *319*
Navicular, 478–479
Neck. *See also* Vertebral column
flexors, 336, 341
Neck, femoral, 375
Negative work, 127, 146–149
Nerve fibers, 87
afferent, 86, 88, 90
in the central nervous system, 89–90
corticospinal tract, 109
injury, 118
perineal, 505
in the peripheral nervous system, 88
types, *89*
Nerve impulses, 85
Nerves, elbow, and forearm complex, *233–238*
Nervous system, 118
central, 86
cerebral palsy and, 118
cerebrovascular accident and, 119
classifications, 86–87
nerve fibers, 87–90
nerve injury and, 118
pathological conditions, 116–119
peripheral, 86, 88–89, 307–310
Nervous tissue physiology, 84–86
Neurological gait, 568–572
Neuromuscular impairments, 113–116
Neuromuscular junction, 94
Neurons, 86
alpha motor, 98
association, 90
autonomic, 88
first order, 90
fusimotor, 104
gamma motor, 89
inter-, 87, 90
lower motor, 90
second order, 90
sensory and motor, 88–89
third order, 90
upper motor, 90
Neurotransmitters, 86
Neutral equilibrium, 55–56
Newtons, 32
Newton's laws of motion, 33–35
9 o'clock phase, fast pitch softball pitching, 643
Nodes of Ranvier, 87
Nonaxial joints, *13*
Nonpalpable structures of the vertebral column, 316–317, *318, 319*
Nonweight-bearing functions of hip muscles, 408
Normal force vector, 47
perpendicular component of, *46,* 48
rotary component of, *46,* 48
Nuclei, 90
Nucleus pulposus, 322
"Nursemaid's elbow," 231
Nutation, 333

O

Oblique cord, *226,* 231
Oblique muscles
abdominal, 347, *348–349, 351*
inferior and superior, *340,* 341
Oblique popliteal ligament, *432*
Observational gait analysis, 563–565
Occipital bone, *319*
Occipital condyle, *319*
Occupational and daily activities, 602–609
Occupational tasks, 606–609
Older adult gait pattern, 567
Olecranon bursa, 228
Olecranon fossa, 220, 228
Olecranon process, 220, *225*
One-joint muscles acting at the knee, 453–456
On-guard position gait, 565
Open kinematic chains (OKC), 16–17, 24
ankle and foot and, *518*
elbow complex and, 247
Open kinetic chain vs. closed kinetic chain, 149–150
Open-chain motions, 39
Open-packed joint positions, 24
Opponens digiti minimi, 279, *282,* 303
Opponens pollicis, 279, *281*
Optimal sufficiency, 145
Oral care, 621–622
Orthopedic gait, 572–574
Osseofibrous tunnels, 277
Osteokinematics, 5, 9–17. *See also* Kinematics
clinical goniometry, 11, 14
defined, 10
degrees of freedom, 11
description of types of motion, 10–11
end feel, 14, 16
finger motions, 290
humeroulnar and humeroradial joints, 221–223
kinematic chains, 16–17
pelvis and hip, 382–385, *386–387*
rotary motion, 10–11
translatory motion, 10
wrist motions, 288–289
Overhead reaching, 618–621
Ovoid joint surfaces, 19

P

Palate, hard, *319*
Palatine process of maxillary bone, *319*
Palmar interossei muscles, 280, *284,* 287, 300
Palmar radioulnar ligament, *227,* 232
Palmaris longus, *268,* 274, 275–276
Palpable structures of the vertebral column, 317–321
Parallel elastic component, 136–137
Parallel force systems, 43, *44, 45*
Paralysis, 54
elbow, 243
pretibial muscles, 510
triceps, 241
Parietal bone, *319*
Parkinson's disease, 116, 119, 570–571
Passive and dynamic stabilization of the glenohumeral joint, 200–203
Passive components in muscle strength, 136–137
Passive elastic component, 136
Passive excursion of muscles, 141–143, *144*
Passive insufficiency, 142, *143*
Passive stabilization of the glenohumeral joint, 201
Passive stretching exercises, 73–74
Passive tension, 137
Patella, *426,* 427–428
alta, 441
as an anatomic pulley, 72–73
baja, 441
leverage and length-tension interactions, 145–146
Patellofemoral joint, *433,* 439–441
forces, 458–460
Patellofemoral pain syndrome (PFPS), 460, 551
Pathologic end feel, 16
Pathological conditions affecting movement system function, 116–119
Patient protective measures, 610–612
Pattern generators, 109
Pectineal line, 375
Pectineus, 390, 391, *394, 396,* 401, *402*
Pectoralis major, *199,* 200
Pectoralis minor, *188,* 190–191, 359
Pelvic balance, 335
Pelvic inclination, *383,* 384–385
Pelvic rotation, *383,* 384–385
transverse plane motion and, 415
Pelvis, 331–335, 371, *375. See also* Hip joint; Hip muscles
acetabulum, 374
angle of inclination, *383,* 384–385
arthrokinematics, 388

factors affecting roles of muscles of, 406–408
frontal plane motion and control at hip and, 411–415, 552–553
hip motion on, 385, *386–387*
ilium, 372
ischium, 372–373
joints, 379–380
muscles, 389–406
osteokinematics, 382–385, *386–387*
running and, 568, 576
sagittal plane motion at hip and, 408–411
transverse plane motion and, 415–417
walking and, 548, 550, 553, 568
Pennate muscles, 136
Perimysium, 90, *92,* 136
Peripheral nervous system, 86
classification of motor and sensory nerve fibers on basis of axonal diameter in, 88–89
classification of motor fibers on basis of fiber destination within, 89
classification of sensory fibers on basis of fiber origin within, 89
nerve fibers in, 88
nerve injury, 118
wrist and hand, 307–310
Peroneals, 561
Peroneus brevis, 505–507
Peroneus longus, 505–507, 522
Peroneus tertius, *508*
Perpendicular component of normal force, *46,* 48
Pes cavus, *524,* 525
Pes planus, 524–525
Phalanges, 259, 479
Phasic muscle fibers, 102
Phosphate, 93, 96
Physiological length of muscle, 137–138
Physiology
of excitable tissue, 84–86
functional applications and clinical considerations of neuromuscular, 113–116
importance of understanding, 83–84
introduction to, 83–84
kinesthesia and proprioception, 106–107
movement or "motor" control, 107–113
muscular system, 90–99
nerve fibers, 87–90
nervous system anatomy overview, 86–90
skeletal muscle structure, 90–96
Piriformis, *398, 398–399,* 405, *406*
Pisiform bone, 258
Pitching
baseball, 636–641
fast pitch softball, 641–644
Pivot joints, 11, *12*
Placing the hand behind the head, 207–208, 248
Plafond, 475–476
Plane(s)
cardinal, 5, *6*
coronal, 6
frontal, 6
horizontal, 6
of motion, 5–6
sagittal, 6
of the scapula, 165
Plantar aponeurosis, 521
Plantar calcaneonavicular ligament, *486*
Plantar interossei, *515*
Plantar ligaments, *487, 488*
Plantarflexion, 9
ankle and foot, 480, *481,* 482, 489, *490,* 494–495, 496, 502–503, 551–552, 560–561
knee extension combined with, 456
knee flexion combined with ankle, 456
Plantaris, *447,* 450, *498,* 501
Platysma, 341
Plumb line, 537
Points of peak forces, 556
Poliomyelitis, 180
Popliteal fossa, 428
Popliteofibular ligament, *432*
Popliteus, *448,* 450, 453
Positive work, 127, 146–149
Posterior ankle and foot muscles, 497–505
Posterior cervical muscles, *340,* 341–342
Posterior cruciate ligament, *431,* 434–435
Posterior femoral ligament, *433*
Posterior inferior iliac spine (PIIS), 372
Posterior longitudinal ligaments (PLL), 323
Posterior lumbar muscles, 342–343
Posterior pelvic tilt, 382, 384
Posterior radioulnar ligament, *227,* 232
Posterior scalene muscles, 336, *339*
Posterior superior iliac spine (PSIS), 372
Posterior talofibular ligament, *485*
Posterior thoracic muscles, 342–343
Posterior transversospinal muscles, *340*
Posterior vertebral joint elements, 324–326
Posterolateral band, 435
Posteromedial bundle, 435
Postural equilibrium, 107
Postural sway, 539–540
Postural tone, 104–105, *106*
Posture, 403
balance of forces occurring in symmetric stance, 540–542
defined, 536
postural sway and, 539–540
recovery strategies, 542–543
stance, 536–543
Potential difference, 84
Pouring, 627, *628*
Power grips, 291–293
Power phase, cycling, 660–662
Practice points
absent clavicle, 172
active and passive stretching, 103
ambulation safety, 548
ankle sprains, 491
antagonist muscles, 130
ATP in live muscle, 96
autogenic inhibition, 101
base of support, 57, 58
biceps tendon, 183
boutonnière deformity, 305
bursitis, 389
carpal bones arrangement, 256
carpal tunnel syndrome, 310
center of gravity, 58
cerebellar lesions, 111
compressive force and stance, 413
concurrent force systems, 47
core stabilization, 355
coxa valga and coxa vara, 378
degenerative disc disease, 329
degrees of freedom, 16
distraction injury, 231
eccentric activities, 147, 148
elbow dislocation, 228
elbow flexors, 232, 239, 240
elbow function, 626
elbow hyperextension, 223
energy conservation, 244
erector spinae, 343
extensor digitorum injuries, 287
extensor tendons of fingers, 286
external resistance, 33
femur, 375, 379
fibrocartilaginous disc, 265
finger deformity, 305
finger extension, 295
finger sprains, 263
flexor digitorum profundus function, 278
foot arches, 521
force arm and resistance arm, 40
forearm pronation and supination, 629
functional activity stabilization, 130
gait, 551, 552, 558, 570, 571, 574
gastrocnemius-soleus strength, 502
glenohumeral impingement, 205, 206
glenohumeral joint, 176
glenohumeral muscles, 196
gluteus maximus weakness, 411
grip strength, 295
ground reaction forces, 556
hamstrings, 404
hand injuries, 631
heel pain, 478
hip abductors and adductors, 404, 412
hip flexors, 409, 551
hip joint, 381, 389
hip muscle nerves, 391
hip rotators, 406, 417
iliopsoas, 409
iliotibial band, 401
inertia, 34, 35
interosseous membrane, 231
intrinsic wrist and hand muscles, 302, 310
ischial tuberosities, 374
isolation of a muscle or tendon from other surrounding structures, 208
joint capsule, 19

joint dislocation vs. subluxation, 21
joint dysfunction, 22
joint forces, 41
lateral collateral ligament injury, 483
leverage factor, 73
lifting, 357
limitations of joint movement, 14
line of gravity, 541
loss of sensation, 119
lumbosacral muscles, 331
manual resistance activities, 74
maximum resistance torque, 69
medial and lateral epicondyle, 220
medial collateral ligament, 228, 434
medial compartment osteoarthritis, 458
meniscus tears, 430, 457
mild joint distraction, 70
modified hinge joint, 223
moment arms, 45
motor skills, 113
motor units, 99
movement of planes, 30
multijoint muscles, 245
muscle atrophy, 115
older persons, 98
olecranon bursitis, 228
orthotics, 75
paralysis, 54, 241, 243
Parkinson's disease, 112
passive insufficiency, 143
passive tension and rebound response, 137
patellofemoral pain syndrome (PFPS), 460
pelvis symmetry, *373*
peroneal muscles, 505
piriformis, 406
plantar fasciitis, 523
posterior tibial shin splint, 525
postural sway, 540
posture, 403, 537, 543
pretibial muscle paralysis, 510
pronation and supination, 518
Q angles, 442
quadriceps muscle paralysis, 455
quadriceps strength, 461
range of motion, 13, 23, 181
reciprocal innervation, 462
recovery strategies, 543
rectus femoris, 452
respiratory muscles, 351
retinacular system, 288, 289
running, 555, 579, 583, 584
scaphoid, 258
scapular rotator strength, 210
scapulothoracic joint, 176
shins, 476
shoulder adduction, 247
shoulder and activities of daily living, 622
SI joint, 380
spasticity, 117
spina strength, 325
spine muscle function, 336
spondylolisthesis, 329
stance, 56, 541
stress and injuries, 147
stroke, 111
supination, 247
swan neck deformity, 305
symphysis pubis pain, 333
tenodesis, 143, 292
tension headaches, 341
tibialis posterior, 505
tibiofibular ligament, 483
torque reduction, 43
traction force, 37, 48
transverse abdominis, 347
trunk movement, 336
ulnar nerve, 221, 309
UMN pathology, 114
upper extremities strengths, 207
wrist extension, 274
wrist flexors and extensors strength, 299–300
Pressure, 74–75
center of, 556
Preswing, 544, 557
Pretibial group function, 509–510
Progression, angle of, 547
Pronation, 9
ankle and foot, 480, *482,* 517–520
forearm, 229–230, *238,* 242–243, 246–247, 629
Pronator quadratus, 243, 246–247, 248, *249*
Pronator teres, 240, 243, 246–247
Prone position, hip extension in, 411
Proprioception, 106–107
Proprioceptors, 99
Propulsion phase in running, 575–576
Protraction, 9, 176
radioulnar joint, *239*
shoulder girdle, 168
Proximal attachments, 128–129
Proximal radioulnar joint, 230
Pterygoid hamulus, *319*
Pubic symphysis, *12,* 380
Pubic tubercle, 374
Pubis, 373–374
Pubofemoral ligament, *386*
"Pulled elbow syndrome," 231
Pulleys, 70–73
flexor, 288
patellofemoral joint forces and, 458–459
Pulling, 208, 248–249
Pull-through phase, freestyle swimming, 648–649
Pyramidal tract, 109
Pythagorean theory, 49, 68–69

Q

Q angle, 441, 442
Quadrate ligament, *226,* 231
Quadratus lumborum, 343, *346*
breathing and, 359
Quadratus plantae, *513*
Quadriceps, *443, 443–444,* 451–452
femoris torque, 460–461
strength, 461
torque ratio, hamstring to, 462
weakness, 572
Qualitative analysis, 635

R

Radial deviation, 9
Radial flexion, 9
Radial fossa, 220
Radial neck, 221, *226*
Radial nerve, *236, 237,* 307–308
Radial notch, 220, *226, 227*
Radial styloid process, 256
Radial tuberosity, 221, *226*
Radiocarpal joint, 259
Radioulnar articulations, 229–232
Radioulnar joint kinematics, 229–230
Radius, 221
distal, 256
Rancho Los Amigos terminology, 544
Range of motion, 14, *15,* 23, 30
elbow joint, 222
requirements of normal gait, 554
Ranvier, Louis, 87
Rate of motion, 31
Rays, 496
Reaching
overhead and backward, 620–621
overhead and forward, 618–620
strategies, 543
Reaction force, joint, 65–66
Reafference, 111
Rearfoot, 477
Receptors
Golgi tendon organs, 100
joint, 99–105
muscle spindles, 89, 100–105
Reciprocal arm swing, 565
Reciprocal inhibition, 103
Reciprocal innervation, 462
Recording muscle activity, 126–127
Recovery phase
cycling, 662–663
freestyle swimming, 651–652
Rectilinear motion, 10
Rectus abdominis, 347, *348, 351*
Rectus capitis anterior muscles, 336, *337*
Rectus capitis lateralis muscles, 336, *337*
Rectus capitis posterior major, *340,* 341
Rectus capitis posterior minor, *340,* 341
Rectus femoris, 390, 391, *393, 401, 443, 449,* 452
Reflex(es)
feedback, 149
force feedback, 149
sensory innervation and, 463
spinal, 109
Reinforcement, glenohumeral joint capsular, 177–180

Relaxation, muscle, 94, 96
Repolarization, 85
Resistance
  applied to the body, 69–70
  arm, 38, 40
  clinical application of externally applied, 33, 70–75
  mechanical advantage and, 39–40
Resolution of forces, 45, *46*
Respiratory muscles, *350,* 351, 359
Response, loading, 557
Resting
  and close-packed positions of the shoulder complex joints, 183
  length of muscles, 137
  position, 24
  potential, 85
  tremor, 116
Reticulospinal tract, 109
Retinacular system, fingers, 287–288
Retraction, 9, 176
  shoulder girdle, 168
Retroversion, 165, 378
Rhomboids, *187,* 190
Rib cage, 321
Right triangle, laws of the, 49–51
Rigidity, muscle, *117*
Rocking motion, 21
Rolling motion, 21, 594–595
  freestyle swimming, 648
Rotary component of normal force, *46,* 48
Rotary distance, 30
Rotary motion, 10–11, 30
Rotation, 9
  axial knee, 437–438
  glenohumeral joint, 181
  hip, 385, *386–387,* 415
  of knee, terminal, 438–439
  lateral, 9
  medial, 9
  pelvic, *383,* 384–385
  scapular tilting, 168–170
  shoulder girdle downward, 168
  shoulder girdle upward, 168
Rotational torque, 63–64
Rotator cuff
  deltoid and, 201–203
  muscles, 179
  stabilization, 201
Rotators, *340,* 341–342, *345*
  deep, 342–343
  hip, *398–399,* 405–406
  tibial, 450–451
Running, 555, 574–575. *See also* Gait
  changes at different speeds, 579–580
  kinematics, 576–578
  kinetics of, 583–584
  muscles activity at hip, knee, and ankle in, 580–583
  phases, 575–576
  sagittal plane motion during, 576–577
  stance phase, 575–576

S

Sacroiliac joint, 331–335
Sacrospinalis muscles, 342
Sacrum, 320–321, 331–335
Saddle joints, 11, *12*
Sagittal plane motion, 6
  at hip and pelvis, 408–411
  during running, 576–577
  during walking, 548, *549*
Sagittal suture, *319*
Sanding wood, 621
Sarcolemma, 91, *92*
Sarcomeres, 91, *92,* 94, 137–138
Sarcoplasmic reticulum, 95
Sartorius, 390, 391, *393, 399, 401, 448,* 449, 452
Scalene muscles, 336, *338, 338–339*
Scaphoid, 256
Scaption, 183
Scapula, 163–165, *320*
  anterior-posterior tilting of, 169–170
  joints, 167–170
  medial-lateral tilting of, 170
  shoulder abduction in the plane of, 183
  synergistic muscle actions, 203–204, *205*
  tilting, 168–170
Scapular dyskinesis, 209
Scapular stabilizer muscles, 185–191
Scapular tilting, 168–170
Scapulohumeral rhythm, 183–185, 209
Scapulothoracic joint, 167–168, 175–176
Scoliosis, 362
Screw home mechanism, 438–439
Second law of motion, 34
Second order neurons, 90
Second-class levers, *38*
Seesaw, 38–39
Segment and body motion, 6, 30
Sellar joint surfaces, 19
Semilunar notch, 220
Semimembranosus, 390, 391, *397,* 403, *446*
Semispinalis capitis, *340,* 342
Semispinalis cervicis, *340*
Semitendinosus, 390, 391, *397,* 403, *446, 448,* 449–450
Sensory fibers, classification on basis of fiber origin, 89
Sensory innervation and reflexes, 463
Sensory neurons, 88–89
Sequence of movement
  clinician activities, 610
  donning socks or pants, 624–625
  driving, 626
  feeding, 623
  household tasks, 604–605
  mobility, 595, 597, 600
  occupational and daily activities, 602–603
  occupational tasks, 607, 608
  oral care, 621–622
  pouring, 627
  reaching overhead and backward, 620
  reaching overhead and forward, 618–619
  turning a key, 628
  using a hammer, 629
  wood sanding activity, 621
Series elastic component, 136–137
Serratus anterior, 185, *186, 190,* 209
Sesamoid bones, 265, 427
Shaft of the femur, 375–376, *376*
Shapes, joint, 22–23
Shins, 476
Short plantar ligament, *487*
Shoulder complex
  activities requiring primarily movement of the, 618–622
  bicipital groove, 183
  bones, 162–166
  defined, 162
  definition of shoulder girdle movements, 167–170
  freestyle swimming and, 648–652
  function of muscles of the, 200–208
  functional deficiency applications, 208–209
  glenohumeral stabilizing muscles, 191–197
  golf swing and, 652–656
  humerus, 165–166
  joints, 166–185, 210
  large muscle movers, 197–200
  manubrium, 163
  muscle activity during functional motions, 207–208
  muscle regions, 185, *186–189*
  placing the hand behind the head motion and, 207–208
  pulling motion and, 208
  resting and close-packed positions of joints of the, 183
  scapula, 163–165
  scapular stabilizer muscles, 185–191
  scapulohumeral rhythm, 183–185
  synergistic muscle actions, 203–204, *205*
  tennis serve and, 656–660
Shoulder complex joints, 166–167, 210
  acromioclavicular, 164, 166–168, 173–175
  definition of shoulder girdle movements and, 167–170
  glenohumeral, 176–183
  scapulothoracic, 167–168, 175–176
  sternoclavicular, 166–168, 170–173
Shoulder complex muscles
  function of, 200–208
  glenohumeral stabilizing, 191–197
  large muscle movers, 197–200
  regions, 185, *186–189*
  scapular stabilizer, 185–191
Shoulder girdle, 162, 167–170
  depression, 168, 174
  downward rotation, 168, 176
  elevation, 168, 174

protraction, 168, 176
retraction, 168, 176
scapulohumeral rhythm, 183–185
upward rotation, 168, 176
SI. *See* International System of Units (SI); Sacroiliac joint
Sigmoid notch, 256
Sine, 49, *50,* 51
Single fixed pulleys, 70, *71*
Single limb support, 544
Sitting
hip extension in, 411
hip flexion in, 409
peroneal nerve and, 505
Sit-to-stand transfer, 599–602
Sit-ups, 409–410
6 o'clock phase, fast pitch softball pitching, 642
Size, muscle, 135
Skeletal muscle, structure of, 90–96
Skull. *See also* Vertebral column
balancing of the vertebral column and, 352
nonpalpable structures, 317, *318, 319*
Sliding filament model, 94, 95–96
Sliding motion, 21
Slow oxidative muscle fibers, 96
Slow-twitch muscle fibers, 96
SO. *See* Slow oxidative muscle fibers
Soccer instep kick, 644–647
Soft tissue
hip joint, 388–389
humeroulnar and humeroradial articulations, 224–228
knee capsule, 435–436
radioulnar joint complex, 230–232
Softball pitching, fast pitch, 641–644
SOH-CAH-TOA, 49–51
Soleus, *498,* 501, 502
Somatosensory inputs, 107
Space diagrams, 60–61
Spasticity, muscle, *117*
Spatial and temporal characteristics of gait, 546–548
Speed of contraction, 139–140
Spherical grasp, 291, *293, 297*
Spinal column. *See* Vertebral column
Spinal cord, 107
motor control in region of, 108–109
pattern generators, 109
Spinal reflexes, 109
Spinales, 342
Spinalis lumborum, *346*
Spinalis thoracis, *346*
Spindles, muscle, 89, 100–105
Spine. *See* Vertebral column
Spinning motion, 21
Splenius capitis, 342, *344*
Splenius cervicis, *344*
Spondylolisthesis, 329
Sports activities. *See also* Leisure activities
baseball pitching, 636–641
fast pitch softball pitching, 641–644
freestyle swimming, 647–652
soccer instep kick, 644–647
Spotting during ambulation, 610–612
Sprinting, 575
"Squat" lift, *60*
Squat lifting, 357, *358*
SR. *See* Sarcoplasmic reticulum
Stabilization of the glenohumeral joint, 200–203
Stabilizing component of muscle force, *46,* 48–49
Stable equilibrium, 55–56
base of support and, 56–57
Stance, 56–57, *58. See also* Gait
balance of forces occurring in symmetric, 540–542
forces required to maintain, 537–539
functional control at ankle joint, 540
functional control at knee joint, 540–541
line of gravity and, 537–539
mid-, 544, 557
phase in running, 575–576
postural sway and, 539–540
posture, 536–543
recovery strategies, 542–543
terminal, 544, 557
Standing
hip extension in, 411
hip flexion in, 409
Static, patellofemoral, 440–441
Static equilibrium, 40
Step
duration, 547
length, 547
width, 547
Stepping strategies, 543
Sternoclavicular joint, 166–168, 170–173
Sternocleidomastoid muscles (SCM), 317, 336, *339,* 341
breathing and, 359
Sternocostal joints, *12*
Sternum, 321
junction, *320*
Stiff leg gait, 570
Stiffness, muscle, 104
"Stoop" lift, *60*
Straight leg raises, 409–410
Strain, hamstring, 151–152
Stratum fibrosum, 18
Stratum synovium, 18
Strength, muscle, 134–135
active tension and, 140–141
age and gender in, 141, *142*
contractions, 98–99
factors affecting maximum isometric muscle force and, 150–152
fiber architecture and, 135–136
grip, 293–299
length-tension relationships and, 137–138
moment arm and, 138–139
muscle size and, 135
passive components in, 136–137
speed of contraction and, 139–140
Stress-strain, 133–134
Stretching vs. joint mobilization, 73–74
Stretch reflex, 102, *103, 104*
Stretch-shortening cycle, 149
Stride, 543
length, 546
phase, baseball pitching, 638–639
Strokes, 119, 569–570
Structure, joint, *13,* 18–20
Styloid process, *319*
Styloid process of the radius, *234*
Subacromial bursa, 180
Subdeltoid bursa, 180
Subluxation, joint, 21
Suboccipital muscles, *340,* 341
Subscapularis, *193,* 195, *196*
Subtalar joint, 489–492, *493,* 518–520
gait and, 553
ligaments, *484–486*
pronation and supination and, 518–519
Sufficiency, optimal, 145
Superior Labrum Anterior to Posterior (SLAP) lesions, 209
Superior nuchal line, *319*
Superior oblique muscles, *340,* 341
Superior ramus, 374
Superior tibiofibular joint, 481–482
Supination, 9
ankle and foot, 480, *482,* 517–520
forearm, 240–242, 246–247, 629
radioulnar joint, *239*
Support, base of, 56–57, *58*
Suprahyoid muscles, 341, 359
Supraspinatus, 191, *192,* 195
outlet, 179
Supraspinous ligament, 325
Surfaces, joint, 19, *20*
Sustentaculum tali, 478
Swan neck deformity, 305
Sway, postural, 539–540
Swimming, freestyle, 647–652
Swing phases
gait, 544–545, 557–558
golf, 652–656
running, 576
Symmetric stance, 540–542
Symphysis pubis, 335, 374, 380
pain, 333
Synapses, 86, 90
Synarthrodial joints, *12, 13,* 18
Synarthrodial surfaces, *12*
Syndesmosis joints, *12, 13,* 18
Synergist muscles, 130
elbow and forearm complex, 244
in movements of the thumb and little finger, 307
Synergistic muscle actions, 203–204, *205*
Synergy, muscle, 107, 115

Synovial fluid, 18
Synovial joints, 18, 19–20

T

Talar dome, 482
Talocrural joint, 482–483, 489, 519–520
  ligaments, *484–485*
Talonavicular joint, 493
  ligament, *486*
Talus, 477–478
Tangent, 49–51
Tangential force vectors, 47, 64
Tarsal bones, 476–479
Tarsometatarsal joints, 495–496, 520
  ligaments, *487*
Temporal bone, 317, *319*
Temporal characteristics of gait, 547
Temporalis, 360
Temporomandibular joint (TMJ), 317, *319,* 359–362
Tendons
  action of muscle, 143, *144*
  biceps, *195*
  wrist and hand, 274–275, 285–287
Tennis serve, 656–660
Tenodesis, 143, *144,* 292
Tension
  active, 140–141
  headaches, 341
  passive, 137
Tensor fascia latae, 390, *394, 398,* 401, *402,* 405, *448*
Teres major, *194,* 200
Teres minor, *193,* 195
Terminal rotation of the knee, 438–439
Terminal stance, 544, 557
Terminal swing, 545, 576
Terminology, kinesiology, 4–9
TFCC. *See* Triangular fibrocartilage complex (TFCC)
Thenar muscle group, 279, *280, 281–282*
Third law of motion, 34–35
Third order neurons, 90
Third-class levers, *38,* 39
  force required by muscles as, 59
Thoracic facet joints, 327, *328*
Thoracic outlet syndrome, 336
Thoracic vertebrae, 320
  joints, 327–329
Thoracis, 342
Thoracolumbar fascia, 329–330
Thorax, 321
Three cuneiforms, 479
3 o'clock phase, fast pitch softball pitching, 643
Three-prong chuck, *294, 298*
Thumbs, 9, 255, 260–262. *See also* Fingers; Wrist and hand complex
  balanced forces, 305–307
  mobility, 306
  motions, 290–291
  muscles, *272,* 277–280, *281–283*
  strength of grip and, 293–297
  synergic action of wrist muscles in movements of the little finger and, 307
  thenar muscle group, 279, *280*
Thyroid cartilage, *320*
Tibia, 426–426, 475–476
Tibial crest, *426,* 427
Tibial rotators, 450–451
Tibial torsion, 482
Tibial tuberosity, *426,* 427
Tibialis anterior, 507–509, *510*
Tibialis posterior, *499,* 503, 504–505
Tibiofemoral joint, 428–430, *431, 431–432*
  arthrokinematics, 439
  forces, 456–458
  kinematics, 436–439
  line, 426
Tibiofibular joints, 480–482
Tilt, pelvic, 382–384
Tilting, scapular, 168–170
Tip-to-tip pinch, *294, 298*
Tissue, physiology of excitable, 84–86
Toes, 479, 522–523, 553. *See also* Ankle and foot
Tone, muscle, 104
  abnormal, 115
  postural, 104–105, *106*
Tonic muscle fibers, 102
Torque, *32*
  defined, 40–43
  forces acting at angles and, 45–47
  joint forces and, 67–68
  laws of the right triangle and, 49–51
  levers and, 44–45
  maximum isometric, 206
  of muscles acting at the knee, 460–462
  parallel force systems, 43, *44, 45*
  resolution of forces and, 45, *46*
  rotational, 63–64
  triceps surae, 502
Torsion
  angle of, 165, 377–378, *378*
  tibial, 482
Tract, 86
Transfer, sit-to-stand, 599–602
Translatory motion, 10, 22, *22,* 29–30
  Newton's first law of motion and, 34
Transverse abdominis, 347, *350*
Transverse arch, 477
Transverse carpal ligament, 265
Transverse plane motion, 6
  at the hip and pelvis, 415–417
  running and, 568
  walking and, 548, *550,* 553–554
Transverse tarsal joint, 492–495, *496*
  ligaments, *486*
Transverse tubular system, 95
Transversospinal muscles, *340,* 341–342, 342–343, *344, 345*
Trapezium, 257
Trapezius, 185, *186,* 190, *190,* 209
  breathing and, 359
Tremors, 116
Trendelenburg sign, 414
Triangular fibrocartilage complex (TFCC), 231–232, 265
Triaxial joints, 11, *12, 13*
Triceps brachii, 195–196, 240, 241, 247
Triceps surae, 502–503
Triplanar axis, 480
Triquetrum, 258
Trochlea, medial, 219
Trochlear groove, 219, 425
Trochlear notch, 220
Trochlear ridge, 220
Tropomyosin, 92–93
Troponin, 93
Trunk. *See also* Head, neck, and trunk region; Vertebral column
  forward bending and lifting, 355–357
  functional activities of muscles of the, 358–359
  motions and stabilization of the vertebrae, 352–355
  muscles and gait, 558–559
  running and, 576
  squat lifting and, 357, *358*
T-system. *See* Transverse tubular system
Tubercle of the radius, 256
Tubercles, greater and lesser, 165–166
Turning a key, 627–629
Turning effect of forces, 43, *44*
12 o'clock phase, fast pitch softball pitching, 643
Two-joint muscles acting at the knee, 453–456
Type I muscle fibers, 96–98, 129
  active tension and, 141
Type II muscle fibers, 96–98, 129
  active tension and, 140–141
Types of forces, 31–37
Types of motion, 29–30

U

Ulna, 220–221
  distal, 256
  elbow flexors, *233*
  ligaments, *225–227*
Ulnar deviation, 9
Ulnar flexion, 9
Ulnar nerve, 221, 309
Ulnar notch, 256
Ulnar styloid process, 256
Ulnar tuberosity, 220, *233*
UMN. *See* Upper motor neurons
Uniaxial joints, 11, *12, 13*
Unipennate muscles, 136
Unstable equilibrium, 55–56
Upper extremities
  activities requiring primarily elbow movement, 623–626

activities requiring primarily shoulder complex movement, 618–622
muscles and gait, 558
resistance, 612–613
Upper motor neurons, 90, 113–114
Upward rotation, shoulder girdle, 168, 176

V

Vacuuming, 604–606
Valgus, 430
Vastus lateralis, *443*
Vastus medialis oblique (VMO), 439–440, 441, 449, *451,* 452
Vectors, force, 35–36, *62*
component, 45
normal, 47
tangential, 47
Velocity, 31, 146, 547
angular, 59, *60*
Vertebrae, cervical
C-7 prominence, 320
first and second, 318–319
third to sixth, 319–320
Vertebrae, lumbar, 320
Vertebrae, thoracic, 320
Vertebral column
anterior and lateral trunk muscles, 343–351
anterior cervical muscles, 336, *337–339,* 341
anterior vertebral joint elements, 322–324
balancing of the head and, 352
bones, 315–321
cervical region joints, 326–327
coccyx, 320–321
coupling motions, 325–326
first and second cervical vertebrae, 318–319
ligaments, 324–325
lumbar region joints, 329–330
muscles, 335–359
nonpalpable structures, 316–317, *318*
normal curves, 315–316
palpable structures, 317–321
posterior cervical muscles, *340,* 341–342
posterior thoracic and lumbar muscles, 342–343
posterior vertebral joint elements, 324–326
primary neck flexors, 336, 341
sacrum, 320–321, 331–335
sternum and, *320,* 321
third to sixth cervical vertebrae, 319–320
thoracic and lumbar vertebrae, 320
thoracic region joints, 327–329
thorax and, 321
trunk motions and stabilization of the, 352–355
vertebral motions, 321
Vertebral endplates, 322
Vertebral motions, 321
Vestibulospinal tract, 109
Viscoelasticity, 133
Viscosity, 131

W

Walking. *See also* Gait
angular joint displacements and, 548
ankle and foot during, 551–552, 554, 568
ankle dorsiflexion and, 560
ankle plantarflexion and, 560–561
assistive devices and, 574
ataxia and, 571–572
cerebral palsy and, 568–569
cerebrovascular accident and, 569–570
challenges to efficiency of, 568–574
changes in older adults, 567
crouch, 570
hip during, 550, 553–554, 559–560, 568
intrinsic muscles of foot and, 561
kinematics, 546–554
kinetics of, 554–556
knee during, 550–551, 553, 554, 560–561, 568
knee motion restriction and, 572–573
lower extremity muscles and, 559–561
pelvis during, 548, 550, 553
swing phase, 544–545, 557–558
transverse plane motion and, 553–554
trunk muscles and, 558–559
upper extremity muscles and, 558–559
Wasting, muscle, 114–115
Weakness, muscle, 113–115
Weight, 31, *32, 62*
applied to joint structures, 69
bearing functions of hip muscles, 408
loading of the foot and, 523–524
Wheelbarrow, 39
Windlass mechanism, 521
Windup phase
baseball pitching, 636–637
fast pitch softball pitching, 641–642
golf swing, 652–655
tennis serve, 656–657
Women
center of gravity in, 53
muscle strength in, 141
Wood sanding, 621
Work, positive and negative, 127, 146–149
Wrist and hand complex, 9
abduction and adduction, 302–303
activities requiring primarily movement of the, 629–631
balanced forces, 303–307
bones, 255–259
freestyle swimming and, 648–652
functional movements, 291–303
grasping, 295–302
intrinsic-plus and intrinsic-minus positions, 302
introduction to, 255
joints, 259–262, 290–291, 300–302, 305
ligaments, 263–266
median nerve, *235, 238*
muscles, 266–288
muscles acting on the digits, *270–274,* 276–280
peripheral nerve injuries, 308–310
peripheral nerves, 307–310
radial nerve, *236, 237,* 307–308
strength of grip, 293–297
synergic action of the wrist muscles in movements of the thumb and little finger, 307
tendinous system, 285–287
thumb muscles, *272,* 277–280, *281–283*
types of grasp, 291–293
wrist motions, 288–290
wrist muscles, 266–276
Wrist and hand complex joints
carpometacarpal, 260, *261, 261–262,* 305
finger motion and, 290–291
interphalangeal, 262–263
metacarpophalangeal, 260–262, 290–291, 300–302, 305
midcarpal, 259
radiocarpal, 259
Wrist and hand complex muscles, 266
finger, *270–274,* 276–280
midpalm, 280, *284,* 300
thumb, *272,* 277–280, *281–283*
wrist extensors, 266, *267–268, 274*
wrist flexors, *268–269,* 274–276

X

Xiphoid process, *320,* 321

Z

Zygomatic arch, *319*